Brain and Spinal Tumors
of Childhood

Brain and Spinal Tumors of Childhood

Edited by

DAVID A. WALKER BMedSci BM BS FRCP FRCPCH

Reader and Honorary Consultant in Paediatric Oncology
Children's Brain Tumour Research Centre
Division of Child Health, School of Human Development
University of Nottingham, Queen's Medical Centre
Nottingham, UK

GIORGIO PERILONGO MD

Pediatric Oncologist, Neuro-oncology Program
Division of Hematology/Oncology, Department of Pediatrics
University Hospital of Padua, Italy

JONATHAN A. G. PUNT MB BS FRCS FRCPCH

Formerly Senior Lecturer in Paediatric Neurosurgery and
Consultant Paediatric Neurosurgeon
Children's Brain Tumour Research Centre, Nottingham, UK

and

ROGER E. TAYLOR MA MB BS FRCP(Edin) FRCP FRCR

Consultant Clinical (Radiation) Oncologist
Department of Clinical Oncology
Cookridge Hospital, Leeds, UK

ARNOLD
A member of the Hodder Headline Group
LONDON

First published in Great Britain in 2004 by
Arnold, a member of the Hodder Headline Group,
338 Euston Road, London NW1 3BH

http://www.arnoldpublishers.com

Distributed in the United States of America by
Oxford University Press Inc.,
198 Madison Avenue, New York, NY10016
Oxford is a registered trademark of Oxford University Press

Whilst the advice and information in this book are believed to be true and
accurate at the date of going to press, neither the authors nor the publisher
can accept any legal responsibility or liability for any errors or omissions
that may be made. In particular (but without limiting the generality of the
preceding disclaimer) every effort has been made to check drug dosages;
however, it is still possible that errors have been missed. Furthermore,
dosage schedules are constantly being revised and new side effects
recognized. For these reasons the reader is strongly urged to consult the
drug companies' printed instructions before administering any of the drugs
recommended in this book.

British Library Cataloguing in Publication Data
A catalogue record for this book is available from the British Library

Library of Congress Cataloging-in-Publication Data
A catalog record for this book is available from the Library of Congress

ISBN 0 340 76260 8

1 2 3 4 5 6 7 8 9 10

Commissioning Editor: Joanna Koster
Development Editor: Sarah Burrows
Project Editor: Zelah Pengilley
Production Controller: Lindsay Smith
Cover Design: Lee-May Lim

Typeset in 10/12 pt Minion by Charon Tec Pvt. Ltd., Chennai, India
Printed and bound in the UK by Butler & Tanner Ltd.

What do you think about this book? Or any other Arnold title?
Please send your comments to **feedback.arnold@hodder.co.uk**

Acknowledgments

We would like to take this opportunity to thank our wives – Gill, Nina, Alessandra and Angie – who have held home and family together while we have been advancing the cause of pediatric neuro-oncology.

We would like to thank the children and families who have encouraged us to promote research through sharing their experiences and through their tangible support of finance of our national studies groups and research charities.

We would also like to acknowledge the support of the Children's Brain Tumour Research Centre at the University of Nottingham in providing the funding for secretarial support that has helped to bring the book together. This book would not have been assembled without the skilled, good-humored and dedicated work of Sue Franklin, for whom we have developed a great respect and to whom we are extremely grateful.

Finally, we would like to thank all the outstanding authors who have contributed to the book, without whom this project would never have been possible.

The editors

Contents

Contributors

Christine Abercrombie
Consultant Paediatric Anaesthetist
Queen's Medical Centre
Nottingham, UK

Vanessa J. Appleby PhD
Department of Anatomy
University of Bristol
School of Medical Sciences
University Walk
Bristol, UK

Cliff Bailey
Professor and Regional Director of Research and Development
Research School of Medicine
Leeds, UK

Stacey L. Berg MD
Associate Professor of Pediatrics
Texas Children's Cancer Center
Baylor College of Medicine
Houston, TX, USA

Susan M. Blaney MD
Associate Professor of Pediatrics
Texas Children's Cancer Center
Baylor College of Medicine
Houston, TX, USA

W. Archie Bleyer
Professor of Pediatrics
University of Texas
MD Anderson Cancer Center
Houston, TX, USA

Alan V. Boddy
Northern Institute for Cancer Research
University of Newcastle
Newcastle upon Tyne, UK

Jane Bond
Lichfield, Staffordshire, UK

Eric Bouffet MD
Section Head of Pediatric Neuro-Oncology
Professor of Pediatrics
Division of Hematology/Oncology
Hospital for Sick Children
University of Toronto
Toronto, Canada

Michael Brada
Reader and Consultant in Clinical Oncology
The Institute of Cancer Research and
The Royal Marsden Hospital
Sutton, Surrey, UK

Gabriele Calaminus MD
Consultant Pediatric Oncologist
Department of Pediatric Hematology/Oncology/Immunology
Heinrich Heine University Children's Hospital
Dusseldorf, Germany

Pascal Chastagner MD PhD
Professor of Paediatrics
Hôpital D'Enfants
Service de Medicine Infantile 2
Nancy, France

Paul D. Chumas MD FRCS(SN)
Consultant Neurosurgeon
Department of Neurosurgery
The General Infirmary
Leeds, UK

Maureen Dennis PhD
Department of Psychology
Research Institute Brain and Behavior Program
Hospital for Sick Children
and Department of Surgery
Faculty of Medicine
University of Toronto
Toronto, Canada

Catherine DeVile
Consultant Paediatric Neurologist
Great Ormond Street Hospital for Children NHS Trust
London, UK

François Doz
Pediatric Oncologist
Institut Curie
Paris, France

James M. Drake FRCS(C)
Professor of Surgery
Division of Neurosurgery
Hospital for Sick Children
University of Toronto
Toronto, Canada

Jonathan L. Finlay MB ChB
Professor of Pediatrics and
Director, Neural Tumors Program
Children's Center for Cancer and Blood Disorders
Children's Hospital Los Angeles
Keck School of Medicine
University of Southern California, CA, USA

Carolyn R. Freeman MB BS FRCP(C)
McGill University Health Centre
Montreal General Hospital
Department of Radiation Oncology
Montreal, Canada

Maria Luisa Garré
Department of Pediatric Hematology and Oncology
Giannina Gaslini Children's Research Hospital
Genoa, Italy

Felice Giangaspero MD
Associate Professor of Pathology
Department of Experimental Medicine and Pathology
University of Rome "La Sapienza"
Rome, Italy

Richard Gilbertson MRCP PhD
Assistant Professor
Department of Developmental Neurobiology
St Jude Children's Research Hospital
Memphis, TN, USA

Adam Glaser DM MRCP(UK) FRCPCH
Yorkshire Regional Centre for Paediatric Oncology and
Haematology
Children's Day Hospital
St James's Hospital
Leeds, UK

Astrid K. Gnekow
Pediatric Oncologist
Hospital for Children and Adolescents
Augsburg, Germany

Mark L. Greenberg MBChB FRCP(C)
Professor of Pediatrics and Surgery
POGO Chair in Childhood Cancer Control and Senior Staff
Oncologist
Hospital for Sick Children
University of Toronto
Toronto, Canada

Paul D. Griffiths
Professor of Radiology
Academic Unit of Radiology
University of Sheffield
Sheffield, UK

Michael A. Grotzer MD
Division of Oncology
University Children's Hospital
Zurich, Switzerland

Richard Grundy
Clinical Senior Lecturer in Paediatric Oncology
Department of Oncology
Birmingham Children's Hospital
Birmingham, UK

Darren Hargrave
Consultant Paediatric Oncologist
The Royal Marsden Hospital
Sutton, Surrey, UK

Richard D. Hayward
Consultant Paediatric Neurosurgeon
Great Ormond Street Hospital for Children NHS Trust
London, UK

Anne Ingle
Play Specialist
Children's Services
Queen's Medical Centre
Nottingham, UK

Timothy Jaspan BSc FRCR FRCP
Consultant Neuroradiologist
Department of Neuroradiology
Imaging Centre
University Hospital
Nottingham, UK

Colin Kennedy MD FRCP FRCPCH
Consultant and Reader in Paediatric Neurology
Department of Paediatric Neurology
Child Health
Southampton General Hospital
Southampton, UK

Fenella J. Kirkham
Consultant Paediatric Neurologist
London Centre for Paediatric Endocrinology
Middlesex Hospital and Neurosciences Unit
Institute of Child Health (University College London)
London, UK

Rolf D. Kortmann
Department of Radiooncology
University of Tübingen
Germany

Joachin Kühl (dec.)
Padiatrische Onkologie und Hamatologie
Leiter der Hirntumorstudie HIT 2000
Universitats-Kinderlink Wurzburg
Oberarzt der Klinik
Wurzburg, Germany

Abhaya V. Kulkarni MD PhD FRCSC
Consultant Neurosurgeon
Division of Neurosurgery
Hospital for Sick Children
University of Toronto
Toronto, Canada

Daune L. MacGregor MD FRCPC
Professor of Pediatrics (Neurology)
University of Toronto
Associate Pediatrician-in-Chief
Hospital for Sick Children
Toronto, Canada

Conor Mallucci
Paediatric Neurosurgeon
Alder Hey Children's Hospital
Liverpool, UK

Lindy May RGN RSCN MSc
Sister, Neurosurgery
Great Ormond Street Hospital for Children NHS Trust
London, UK

Virginia McGivern RGN RM RSCN MGPP
Complementary Therapy Nurse
Specialist Children's Services
Queen's Medical Centre
Nottingham, UK

Antony Michalski
Consultant Paediatric Oncologist
Great Ormond Street Hospital for Children NHS Trust
London, UK

Trimurti D. Nadkarni MCh
Associate Professor
Department of Neurosurgery
King Edward Memorial Hospital and
Honorary Consultant Neurosurgeon
Tata Memorial Hospital
Mumbai, India

Donald M. O'Rourke MD
Associate Professor
Departments of Neurosurgery and Pathology and
Laboratory Medicine
University of Pennsylvania School of Medicine
USA

Roger J. Packer
Executive Director
Neuroscience and Behavioral Medicine
Children's National Medical Center
Professor, Neurology and Pediatrics
George Washington Unit
Washington, DC, USA

Giorgio Perilongo MD
Consultant Pediatric Oncologist, Neuro-oncology Program
Division of Hematology/Oncology
Department of Pediatrics
University Hospital of Padua
Padua, Italy

Jonathan A. G. Punt MB BS FRCS FRCPCH
Formerly Senior Lecturer in Paediatric Neurosurgery and
Consultant Paediatric Neurosurgeon
Children's Brain Tumour Research Centre
Nottingham, UK

Harold L. Rekate MD FACS FAAP
Clinical Professor of Neurosurgery
University of Arizona School of Medicine, Tucson, and
Chief, Pediatric Neurosciences
Barrow Neurological Institute
Phoenix, AZ, USA

Daria Riva
Chief Developmental Neurology Division
Istituto Nazionale
Neurologico C. Besta
Milan, Italy

Bradford J. Ross PhD
Coordinator of Neuropsychology
Children's Specialized Hospital
Mountainside, NJ
USA

Ronald C. Savage
Executive Vice President
Bancroft NeuroHealth
Haddonfield, NJ, USA

Paul J. Scotting PhD
Senior Lecturer in Genetics
Institute of Genetics
School of Biology
University of Nottingham
Queen's Medical Centre
Nottingham, UK

Michael Sokal
Consultant Clinical Oncologist
Department of Oncology
City Hospital
Nottingham, UK

Carlos de Sousa MD BSc FRCP FRCPCH
Consultant Paediatric Neurologist
Great Ormond Street Hospital for Children NHS Trust
London, UK

Brenda J. Spiegler PhD ABPP(cn)
Assistant Professor of Pediatrics
Department of Psychology and
Division of Hematology/Oncology
Hospital for Sick Children
University of Toronto
Toronto, Ontario, Canada

Richard Sposto PhD
Group Statistician, Children's Oncology Group,
Associate Professor of Research
Department of Preventive Medicine,
University of Southern California
Arcadia, CA, USA

Helen Spoudeas
Consultant Endocrinologist
UCH/Middlesex Hospital
London, UK

Charles A. Stiller
Childhood Cancer Research Group
Department of Paediatrics
University of Oxford
Oxford, UK

Roger E. Taylor MA MB BS FRCP(Edin) FRCP FRCR
Consultant Clinical (Radiation) Oncologist
Department of Clinical Oncology
Cookridge Hospital
Leeds, UK

Atul Tyagi MS FRCS(SN)
Consultant Neurosurgeon
Department of Neurosurgery
The General Infirmary
Leeds, UK

David A. Walker BMedSci BM BS FRCP FRCPCH
Reader and Honorary Consultant in Paediatric Oncology
Children's Brain Tumour Research Centre
Division of Child Health
School of Human Development
University of Nottingham
Queen's Medical Centre
Nottingham, UK

Sue Walker
Educational Psychologist
Treloar School
Alton, Hampshire, UK

Beth Wicks
Education Consultant
Nottingham, UK

Otmar D. Wiestler MD
Head, German Cancer Research Center
Heidelberg, Germany

Johannes E. A. Wolff MD PD
Department of Pediatrics and Oncology
University of Calgary
Canada; and
St Hedwig's Hospital Regensburg
Germany

Foreword

Readers who scan the list of contributors to this timely volume will know it promises to contain much needed fresh insights and new approaches to *The Brain And Spinal Tumors Of Childhood*. The deceptively simple title encompasses a complex set of clinical, biologic and genetic problems.

One of the immediate and obvious difficulties is inherent if one considers the word tumors. Not long ago, patients being seen at a major center for a variety of oncologic problems were asked whether they had been told they had cancer. Most answered yes, but many with brain tumors answered no. This was reported with a figurative cluck of the tongue. Had these patients been denied the truth, or – in truth – did these many not have cancer?

Conflating brain tumor with malignant disease establishes a mindset. The American Cancer Society (ACS) compilation of cancer survival rates for children includes in its table the category "brain and other nervous systems"[1]. However, benign tumors account for about half the central nervous system (CNS) tumors listed by the Surveillance, Epidemiology and End Results (SEER) program, which provides the database for the ACS reports[2]. Careful perusal of Chapter 5 will reward the reader in this connection.

To be sure, many such benign masses can be lethal, in the same way that an enlarging hemangioma of the larynx can throttle an infant. There is too much of a not very bad thing in a very bad, very tight, vitally important space. This mindset has important clinical consequences. Despite their frankly benign or quasi-benign histologic appearance (i.e. low-grade characteristics) most enlarging CNS masses are treated as though they were malignant. This is done perhaps partly in frustration, but also because the treatments used for malignant diseases are familiar, tolerance doses are established, and nothing better is available. It calls to mind the intrathecal drugs used for prophylaxis and therapy of the meninges threatened by cancerous cells of epithelial or mesodermal origin. Methotrexate, cytarabine and hydrocortisone are commonly employed not because these nonleukemic cell types are known to be sensitive to those particular topically applied drugs. They are adopted largely because they have been used in thousands of patients with leukemia, and oncologists are thoroughly familiar and comfortable with them.

The thought evokes the old joke having to do with the drunk seen in the dead of night on all fours looking for his car keys under the street lamp, "Because," he explains, "the light is better here than in the dark alley back there where I dropped them."

The point is that such conflation of the very disparate benign lesions with the malignant is bound to dull the thrust towards needed different, novel means of managing this important portion of the total CNS tumor number.

Certainly, adjuvant antimitotic therapies have been successful, as might be expected in the management of clearly cancerous CNS neoplasms like the medulloblastoma. But CNS tumors defy the rules. The very undifferentiated glioblastoma multiforme with its high mitotic index should be very responsive to chemo radiotherapy, yet it continues on its lethal trajectory despite adjuvant treatments. By contrast, the craniopharyngioma – basically a wen – can be irradiated successfully (Chapter 20), and the bland-appearing optic nerve gliomas, with few if any visible mitoses, can be controlled for varying periods of time by chemotherapy and/or radiotherapy[3].

Such broad statements obscure some critical facts in individual cases and in wider discussions of CNS tumors. One of them is that the written histopathologic report may reflect a compromise position taken by the neuropathologist when reviewing the all too often scant biopsy material derived from a particular patient. The nuances that affect decision-making cannot be imparted in the bald written report. These remarks serve only to emphasize the obvious; namely, the neuropathologist plays a central role in all these discussions. Not only must that specialist be included in strategy planning sessions, but should also be consulted when the therapy to be adopted for individual patients is being considered. Indeed, a regularly scheduled, periodic combined clinicopathologic review session is critically important in any neuro-oncology center. All members of the team should be present. There is no better way for the continually evolving concepts in neuropathologic diagnosis of CNS tumors to be brought forward and made palpable.

That classifications and categorizations of these lesions are being changed and rethought is well brought out in

Chapters 3 and 5. They also make evident the need for the neuropathologist to be part of the planning team when clinical trials are being evolved.

Major advances have nonetheless been made in local control measures. The operating microscope and the Cavitron® have made it possible for neurosurgeons to remove tumors completely and safely.

Radiation therapy (RT) methods are improving at a rapid pace. Means of delivering RT to the tumor volume with very little dose to adjoining normal cells have been notable. Included in such techniques are radiosurgery, intensity modulated radiation therapy (IMRT) and three-dimensional conformal RT. On the horizon is an expanding number of proton irradiation facilities. They will build on the pioneering clinical studies started decades ago at MIT and Uppsala to name but two. Even heavier charged ion beams are being explored for clinical use. These particulate forms will mean that long-term survivors will suffer fewer of the late delayed damage seen after conventional photon RT, as explained in Chapter 10.

The sharp edges of these more localized therapies have their disadvantages, however. They are so sharp there is the real hazard of geographic misses, i.e. unaccounted-for cells just beyond the designated volume at risk might be excluded from the beam.

Here, the extraordinary improvements in imaging methods can play a role. Certainly, the advent of magnetic resonance imaging (MRI) has made possible unimaginable accuracy in the pre- and post-operative assessment of tumor extent. More recent innovations such as positron emission tomography (PET) and single photon emission computed tomography (SPECT) identify active tumor cells. Magnetic resonance spectroscopy (MRS) can even suggest the histologic tumor type.

There is still room for improvement in the therapy of CNS tumors that have been shown to be chemo-responsive. With other cancers, many of the recent advances have been achieved through the better combination of existing drugs. This can be done with CNS tumors too, with the occasional addition of new and promising agents like the imidazotetrazine derivative temozolomide.

The approaches being taken with a kindred neoplasm of neural crest origin, the neuroblastoma (NBL), offer encouragement. These entail, for example, the addition of biologic modifiers to bring under control the few remaining cells after more standard treatments. It was found that 13-*cis*-retinoic acid, an inducer of differentiation, was effective in improving survival rates when added after the aggressive treatments used in stem cell transplant regimens. Might a similar approach be beneficial in the embryologically and morphologically similar medullo- and retinoblastoma? The latter resembles neuroblastoma even in having its benign counterpart (the retinocytoma), and – albeit rarely – appearing to have the capacity for spontaneous regression.

No less cogent, the molecular genetic pathways that lead to the malignant transformation of the anlage cells are under intense investigation. Elegant laboratory studies by Tang *et al.*[4] have shown that transfection of *EPHB6* (a tyrosine kinase family receptor) with cDNA into a human NBL cell line can transform the malignant cells into their benign phenotype both *in vitro* and in an *in vivo* murine model. Modification of CNS cell tumor behavior rather than cell kill techniques through molecular genetic manipulations beckon. Chapter 23 offers some insights.

It remains for the neuro-oncologists to orchestrate these many strains. This can only be done through genuine collaboration among all the principal players, each with his or her instrument ready to join the concerted effort that is needed. This concerto, until recently played *lento* and only in a minor key, is now enlivened by much happier notes and a rising *tempo*.

Giulio J. D'Angio, MD
Professor Emeritus
University of Pennsylvania School of Medicine
Philadelphia, PA, USA
October 2003

REFERENCES

1. Greenlee RT, Murray T, Bolden S, *et al.* Cancer Statistics. *CA Cancer J Clin* 2000; **50**:7–33.

2. Prados MD, Berger MS, Wilson CB. Primary central nervous system tumors: Advances in knowledge and treatment. *CA Cancer J Clin* 1998; **48**:331–60.

3. Packer RJ, Lange B, Ater J, *et al.* Carboplatin and vincristine for recurrent and newly diagnosed low-grade gliomas of childhood. *J Clin Oncol* 1993; **11**:850–6.

4. Tang XX, Zhao H, Robinson ME, *et al.* Implications of *EPHB6*, *EFNB2* and *EFNB3* expressions in neuroblastoma. *Proc Natl Acad Sci USA* 2000; **97**:10936–41.

Joachin Kühl

A few months before the publication of this book, Joachin Kühl succumbed to a brain tumour. It is an absurd fate for a physician to die of the disease against which he dedicated a great part of his professional life and his research.

Joachin Kühl graduated at the University of Wurzburg where he became responsible physician for the paediatric oncology department in 1979. In 1981 he completed his training in paediatrics, becoming a professor of paediatrics in 1994 and Extraordinary Professor in 2002.

In 1987 Joachin Kühl founded the German Brain Tumour Study Group. He chaired various national cooperative trials in malignant brain tumours in children and young adults. He initiated the Brain Tumour Network in Germany, coordinating research activities in the field of paediatric neuro-oncology. This project was financially supported by the German Children's Cancer Foundation and served as a model for cancer care and research in children throughout Europe. Joachin was awarded the Bundesverdienstkreuz Cross in recognition of service to the state in August 2003.

The colleagues who worked closely with him say that Joachin Kühl was a fair, enthusiastic, critical partner. He gave a cohort of young doctors the chance to realise their potential; he was always capable of transferring responsibility to the young chairmen without backing away when discussion was needed.

He distinguished himself by his perennial enthusiastic, extremely serious, consistent and determined scientific attitude. He was everybody's highly appreciated German friend. The paediatric neuro-oncology community will miss him.

The editors

Abbreviations

17-AAG	17-allylamino-17-dematheoxygel-danamycin	CISS	constructive interference in the steady state
ACS	American Cancer Society	CNS	central nervous system
ACTH	adrenocorticotropic hormone	COG	Children's Oncology Group
ADH	antidiuretic hormone	CPA	cerebellar pontine angle
AFP	alpha-fetoprotein	CPC	choroid plexus carcinoma
AGT	alkylguanyl-DNA alkyltransferase	CPP	choroid plexus papilloma
ALL	acute lymphatic leukemia	CRM	continual reassessment method
ALL	acute lymphoblastic leukemia	CSF	cerebrospinal fluid
ALT	alternative lengthening of telomeres	CSI	chemical shift imaging
ANC	absolute neutrophil count	CSRT	craniospinal radiotherapy
APC	antigen-presenting cell	CT	computed tomography
AT/RT	atypical teratoid/rhabdoid tumor	CTV	clinical target volume
ATP	adenosine triphosphate	CUSA	cavitron ultrasonic aspirator
BBB	blood–brain barrier	DEXA	dual energy x-ray absorptiometry
BCNU	carmustine	DIA	desmoplastic infantile astrocytoma
BDNF	bone-derived neurotrophic factor	DIG	desmoplastic infantile ganglioglioma
bFGF	basic fibroblast growth factor	DLT	dose-limiting toxicity
β-HCG	beta-human chorionic gonadotrophin	DMC	data monitoring committee
bHLH	basic helix–loop–helix	DNT	dysembryoplastic neuroepithelial tumor
BIH	benign intracranial hypertension	DSMB	data and safety monitoring board
BMD	bone mineral density	DTIC	Temazolamide, dacarbazine
BMI	body mass index		
BMP	bone morphogenetic protein	ECG	electrocardiography
BSG	brainstem glioma	ECM	extracellular matrix
BTB	blood–tumor barrier	EEG	electro-encephelogram
BTP	brain tumor–polyposis	EFS	event-free survival
		EGF	epidermal growth factor
CAM	cell adhesion molecule	EGFR	epidermal growth factor receptor
CBF	cerebral blood flow	EGL	external granule layer
CBV	cerebral blood volume	EMA	epithelial membrane antigen
CCG	Children's Cancer Group	EMF	electromagnetic field
CCNU	lomustine	ENT	ear, nose and throat
CCSG	Children's Cancer Study Group	EST	endodermal sinus tumor
CDDP	cysplatin	EVD	external ventricular drain
CDK	cyclin-dependent kinase		
CEA	carcinoembryonic antigen	FDA	Food and Drug Administration
CGE	cobalt gray transporters	FGF	fibroblast growth factor
CGH	comparative genomic hybridization	FISH	fluorescence in situ hybridization
CHART	continuous hyperfractionated accelerated radiotherapy	FLAIR	fluid attenuated inversion recovery
		fMRI	functional magnetic resonance imaging
CHC	choriocarcinoma	FOG	^{18}F-flourodeoxyglucose
CI	confidence interval	FPP	farnesyl pyrophosphate
		FTase	farnesyl transferase

FTIs	Ftase inhibitors	MMT	malignant mesenchymal tumor
5-FU	5-fluorouracil	MNGGCT	malignant non-germinomatous germ-cell tumor
GAG	glycosaminoglycan	MNTIs	melanotic neuroectodermal tumors of infancy
GAP	GTPase-activating protein	MOPP	methocholorethamine, prednisone, procarbazine and vincristine
GBM	glioblastoma multiforme		
GCS	Glasgow Coma Scale	MRA	magnetic resonance angiography
GCT	germ-cell tumor	MRI	magnetic resonance imaging
GDP	guanosine diphosphate	MRP	multidrug resistance-associated proteins
GFAP	glial fibrillary acid protein	MRS	magnetic resonance spectroscopy
GH	growth hormone	MRSI	magnetic resonance spectroscopic imaging
GHRH	growth-hormone releasing hormone	MRT	magnetic resonance tomography
GnRH	gonadotrophin-releasing hormone	MRV	magnetic resonance venography
GPOH	Gesellschaft Pädiatrische Onkologie und Hämatologie	MSD	mutism with subsequent dysarthria
		MTD	maximum tolerated dose
GRP94	glucose-related protein-94	MTIC	methyl-triaxenyl imidazole carboximide
GTP	guanosine triphosphate	mTOR	mammalian target of rapamycin
GTR	gross total resection	MVD	microvessel density
GTV	gross tumor volume		
		NAA	N-acetyl aspartate
HART	hyperfractionated accelerated radiotherapy	NAWM	normal-appearing white matter
HCG	human chorionic gonadotrophin	NBCCS	nevoid basal cell carcinoma syndrome
HDAC	histone deacetylase complexes	NBL	neoblastoma
HIT	hirntumoren	NCA	nurse-controlled analgesia
HGF	hepatocyte growth factor	NCAM	neural cell adhesion molecule
HGG	high-grade glioma	NCM	neurocutaneous melanosis
HFRT	hyperfractionated radiotherapy	NF-1	neurofibromatosis type 1
HPA	hypothalamo-pituitary axis	NF-2	neurofibromatosis type 2
HPF	high-power field	NGF	nerve growth factor
HRQL	health-related quality of life	NMDA	N-methyl-D-aspartate
HSP90	heat shock protein-90	NMR	nuclear magnetic resonance
HUI	Health Utility Index	NRCT	National Registry of Childhood Tumours
		NSE	non-specific enolase
ICAM	intercellular cell adhesion molecule	NSTs	nerve sheath tumors
ICCC	International Classification of Childhood Cancer	NTV	neuroendoscopic third ventriculostomy
		OARs	organs at risk
ICRU	International Commission for Radiation Units	O^6BG	O^6-benzylguanine
		ONG	optic-nerve glioma
IGF	insulin-like growth factor	OS	overall survival
IGL	inner granule layer		
IL-10	interleukin 10	PAS	periodic acid-Schiff
		PBTC	Pediatric Brain Tumor Consortium
IMRT	intensity-modulated radiotherapy	PCA	patient-controlled analgesia
		PCNA	proliferating cell nuclear antigen
JC	Jamestown Canyon	PCV	Prednisone, CCNU, vincristine
JPA	juvenile pilocytic astrocytoma	PDGF	platelet-derived growth factor
		PDGF-R	platelet-derived growth factor receptor
LEDs	light-emitting diodes	PEI	cisplatin, etoposide and ifosfamide
LEF	lymphoid enhancer factor	PET	positron-emission tomography
LOH	loss of heterozygosity	PFS	progression-free survival
		PGP	p-glycoprotein
mAbs	monoclonal antibodies	PH	proportional hazard
MAPK	mitogen-activated protein kinase	PICU	pediatric intensive care unit
MDM2	murine double minute 2	PLAGA	poly(D,L, lactide-co-glycolide)
MEPs	motor-evoked potentials		
MIBG	meta-iodobenzylgluanidine		
MMP	matrix metalloproteinase		
MMPIs	matrix metalloproteinase inhibitors		

PLAP	placental alkaline phosphatase
pMRI	perfusion magnetic resonance imaging
PNET	primitive neuroectodermal tumor
POG	Pediatric Oncology Group
PRESS	point-resolved spectroscopy
PTV	planning target volume
PXAs	pleomorphic xanthoastrocytomas
QARC	Quality Assurance Review Center
r-HGH	recombinant hormone growth hormone
Rb	retinoblastoma
RCTs	randomized controlled trials
RECIST	response evaluation criteria in solid tumors
RFLP	restriction fragment length polymorphism
RFR	relative failure rate
RNA	ribonucleic acid
RRT	reduced-dose neuraxial radiotherapy
RT	radiation therapy
RT/ATT	rhabdoid/atypical teratoid tumor
RTS	Rubinstein–Taybi syndrome
SCEP	spinal cord evoked potential
SCF	stem cell factor
SD	standard deviation
SEARCH	Surveillance of Environmental Aspects Related to Cancer in Humans
SEER	Surveillance, Epidemiological, and End Results
SEP	somatosensory evoked potential
SF	scatter factor
SF/HGF	scatter factor/hepatocyte growth factor
SFOP	Société Francaise d'Oncologie Pédiatrique
shh	sonic hedgehog
SIOP	Société Internationale d'Oncologie Pédiatrique

SIR	standardized incidence ratio
SLD	sum of the largest diameter
SMN	second malignant neoplasm
SPECT	single-photon-emission computed tomography
SRT	standard-dose radiotherapy
SSEPs	somatosensory evoked potentials
STAT	signal transduction and activation of transcription
STEAM	stimulated-echo acquisition mode
SV40	simian virus 40
TCF	t-cell factor
TGF	tumor growth factor
TGF-α	transforming growth vector alpha
TGF-β	transforming growth factor beta
TIA	transient ischemic attack
TNF	tumor necrosis factor
t-PA	tissue plasminogen activator
TRAIL	tumor necrosis factor-related apoptosis-inducing ligand
TSH	thyroid-stimulating hormone
TUNEL	terminal UTP nick-end labeling
UBO	unidentified bright object
UKCCSG	UK Children's Cancer Study Group
VCAM	vascular cell adhesion molecule
VEGF	vascular endothelial growth factor
VM-26	teniposide
VP-16	etoposide
YST	yolk-sac tumor
WHO	World Health Organization

PART I

Introduction

Introduction

DAVID A. WALKER, GIORGIO PERILONGO, JONATHAN A. G. PUNT AND ROGER E. TAYLOR

The idea for this book arose during the mid-1990s, when the editors and authors were meeting each other in the specialized neuro-oncology multidisciplinary teams that were developing in children's hospitals, the national and international meetings where advances in clinical practice and applied research were reported, and the strengthening national and international clinical trials groups developing in Europe and the USA. The first editorial meeting took place in a bar in Leuven, Belgium – so it could be said that Belgian beer was an important source of inspiration!

Until now, most books concerned with pediatric oncology have placed the information about primary central nervous system (CNS) tumors within a single chapter, national trials groups have discussed the many tumor entities under a single agenda item, and neurosurgical collaboration in the design of trials has been a rare event. The European and international communities of pediatric neurosurgeons had done their best to promote the needs of these children through their own meetings and literature. However, standard use of radiotherapy after resection, whilst deliverable in the majority, was technically the most difficult radiotherapy to give, and it was seen to be damaging to the developing brain. Most reports of such approaches were institution-based, with small numbers of patients recruited over prolonged time periods. The closer involvement of pediatric oncologists in this field started to give access to the organizational infrastructure and expertise for the conduct of clinical trials, which had been applied to childhood leukemia and other solid tumors.

All of us were unhappy that, despite a small number of clinical trials in Europe and the USA investigating chemotherapy in medulloblastoma, the results of treatment were improving only slowly, if at all. We were all starting to see increasing numbers of children with rarer malignant tumors, as well as substantial numbers of children with so-called benign tumors. There were very few topics upon which there was clear consensus about diagnostic criteria, staging procedures, treatment strategies, and outcome measures, let alone methods for measuring long-term quality of survival. The overall survival for all brain tumors, when assessed together, had not improved noticeably in more than a decade, only half the patients were being seen at diagnosis by specialist neuro-oncology teams, and the quality of survival for those who were treated and survived from the previous era was seen to be very poor for some. There were regions in Europe where there were few specialist pediatric neurosurgeons; even among pediatric neurosurgeons, very few were prepared to work with pediatric oncologists in multidisciplinary clinical teams and research groups. Nihilistic attitudes towards adults with malignant brain tumors undoubtedly influenced philosophy towards children. Pediatric oncologists found themselves being drawn into delivering complex anticancer treatments, in parallel with trying to achieve complex neuro-rehabilitation, within health systems where child-focused resources are insufficient, fragmented, and poorly organized for someone with acquired brain injury. Pediatric oncologists found themselves inadequately trained for this; what is more, they found that their colleagues in the educational system were unaware of the impact of acquired brain injury on a child's subsequent capacity for education and personality development.

The publications and meetings during the 1990s were focused upon reporting pilot data from institutional studies, literature reviews, survival data from the cancer registries, preliminary information on the biology of these tumors, and the results of a small number of cooperative trials as they matured. This led to the establishment of new consensus views on diagnostic and therapeutic approaches. It was very important at this time that we worked separately from our colleagues in adult neuro-oncology, as the spectrum of disease in childhood was markedly different, high-grade glioma being, in contrast, the rarest of the childhood tumor categories. Furthermore, new tumor entities specific to the childhood age range were emerging, such as desmoplastic infantile ganglioglioma (DIG), dysembryoplastic neuroepithelial tumor (DNT), and the monomorphous polymyxoid astrocytoma. Finally, the balance of risks considered for any clinical intervention was influenced heavily by the age and stage of physical growth and development of the young patient. As these new, child-focused consensus views emerged, it became clear that there were questions that needed answering through clinical and basic research, as well as the need to test new ideas for therapy in clinical trials. Attempting a clinical trial in almost any of the tumor groups required international (in Europe) and cooperative group (in the USA) collaboration if sufficient numbers were to be recruited for statistical analysis. International cancer registry data at the beginning of the new millennium now show that the survival rates for primary CNS tumors are rising, giving reward for the efforts of those involved in these early cooperative efforts. However, mysteriously, it would seem that the incidence rates are rising too. Reliable explanations for this phenomenon are awaited.

Leading up to and since the beginning of the new millennium, the observations in the clinic have generated a variety of hypotheses that are testable through scientific and clinical research. They are likely to be highly informative. There is now a great need to establish links with neuroscientists, experts in the biology of brain development, tumor biology, mechanisms of brain injury, and techniques of neuroprotection, as well as the complex processes of neurodegeneration that have been the focus of so much adult research. These scientists have found the links to pediatric neuro-oncology fascinating and tempting. However, the complex ethics of childhood research as well as the rarity of spare biological material pose special problems requiring multicenter research group methodologies, which are inevitably slow. The era of the international clinical trial (in Europe) and the cooperative group clinical trial (in the USA) for CNS tumors has opened in earnest. New ideas are being tested, multicenter collaboration is established, and, as a result, the future looks good for the child and family as well as the clinical and scientific investigator.

The comprehensive care of a child with a primary CNS tumor requires specialized knowledge and a broad range of technical expertise, specialist equipment, and facilities, as well as established care pathways to lead the child and family through the complexities of modern health, education, and social care services. A child with a brain tumor, and their family, may encounter a wide variety of individuals fulfilling up to 55 different clinical, social, educational, and even political roles, each critical to the child's care at some time in their journey. In addition, each role may be played by more than one person. It is hardly surprising, therefore, that children, their families, and even the professionals involved can have some difficulties with team working and "joined-up thinking." This book is an attempt to bring together the issues related to decision-making in this complex patient journey so that a greater level of mutual understanding about the needs of the child can be achieved between us all.

Much of this knowledge is not part of conventional medical, nursing, educational, or social professional training, at either undergraduate or postgraduate level. Within the childhood cancer specialties, neuro-oncology is emerging as an independent subspecialty, further justifying a systematic review of what is known about this area of clinical practice, which we hope will inform established specialists and trainees alike but also, most importantly, will facilitate further service development.

This book is an attempt, therefore, to bring together in a single volume the conclusions of the debates of the 1990s. We hope that it will herald the beginning of an era where standard pediatric oncology textbooks either devote a chapter to each group of primary CNS tumor entities and explain the basic principles of clinical neuroscience practice relevant to CNS tumors, or omit them altogether so that specialist books such as this can give the subject the emphasis it deserves. The cooperative groups are already considering the needs of each primary CNS tumor entity under their own agenda headings. Collaboration with our neurosurgical colleagues in designing trials is now the routine.

The authors of this book are from Europe and North America because we met each other at these meetings. We have tried to make the text relevant by including illustrations, images, summary boxes, and clinical scenarios to keep the needs of patients central in the reader's mind. We anticipate, therefore, that the readership will come from a wide range of professional and scientific backgrounds, including children's medicine and nursing, diagnostic imaging, neurosurgery, neuropathology, and radiotherapy (clinical oncology) rehabilitation specialists in health, social, and educational services. This book is intended to be not a "bible" but an expanded handbook providing accessible information for all of these specialists.

Finally, the focus in this book of our efforts as neuro-oncologists is not simply to describe how to cure children with primary CNS tumors but to describe, comprehensively, how to care for them with attempted cure being the objective for each patient at the outset of therapy. This idealized approach can be achieved only by integrating the acquisition of data from research-based clinical practice and the timely application of these new data back to research-based clinical practice as soon as they are reliable. By this method, the possibility of *cure for all* can be pursued whilst ensuring that *care for all* is delivered to the highest possible standard.

Historical basis of neuro-oncology

JONATHAN A. G. PUNT, GIORGIO PERILONGO, ROGER E. TAYLOR, CLIFF BAILEY AND DAVID A. WALKER

INTRODUCTION

It is now clear that pediatric neuro-oncology has emerged as a separate subspecialty as a result of the fusion of skills, knowledge, and attitudes from neuroscience, surgical practice, radiotherapy, the clinical practices and science of medical oncology, and pediatric subspecialty practice. In this chapter, we have tried to tell the story using a time-line, which details the drawing together of the different threads of the story and a textual account of our memories of events over the past two decades that have been reported and debated and have therefore modified our thinking about child-centered clinical practice, clinical and scientific research, and the translation of these ideas into new prac-tice through clinical training.

PATHOLOGY

The modern classification of central nervous system (CNS) tumors was initiated by an American neurosurgeon, Harvey Cushing (1870–1939). Cushing asked Percival Bailey, a resident who was working with him at the Peter Bent Brigham Hospital in Boston, to classify more than 400 tumors that he had operated on. Based on this pio-neering work in 1926, Bailey and Cushing published their landmark work entitled "A classification of the tumors of the glioma group on a histogenetic basis with a correlation study on prognosis."[1] According to this scheme, 14 groups were defined on a cytogenetic basis. Although Bailey based

his concepts of tumor classification on those of a German pathologist Ribbert,[2] who asserted that each tumor type was derived from a particular cell line, with cells under-going developmental arrest during neuronal or glial histo-genesis, an embryogenetic significance was not attributed. However, before this seminal work, James Homer Wright in 1910 had already described the separate pathological entity we now know as medulloblastoma.[3] Bailey and Cushing recognized this tumor, which was made up of poorly differentiated, primitive-appearing cells arising from the cerebellar vermis primarily in children. They recorded some 29 cases of this condition. Medulloblas-tomas had previously been included in the category of sarcomas, but the new classification system recognized that these tumors in the CNS were of neuroepithelial ori-gin. Wright thought that they were derived from neuro-blasts, the precursor cells of neurons, while Cushing and Bailey originally thought that these tumors derived from glial progenitor cells called spongioblasts. Consequently, the name "spongioblast cerebelli" was chosen, although, unfortunately, this had already been used by Globus and Strauss to describe the tumor now known as "glioblastoma multiforme."[4] Cushing and Bailey, therefore, adopted an alternative name – "medulloblastoma cerebelli" – as they proposed that the tumor derived from a totipotential cell known as the medulloblast, which was capable of differ-entiating into astrocytes, oligodendrocytes, and neurons. It is of interest that in the footnote of the original paper describing the medulloblastoma, Bailey and Cushing reported that they had encountered five tumors with a similar histology in the supratentorial compartment. They therefore never addressed the issue of the cell or origin for tumors in this area, as the medulloblastoma was thought to be a unique tumor of the cerebellum. It was not until 1973 that Hart and Earle introduced the term "primitive neuroectodermal tumor" (PNET) as a generic title to include all these primitive-looking tumors.[5]

The concept of grading astrocytic tumors according to numerical grade was introduced by Kernohan in 1949;[6] it adopted a similar system proposed previously by Broders in the 1920s for grading adult carcinoma.[7] The grading system proposed by Kernohan has been the subject of many discussions, and, in consequence, many grading systems now exist.

Fifty years after the original work of Bailey and Cushing, a new comprehensive classification on human CNS tumors was developed. Known as the "Blue Book," the new system was developed by a group of neuropathologists on behalf of the World Health Organization (WHO). The neuropathologists felt subsequently, however, that there was a need to understand more about the histological prognostic features for childhood brain tumors and consequently highlighted the need for a classification system based upon histological features rather than the putative predominant cell type. A neuropathology working group reviewed the diagnosis of 3300 childhood brain tumors and proposed a further WHO classification system. The classification system was adequate for many tumors, although some of the more complex cerebral neoplasms did not fit into the system easily. Based on these observations, the committee was then invited to develop a new, revised WHO classification only for childhood brain tumors; this was subsequently published in 1985.[8] Further revisions have followed, and these are expected to improve our knowledge of childhood tumors.

IMAGING

Until the 1970s, most diagnostic tools were invasive, inexact, and time-consuming. Plain skull radiography could note intracranial calcification, suture widening, copper-beaten appearance, and the erosion of the sella turcica. The pneumoencephalogram was a commonly used diagnostic tool, apparently discovered serendipitously by William H. Luckett in 1913.[9] Luckett was studying a patient with a frontal fracture and spontaneous pneumoencephaly; he noted that this seemed to outline a tumor and gave information on the ventricular sizes. Pneumoencephalography was usually carried out through a ventricular burr hole, as the use of a lumbar spinal needle in the presence of raised intracranial pressure was considered inherently dangerous. These techniques were developed by a neurosurgeon, Walter Dandy (1883–1947), and a pediatrician, Kenneth D. Blackfan.[10] Initially, they

were used to study hydrocephalus, but they soon became the standard for investigating brain tumors. Neurosurgeons were able to localize the tumor by noting the shift it produces by lesions on the pneumoencephalogram. Cannulation of the femoral artery and retrograde threading of the cannula into the appropriate cranial artery produced arteriograms, which could allow localization and extent of any tumors. This idea of introducing a nontoxic contrast agent into human arteries was pioneered by a Portuguese physician Antonio Caetano Abrev Friere Egas Moniz in the late 1920s.[11] It is interesting to note that Moniz was awarded the Nobel Prize for his studies on the use of technetium-99 radioisotope scans in patients following frontal lobotomy rather than the more ubiquitous and informative angiography.

The development of the computed tomography (CT) scan and its widespread availability from the 1970s onwards saw the beginning of the modern era in neuroimaging. Godfrey Hounsfield was awarded the 1979 Nobel Prize in Medicine (the first engineer to be awarded a Nobel Prize in Medicine) for his discovery and development of the computerized tomogram.[12] He was particularly interested in pattern recognition, and he developed research projects to recognize objects contained in closed containers. He developed multiplanar images by using X-rays passing through containers and then integrating the images. The first experiment took more than a week to be completed. The first image of the human brain was obtained in 1971.

Nuclear magnetic resonance (NMR) was the next significant development in neuroimaging. The impact of this diagnostic technology is such that it deserves a wide review of the steps of development.

In the 1950s, Felix Block, working at Stanford University, and Edward Purcell, from Harvard University, found that certain nuclei absorbed and emitted energy when placed in a magnetic field. The strength of the magnetic field and the radiofrequency matched each other, as demonstrated earlier by Sir Joseph Larmor, an Irish physicist (1857–1942); this is known as the Larmor relationship, i.e. the angular frequency of precession of the nuclear spins is proportional to the strength of the magnetic field. This phenomenon was termed "nuclear magnetic resonance" as follows:

- *Nuclear*, because only the nuclei of certain atoms reacted in that way.
- *Magnetic*, because a magnetic field was required.
- *Resonance*, because of the direct frequency dependence of the magnetic and radiofrequency fields.

Bloch and Purcell were awarded the Nobel Prize for Physics in 1952 for this discovery.

However, it was Dr Isidor Rabi in the late 1930s who first recorded the phenomenon of NMR when working as a physicist at Columbia University. He was awarded the Nobel Prize for Physics in 1944 for his development of the atomic and molecular beam magnetic resonance method for observing atomic spectra. At that time, he considered it to be an artifact of his apparatus and disregarded its importance. During the 1950s and 1960s, NMR spectroscopy became a widely used technique for the non-destructive analysis of small samples.

In the late 1960s, Raymond Damadian, working at New York State University, demonstrated that different kinds of animal tissue emit response signals of variable length. He noticed that cancer tissue emitted response signals that were much longer than those emitted by normal tissue. Consequently, he brought NMR technologies into clinical practice.

In 1973, a short paper was published by Paul Lauterbur in *Nature*.[13] This paper was initially rejected by the editor of the journal as he thought its significance was not sufficiently wide for inclusion in *Nature*. In this seminal paper, Lauterbur described a new imaging technique that he termed "zeugmatography" (from the Greek *zeugmo* meaning yoke or a joining together). This described the joining together of a weak gradient magnetic field with the stronger main magnetic field, thus allowing spatial localization of two test-tubes of water. He used a back-projection method to produce the image of the two test-tubes. This imaging experiment moved NMR technology away from the single dimension, seen in spectroscopy, to the two-dimensional spatial orientation that was the foundation of NMR imaging.

In 1974, Damadian patented the idea of using MRI as a tool for medical diagnosis in the USA. By 1977, he had completed the construction of the first whole-body MRI scanner, which he named the "Indomitable." MRI technology had finally reached the patient, and its diagnostic advantages were clearly applicable. The first commercial magnetic resonance scanner in Europe (from Picker Ltd) was installed in 1983 at the University of Manchester Medical School.[14]

SURGERY

The evolution of the surgical aspects of neuro-oncology has inevitably been linked to, and benefited from, general developments that pervade many areas of neurosurgery and beyond. This brief review touches on these vital interactions and highlights those at the heart of the subject.

From the outset of the modern era, the vulnerability of neural tissue and its coverings to bacterial infection predicated that aseptic practice was of the highest order. Minimal touch techniques were de rigueur from an early stage; the conditions imposed by operating in cavities, and at a depth, dictated the development of improved methods of illumination and the design of special instruments. The

risks posed by postoperative hemorrhage were addressed only by the highest standards of intraoperative hemostasis. Electrodiathermy was rapidly embraced by Cushing, who collaborated with Bovie in the 1920s to develop an electrosurgical unit both for hemostasis and also as a method to facilitate the removal of intracranial tumors, especially meningiomas.[15,16]

Perioperative and supportive care has always played a special part in neurosurgery because of the importance of maintaining optimal physiological parameters and the need to detect adverse clinical changes in a timely manner. Cushing introduced the "ether chart" as the precursor of modern anesthetic records[17] and imported blood pressure monitoring, having encountered the Riva–Rocci device in Padua, Italy.[18] A much later generation of neurosurgeons in Glasgow, UK, introduced the Glasgow Coma Scale (GCS) as a dependable and reproducible method of describing levels of consciousness.[19,20] The special needs of the patient with impaired consciousness, paralysis, or bulbar palsy led to the development of specialist nursing techniques. It was the need to optimize intracranial operating conditions, and to maximize patient safety, that promoted a move away from using the good offices of medical students and interns in favor of full-time anesthesia specialists and even nurse anesthetists.[21] Insufflation anesthesia flowed from the neurosurgical practice of Elsberg in New York.[22] Mennell in London became the first dedicated neuroanesthetist, and in 1922 he was able to report on his experiences with 129 intracranial tumors.[23] The concepts and practice of neurological intensive care developed from the perceived needs of patients suffering from head injuries and from reports, such as that in 1958 from Newcastle upon Tyne, UK, that suggested improved outcomes were the result.[24] As pediatric neuro-oncology becomes more complex and more intensive, and as the prospects of good-quality outcomes increase this aspect of supportive care, already embodied in general pediatric oncology practice, will become more commonplace for children and young people with CNS tumors.

The significance of raised intracranial pressure as a cause of neurological symptoms, the need to recognize its presence, and the requirement to take appropriate action are core issues of management throughout the care of a patient with an intracranial tumor. The fundamental concept of the effect of incompressible blood and brain within the closed cranium was suggested in 1783 by a Scottish physiologist, Monro.[25] The role of cerebrospinal fluid (CSF) was inserted into the equation by Burrows in 1846. However, it was not until surgery for intracranial space-taking lesions became a realistic prospect that the true clinical significance was appreciated through the laboratory and clinical research of Kocher, a surgeon working in Bern, Switzerland. Kocher incidentally reported the lethal effects of cerebellar tonsillar herniation following lumbar puncture in the face of intracranial hypertension, a message that neurosurgeons have tried to propagate with variable success through successive generations of doctors.[26,27] The need to intervene promptly and effectively emerged.[28] The importance of brain shifts and internal herniae was developed further by Jefferson, working in Manchester, UK, who described the phenomenon of tentorial herniation in 1938.[29] The complexity of the physiology became clearer when a group of workers led by Lundberg in the 1960s reported the insights that could be gained from continuous intracranial pressure monitoring[30] and discovered that there were three distinct patterns of intracranial pressure.[31] This paved the way for Langfitt in the USA to devise the theory of cerebral compliance.[32]

Early techniques for the control of intracranial pressure were surgical and fell into the category of external decompression. The term "decompressive trephining" is attributed to a French surgeon Jaboulay.[33] In 1919, Weed and McKibben described the reduction of brain bulk and CSF pressure by intravenous infusion of hypertonic solutions in experimental settings.[34,35] In the same year, Haden reported the clinical use of intravenous 25 per cent glucose.[36] These temporizing measures were not favored universally. It also became apparent that external decompression in cases of cerebral tumor, as opposed to trauma, led to a protracted and dismal terminal phase. In 1936, a Canadian neurosurgeon McKenzie made a clear and humane case for internal decompression by maximal debulking in cases of malignant cerebral glioma.[37] The management of raised intracranial pressure in association with brain tumors, and the treatment of brain swelling in several other settings such as during radiation therapy, was assisted greatly by the introduction of the glucocorticoid dexamethasone for this purpose in 1960.[38]

The predilection of brain tumors in children for the cerebral midline makes the management of hydrocephalus a major issue. In 1952 there was a considerable advance with the introduction by Spitz and Holter in Philadelphia, USA, of the implanted, valve-regulated ventricular shunt for the management of hydrocephalus. This made the effective management of hydrocephalus an achievable objective. Unfortunately, hydrocephalus shunts brought their own catalog of complications.[39] The reintroduction of neuroendoscopic third ventriculostomy by Jones in Sydney,[40] followed by Sainte-Rose in Paris[41] and Punt in Nottingham, UK,[42] has been particularly beneficial in neuro-oncology surgery.[43] Furthermore, the use of neuroendoscopic third ventriculostomy to treat shunt complications has reduced one particularly tiresome type of late surgical morbidity.[44]

The confirmation of the presence of an intracranial or intraspinal mass lesion, and its accurate localization, has been, and remains, a matter of the greatest importance in neuro-oncology. It is therefore hardly surprising that practice and progress in neurosurgery have always been bound inextricably to developments in imaging, as described above. It is noteworthy, in passing, that it was the success of the combined efforts of Bennett and Godlee in London to localize and then remove a cerebral glioma in 1884[45] that put an end to debates about the morality of investigating localization of cerebral function. Preoperative prediction of histology and grade has been, and remains, the Holy Grail of neuroimaging ever since a German neurologist, Oppenheim, identified the presence of a brain tumor on plain skull radiographs in 1899.[46] Each new modality of imaging has been hailed as holding the key, only to be ultimately frustrated in this ambition. It remains to be seen whether the expectations for magnetic resonance spectroscopy (MRS) and positron-emission tomography (PET) fulfil the high expectations currently held for them. In any event, those managing children with CNS tumors are now substantially advantaged over their predecessors in that localization is generally excellent; there is the ability to assess more fully the extent of neuraxial disease, and of residual tumor after surgical resection; and there is a far greater ability than ever existed previously to distinguish complications of therapy from tumor recurrence.

For most brain tumors, the first step towards curative therapy is usually surgical removal. In this regard, the technical aids to excision have probably played a part in achieving more extensive resection and possibly in reducing surgical morbidity and mortality. The toxicity of neurosurgery awaits formal investigation in prospective studies, but this is under consideration in some multidisciplinary groups. The operating microscope, the ultrasonic aspirator,[47] and the surgical laser have all found their roles. In the sphere of minimally invasive neurosurgery,[48] image-guided stereotactic surgery[49] and neuroendoscopy[43] have also been applied successfully. It is unfortunate that there have been very view structured attempts to undertake studies designed to demonstrate whether, and to what extent, the use of these adjuncts has actually resulted in reduced surgical toxicity and more extensive surgical resection.

The first 100 years of modern neurosurgery were inevitably concerned with exciting technological advances. Of the utmost importance have been the outwardly less glamorous organizational developments that have brought pediatric neurosurgeons together at national and international levels. The formation of specialist societies such as the European Society for Pediatric Neurosurgery (in 1967) and the International Society for Pediatric Neurosurgery (in 1972) have been seminal events. The production of specialist textbooks concerning children's neurosurgery by founding fathers of the specialty, such as Ingraham and Matson[50] and Till,[51] and the launching of specialist journals such as Child's Brain (in 1975) and Child's Nervous System (in 1985) have been further sentinel milestones. More recently, the neurosurgical establishments of some countries have accepted that children have special requirements that justify provision of dedicated neurosurgical services[52] and due consideration of the multidisciplinary approach that is essential, especially in neuro-oncology.[53] Hopefully, the third millennium will bring child-centered pediatric neurosurgery rather than neurosurgeon-centered pediatric neurosurgery.

Of even greater significance has been the much more recent integration of active pediatric neurosurgeons into national and international cancer study groups, such as the United Kingdom Children's Cancer Study Group (UKCCSG), the Société Internationale d'Oncologie Pédiatrique (SIOP), and the Children's Cancer Group (CCG). The introduction of surgical questions into prospective protocols should be a further step in achieving increased efficacy and decreased morbidity for children and young people with CNS tumors.

RADIOTHERAPY

Compared with surgery, radiotherapy is a relatively new modality. X-rays were discovered by Roentgen in 1895 and used in the treatment of cancer only a few years later. The history of the radiotherapeutic management of children with CNS tumors parallels the development of radiotherapy in general.

In 1936, it was reported that radiotherapy had been used to treat medulloblastoma.[54] Subsequently, it emerged that for many children with tumors of the CNS, adjuvant radiotherapy following surgical excision or to treat macroscopic residual disease improved the chances of long-term survival. Radiotherapists in the early years encountered many of the same problems experienced by their surgical colleagues. The lack of appropriate imaging, poor supportive care, and relatively unsophisticated technology all limited the impact of radiotherapy on management of these CNS tumors.

Edith Patterson in the 1950s realized that biological behavior of certain tumors, such as medulloblastoma and malignant ependymoma, required radiotherapy to include the cranial contents and the spine.[55] She realized that although no tumor could be recognized in some of these areas, relapse was highly likely if treatment was not directed to these regions. The doses required to prevent subsequent metastatic disease in these areas was unknown but was limited by the tolerance of the spinal cord.

A standard dose in the region of 24 Gy was accepted. This dramatically reduced the occurrence of metastatic disease. Following recognition of the propensity for leptomeningeal spread, techniques for the irradiation of the entire craniospinal axis evolved. Initially, these were with the technology of the day, namely orthovoltage radiation.[55] However, even then the importance of precision was recognized. Since the 1950s, with the advent of machines producing gamma rays, from cobalt-60 sources, and later linear accelerators, techniques have been modified and refined further.[56,57]

Higher doses of radiation were usually necessary to obtain cure in those areas where tumor remained visible after surgery. However, this dose was also limited by the tolerance of normal brain tissue. Long-term follow-up continued to demonstrate that despite the dose being administered to the tolerable limits of normal tissue, local relapse remained a common problem. Furthermore, patients developed a variety of growth, endocrine, and intellectual deficits, which were likely to be the result of radiotherapeutic damage to the still-developing brain.

Radiotherapy techniques continued to advance. Megavoltage radiation therapy equipment and the use of custom-made immobilizing shells made the delivery of radiotherapy a more precise science. In the 1940s, Spiegel and Wycis developed a system that correlated the internal structure of the brain to an external coordinate system. Since then, many different stereotactic systems have been developed, all based on the concept of a rigid frame attached to the skull in such a way that axes can be fixed relative to the brain. Leksell in Sweden was the first to apply these techniques to the delivery of radiation at two circumscribed targets within the brain using orthovoltage X-rays, proton beams, and finally cobalt-60 gamma radiation.[58] In the late 1960s, Leksell, Larsson and coworkers developed the gamma knife, a set of highly collimated cobalt-60 sources; they used this to treat a variety of human tumors.[59] Subsequently, heavy charged particles were introduced, and a number of groups adopted conventional radiotherapy linear accelerators to produce narrow collimated beams of X-rays.

In the past three decades, advances in computing technology have been incorporated into radiotherapy planning and delivery. The use of radiotherapy-planning computers was first reported in 1955,[60] but it did not come into routine use until the late 1970s. Planning using three-dimensional technology was first reported in 1965[61] and was introduced widely in the 1980s.[62] Three-dimensional planning and delivery techniques have become used widely in the treatment of children with brain tumors since the 1980s and 1990s.

In the 1990s, we saw further refinements, with the advent of intensity-modulated radiotherapy (IMRT). This allows a further matching of the target volume to the tumor.[63] Refinements in planning cannot be implemented without precise patient positioning, and newer techniques for immobilization and verification of patient position with online electronic portal imaging have become important.

Radiotherapy fractionation evolved over many decades as being given in daily fractions, Mondays to Fridays. However in the 1970s and 1980s, it became clear from clinical and radiobiological studies that the long-term effects of radiation on normal tissues were enhanced when radiotherapy was given in high doses per fraction.[64] This linear quadratic model predicted that the therapeutic ratio could potentially be improved by giving smaller doses per fraction. Hyperfractionation involves giving a larger than conventional number of fractions, but with smaller doses per fraction, usually twice daily. During the 1980s and 1990s, this was investigated extensively in the treatment of brainstem glioma, with no benefit. However, its potential role in the treatment of medulloblastoma and ependymoma remains to be clarified.

In 1980, the North American Pediatric Oncology Group (POG) and, in a parallel development, the radiotherapy Quality Assurance Review Center (QARC) were established. Amongst other quality assurance functions, the QARC has played a key role in reviewing quality assurance data from several pediatric trial groups, including the POG and the Children's Oncology Group (COG).

In the past decade, prescribing and reporting have been standardized in the International Commission on Radiation Units (ICRU) documents 50[65] and 62.[66] In the 1990s, radiotherapy groups within the POG, the CCG (later the COG), and the SIOP have evolved. These groups have evolved to provide valuable opportunities for discussion and development of pediatric radiotherapy protocols and technical issues within these parent pediatric oncology organizations.

CHEMOTHERAPY

In 1943, an American battleship Jon Harvey was bombed in the harbor of Bari, Italy, by a German aeroplane. It was noted subsequently that many hundreds of service personnel died of aplastic anemia. The investigation into this incident highlighted that an ipride derivative (nitrogen mustard) was responsible for causing the aplastic anemia. In the same year, Goodman and Gilman injected nitrogen mustard into patients with malignant lymphoma and obtained the first short-lasting remissions.[67] This was the start of the modern history of chemotherapy. Since then, there has been a continued development of new chemotherapy agents. Wilms' tumor was one of the early solid tumors to be treated with chemotherapy through the pioneering work of Farber and colleagues.[68] In 1970, multiagent chemotherapy was introduced for the treatment of human cancer, with the development of the methochlorethamine, prednisone, procarbazine, and vincristine (MOPP) regime in patients affected by Hodgkin's disease.

The use of chemotherapy for intracranial tumors was limited initially by the belief that drugs needed to cross the blood–brain barrier to be effective. Much emphasis was placed on the need for a highly lipid-soluble non-ionized molecule that did not have significant protein bindings. Research demonstrated that the blood–brain barrier was absent at the center of the tumor but was apparently intact at the tumor–brain interface, and it was here that the cell activity was greatest. In consequence, the clinicians felt that the tumor in the CNS was relatively well protected from the effects of chemotherapy. More recent work has shown, however, that tissue transport is increased in brain tumors and consequently water-soluble chemotherapy agents may have a greater role in the treatment of these tumors than was originally supposed.

Early studies on the value of chemotherapy in brain tumors involved a series of single phase II studies aimed at investigating the chemosensitivity of neoplasms to different agents. Based on these studies, a large number of drugs have been shown to be active against brain tumors, including vincristine, procarbazine, etoposide, carmustine, cyclophosphamide, dibromodulcitol, cisplatin, carboplatin, and thiotepa. The comparative rarity of childhood brain tumors makes multi-institutional or international studies imperative for proper assessment. Various collaborative groups, including the South West Oncology Group, the Children's Cancer Study Group (CCSG), the POG, and the SIOP, have all developed cooperative groups to initiate large-scale brain tumor clinical research programs. Bloom and Neidhardt designed and coordinated the first multicenter trial in Europe for the SIOP,[69] while Evans and Krischer led the early initiatives for the CCSG and POG.[70] These early trials looked to improve the survival rate for children with medulloblastoma and malignant astrocytic tumors by introducing chemotherapy to surgery and conventional radiotherapy.

Since then, a number of randomized trials have been completed in both Europe and the USA and have contributed to defining and refining the present treatment strategies for curing children with medulloblastoma. Further multicenter, randomized studies, however, have been slow to develop and reflect the difficulties in promoting large cooperative studies in childhood neuro-oncology.

LATE EFFECTS OF TREATMENT

Many studies have looked at the quality of life in long-term surviving children with brain tumors. The importance of these studies reflects the fact that most children who do survive their tumors rarely escape without some long-term consequences. The problems of radiotherapy have been particularly highlighted. The younger the child at the time of radiotherapy, the greater the resulting damage. The experience of the child cured of their tumor but severely brain-injured by the effects of the tumor, surgery, radiotherapy, and, to a lesser extent, chemotherapy, was deeply shocking to those exploring multimodality treatments. Investigations into brain-sparing therapies using chemotherapy and reduced-dose field or delayed radiotherapy in very young children comprised the first group of patients where it was thought ethical to explore such approaches. A view was taken that quality of survival was more important than pursuing survival alone at any cost. Investigators in the USA treated children under the age of two years with chemotherapy in an attempt to avoid, or at least delay, the use of radiotherapy. This strategy in the 1990s led to a series of catch-all chemotherapy-based infant and early childhood studies offering all histological types similar dose intensity, brain-sparing chemotherapy, and delaying, reducing, or omitting radiotherapy. The damaging effects of the tumor and the surgical consequences of interventions or critical neurological incidents (hydrocephalus, fitting, encephalopathy, hemorrhage, necrosis) were identified increasingly as the main villains, and will remain so.

Other late effects of treatment have been noted. Cognitive function, endocrine damage, and neurological sequelae are all well recognized following treatment for children with brain tumors. Intellectual damage may result from a variety of causes but is particularly noticeable following radiotherapy. Observation and measurement of these problems have resulted in the development of alternative therapies aimed at minimizing the impact. However, there are concerns that replacing radiotherapy with chemotherapy would not be without problems, and close observations of these patients must be built into care plans. Properly constructed follow-up studies will need to be undertaken for many years to ensure that the impact of treatment is well understood.

CONCLUSIONS

The emergence of the subspecialty has been a long time coming. It has relied on the unique fusion of scientific and clinical observation and description, judicious planned and serendipitous experimentation, bold clinical trials of novel approaches to treatment, government backing of scientific endeavors, the application of startling technical advances, individual heroic acts by those affected by the loss of life and abilities of children, and committed clinicians prepared to put the child and family at the center of their clinical decision-making, often throwing down long-held professional barriers to change at critical moments. This history is fresh and ongoing. There is a lot more to come. The rest of this book is an attempt to put this into some perspective.

REFERENCES

1 Bailey P, Cushing H. *A classification of the tumors of the glioma group on a histogenetic basis with a correlation study on prognosis.* Philadelphia: JB Lippincott. 1926.

2 Ribbert H. Ueber das spongioblastoma und das gliom. *Virchows Arch Pathol Anat* 1918; **225**:195–213.

3 Wright JS. Neurocytoma or neuroblastoma, a kind of tumour not generally recognized. *J Exp Med* 1910; **12**:556–61.

4 Globus JH, Strauss I. Spongioblastoma multiforme, primary malignant form of neoplasm (its clinical and anatomical features). *Arch Neurol Psychiatr* 1925; **14**:39.

5 Hart MN, Earle KM. Primitive Neuroectodermal tumours of the brain in children. *Cancer* 1973; **32**:890–7.

6 Kernohan JW, Mabon RF, Svien HJ *et al.* A simplified classification of gliomas. *Proc Staff Meet Mayo Clinic* 1949; **24**:71–5.

7 Broders AC. Carcinoma grading and practical application. *Arch Pathol Lab Med* 1926; **2**:376–81.

8 Rorke LB, Gilles FH, Davis RL, Becker LE. Revision of the World Health Organization Classification of brain tumors for childhood brain tumors. *Cancer* 1985; **56**:1869–86.

9 Luckett WH. Air in the ventricles following a fracture of the skull. *Surg Gynecol Obstet* 1913; **17**:237–40.

10 Dandy WE, Blackfan KN. An experimental and clinical study of internal idrocephalus. *JAMA* 1913; **61**:2216–17.

11 Moniz CE. L'enecéphalographie artérielle, son importance dans la localisation des tumeurs cérébrales. *Rev Neurol* 1927; **2**:72–90.

12 Hounsfield GN. Computerized transverse axial scanning (tomography). *Br J Radiol* 1973; **46**:1016–22.

13 Lauterbur P. Image formation by induced local interaction; examples employing magnetic resonance. *Nature* 1973; **242**:190–1.

14 Isherwood I. The golden age: a shifting spectrum. British Institute of Radiology Presidential Address 1985. *Br J Radiol* 1986; **59**:643–52.

15 Cushing H. Macewen memorial lecture on the meningiomas arising from the olfactory groove and their removal by the aid of electro-surgery. *Lancet* 1927; **1**:1329–39.

16 Cushing H. Electro-surgery as an aid to the removal of intracranial tumors. With a preliminary note on a new surgical-current generator (by W.T. Bovie). *Surg Gynecol Obstet* 1928; **47**:751–84.

17 Tracy PT, Hanigan WC. History of neuroanesthesia. Greenblatt SH (ed.). *A History of Neurosurgery in its Scientific and Professional Contexts.* Park Ridge, IL: American Association of Neurological Surgeons, 1997, pp. 213–21.

18 Cushing H. On routine determination of arterial tension in operating room and clinic. *Boston Med Surg J* 1903; **148**:250–6.

19 Teasdale G, Jennett B. Assessment of coma and impaired consciousness. *Lancet* 1974; **ii**:81–4.

20 Teasdale G, Knill-Jones R, Van der Sande J. Observer variability in assessing impaired consciousness and coma. *J Neurol Neurosurg Psychiatry* 1978; **41**:603–10.

21 Bingham WF. The early history of neurosurgical anesthesia. *J Neurosurg* 1973; **39**:568–84.

22 Elsberg CA. Anesthesia by intratracheal insufflation. In: Gwathmey JT (ed.). *Anesthesia*, 2nd edn. New York: Macmillan, 1924.

23 Hunter AR, Mennell Z. A pioneer of neurosurgical anaesthesia. *Anaesthesia* 1983; **38**:1214–16.

24 MacIver IN, Frew IFC, Matheson JG. The role of respiratory insufficiency in the mortality of severe head injuries. *Lancet* 1958; **1**:390–3.

25 Monro AS. *Observations on the Structure and Function of the Nervous System*. Edinburgh: W. Creech & Johnson, 1783.

26 Kocher T. *Chirurgische Operationslehre*. Jena: G. Fischer, 1892.

27 Kocher T. *Text-book of Operative Surgery*, 3rd English edn. Authorised translation from the 5th German edn. New York: Macmillan, 1911.

28 Weisenburg TH. *Manual of Neuro-Surgery*. Washington, DC: Government Printing Office, 1919.

29 Jefferson G. The tentorial pressure cone. *Arch Neurol Psychiatry* 1938; **40**:857–76.

30 Lundberg N. Continuous recording and control of ventricular fluid pressure in neurosurgical practice. *Acta Psychiatr Neurol Scand* 1960; **36** (suppl. 149):1–193.

31 Lundberg N. Monitoring of the intracranial pressure. In: Critchley M, O'Leary JL, Jennett B (eds). *Scientific Foundations of Neurology*. London: William Heinemann Medical, 1972, pp. 356–71.

32 Miller JD, Adams H. Physiology and management of increased intracranial pressure. In: Critchley M, O'Leary JL, Jennett B (eds). *Scientific Foundations of Neurology*. London: William Heinemann Medical, 1972, pp. 308–24.

33 Elsberg CA. Operations on the brain and its membranes. In: Johnson AB (ed.). *Operative Therapeusis*. New York: D Appleton & Co, 1921, pp. 659–736.

34 Weed LH, McKibben PS. Pressure changes in the cerebrospinal fluid following intravenous injections of solutions of various concentrations. *Am J Physiol* 1919; **48**:512–30.

35 Weed LH, McKibben PS. Experimental alterations of brain bulk. *Am J Physiol* 1919; **48**:531–55.

36 Haden RL. Therapeutic applications of the alteration of brain volume by the intravenous injection of glucose. *J Am Med Assoc* 1919; **73**:983–4.

37 McKenzie KG. Glioblastoma. A point of view concerning treatment. *Arch Neurol Psychiatry* 1936; **36**:542–6.

38 Galichich JH, French LA. Use of dexamethasone in the treatment of cerebral edema resulting from brain tumors and brain surgery. *Am Pract* 1961; **12**:169–74.

39 Punt J. Principles of CSF diversion and alternative treatments. In: Schurr PH, Polkey C (eds). *Hydrocephalus*. Oxford: Oxford Medical Publications, 1993, pp. 139–60.

40 Jones RFC, Stening WA, Brydon M. Endoscopic third ventriculostomy. *Neurosurgery* 1990; **26**:86–92.

41 Sainte-Rose C. Third ventriculostomy. In: Manwaring K, Crone KR, Dante MD (eds). *Neuroendoscopy*. New York: Liebert, 1992, pp. 47–62.

42 Punt J, Wilcock D, Jaspan T, Worthington B. Neuroendoscopy in the management of hydrocephalus. *Eur J Pediatr Surg* 1995; **5** (suppl. 1):3921.

43 Macarthur DC, Buxton N, Vloeberghs M, Punt J. The effectiveness of neuroendoscopic interventions in children with brain tumours. *Childs Nerv Syst* 2001; **17**:589–94.

44 Mallucci CL, Vloeberghs M, Punt JA. Neuroendoscopic third ventriculostomy: the first-line treatment for blocked ventriculo-peritoneal shunts? *Child Nerv Syst* 1997; **13**:498.

45 Bennett AE, Godlee R. Excision of a tumour of the brain. *Lancet* 1884; **2**:1090–1.

46 Oppenheim H. Discussion at Berliner Gesellschaft fur Psychiatrie und Nervenkrankenheiten, November 13, 1899. *Arch Psychiatry* 1901; **34**:303–4.

47 Fasano VA, Zeme S, Frego L, Gunetti R. Ultrasonic aspiration in the surgical treatment of intracranial tumors. *J Neurosurg Sci* 1981; **25**:35–40.

48 Punt J. Minimally invasive neurosurgery as a strategy for minimising brain damage. Presented at The Developing Brain in Paediatric Oncology: Second Congress of the European Association for Neuro-Oncology, Wurzburg, 1996.

49 Perry JH, Rosenbaum AE, Lunsford LD, Swink CA, Zorub DS. Computed tomography-guided stereotactic surgery: conception and development of a new stereotactic methodology. *Neurosurgery* 1980; **7**:376–81.

50 Ingraham FD, Matson DD. *Neurosurgery of Infancy and Childhood*. Springfield, IL: Charles C. Thomas, 1954.

51 Till K. *Paediatric Neurosurgery for Paediatricians and Neurosurgeons*, 1st edn. Oxford: Blackwell Scientific Publications, 1975.

52 Society of British Neurological Surgeons. *Safe Paediatric Neurosurgery*. London: Society of British Neurological Surgeons, 1998.

53 Walker DA, Hockley A, Taylor R, *et al. Guidance for Services for Children and Young People with Brain and Spinal Tumours*. London: Royal College of Paediatrics and Child Health, 1997.

54 Cutler EC, Sosman MC, Vaughan WW. Place of radiation in treatment of cerebellar medulloblastoma: report of 20 cases. *Am J Roentgenol Radium Ther Nucl Med* 1936; **35**:429–53.

55 Paterson E, Farr RF. Cerebellar medulloblastoma: treatment by radiation of the whole central nervous system. *Acta Radiologica* 1953; **39**:323–36.

56 Bloom HJ, Wallace EN, Henk JM. The treatment and prognosis of medulloblastoma in children. A study of 82 verified cases. *Am J Roentgenol Radium Ther Nucl Med* 1969; **105**:43–62.

57 Van Dyk J, Jenkin RTD, Leung PMK, Cunningham JR. Medulloblastoma: treatment technique and radiation dosimetry. *Int J Radiat Oncol Biol Phys* 1977; **2**:993–1005.

58 Leksell L. The stereotaxic method and radiosurgery of the brain. 1951; *Acta Chir Scan* **102**:316–19.

59 Arndt J. Focussed gamma radiation; the Gamma Knife. In: Phillips MH (ed.). *Physical Aspects of Stereotactic Radiosurgey*. New York, NY: Plenum, 1993, 87–128.

60 Tsien KC. The application of automatic computing machines to radiation treatment planning. *Br J Radiol* 1955; **28**:432–9.

61 Sterling TD, Perry H, Katz L. Automation of radiation treatment planning V. Calculation and visualisation of the total treatment volume. *Br J Radiol* 1965; **38**:906–13.

62 Goietin M, Abrams M, Rowell D *et al.* Multi-dimensional treatment planning: II. Beam's eye view, back projection, and projection through CT sections. *Int J Radiat Oncol Biol Phys* 1983; **9**:789–97.

63 Intensity Modulated Radiation Therapy Collaborative Working Group. Intensity-modulated radiotherapy: current status and issues of interest. *Int J Radiat Oncol Biol Phys* 2001; **51**:880–914.

64 Thames HD, Withers HR, Peters LJ, Fletcher GH. Changes in early and late radiation responses with altered dose fractionation: implications for dose survival relationships. *Int J Radiat Oncol Biol Phys* 1982; **8**:219–26.

65 ICRUa. International commission on radiation units and measurements. Prescribing, recording, and reporting photon beam therapy. *ICRU Report* 1993; **50**. Bethesda.

66 ICRUb. International commission on radiation units and measurements. Prescribing, recording, and reporting photon beam therapy. Supplement to ICRU report 50, *ICRU Report* 1999; **62**. Bethesda.

67 Bonadonna, G. Principi di chemioterapia. In: Bonadonna G, Robustelli della Cuna G and Valagussa P (eds) *Medicina Oncologica.* Milan: Masson, 1999.

68 Farber S. Chemotherapy in the treatment of leukemia and Wilms' tumour. *JAMA* 1966; **198**:826–36.

69 Tait DM, Thornton-Jones H, Bloom HJ. Adjuvant chemotherapy for medulloblastoma, the first multi-centre controlled trial of the International Society of Paediatric Oncology (SIOP I). *Eur J Cancer* 1990; **26**:464–9.

70 Fisher PG, Fry TJ, Wharam MD. Lessons learned from the clinical cooperative trials groups for childhood brain tumors. *Neurosurgery Quarterly* 1998; **8**:216–31.

APPENDIX: TIMELINE

Writing a commentary about the evolution of a subject as new as pediatric neuro-oncology is a hazardous task. Things are currently happening so fast that, as you write your perspective of events, your interpretation may be shown to be wide of the mark when reviewed a few years later. The timeline that we have produced is an attempt to show how the subject of pediatric neuro-oncology has emerged from wide-ranging clinical developments and the translation of scientific understanding into surgery, imaging, infections and cancer, epidemiology, and neuroscience. It is the integration of developmental neuroscience component of this pot pourri that is pediatric neuro-oncology that makes the subject uniquely challenging. Survival alone for these children was rapidly seen to be an inadequate end point for the evaluation of new treatments. The definition of cure has increasingly included holistic themes where not only should life be extended but also disability should be minimized and the capacity for growth, development, learning, and reproduction optimized. These are big objectives that emerged quickly from discussions of the first institutional series and multicenter trials that were reported at a time when drug treatment of leukemia and lymphoma was being seen to offer true cures, and the combination of chemotherapy and modified surgical and radiotherapeutic techniques in solid tumors of childhood was being seen to avoid the need for high-risk, mutilating interventions. Parallel developments in neonatology focused upon brain-sparing methods in small children: these are still being developed and are based primarily upon meticulous attention to detail regarding intensive and supportive care. Neuroprotective agents are hoped for. However, they are yet to become established in clinical practice. What we have not been able to identify in this timeline is the provision of rehabilitation services/priorities in children's health services around the world. There is no doubt that such national strategies make a massive difference for the recovery of the child and family. The technology required is frequently low-tech, concentrating on communication, liaison, provision of home aids, and assessment for appropriate educational provision. However low-tech, it is the final pathway along which each child and their family must travel if they are to derive benefit from the application of high-tech solutions that cause so much excitement in the research-focused world of neuro-oncology. We look forward to adding to this timeline as developments occur. It may be that previous discoveries not identified here will prove to be critical for future developments in the field, such is the excitement of working and assisting with the development of modern medicine at this time.

David Walker
July 2004

Year	Neuroscience		Oncology	
	Neurosurgery	Imaging	Radiotherapy	Chemotherapy
2500–1600 BC	"Edwin Smith" papyrus from Ancient Egypt: earliest description of surgical treatment of cancer.			"George Elbers" papyrus from Luxor, Ancient Egypt, outlines pharmacological, mechanical, and magical treatments for cancer. 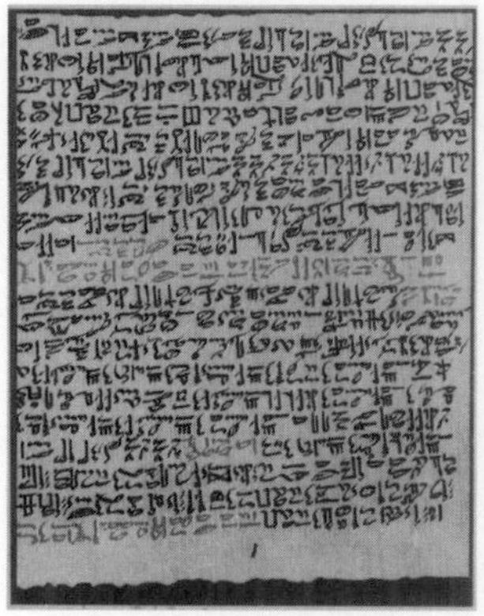
1802	L'Hôpital des Enfants Malades, Paris, founded. 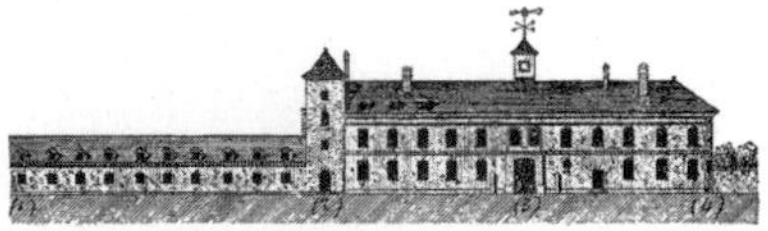			
1821		Babbage designs an ophthalmoscope, which he later (1848) constructs following an observation by a medical student.		
1830			Domenico Rigoni-Stern concludes that incidence of cancer increases with age, city living, and unmarried status.	

Image courtesy of the National Library of Medicine

Abb. 33   Das Pariser Hôpital des enfants malades im Jahre 1802.

Image courtesy of the Wellcome Library, London

Year	Neuroscience		Oncology	
	Neurosurgery	Imaging	Radiotherapy	Chemotherapy
1838			Muller's book introduces histology to oncology.	
1842	Dr Crawford Long first uses ether anesthesia for cancer operation.			

Image courtesy of Mary Evans Picture Library

| 1851 | Von Helmholtz (Konigsberg, Prussia) rediscovers the ophthalmoscope.[1] |

Image courtesy of the Welllcome Library, London

| Year | Neuroscience | | Oncology | |
	Neurosurgery	Imaging	Radiotherapy	Chemotherapy
1854	Hospital for Sick Children, London, founded.			

Image courtesy of Mary Evans Picture Library

Year	Neurosurgery	Imaging	Radiotherapy	Chemotherapy
1855	Children's Hospital of Philadelphia founded.			
1863	Jackson (London, UK) recognizes papilledema;[2] Seguin (Columbia, USA) subsequently notes association with headache and brain tumor.			
1875	Hospital for Sick Children, Toronto, founded.			

Year	Neuroscience		Oncology	
	Neurosurgery	Imaging	Radiotherapy	Chemotherapy
1879	First successful removal of a brain tumor when Macewen (Glasgow, UK) operates on meningeal tumour in 14-year-old girl.[3]			

Image courtesy of the Wellcome Library, London

Year	Neuroscience		Oncology	
1879	Naunyn and Schreiber (Bern, Switzerland) note relationship between intracranial pressue (ICP), blood pressure (BP) and heart rate (HR).[4]			
1881	Wernicke (Breslau, Germany) performs external ventricular drainage.[5]			

	Neuroscience		Oncology	
Year	Neurosurgery	Imaging	Radiotherapy	Chemotherapy
1884	Godlee (London, UK) removes glioma from 25-year-old man localized by abnormal neurology and analyzed by Bennett.[6]			

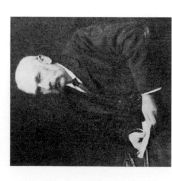

Image courtesy of the Wellcome Library, London

1887	Horsley (London, UK) removes spinal neurofibroma, localized clinically by Gowers.[7]			

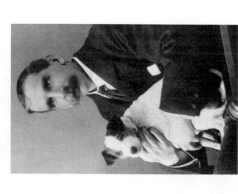

Image courtesy of the Wellcome Library, London

Year	Neuroscience		Oncology	
	Neurosurgery	Imaging	Radiotherapy	Chemotherapy
1888	Keen (Philadelphia, USA) performs first ventricular tap of modern era.[8]			
1889	Wynter (London, UK) employs therapeutic lumbar puncture.			
1889	Wagner introduces osteoplastic craniotomy.[9]			
1891	Spontaneous electrical activity of the brain detected by Gotch and Horsley (London, UK).[10]			
1895			Roentgen (Wuerzberg, Germany) discovers X-rays.[11]	
1896	Chipault (Paris, France) starts *Travaux de Neurologie Chirurgicale*, the first neurosurgical journal.		E. H. Grubbe, a Chicago researcher, becomes first person known to administer X-rays to a cancer patient.	

Image © Bettmann/Corbis

Year	Neuroscience		Oncology	
	Neurosurgery	Imaging	Radiotherapy	Chemotherapy
1896		Cushing (Baltimore, USA) demonstrates bullet in cervical spine on X-ray.[12] *Image courtesy of akg-images*		
1899		Oppenheim diagnoses brain tumor on plain skull radiograph.[13]		
1900				Theodor Boveri, Professor of Zoology at Wurzberg, Germany, promotes a genetic explanation for cancer.
1905	Cushing (Baltimore, USA) defines importance of raised ICP.[14]			
1906	Horsley (London, UK) introduces operating headlight.[15]			

| | Neuroscience | | Oncology | |
Year	Neurosurgery	Imaging	Radiotherapy	Chemotherapy
1907	Von Eiselsberg (Vienna, Austria) performs first successful removal of intramedullary spinal cord tumor.[16] 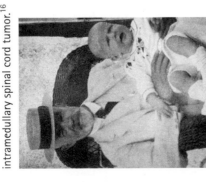 *Image courtesy of the Wellcome Library, London*			
1911			Alexis Carrel and Montrose Burrows develop the first long-term tissue cultures of cancer cells. 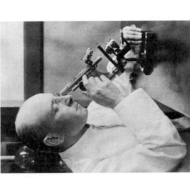 *Image © Corbis*	

Year	Neuroscience		Oncology	
	Neurosurgery	Imaging	Radiotherapy	Chemotherapy
1911				Peyton Rous transmits cancer between chickens in a cell-free filtrate, concluding that a virus is the cancer agent. Awarded Nobel Prize in 1966.

Image © Robert Dowling/Corbis

Year	Neurosurgery	Imaging	Radiotherapy	Chemotherapy
1914	Dandy and Blackfan (Baltimore, USA) publish classic paper on hydrocephalus.[17]			
1916		Hever and Dandy (Baltimore, USA) appreciates limitations of non-contrast radiographs in diagnosis of brain tumors.[18]	Frederick L. Hoffman, insurance statistician, compiles world cancer statistics, persuading US government to analyze cancer mortality.	
1918		Dandy (Baltimore, USA) describes air ventriculography.[19]		
1919	Haden (USA) describes use of intravenous 25% glucose to decrease brain volume.[21]	Dandy (Baltimore, USA) describes air encephalography.[22]	Frazier (Philadelphia, USA) implants radium sources directly into brain tumors.[23] Cushing (Boston, USA) treats medulloblastomas with radiation therapy.[20]	
1920	Mixter (Boston, USA) performs first endoscopic third ventriculostomy.[24]			
1923	Cushing and Martin (Boston, USA) describe optic nerve glioma.[25]			
1924	Berger (Jena, Germany) records spontaneous electrical activity from skin over a skull defect, and coins EEG.[26]	Moniz (Lisbon, Portugal) makes first successful cerebral angiogram in living patient.[28]		

Year	Neuroscience		Oncology	
	Neurosurgery	Imaging	Radiotherapy	Chemotherapy
1924 (contd.)	Bailey and Cushing (Boston, USA) classify gliomas, identifying those found typically in children.[27]			
1926	Cushing (Boston, USA) introduces electrocautery.[29]		Bailey and Cushing describe first use of radiotherapy to treat four cases of medulloblastoma.[27]	
1927	Cushing (Boston, USA) presents case of complete excision of intramedullary spinal cord tumor in 11-year-old girl at combined meeting with pediatricians.[30]			
1929	Ingraham (Boston, USA) specializes in pediatric neurosurgery.			
1930	Cushing (Boston, USA) publishes series of 61 cases of medulloblastoma.[20]			
1936			Cutler publishes 20 cases of medulloblastoma treated with radiotherapy.[31]	
1939	Mortality figures published (Boston, USA) for cerebellar astrocytoma (5%), medulloblastoma (15.4%), and fourth ventricle ependymoma (50%).[32]			National Cancer Institute founded in USA. The first director (1938–1945) is Dr Carl Voegtlin, a Swiss-born pharmacologist.

Image courtesy of the National Cancer Institute

| Year | Neuroscience | | Oncology | |
	Neurosurgery	Imaging	Radiotherapy	Chemotherapy
1940s			Linear accelerators developed during the 1940s.	

Image © Hulton–Deutsch Collection/Corbis

Year	Neuroscience		Oncology	
	Neurosurgery	Imaging	Radiotherapy	Chemotherapy
1948		Moore (Minneapolis, USA) localizes brain tumor with ^{131}I scanning.[33]	Ralston Paterson proposes role of craniospinal radiotherapy for medulloblastoma.[34]	Sidney Farber finds that a folic "antagonist" developed by Yellapragada SubbaRow inhibits tumor growth in mice and children with leukemia.[35]
1952	Spitz and Holter (Philadelphia, USA) devise the valved shunt.[36]			
1953			James Watson and Francis Crick unveiled their model of the structure of DNA.[37]	

Image courtesy of Associated Press

Year	Neuroscience		Oncology	
	Neurosurgery	Imaging	Radiotherapy	Chemotherapy
1953			Edith Paterson (Christie Hospital, Manchester, UK) reports 21% five-year survival in medulloblastoma treated with craniospinal radiation therapy.[38] Talairach (Paris, France) performs stereotactic brachytherapy of brain tumors.[39]	
1954	Ingraham and Matson (Boston, USA) publish the first textbook devoted to pediatric neurosurgery, *Neurosurgery of Infancy and Childhood*.			
1955			Use of computers for radiotherapy planning first described.	US Congress funds national chemotherapy program devoted to testing chemicals that might be effective against cancer.
1955			Children's Cancer Study Group (CCSG) founded.[40]	
1956	Leksell (Stockholm, Sweden) introduces ultrasound in neurosurgery.[41]			
1958			Larsson (Uppsala, Sweden) pioneers proton beam.[42]	
1960	Dexamethasone introduced for treatment of tumoral brain edema.[43]			
1960s			Introduction of linear accelerators for megavoltage radiotherapy.	
1962			St Jude Children's Research Hospital, Memphis, USA, opens as a result of fundraising initiated by the dream of comedian Danny Thomas.	
1964				MOPP combination chemotherapy for Hodgkin's disease introduced and outstanding results published.[44]
1965			Three-dimensional radiotherapy planning first described.	

Year	Neuroscience		Oncology	
	Neurosurgery	Imaging	Radiotherapy	Chemotherapy
1967	European Society for Pediatric Neurosurgery founded.			
1968			Leksell (Stockholm, Sweden) installs first gamma-knife unit.[45]	
1969				First International Meeting of Société Internationale d'Oncologie Pédiatrique (SIOP) in Madrid, Spain.
1969			Importance of precision and dose in radiotherapy for medulloblastoma reported by Bloom (Royal Marsden Hospital, London, UK).[46]	
1970				Howard Temin and David Baltimore independently discover the enzyme reverse transcriptase, making genetic engineering possible.
1971	Pediatric section of American Association of Neurological Surgeons founded.		Donald Pinkel describes total therapy including cranial radiotherapy for acute lymphatic leukemia in children and reports cures.[47]	Knudson and Strong propose two mutation hypothesis for inherited retinoblastoma (chromosome 13q14). December 23, 1971, President Nixon signs the National Cancer Act.
1972	International Society for Pediatric Neurosurgery founded.			
1972	University of California, San Francisco Neurosurgery Brain Tumor Research Center founded.	Hounsfield and Ambrose (London, UK) demonstrate cystic brain mass on CT.[48]		
1973	Japanese Society for Pediatric Neurosurgery founded.			
1974	Club de Neurochirurgie Pédiatrique founded.[49]			
1975				Cesar Milstein and George Kohler developed hybridoma technology permitting mass production of "monoclonal antibody," revolutionizing cancer diagnosis and treatment.[50]
1975		Ter-Pogossian constructs PET scanner.[51]	Survival advantage for patients with low-grade glioma treated by radiotherapy described by Leibel.[52]	
1977			Van Dyk describes the "modern" technique of craniospinal radiotherapy.[53]	UK Children's Cancer Study Group (UKCCSG) founded.

Year	Neuroscience		Oncology	
	Neurosurgery	Imaging	Radiotherapy	Chemotherapy
1978	American Society of Pediatric Neurosurgery founded.[54] Jones (Sydney, Australia) introduces the modern era of neuroendoscopic treatment of hydrocephalus.[55]			
1980		First clinical magnetic resonance images acquired at Nottingham[57] and Aberdeen[26], UK.		
1980s			Three-dimensional conformal radiotherapy implemented.	
1981	Ultrasonic aspirator introduced as adjunct in removal of brain and spinal tumors.[58]			
1982				First annual meeting of the Nordic Society of Pediatric Haematology and Oncology. Pediatric Oncology Group (POG) founded.
1983	CT-guided stereotactic brain tumor biopsy.[56]		Webster Cavenee shows that both copies of chromosome 13 in inherited retinoblastoma have DNA deletions, supporting Knudson's "two-hit" process and the idea of tumor suppressor genes.[59]	Gesellschaft für Pädiatrische Onkologie und Hämatologie (GPOH) established.
1984				Emil Frei describes scientific model for investigation of treatments in childhood leukemia.[60] Société Française d'Oncologie Pédiatrique (SFOP) created.
1985				First International Symposium in Paediatric Neuro-oncology (ISPNO) held in Tokyo.

	Neuroscience		Oncology	
Year	Neurosurgery	Imaging	Radiotherapy	Chemotherapy
1986			Winston and Lutz (Boston, USA) produce first true CT-guided stereotactic LINAC device.[61]	
1987	British Paediatric Neurosurgery Group of Society of British Neurological Surgeons founded.		Intensity-modulated radiotherapy (IMRT) first described.	
1989				CCG trial of adjuvant chemotherapy in high-grade glioma.[62]
1990			SIOP radiotherapy group founded.	First multicenter controlled trial of SIOP in medulloblastoma published.[63] CCG randomized trial in medulloblastoma.[64]
1990s			Commencement of the clinical implementation of IMRT.	
1993			International Commission on Radiation Units (ICRU) publishes the ICRU-50 document defining target volumes and dose specification for radiotherapy planning.	
1996	Société Française de Neurochirurgie Pédiatrique founded.[65]			Kenneth Culver and Michael Blaese insert a gene that confers sensitivity to an anti-viral drug into a brain tumor.[66]
1997		Royal College of Paediatrics and Child Health (UK) publishes guidance document on services for children with CNS tumors.[67]		Second multicenter controlled trial of SIOP and GPOH in medulloblastoma published.[68]
1998				SIOP/GPOH/UKCCSG Low Grade Glioma Study launched.[69]
2000s				CCG and POG merge to form Children's Oncology Group (COG).[70]
2003				Third multicenter SIOP/UKCCSG PNET study.[71]

REFERENCES FOR APPENDIX

1 Sachs E. *Fifty Years of Neurosurgery. A Personal Story*. New York: Vantage Press, 1958.

2 Jackson JH. On the use of the ophthalmoscope in affections of the nervous system. *Med Times Gaz* 1863; **ii**:359.

3 Macewen W. Tumour of the dura mater – convulsions – removal of tumour by trephining – recovery. *Glasgow Med J* 1879; **12**:210–13.

4 Naunyn B, Schreiber J. *Ueber Gehirndruck*. Leipzig: Vogel, 1881, p. 112.

5 Wernicke C. *Lehrbuch der Gehirnkrankheiten fur Aerzte und Studirende*, Vol. 3. Berlin: Fischer, 1881, pp. 253–572.

6 Bennett AE, Godlee R. Excision of a tumour from the brain. *Lancet* 1884; **2**:1090–1.

7 Gowers WR, Horsley VH. A case of tumour of the spinal cord. Removal: recovery. *Med Chir Trans (2nd ser)* 1888; **71**:377–430.

8 Keen WW. Exploratory trephining and puncture of the brain almost to the lateral ventricle, for intracranial pressure supposed to be due to an abscess in the tempero-sphenoidal lobe. Temporary improvement; death on the fifth day; autopsy; meningitis with effusion into the ventricles, with a description of a proposed operation to tap and drain the ventricles as a definite surgical procedure. *M News* 1888; **53**:603–9.

9 Wagner W. Die temporare Resektion des Schadeldaches an Stelle der Trepanation. *Zentralbl Chir* 1889; **16**:833–8.

10 Gotch F, Horsley V. On the mammalian nervous system, its functions and their localisation determined by an electric method. *Philos Trans Lond* 1891; **182B**:267–526.

11 Oldendorf WH. *The Quest for an Image of Brain*. New York: Raven Press, 1980.

12 Cushing H. Haematomyelia from gunshot wounds of the spine. A report of two cases with recovery following symptoms of hemilesion of the cord. *Am J Med Sci* 1898; **115**:654–83.

13 Oppenheim H. Discussion at Berliner Gesellschaft fur Psychiatrie und Nervenkrankheiten, November 13, 1899. *Arch Psychiatry* 1901; **34**:303–4.

14 Cushing H. The special field of neurological surgery. *Bull Johns Hopkins Hosp* 1905; **16**:77–87.

15 Horsley V. On the technique of operations on the central nervous system. *Br Med J* 1906; **2**:411–23.

16 Von Eiselsberg AF, Ranzi E. Ueber die chirurgische Behandlung der Hirn- und Ruckenmarkstumoren. *Arch Klin Chir* 1913; **102**:309–468.

17 Dandy WE, Blackfan KD. Internal hydrocephalus, an experimental, clinical, and pathological study. *Am J Dis Child* 1914; **8**:406–82.

18 Heuer G, Dandy W. Roentgenography in the localization of brain tumor, based upon one hundred consecutive cases. *Bull Johns Hopkins Hosp* 1916; **27**:311–22.

19 Dandy WE. Ventriculography following the injection of air into the cerebral ventricles. *Ann Surg* 1918; **68**:5–11.

20 Cushing H. Experiences with the cerebellar medulloblastomas. A critical review. *Acta Pathol Microbiol Scand* 1930; **7**:1–86.

21 Haden RL. Therapeutic application of the alteration of brain volume by the intravenous injection of glucose. *J Am Med Assoc* 1919; **73**:983–4.

22 Dandy WE. Roentgenography of the brain after the injection of air into the spinal canal. *Ann Surg* 1919; **70**:397–403.

23 Frazier CH. The effects of radium emanations upon brain tumors. *Surg Gynecol Obstet* 1920; **31**:236–9.

24 Mixter WJ. Ventriculoscopy and puncture of the floor of the third ventricle. *Boston Med Surg J* 1923; **188**:277–8.

25 Cushing H, Martin P. Primary gliomas of the chiasm and optic nerves in their intracranial portion. *Arch Ophthalmol* 1923; **52**:209–41.

26 Mallard J, Hutchison JM, Edelstein WA, Ling CR, Foster MA, Johnson G. In vivo n.m.r. imaging in medicine: the Aberdeen approach, both physical and biological. *Philos Trans R Soc Lond B Biol Sci* 1980; **289**:519–33.

27 Bailey P, Cushing H. *A Classification of the Tumors of the Glioma Group on a Histogenetic Basis with a Correlated Study of Prognosis*. Philadelphia: JB Lippincott, 1926.

28 Moniz E. L'encephalographie arterielle, son importance dans la localisation des tumeurs cerebrales. *Rev Neurol* 1927; **2**:72–90.

29 Cushing H. Electro-surgery as an aid to the removal of intracranial tumors. With a preliminary note on a new surgical-current generator (by W.T. Bovie). *Surg Gynecol Obstet* 1928; **47**:751–84.

30 Cushing H. The intracranial tumors of preadolescence. Report of a clinic for the combined meeting of the Pediatric Section of the New York Academy of Medicine, the Philadelphia Pediatric Society and the New England Pediatric Society, held at the Peter Bent Brigham Hospital, Boston, October 16, 1926. *Am J Dis Child* 1927; **33**:551–84.

31 Cutler EC, Sosman MC, Vaughan WW. Place of radiation in treatment of cerebellar medulloblastoma: report of 20 cases. *Am J Roentgenol Radium Ther Nucl Med* 1936; **35**:429–53.

32 Bailey P, Buchanan D, Bucy PC. *Intracranial Tumors of Infancy and Childhood*. Chicago: University of Chicago Press, 1939.

33 Moore GE. Use of radioactive diiodofluorescein in the diagnosis and localization of brain tumors. *Science* 1948; **107**:569.

34 Paterson R. *The Treatment of Malignant Disease by Radium and X-rays Being a Practice of Radiotherapy*. London: Edward Arnold, 1948.

35 Farber S, Diamond LK, Mercer RD, Sylvester RF, Jr, Wolff JA. Temporary remissions in acute leukemia in children produced by folic acid antagonist, 4-aminopteroyl-glutamic acid (aminopterin). *N Engl J Med* 1948; **238**:787–93.

36 Nulsen FE, Spitz EB. Treatment of hydrocephalus by direct shunt from ventricle to jugular vein. *Surg Forum* 1952; **2**:399–403.

37 Watson JD, Crick FHC. Molecular structure of nucleic acids. *Nature* 1953; **171**:737.

38 Paterson E, Parr RF. Medulloblastoma. Treatment by irradiation of the whole central nervous system. *Acta Radiol* 1953; **39**:323–36.

39 Talairach J, Aboulker P, Ruggiero G, *et al*. Utilization de la methode radiostereotaxique pour le traitement radioactif in situ des tumeurs cerebrales. *Rev Neurol* 1953; **90**:656–8.

40 Bleyer WA. The US pediatric cancer clinical trials programmes: international implications and the way forward. *Eur J Cancer* 1997; **33**:1439–47.

41 Leksell L. Echo-encephalography. I. Detection of intracranial complications following head injury. *Acta Chir Scand* 1956; **110**:301.

42 Larsson B. On the application of a 185 MeV proton beam to experimental cancer therapy and neurosurgery: a biophysical study. *Acta Univ Uppsala* 1962; **9**:7–23.

43 Galicich JH, French LA. Use of dexamethasone in the treatment of cerebral edema resulting from brain tumors and brain surgery. *Am Pract* 1961; **12**:169–74.

44 Devita Jr VT, Serpick A, Carbone PP. Combination chemotherapy in the treatment of advanced Hodgkin's disease. *Ann Intern Med* 1970; **73**:881.

45 Leksell DG. Special stereotactic techniques: stereotactic radiosurgery. In: Heilbrun MP (ed.) *Stereotactic Neurosurgery*. Baltimore, MD: Williams & Wilkins, 1988.

46 Bloom HJ, Wallace EN, Henk JM. The treatment and prognosis of medulloblastoma in children: a study of 82 verified cases. *Am J Roentgenol* 1969; **105**:43–62.

47 Pinkel D. Five-year follow-up of "total therapy" of childhood lymphocytic leukemia. *J Am Med Assoc* 1971; **216**:648–52.

48 Ambrose J. Computerized transverse axial scanning (tomography). Part 2. Clinical application. *Br J Radiol* 1973; **46**:1023–47.

49 Choux M. Personal communication. 2000.

50 Milstein C, Kohler G. Continuous cultures of fused cells secreting antibody of pre-defined specificity. *Nature* 1975 **256**:495–7.

51 Ter-Pogossian MM, Phelps ME, Hoffman EJ, Mullani NA. A positron-emission transaxial tomograph for nuclear imaging (PETT). *Radiology* 1975; **14**:89–98.

52 Leibel SA, Sheline GE, Wara WM, *et al.* The role of radiation therapy in the treatment of astrocytomas. *Cancer* 1975; **35**:1551–7.

53 Van Dyk J, Jenkin RTD, Leung PMK, Cunningham JR. Medulloblastoma: treatment technique and radiation dosimetry. *Int J Radiat Oncol Biol Phys* 1977; **2**:993–1005.

54 McClone DG. Personal communication. 2000.

55 Jones RFC, Kwok BCT, Stening WA, Vonau M. Neuroendoscopic third ventriculostomy. A practical alternative to extracranial shunts in non-communicating hydrocephalus. *Acta Neurochir Suppl* 1994; **61**:79–83.

56 Perry JH, Rosenbaum AE, Lunsford LD, Swink CA, Zorub DS. Computed tomography-guided stereotactic surgery: conception and development of a new stereotactic methodology. *Neurosurgery* 1980; **7**:376–81.

57 Hawkes RC, Holland GN, Moore WS, Worthington BS. Nuclear magnetic resonance (NMR) tomography of the brain: a preliminary clinical assessment with demonstration of pathology. *J Comput Assist Tomogr* 1980; **4**:577–86.

58 Fasano VA, Zeme S, Frego L, Gunetti R. Ultrasonic aspiration in the surgical treatment of intracranial tumors. *J Neurosurg Sci* 1981; **25**:35–40.

59 Cavenee W, Dryja TP, Philips RA, *et al.* Expression of recessive alleles by chromosomal mechanisms in retinoblastoma. *Nature* 1983; **305**:779–84.

60 Frei E. Acute leukaemia in children. Model for the development of scientific methodology for clinical therapeutic research in cancer. *Cancer* 1984; **53**:2013–25.

61 Lutz W, Winston KR, Maleki N. A system for stereotactic radiosurgery with a linear accelerator. *Int J Radiat Oncol Biol Phys* 1988; **14**:373–81.

62 Sposto R, Ertel IM, Jenkin RDT, *et al.* The effectiveness of chemotherapy for treatment of high-grade astrocytoma in children: results of a randomized trial. *J Neuro-Oncol* 1989; **7**:165–77.

63 Tait DM, Thornton-Jones H, Bloom HJ. Adjuvant chemotherapy for medulloblastoma, the first multi-centre controlled trial of the International Society of Paediatric Oncology (SIOP I). *Eur J Cancer* 1990; **26**:464–9.

64 Evans AE, Jenkin RDT, Sposto R, *et al.* The treatment of medulloblastoma: results of a prospective randomized trial of radiation therapy with and without CCNU, vincristine, and prednisone. *J Neurosurg* 1990; **72**:572–82.

65 Choux M. Personal communication. 2002.

66 Ram Z, Culver KW, Warbridge J, Frank JA, Blaese RM, Oldfield EH. Toxicity studies of retroviral-mediated gene transfer for the treatment of brain tumors. *J Neurology* 1993; **79**:400–7.

67 Walker DA, Hockley A, Taylor R, *et al. Guidance for Services for Children and Young People with Brain and Spinal Tumours. A Report of a working party of the United Kingdom Children's Cancer Study Group (UKCCSG) and the Society of British Neurological Surgeons (SBNS).* London: Royal College of Paediatric and Child Health, 1997.

68 Bailey CC, Gnekow A, Wellek S, *et al.* Prospective randomised trial of chemotherapy given before radiotherapy in childhood medulloblastoma. International Society of Paediatric Oncology (SIOP) and the German Society of Paediatric Oncology (GPO): SIOP II. *Med Pediatr Oncol* 1997; **25**:16–178.

69 Taylor RE, Walker D, Gnekow AK, *et al.* A preliminary report of the SIOP/GPOH/UKCCSG Low Grade Glioma Study. *Med Pediatr Oncol* 1998; **31**:242.

70 Packer RJ, Sposto R, Friedman, Perilongo G. Cooperative group trials. In: Keating RF, Goodrich JT, Packer RJ (eds) *Tumors of the Pediatric Central Nervous System*. New York: Thieme, 2001, pp. 511–23.

71 Taylor RE, Bailey CC, Robinson K, *et al.* Results of a randomised study of pre-radiation chemotherapy vs radiotherapy alone for non-metastatic (M0-1) medulloblastoma the SIOP/UKCCSG PNET-3 study. *J Clin Oncol* 2003; **21**:1581–91.

Epidemiology

Epidemiology

CHARLES A. STILLER AND W. ARCHIE BLEYER

INTRODUCTION

Brain and spinal cord tumors are the most frequent type of solid tumor in children under 15 years of age and second only to leukemias among all malignancies. In most populations, they represent upwards of 20 per cent of all childhood cancers.[1] These tumors cannot be considered together as a single entity, however, as they are of several distinct histological types, with their own patterns of incidence, and cannot be assumed to have a common etiology. In the International Classification of Childhood Cancer (ICCC),[2] which groups childhood tumors mainly on the basis of morphology, diagnostic group III, "CNS and Miscellaneous Intracranial and Intraspinal Neoplasms," contains six subgroups, namely (a) ependymomas (including choroid plexus tumors), (b) astrocytomas, (c) primitive neuroectodermal tumors (PNETs), (d) other gliomas, (e) other specified neoplasms (including pituitary adenomas, craniopharyngiomas, pineal parenchymal tumors, gangliogliomas, and meningiomas), and (f) unspecified neoplasms. The non-malignant tumors are concentrated in subgroups a, e, and f. A further ICCC subgroup, Xa, comprises intracranial and intraspinal germ-cell tumors and also includes a sizeable proportion of non-malignant tumors. Non-malignant tumors of blood vessels and peripheral nerves, including haemangiomas, haemangioblastomas, and schwannomas, are not included in the ICCC.

INCIDENCE

Table 3.1 shows age-standardized annual incidence rates for ICCC groups III and Xa from more than 30 countries.[1]

The data relate mainly to the 1980s and are drawn from population-based cancer registries with reasonably large numbers of cases and high levels of completeness of ascertainment. Tumors of other types, including soft-tissue sarcomas and non-Hodgkin lymphomas, can occur with intracranial or intraspinal primary site, but they are very rare and are not shown in this table.

Many cancer registries, while generally restricting their coverage to malignant neoplasms, also include benign and unspecified intracranial and intraspinal tumors. Others, as noted in Table 3.1, include only malignant tumors of these sites. Total incidence of malignant central nervous system (CNS) tumors falls steadily from age 0–4 years to a minimum at age 15–19 years, before rising steadily through adulthood (Figure 3.1). In the USA, it has been estimated that the inclusion of non-malignant tumors increases the incidence among children under 15 years of age by 22 per cent overall; for age groups 0–4 years and 5–9 years, the increase is 17 per cent, but for age 10–14 years it is 31 per cent.[3]

Among the mainly white populations of western industrialized countries, total incidence is nearly always in the range 25–40 per million; the male/female ratio is typically 1.2 to one. The highest incidence rates are observed in the Nordic countries. Japan and Israeli Jews have comparable incidence rates above 25 per million.

In developing countries, brain and spinal tumors are usually outnumbered not only by leukemias but also by lymphomas, and the recorded incidence of brain and spinal tumors is often no more than 15 per million. The true incidence is not necessarily that low, since there is almost certainly considerable underdiagnosis and underascertainment in areas that are not served by neurological

Table 3.1 *Brain and spinal neoplasms of childhood: age-standardized annual incidence rates per million children aged 0–14 years for International Classification of Childhood Cancer (ICCC) subgroups*

	IIIa (ependymoma)	IIIb (astrocytoma)	IIIc (PNET)	IIId (other gliomas)	IIIe (other specified)	IIIf (unspecified)	IIIa–f (total)	Xa (germ–cell)
*Zimbabwe, Harare, African	–	3.1	1.1	–	–	7.8	12.0	–
*Colombia, Cali	1.3	4.7	3.1	1.2	–	6.6	16.8	0.4
*Costa Rica	1.8	8.3	3.9	2.7	0.1	0.5	17.4	0.8
*Puerto Rico	3.3	10.0	4.8	3.7	0.4	0.8	22.8	0.3
Uruguay	2.1	3.2	6.2	2.0	1.4	8.1	23.0	0.5
*Canada	3.0	13.8	5.6	3.4	0.3	2.9	29.0	1.0
*USA, SEER, white	3.2	16.0	6.5	5.1	0.4	0.5	31.8	0.6
*USA, SEER, black	3.6	13.5	3.9	5.1	0.7	0.6	27.4	0.6
USA, LA, Hispanic	3.8	11.5	7.1	4.1	2.5	0.6	29.6	1.3
USA, LA, other white	2.8	16.6	9.0	3.6	3.5	1.1	36.6	1.2
USA, LA, black	2.0	13.5	4.7	2.7	0.8	0.5	24.2	0.8
China, Tianjin	0.5	0.5	0.5	1.7	1.5	12.5	17.3	–
*Hong Kong	1.5	6.9	3.2	0.9	0.1	4.3	16.9	0.4
*India, Bombay and Madras	0.6	3.9	2.9	0.8	0.1	2.2	10.5	0.0
Israel, Jewish	2.3	9.5	7.9	3.3	2.0	4.9	29.9	0.3
Israel, non-Jewish	1.5	4.8	4.6	2.7	0.9	3.6	18.1	–
Japan, Osaka	1.6	5.1	3.5	1.8	1.7	12.8	26.5	2.7
Korea, Seoul	0.6	4.8	3.6	0.7	0.2	6.7	16.6	1.0
Singapore, Chinese	2.3	6.8	6.1	0.8	0.8	2.4	19.1	2.1
Thailand	0.9	2.7	2.4	0.4	0.4	3.3	10.9	0.1
Czech Republic	2.9	9.7	4.7	1.6	1.0	3.0	23.0	–
Denmark	2.3	15.1	7.0	1.5	3.8	9.1	38.8	1.9
Estonia	2.1	9.6	4.0	0.6	0.8	8.5	25.6	–
Finland	4.9	23.3**	4.6	–	2.7	3.8	39.2	0.6
France	4.1	10.7	6.0	4.1	1.9	1.4	28.2	0.8
Germany, ex-GDR	6.0	13.7	5.7	0.9	2.6	3.3	32.2	1.2
Italy	3.4	13.0	5.1	1.9	1.5	5.5	30.3	1.0
*Netherlands	4.3	14.1	7.4	1.3	0.5	2.6	30.2	1.0
Norway	2.8	14.4	5.8	4.2	1.4	5.4	34.0	0.7
Slovakia	3.5	11.1	6.3	3.8	0.9	3.3	28.9	0.2
*Slovenia	3.3	7.6	4.1	1.9	0.7	2.2	19.8	1.1
Spain	2.9	10.2	5.3	4.2	0.7	2.8	26.2	0.8
Sweden	4.3	22.2**	7.1	–	2.2	5.2	41.0	1.0
Switzerland	3.3	12.4	6.2	1.3	2.2	1.9	27.2	0.7
UK, England and Wales	3.0	10.3	5.8	4.1	2.2	1.6	27.0	1.0
UK, Scotland	3.6	12.5	8.7	4.0	1.7	0.6	31.0	1.5
Australia	2.9	13.7	6.4	3.3	2.2	1.1	29.6	1.1
*New Zealand, Maori	2.0	9.1	12.0	3.9	–	4.7	31.6	1.6
*New Zealand, non-Maori	1.9	15.8	6.6	3.0	0.6	4.2	32.0	1.0
*USA, Hawaii, Hawaiian	3.2	10.7	11.8	2.8	–	–	28.5	2.1

PNET, primitive neuroectodermal tumor; SEER, Surveillance, Epidemiological, and End Results.
* Series including only malignant tumors. ** In Finland and Sweden, rates for IIIb (astrocytoma) include those for IIId (other gliomas) because they have the same morphology code.
Data from Parkin *et al.*[1]

facilities. Registries that depend substantially on pathology departments for notification of cases will suffer a further deficit if autopsies are rarely performed. In the developing countries of Asia, but not in Africa or Latin America, there is a larger excess of boys affected than in industrialized countries, with a male/female ratio of around 1.4 to one.

Incidence by ethnic group

Comparison of incidence rates within the same country suggests that risk may vary between ethnic groups. In the USA, incidence among blacks is lower than among whites, most markedly so in early childhood. Incidence among Hispanic children in Los Angeles is slightly lower than

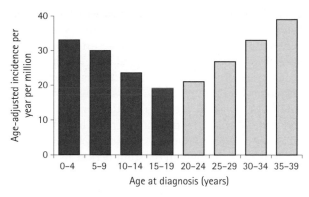

Figure 3.1 *Incidence of malignant central nervous system tumors according to the International Classification of Childhood Cancers (ICCC), 1975–1998, USA: Surveillance, Epidemiology and End Results (SEER) program.*
(*Data from Ries LAG, Eisner MP, Kosary CL, et al. SEER Cancer Statistics Review, 1973–1997: Tables and Graphs.* Bethesda, MD: National Cancer Institute, 2000.)

among non-Hispanic whites, and this difference is more marked in California as a whole.[4] In Britain, incidence among children of southern Asian ethnic origin is low, apparently because of a marked deficit among those of Indian rather than Pakistani origin.[5] Children of West Indian ethnic origin have a low relative frequency of CNS tumors,[6] suggesting that their incidence is also low. In Israel, incidence is much lower in non-Jews than in Jews. In Singapore, the Malay population has only about half the incidence of the Chinese. In New Zealand, however, the Maori have a very similar incidence to the overwhelmingly white, non-Maori, population. In most instances, it is the economically disadvantaged ethnic groups that have the lower incidence, and so differential access to medical care might be a contributing factor. This appears less likely in Britain, where there is a universal free health service and, moreover, children of Indian origin tend to be of higher socioeconomic status than those of Pakistani ancestry.

Incidence by histology

Ependymomas (including choroid plexus tumors) hardly ever have an incidence above four per million. In most series, they account for 10–15 per cent of CNS tumors of specified type. In the German Childhood Cancer Registry, 60% of ependymomas of known site were infratentorial.[7] Ependymoma is more than twice as common at age 0–4 years as it is in the next decade. The male/female ratio is around 1.2–1.3 to one.

Astrocytomas collectively are by far the most common childhood CNS tumors, usually accounting for 40–55 per cent of those of specified type. They cover a wide spectrum of degrees of malignancy, ranging from the often slow-growing pilocytic or juvenile astrocytoma to the highly malignant glioblastoma multiforme, but

low-grade tumors predominate.[7] Among astrocytomas of known site in the German registry, 53 per cent were supratentorial.[7] The highest incidence rates were recorded in predominantly white populations in North America, Europe, and Oceania. In California, incidence among Hispanic children is about half that among non-Hispanic whites of both sexes and in all three of the five-year age groups.[4] The incidence in Osaka, Japan, is lower, but this registry has a high proportion of tumors of unspecified type, and the relative frequency of astrocytoma out of all specified tumors is similar to that in western populations, suggesting that this may also be true of incidence. Elsewhere in the world, incidence is lower, but the relative frequency as a proportion of all CNS tumors is similar to that in western countries. Incidence is fairly constant throughout childhood, and the male/female ratio is usually 1–1.1 to one.

Primitive neuroectodermal tumor (PNETs) are the second most frequent subgroup in most populations, typically accounting for 20–30 per cent of all specified CNS tumors. In the German registry, 73 per cent of PNETs were infratentorial,[7] and nearly all of these would have been cerebellar medulloblastomas. The highest incidence rates, around 12 per million, have been recorded in two indigenous Pacific populations, the Hawaiians of Hawaii and the Maori of New Zealand. In mainly white populations, the incidence is commonly five to nine per million, and the similarity of relative frequencies across other registries suggests that there is little international or ethnic variation in underlying risk outside the Pacific region. The incidence is highest at age 1–4 years, slightly lower among infants and at age 5–9 years, but falls to around half its peak by age 10–14 years. The male/female ratio is 1.6–1.7 to one.

Other gliomas tend to have a similar incidence and relative frequency to ependymomas. Most of these tumors were not specified further in the literature, but there were also substantial numbers of oligodendrogliomas.

The incidence of other specified tumors (other than germ-cell) is nearly always below three per million. As many of these tumors are non-malignant, some of the differences in rates between registries must be due to variations in ascertainment of non-malignant tumors. The most frequent histological type is craniopharyngioma, which has an incidence of one to two per million in children in the USA.[8] This is followed by pineal parenchymal tumors and meningiomas.

Childhood germ-cell tumors of any site are most common in eastern Asian populations. The highest incidence of intracranial and intraspinal germ-cell tumors is found in Japan and among Singapore Chinese. The next highest rate is in Denmark, but over half of the cases there are non-malignant.

Two rare tumors that have been consistently diagnosed and registered only fairly recently are not included in Table 3.1: dysembryoplastic neuroepithelial tumor

(DNT) and atypical teratoid rhabdoid tumor (AT/RT). During the period 1995–1999, the National Registry of Childhood Tumours (NRCT) in Great Britain recorded 30 children with DNT and 15 with ATRT, in both cases giving annual incidence rates well below one per million.

Table 3.2 shows incidence rates among adolescents aged 15–19 years from the few population-based studies with information on histological subgroup.[9–11] Total incidence is lower than for children overall but fairly similar to that observed at age 10–14 years. Astrocytoma is the most frequent histological subtype and PNET is quite rare. Elsewhere in the world, only site-specific incidence rates are available. Table 3.3 shows incidence in selected cancer registries around 1990.[12] Incidence is generally somewhat lower than during the first 15 years of life, although it should be remembered that, unlike in Tables 3.1 and 3.2, the rates in Table 3.3 refer only to malignant tumors.

Trends in incidence of brain and spinal tumors

Reported incidence of childhood CNS tumors in almost every country for which data are available rose between the 1970s and 1980s, often by more than 20 per cent. Annual increases for malignant CNS tumors in the USA between 1975 and 1998 have been estimated from the Surveillance, Epidemiological, and End Results (SEER) program and are shown in Figures 3.2 (overall) and 3.3 (by histological subgroup). Smith and colleagues[13] analyzed data from the SEER program for the period 1973–1994 and found that a jump from a lower to a higher constant incidence at 1985 produced a significantly better fit than a linear increase throughout the study period. As the timing of the jump coincided with the start of wide-scale availability of magnetic resonance imaging (MRI) in the USA, they hypothesized that the increase in recorded incidence was an artifact of improved diagnosis and reporting. Smith and colleagues[13] suggested that this was supported by the absence of a similar stepwise increase in mortality from CNS tumors in childhood. Much of the increased incidence, however, was in low-grade astrocytomas and gliomas; these have high survival rates, and even fatal CNS tumors can have a protracted course. Therefore, any increase in mortality resulting from a sudden increase in risk would probably be relatively small and gradual and thus hard to detect. Against the hypothesis that the

Table 3.2 *Brain and spinal neoplasms at age 15–19 years: annual incidence per million for International Classification of Childhood Cancer (ICCC) subgroups*

	IIIa (ependymoma)	IIIb (astrocytoma)	IIIc (PNET)	IIId (other gliomas)	IIIe (other specified)	IIIf (unspecified)	IIIa–f (total)	Xa (germ-cell)
Nordic countries[9]	1.3	9.5	2.1	1.6	14.2**	?	28.7	?
England, northern region[10]	2.1	7.5	1.0	3.4	6.1	2.6	22.6	0.6
*USA, SEER[11]	1.1	12.3	2.5	?	?	?	20.2	?

PNET, primitive neuroectodermal tumor; SEER, Surveillance, Epidemiological, and End Results.
* Series including only malignant tumors. ** Including unspecified tumors and non-malignant germ-cell tumors.

Table 3.3 *Malignant brain and nervous system tumors: annual incidence per million at age 15–19 years*

Puerto Rico	9.9
Costa Rica	11.8
Japan, Osaka	10.6
Hong Kong	16.2
Singapore, Chinese	9.2
India, Bombay and Madras	9.3
Israel, Jewish	18.7
Israel, non-Jewish	17.7
Slovakia	21.7
Slovenia	15.1
Netherlands	17.1
Australia, NSW	23.4

Data from Parkin *et al.*[12]

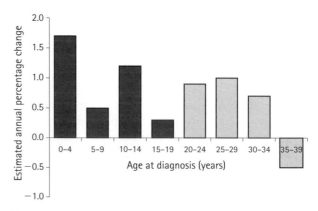

Figure 3.2 *Increase in incidence of malignant central nervous system tumors according to the International Classification of Childhood Cancers (ICCC), 1975–1998, USA: Surveillance, Epidemiology and End Results (SEER) program. The ordinate represents the average annual percentage change over the 23-year interval from 1975 to 1998. (Data from Ries LAG, Eisner MP, Kosary CL, et al. SEER Cancer Statistics Review, 1973–1997: Tables and Graphs. Bethesda, MD: National Cancer Institute, 2000.)*

increase resulted from improved diagnosis, and perhaps in particular earlier detection of slow-growing tumors, is the fact that there is no sign of the fall in recorded incidence that might have been expected within a few years of accelerated diagnosis of any "backlog" of low-grade tumors. An increase in the incidence of astrocytoma has also been found in Sweden.[14] However, while it has been suggested that the "jump" model would again be a better fit than a continuous linear trend,[15] this has yet to be tested. During the period 1954–1998 in north-west England, the incidence rates of both pilocytic astrocytoma and PNET increased by one per cent per annum.[16] These increases could not be accounted for by changes in reporting practice or diagnosis. In the Greater Delaware Valley, a part of the USA not covered by the SEER program, incidence of all CNS tumors and of glioma and PNET increased during the period 1970–1989.[17] The end of the study period was too early to provide evidence of trends following changes in diagnostic technology in the mid-1980s.

Comparison with adults

The main variations in age-specific incidence during the first 20 years of life have been described, but the contrast with the pattern of incidence at older ages is much greater. Although CNS tumors are outnumbered only by leukemias among children and adolescents in many regions of the world, they are less common than in any other age group.[18] Infratentorial tumors are at least as frequent as supratentorial tumors in children,[7,11] but they account for only a small minority of CNS neoplasms among adults.[18] Whereas low-grade astrocytomas and PNETs are the most numerous CNS tumors in children, glioblastoma and meningioma are the predominant types in adults.[18]

SURVIVAL AND FOLLOW-UP

Compared with most other types of childhood cancer, improvements in survival from CNS tumors have been modest, although some subtypes, notably astrocytoma, have long had a relatively good prognosis.

Table 3.4 shows population based five-year survival rates for children with the main types of CNS tumor diagnosed during the 1980s.[19–25] In North America, western Europe, and Australia, there was little international variation. Five-year survival was generally slightly over 70 per cent for astrocytoma and around 50 per cent for PNET. Italy had markedly higher survival from PNET, but the data covered only part of the country and the numbers were small. In Eastern Europe, Slovakia had a somewhat lower survival rate for astrocytoma. In Bangalore, India, survival from astrocytoma was still lower, whereas for PNET it was similar to that observed in western countries, but the numbers of cases were, again, small. It seems likely that lower survival in socioeconomically disadvantaged countries is due partly to a lack of specialist facilities for the treatment of children with CNS tumors. There is, however, some evidence that survival is lower even within specialist centers in developing countries; for example, the five-year survival rate for children with cerebellar juvenile (pilocytic) astrocytoma at a tertiary center for pediatric neurosurgery in India during the period 1984–1999 was 67 per cent,[26] compared with a population-based rate of 84 per cent in north-west England during the period 1954–1984.[27]

Few population-based data are available on survival beyond five years from diagnosis. In Britain, among children diagnosed during the period 1971–1985, the actuarial

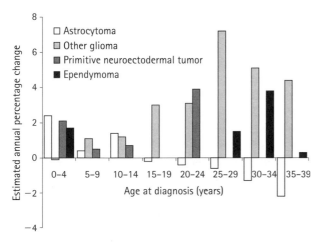

Figure 3.3 *Increase in incidence of malignant central nervous system tumors by International Classification of Childhood Cancers (ICCC) type, 1975–1998, USA: Surveillance, Epidemiology and End Results (SEER) program. The ordinate represents the average annual percentage change over the 23-year interval from 1975 to 1998.*
(Data from Ries LAG, Eisner MP, Kosary CL, et al. SEER Cancer Statistics Review, 1973–1997: Tables and Graphs. Bethesda, MD: National Cancer Institute, 2000.)

Table 3.4 *Population-based five-year actuarial survival rates (%) for children aged 0–14 years diagnosed during the 1980s*

Country	Period	Ependymoma	Astrocytoma	PNET
USA, SEER[19]	1983–87	47	74	49
*Canada[20]	1985–88	56	71	50
Great Britain[21]	1986–88	50	71	42
Italy[22]	1986–89	75	76	85
Slovakia[23]	1983–87	–	56	–
Australia, Victoria[24]	1980–89	64	80	52
India, Bangalore[25]	1982–89	–	40	43

PNET, primitive neuroectodermal tumor; SEER, Surveillance, Epidemiological, and End Results.
* Age 0–19 years.

probability of surviving a further ten years after five-year survival was 89 per cent for all CNS tumors and for ependymoma, 92 per cent for astrocytoma, but only 81 per cent for PNET.[28] In a recent study of five-year survivors diagnosed under age 20 years throughout the five Nordic countries during the period 1960–1989, survival rates were not quoted but there was a borderline significant reduction of 19 per cent in the risk of death for those who had a CNS tumor diagnosed in the period 1980–1989 compared with the period 1960–1969.[29] Recurrent tumor was the most frequent cause of death in both series, accounting for over 80 per cent of deaths at five to nine years after diagnosis and over 60 per cent at 10–14 years after diagnosis, in both series. In the Nordic countries, recurrent tumor was still the most frequent cause of death at 30 years after diagnosis. Treatment-related causes accounted for around 10–15 per cent of deaths in both series, while second primary tumors accounted for three to four per cent of deaths. Similar results were observed in a large multi-institutional study in North America;[30] there was a 20 per cent chance of death between five and 25 years after diagnosis of a CNS tumor. The cumulative risk of developing a second primary tumor within 20 years of diagnosis of a childhood CNS tumor in large population-based series from Britain and the Nordic countries was around two to three per cent, representing a relative risk of three to five.[31,32] Both series included patients diagnosed from the 1940s onwards. Risk estimates were not presented for calendar period of diagnosis or age at follow-up, although most of the second primary tumors may be assumed to have occurred in adulthood. In a study in Germany of children diagnosed since 1980, the relative risk of developing a second primary cancer in childhood following a CNS tumor was much higher, at 18.3.[33] It is not yet known whether this reflects greater susceptibility among younger survivors or a higher risk following more aggressive therapy for the original tumor, but it should be noted that CNS tumors were ascertained incompletely by the registry, with the deficit being most marked during the earlier years and for less malignant tumors, which would tend to be treated less intensively.

Two large, population-based studies have included analyses of prognostic factors for childhood CNS tumors. These are the SEER Pediatric Monograph in the USA[11] and the EUROCARE study in Europe.[34] Their conclusions are broadly similar. There was very little difference in survival between boys and girls. Age, however, was an important prognostic factor. In both series, children aged under five years of age had lower survival rates from PNET. Poor survival among this age group was also found for ependymoma, but not for astrocytoma, in the USA and for a combined group of ependymoma, astrocytoma, and other glioma in Europe. In the USA and Britain, there is little evidence for differences in survival between ethnic groups.[11,35,36]

As described above, long-term survival after childhood CNS tumor is well documented in several large, mostly population-based, series. The same is true to a slightly lesser extent of the patterns and risks of occurrence of second primary neoplasms and deaths from non-neoplastic causes. By contrast, there is very little published information on non-fatal morbidity among survivors based on substantial numbers of patients. Large population-based or multicenter questionnaire studies are in progress in the UK and North America, however, in which survivors are asked for detailed information about many aspects of their present state of health and their personal and social circumstances. A preliminary report from the North American study has shown that fewer survivors of CNS tumors have been married compared with survivors of other types of cancer.[37] Many more results should become available from both studies during the next few years.

MORTALITY

The crude annual mortality rate for cancer of the brain and nervous system among children aged 0–14 years in western, industrialized countries in 1990 was in the range 9–11 per million.[38] Worldwide, among countries with more than ten deaths from childhood cancers of the brain and nervous system, both the highest and the lowest mortality rates were in developing countries, respectively Haiti (32.2 and 37.2 per million in males and females, respectively) and Bangladesh (1.1 and 0.8 per million in males and females, respectively).[38] These extremes presumably reflect on the one hand very poor survival combined with a high rate of diagnosis, or possibly a low level of accuracy in death certification, and on the other hand a low rate of diagnosis due to lack of specialist facilities for treatment combined with a low autopsy rate.

In the USA, mortality from childhood CNS cancer decreased by only 20 per cent between 1975–1977 and 1993–1995, compared with declines of 52 per cent for leukemia and 59 per cent for all other cancers.[39] This modest decrease in the mortality rate reflects improvements in survival that were small compared with those for many other childhood cancers, together with the increase in incidence described earlier. As a result, the proportion of childhood cancer mortality accounted for by CNS tumors rose from around 22 per cent to 30 per cent over the same period. Similar patterns can be observed in other industrialized countries.

ORGANIZATION OF SERVICES

Treatment of CNS tumors is bound to be specialized to the extent that surgery will invariably be performed in a neurosurgical unit. The routine referral of children with CNS tumors to pediatric oncology centers has, however, lagged behind that for other common childhood cancers. In the USA in the 1980s, data on registration with cooperative trials groups were published from Los Angeles County, California,[40] and from Florida.[41] In Los Angeles during the period 1980–1987, 44 per cent of children aged under 15 years and with CNS tumors were registered with cooperative groups compared with 62 per cent of those with other cancers. In Florida during the period 1981–1986, the proportions registered were 74 per cent and 83 per cent, respectively. By the early 1990s, however, not only did referral rates appear to have increased greatly, but they had also caught up with those for other childhood cancers. Results based on comparison of individual case records have not been published, but expected national numbers of cases were calculated from incidence rates provided by SEER program cancer registries, which cover about a tenth of the population; these results were compared with numbers registered by the CCG and the POG.[42] It is estimated that during the period 1989–1991, 96 per cent of children with malignant CNS tumors and 94 per cent of those with other cancers were registered with one of the two cooperative groups.

In Great Britain, referral of children with CNS tumors to pediatric oncology centers increased from 36 per cent in the period 1981–1984 to 73 per cent in the period 1993–1995, compared with an increase from 64 per cent to 81 per cent for all childhood cancers combined.[43] In Italy, as in the USA, expected national numbers of cases could be calculated only on the basis of regional registration data. For the period 1989–1994, an estimated 36 per cent of children with a CNS tumor were referred to a pediatric oncology center, compared with 78 per cent of all children with any type of cancer.[44]

While there is a long and established tradition in many countries of entering children with leukemia and most of the principal types of solid tumor into clinical trials and studies, CNS tumors have often been an exception. In part, this can be explained by lack of protocols, particularly for tumors where chemotherapy is not used widely, and by low referral rates to pediatric oncology centers. Even among children treated at these centers for types of tumor for which protocols do exist, however, entry rates have often been low. In Florida during the period 1981–1986, only 14 per cent of eligible children with brain tumors at centers with protocols available were entered, compared with 55 per cent for all cancers.[41] In Italy, 66 per cent of children with cancer diagnosed in the period 1989–1991 at pediatric oncology centers were treated with protocols of the Italian Association of Pediatric Hematology–Oncology and the Italian Task Force for Pediatric Oncology; for the period 1992–1994, this figure was 73 per cent. For CNS tumors, the corresponding figures were 20 per cent and 27 per cent.[44]

Studies of survival in relation to patterns of care for CNS tumors have concentrated on medulloblastoma. During the 1970s, survival in Connecticut and the Greater Delaware Valley, USA, was significantly higher among children treated at cancer centers than at other hospitals.[45,46] Both series were rather small, however, and possible confounding with other prognostic factors was not taken into account. In Britain, over a similar period, survival did not vary between neurosurgical or radiotherapy centers with different numbers of patients; this series was somewhat larger, but again other prognostic factors were not controlled for.[47] In Ontario, Canada, between 1977 and 1987, children treated outside metropolitan Toronto had nearly twice the risk of recurrence or death of those seen in Toronto.[48] After controlling for tumor stage, sex, extent of surgery, and meningitis, the difference was no longer statistically significant. The Toronto group tended to be of lower tumor stage and contained higher proportions of girls and of children with total rather than near-total resection, all of which were favorable prognostic factors; the Toronto group also included all the children with meningitis, which had an adverse effect on survival. In the Connecticut study, children with brainstem glioma treated at cancer centers had higher survival than those treated at other hospitals, but there was no difference between the two groups for ependymoma or other astrocytomas.[45]

Data from the Société International de Oncologie Pédiatrique (SIOP) randomized trial of treatment for medulloblastoma, also in the 1970s, were analyzed according to size of treatment center.[49] The 124 patients from centers entering at least 20 patients in the trial had a significantly higher disease-free survival rate than the 162 patients from other centers. Within CCG studies of medulloblastoma and high-grade glioma during the period 1985–1992, children operated on by pediatric rather than general neurosurgeons had a higher proportion of radical resection.[50] Complete tumor removal tends to be associated with a better prognosis, but survival rates were not reported by type of surgeon.

ETIOLOGY AND RISK FACTORS

In common with most childhood cancers, established risk factors almost certainly account for only a small proportion of CNS tumors in young people. The literature up to the mid-1990s has been reviewed in detail by Little;[51] therefore, this section aims largely to review studies published since then. The SEER Pediatric Monograph[11] contains a useful summary of knowledge on the causes of CNS tumors in children as of 1998 in the form of a table of known, potential, and refuted risk factors. A modified version is given here (Table 3.5).

Table 3.5 *Current knowledge on causes of childhood central nervous system (CNS) tumors*

Factor	Current knowledge
Known risk factors	
Sex	Boys at higher risk of PNET
Neurofibromatosis 1 and 2, tuberous sclerosis 1 and 2, Gorlin (basal-cell nevus) syndrome, brain tumor polyposis syndrome, germ–line mutations of TP53 (giving rise to Li–Fraumeni syndrome) and of *hSNF5/INI1*	Children with any of these genetic conditions have an increased risk of brain tumors. Children with Down's syndrome are at increased risk of intracranial germ-cell tumors
Parent or sibling with CNS tumor	Associated with a three- to nine-fold increased risk. Probably explained almost completely by the specific genetic conditions listed above
Family history of leukemia or sarcoma	Probably explained by Li–Fraumeni syndrome
Therapeutic doses of ionizing radiation to the head	The only conclusively established environmental risk factor. Children treated in the past for tinea capitis experienced a 2.5- to six-fold increased risk. Those now at risk are children treated with radiation to the head for leukemia or a previous brain tumor
Factors for which evidence is suggestive but not conclusive	
Maternal diet during pregnancy	Frequent consumption of cured meat associated with increased risk in several studies. Consumption of multivitamin supplements appears to be protective
Paternal smoking	Meta-analysis of ten studies showed a significantly raised relative risk of 1.2 with child's exposure to paternal tobacco smoke. Maternal passive smoking during pregnancy may also be a risk factor
Factors for which evidence is limited or inconsistent	
Other products containing N-nitroso-compounds or precursors	Associations seen in one study have generally not been repeated in later studies
Father's occupation and related exposures	Many associations have been reported, but few have been replicated
Pesticides	Many studies have reported associations, but with limited consistency between them. Exposure is confounded with farm residence and exposure to animals
Farm residence and exposure to farm animals	Heavily confounded with exposure to pesticides
Characteristics of pregnancy and birth	Raised risk of astrocytoma with high birthweight in early studies has not been found in more recent studies. Many other associations found in only one or two studies
Power-frequency electromagnetic fields	Associations found in early, small studies not confirmed more recently
Virus infection	Large cohort studies generally have not found raised risk among those exposed to polio vaccine contaminated with SV40
Factor on which there is public concern but no evidence relating specifically to childhood tumors	
Wireless frequency electromagnetic fields	All studies of mobile telephone exposure and CNS tumors have related to adults

PNET, primitive neuroectodermal tumor.

Cancer-predisposing syndromes

Genetic predisposition is undoubtedly a risk factor in some cases. For nearly all the syndromes discussed below, the specific genetic loci have been identified.

Neurofibromatosis type 1 (NF-1) confers an excess risk of CNS tumors, particularly optic nerve gliomas and other astrocytomas.[52] In a series of over 500 NF-1 patients from north-west England, the actuarial risk of optic nerve glioma was 4.4 per cent by age 15 years and 5.2 per cent by age 20 years.[53] In a population-based mortality study covering the whole of the USA, the relative risk of death from a malignant brain tumor among people with NF-1 was 3.94 at age 0–9 years and 11.4 at age 10–19 years.[54] In a population-based series of 3872 British children with CNS tumors in the NRCT, 60 (1.5 per cent) had neurofibromatosis;[55] with the exception of three children with meningiomas, these were probably all NF-1. Neurofibromatosis type 2 (NF-2) is also associated with an increased risk of CNS tumors,[52] but since it occurs with only one-tenth of the frequency of NF-1 and the tumors are most commonly meningiomas and spinal cord ependymomas, it must account for far fewer childhood CNS tumors than NF-1.

There are two types of tuberous sclerosis, which occur with approximately equal frequency.[52] In patients with either type, the incidence of childhood brain tumors has been reported as 5–14 per cent, of which 90 per cent are subependymal giant-cell astrocytomas.[52] Among a population-based series of 131 patients with tuberous sclerosis, nine (seven per cent) had developed giant-cell astrocytoma.[56] In four cases, the astrocytoma was diagnosed before age 20 years, giving a cumulative incidence of three per cent in childhood and adolescence, but this is probably an underestimate, since some subjects were still children when the data were collected. In the NRCT series, 18 of 3872 (0.5 per cent) CNS tumors were associated with tuberous sclerosis.[55]

Cerebellar or spinal-cord hemangioblastomas occur in around half of all patients with von Hippel–Lindau disease, and frequently cause the first symptoms of the disorder, but they are found in adulthood more often.[52]

In a population-based series of 173 consecutive cases of medulloblastoma, four (2.3 per cent) were in children with Gorlin (basal-cell nevus) syndrome.[57] All four tumors were desmoplastic medulloblastoma on pathology review and occurred before age three years. An additional child with Gorlin syndrome died of a presumed, but unverified, medulloblastoma, suggesting that the actual proportion of cases due to Gorlin syndrome may exceed three per cent.

Brain tumors are a recognized component of the Li–Fraumeni family cancer syndrome. In a large series of classic Li–Fraumeni and Li–Fraumeni-like families, most of the brain tumors were high-grade astrocytomas and medulloblastomas;[58] 13 of 16 (81 per cent) were in patients with a germ-line mutation of the *TP53* tumor suppressor gene, which is located on chromosome 17p13. In a cohort study of members of 28 Li–Fraumeni families with germ-line *TP53* mutations, 14 of 148 cancers were brain and spinal-cord tumors. This was 22 times the number expected from population incidence rates and twice the number predicted if all cancers were to have had a uniformly elevated risk, indicating that CNS tumors are associated strongly with *TP53* mutations.[59] A review of 91 families with *TP53* germ-line mutations revealed a bimodal age distribution for associated brain tumors, with the more marked peak in the first ten years of life and a second peak at age 20–40 years.[60] Among tumors of specified morphology, 69 per cent were astrocytomas and 17 per cent were PNET. There have been several reports of choroid plexus carcinoma in Li–Fraumeni syndrome,[61,62] indicating that the relative risk may be especially high for this usually rare tumor.

Choroid plexus tumors and atypical teratoid rhabdoid tumors have been found in association with germ-line mutations of the *hSNF5/INI1* gene, which is located on chromosome 22q11.[63–65] This raises the possibility that *hSNF5/INI1* is a tumor suppressor gene that may provide the basis for some cases of Li–Fraumeni syndrome without *TP53* germ-line mutation.[64]

The term "Turcot's syndrome" has been applied generally to the association of brain tumors and colorectal polyposis or cancer in the same person.[52] In a review of 151 published cases of brain tumor–polyposis (BTP) syndrome,[66] two distinct groups were identified. The first, which the authors called BTP syndrome type 1, consisted of patients with glioma and colorectal adenomas without polyposis and their siblings with glioma and/or colorectal adenomas. The gliomas were usually high-grade astrocytomas and occurred during childhood and adolescence. BTP syndrome type 2 consisted of patients with a CNS tumor occurring within a familial adenomatous polyposis kindred. The CNS tumors were predominantly medulloblastomas. In a study of 1321 members of 50 families in the Dutch registry for hereditary nonpolyposis colorectal cancer, which in combination with brain tumors would correspond to BTP syndrome type 1, the risk of a brain tumor was four to six times that in the general population.[67]

There appears to be an overall deficit of CNS tumors in people with Down's syndrome, but the risk of intracranial germ-cell tumors in Down's syndrome is increased.[68]

After the exclusion of neurofibromatosis, tuberous sclerosis, Down's syndrome, and other known chromosomal defects, the incidence of congenital anomalies in a large population-based series from the NRCT was lower for CNS tumors than for most other diagnostic groups.[69] Hydrocephalus, spina bifida, and other spinal anomalies, however, were more common than expected. The excess of hydrocephalus might be accounted for as a symptom of a brain tumor. The association with spina bifida may indicate a common environmental risk factor rather than a common genetic basis, a possibility that is discussed later in this chapter. Only two children with any type of cancer were diagnosed with Rubinstein–Taybi syndrome (RTS), and both had medulloblastoma. The international RTS registry contained two cases of medulloblastoma, including one of the NRCT cases, among 724 individuals with RTS, but there were also an oligodendroglioma, an oligoastrocytoma, and an ectopic pinealoma in addition to various non-CNS tumors.[70]

Familial aggregations of CNS tumors may be expected to occur in some of the syndromes described above, especially NF-1, Turcot's syndrome, and Li–Fraumeni syndrome. In the population-based Swedish Family Cancer Database, only 1.3 per cent of children with a brain tumor had a parent with a nervous-system cancer.[71] The standardized incidence ratio (SIR) for brain tumors in the offspring of a parent with a brain tumor was 2.54 for the first five years of life and 1.88 for the first 15 years. This was accounted for entirely by children with astrocytomas. The SIR was particularly high, being 10.26 in the first five years of life and 4.29 in the first 15 years of life, for astrocytoma in the children of parents with meningioma, possibly due to NF-2. An excess of ependymoma (SIR 3.70) in offspring of parents with colon cancer may represent a variant of BTP syndrome. There was a significantly raised SIR of 13.33 for medulloblastoma with parental salivary gland cancer, but this was based on only two cases and had not been reported previously. In a population-based study in the five Nordic countries, there was no excess of CNS tumors or of cancer overall in the siblings of children with CNS tumors after the exclusion of sibling pairs with known genetic aetiology.[72] This need not imply that other childhood CNS tumors do not have a genetic etiology, however; it is possible that as yet unidentified low-penetrance germ-line mutations of *TP53* or other genes could be involved, as appears to be the case with some childhood adrenocortical tumors.[73]

Environmental and exogenous factors

The only established environmental risk factor for CNS tumors is ionizing radiation.[51] The sharp reduction in obstetric irradiation since the introduction of ultrasound examination should mean that fewer cases are now attributable to this cause than previously. Radiation treatment in the past for benign conditions such as tinea capitis carried an increased risk of CNS tumors,[74] but the abandonment of this practice should mean that it does not account for any newly diagnosed childhood tumors. Radiotherapy for cancer is a significant risk factor in the development of a subsequent primary CNS tumor,[75] although many of the radiation-induced tumors occur in adulthood.

There has been much public concern about the possible carcinogenic effect of extremely low-frequency electromagnetic fields (EMFs) emitted by electrical sources, such as power-transmission lines and domestic wiring. Consistently elevated risks of leukemia have been found at the high EMF exposure levels experienced by a small minority of children, but the reasons for this are unknown and it may be attributable in part to selection bias. There is, however, no evidence of a comparable association with EMF for CNS tumors.[76,77] A German case–control study agreed with earlier studies in finding no effect.[78] When the available studies were reviewed by Little,[51] there was no consistent evidence for a raised risk of childhood CNS tumors with parental exposure to EMF from domestic appliances or at work. Two further occupational studies, one each of fathers[79] and of mothers,[80] do nothing to change this conclusion. There has also been considerable public concern about the possible association between radiofrequency radiation from mobile telephones and brain tumors. Several studies, including the largest case–control study[81] and the largest cohort

study,[82] found no evidence of increased risk. The subjects were exclusively adults, however, and this topic has yet to be investigated formally among children.

Following experimental evidence that transplacental exposure to several N-nitroso-compounds can induce nervous-system tumors, the possible risk associated with exposure to preformed N-nitroso-compounds and their precursors has been a principal focus of epidemiological studies of childhood brain tumors. Nine published studies have investigated a possible association with maternal consumption of cured meats during pregnancy. Most found an association with frequent consumption,[83] but numbers of cases in some studies were small, the validity of the dietary information appears not to have been evaluated, and selection bias cannot be ruled out.[51] Three of the studies were part of the Surveillance of Environmental Aspects Related to Cancer in Humans (SEARCH) collaboration, but no pooled analysis of the SEARCH data on dietary factors other than vitamin supplements has yet been published.

Tobacco smoke is a potent source of N-nitroso-compounds, although of course other constituents are also carcinogenic. A meta-analysis of 12 studies published up to 1997 found no evidence of association between maternal smoking and childhood CNS tumors.[84] Meta-analysis of the ten studies with data on children's exposure to paternal tobacco smoke showed a significantly raised relative risk of 1.22 (95 per cent confidence interval 1.05–1.40), but confounding with other potential risk factors could not be ruled out. A significantly raised risk of CNS tumors in children whose non-smoking mothers were exposed regularly to tobacco smoke in pregnancy was found in a study in Lombardy, Italy,[85] and confirmed in a later, non-overlapping study in the same region.[86] A case–control study in China produced no evidence of association between parental smoking before or during pregnancy and childhood brain tumors, but it was based on only 82 cases in total and fewer than 25 of any one type.[87] In the same study, there was a fourfold odds ratio with paternal consumption of spirits, but this finding has yet to be replicated.

Other products that are sources of N-nitroso-compounds, including beer, incense, cosmetics, rubber teats, and some categories of drugs, including diuretics and antihistamines, have been investigated less frequently. There is little consistency of results between studies.[51] In the US West Coast Childhood Brain Tumor Study, no consistent associations were found with the source of residential drinking water during the index pregnancy nor, where available, with measurements of nitrates or nitrites in tap water.[88]

By 1998, exposure to pesticides in relation to childhood CNS tumors had been analyzed in 17 studies,[89] and exposure to animals and residence on farms had been investigated in seven studies, including five that also dealt with pesticides.[90] Elevated risks for at least one measure of pesticide exposure were found in half the studies and tended to be greater for domestic rather than occupational exposure and for exposure prenatally rather than during childhood. In most studies, there were also several non-significant results, and risks were seldom calculated for specific histological types. Childhood farm residence and maternal or child exposure to farm animals tended to be associated with a raised risk. In studies of specified histological types, the increased risks were usually for PNET rather than astrocytoma. If the excess risk with exposure to animals and farm life is real, then it might be related to animal viruses that are oncogenic, but these exposures are also likely to be highly confounded with exposure to pesticides.

Several studies up to the mid-1990s indicated a protective effect of maternal consumption of vitamin supplements during pregnancy. This has been corroborated by a pooled analysis of data from most participating centers of the SEARCH collaboration.[91] There was a significantly reduced risk of brain tumors for children whose mothers used vitamin supplements for at least two trimesters, with a highly significant trend of less risk with longer duration of use. The effect did not vary between astrocytoma, PNET, and other tumors. No effect was found for supplements taken before conception or during breast-feeding. As neural-tube defects can result from folate deficiency during pregnancy, the possibly raised risk of CNS tumors in children with spina bifida may also be a consequence of insufficient folate intake. Only limited data are available on other aspects of maternal diet, but there are suggestions of a protective effect of vegetables.[83]

Childhood diet has been examined much less intensively, and no clear relationship with CNS tumors has been identified. In a comprehensive analysis of maternal and child dietary factors from the Israel component of the SEARCH study,[92] the only significant associations were with potassium intake during gestation and vegetable fat in the child's diet, both with raised odds ratios. No associations were found with nitrate, nitrite, or vitamin C.

Paternal and, less frequently, maternal employment in many different occupations has been linked to the development of CNS tumors in offspring, as has parental occupational exposure to a wide range of chemicals. Paternal exposure to paints, inks, and pigments has tended to be associated with a raised relative risk, although the numbers of exposed fathers have been small.[93] There has, however, been little overall consistency in findings between studies.[51,93] In a pooled analysis from the SEARCH collaboration, the increased risks were for either parent working in agricultural, motor-vehicle-related, or electrical occupations, and for mothers working in textile-related occupations.[94] Previous associations with other employment sectors, including the aerospace, chemical, and food industries, were not confirmed.

There is little evidence that any childhood infection is a risk factor for CNS tumors.[51] Polio vaccines administered during the period 1955–1963 were contaminated with simian virus 40 (SV40), which was shown soon afterwards to be carcinogenic in rodents. In laboratory studies, SV40 DNA sequences have been detected in large proportions of human choroid plexus tumors and ependymomas, raising the possibility of a role for SV40 in the etiology of tumors.[95] Population studies in Germany, the USA, and Sweden, however, showed no differences in incidence of choroid plexus tumors[96] or ependymoma[96–98] among cohorts exposed to SV40-contaminated vaccine and those not so exposed. A recent analysis of medulloblastoma incidence in the USA[99] did not support earlier suggestions of an increase among children exposed to SV40 in infancy in Connecticut.[100] The Connecticut study found a significantly higher rate of maternal polio vaccination in pregnancy during the period of SV40 contamination among medulloblastoma patients compared with control children, but only 62 cases were born during the relevant period and maternal vaccination status was missing for 40 per cent of cases and controls.[100]

Raised risks of brain tumor have been found in association with epilepsy and its treatment, but epilepsy can also be an early symptom of brain tumor. In a recent study, the risk was elevated even for epilepsy more than ten years before diagnosis of the brain tumor, but the overall odds ratio was much higher for astroglial tumors, which tend to be slow-growing, than for PNET, which develop more rapidly.[101]

There is no consistent evidence that head injury is a risk factor for childhood CNS tumors. A national population-based cohort study of head injury and intracranial tumors among people of all ages in Denmark used record linkage between the hospital discharge registry and the cancer registry and was therefore not subject to recall bias.[102] Raised risk of brain tumors was found only in the first year after head injury and was particularly high for people who also had epilepsy, suggesting that the association was in fact due to an elevated risk of head injury in the presence of an as yet asymptomatic brain tumor.

A wide range of factors related to pregnancy and birth has been studied in relation to the risk of childhood CNS tumors. In the past, there has been no consistent evidence for any effect of parental age. Maternal and paternal age effects were investigated among 1617 children in the Swedish Family Cancer Database with a brain tumor diagnosed during the period 1958–1994 and for whom the ages of both parents were known.[103] As in previous, smaller, studies, no maternal age effect was found. There was a raised risk of brain tumors in children of older fathers, which remained after adjustment for maternal age; fathering a child after age 40 years conferred a 24 per cent increase in relative risk. It was suggested that the trend towards older parenthood could explain in part the increase in incidence of childhood brain tumors. That increase was largely in astrocytomas,[14,103] but unfortunately parental age was not studied for different types of brain tumor.[103] In a cohort study of 459 childhood brain tumors using the Medical Birth Registry in the neighboring country of Norway, there was a decreasing trend in risk with father's age, which just failed to reach statistical significance for all brain tumors combined.[104] A large record-based case–control study in Great Britain that included over 2300 children with CNS tumors found no evidence of association with age of either parent.[105]

There is little consistent evidence for association of CNS tumors with prior fetal loss, complications of the index pregnancy, or mode of delivery. Overall, use of anesthetics in labor does not appear to affect the risk of CNS tumor in the child. In the Swedish record linkage study, however, there were raised risks with the use of pentane for all CNS tumors combined, high-grade astrocytoma, and medulloblastoma, and with the use of narcotics for all CNS tumors combined, high-grade astrocytoma, and a heterogeneous group of other CNS tumors.[106] In the SEARCH study, use of anesthetic gas was associated with a raised risk of CNS tumors overall, but especially astrocytoma.[107]

A consistent association of astrocytoma with high birthweight in earlier studies[51] has not been borne out more recently. In the Norwegian cohort study, high birthweight was a risk factor for medulloblastoma, while for astrocytoma there was a non-significant reduced risk.[104] In the international SEARCH case–control study of 1218 cases, there was little evidence of any variation in risk with birthweight.[107] In a German case–control study of 466 cases, CNS tumors were not associated with high birthweight, but there was a significantly raised risk for low birthweight (less than 2500 g) for all CNS tumors combined.[78] Case numbers were too small to give reliable estimates of risk for the main histological subgroups.

Condition at birth as measured by the Apgar score was investigated in two Scandinavian record linkage studies. In Sweden, a score of less than seven was associated with increased risk of CNS tumors;[106] in Norway, no effect was found,[104] but all scores below nine were considered together. Of two case–control studies in the UK that obtained information from obstetric, delivery, and neonatal records, but each of which contained fewer than 100 CNS tumors, one found a borderline significant raised risk with Apgar score below seven[108] and one found no effect.[109]

REFERENCES

1 Parkin DM, Kramarova E, Draper GJ et al (eds) International Incidence of Childhood Cancer, vol. II. IARC Scientific Publications no.144. Lyon: IARC, 1998.

2 Kramarova E, Stiller CA. The International Classification of Childhood Cancer. Int J Cancer 1996; **68**:759–65.

3 Gurney JG, Wall DA, Jukich PJ, Davis FG. The contribution of nonmalignant tumors to CNS tumor incidence rates among children in the United States. Cancer Causes Control 1999; **10**:101–5.

4 Glazer ER, Perkins CI, Young JL, Schlag RD, Campleman SL, Wright WE. Cancer among Hispanic children in California, 1988–1994: comparison with non-Hispanic children. Cancer 1999; **86**:1070–9.

5 Powell JE, Kelly AM, Parkes SE, Cole TRP, Mann JR. Cancer and congenital abnormalities in Asian children: a population-based study from the West Midlands. Br J Cancer 1995; **72**:1563–9.

6 Stiller CA, McKinney PA, Bunch KJ, Bailey CC, Lewis IJ. Childhood cancer and ethnic group in Britain: a United Kingdom Children's Cancer Study Group (UKCCSG) study. Br J Cancer 1991; **64**:543–8.

7 Kaatsch P, Rickert CH., Kuhl J, Schuz J, Michaelis J. Population-based epidemiologic data on brain tumors in German children. Cancer 2001; **92**:3155–64.

8 Bunin GR, Surawicz TS, Witman PA, Preston-Martin S, Davis F, Bruner JM. The descriptive epidemiology of craniopharyngioma. J Neurosurg 1998; **89**:527–51.

9 Tulinius H, Storm HH, Pukkala E, Andersen A, Ericsson J. Cancer in Nordic countries 1981–86. A joint publication of the five Nordic cancer registries. APMIS 1994; **100** (suppl. 31):1–194.

10 Cotterill SJ, Parker L, Malcolm AJ, Reid M, More L, Craft AW. Incidence and survival for cancer in children and young adults in the North of England, 1968–1995: a report from the Northern Region Young Persons Malignant Disease Registry. Br J Cancer 2000; **83**:397–403.

11 Gurney JG, Smith MA, Bunin GR. CNS and miscellaneous intracranial neoplasms. In: Ries LAG, Smith MA, Gurney JG, et al (eds) Cancer Incidence and Survival among Children and Adolescents: United States SEER Program 1975–1995. Bethesda, MD: National Cancer Institute, SEER Program, 1999, pp. 51–63.

12 Parkin DM, Whelan SL, Ferlay J, Raymond L, Young J (eds). Cancer Incidence in Five Continents, vol. VII. IARC Scientific Publication No. 143. Lyon: IARC, 1997.

13 Smith MA, Freidlin B, Ries LAG, Simon R. Trends in reported incidence of primary malignant brain tumors in children in the United States. J Natl Cancer Inst 1998; **90**:1269–77.

14 Hjalmars U, Kulldorff M, Wahlquist Y, Lannering B. Increased incidence rates but no space–time clustering of childhood astrocytoma in Sweden, 1973–1992. Cancer 1999; **85**:2077–90.

15 Smith MA, Freidlin B, Ries LAG, Simon R. Increased incidence rates but no space–time clustering of childhood astrocytoma in Sweden, 1973–1992. A population-based study of pediatric brain tumours. Cancer 2000; **88**:1492–3.

16 McNally RJQ, Kelsey AM, Cairns DP, Taylor GM, Eden OB, Birch JM. Temporal increases in the incidence of childhood solid tumours seen in north-west England (1954–1998) are likely to be real. Cancer 2001; **92**:1967–76.

17 Bunin GR, Feuer EJ, Witman PA, Meadows AT. Increasing incidence of childhood cancer: report of 20 years experience from the Greater Delaware Valley Pediatric Tumor Registry. Paediatr Perinatal Epidemiol 1996; **10**:319–38.

18 Surawicz TS, McCarthy BJ, Kupelian V, et al. Descriptive epidemiology of primary brain and CNS tumors: results of the

Central Brain Tumor Registry of the United States, 1990–1994. *Neuro-oncology* 1999; **1**:14–25.

19 Miller RW, Young JL, Novakovic B. Childhood Cancer. *Cancer* 1995; **75**:395–405.

20 Villeneuve PJ, Raman S, Leclerc J-M, Huchcroft S, Dryer D, Morrison H. Survival rates among Canadian children and teenagers with cancer diagnosed between 1985 and 1988. *Cancer Prev Control* 1998; **2**:15–22.

21 Stiller CA. Population-based survival rates for childhood cancer in Britain, 1980–91. *BMJ* 1994; **309**:1612–16.

22 Magnani C, Pastore G, ITACARE Working Group. Survival of childhood cancer patients in Italy, 1978–1989. *Tumori* 1997; **83**:426–89.

23 Kramarova E, Plesko I, Black RJ, Obsitnikova A. Improving survival for childhood cancer in Slovakia. *Int J Cancer* 1996; **65**:594–600.

24 Giles G, Waters K, Thursfield V, Farrugia H. Childhood cancer in Victoria, Australia, 1970–89. *Int J Cancer* 1995; **63**:794–7.

25 Nandakumar A, Anantha N, Appaji L, *et al.* Descriptive epidemiology of childhood cancers in Bangalore, India. *Cancer Causes Control* 1996; **7**:405–10.

26 Desai KI, Nadkarni TD, Muzumdar DP, Goel A. Prognostic factors for cerebellar astrocytoma in children: a study of 102 cases. *Pediatr Neurosurg* 2001; **35**:311–17.

27 Kibirige MS, Birch JM, Campbell RHA, Gattamaneni HR, Blair V. A review of astrocytoma in childhood. *Pediatr Hematol Oncol* 1989; **6**:319–29.

28 Robertson CM, Hawkins MM, Kingston JE. Late deaths and survival after childhood cancer: implications for cure. *BMJ* 1994; **309**:162–6.

29 Moller T, Garwicz S, Barlow L, *et al.* Decreasing late mortality among five-year survivors of cancer in childhood and adolescence: a population-based study in the Nordic countries. *J Clin Oncol* 2001; **19**:3173–81.

30 Mertens AC, Yasui Y, Neglia JP, *et al.* Late mortality experience in five year survivors of childhood and adolescent cancer: the Childhood Cancer Survivor Study. *J Clin Oncol* 2001; **19**:3163–72.

31 Hawkins MM, Draper GJ, Kingston JE. Incidence of second primary tumours among childhood cancer survivors. *Br J Cancer* 1987; **56**:339–47.

32 Olsen JH, Garwicz S, Hertz H, *et al.* Second malignant neoplasms after cancer in childhood or adolescence. *BMJ* 1993; **307**:1030–6.

33 Westermeier T, Kaatsch P, Schoetzau A, Michaelis J. Multiple primary neoplasms in childhood: data from the German Children's Cancer Registry. *Eur J Cancer* 1998; **34**:687–93.

34 Magnani C, Aareleid T, Viscomi S, *et al.* Variation in survival of children with central nervous system malignancies diagnosed in Europe between 1978 and 1992: the EUROCARE study. *Eur J Cancer* 2001; **37**:711–21.

35 McKinney PA, Feltbower RG, Parslow RC, *et al.* Survival from childhood cancer in Yorkshire, UK: effect of ethnicity and socio-economic status. *Eur J Cancer* 1999; **35**:1816–23.

36 Stiller CA, Bunch KJ, Lewis IJ. Ethnic group and survival from childhood cancer: report from the UK Children's Cancer Study Group. *Br J Cancer* 2000; **82**:1339–43.

37 Rauck AM, Green DM, Yasui Y, Mertens A, Robison LL. Marriage in the survivors of childhood cancer: a preliminary description from the Childhood Cancer Survivor Study. *Med Pediatr Oncol* 1999; **33**:60–3.

38 Ferlay J, Parkin DM, Pisani P. *GLOBOCAN*, vol. 1: cancer incidence and mortality worldwide (CD-ROM). Lyon: IARC, 1998.

39 Linet MS, Ries LAG, Smith MA, Tarone RE, Devesa SS. Cancer surveillance series: recent trends in childhood cancer incidence and mortality in the United States. *J Natl Cancer Inst* 1999; **91**:1051–8.

40 Bernstein LG, Sullivan-Halley J, Krailo MD, Hammond GD. Trends in patterns of treatment of childhood cancer in Los Angeles County. *Cancer* 1993; **71**:3222–8.

41 Krischer JP, Roush SW, Cox MW, Pollock BH. Using a population-based registry to identify patterns of care in childhood cancer in Florida. *Cancer* 1993; **71**:3331–6.

42 Ross JA, Severson RK, Pollock BH, Robison LL. Childhood cancer in the United States. A geographical analysis of cases from the pediatric cooperative clinical trials groups. *Cancer* 1996; **77**:201–7.

43 Mott MG, Mann JR, Stiller CA. The United Kingdom Children's Cancer Study Group – the first 20 years of growth and development. *Eur J Cancer* 1997; **33**:1448–52.

44 Pession A, Rondelli R, Haupt R, *et al.* Sistema di rilevazione dei casi di tumore maligno in eta pediatrica in Italia su base ospedaliera. The Italian hospital-based registry of pediatric cancer. *Riv Ital Pediatr* 2000; **26**:333–41.

45 Duffner PK, Cohen ME, Flannery JT. Referral patterns of childhood brain tumors in the state of Connecticut. *Cancer* 1982; **50**:1636–40.

46 Kramer S, Meadows AT, Pastore G, Jarrett P, Bruce D. Influence of place of treatment on diagnosis, treatment and survival in three pediatric solid tumors. *J Clin Oncol* 1984; **2**:917–23.

47 Stiller CA, Lennox EL. Childhood medulloblastoma in Britain 1971–77: analysis of treatment and survival. *Br J Cancer* 1983; **48**:835–41.

48 Danjoux CE, Jenkin RDT, McLaughlin J, *et al.* Childhood medulloblastoma in Ontario, 1977–87: population-based results. *Med Pediatr Oncol* 1996; **26**:1–9.

49 Tait DM, Thornton-Jones H, Bloom HJG, Lemerle J, Morris Jones P. Adjuvant chemotherapy for medulloblastoma: the first multi-centre control trial of the International Society of Paediatric Oncology (SIOP I). *Eur J Cancer* 1990; **26**:464–9.

50 Albright AL, Sposto R, Holmes E, *et al.* Correlation of neurosurgical subspecialization with outcomes in children with malignant brain tumors. *Neurosurgery* 2000; **47**:879–87.

51 Little J. *Epidemiology of Childhood Cancer*. IARC Scientific Publication No. 149. Lyon: IARC, 1999.

52 Lindor NM, Greene MH. Mayo Familial Cancer Program. The concise handbook of family cancer syndromes. *J Natl Cancer Inst* 1998; **90**:1039–71.

53 McGaughran JM, Harris DI, Donnai E, *et al.* A clinical study of type 1 neurofibromatosis in north west England. *J Med Genet* 1999; **36**:197–203.

54 Rasmussen SA, Young Q, Friedman JM. Mortality in neurofibromatosis 1: an analysis using US death certificates. *Am J Hum Genet* 2001; **68**:1110–18.

55 Narod SA, Stiller C, Lenoir GM. An estimate of the heritable fraction of childhood cancer. *Br J Cancer* 1991; **63**:993–9.

56 Webb DW, Fryer AE, Osborne JP. Morbidity associated with tuberous sclerosis: a population study. *Dev Med Child Neurol* 1996; **38**:146–55.

57 Cowan R, Hoban P, Kelsey A, Birch JM, Gattamaneni HR, Evans DGR. The gene for the naevoid basal cell carcinoma

syndrome acts as a tumour-suppressor gene in medulloblastoma. *Br J Cancer* 1997; **76**:141–5.

58 Varley JM, Evans DGR, Birch JM. Li–Fraumeni syndrome – a molecular and clinical review. *Br J Cancer* 1997; **76**:1–14.

59 Birch JM, Alston RD, McNally RJQ, *et al.* Relative frequency and morphology of cancers in carriers of germline TP53 mutations. *Oncogene* 2001; **20**:4621–8.

60 Kleihues P, Schauble B, zur Hausen A, Esteve J, Ohgaki H. Tumors associated with p53 germline mutations: a synopsis of 91 families. *Am J Pathol* 1997; **150**:1–13.

61 Garber JE, Burke EM, Lavally BL, *et al.* Choroid plexus tumors in the breast cancer-sarcoma syndrome. *Cancer* 1990; **66**:2658–60.

62 Sedlacek Z, Kodet R, Kriz V, *et al.* Two Li–Fraumeni syndrome families with novel germline p53 mutations: loss of the wild-type p53 allele in only 50% of tumours. *Br J Cancer* 1998; **77**:1034–9.

63 Biegel JA, Zhou J-Y, Rorke LB, Stenstrom C, Wainwright LM, Fogelgren B. Germ-line and acquired mutations of *INI1* in atypical teratoid and rhabdoid tumours. *Cancer Res* 1999; **59**:74–9.

64 Sevenet N, Sheridan E, Amran D, Schneider P, Handgretinger R, Delattre O. Constitutional mutations of the *hSNF5/INI1* gene predispose to a variety of cancers. *Am J Hum Genet* 1999; **65**:1342–8.

65 Taylor MD, Gokgoz N, Andrulis IL, Mainprize TG, Drake JM, Rutka JT. Familial posterior fossa brain tumors of infancy secondary to germline mutation of the *hSNF5* gene. *Am J Hum Genet* 2000; **66**:1403–6.

66 Paraf F, Jothy S, van Meir EG. Brain tumor – polyposis syndrome: two genetic diseases? *J Clin Oncol* 1997; **15**:2744–58.

67 Vasen HFA, Sanders EACM, Taal BG, *et al.* The risk of brain tumours in hereditary non-polyposis colorectal cancer (HNPCC). *Int J Cancer* 1996; **65**:422–5.

68 Hasle H. Patterns of malignant disorders in individuals with Down's syndrome. *Lancet Oncol* 2001; **2**:429–36.

69 Narod SA, Hawkins MM, Robertson CM, Stiller CA. Congenital anomalies and childhood cancer in Great Britain. *Am J Hum Genet* 1997; **60**:474–85.

70 Miller RW, Rubinstein JH. Tumors in Rubinstein–Taybi syndrome. *Am J Med Genet* 1995; **56**:112–15.

71 Hemminki K, Kyyronen P, Vaittinen P. Parental age as a risk factor of childhood leukemia and brain cancer in offspring. *Epidemiology* 1999; **10**:271–5.

72 Falck Winther J, Sankila R, Boice JD, *et al.* Cancer in siblings of children with cancer in the Nordic countries: a population-based cohort study. *Lancet* 2001; **358**:711–17.

73 Varley JM, McGown G, Thorncroft M, *et al.* Are there low-penetrance *TP53* alleles? Evidence from childhood adrenocortical tumors. *Am J Hum Genet* 1999; **65**:995–1006.

74 Ron E, Modan B, Boice JD, *et al.* Tumors of the brain and nervous system after radiotherapy in childhood. *N Engl J Med* 1988; **319**:1033–9.

75 Garwicz S, Anderson H, Olsen JH, *et al.* Second malignant neoplasms after cancer in childhood and adolescence: a population-based case–control study in the 5 Nordic countries. *Int J Cancer* 2000; **88**:672–8.

76 NRPB Advisory Group on Non-ionising Radiation. ELF electromagnetic fields and the risk of cancer. *Doc NRPB* 2001; **12**:3–179.

77 Kheifets LI. Electric and magnetic field exposure and brain cancer: a review. *Bioelectromagnetics* 2001; **suppl 5**:S120–31.

78 Schuz J, Kaletsch U, Kaatsch P, Meinert R, Michaelis J. Risk factors for pediatric tumors of the central nervous system: results from a German population-based case–control study. *Med Pediatr Oncol* 2001; **36**:274–82.

79 Williams JR, Wellage LC. Brain tumor risk in offspring of men occupationally exposed to electric and magnetic fields. *Scand J Work Environ Health* 1996; **22**:339–45.

80 Sorahan T, Hamilton L, Gardner K, Hodgson JT, Harrington JM. Maternal occupational exposure to electromagnetic fields before, during and after pregnancy in relation to risks of childhood cancers: findings from the Oxford Survey of Childhood Cancers, 1953–1981 deaths. *Am J Ind Med* 1999; **35**:348–57.

81 Inskip PD, Tarone RE, Hatch EE, *et al.* Cellular-telephone use and brain tumors. *N Engl J Med* 2001; **344**:79–86.

82 Johansen C, Boice J, McLaughlin J, Olsen J. Cellular telephones and cancer – a nationwide cohort study in Denmark. *J Natl Cancer Inst* 2001; **93**:203–7.

83 Bunin GR. Maternal diet during pregnancy and risk of brain tumors in children. *Int J Cancer Suppl* 1998; **11**:23–5.

84 Boffetta P, Tredaniel J, Grew A. Risk of childhood cancer and adult lung cancer after childhood exposure to passive smoke: a meta-analysis. *Environ Health Perspect* 2000; **108**:73–82.

85 Filippini G, Farinotti M, Lovicu G, Maisonneuve P, Boyle P. Mothers' active and passive smoking during pregnancy and risk of brain tumours in children. *Int J Cancer* 1994; **57**:769–74.

86 Filippini G, Farinotti M, Ferrarini M. Active and passive smoking during pregnancy and risk of central nervous system tumours in children. *Paediatr Perinatal Epidemiol* 2000; **14**:78–84.

87 Hu J, Mao Y, Ugnat A–M. Parental cigarette smoking, hard liquor consumption and the risk of childhood brain tumors. A case–control study in north east China. *Acta Oncol* 2000; **39**:979–84.

88 Mueller BA, Newton K, Holly EA, Preston-Martin S. Residential water source and the risk of childhood brain tumors. *Environ Health Perspect* 2001; **109**:551–6.

89 Zahm SH, Ward MH. Pesticides and childhood cancer. *Environ Health Perspect* 1998; **106** (suppl 3):893–908.

90 Yeni-Komshian H, Holly EA. Childhood brain tumours and exposure to animals and farm life: a review. *Paediatr Perinatal Epidemiol* 2000; **14**:248–56.

91 Preston-Martin S, Pogoda JM, Muller BA, *et al.* Prenatal vitamin supplementation and risk of childhood brain tumors. *Int J Cancer Suppl* 1998; **11**:17–22.

92 Lubin F, Farbstein H, Chetrit A, *et al.* The role of nutritional habits during gestation and child life in pediatric brain tumor etiology. *Int J Cancer* 2000; **86**:139–43.

93 Colt JS, Blair A. Parental occupational exposure and risk of childhood cancer. *Environ Health Perspect* 1998; **106** (suppl 3):909–25.

94 Cordier S, Mandereau L, Preston-Martin S, *et al.* Parental occupations and childhood brain tumors: results of an international case–control study. *Cancer Causes Control* 2001; **12**:865–74.

95 Bergsagel DJ, Finegold MJ, Butel JS, Kupsky WJ, Garcea RL. DNA sequences similar to those of simian virus 40 in ependymomas and choroid plexus tumors of childhood. *N Engl J Med* 1992; **326**:988–93.

96   Geissler E. SV40 and human brain tumors. *Prog Med Virol*
     1990; **37**:211–22.

97   Strickler HD, Rosenberg PS, Devesa SS, Hertel J, Fraumeni JF,
     Goedert JJ. Contamination of poliovirus vaccines with simian
     virus 40 (1955–1963) and subsequent cancer rates. *JAMA*
     1998; **279**:292–5.

98   Olin P, Giesecke J. Potential exposure to SV40 in polio
     vaccine used in Sweden during 1957: no impact on cancer
     incidence rates 1960–1993. *Dev Biol Stand* 1998;
     94:227–33.

99   Strickler HD, Rosenberg PS, Devesa SS, Fraumeni JF,
     Goedert JJ. Contamination of poliovirus vaccine with SV40
     and the incidence of medulloblastoma. *Med Pediatr Oncol*
     1999; **32**:77–8.

100 Farwell JR, Dohrmann GJ, Flannery JT. Medulloblastoma in
     childhood: an epidemiological study. *J Neurosurg* 1984;
     61:657–64.

101 Gurney JG, Mueller BA, Preston-Martin S, *et al.* A study of
     pediatric brain tumors and their association with epilepsy
     and anticonvulsant use. *Neuroepidemiology* 1997;
     16:248–55.

102 Inskip PD, Mellenkjaer L, Gridley G, Olsen JH. Incidence
     of intracranial tumors following hospitalization for head
     injuries (Denmark). *Cancer Causes Control* 1998;
     9:109–16.

103 Hemminki K, Kyyronen P, Vaittinen P. Parental age as a risk
     factor of childhood leukemia and brain cancer in offspring.
     Epidemiology 1999; **10**:271–5.

104 Heuch JM, Heuch I, Akslen LA, Kvale G. Risk of primary
     childhood brain tumors related to birth characteristics: a
     Norwegian prospective study. *Int J Cancer* 1998; **77**:498–503.

105 Dockerty JD, Draper G, Vincent T, Rowan SD, Bunch KJ.
     Case–control study of parental age, parity and socioeconomic
     level in relation to childhood cancers. *Int J Epidemiol* 2001;
     30:1428–37.

106 Linet MS, Gridley G, Cnattingius S, *et al.* Maternal and
     perinatal risk factors for childhood brain tumors (Sweden).
     Cancer Causes Control 1996; **7**:437–48.

107 McCredie M, Little J, Cotton S, *et al.* SEARCH international
     case–control study of childhood brain tumours: role of index
     pregnancy and birth, and mother's reproductive history.
     Paediatr Perinatal Epidemiol 1999; **13**:325–41.

108 Fear NT, Roman E, Ansell P, Bull D. Malignant neoplasms of
     the brain during childhood: the role of prenatal and neonatal
     factors (United Kingdom). *Cancer Causes Control* 2001;
     12:443–9.

109 McKinney PA, Juszczak E, Findlay E, Smith K, Thomson CS.
     Pre- and perinatal risk factors for childhood leukaemia and
     other malignancies: a Scottish case control study. *Br J Cancer*
     1999; **80**:1844–51.

Neuroembryology

PAUL J. SCOTTING AND VANESSA J. APPLEBY

DEFINITIONS

Basic helix–loop–helix (bHLH) Large family of transcription factors (many of which are neurogenic) that dimerize through a helix–loop–helix motif and then bind DNA via the adjacent basic domain. Includes *HES, neurogenin, NeuroD, ASH, MASH, ATH,* and *MATH.*

Bone morphogenetic proteins (BMPs) Members of the tumor growth factor beta (TGFb) superfamily of signal peptides. Roles include pushing ectodermal cells towards an epidermal rather than a neural fate.

Chordin Inhibitor of *bone morphogenetic proteins (BMPs).* Appears to play a role in neural induction.

Cyclins Components of kinase complexes that regulate transitions throughout the cell cycle.

ErbB Receptor family for neuregulins.

Fibroblast growth factor (FGF) Family of small signal peptides, different members implicated in inhibiting and stimulating neural differentiation.

Lateral inhibition Phenomenon whereby neighboring cells inhibit each other from following certain developmental pathways via the Notch signaling pathway:

- **Delta** – Cell-surface ligand for Notch.
- **Serrate** – Cell-surface ligand for Notch.
- **Notch** – Cell-surface receptor.

Neural Term applied to tissue capable of producing cells of the nervous system.

Neural induction Process by which tissues signal to ectoderm to become neural.

Neural plate Axial region of ectoderm initially set aside to form the *central nervous system (CNS).*

Neural tube Early tube structure formed by the rolling up of the neural plate.

Neuregulins Epidermal growth factor (EGF)-related peptide signal molecules.

Neurogenesis Process of forming neuronal cells from proliferating precursors.

Neurotrophins Peptide factors that function in the survival, proliferation, and differentiation of nerve cells, including nerve growth factor (NGF) and brain-derived neurotrophic factor (BDNF).

Noggin Inhibitor of *bone morphogenetic proteins (BMPs)* that appears to play a role in neural induction.

P27/KIP Cyclin-dependent kinase inhibitor.

Patched Twelve-pass transmembrane protein that appears to act as a cell-surface receptor for the *shh* signaling molecule. When no *shh* is bound, the Patched protein inhibits the associated smoothened protein from activating a downstream signaling pathway. Two distinct Patched receptors have now been defined.

Sonic hedgehog (shh) Signaling peptide that plays a role in an amazing diversity of processes during embryonic development, including granule cell proliferation, dorsoventral patterning in the *central nervous system (CNS),* anteroposterior patterning in the limb, and radial organization of the gut. So-called due to homology with the *Drosophila melanogaster* gene *hedgehog.*

Smoothened Seven-pass G-protein-related receptor molecule inhibited by Patched. When active (e.g. when Patched is absent or inhibited by binding of shh), Smoothened signals to activate gene expression by activating Gli proteins. Can also affect cell cycle by direct effects on cyclinB1.

Transcription factors Proteins that function to regulate the transcription and thus the expression of other genes. The vertebrate genome contains hundreds of genes encoding these factors, and these are usually grouped according to the structural motifs they contain, often responsible for the ability of the factors to bind to their target genes in a sequence-specific manner.

Trk (tropomyosin-related kinase family of receptors) Receptors for the neurotrophins.

Wnt Large family of soluble signal peptides involved in a wide range of embryonic processes. Act via the frizzled family of receptors, the antigen-presenting cell (APC) protein, and the LEF/TCF family of transcription factor effector proteins.

INTRODUCTION

For many years, it has been clear that there is a fundamental link between cancer cells and embryonic cells. Many genes first identified through their roles as oncogenes have been shown subsequently to be key regulators of normal developmental events. Likewise, genes first studied with respect to their involvement in embryonic processes have also been shown to play direct roles in tumor etiology. In the case of brain tumors, the similarity between tumor cells and embryonic cells is particularly pronounced, such that a major class of pediatric brain tumors is classified as "embryonic tumors." It is these embryonic tumors that are the focus of this chapter. Particular attention will be devoted to development of the cerebellum and processes relevant to the most common pediatric brain tumor, medulloblastoma.

In this chapter, we will consider the early development of the central nervous system (CNS), with particular emphasis on those aspects that we believe are most likely to shed light on the process of tumor development. In the following sections, we will describe briefly the developmental processes through which the normal CNS is formed in order to provide a biological framework within which pediatric CNS tumors can be better understood. This discussion will be limited to the early events when decisions regarding proliferation, migration, and initial differentiation take place (thus not necessarily including events involved in terminal differentiation, such as synapse formation and neuronal signaling). Through knowledge of their relationship to the normal tissue from which they arise, particularly aspects that appear disrupted in such tumors, it is hoped that the etiology of these tumors will become clear. We will pay particular attention to processes that have been studied in the tumors themselves. However, many processes controlling development of the CNS

have been elucidated only over the past few years and have not yet made the transition to the field of neuro-oncology. We will, therefore, also present data on these other developmental processes that we believe are likely to be of relevance to this class of tumor. Although the general development of the CNS, including both neuronal and glial components, will be discussed, detailed discussion of glial development with respect to glioma and the genes implicated through identification of genetic lesions in gliomas is reviewed beautifully by Maher and colleagues[1] and will not be included here. The first half of this chapter will consider control of cell proliferation, control of cell maturation, cell migration, and cell-type specification. In each section, the developmental process will be described, followed by a discussion of the possible or known relevance to tumor biology. In the latter half of the chapter, we will review the process of cerebellum development with particular reference to the molecular control of granule cell proliferation and maturation, since this is believed to be the cellular origin of the most common pediatric brain tumor, medulloblastoma.

In general, the studies of both cellular and molecular mechanisms described here have been carried out predominantly in developing rodents and chickens. For those outside the field of developmental biology, this may seem somewhat removed from the human state. We would therefore like to stress that, while there are some details of CNS development that differ between organisms such as chickens, mice, and humans, there is no doubt that much of what will be described is true for all of these. The expression of many genes and description of morphological processes has often been confirmed in human samples, but of course the experimental proofs of function are often possible only using animal models.

OVERVIEW OF CENTRAL NERVOUS SYSTEM DEVELOPMENT

At all stages of development, events are regulated at several levels. In general, cells alter their behavior in response to signals from outside of the cell. During the early period of CNS formation, the families of signaling molecules most frequently seen in this context are members of the bone morphogenetic proteins (BMPs), fibroblast growth factors (FGFs), and Wnt proteins. The effects of these signals frequently include changes in gene expression, and much research has therefore centered on understanding how these transcriptional changes are achieved. Such changes are mediated by transcription factors, proteins that bind to the regulatory elements of genes and either activate or repress their expression. Thus, each regulatory process often includes specific external signals, their receptors, and a cascade of internal signaling events that finally changes the expression of genes via alteration of the function of transcription factors. Several such pathways will be described in this chapter.

Formation of the neural tube

In developmental biology, one of the most studied but least well understood processes has been the mechanisms through which tissue is set aside as neural via a phenomenon called neural induction. The past decade has seen the elucidation of much of the cellular and molecular mechanism controlling this phenomenon (Figure 4a.1) (reviewed by Harland[2] and Scotting and Rex[3]). It has been known for some time that the position of the CNS, running along the midline of the embryo, is achieved through its induction by axial mesodermal tissue lying below the ectoderm. This inductive signaling results in restricted regions of ectoderm adopting a neural fate while the rest becomes the epidermis that will cover the outer surface of the embryo.

The earliest evidence of a response to neural induction is the expression of the genes *Sox2* and *Sox3*,[4,5] which are themselves transcription factors. As such, the proteins encoded by these *Sox* genes may function to convert the initial signal to changes in gene expression necessary for the cells to behave as neural cells. These changes include morphological thickening, which gives rise to the neural plate (Figure 4a.1b) and folding of the ectoderm, probably mediated by changes in cell adhesion. The end result is the formation of the neural tube that will give rise to all parts of the CNS (Figure 4a.1c).

TUMORS

While the events described above clearly occur well before the initiation of tumorigenic processes, which are likely to present postnatally, investigating these processes may yet be of value to neuro-oncologists. These studies provide insight into the molecular mechanisms by which cells are specified to be neural, processes that might be disrupted in tumorigenesis, leading to the presence of non-neural cell types in a neural site, as seen for example in teratoid/rhabdoid tumors.[6] Indeed, *Sox* gene expression is now being considered as one of the best markers of the neural stem cell,[7] from which many CNS embryonic tumors may well originate.[8] In addition, studies of these early events provide an understanding of the molecular pathways, and links between pathways, that are also found to be active in later stages of development and in tumor etiology.

Neurogenesis

Once the tissue of the nervous system has been set aside, it grows through maintained proliferation. However, production of the mature cells of the nervous system is initiated very early during its development. Thus, there must be very effective control of these two processes, such that the cells of the CNS are produced in the correct temporal and spatial manner while sufficient cells are maintained in proliferation to achieve the required size and complexity of the nervous tissue. Not surprisingly for this most complex of tissues, it seems that there are very many genes involved in controlling this choice, and there appear to be many safeguards against errors.

Figure 4a.1 *Diagrammatic representation of central nervous system (CNS) development in higher vertebrates. Transverse section views of the developing CNS in progressively later stages of development. (a) Prior to neural induction, the three germ tissue layers (ectoderm, mesoderm, endoderm) are formed via gastrulation. Cells along the midline of the ectoderm (at this stage called the epiblast) migrate ventrally and spread out beneath the ectoderm to form the endoderm (which will go on to form the internal lining of the inner organs such as gut and lung) and the mesoderm (which forms between the ectoderm and endoderm and gives rise primarily to muscle and bone). (b) Signals from the midline mesoderm cause the more medial ectoderm to thicken and fold and express markers of neural fate such as Sox2; this is the process of neural induction; the thickened ectoderm is called the neural plate. (c) The neural plate rolls up and fuses dorsally to form the neural tube from which all CNS structures arise. (d) For simplicity, only the spinal cord is shown at this later stage. The spinal cord is thickening through continued proliferation of the neuroepithelium. The bulk of the spinal cord is now made up of cells that have stopped dividing and migrated laterally, first to the subventricular zone, and later to be pushed further outwards as they differentiate. The outermost part is the white matter, where axons run along the spinal cord.*

Neural induction is the phenomenon by which the axial mesoderm causes the neural plate to form. Work from many groups has now shown that bone morphogenetic proteins (BMPs) drive away ectoderm from a neural fate and that BMP-blocking molecules, such as noggin and chordin (derived from the inducing tissue), cause the midline ectoderm to become neural by relieving this inhibition. In higher vertebrates (birds, mice, and, presumably, humans), very recent work has shown that fibroblast growth factor (FGF) signals also play a role in driving cells towards a neural fate and that Wnt signals may override these FGF signals. Thus, coordinated activity of all three of these signaling systems results in restricted regions of ectoderm adopting a neural fate while the rest becomes the epidermis, which will cover the outer surface of the embryo. In summary, a current model suggests that BMPs inhibit cells from becoming neural, while FGFs inhibit BMP signaling and drive cells towards a neural state and Wnts might block the positive effects of the FGFs. Thus, absence of Wnts and presence of FGFs, as seen where the CNS develops, causes activation of transcriptional changes, at least in part, through the activation of Sox proteins.

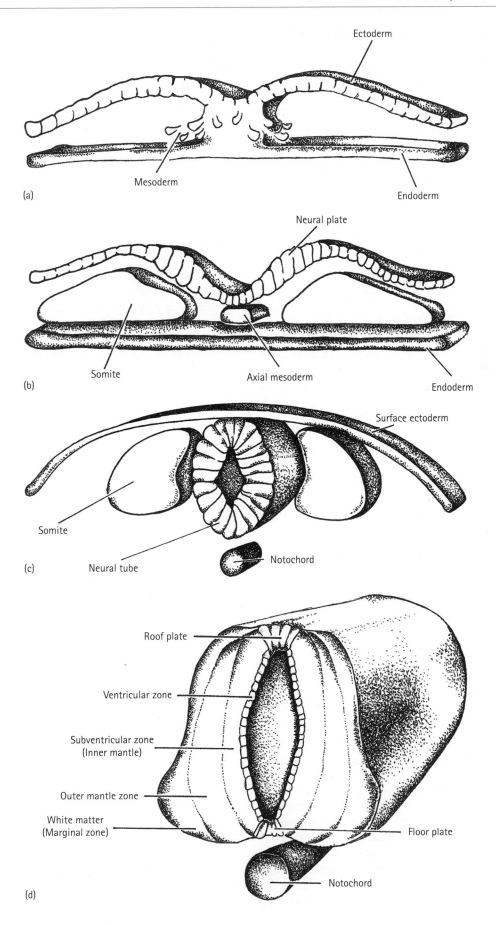

However, it is this very choice that is disrupted in the cancers that are the focus of this book.

The neural tube is initially a single-layered neuro-epithelium, still expressing early markers such as *Sox2* and *Sox3*, from which all cell types of the mature CNS will eventually arise. In fact, *Sox3* and *Sox2* remain expressed in the proliferating population of the neuroepithelium throughout development.[9] As such, these two genes provide excellent markers of the most primitive cells of the nervous system. Neurogenesis, the production of functional neurons, begins anteriorly and moves as a wave from anterior to posterior. Neurogenesis is controlled by both positive and repressive influences. Recent experiments suggest that FGF-8, produced in the mesoderm adjacent to the immature part of the neural tube, inhibits this process, while another, as yet undefined, factor produced by more mature anterior mesoderm is required to promote differentiation.[10]

Once neurogenesis begins, individual cells in the neural tube sequentially express a series of neurogenic transcription factors, most from the basic helix–loop–helix (bHLH) gene family (Figure 4a.2).[11,12] Concomitantly, the cells stop dividing and migrate laterally away from the lumen of the CNS to differentiate fully in a more lateral position within the CNS. It seems clear from many studies that it is these bHLH genes that are the master control factors regulating the first steps in the neurogenesis program. However, the details of cell movements and the precise series of transcription factors expressed vary in different regions of the CNS, thus a simplified general scheme will be discussed here. At later stages, gliogenesis seems to follow a similar series of events.

When cells undergo the transition from a proliferating to a post-mitotic state, they also initiate the first events of differentiation. It therefore seems that the same signal(s) cause cells to stop dividing and to initiate differentiation. A complex series of events then regulates the actual differentiation program as post-mitotic neurons mature. We will therefore first consider the control of proliferation, including the decision of whether to exit the cell cycle and initiate differentiation, after which we will consider the control of cell maturation as post-mitotic cells mature.

CONTROL OF CELL PROLIFERATION

The regulation of cell proliferation can be considered at several levels. As described above, there are signals that lead to a cell remaining proliferative and those that antagonize these signals, thus driving neuronal and glial differentiation. Cytoplasmic events include effects on components of signaling pathways that mediate the transfer of cell-surface signals to nuclear changes. Finally, events in the nucleus represent the effectors of those signaling pathways.

In general, the proliferating ventricular zone appears quite similar in all brain regions. As cells exit mitosis, they migrate laterally. Once they have exited the ventricular zone, they enter the subventricular zone and then move out to their final location (Figure 4a.1d). But what actually regulates the proliferation of these cells? As mentioned above, it has been shown that FGF signals from the mesoderm seem to inhibit early neurogenesis. Likewise, recent data suggest that the sonic hedgehog (shh) signal peptide acts as a mitogen in several regions of the brain, including the cerebellum (Figure 4a.3) (see p. 61 for a detailed description of the shh pathway).[13] However, extracellular signals that drive neurogenesis have not yet been identified. It may be that neurogenesis is simply the result of cells becoming immune to mitogenic stimuli via cell autonomous changes. Once neurogenesis has begun within the nervous system as a whole, a process termed "lateral inhibition" appears to play a dominant role in the choice between proliferation and differentiation (Figure 4a.2).[12,14] This is a phenomenon by which differentiating cells express on their surface a protein (a member of the Delta/ Serrate/-Jagged family) that interacts with a receptor of the Notch family on the surface of neighboring cells. The result of this interaction is that the cell receiving the signal is inhibited from that pathway of differentiation. It is believed that this is a central mechanism to ensure that the correct balance between proliferation and differentiation is maintained. In the CNS, experimental interference with this pathway can result in a mass differentiation of cells at the expense of proliferation,[15] while experimentally activating this pathway inhibits any differentiation.[15] The signaling that results from lateral inhibition is effected at a transcriptional level, by activating the HES family of transcription factors.[12,16] HES proteins repress genes that promote differentiation (Figure 4a.2).[16]

The final step in any pathway that promotes proliferation must be to regulate the cell-cycle machinery. A great deal of the molecular detail of this machinery has been elucidated (Figure 4a.4) (reviewed in detail by Ross[17] and Ohnuma *et al.*[18]). However, the specific mechanisms by which this machinery is regulated in the CNS is less clear. It is striking, however, that CNS tumors rarely exhibit mutations in genes such as those encoding the retinoblastoma (Rb) and p53 tumor suppressor proteins,[19–21] which are frequent oncogenic targets in tumors of other tissue types. It is likely, therefore, that the fundamental cell-cycle control programs are regulated by other mechanisms in the CNS. Some of these are discussed in more detail below, in the context of cerebellum development. As for the trophic support of nerve cells, several growth factors, including epidermal growth factor (EGF) and platelet-derived growth factor (PDGF), have been shown to be important for their survival in vitro and in vivo.[22–24] Thus, the expression of receptors for these families could be an important feature of the maintenance of proliferation.

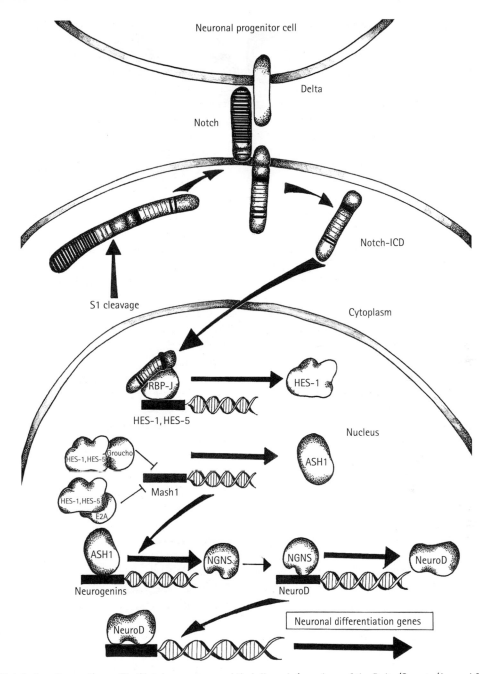

Figure 4a.2 *Notch signaling pathway. The Notch receptors and their ligands (members of the Delta/Serrate/Jagged families) mediate the process of lateral inhibition. In this process, a ligand for Notch expressed on the surface of one cell interacts with its Notch receptor on a neighboring cell and thus alters the behavior of that second cell. In the developing central nervous system, cells that have only recently stopped dividing that express the ligand, and this allows them to inhibit their immediate neighbors from initiating neuronal differentiation. This is believed to regulate the number of cells undergoing neurogenesis at any one time.*

Both ligands and receptors have a similar structure, spanning the membrane once and containing a series of EGF-like repeats in their extracellular domain. When Notch binds a ligand, this triggers its cleavage such that its intracellular domain (Notch-ICD) is released into the cytoplasm and subsequently enters the nucleus. In association with a cofactor RBP-J, the Notch-ICD acts as a transcription factor activating expression of a HES gene. HES proteins (e.g. HES-1, HES-5) are members of the bHLH family of transcription factors, but, unusually, most HES factors repress rather than activate their gene targets. Thus, HES proteins inhibit the expression of genes that activate neuronal maturation, and the activated Notch therefore blocks cells from becoming neurons. The sequence of events that is inhibited by HES factors represents a neurogenic cascade. Although the precise factors involved vary between different regions of the nervous system, the basic principles are generally true. When HES expression is off, other classes of bHLH transcription factors such as the ASH genes (MASH1 in mice) can be expressed. ASH proteins can activate expression of neurogenins, which can activate expression of genes such as NeuroD. All of these are bHLH factors, and each is capable of inducing some aspects of neuronal differentiation.

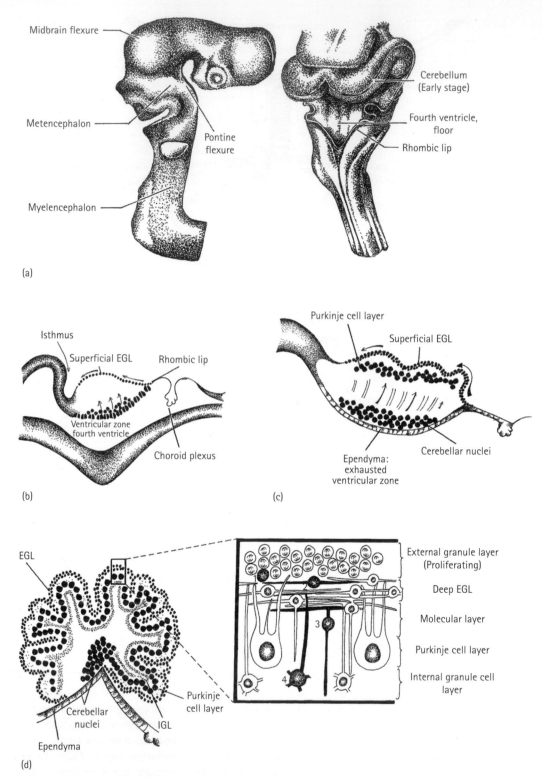

Figure 4a.3 *Development of the cerebellum. (a) Side and dorsal views of the developing human brain at three months' gestation. (b)–(d) Diagrammatic representations of sagittal sections through developing cerebellum (anterior to the left). The rhombic lip, located between the fourth ventricle and the roof plate of the metencephalon, is formed due to a failure in neural-tube closure (a), which results in the formation of a gap along the dorsal neural tube. As the embryo continues to grow, the pontine flexure is established, causing this gap to distort into a mouth-like structure. As the flexure deepens, the mesencephalon is brought closer to the metencephalon, displacing the lips laterally. The most dorsal aspects of these displaced neural tube lips are known as the rhombic lips,*

Consistent with this idea, amplification of epidermal growth factor receptor (EGFR) is seen in tumors of the CNS, particularly in gliomas. A large body of work has studied the dependence of post-proliferative cells on these factors, which has identified the importance of the EGF-related neuregulins and their erbB receptors (reviewed in Buonanno and Fischbach[25]) and the tropomyosin related kinase (Trk) family of receptors for the neurotrophins (such as nerve growth factor (NGF), reviewed in Huang and Reichardt[26]). Interestingly, TrkC is one of the few factors expressed in medulloblastomas that might provide an indication of the prognostic outcome for these tumors.[27,28]

Tumors

Of the above systems regulating proliferation, few have been identified as significant in tumors of the CNS. The ability of Notch to affect whether a cell differentiates or proliferates makes it an obvious candidate as a target for mutations that would result in tumor like behavior. However, the effects of Notch activation might be tissue- and stage-specific. Overexpression of activated Notch receptor has been shown to be able to block differentiation of small-cell lung-carcinoma cell lines,[29] while it can activate differentiation of neuroblastoma cells.[30] Notch activation has also been implicated in a number of other tumor types, including mammary tumors[31] and lymphomas.[32] Given the ability of Notch activation to block differentiation in the CNS in some contexts, this pathway remains a significant area for study in CNS tumors. Indeed, a recent study demonstrated that experimental activation of Notch2 or its target, *HES-1*, could block the differentiation of cerebellar granule cells, from which medulloblastomas arise.[33] Elucidating the full details of the downstream consequences of Notch signaling may provide insight into elements of these control processes that are indeed altered in CNS tumor development.

Although many elements of the basic control of the cell cycle are seen in all cell types, some components of the regulatory machinery that controls whether cells progress through the cycle or stop are more tissue-specific.

To date, study of this process with particular relevance to neurons is somewhat limited. An elegant study in mice has demonstrated clearly that such tissue-specificity is likely to be of central relevance to the role of such genes in tumorigenesis. Yu and colleagues[34] showed that specific members of the cyclinD protein family are involved in tumor development in particular tissues. Loss of cyclinD1 resulted in immunity to breast tumors induced by the oncogenes *neu* and *ras*. These same oncogenes were still able to induce salivary tumors, and other oncogenes were still able to induce breast tumors. Overall, it seems that different oncogenic pathways might activate the cell cycle via different cyclins, and this might also vary depending on the tissue involved. Clearly, knowledge of the components able to control these processes in normal development will provide more directed target genes for analysis in tumors of the nervous system.

CONTROL OF CELL MATURATION

Control of the events that occur immediately after a cell leaves the cell cycle is related directly to the signaling pathways that control proliferation, since the trigger to continue or cease proliferating appears to be the same as the trigger to initiate a differentiation program. These have been described above, so this discussion will be limited to the events that occur during the cell's subsequent maturation.

The decision to undergo neuronal differentiation is effected through the activation of neurogenic genes. Although the precise details of the genes expressed vary between different regions and cell types in the CNS, some features are generally true. First, *Sox3* and *Sox2* expression is lost (except in glia).[4,9] Also, as described above, expression of the *HES* family of repressor genes is lost and Notch ligands are upregulated transiently. The first of the neurogenic transcription factors to be upregulated are members of the bHLH gene family. These genes function in a cascade of activation (Figure 4a.2).[12] Thus, following the decision to exit the cell cycle, particular

from which cells migrate tangentially across the surface of the cerebellar anlage beneath the pia mater (b). These cells form the external granule layer (EGL) and are the precursors of granule neurons.

The first cells to stop dividing and begin differentiation migrate outwards from the ventricular zone of the roof of the fourth ventricle (shown as large cells in (b)). Soon afterwards, the secondary germinal zone (the EGL) forms through migration of cells over the dorsal cerebellar surface (shown as small cells in (b)). During early stages of cerebellar maturation, cells continue to migrate laterally from the ventricular zone, producing all cells of the cerebellum except for the granule cells (c). Cells of the EGL proliferate to form a layer that is several cells thick. Cells from the EGL then begin to exit mitosis and move inwards (d). The sequential stages of granule cell development are shown as black cells numbered 1–4 in detail. On reaching the premigratory EGL, the granule cells begin to differentiate, extending processes parallel to the surface (2). The granule cells then extend another process through the molecular layer and Purkinje cell layer towards the inner granule layer (IGL). Finally, the soma of the cell translocates along this last process (3) to produce a cell with its body in the IGL and a T-shaped process projecting out towards the surface (4).

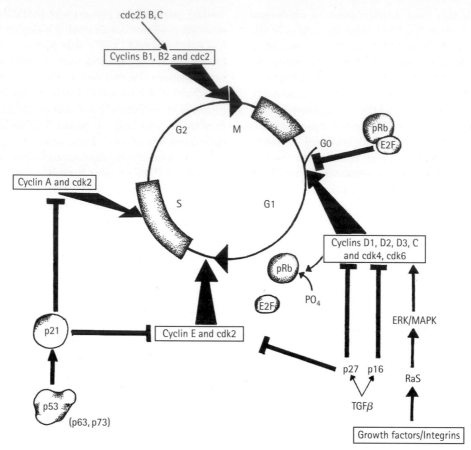

Figure 4a.4 *Cell-cycle control. The proteins responsible for cell-cycle progression are the cyclin-dependent serine/threonine kinases (cdks), which are present throughout the cell cycle, and the cyclins, which bind to and regulate the specific activity of the cdks, targeting these molecules to the correct location within a cell and to the correct substrates. The cyclins are synthesized (unlike the cdks) at specific stages in the cell cycle and appear to be regulated primarily at the level of translation. All cyclins contain a destruction box that targets the proteins for ubiquitination and subsequent proteolysis. The turnover rate of cyclins is very rapid, a feature required for the progressive stages of the cell cycle to occur. Passage through the G1 restriction point of the cell cycle commits cells to divide. This passage is blocked by the retinoblastoma protein (pRb), which binds to E2F-like transcription factors and inhibits their activation of genes required for cell-cycle progression, including S-phase regulators such as c-Myc and DNA polymerase alpha, and also the D-type cyclins that are necessary for G1–S phase progression. CyclinD proteins are upregulated in response to growth factor stimulus, peaking at the G1–S phase boundary. Progression through G1–S is achieved when cdks 4 and 6 bind to the regulatory cyclinD subunit. CyclinD levels have to reach a threshold level to achieve this binding, as the inhibitor p27 competes with cyclinD for cdk binding. Once an active cyclinD-cdk4/6 complex is formed, it phosphorylates pRb, allowing E2F to dissociate. Another inhibitor, p16, displaces p27 and allows it to bind in turn to cdk2, the cdk that is activated by cyclinE, which reaches maximal protein levels at the G1–S phase boundary and is also required for entry into S phase. CyclinE is degraded early in S phase, allowing cdk2 to bind to cyclinA, which in turn is required for progression through S phase. Both cyclinE and cyclinA are inhibited by the binding of many p21 molecules. P21, an inhibitor activated by p53 in response to DNA damage, also binds to proliferating cell nuclear antigen (PCNA), a cofactor required for DNA polymerase activity. The last stage in the cell cycle is mitosis; the B-type cyclins and cdc2 are required for cells to progress from G2 into this phase. Activity of cyclinB-cdc2 is in turn regulated by the phosphatase cdc25, which removes a critical phosphate that blocks activation. Degradation of the B-type cyclins is necessary for completion of mitosis, which continues until late into G1 to prevent mitosis of the next cycle occurring before the next S phase has taken place. Cyclin–cdk partners have also been shown to be regulated by cdk-activating kinases, which phosphorylate residues essential for activity of the complexes.*

bHLH genes are expressed, often *neurogenins*. This results in activation of other bHLH genes, such as *NeuroD1*, which then activates later genes, which might also include transcription factors. Although it is likely that many of the genes involved are yet to be identified, experimental evidence shows that it is this sequential activation of transcription factors that mediates the maturational changes that neurons undergo.

Tumors

In the context of tumors, it is of particular note that these factors are all expressed in slightly different temporal ways during the time when cells are escaping the proliferating epithelium and migrating. Their presence in tumor cells may therefore reflect not only the very precise maturational state of those cells but also some aspects of their cellular behavior. The genes that regulate the earliest steps of neuronal maturation also provide candidates targets for mutations that disrupt that maturation, such changes perhaps representing secondary or later alterations as cells undergo tumor progression. However, it has also been shown that some of the genes described above can have direct dominant effects on the decision to exit the cell cycle and so could be involved in tumor initiation (reviewed by Ohnuma et al.[18]).

CELL MIGRATION

As stated earlier, migration of newly born neuronal cells is a fundamental feature of CNS development (reviewed by Gleeson and Walsh[35] and Lambert de Rouvroit and Goffinet[36]). Clearly, in the context of tumors, the ability of cells to migrate through surrounding tissue is an important biological problem. The molecular basis of cell migration varies depending on the site and cell type. In general, neurons move via extension of a long cellular process, followed by displacement of the nucleus along that process. They also frequently move along the surface of the extended fibers from other cells. Thus, in the cortex, early cells, the radial glia, extend processes to the outer surface of the cortex, and newly born neurons then migrate outwards along those processes. In general, however, the highly organized movements of neurons during normal development seem quite different to the events that are likely to trigger tumor cell dispersion. Although several genetic mutations have been found where the ability to migrate or the directional control of that migration is disrupted, the genes implicated generally regulate cytoskeletal organization and directional movements, resulting in a disorganized CNS. The movements seen during metastasis represent an abnormal escape of cells from the CNS tissue that is not seen in the above cases, hence study of such normal events may have little bearing on tumor cell biology.

Tumors

One aspect of normal migration may be of particular relevance. In a relatively rare, X-linked disorder, periventricular heterotopia,[36] cells fail to escape from the neuroepithelium. This disorder manifests in females (males die prenatally) such that affected cell populations remain in the ventricular zone. The genetic basis of this disease is mutation of an actin-binding protein, filamin 1. Thus, these mutations are likely to interfere with the necessary changes in cytoskeletal organization for delamination from the neuroepithelium. Clearly, understanding this biological process might shed light on some of the changes necessary for neuroepithelial-like cells of primitive neuroectodermal tumors (PNETs) to undergo migration.

CELL-TYPE SPECIFICATION

Within the CNS, the type of cell, neuron, or glia, and subtypes thereof, is determined by the time of birth and position within the anteroposterior, dorsoventral, and mediolateral axes (reviewed by Scotting and Rex[3], Jessell[37], Goulding and Lamar[38], and Lumsden and Krumlauf[39]).

In the anteroposterior axis of the spinal cord, little variation in cell type is seen, most cell types being represented along its entire length. However, there is extensive variation in cell populations throughout the brain. The molecular basis underlying the specification of these cells is effected by a combination of transcription factors, many of which are within the homeodomain family (particularly the Hox, Otx, and Etx families). Thus, each cell expresses an appropriate set of genes for its correct morphology and biological function as a result of the activity of the specific set of transcription factors it expresses. Control of the correct set of transcription factors seems to be regulated by signaling through retinoid-related signal molecules and their receptors.

The dorsoventral axis exhibits a high level of variation in cellular subtypes throughout the entire CNS. The effectors of these differences are again transcription factor codes, but in this case different subtypes of homeodomain factors (Pax, Nkx, and Irx subfamilies) are involved. The correct set of these genes is established by signals arising from the tissues dorsal (ectoderm-producing BMPs) and ventral (notochord-producing shh) to the neural tube.

Position in the mediolateral axis is regulated primarily by the time at which a cell is "born" from the ventricular zone. As described earlier, cells migrate outwards from the ventricular zone to defined sites. The fate of the cells is, in some cases at least (such as cor-tex), determined around the time of the cell's "birth" (when the cell exits mitosis) rather than being influenced later by the environment it experiences once it has migrated.

Tumors

This is one of the least studied aspects of study in neuro-oncology, and yet it is one of immense breadth and depth of data from developmental systems. Classically, a major criterion upon which tumors have been categorized has been according to the types of cell they contain. However, this has been based largely on morphological features and a small range of markers of differentiated cell types. Such classification has proven to be of limited value in prognostic evaluation. Since the most differentiated cells of a tumor are generally no longer a threat to the patient, it is not surprising that the biology of these cells seems to have little bearing on the prognosis for that patient. The main value of studying these more mature cells is to provide clues as to the biology or cellular origin of the proliferative tumor cells from which they have arisen. Clearly, knowledge of the genes expressed when cells first acquire their positional identity provides markers that allow detailed classification of proliferating precursors. It might be hoped that such a classification of pediatric brain tumors will identify subgroups of different prognostic outcomes.

Since the means of classification used to date provide only limited prognostic value, it may be that only a detailed molecular characterization of the tumors into small subgroups based on features such as cell type will identify those groups that respond to specific therapeutic regimes.

CEREBELLUM DEVELOPMENT: A SPECIAL CASE

Since the cerebellum is a predominant site of pediatric brain tumors and exhibits unique developmental features, it is discussed in detail here (see also Figure 4a.3 and the reviews of Wang and Zoghbi[40], Hatten and Heintz[41], and Hanway[42]).

Although the formation of the cerebellum begins early during embryonic development, it does not achieve maturity until several months after birth, resulting in a prolonged formative period with an increased vulnerability to developmental aberrations and neoplasia. The cerebellum is derived from the dorsal neural tube of the fourth ventricle, with elements originating from both the mesencephalon and metencephalon. The early cerebellum develops through a complex series of morphogenetic movements under the control of signals released from the isthmus organizer (a narrow region at the border of the mid- and hindbrain (reviewed by Wang and Zoghbi[40]).

One of the most unusual features of the cerebellum is that its constituent cells arise from two separate germinal regions. The first is a typical epithelial ventricular zone, which lies beneath the developing cerebellar plate, between the isthmus and choroid plexus. The first group of precursors to leave the ventricular zone, at E10–11 in mice and week eight in human embryogenesis, are fated to give rise to the deep cerebellar nuclei, which form a mantle above the initial ventricular zone (Figure 4a.3a). From

E13 in mice and week nine in humans, cells fated to generate the interneurons of the molecular layer, the Purkinje cells, and the glial cells of the cortex arise via radial migration away from the germinal epithelium, along glial fibers (Figure 4a.3b). The Purkinje cells form a plate-like structure that is suspended beneath the later-forming external granule layer. These events seem to occur via similar mechanisms to those seen in most other brain regions. The second germinal matrix, the external granule layer (EGL), is derived, at E13–15 in mice and at week 11 in humans, from cells migrating exclusively from the metencephalic rhombic lip (Figure 4a.5).

Granule cell precursors in the EGL are marked in mice by expression of the bHLH transcription factor, Math1.[43] Math1 is expressed in the mid-hindbrain region from E9.5 onwards and persists throughout the early migration of the proliferating granule cell precursors and their post-natal proliferation in the EGL.[43] During the tangential migration to form the EGL, a number of other genes are expressed, including *nestin* and the granule cell marker *RU49/Zipro1*.[44] This second germinal layer of the cerebellum, the EGL, is unusual in several respects. In particular, unlike most other germinal regions, it no longer exhibits an epithelial structure and, also unlike most other regions, most or all cells of the EGL are specified while still actively proliferating, to give rise only to one type of neuron, the granule neuron.[45,46]

The EGL eventually forms a thin layer of granule cell precursors covering the entire surface of the cerebellum. The EGL proliferates postnatally to generate a layer up to eight cells thick. Cells on the outer surface of the EGL continue to proliferate, while cells moving inward to the deep EGL (or premigratory zone) become post-mitotic. Tight regulation of the number of EGL cells produced is essential in generating a fully functional mature cerebellum, both at the level of maintaining EGL cells in a proliferative state and specifying when a cell should stop dividing and start differentiating.

Differentiation occurs as post-mitotic cells move into the inner EGL. Granule cells first extend parallel fibers horizontally to the pial surface and the cell bodies move along the axons. The granule cells then extrude a third process inwards and, after turning through 90 degrees, descend into the inner granule layer (IGL), leaving behind a trailing process, still attached to the horizontal parallel fibers, which will eventually contact the processes of the Purkinje neurons (Figure 4a.3c). Several genes are expressed during the initial polarization of the post-mitotic granule cells, including those that code for Tag1, class 3β tubulin, and components of the Dcc/netrin pathway.[40] Studies of granule cells in culture demonstrate that this polarization is a cell autonomous activity independent of spatial cues; a candidate molecule for initiating this behavior is Pax6. Mouse mutants lacking functional Pax6 put out irregular and sometimes multiple processes and migrate in a disorganized manner.[47] It has therefore been suggested that Pax6 may be involved in a vital regulatory process of cytoskeletal organization during the polarization and migration of CNS neurons.[47]

Molecular regulation of granule cell proliferation and maturation

Several molecules have been suggested to play a role in maintaining the proliferative state of granule cell precursors. Some of these molecules are released from the underlying Purkinje neurons, while others are expressed as a result of homotypic interactions between the proliferating granule cell precursors.[48] The importance of Purkinje cells in stimulating the proliferation of granule cells has been shown in several studies, and the soluble signaling molecule, shh, is the likely candidate factor mediating this effect. Shh acts via a cell-surface receptor, Patched-1, which leads to activation of transcriptional events via the zinc-finger transcription factors Gli1-3. Many downstream components of the shh signaling pathway are expressed in granule cells, including its proposed receptor Patched-1 and the effectors of the activated pathway, Gli1 and Gli2 (Figure 4a.5). These genes are expressed in granule cells at the same time that shh is produced by the underlying Purkinje cells; it has been demonstrated in vitro that shh induces expression of these genes in cerebellar cells, indicating that the pathway is active in this population. Blocking shh signaling in vivo results in the formation of hypoplastic cerebella with resultant folial abnormalities due to a gross reduction or absence in the number of granule neurons present.[49] Several overexpression studies have indicated that shh can maintain granule cell precursors in a proliferative state, indicating that shh is a potent mitogen for granule cell precursors.[49–51] A similar effect is seen when the granule cell marker *RU49/Zipro1* (a zinc-finger transcription factor) is overexpressed, indicating that this gene may participate in the same or related signaling pathway. It is interesting to note that although shh is a mitogen for granule cells, it has alternative roles in other cell populations of the cerebellum; for instance, it promotes the differentiation of Bergmann glia. It seems probable, therefore, that other factors in addition to shh are required in order to specify the precise mitogenic response of granule cells to this signaling molecule. Also, mice lacking a functional *Gli1* gene show no obvious phenotype, including no behavioral abnormalities, to suggest a defective cerebellum.[52] It seems, therefore, that it is more than just Gli1 that mediates the effects of shh in the cerebellum. This proposition is supported by the observation that lack of Gli1 has not yet been shown to arrest tumor growth.[8]

In addition to the shh activated pathway described in Figure 4a.5, an alternative mechanism by which shh could affect the cell cycle has been suggested. Patched-1, the proposed receptor of the shh signaling molecule, has been found to be involved in blocking G2-M phase progression of the cell cycle. This inhibition is the result of Patched-1 binding to and retaining cyclinB1 in the cytoplasm/plasma membrane so that it cannot phosphorylate and activate essential components of the mitotic machinery in the nucleus.[53] Addition of shh disrupts this interaction, allowing cyclinB1 to localize to the nucleus and drive mitosis. Therefore, shh may control activation of granule cell proliferation through both cyclinB1/cdc2 and Gli1.

In contrast to the regulation of granule cell proliferation described above, in which the stimulus is largely from the Purkinje cells, a homotypic stimulus of granule cell proliferation has been suggested to occur. This system involves granule cells interacting via the Notch receptor on their surface and a ligand on the surface of adjacent granule cells. As described earlier, such signaling is important in maintaining neural precursor populations in many CNS regions during embryogenesis through the process of lateral inhibition (Figure 4a.2). Experimental data suggest that activation of Notch2, which is expressed specifically in the granule cell precursor population, leads to increased expression of the transcription factor HES1, with a concomitant increase in EGL proliferation and inhibition of differentiation.[33]

As granule cells in the EGL become post-mitotic, they express several genes specific to this stage of maturation, including those encoding the transcription factor NeuroD, which is required for the survival of post-mitotic granule cell neurons,[54] and the cell-cycle inhibitor p27/KIP. There is some evidence that it is accumulation of p27/KIP that allows granule cells to stop proliferating and start differentiating, even in the presence of high concentrations of shh.[55] At this same time, expression of *MATH1*, which is expressed strongly in proliferating granule cell precursors, is lost. Interestingly, mice lacking functional *MATH1* exhibit an almost complete loss of granule cells,[43] while overexpression disrupts normal granule cell differentiation.[56]

Although few studies have addressed the roles of cell-cycle control machinery specifically in granule cell development, there are some very interesting data that might provide insight into targets for disruption of the cell cycle in tumors derived from granule cells. The D-type cyclins are expressed in a cell-specific manner in the developing brain, which provides opportunity for modulation of the cell cycle in a region-specific manner during CNS development. Expression of these cyclins also appears to be specific to the developmental stage of a particular cell type. For instance, the splice form of cyclinD2, *MN20*, a cyclin subtype highly restricted to brain, is expressed in the

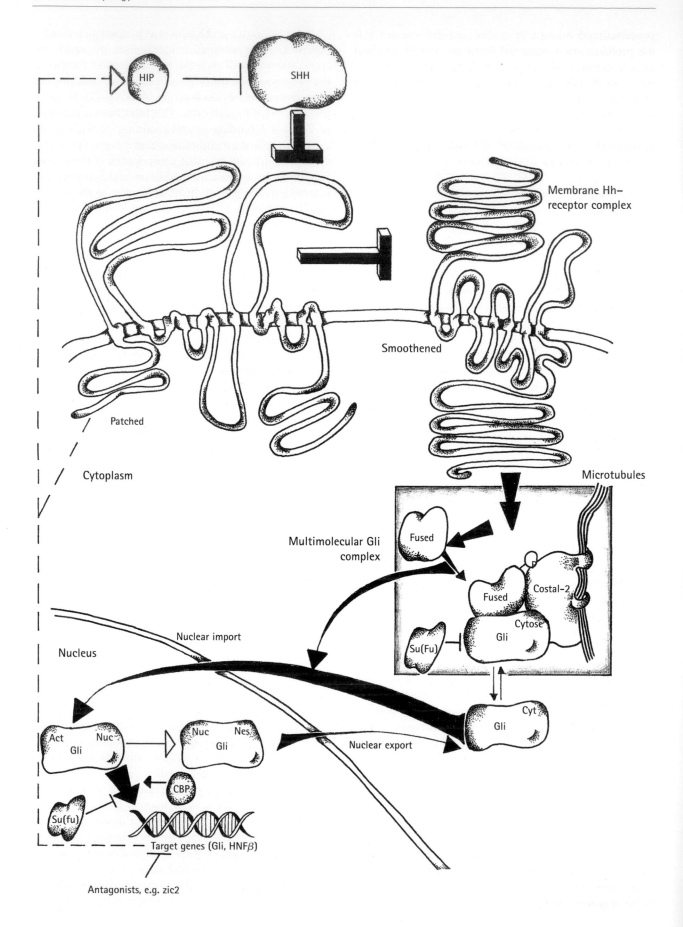

proliferating EGL, but only during the transition between the proliferating granule cells and assumption of their mature neuronal phenotype.[17,57] It has been suggested, therefore, that the role of cyclinD2 may be to signal that cells have reached their final division cycle before the initiation of terminal differentiation.[17]

Loss of cyclinD1 or D2 separately (in knockout mice) does not affect the mitogenic effects of shh, even though shh causes increased expression of both genes.[50] However, cyclinD2 knockout mice, but not cyclinD1 knockout mice, do have fewer granule cells than wild-type mice.[50,58] In the cerebellum, the effect of cyclinD2 appears to be quite specific to granule cells and stellate interneurons. Interestingly, it appears that cyclinD2 is necessary for granule cells to initiate differentiation. However, lack of cyclinD2 results in only a 50 per cent decrease in granule cell numbers, suggesting that there are subsets of granule cells as defined by their susceptibility to lack of cyclinD2. It is noteworthy that alteration of Notch2/-HES1 signaling also affects only a subset of granule cells, although this may be due to the experimental methodology.[33]

The data described above demonstrate that certain pathways and cell-cycle control elements are central to determining whether granule cells divide or differentiate. It is also clear that not all granule cells may behave the same and that no one pathway is sufficient or necessary for the proliferation of all granule cells. Hence, elucidating the full complexity of these regulatory events is likely to provide many clues and targets for research into the events that cause such cells to behave abnormally in cerebellar tumors.

TUMORS

Unsurprisingly, given the role for the shh/Patched pathway in regulating granule cell proliferation described above, the same pathway has been implicated in granule cell tumors (reviewed by Taipale and Beachy,[8] Scotting et al.,[59] and Ingham[60]). In 1996, mutations in the Patched gene were identified in patients suffering from Gorlin's syndrome, a small percentage of whom develop both basal cell carcinomas and medulloblastomas.[61,62] Since then, mutations have also been found in 5–12 per cent of sporadic medulloblastomas.[61,63–66] These data suggest that loss of function of the Patched protein leads to a predisposition to develop medulloblastoma (and basal cell carcinoma) and that such mutations are involved in the etiology of a small proportion of these tumors. This proposition is supported by the finding that mice in which one copy of the Patched gene has disrupted also show a predisposition to form such tumors.[67] Thus, it seems that having only one fully functional copy of the Patched gene is sufficient to increase the probability of developing medulloblastoma. Although subsequent insults are necessary for the tumors to form, it seems very probable that tumors developing due to this initial genetic defect are likely to have a characteristic phenotype.[68] Given the many steps involved in the Patched pathway, it seems likely that mutations in other components of this pathway will be found to be causative in additional cases of medulloblastoma.

While Patched-1 mutant mice do exhibit an increased tendency to develop medulloblastoma, a more reproducible model for this class of tumor comes from a surprising route. Although there seems to be no association between medulloblastoma and mutations of the Rb gene, and only a weak association with p53 mutations,[19–21] these two genes have provided a powerful model for medulloblastoma. The study of Marino and colleagues[19] showed that loss of function of both Rb and p53, but neither alone, produced medulloblastoma in almost all affected mice. Despite the fact that this clearly does not directly reflect the normal etiology of such tumors in humans, the tumors seen are remarkably similar to the human tumor and have already provided strong evidence in support of the EGL as the origin of the medulloblastoma. One possible link between the human tumor and this model comes from the observation that cells treated with shh exhibit inactivation (via hyperphosphorylation) of the Rb protein.[50] Thus, Patched-1 mutations may lead to tumor formation at least in part via inhibition of Rb function. Such a model is likely to provide a system in which detailed molecular studies of the developing tumors can be dissected.

The Wnt signaling pathway (reviewed by Ho et al.[6]) has also been implicated directly in medulloblastomas. Mutations in the APC gene, a key intermediate in this pathway, are a common event in Turcot's syndrome. This disorder is characterized by the occurrence of brain tumors and colorectal adenomas, with mutations in several different genes implicated in its etiology. In a large

Figure 4a.5 *The sonic hedgehog/Patched signaling pathway. This pathway affects the transcription of several genes via activation of the Gli family of transcription factors. Target genes include* N-Myc *and* Gli-1 *and* Patched *themselves. In the absence of sonic hedgehog (shh), the pathway is inactive. This is due to the ability of the Patched protein to inhibit the Smoothened protein. Lack of activity of smoothened results in Gli-1 being sequestered to the cytoplasmic complex containing Fused and Costal-2. If shh binds to its receptor Patched, then the repression of Smoothened is relieved and Smoothened triggers the release of Gli-1, which translocates to the nucleus and activates expression of its target genes.*

Additional levels of control of the pathway are possible through HIP, which inhibits shh, Su(fu), which inhibits Gli, and antagonists of Gli target genes such as Zic2.

study, medulloblastomas were found in 11 of 14 Turcot's syndrome patients with mutated *APC* genes.[69] Turcot's syndrome patients with other genetic bases developed glioblastoma multiformae.[69] Mutations in the *APC* gene (four per cent),[70] the β-*catenin* gene (8–15 per cent) (an effector of the Wnt pathway), and other components of the Wnt signaling pathway have also been identified in sporadic medulloblastomas cases.[71–74] This is strong evidence, therefore, for a role of the Wnt pathway in medulloblastoma etiology. In embryonic development, Wnts (of which there are more than ten members) are involved in a diverse range of processes in many tissues. In the nervous system, they appear to be involved in the initial formation of the neural ectoderm (as described above) and brain patterning (including regulation of proliferation of many cells of the hippocampus).[75] In the cerebellum, Wnts have been implicated in the postnatal development of Purkinje cells and granule cells,[76] but little is known of their role in decisions regarding granule cell maturation.

As is clear from several examples described above, the use of developmental systems to study the biology of processes shown to be involved in tumor etiology has proven to be very informative. The case of the shh/Patched pathway is a good example of this. However, once identified as a pathway active in both developmental and oncogenic processes, developmental systems may again provide the ideal situation in which to study these processes. In particular, when one component of a pathway has been implicated in the etiology of a cancer, then understanding the other components of that pathway allows each step to be analyzed independently as additional oncogenic candidates. It is also becoming increasingly clear that multiple pathways are utilized in regulating the critical steps from proliferation to differentiation. Understanding these relationships is also likely to provide clues to the multiple oncogenic events necessary to lead to a fully transformed cancer cell. Once again, the role of the shh pathway in medulloblastoma provides an illustration of this phenomenon.[77] The recent study of *Patched* mutant mice shows that there appear to be two stages of tumor development even after loss of one *Patched* allele, such that only 50 per cent of mice develop abnormal growths in their cerebellum and only 14 per cent develop full-blown medulloblastomas. Such studies provide the exciting possibility of identifying the second and third events needed for full tumor development.

RECENT ADVANCES IN MOLECULAR ANALYSIS

The completion of the human genome sequence and the advent of new genome-wide technologies provide the means to massively expand analysis of tumors and normal developmental processes. In particular microarrays allow the transcriptosome (the complete set of expressed genes) of any cell population to be determined. Thus, the genes expressed by tumors and embryonic cells can be compared. This should allow the relationship between the tumors and their normal developmental counterparts to be determined more precisely. This technology will also allow researchers to determine exactly which genes are turned on and off by the transcription factors that regulate the switch between proliferation and differentiation. It is now possible, therefore, to describe tumors in terms of large, objective sets of the genes they express. One of the first examples of this demonstrates the amazing power of this approach: Pomeroy and colleagues[68] used microarrays to compare a range of CNS tumors according to their gene expression. Using a chip carrying just under 7000 genes, they analyzed 99 tumors comparing different classes (medulloblastoma, other PNETs, glioma, rhabdoid and normal cerebellum). This analysis identified specific groups of genes, the expression of which could be used as an objective basis on which to classify the type and subtypes of tumor (classical medulloblastoma versus desmoplastic). Possibly the most striking result was the ability to define a small subset of genes (as few as eight) that could be used to predict good and poor response to therapy with a relatively high level of confidence. The most obvious use of these results, in which only about a fifth of the total gene pool has been studied, is to provide new criteria with which to classify tumors in order to better allocate patients to specific treatment. However, this huge increase in knowledge of the genes expressed in different circumstances also provides a dataset that can now be compared with the genes expressed when tumor cells or their normal counterparts are manipulated experimentally. Thus, the steps in tumor development can be analyzed sequentially in order to determine how such tumors have finally acquired the gene expression profiles that Pomeroy and colleagues describe. It is to be hoped that such detailed understanding might finally provide more directed approaches to the design of new therapies.

REFERENCES

1 Maher EA, Furnari FB, Bachoo RM, *et al.* Malignant glioma: genetics and biology of a grave matter. *Genes Dev* 2001; **15**:1311–33.

2 Harland R. Neural Induction. *Curr Opin Gen Dev* 2000; **10**:357–62.

3 Scotting P, Rex M. Transcription factors in early development of the central nervous system. *Neuropathol Appl Neurobiol* 1996; **22**:469–81.

4 Rex M, Orme A, Uwanogho D, *et al.* Dynamic expression of the chicken *Sox2* and *Sox3* genes in ectoderm induced to form neural tissue. *Dev Dyn* 1997; **209**:323–32.

5   Streit A, Sockanathan S, Perez L, *et al.* Preventing the loss of competence for neural induction: HGF/SF, L5 and *Sox-2*. *Development* 1997; **124**:1191–202.

6   Ho D, Hsu C, Wong T, *et al.* Atypical teratoid/rhabdoid tumor of the central nervous system: a comparative study with primitive neuroectodermal tumor/medulloblastoma. *Acta Neuropathol* 2000; **99**:482–8.

7   Zappone M, Galli R, Catena R, *et al. Sox2* regulatory sequences direct expression of a beta-geo transgene to telencephalic neural stem cells and precursors of the mouse embryo, revealing regionalization of gene expression in CNS stem cells. *Development* 2000; **127**:2367–82.

8   Taipale J, Beachy PA. The hedgehog and Wnt signaling pathways in cancer. *Nature* 2001; **411**:349–54.

9   Uwanogho D, Rex M, Cartwright E, *et al.* Embryonic expression of the chicken *Sox2*, *Sox3* and *Sox11* genes suggests an interactive role in neuronal development. *Mech Dev* 1995; **49**:23–36.

10 Bertrand N, Medevielle F, Pituello F. FGF signalling controls the timing of Pax6 activation in the neural tube. *Development* 2000; **127**:4837–43.

11 Kageyama R, Nakanishi S. Helix–loop–helix factors in growth and differentiation of the vertebrate nervous system. *Curr Opin Genet Dev* 1997; **7**:659–65.

12 Lee J. Basic helix–loop–helix genes in neural development. *Curr Opin Neurobiol* 1997; **7**:13–20.

13 Dahmane N, Sanchez P, Gitton Y, *et al.* The sonic hedgehog-Gli pathway regulates dorsal brain growth and tumorigenesis. *Development* 2001; **128**:5201–12.

14 Lewis J. Neurogenic genes and vertebrate neurogenesis. *Curr Opin Neurobiol* 1996; **6**:3–10.

15 Henrique D, Hirsinger E, Adam J, *et al.* Maintenance of neuroepithelial progenitor cells by delta-notch signalling in the embryonic chick retina. *Curr Biol* 1997; **7**:661–70.

16 Kageyama R, Ohtsuka T. The Notch-Hes pathway in mammalian neural development. *Cell Res* 1999; **9**:179–88.

17 Ross M. Cell division and the nervous system: regulating the cycle from neural differentiation to death. *Trends Neurosci* 1996; **19**:62–8.

18 Ohnuma S, Philpott A, Harris W. Cell cycle and cell fate in the nervous system. *Curr Opin Neurobiol* 2001; **11**:66–73.

19 Marino S, Vooijs M, van Der Gulden H, *et al.* Induction of medulloblastomas in p53-null mutant mice by somatic inactivation of Rb in the external granular layer cells of the cerebellum. *Genes Dev* 2000; **14**:994–1004.

20 Cogen P, McDonald J. Tumor suppressor genes and medulloblastoma. *J Neuro-Oncol* 1996; **29**:103–12.

21 Malkin D, Li F, Strong L, *et al.* Germ line P53 mutations in a familial syndrome of breast-cancer, sarcomas, and other neoplasms. *Science* 1990; **250**:1233–8.

22 Whittemore SR, Morassutti DJ, Walters WM, *et al.* Mitogen and substrate differentially affect the lineage restriction of adult rat subventricular zone neural precursor cell populations. *Exp Cell Res* 1999; **252**:75–95.

23 Erlandsson A, Enarsson M, Forsberg-Nilsson K. Immature neurons from CNS stem cells proliferate in response to platelet-derived growth factor. *J Neurosci* 2001; **21**:3483–91.

24 Caldwell MA, He XL, Wilkie N, *et al.* Growth factors regulate the survival and fate of cells derived from human neurospheres. *Nat Biotechnol* 2001; **19**:475–9.

25 Buonanno A, Fischbach G. Neuregulin and erbB receptor signalling in the nervous system. *Curr Opin Neurobiol* 2001; **11**:287–96.

26 Huang EJ, Reichardt LF. Neurotrophins: roles in neuronal development and function. *Annu Rev Neurosci* 2001; **24**:677–736.

27 Grotzer M, Fung K, Janss A, *et al.* Expression of trk-C receptors in primitive neuroectodermal tumor medulloblastoma correlates with the expression of neurofilament proteins and is associated with favorable prognosis. *J Neuropathol Exp Neurol* 1999; **58**:139.

28 Grotzer M, Janss A, Fung K, *et al.* TrkC expression predicts good clinical outcome in primitive neuroectodermal brain tumors. *J Clin Oncol* 2000; **18**:1027–35.

29 Sriuranpong V, Borges MW, Ravi RK, *et al.* Notch signaling induces cell cycle arrest in small cell lung cancer cells. *Cancer Res* 2001; **61**:3200–5.

30 Grynfeld A, Pahlman S, Axelson H. Induced neuroblastoma cell differentiation, associated with transient HES-1 activity and reduced HASH-1 expression, is inhibited by Notch1. *Int J Cancer* 2000; **88**:401–10.

31 Dievart A, Beaulieu N, Jolicoeur P. Involvement of Notch1 in the development of mouse mammary tumors. *Oncogene* 1999; **18**:5973–81.

32 Anderson A, Robey EA, Huang YH. Notch signaling in lymphocyte development. *Curr Opin Genet Dev* 2001; **11**:554–60.

33 Solecki DJ, Liu XL, Tomoda T, *et al.* Activated Notch2 signaling inhibits differentiation of cerebellar granule neuron precursors by maintaining proliferation. *Neuron* 2001; **31**:557–68.

34 Yu QY, Geng Y, Sicinski P. Specific protection against breast cancers by cyclin D1 ablation. *Nature* 2001; **411**:1017–21.

35 Gleeson J, Walsh CA. Neuronal migration disorders: from genetic diseases to developmental mechanisms. *Trends Neurosc* 2000; **23**:352–9.

36 Lambert de Rouvroit C, Goffinet A. Neuronal migration. *Mech Dev* 2001; **105**:47–56.

37 Jessell T. Neuronal specification in the spinal cord: Inductive signals and transcriptional codes. *Nat Rev Genet* 2000; **1**:20–29.

38 Goulding M, Lamar E. Neuronal patterning: making stripes in the spinal cord. *Curr Biol* 2000; **10**:R565–8.

39 Lumsden A, Krumlauf R. Patterning the vertebrate neuraxis. *Science* 1996; **274**:1109–15.

40 Wang V, Zoghbi H. Genetic regulation of cerebellar development. *Nat Rev Neurosci* 2001; **2**:484–91.

41 Hatten M, Heintz N. Mechanisms of neural patterning and specification in the developing cerebellum. *Annu Rev Neurosci* 1995; **18**:385–408.

42 Hanaway J. Formation and differentiation of the external granular layer of the chick cerebellum. *J Comp Neurosci* 1967; **131**:1–14.

43 Ben-Arie N, Bellen H, Armstrong D, *et al.* Math1 is essential for genesis of cerebellar granule neurons. *Nature* 1997; **390**:169–72.

44 Yang X, Zhong R, Heintz N. Granule cell specification in the developing mouse brain as defined by expression of the zinc finger transcription factor RU49. *Development* 1996; **122**:555–66.

45 Ryder EF, Cepko CL. Migration patterns of clonally related granule cells and their progenitors in the developing chick cerebellum. *Neuron* 1994; **12**:1011–29.

46 Lin J, Cai L, Cepko C. The external granule layer of the developing chick cerebellum generates granule cells and cells of the isthmus and rostral hindbrain. *J Neurosci* 2001; **21**:159–68.

47 Yamasaki T, Kawaji K, Ono K, *et al.* Pax6 regulates granule cell polarization during parallel fiber formation in the developing cerebellum. *Development* 2001; **128**:3133–44.

48 Gao W-Q, Heintz N, Hatten ME. Cerebellar granule cell neurogenesis is regulated by cell–cell interactions in vitro. *Neuron* 1991; **6**:705–15.

49 Dahmane N, Altaba ARI. Sonic hedgehog regulates the growth and patterning of the cerebellum. *Development* 1999; **126**:3089–100.

50 Kenney A, Rowitch D. Sonic hedgehog promotes G(1) cyclin expression and sustained cell cycle progression in mammalian neuronal precursors. *Mol Cell Biol* 2000; **20**:9055–67.

51 Wechsler-Reya R, Scott M. Control of neuronal precursor proliferation in the cerebellum by sonic hedgehog. *Neuron* 1999; **22**:103–14.

52 Park HL, Bai C, Platt KA, *et al.* Mouse Gli1 mutants are viable but have defects in SHH signaling in combination with a Gli2 mutation. *Development* 2000; **127**:1593–605.

53 Barnes EA, Kong M, Ollendorff V, Donoghue DJ. *Patched1* interacts with cyclin B1 to regulate cell cycle progression. *EMBO Journal* 2001; **20**:2214–23.

54 Miyata T, Maeda T, Lee JE. NeuroD is required for differentiation of granule cells in the cerebellum and hippocampus. *Genes Dev* 1999; **13**:1647–52.

55 Miyazawa K, Himi T, Garcia V, *et al.* A role for p27/Kip1 in the control of cerebellar granule cell precursor proliferation. *J Neurosci* 2000; **20**:5756–63.

56 Helms A, Gowan K, Abney A, *et al.* Overexpression of *MATH1* disrupts the coordination of neural differentiation in cerebellum development. *Mol Cell Neurosci* **2001**:671–82.

57 Ross ME, Risken M. Mn20, a D2 cyclin found in brain, is implicated in neural differentiation. *J Neurosci* 1994; **14**:6384–91.

58 Huard J, Forster C, Carter M, *et al.* Cerebellar histogenesis is disturbed in mice lacking cyclin D2. *Development* 1999; **126**:1927–35.

59 Scotting P, Thompson S, Punt J, Walker D. Paediatric brain tumours: an embryological perspective. *Child Nerv Syst* 2000; **16**:261–8.

60 Ingham P. The patched gene in development and cancer. *Curr Opin Genet Dev* 1998; **8**:88–94.

61 Hahn H, Wicking C, Zaphiropoulos P, *et al.* Mutations in the human homolog of *Drosophila* patched in the nevoid basal cell carcinoma syndrome. *Cell* 1996; **85**:841–51.

62 Johnson RL, Rothman AL, Xie J, *et al.* Human homolog of patched, a candidate gene for the basal cell nevis syndrome. *Science* 1996; **272**:1668–71.

63 Pietsch T, Waha A, Koch A, *et al.* Medulloblastomas of the desmoplastic variant carry mutations in the human homologue of *Drosophila* patched. *Cancer Res* 1997; **57**:2085–8.

64 Raffel C, Jenkins R, Frederick L, *et al.* Sporadic medullo-blastomas contain PTCH mutations. *Cancer Res* 1997; **57**:842–5.

65 Vorechovsky I, Tingby O, Hartman M, *et al.* Somatic mutations in the human homologue of *Drosophila* patched in primitive neuroectodermal tumours. *Oncogene* 1997; **15**:361–6.

66 Wolter M, Reifenberger J, Sommer C, *et al.* Mutations in the human homologue of the *Drosophila* segment polarity gene patched (PTCH) in sporadic basal cell carcinomas of the skin and primitive neuroectodermal tumors of the central nervous system. *Cancer Res* 1997; **57**:2581–5.

67 Goodrich L, Milenkovic L, Higgins K, Scott M. Altered neural cell fates and medulloblastoma in mouse patched mutants. *Science* 1997; **277**:1109–13.

68 Pomeroy S, Tamayo P, Gaasenbeek M, *et al.* Prediction of central nervous system embryonal tumour outcome based on gene expression. *Nature* 2002; **415**:436–42.

69 Hamilton SR, Liu B, Parsons RE, *et al.* The molecular basis of Turcot's syndrome. *N Engl J Med* 1995; **332**:839–47.

70 Huang HT, Mahler-Araujo BM, Sankila A, *et al.* APC mutations in sporadic medulloblastomas. *Am J Pathol* 2000; **156**:433–7.

71 Zurawel RH, Chiappa SA, Allen C, Raffel C. Sporadic medullo-blastomas contain oncogenic beta-catenin mutations. *Cancer Res* 1998; **58**:896–9.

72 Eberhart CG, Tihan T, Burger PC. Nuclear localization and mutation of beta-catenin in medulloblastomas. *J Neuropathol Exp Neurol* 2000; **59**:333–7.

73 Koch A, Waha A, Tonn JC, *et al.* Somatic mutations of WNT/wingless signaling pathway components in primitive neuroectodermal tumors. *Int J Cancer* 2001; **93**:445–9.

74 Dahmen RP, Koch A, Denkhaus D, *et al.* Deletions of AXIN1, a component of the WNT/wingless pathway, in sporadic medulloblastomas. *Cancer Res* 2001; **61**:7039–43.

75 Wilson SI, Rydstrom A, Trimborn T, *et al.* The status of Wnt signalling regulates neural and epidermal fates in the chick embryo. *Nature* 2001; **411**:325–30.

76 Patapoutian A, Reichardt LF. Roles of Wnt proteins in neural development and maintenance. *Curr Opin Neurobiol* 2000; **10**:392–9.

77 Corcoran R, Scott M. A mouse model for medulloblastoma and basal cell nevus syndrome. *J Neuro-Oncol* 2001; **53**:307–18.

4b

Tumor biology

MICHAEL A. GROTZER

INTRODUCTION

Over the past 30 years, progress in molecular biology and genetics has yielded an enormous amount of information on the genes involved in nervous system development and the development of various types of brain tumors. Cancer research has generated a rich and complex body of knowledge, revealing cancer to be a disease involving dynamic changes in the genome. In the near future, new high-throughput technologies, including DNA chip technology, tissue microarrays, and proteomics, will bring further knowledge but also increase the difficulty of keeping track of an increasing bank of data that is already dauntingly complex.

However, the complexities of the disease described in the laboratory and clinic will become understandable in terms of a small number of underlying principles.[1] Important acquired capacities of cancer include self-sufficiency in growth signals, insensitivity to antigrowth signals, avoidance of apoptosis, sustained angiogenesis, tissue invasion and metastasis, and unlimited replicative potential. In this chapter, the molecular genetic events and the biological consequences associated with these tumor-related phenotypes are discussed in relation to pediatric brain tumors.

SELF-SUFFICIENCY IN GROWTH SIGNALS

Cellular proliferation and increased mitotic activity are general hallmarks of most malignant tumors, and their quantification by flow cytometry, mitotic counting, or immunohistochemical analysis of proliferation-related antigens (e.g. Ki-67 (MIB-1)) is a valuable source of diagnostic and prognostic information for a number of human tumors.[2,3] For brain tumors, the following generalizations can be made: the Ki-67 (MIB-1) proliferation index has been shown to correlate with the histological grade in gliomas[4–6] and with survival outcome in subgroups such as pilocytic astrocytomas[7] and WHO grade II gliomas.[8] In ependymoma[9] and medulloblastoma,[10] the Ki-67 (MIB-1) proliferation index correlates with survival outcome.

Normal cells require mitogenic growth signals before they can move from a quiescent state into an active proliferative state. These signals are transduced into the cell by transmembrane receptors that bind soluble growth factors, extracellular matrix components, and cell–cell adhesion/interaction molecules.[1] Dependence on growth signaling is apparent when normal cells are propagated in culture. These cells typically proliferate only when supplied with appropriate diffusible mitogenic factors and a proper substratum for their integrins. Such behavior contrasts strongly with that of tumor cells, which invariably show a greatly reduced dependence on exogenous growth stimulation.

Common molecular strategies for achieving growth-signaling autonomy include (i) alteration of extracellular growth signals, (ii) alteration of transcellular transducers of those signals, and (iii) alterations in the intracellular circuits that translate those signals into action.[11] Many cancer cells acquire the ability to synthesize soluble growth factors to which they themselves respond, resulting in autocrine/paracrine stimulation.[12] This is illustrated by the production of platelet-derived growth factor (PDGF) in medulloblastoma,[13,14] ependymoma,[13] and gliomas;[12] tumor growth factor alpha (TGF-α) in gliomas;[15] and insulin-like growth factor I (IGF-I) in medulloblastoma[16] and glioma.[17]

The transmembrane receptors that transduce growth-stimulatory signals into the cell interior are themselves targets of deregulation during tumor pathogenesis. Growth factor receptors, often carrying tyrosine kinase activities in their cytoplasmic domains, are overexpressed in many cancers. Growth factor receptor overexpression may allow the cancer cell to become hyperresponsive to ambient levels of growth factor that normally would not trigger proliferation. For example, the epidermal growth factor receptor (EGFR) is amplified/overexpressed in more than a third of adult glioblastomas but not in lower-grade tumors, and the platelet-derived growth factor receptor (PDGF-R) is overexpressed in glial tumors and meningiomas.[18,19] In medulloblastoma, elevated expression of the EGFR family members ErbB2 and ErbB4 was found to correlate with high mitotic index, advanced metastatic stage, and reduced survival.[20] In addition, structural alterations of growth factor receptors can elicit ligand-independent signaling. For example, truncated versions of the EGFR lacking much of the cytoplasmic domain are constitutively active.[21]

Cancer cells can also switch the types of extracellular matrix (ECM) receptors (integrins) they express, favoring those that transmit pro-growth signals.[22,23] Binding to specific moieties of the ECM enables the integrin receptors to transduce signals into the cytoplasm that influence cell behavior, switching from quiescence in normal tissue to motility, and entry into the active cell cycle.

Both ligand-activated growth factor receptors and pro-growth integrins bound to ECM components can activate the SOS–Ras–Raf–MAP kinase pathway that plays a central role as a downstream cytoplasmic circuitry, receiving and processing the signals emitted by ligand-activated growth factor receptors and integrins.[23,24] Components of the SOS–Ras–Raf–MAP kinase cascade can be altered in several ways. In about 25 per cent of human tumors, Ras proteins are present in structurally altered forms that enable them to release a flux of mitogenic signals into cells, in the absence of ongoing stimulation by their normal upstream regulators.[25] In brain tumors, the incidence of Ras oncogenes mutations is lower,[26–28] and amplification of Ras oncogenes is also uncommon.[29] However, overexpression of Ras relative to histological grade has been noted in gliomas.[30] In addition, expression profiling of medulloblastoma showed upregulation of members of the downstream Ras-MAP kinase signal transduction pathway in metastatic tumors.[31] New downstream effector pathways that radiate from the central SOS–Ras–Raf–MAP kinase mitogenic cascade are being elucidated.[32,33] A variety of cross-talking connections also links this cascade with other pathways; these connections enable extracellular signals to elicit multiple cell biological effects. For example, the direct interaction of the Ras protein with the survival-promoting phosphatidylinositol-3 (PI-3) kinase enables growth signals to evoke survival signals concurrently within the cell.[34]

The neurofibromatoses types 1 and 2 (NF-1 and NF-2, respectively) are cancer-predisposition syndromes in which patients are prone to development of mostly benign but occasionally malignant tumors. Clinical NF-1 can result from a variety of inactivating mutations in the tumor suppressor gene NF-1.[35] The neurofibromatosis NF-1 gene product, a protein called neurofibromin, is expressed in neurons, oligodendrocytes, and Schwann cells. Sequence analysis of neurofibromin has revealed a region of homology with p120-GAP, the GTPase-activating protein (GAP) for the Ras family of proto-oncogenes. The inactivation of Ras by neurofibromin GAP activity leads to regulated cell growth. However, loss of neurofibromin in tumors as a result of NF-1 gene inactivation leads to increased Ras activity and increased cell growth. The neurofibromatosis NF-2 tumor suppressor gene is mutated in patients with clinical NF-2. The protein product of NF-2 – termed merlin or schwannomin – is also a negative growth regulator.[35] However, unlike neurofibromin, it remains to be elucidated how merlin regulates cell growth.

In normal tissue, cells receive growth instructions predominantly from their neighbors (paracrine signals) or via systemic (endocrine) signals. Cell–cell growth signaling is likely to operate in the vast majority of human tumors as well; virtually all brain tumors are composed of several distinct cell types that appear to communicate via heterotypic signaling.[15] Heterotypic signaling between the diverse cell types within a tumor may ultimately prove to be as important in explaining tumor cell proliferation as the cancer cell autonomous mechanisms enumerated above.[1]

INSENSITIVITY TO ANTIGROWTH SIGNALS

Normal cells possess a series of checks and balances to control proliferation.[36] Growth factor receptor interactions activate cytoplasmic intermediates, which transduce the signal into the nucleus, where the decision to divide is regulated by positive effectors and negative regulators. The positive effectors include the cyclin-dependent kinase (CDK)–cyclin complexes,[37,38] the proto-oncogenes murine double minute 2 (MDM2), and the paired box gene 5 (PAX5). MDM2 interacts with the tumor suppressor p53, resulting in a reduction in p53 protein levels through enhanced proteosome-dependent degradation.[39] The transforming capability of MDM2 was demonstrated by its overexpression in neonatal rat astrocytes.[40] In a study examining the correlation between *p53* mutations and *MDM2* overexpression, none of the *MDM2*-amplified glioblastomas had *p53* mutations, supporting the hypothesis that *MDM2* overexpression is an alternative mechanism for *p53* inactivation.[41] While *MDM2* amplification and overexpression are reported to be present in a substantial proportion of glioblastomas,[19] ependymomas,[42] and intracranial germ-cell tumors,[43] they are relatively uncommon in medulloblastoma.[44]

PAX5 represses the transcriptional activation of the *p53* gene.[45] Thus, overexpression of the *PAX5* gene could eliminate the *p53* signal, thereby promoting tumor initiation or progression. Indeed, increased expression of *PAX5* has been found to correlate with increased malignancy in astrocytomas.[46] In medulloblastoma, upregulated expression of *PAX5* correlates positively with cell proliferation,[47] but overexpression of *PAX5* is not sufficient for neoplastic transformation of mouse neuroectoderm.[47,48]

The negative regulators include the CDK inhibitors p16, p15, and p21 and the tumor suppressors retinoblastoma (*Rb*) and *p53*. *p16* and the neighboring gene *p15* are inactivated by homozygous deletion in diffuse astrocytic tumors, but not in medulloblastomas or ependymomas.[49,50] In high-grade gliomas, Ki-67 proliferation indices are significantly higher in tumors with *p16* deletions than in those without deletions, underscoring the importance of *p16* in cell-cycle control.[51]

Antigrowth signals can block proliferation by two distinct mechanisms. Cells may be forced out of the active proliferative cycle into the quiescent (G_0) state, from which they may re-emerge at some future point when extracellular signals permit. Alternatively, cells may be induced to relinquish their proliferative potential permanently by entering into post-mitotic states usually associated with terminal differentiation.

Many of the antiproliferative signals are channeled through the *Rb* and *p53* pathways.[52,53] Hypophosphorylated Rb protein blocks proliferation by sequestering and modifying the E2F transcription factors that regulate the expression of genes essential for G_1 to S transition.[53] If *Rb* is phosphorylated by CDK4, then E2Fs are released and proliferation is allowed. CDK4 is inhibited by *p16INK4A*. Therefore, loss of function mutations in *Rb* or *p16INK4A*, or amplification/overexpression of CDK4, allows uncontrolled cell growth.[54] In fact, alterations of all these genes occur in astrocytoma.[55] Interestingly, somatic inactivation of *Rb* in cells of the external granular layer of the cerebellum of *p53*-null mutant mice resulted in the development of medulloblastomas.[56]

For cells to proliferate, however, they must do more than simply escape cytostatic antigrowth signals. Tissues also block cell multiplication by instructing cells to enter post-mitotic, differentiated states; this differentiation is irreversible. Tumor cells have a range of strategies through which they avoid terminal differentiation. For example,

during normal development, the growth-stimulating action of the *MYC* (*c-myc*) oncogene, which encodes a transcription factor that associates with *Max*, can be replaced as alternative complexes of *Max* form with a group of Mad transcription factors. The Mad–Max complexes elicit differentiation-inducing signals.[57] However, overexpression of the MYC oncoprotein can reverse this process, shifting the balance back to favor MYC–Max complexes, thereby impairing differentiation and promoting growth.

MYC gene amplification is rare in medulloblastoma, with an incidence of about eight per cent in primary tumors.[29,58–61] The incidence of *MYC* gene amplification in medulloblastoma cell lines and xenografts is higher, suggesting that *MYC* gene amplification correlates with cell-line establishment and tumorigenicity.[62,63] *MYC* gene amplification has been suggested as an indicator of poor prognosis in case reports[64–66] and in a study of 29 medulloblastoma patients.[60] *MYC* mRNA expression varies widely and does not correlate with the presence of *MYC* gene amplification in primitive neuroectodermal tumor (PNET) cell lines or primary medulloblastomas.[67,68] Mechanisms to activate *MYC* other than gene amplification are well recognized in a variety of solid tumors. In PNET, transcriptional regulation of *MYC* may involve the adenomatous polyposis coli (*APC*) or β-catenin (*CTNNB1*) pathways.[69–73] In a recent study, we found that high levels of *MYC* mRNA expression correlated strongly, and independently of any clinical factors, with an unfavorable survival outcome in medulloblastoma patients.[67]

EVASION OF APOPTOSIS

The ability of tumor cell populations to increase in number is determined not only by the rate of cell proliferation but also by the rate of cell death. Programmed cell death – apoptosis – represents a major source of cell death. The apoptotic program is present in latent form in virtually all cell types throughout the body. Once triggered by a variety of physiological signals, this program unfolds in a precisely choreographed series of steps. Several morphological features of apoptotic cells distinguish them from cells that die in response to trauma or hypoxia.[74] Necrotic cell death is characterized by cell swelling and gross disruption of organelles and the cell membrane. In contrast, apoptotic cell death is characterized by cell contraction, blebbing of the cytoplasmic membrane, dense condensation of the nucleus, and autodigestion of the genome into 180–200-base-pair (bp) fragments, a size that corresponds to multiples of the amount of DNA found in individual nucleosomes (Figure 4b.1). Characteristically, apoptotic cells will neither injure neighboring cells nor elicit any inflammatory reaction.[75]

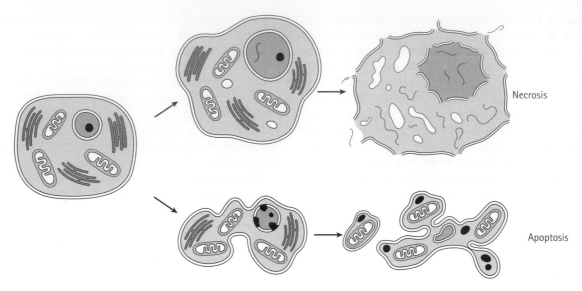

Figure 4b.1 *Schematic representation of apoptosis and necrosis. Necrosis is characterized by cell swelling and gross disruption of organelles and the cell membrane, whereas apoptosis is associated with cell contraction, dense condensation of the nucleus, and the ultimate formation of apoptotic bodies.*

Methods of detecting apoptosis-associated DNA fragmentation include gel-based DNA fragmentation assays and *in situ* end-labeling assays, which use enzymes such as DNA polymerase and terminal deoxynucleotidyl transferase (Tdt) (terminal UTP nick-end labeling, TUNEL) to insert labeled nucleotides at the 3′-hydroxyl terminal of endonuclease-induced DNA breaks.[76]

In central nervous system (CNS) tumors, the abundance of apoptotic neoplastic cells has been reported to correlate with the histological grade of malignancy and clinical outcome in oligodendrogliomas and astrocytomas.[77,78] In medulloblastoma, spontaneous apoptosis shows large inter- and intratumoral variability in primary tumors.[79–81] In one study of 43 medulloblastoma patients, the apoptotic index was suggested as a prognostic factor.[82] In contrast, we found no correlation of apoptotic index and survival outcome probabilities in 78 PNET patients.[83]

The apoptotic machinery can be divided broadly into sensors and effectors. The sensors are responsible for monitoring the extra- and intracellular environments for conditions of normality or abnormality that influence whether a cell should live or die. The sensors include cell-surface receptors that bind survival or death factors. An example of these ligand/receptor pairs is the survival signals conveyed by IGF-I through its receptor IGF-IR.[84] Death signals are conveyed by the Fas ligand (CD95) binding the Fas receptor, tumor necrosis factor (TNF) alpha binding TNF-R1, and TNF-related apoptosis-inducing ligand (TRAIL) binding DR4 and DR5.[85–87] An intracellular region called the death domain, which is required for the transmission of the apoptotic signal, characterizes these death receptors.[88]

Intracellular sensors activate the death pathway when abnormalities are detected, such as DNA damage, signaling imbalance provoked by oncogene action, survival factor insufficiency, and hypoxia.[89] Many of the signals that elicit apoptosis converge on the mitochondria, which respond to pro-apoptotic signals by releasing cytochrome C, a potent catalyst of apoptosis.[90] Members of the Bcl-2 family of proteins, whose members have either pro-apoptotic (Bax, Bak, Bid, Bim) or anti-apoptotic (Bcl-2, Bcl-XL, Bcl-W) function, act in part by governing mitochondrial death signaling through cytochrome C release. Brain tumor types in which expression of proteins of the Bcl-2 family have been studied include glioma,[91] medulloblastoma,[92] ganglioglioma,[93] and dysembryoplastic neuroepithelial tumors (DNTs).[94] The p53 tumor suppressor protein can elicit apoptosis by upregulating expression of pro-apoptotic Bax in response to sensing DNA damage; Bax in turn stimulates mitochondria to release cytochrome C.

The ultimate effectors of apoptosis include an array of intracellular proteinases termed caspases.[95] Two initiator caspases, 8 and 9, are activated by death receptors and by cytochrome C released from mitochondria, respectively. These proximal caspases trigger the activation of effector caspases that execute the death program through selective destruction of subcellular structures and organelles and of the genome.

Resistance to apoptosis can be acquired by cancer cells through a variety of strategies. The most commonly occurring loss of a pro-apoptotic regulator through mutation involves the *p53* tumor suppressor gene. Mutational frequencies are high in adult anaplastic astrocytoma

(67 per cent) and glioblastoma multiforme (41 per cent) but much lower in oligodendroglioma (13 per cent), medulloblastoma (11 per cent), and pilocytic astrocytoma (less than 5 per cent), and virtually absent in other CNS tumors.[96] Early studies on pilocytic and malignant astrocytomas in children suggested that *p53* mutations were rare; however, more recent series have found frequent *p53* mutations in children with these tumors.[54] The resulting functional inactivation of the p53 protein removes a key component of the DNA damage sensor that can induce the apoptotic effector cascade.[97] Signals evoked by other abnormalities, including hypoxia and oncogene overexpression, are also funneled in part via p53 to the apoptotic machinery; these too are less able to elicit apoptosis when p53 function is lost.[98] Additionally, the Akt pathway is likely to be involved in inhibiting apoptosis in malignant glioma.[98] This survival signaling circuit can be activated by extracellular signals such as IGF-I,[88] by intracellular signals from Ras,[99,100] and by loss of the *pTEN* tumor suppressor.[101]

Resistance to apoptosis induced by death receptors is mediated by downregulation of death receptors, presence of decoy receptors, or loss of downstream signaling elements. A mechanism for abrogating the Fas death signal has been revealed in glioblastoma: DcR3, a non-signaling decoy receptor for Fas ligand, is upregulated, titrating the death-inducing signal away from the Fas death receptor.[102] In medulloblastoma, loss of caspase-8 has been identified as a mechanism for inhibiting the TRAIL death pathway.[103,104]

Another way of mediating resistance to apoptosis in PNET may involve downregulation of the neurotrophin receptor TrkC. Although the role of neurotrophins in the induction and progression of tumors remains speculative, it is conceivable that at least some PNETs may respond to endogenous neurotrophins. PNETs with high TrkC mRNA expression have been found to have high apoptotic indices (unpublished data). This finding is consistent with that of Kim and colleagues,[105] who reported that TrkC activation induces apoptosis in DAOY human PNET cells. They also found that overexpression of TrkC inhibits the growth of intracerebral DAOY xenografts and that the rate of apoptosis is increased significantly in these xenografts compared with DAOY wild-type xenografts. Therefore, PNET cells with low expression of functional TrkC may be less susceptible to programmed cell death. This might be one explanation for the prognostic significance of TrkC in PNETs.[105–107]

Most regulatory and effector components of the apoptotic signaling circuitry are present in redundant form. This redundancy has important implications for the development of novel types of anti-tumor therapy, since tumor cells that have lost pro-apoptotic components are likely to retain other, similar ones. New high-throughput technologies will be able to reveal the apoptotic pathways still operative in specific types of brain tumors, and we anticipate that new drugs will enable the apoptotic mechanism to be restored, with substantial therapeutic benefit.

SUSTAINED ANGIOGENESIS

The microvessel density (MVD) of many brain tumors is high, and it has been recognized that glioblastomas are among the best vascularized human tumors.[55,108] While the vasculature of low-grade gliomas closely resembles that of normal brain, malignant gliomas show prominent microvascular proliferation. Moreover, a correlation of MVD with survival outcome has been reported for gliomas.[109] In childhood medulloblastoma, MVD has been found to show substantial intertumoral variability, with ranges of MVD values comparable to those observed in adult malignant glioma.[92,110,111]

Angiogenesis, the formation of new blood vessels from existing vasculature, is a tightly regulated process.[112,113] Counterbalancing positive and negative signals enhances or blocks angiogenesis. Endothelial cell activation, proliferation, migration, and tissue infiltration from preexisting blood vessels are triggered by specific angiogenic growth factors produced by tumor cells and the surrounding stroma.[114–116] Angiogenic growth factors include vascular endothelial growth factor (VEGF), basic fibroblast growth factor (bFGF), angiopoetin-1 and -2, transforming growth factors, and PDGF.[117,118] Endogenous inhibitors of angiogenesis include thrombospondin-1, platelet-derived factor 4, angiostatin, and endostatin.[119]

The ability to induce and sustain angiogenesis seems to be acquired during tumor development via an angiogenic switch from vascular quiescence. Tumors appear to activate the angiogenic switch by changing the balance of angiogenesis inducers and countervailing inhibitors.[115] This can be accomplished by increasing the expression of angiogenic factors or by the loss of their inhibitors (Figure 4b.2).

Anaplastic astrocytoma and glioblastoma multiforme often produce high levels of bFGF, TGF-α, angiopoetins, and VEGF.[120–125] Moreover, expression of VEGF mRNA has been shown to correlate with vascularity in both gliomas and meningiomas.[126] Medulloblastomas produce a wide range of angiogenic factors[110] and show strong immunoreactivity for VEGF and bFGF.[126,127]

VEGF has been recognized as one of the most potent angiogenic factors for many solid tumor systems, including malignant gliomas[128–131] and medulloblastomas.[14] The VEGF receptors are endothelial-specific; although they are expressed very rarely in endothelial cells of the normal vasculature, they are overexpressed in the vascular supply of neoplastic tissue. Hence, it has been proposed that the inhibition of this factor may result in the inhibition of

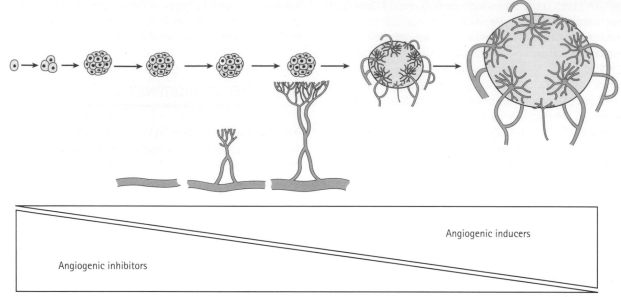

Figure 4b.2 *Schematic representation of tumor growth depending on angiogenesis, which results from a shift in the balance between angiogenesis inhibitors and stimulators during tumor progression.* (Modified from Folkman.[184])

angiogenesis, and a number of agents have been developed to inhibit VEGF.[132–134]

Thrombospondin-1 is a potent angiogenesis inhibitor expressed in normal brain tissue and low-grade astrocytomas.[135] Its expression is regulated by a gene on chromosome 10, and it has been shown that returning wild-type chromosome 10 to glioblastoma cell lines or overexpression of thrombospondin-1 results in an anti-angiogenic phenotype and inhibits tumor growth.[135,136] Thus, the increased angiogenesis observed in high-grade gliomas can be correlated with the loss of chromosome 10 and the resultant lack of thrombospondin-1. Additionally, aberrant promoter methylation of thrombospondin-1 has been documented in a third of primary glioblastoma multiforme as an alternative way of silencing this important angiogenesis inhibitor.[137]

Clearly, both upregulation of angiogenic factors and downregulation of angiogenic inhibitors may be linked in some tumors.[138,139] Another dimension of regulation is emerging in the form of proteinases, which can control the bioavailability of angiogenic activators and inhibitors.[140]

The ubiquitous expression of several angiogenesis stimulators in brain tumors suggests that anti-angiogenesis therapy may provide a novel strategy, especially against highly vascularized tumors. In contrast to traditional cancer treatments that attack tumor cells directly, angiogenesis inhibitors target the formation of tumor-feeding blood vessels that provide supply of nutrients and oxygen.[119] Tumor vasculature is morphologically abnormal, and various cell-surface and extracellular matrix (ECM) proteins can be used as markers to distinguish tumor vessels from normal vasculature.[141] Therefore, tumor blood vessels are prime targets for suppressing tumor growth because they are distinct from normal resting vessels and

can be destroyed selectively without affecting normal vessels significantly. With respect to brain tumor therapy, inhibitors of angiogenesis display unique features, including independence of the blood–brain barrier, cell-type specificity, and reduced resistance.

TISSUE INVASION AND METASTASIS

The processes of invasion of host cellular and ECM barriers and metastasis are related closely. Both use similar operational strategies, changing the physical coupling of cells to their microenvironment and activating extracellular proteinases. For reasons that are poorly understood, most primary brain tumors do not metastasize and rarely disseminate through CSF (an exception is primitive neuroectodermal tumors).[142] However, they do invade the surrounding normal brain. Individual glioma cells can migrate more than 4–7 cm from the gross tumor into the surrounding normal brain tissue.[143,144] The characteristic local invasiveness of gliomas contributes substantially to the inability to achieve total resection by surgery and often results in recurrences at the primary site and at locations on the opposite side of the brain.[145]

Tumor cell invasion is a multistep process that involves (i) adhesion of tumor cells to the ECM, (ii) proteolysis of matrix barriers, and (iii) migration of tumor cells into the newly created space. The ECM of the CNS consists of the glial external limiting membrane (made of types I, III, and IV collagen, fibronectin, laminin, and heparan sulfate), the vascular basement membrane (made of types IV and V collagen, laminin, entactin, fibronectin, vitronectin, and heparan sulfate), and the amorphous matrix of the brain parenchyma (consisting mainly of glycosaminoglycans (GAGs)).[145,146]

Cell-matrix adhesion molecules at the cell surface specifically recognize and bind the ECM components, thereby mediating the ability of cells to adhere and migrate. The integrins,[147] as a class of cell-surface receptors that bind to components of the ECM, and the hyaluronate receptor CD44 both play major roles in glioma cell-matrix adhesion.[148–150] The majority of glioma cells appear to migrate preferentially on laminin, tenascin, or fibronectin, and to lesser degrees on collagen and vitronectin.[151] PNETs appear to be more restricted, with migration limited to laminin, fibronectin, and type IV collagen.[152] Tumor cells can synthesize and deposit alternative ECM constituents, such as tenascin, which is not present in normal brain. Tenascin expression has been reported to correlate with malignancy in gliomas and ependymoma, and with lepto-meningeal dissemination in medulloblastoma.[153–155]

Tumor cell motility is enhanced further by the loss of cell–cell contacts, which are modulated by cell–cell adhesion proteins. The most important receptors for cell–cell interaction are the cadherins, the selectins, and certain members of the immunoglobulin superfamily, including neural cell adhesion molecule (NCAM), intercellular cell adhesion molecule (ICAM), and vascular cell adhesion molecule (VCAM).[148] The processes of adhesion and migration require mediation by these receptors and the proteinases involved.

In invasive tumors, proteinase genes are upregulated, proteinase inhibitor genes are downregulated, and inactive zymogen forms of proteinases are converted into active enzymes. Matrix-degrading proteinases are characteristically associated with the cell surface, by containing a transmembrane domain, by binding to specific proteinase receptors, or by association with integrins.[156,157] One imagines that docking of active proteinases on the cell surface can facilitate invasion by cancer cells into nearby stroma, across blood vessel walls, and through nearby normal cell layers. Nevertheless, it is difficult to ascribe the functions of particular proteinases unambiguously to this capability, given their evident roles in angiogenesis and growth signaling, which in turn contribute directly or indirectly to the invasive/metastatic ability.[156,158]

The matrix metalloproteinases (MMPs) are a family of zinc-dependent proteinases that collectively are capable of degrading essentially all the components of the extracellular matrix.[159,160] Because cells have receptors for structural ECM components, cleavage of ECM proteins by MMPs also affects cellular signaling and functions, explaining why MMPs are involved not only in invasion and metastasis but also in several steps of cancer development. The human MMP gene family consists of more than 21 structurally related members that fall into eight classes, three of which are membrane-bound, according to their primary structure and substrate specificity. Although gliomas express other proteinases, MMPs seem to be responsible for much of the degradation of a broad range of ECM components. In particular, gliomas contain elevated levels of MMP-2, MMP-9, and MT1-MMP compared with normal brain tissue.[161] In medulloblastoma, MMP-9 protein is expressed by tumor and endothelial cells.[162] However, strong immunoreactivity for MMP-9 in benign lesions such as neurinomas and meningiomas,[163] together with the lack of correlation between MMP-9 expression and the regional proliferative activity, and the strong signal around endothelial cells, has raised doubt about the direct proteolytic significance of MMP-9 in tissue degradation during tumor progression and invasion. It has been proposed that MMP-9 plays a role in the activation of VEGF during angiogenesis[164] and growth signaling.[156,158]

While it is clear that the activation of extracellular proteinases and modified binding specificities of cadherins, cell adhesion molecules (CAMs), and integrins are central to acquiring invasiveness, the regulatory circuits and molecular mechanisms involved remain unclear. Evolving analytical techniques should soon make it possible to construct comprehensive tumor-type specific profiles of the expression and functional activities of proteinases, integrins, and CAMs. In a pilot study, MacDonald and colleagues[31] derived expression profiles of 23 primary medulloblastomas clinically designated as either metastatic or non-metastatic, and identified 85 genes whose expression differed significantly between the two groups. The challenge is now to apply the new molecular insights about tissue invasiveness to the development of effective therapeutic strategies.

UNLIMITED REPLICATIVE POTENTIAL

The proliferative ability of normal somatic cells is highly restricted, with cells becoming senescent after a certain number of division cycles. Cancer cells must therefore overcome the normal mechanisms regulating cellular senescence.[165] Experimental data from cultured human fibroblasts indicate that two checkpoints must be bypassed before immortalization can occur: mortality stage 1 (M_1) and mortality stage 2 (M_2).[166] The M_1 stage is considered equivalent to normal cellular senescence. Oncogene activation or tumor suppressor gene inactivation may overcome the M_1 mechanism, endowing the cells with additional proliferative capacity until the second independent mechanism (M_2) occurs. Only cells surviving M_2 acquire the ability to proliferate indefinitely in vitro.[167]

Human telomeres consist of tandem hexametric $(TTAGGG)_n$ repeats at the ends of chromosomes. Most normal somatic cells lose approximately 50–100 bp of the terminal telomeric repeat DNA with each cycle of cell division. This shortening of telomeres is considered to be the mitotic clock with which cells count their divisions, and very short telomeres are likely to induce the onset of cellular senescence, M_1, in somatic cells. Shortened telomeres have a dual effect: they initiate checkpoint signals that provoke a cell-cycle arrest or trigger apoptosis, but they can also cause chromosomal instability. Thus, whereas the checkpoint signals protect against tumor formation, increased genetic instability is likely to speed up the multistep tumorigenic process.[167,168]

Telomere maintenance is evident in virtually all types of malignant cells: 85–90 per cent show upregulated expression of the enzyme telomerase, which adds hexanucleotide repeats on to the ends of telomeric DNA,[169,170] while the remaining cells have invented a way of activating a mechanism, alternative lengthening of telomeres (ALT), which appears to maintain telomeres through recombination-based interchromosomal exchanges of sequence information.[171]

Telomerase, or telomere terminal transferase, is a ribonucleoprotein that catalyzes the de novo synthesis and elongation of telomeric repeats at chromosomal ends by using the RNA segment within its molecule as a template.[172,173] While functionally immortal germ-line cells express telomerase and maintain adequate telomeric repeats, most human somatic cells do not express telomerase. They fail to acquire telomerase activity in successive cultures and become senescent. In contrast, telomerase activity has been detected in numerous cancer cells and tissues.[174] Brain tumors in which telomerase activity has been detected include medulloblastoma, glioblastoma, anaplastic astrocytoma, and oligodendroglioma.[175–177] Increased expression of the telomerase RNA component has been found to be associated with increased cell proliferation in astrocytomas and ependymomas.[178] Malignant brain tumors have a higher positive rate of telomerase activity than benign tumors.[177] Moreover, telomerase activity in meningiomas has been found to correlate with poor survival outcome, indicating that these apparently benign tumors may contain a population of immortal cells.[179] The finding that at least 90 per cent of human tumors express high levels of telomere activity, whereas most normal somatic cells do not, makes telomerase activity a potentially useful diagnostic marker as well as a therapeutic target.[180]

Signals other than shortening telomeres can trigger a senescent phenotype. These include Ras signaling, which induces cell-cycle arrest in the presence of functional *p53*. Reactivating *p53* in tumor cells – for example by the use of small molecules that have been shown to "normalize" mutant *p53* activity[181] – might therefore be a therapeutic route to the induction of senescence in tumor cells.

SUMMARY

Important acquired capacities of malignant brain tumors include self-sufficiency in growth signals, insensitivity to antigrowth signals, avoidance of apoptosis, sustained angiogenesis, tissue invasion, and unlimited replication potential. These hallmark abilities may be acquired at different times during tumor progression. Any given cancer type may show alterations of particular target genes in only a subset of otherwise histologically identical tumors. Moreover, alterations of target genes may occur at an early stage of some tumor progression pathways and later in others.

Much of the information that we currently have about the molecular processes of carcinogenesis has been obtained from cancer cells propagated in culture and then dissected into their molecular components. Yet by reducing cancer to a cell-autonomous process intrinsic to the cancer cell, experimental models like these ignore a central biological reality of tumor formation in vivo: cancer development is also dependent on changes in the heterotypic interactions between tumor cells and their normal neighbors.[1] The interactions between cancer cells and their macro- and microenvironments create a context that promotes tumor growth and change as

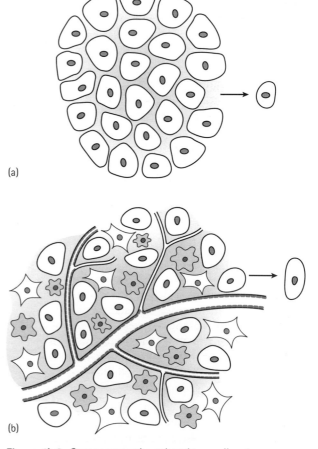

(a)

(b)

Figure 4b.3 *Cancer cannot be reduced to a cell-autonomous process intrinsic to the cancer cell (a). It is a complex process in which cancer cells conscript and subvert normal cells to serve as active collaborators in tumor growth (b).*

malignancy progresses (Figure 4b.3).[182] Looking at cancer cell biology in this way has begun to change profoundly how we study this disease experimentally. A continuing understanding of cancer pathogenesis will increasingly require heterotypic organ culture systems in vitro and ever more refined animal models in vivo.[183]

Dramatic advances in the understanding of normal and malignant cell biology combined with better in vitro and in vivo models and the use of novel high-throughput technologies will elucidate significant circuitries of pediatric brain tumors in the next decade. This will lead to the development of new drugs that are directed at specific differences between host and tumor.

ACKNOWLEDGMENTS

I am indebted to Dr Tarek Shalaby for helping to prepare the manuscript and to Susanne Staubli for artwork. Supported by the Schweizer Forschungsstiftung Kind und Krebs.

REFERENCES

1 Hanahan D, Weinberg RA. The hallmarks of cancer. *Cell* 2000; **100**:57–70.

2 Gerdes J. Ki-67 and other proliferation markers useful for immunohistological diagnostic and prognostic evaluations in human malignancies. In: Osborn M (ed.) *Cancer Biology*, vol. 1. London: Saunders Scientific Publications, 1990, pp. 99–206.

3 Hall PA, Woods AL. Immunohistochemical markers of cellular proliferation: achievements, problems and prospects. *Cell Tissue Kinet* 1990; **23**:505–22.

4 Jaros E, Perry RH, Adam L, *et al*. Prognostic implications of p53 protein, epidermal growth factor receptor, and Ki-67 labeling in brain tumours. *Br J Cancer* 1992; **66**:373–85.

5 Montine TJ, Vandersteenhoven JJ, Aguzzi A, *et al*. Prognostic significance of Ki-67 proliferation index in supratentorial fibrillary astrocytic neoplasms. *Neurosurgery* 1994; **34**:674–8.

6 Khalid H, Shibata S, Kishikawa M, Yasunaga A, Iseki M, Hiura T. Immunohistochemical analysis of progesterone receptor and Ki-67 labeling index in astrocytic tumors. *Cancer* 1997; **80**:2133–40.

7 Dirven CMF, Koudstaal J, Mooij YYA, Molenaar WM. The proliferative potential of the pilocytic astrocytoma; the relation between MIB-1 labeling and clinical and neuro-radiological follow-up. *J Neuro-Oncol* 1998; **37**:9–16.

8 McKeever PE, Strawderman MS, Yamini B, Mikhail AA, Blaivas M. MIB-1 proliferation index predicts survival among patients with grade II astrocytoma. *J Neuropathol Exp Neurol* 1998; **57**:931–6.

9 Ritter AM, Hess KR, McLendon RE, Langford LA. Ependymoma: MIB-1 proliferation index and survival. *J Neuro-Oncol* 1998; **40**:51–7.

10 Grotzer MA, Geoerger B, Janss AJ, Zhao H, Rorke LB, Phillips PC. Prognostic significance of Ki-67 (MIB-1) proliferation index in childhood primitive neuroectodermal tumors of the central nervous system. *Med Ped Oncol* 2001; **36**:268–73.

11 Hamel W, Westphal M. Growth factors in gliomas revisited. *Acta Neurochir* 2000; **142**:113–37.

12 Hermanson M, Funa K, Hartman M, *et al*. Platelet-derived growth factor and its receptors in human glioma tissue: expression of messenger RNA and protein suggests the presence of autocrine and paracrine loops. *Cancer Res* 1992; **52**:3213–19.

13 Black P, Carroll R, Glowacka D. Expression of platelet-derived growth factor transcripts in medulloblastomas and ependymomas. *Pediatr Neurosurgi* 1996; **24**:74–8.

14 Huber H, Eggert A, Janss AJ, *et al*. Angiogenic profile of childhood primitive neuroectodermal brain tumors. *Eur J Cancer* 2001; **37**:2064–72.

15 Van der Valk P, Lindeman J, Kamphorst W. Growth factor profiles of human gliomas. Do non-tumour cells contribute to tumour growth in glioma? *Ann Oncol* 1997; **8**:1023–9.

16 Patti R, Reddy CD, Geoerger B, *et al*. Autocrine secreted insulin-like growth factor-I stimulates MAP kinase-dependent mitogenic effects in human primitive neuroectodermal tumor/medulloblastoma. *Int J Oncol* 2000; **16**:577–84.

17 Hirano H, Lopes MB, Laws ER, Jr, *et al*. Insulin-like growth factor-1 content and pattern of expression correlates with histopathologic grade in diffusely infiltrating astocytomas. *Neuro-Oncol* 1999; **1**:109–19.

18 Meuillet EJ, Bremer EG. Growth factor receptors as targets for therapy in pediatric brain tumors. *Pediatr Neurosurg* 1998; **29**:1–13.

19 Kleihues P, Burger PC, Collins VP, Newcomb EW, Ohgaki H, Cavenee WK. Glioblastoma. In: Kleihues P, Cavenee WK (eds) *Pathology and Genetics of Tumours of the Nervous System*. Lyon: IARC Press, 2000, pp. 29–44.

20 Gilbertson RJ, Perry RH, Kelly PJ, Pearson ADJ, Lunec J. Prognostic significance of HER2 and HER4 coexpression in childhood medulloblastoma. *Cancer Res* 1997; **57**:3272–80.

21 Ekstrand AJ, Liu L, He J, *et al*. Altered subcellular location of an activated and tumour-associated epidermal growth factor receptor. *Oncogene* 1995; **10**:1455–60.

22 Lukashev ME, Werb Z. ECM signalling: orchestrating cell behaviour and misbehaviour. *Trends Cell Biol* 1998; **8**:437–41.

23 Giancotti FG, Ruoslahti E. Integrin signaling. *Science* 1999; **285**:1028–32.

24 Aplin AE, Howe A, Alahari SK, Juliano RL. Signal transduction and signal modulation by cell adhesion receptors: the role of integrins, cadherins, immunoglobulin-cell adhesion molecules, and selectins. *Pharmacol Rev* 1998; **50**:197–263.

25 Medema RH, Bos JL. The role of p21ras in receptor tyrosine kinase signaling. *Crit Rev Oncol* 1993; **4**:615–61.

26 Iolascon A, Lania A, Badiali M, *et al*. Analysis of N-ras gene mutations in medulloblastomas by polymerase chain reaction and oligonucleotide probes in formalin-fixed, paraffin-embedded tissues. *Med Pediatr Oncol* 1991; **19**:240–5.

27 Maltzman TH, Mueller BA, Schroeder J, *et al*. Ras oncogene mutations in childhood brain tumors. *Cancer Epidemiol Biomarkers Prev* 1997; **6**:239–43.

28 Gomori E, Doczi T, Pajor L, Matolcsy A. Sporadic p53 mutations and absence of ras mutations in glioblastomas. *Acta Neurochir* 1999; **141**:593–9.

29 Wasson JC, Saylors RL, III, Zeltzer P, *et al.* Oncogene amplification in pediatric brain tumors. *Cancer Res* 1990; **50**:2987–90.

30 Orian JM, Vasilopoulos K, Yoshida S, Kaye AH, Chow CW, Gonzales MF. Overexpression of multiple oncogenes related to histological grade of astrocytic glioma. *Br J Cancer* 1992; **66**:106–12.

31 MacDonald TJ, Brown KM, LaFleur B, *et al.* Expression profiling of medulloblastoma: PDGFRA and RAS/MAPK pathway as therapeutic targets for metastatic disease. *Nat Genet* 2001; **29**:143–52.

32 Hunter T. Oncoprotein networks. *Cell* 1997; **88**:333–46.

33 Rommel C, Hafen E. Ras – a versatile cellular switch. *Curr Opin Genet Dev* 1998; **8**:412–18.

34 Downward J. Mechanisms and consequences of activation of protein kinase B/Akt. *Curr Opin Cell Biol* 1998; **10**:262–7.

35 Reed N, Gutmann DH. Tumorigenesis in neurofibromatosis: new insights and potential therapies. *Trends Mol Med* 2001; **7**:157–62.

36 Sherr CJ. Cancer cell cycles. *Science* 1996; **274**:1672–7.

37 Dirks PB, Rutka JT. Current concepts in neuro-oncology: the cell cycle – a review. *Neurosurgery* 1997; **40**:1000–13.

38 Malumbres M, Barbacid M. To cycle or not to cycle: a critical decision in cancer. *Nat Rev Cancer* 2001; **1**:222–31.

39 Kubbutat MH, Jones SN, Vousden KH. Regulation of p53 stability by Mdm2. *Nature* 1997; **387**:299–303.

40 Kondo S, morimura T, Barnett GH, *et al.* The transforming activities of *MDM2* in cultured neonatal rat astrocytes. *Oncogene* 1996; **13**:1773–9.

41 Schiebe M, Ohneseit P, Hoffman W, Meyermann R, Rodenmann HP, Bamberg M. Analysis of *mdm2* and *p53* gene alterations in glioblastomas and its correlation with clinical factors. *J Neuro-Oncol* 2000; **49**:197–203.

42 Suzuki SO, Iwaki T. Amplification and overexpression of *mdm2* gene in ependymomas. *Mod Pathol* 2000; **13**:548–53.

43 Iwato M, Tachibana O, Tohma Y, Nitta H, Hayashi Y, Yamashita J. Molecular analysis for *p53* and *mdm2* in intracranial germ cell tumors. *Acta Neuropathol* 2000; **99**:21–5.

44 Adesina AM, Nalbantoglu J, Cavenee WK. *p53* gene mutation and *mdm2* gene amplification are uncommon in medulloblastoma. *Cancer Res* 1994; **54**:5649–51.

45 Stuart ET, Haffner R, Oren M, Gruss P. Loss of *p53* function through PAX-mediated transcriptional repression. *EMBO J* 1995; **14**:5638–45.

46 Stuart ET, Kioussi C, Aguzzi A, Gruss P. *PAX5* expression correlates with increasing malignancy in human astrocytomas. *Clin Cancer Res* 1995; **1**:207–14.

47 Kozmik Z, Sure U, Ruedi D, Busslinger M, Aguzzi A. Deregulated expression of *PAX5* in medulloblastoma. *Proc Natl Acad Sci U S A* 1995; **92**:5709–13.

48 Steinbach J.P, Kozmik Z, Pfeffer P, Aguzzi A. Overexpression of *Pax5* is not sufficient for neoplastic transformation of mouse neuroectoderm. *Int J Cancer* 2001; **93**:459–67.

49 Jen J, Harper JW, Bigner SH, *et al.* Deletion of *p16* and *p15* genes in brain tumors. *Cancer Res* 1994; **54**:6353–8.

50 Barker FG, Chen P, Furman F, Aldape KD, Edwards MS, Israel MA. *P16* deletion and mutation analysis in human brain tumors. *J Neuro-Oncol* 1997; **31**:17–23.

51 Ono Y, Tamiya T, Ichikawa T, *et al.* Malignant astrocytomas with homozygous *CDKN2/p16* gene deletions have higher Ki-67 proliferation indices. *J Neuropathol Exp Neurol* 1996; **55**:1026–31.

52 Sherr CJ. Tumor surveillance via the ARF-p53 pathway. *Genes Dev* 1998; **12**:2984–91.

53 Weinberg RA. The retinoblastoma protein and cell cycle control. *Cell* 1995; **81**:323–30.

54 Weiss WA. Genetics of brain tumors. *Curr Opin Pediatr* 2000; **12**:543–8.

55 Cavenee WK, Furnari FB, Nagane M, *et al.* Diffusely infiltrating astrocytomas. In: Kleihues P, Cavenee WK (eds) *Pathology and Genetics. Tumours of the Nervous System.* Lyon: IARC Press, 2000, pp. 10–21.

56 Marino S, Vooijs M, van Der Gulden H, Jonkers J, Berns A. Induction of medulloblastomas in *p53*-null mutant mice by somatic inactivation of Rb in the external granular layer cells of the cerebellum. *Genes Dev* 2000; **14**:994–1004.

57 Foley KP, Eisenman RN. Two MAD tails: what the recent knockouts of Mad1 and Mxi1 tell us about the MYC/MYC/MAD network. *Biochim Biophys Acta* 1999; **1423**:M37–47.

58 Raffel C, Gilles FE, Weinberg KI. Reduction to homozygosity and gene amplification in central nervous system primitive neuroectodermal tumors of childhood. *Cancer Res* 1990; **50**:587–91.

59 Batra SK, McLendon RE, Koo JS, *et al.* Prognostic implications of chromosome 17p deletions in human medulloblastoma. *J Neuro-Oncol* 1995; **24**:39–45.

60 Scheurlen WG, Schwabe GC, Joos S, Mollenhauer J, Sorensen N, Kuhl J. Molecular analysis of childhood primitive neuroectodermal tumors defines markers associated with poor outcome. *J Clin Oncol* 1998; **16**:2478–85.

61 Herms J, Neidt I, Luscher B, *et al.* C-myc expression in medulloblastoma and its prognostic value. *Int J Cancer* 2000; **89**:395–402.

62 Bigner SH, Friedman HS, Vogelstein B, Oakes WJ, Bigner DD. Amplification of the c-myc gene in human medulloblastoma cell lines and xenografts. *Cancer Res* 1990; **50**:2347–50.

63 Batra SK, Rasheed BK, Bigner SH, Bigner DD. Oncogenes and anti-oncogenes in human central nervous system tumors. *Lab Invest* 1994; **71**:621–37.

64 Badiali M, Pession A, Basso G, Andreini L, Rigobello L, Galassi E, Giangaspero F. N-myc and c-myc oncogenes amplification in medulloblastomas. Evidence of particularly aggressive behavior of a tumor with c-myc amplification. *Tumori* 1991; **77**:118–21.

65 Giangaspero F, Rigobello L, Badiali M, *et al.* Large-cell medulloblastomas: a distinct variant with highly aggressive behavior. *Am J Surg Pathol* 1992; **16**:687–93.

66 Jay V, Squire J, Bayani J, Alkhani AM, Rutka JT, Zielenska M. Oncogene amplification in medulloblastoma: analysis of a case by comparative genomic hybridization and fluorescence *in situ* hybridization. *Pathology* 1999; **31**:337–44.

67 Grotzer MA, Hogarty MD, Janss AJ, *et al.* MYC messenger RNA expression predicts survival outcome in childhood primitive neuroectodermal tumor/medulloblastoma. *Clin Cancer Res* 2001; **7**:2425–33.

68 Bruggers CS, Tai KF, Murdock T, *et al.* Expression of the c-myc protein in childhood medulloblastoma. *J Pediatr Hematol Oncol* 1998; **20**:18–25.

69 Hamilton SR, Liu B, Parsons RE, *et al*. The molecular basis of Turcot's syndrome. *N Engl J Med* 1995; **332**:839–47.

70 Zurawel RH, Chiappa SA, Allen C, Raffel C. Sporadic medulloblastomas contain oncogenic beta-catenin mutations. *Cancer Res* 1998; **58**:896–9.

71 Bullions LC, Levine AJ. The role of beta-catenin in cell adhesion, signal transduction, and cancer. *Curr Opin Oncol* 1998; **10**:81–7.

72 Eberhart CG, Tihan T, Burger PC. Nuclear localization and mutation of beta-catenin in medulloblastomas. *J Neuropathol Exp Neurol* 2000; **59**:333–7.

73 He TC, Sparks AB, Rago C, *et al*. Identification of c-MYC as a target of the APC pathway. *Science* 1998; **281**:1509–12.

74 Wyllie AH, Kerr JF, Currie AR. Cell death: the significance of apoptosis. *Int Rev Cytol* 1980; **68**:251–306.

75 Soini Y, Paako P, Lehto V-P. Histopathological evaluation of apoptosis in cancer. *Am J Pathol* 1998; **153**:1041–53.

76 Wikstrand CJ, Fung K-M, Trojanowski JQ, McLendon RE, Bigner DD. Antibodies and molecular immunology. In: Bigner DD, McLendon RE, Bruner JM (eds) *Russell and Rubinstein's Pathology of Tumors of the Nervous System*. London: Arnold, 1998, pp. 251–304.

77 Schiffer D, Dutto A, Cavalla P, Chio A, Migheli A, Piva R. Role of apoptosis in the prognosis of oligodendrogliomas. *Neurochem Int* 1997; **31**:245–50.

78 Carroll RS, Zhang J, Chauncey BW, Chantziara K, Frosch MP, Black PML. Apoptosis in astrocytic neoplasms. *Acta Neurochir* 1997; **139**:845–50.

79 Schiffer D, Cavalla P, Chio A, *et al*. Tumor cell proliferation and apoptosis in medulloblastoma. *Acta Neuropathol* 1994; **87**:362–70.

80 Schiffer D, Cavalla P, Migheli A, *et al*. Apoptosis and cell proliferation in human neuroepithelial tumors. *Neurosci Lett* 1995; **195**:81–4.

81 Schubert TE, Cervos-Navarro J. The histopathological and clinical relevance of apoptotic cell death in medulloblastoma. *J Neuropathol Exp Neurol* 1998; **57**:10–15.

82 Haslam RHA, Lamborn KR, Becker LE, Israel MA. Tumor cell apoptosis present at diagnosis may predict treatment outcome for patients with medulloblastoma. *J Pediatr Hematol Oncol* 1998; **20**:520–7.

83 Grotzer MA, Janss AJ, Fung K-M, *et al*. Abundance of apoptotic neoplastic cells in diagnostic biopsy samples is not a prognostic factor in childhood primitive neuroectodermal tumors of the central nervous system. *J Pediatr Hematol Oncol* 2001; **23**:25–9.

84 Wang JY, Del Valle L, Gordon J, *et al*. Activation of the IGF-IR system contributes to malignant growth of human and mouse medulloblastomas. *Oncogene* 2001; **20**:3857–68.

85 Wiley SR, Schooley K, Smolak PJ, *et al*. Identification and characterization of a new member of the TNF family that induces apoptosis. *Immunity* 1995; **3**:673–82.

86 Frank S, Kohler U, Schackert G, Schackert HK. Expression of TRAIL and its receptors in human brain tumors. *Biochem Biophys Res Commun* 1999; **257**:454–9.

87 Nakamura M, Rieger J, Weller M, Kim J, Kleihues P, Ohgaki H. APO2L/TRAIL expression in human brain tumors. *Acta Neuropathol* 2000; **99**:1–6.

88 Schulze-Osthoff K, Ferrari D, Los M, Wesselborg S, Peter ME. Apoptosis signaling by death receptors. *Eur J Biochem* 1998; **254**:439–59.

89 Evan G, Littlewood T. A matter of life and cell death. *Science* 1998; **281**:1317–22.

90 Green DR, Reed JC. Mitochondria and apoptosis. *Science* 1998; **281**:1309–12.

91 Martin S, Toquet C, Oliver L, *et al*. Expression of bcl-2, bax and bcl-xl in human gliomas: a re-appraisal. *J Neuro-Oncol* 2001; **52**:129–39.

92 Miralbell R, Tolnay M, Bieri S, *et al*. Pediatric medulloblastoma: prognostic value of p53, bcl-2, Mib-1, and microvessel density. *J Neuro-Oncol* 1999; **45**:103–10.

93 Prayson RA. Bcl-2 and Bcl-X expression in gangliogliomas. *Hum Pathol* 1999; **30**:701–5.

94 Prayson RA. Bcl-2, bcl-x, and bax expression in dysembryo-plastic neuroepithelial tumors. *Clin Neuropathol* 2000; **19**:57–62.

95 Thornberry NA, Lazebnik Y. Caspases: enemies within. *Science* 1998; **281**:1312–16.

96 Fulci G, Ishii N, Van Meir EG. *p53* and brain tumors: from gene mutations to gene therapy. *Brain Pathol* 1998; **8**:599–613.

97 Harris CC. *p53* tumor suppressor gene: from the basic research laboratory to the clinic – an abridged historical perspective. *Carcinogenesis* 1996; **17**:1187–98.

98 Levine AJ. *p53*, the cellular gatekeeper for growth and division. *Cell* 1997; **88**:323–31.

99 Sonoda Y, Ozawa T, Aldape KD, Deen DF, Berger MS, Pieper RO. Akt pathway activation converts anaplastic astrocytoma to glioblastoma multiforme in a human astrocyte model of glioma. *Cancer Res* 2001; **61**:6674–8.

100 Downward J. Mechanisms and consequences of activation of protein kinase B/Akt. *Curr Opin Cell Biol* 1998; **10**:262–7.

101 Cantley LC, Neel BG. New insights into tumor suppression: PTEN suppresses tumor formation by restraining the phosphoinositide 3-kinase/AKT pathway. *Proc Natl Acad Sci U S A* 1999; **96**:4240–5.

102 Roth W, Isenmann S, Nakamura M, *et al*. Soluble decoy receptor 3 is expressed by malignant gliomas and suppresses CD95 ligand-induced apoptosis and chemotaxis. *Cancer Res* 2001; **61**:2759–65.

103 Grotzer MA, Eggert A, Zuzak TJ, *et al*. Resistance to TRAIL-induced apoptosis in primitive neuroectodermal brain tumor cells correlates with a loss of caspase-8 expression. *Oncogene* 2000; **19**:4604–10.

104 Zuzak TJ, Steinhoff DF, Sutton LN, Phillips PC, Eggert A, Grotzer MA. Loss of caspase-8 gene expression is common in childhood primitive neuroectodermal brain tumour/medulloblastoma. *Eur J Cancer* 2002; **38**:92–8.

105 Kim JY, Sutton ME, Lu DJ, *et al*. Activation of neurotrophin-3 receptor TrkC induces apoptosis in medulloblastoma. *Cancer Res* 1999; **59**:711–19.

106 Segal RA, Goumnerova LC, Kwon YK, Stiles CD, Pomeroy SL. Expression of the neurotrophin receptor trkC is linked to a favorable outcome in medulloblastoma. *Proc Natl Acad Sci U S A* 1994; **91**:12867–71.

107 Grotzer MA, Janss AJ, Fung K-M, *et al*. TrkC expression predicts good clinical outcome in primitive neuroectodermal brain tumors. *J Clin Oncol* 2000; **18**:1027–35.

108 Li VW, Folkerth RD, Watanabe H, *et al.* Microvessel count and cerebrospinal fluid basic fibroblast growth factor in children with brain tumours. *Lancet* 1994; **344**:82–6.

109 Leon SP, Folkerth RD, Black PM. Microvessel density is a prognostic indicator for patients with astroglial brain tumors. *Cancer* 1996; **77**:362–72.

110 Assimakopoulou M, Sotiropoulou-Bonikou G, Maraziotis T, Papadakis N, Varakis I. Microvessel density in brain tumors. *Anticancer Res* 1997; **17**:4747–54.

111 Grotzer MA, Wiewrodt R, Janss AJ, *et al.* High microvessel density in primitive neuroectodermal brain tumors of childhood. *Neuropediatrics* 2001; **32**:75–9.

112 Folkman J. How is blood vessel growth regulated in normal and neoplastic tissue? *Cancer Res* 1986; **46**:467–73.

113 Folkman J. What is the evidence that tumors are angiogenesis dependent? *J Natl Cancer Inst* 1989; **82**:4–6.

114 Folkman J. Clinical applications of research on angiogenesis. *N Engl J Med* 1995; **333**:1757–63.

115 Hanahan D, Folkman J. Patterns and emerging mechanisms of the angiogenic switch during tumorigenesis. *Cell* 1996; **86**:353–64.

116 Folkman J, D'Amore PA. Blood vessel formation: what is its molecular basis? *Cell* 1996; **87**:1153–5.

117 Folkman J. Angiogenesis in cancer, vascular, rheumatoid and other disease. *Nat Med* 1995; **1**:27–31.

118 Hanahan D. Signaling vascular morphogenesis and maintenance. *Science* 1997; **277**:48–50.

119 Kirsch M, Schackert G, Black PM. Anti-angiogenic treatment strategies for malignant brain tumors. *J Neuro-Oncol* 2000; **50**:149–63.

120 Stefanik DF, Rizkalla LR, Soi A, Goldblatt SA, Rizkalla WM. Acidic and basic fibroblast growth factors are present in glioblastoma multiforme. *Cancer Res* 1991; **51**:5760–5.

121 Takahashi JA, Mori H, Fukumoto M, *et al.* Gene expression of fibroblast growth factors in human gliomas and meningiomas: demonstration of cellular source of basic fibroblast growth factor mRNA and peptide in tumor tissues. *Proc Natl Acad Sci U S A* 1990; **87**:5710–14.

122 Plate KH, Breier G, Weich HA, Risau W. Vascular endothelial growth factor is a potential tumour angiogenesis factor in human gliomas in vivo. *Nature* 1992; **359**:845–8.

123 Samoto K, Ikezaki K, Ono M, Shono T, Kohno K, Kuwano M, Fukui M. Expression of vascular endothelial growth factor and its possible relation with neovascularization in human brain tumors. *Cancer Res* 1995; **55**:1189–93.

124 Bjerkvig R, Lund-Johansen M, Edvardsen K. Tumor cell invasion and angiogenesis in the central nervous system. *Curr Opin Oncol* 1997; **9**:223–9.

125 Zagzag D, Hooper A, Friedlander DR, *et al.* In situ expression of angiopoietins in astrocytomas identifies angiopoietin-2 as an early marker of tumor angiogenesis. *Exp Neurol* 1999; **159**:391–400.

126 Samato K, Ikezaki K, Ono M, *et al.* Expression of vascular endothelial growth factor and its possible relation with neovascularization in human brain tumors. *Cancer Res* 1995; **55**:1189–93.

127 Brem S, Tsanaclis AMC, Gately S, Gross JL, Herblin WF. Immunolocalization of basic fibroblast growth factor to the microvasculature of human brain tumors. *Cancer* 1992; **70**:2673–80.

128 Pietsch T, Valter MM, Wolf HK, *et al.* Expression and distribution of vascular endothelial growth factor protein in human brain tumors. *Acta Neuropathol* 1997; **93**:109–17.

129 Weindel K, Moringlane JR, Marme D, Weich HA. Detection and quantification of vascular endothelial growth factor/vascular permeability factor in brain tumor tissue and cyst fluid: the key to angiogenesis? *Neurosurgery* 1994; **35**:439–48.

130 Millauer B, Shawver LK, Plate KH, Risau W, Ullrich A. Glioblastoma growth inhibited in vivo by a dominant-negative Flk-1 mutant. *Nature* 1994; **367**:576–9.

131 Wesseling P, Ruiter DJ, Burger PC. Angiogenesis in brain tumors: pathobiological and clinical aspects. *J Neuro-Oncol* 1997; **32**:253–65.

132 Presta LG, Chen H, O'Connor SJ, *et al.* Humanization of an anti-vascular endothelial growth factor monoclonal antibody for the therapy of solid tumors and other disorders. *Cancer Res* 1997; **57**:4593–9.

133 Witte L, Hicklin DJ, Zhu Z, *et al.* Monoclonal antibodies targeting the VEGF receptor-2 (Flk1/KDR) as an anti-angiogenic therapeutic strategy. *Cancer Metastasis Rev* 1998; **17**:155–61.

134 Fong TA, Shawver LK, Sun L, *et al.* SU5416 is a potent and selective inhibitor of the vascular endothelial growth factor receptor (Flk-1/KDR) that inhibits tyrosine kinase catalysis, tumor vascularization, and growth of multiple tumor types. *Cancer Res* 1999; **59**:99–106.

135 Hsu SC, Volpert OV, Steck PA, *et al.* Inhibition of angiogenesis in human glioblastomas by chromosome 10 induction of thrombospondin-1. *Cancer Res* 1996; **56**:5684–91.

136 Kragh M, Qujistorff B, Tenan M, Van Meir EG, Kristjansen EG. Overexpression of thrombospondin-1 reduces growth and vascular index but not perfusion in glioblastoma. *Cancer Res* 2002; **62**:1191–5.

137 Li Q, Ahuja N, Burger PC, Issa JP. Methylation and silencing of the thrombospondin-1 promoter in human cancer. *Oncogene* 1999; **18**:3284–9.

138 Singh RK, Gutman M, Bucana CD, Sanchez R, Llansa N, Fidler IJ. Interferons alpha and beta down-regulate the expression of basic fibroblast growth factor in human carcinomas. *Proc Natl Acad Sci U S A* 1995; **92**:4562–6.

139 Volpert OV, Dameron KM, Bouck N. Sequential development of an angiogenic phenotype by human fibroblasts progressing to tumorigenicity. *Oncogene* 1997; **14**:1495–1502.

140 Whitelock JM, Murdoch AD, Iozzo RV, Underwood RA. The degradation of human endothelial cell-derived perlecan and release of bound basic fibroblast growth factor by stromelysin, collegenase, plasmin, and heparanes. *J Biol Chem* 1996; **271**:10079–86.

141 Ruoslahti E. Specialization of tumour vasculature. *Nat Rev Cancer* 2002; **2**:83–90.

142 Cohen ME, Duffner PK. Extraneural metastasis in childhood brain tumors. In: Cohen ME, Duffner PK (eds) *Brain Tumors in Children: Principles of Diagnosis and Treatment.* New York: Raven Press, 1994, pp. 423–36.

143 Kelly PJ, Daumas-Duport C, Kispert DB, Kall BA, Scheithauer BW, Illig JJ. Imaging-based stereotaxic serial biopsies in

untreated intracranial glial neoplasms. *J Neurosurg* 1987; **66**:865–74.

144 Silbergeld DL, Chicoine MR. Isolation and characterization of human malignant glioma cells from histologically normal brain. *J Neurosurg* 1997; **86**:525–31.

145 Giese A, Westphal M. Glioma invasion in the central nervous system. *Neurosurgery* 1996; **39**:235–50.

146 Gupta N, Rutka JT. Molecular neuro-oncology. In: Bernstein M, Berger MS (eds) *Neuro-Oncology: The Essentials.* New York: Thieme Medical Publishers, 2000, pp. 30–41.

147 Hood JD, Cheresh DA. Role of integrins in cell invasion and migration. *Nat Rev Cancer* 2002; **2**:91–100.

148 Goldbrunner RH, Bernstein JJ, Tonn JC. Cell-extracellular matrix interaction in glioma invasion. *Acta Neurochir* 1999; **141**:295–305.

149 Uhm JH, Gladson CL, Rao JS. The role of integrins in the malignant phenotype of gliomas. *Front Biosc* 1999; **4**:D188–99.

150 Ranuncolo SM, Ladeda V, Specterman S, *et al.* CD44 expression in human gliomas. *J Surg Oncol* 2002; **79**:30–5.

151 Rempel S.A. Molecular biology of central nervous system tumors. *Curr Opin Oncol* 1998; **10**:179–85.

152 Friedlander DR, Zagzag D, Shiff B, *et al.* Migration of brain tumor cells on extracellular matrix proteins in vitro correlates with tumor type and grade and involves alphaV and beta1 integrins. *Cancer Res* 1996; **56**:1939–47.

153 Higuchi M, Ohnishi T, Arita N, Hiraga S, Hayakawa T. Expression of tenascin in human gliomas: its relation to histological malignancy, tumor differentiation and angiogenesis. *Acta Neuropathol* 1993; **85**:481–7.

154 Korshunov A, Golanov A, Ozerov S, Sycheva R. Prognostic value of tumor-associated antigens immunoreactivity and apoptosis in medulloblastomas. An anylysis of 73 cases. *Brain Tumor Pathol* 1999; **16**:37–44.

155 Korshunov A, Golanov A, Timirgaz V. Immunohistochemical markers for intracranial ependymoma recurrence. An analysis of 88 cases. *J Neuro Sci* 2000; **177**:72–82.

156 Werb Z. ECM and cell surface proteolysis: regulating cellular ecology. *Cell* 1997; **91**:439–42.

157 Stetler-Stevenson WG. Matrix metalloproteinases in angiogenesis: a moving target for therapeutic intervention. *J Clin Invest* 1999; **103**:1237–41.

158 Bergers G, Coussens LM. Extrinsic regulators of epithelial tumor progression: metalloproteinases. *Curr Opin Genet Dev* 2000; **10**:120–7.

159 Hidalgo M, Eckhardt GS. Development of matrix metallo-proteinase inhibitors in cancer therapy. *J Natl Cancer Inst* 2001; **93**:178–93.

160 Egeblad M, Werb Z. New functions for the matrix metallo-proteinases in cancer progression. *Nat Rev Cancer* 2002; **2**:161–74.

161 Chintala SK, Tonn JC, Rao JS. Matrix metalloproteinases and their biological function in human gliomas. *Int J Dev Neurosci* 1999; **17**:495–502.

162 Vince GH, Herbold C, Klein R, *et al.* Medulloblastoma displays distinct regional matrix metalloprotease expression. *J Neuro-Oncol* 2001; **53**:99–106.

163 Costello PC, Del Maestro RF, Stetler-Stevenson WG. Gelatinase A expression in human malignant gliomas. *Ann N Y Acad Sci* 1994; **732**:450–2.

164 Bergers G, Brekken R, McMahon G, *et al.* Matrix metallo-proteinase-9 triggers the angiogenic switch during carcinogenesis. *Nat Cell Biol* 2000; **2**:737–44.

165 Harley CB, Futcher AB, Greider CW. Telomeres shorten during ageing of human fibroblasts. *Nature* 1990; **345**:458–60.

166 Shay JW, Wright WE, Werbin H. Defining the molecular mechanisms of human cell immortalization. *Biochim Biophys Acta* 1991; **1072**:1–7.

167 Mathon NF, Lloyd AC. Cell senescence and cancer. *Nat Rev Cancer* 2001; **1**:203–13.

168 Hastie ND, Dempster M, Dunlop MG, Thompson AM, Green DK, Allshire RC. Telomere reduction in human colorectal carcinoma and with ageing. *Nature* 1990; **346**:866–8.

169 Shay JW, Bacchetti S. A survey of telomerase activity in human cancer. *Eur J Cancer* 1997; **33**:787–91.

170 Bryan TM, Cech TR. Telomerase and the maintenance of chromosome ends. *Curr Opin Cell Biol* 1999; **11**:318–24.

171 Bryan TM, Englezou A, Gupta J, Bacchetti S, Reddel RR. Telomere elongation in immortal human cells without detectable telomerase activity. *EMBO J* 1995; **14**:4240–8.

172 Blackburn EH. Structure and function of telomeres. *Nature* 1991; **350**:569–73.

173 Feng J, Funk WD, Wang SS, *et al.* The RNA component of human telomerase. *Science* 1995; **269**:1236–41.

174 Kim NW, Piatyszek MA, Prowse KR, *et al.* Specific association of human telomerase activity with immortal cells and cancer. *Science* 1994; **266**:2011–15.

175 Langford LA, Piatyszek MA, Xu R, Schold SC, Jr, Shay JW. Telomerase activity in human brain tumours. *Lancet* 1995; **346**:1267–8.

176 Hiraga S, Ohnishi T, Izumoto S, Miyahara E, Kanemura Y, Matsumura H, Arita N. Telomerase activity and alterations in telomere length in human brain tumors. *Cancer Res* 1998; **58**:2117–25.

177 Sano T, Asai A, Mishima K, Fujimaki T, Kirino T. Telomerase activity in 144 brain tumours. *Br J Cancer* 1998; **77**:1633–7.

178 Grosso R, Schiffer D. Prognostic significance of telomerase in brain tumors. *Crit Rev Neurosurg* 1998; **8**:244–7.

179 Langford LA, Piatyszek MA, Xu R, Schold SC, Jr, Wright WE, Shay JW. Telomerase activity in ordinary meningiomas predicts poor outcome. *Hum Pathol* 1997; **28**:416–20.

180 White LK, Wright WE, Shay JW. Telomerase inhibitors. *Trends Biotechnol* 2001; **19**:114–20.

181 Foster BA, Coffey HA, Morin MJ, Rastinejad F. Pharmaco-logical rescue of mutant *p53* confirmation and function. *Science* 1999; **286**:2507–10.

182 Bissell MJ, Radinsky D. Putting tumours in context. *Nat Rev Cancer* 2001; **1**:46–54.

183 Lampson LA. New animal models to probe brain tumor biology, therapy, and immunotherapy: advantages and remaining concerns. *J Neuro-Oncol* 2001; **53**:275–87.

184 Folkman J. Tumor angiogenesis: therapeutic implications. *N Engl J Med* 1971; **285**:1182–6.

Pathology and molecular classification

FELICE GIANGASPERO AND OTMAR D. WIESTLER

Brain tumors in the pediatric age group represent a complex and heterogeneous group of lesions with variable biological behavior. Although neoplasms similar to those in adults can be observed, some specific clinicopathological entities occur predominantly or exclusively in children.

Different classification schemes have been used for primary central nervous system (CNS) tumors in the past. The revised World Health Organization (WHO) classification system for nervous-system tumors represents a major advance in the diagnosis of brain tumors.[1] The classification of brain tumors still relies predominantly on light-microscopic findings, but immunohistochemical and molecular genetics findings have been included as an integral part of the definition of tumor categories. This chapter will follow the WHO guidelines to illustrate the distinct tumor entities in pediatric neuro-oncology (Table 5.1). Neoplasms that occur almost exclusively in adulthood, such as meningeal mesenchymal tumors and lymphomas, will not be discussed.

EMBRYONAL NEOPLASMS

Embryonal tumors represent a large and important portion of CNS tumors in children. They arise from transformation of undifferentiated and immature neuroepithelial cells with divergent capacities for differentiation. The current classification scheme recognizes five tumor entities that can be assigned to this group. Three entities – ependymoblastoma, medulloblastoma, and supratentorial primitive neuroectodermal tumors (PNETs) – have the generic histological features of small round-cell tumors with a variable potential for differentiation. Two other entities – medulloepithelioma and atypical teratoid/ rhabdoid tumor (AT/RT) – exhibit distinct histological features.

Supratentorial primitive neuroectodermal tumors

The term "supratentorial PNET" describes highly malignant embryonal tumors of the cerebral hemispheres that manifest preferentially in children and may differentiate along various neural lineages. Most frequently, these tumors show neuronal and glial differentiation. When advanced neuronal differentiation is present, the terms "cerebral neuroblastoma" and/or "ganglioneuroblastoma" are used.[2] In contrast to medulloblastomas, few studies are available on the cytogenetic and molecular genetic findings in supratentorial PNET. Non-random cytogenetic gains and losses have been reported in two series for a total of 18 cases.[3,4] Germ-line mutations of *TP53* have been demonstrated in hemispheric PNET occurring in two siblings.[5]

Ependymoblastoma

Ependymoblastoma is a rare tumor that usually presents in young children and occurs preferentially in the cerebral

Table 5.1 *World Health Organization grading of central nervous system tumors*

Tumor family	Tumor entity	Grade I	Grade II	Grade III	Grade IV
Astrocytomas	Pilocytic astrocytoma	●			
	Diffuse astrocytoma		●		
	Anaplastic astrocytoma			●	
	Glioblastoma				●
Oligodendrogliomas	Oligodendroglioma		●		
	Anaplastic oligodendroglioma			●	
Mixed gliomas	Oligoastrocytoma		●		
	Anaplastic oligoastrocytoma			●	
Ependymomas	Myxopapillary ependymoma	●			
	Subependymoma	●			
	Ependymoma		●		
	Anaplastic ependymoma			●	
Choroid plexus tumors	Plexus papilloma	●			
	Plexus carcinoma			●	
Glioneuronal/neuronal tumors	Ganglioglioma	●	●		
	DNT	●			
	Central neurocytoma		●		
	Cerebellar liponeurocytoma	●	●		
Pineal neoplasms	Pineocytoma		●		
	Pineoblastoma				●
	Pineal parenchymal tumor of intermediate differentiation			●	
Embryonal tumors	Medulloblastoma				●
	AT/RT				●
	Supratentorial PNET				●
	Neuroblastoma				●
	Ependymoblastoma				●
Tumors of peripheral nerves	Schwannoma	●			
	Neurofibroma	●			
	MPNST			●	●
Tumors of the meninges	Meningioma	●			
	Atypical meningioma		●		
	Clear-cell meningioma		●		
	Chordoid meningioma		●		
	Anaplastic meningioma			●	
	Papillary meningioma			●	
	Rhabdoid meningioma			●	
	Hemangiopericytoma		●	●	

AT/RT, atypical teratoid/rhabdoid tumor; DNT, dysembryoplastic neuroepithelial tumor; MPNST, malignant peripheral nerve sheath tumors; PNET, primitive neuroectodermal tumor.

hemispheres. Its histological appearance is characterized by solidly packed, darkly staining primitive cells forming stratified ependymoblastic rosettes and tubules. These rosettes are commonly pseudostratified with juxtaluminal mitoses. Unlike anaplastic ependymomas, these tumors are composed of relatively uniform, poorly differentiated cells without significant pleomorphism. So far, no significant molecular genetic findings have been reported.[6] An unusual embryonal CNS neoplasm with combined features of both cerebral neuroblastoma and ependymoblastoma has been reported.[7]

Medulloblastoma

Medulloblastoma is the most frequent malignant CNS neoplasm in children. It occurs in the cerebellum. At least 75% of childhood medulloblastomas arise in the vermis and extend into the fourth ventricle. Several histological variants are recognized.[8] *Classic medulloblastoma* is composed of densely packed cells with round to oval or carrot-shaped, highly hyperchromatic nuclei surrounded by scanty cytoplasm (Plate 1). However, round cells with less condensed chromatin are frequently intermingled, and occasionally they form the main population. Neuroblastic rosettes, which consist of tumor-cell nuclei arranged in a circular fashion around tangled cytoplasmic processes, are observed in less than 40% of cases. Occasionally, ganglion cells are seen. Neuroblastic rosettes are frequently associated with marked nuclear polymorphism and high mitotic activity. Although usually numerous, in approximately 25 per cent of cases, mitoses are infrequent. Apoptosis is frequent, whereas geographic areas of necrosis are less common. Pseudopalisading may be observed.

Desmoplastic/nodular medulloblastoma shows nodular, reticulin-free zones ("pale islands") surrounded by densely packed, highly proliferative cells that produce a dense intercellular reticulin fiber network (Plate 1). The nodules exhibit reduced cellularity, a fibrillary matrix, and marked nuclear uniformity. The nuclei of cells between nodules are usually more irregular and hyperchromatic. Medulloblastomas showing only an increased amount of collagenous and reticulin fibers without the nodular pattern are not classified as desmoplastic/nodular variant.

Medulloblastomas with extreme nodularity, intranodular nuclear uniformity, and cell streaming in a fine fibrillary background are also denominated as cerebellar neuroblastoma.[9] The intranodular round cells resemble the neurocytes of central neurocytoma. These neoplasms occur predominantly in children under three years of age. Their extreme nodularity is appreciable by neuroimaging as a nodular, grape-like appearance. Neoplasms of this type occasionally undergo maturation to more differentiated ganglion cell tumors and carry a better prognosis.

The *large-cell/anaplastic variant* represents approximately four per cent of medulloblastomas. It is composed of cells with large, round, and/or pleomorphic nuclei with prominent nucleoli. Large areas of necrosis, high mitotic activity, and high apoptotic rate are common findings.[10–12]

Very rare variants are the medullomyoblastoma[12,13] and the melanotic medulloblastoma.[14] The former contains neoplastic cells with skeletal muscle differentiation, while the latter shows melanin-containing pigmented cells.

The most common specific chromosomal abnormality in medulloblastomas, present in about 50 per cent of cases, is isochromosome 17q [i(17q)]. Isochromosome 17q has been demonstrated in interphase nuclei using fluorescence *in situ* hybridization (FISH). Although i(17q) accounts for 17p loss in most medulloblastomas, in a small number of cases partial or complete loss of 17p occurs through interstitial deletion, unbalanced translocation, or monosomy 17.[4,15]

Chromosome 1 is also involved frequently in medulloblastoma. The types of abnormality are variable, including unbalanced translocations, deletions, and duplications. In contrast to the chromosome 17 defects, rearrangements of chromosome 1 often result in trisomy 1q without loss of the p-arm.[4]

Studies using comparative genomic hybridization (CGH) have demonstrated a greater degree of genomic imbalance in medulloblastoma than recognized previously. Among other non-random changes, the most frequently observed were losses on chromosomes 10q (41 per cent) and 11 (41 per cent), and gain of chromosome 7 (44 per cent).[16]

In most samples of medulloblastoma with double minutes, amplification of *c-myc* or, less often, the *N-myc* gene has been found. The true incidence of *myc* gene amplification is difficult to determine in these tumors because the observed incidence differs according to the method of analysis. However, a recent analysis by CGH suggested that it may be as high as 20 per cent. Interestingly, the large-cell/anaplastic variant shows a high incidence of *c-myc* amplification.[11,12]

Studies for loss of heterozygosity (LOH) by both restriction fragment length polymorphism (RFLP) and microsatellite analysis have shown loss of genetic material on the chromosomal arm 17p in 30–45 per cent of cases as the most frequent molecular genetic alteration in medulloblastomas.[17] This indicates a medulloblastoma-related tumor suppressor gene located on chromosome 17p that has not yet been identified. As *TP53* is located on 17p13 and is mutated in a variety of human tumors, this gene was initially considered as a candidate gene. However, *TP53* mutations have been demonstrated in only a small subset of medulloblastomas (five to ten per cent of cases).[18–20]

Another putative tumor suppressor locus maps to the long arm of chromosome 9q31, where allelic losses have been described in 10–18 per cent of cases.[21,22] The *PATCHED* gene, which is affected in the nevoid basal cell carcinoma syndrome (NBCCS), has been identified as the target on 9q.[23] Patients with NBCCS are predisposed to develop basal cell carcinoma and medulloblastomas mainly of the desmoplastic/nodular variant.[22] Inactivating germ-line mutations in the human homolog of the *Drosophila* segment polarity gene *patched*, *PTCH*, have been demonstrated in NBCCS. Inactivating mutations of the *PTCH* gene have been identified in sporadic medulloblastomas by several groups.[24–26] LOH 9q and *PTCH* mutations are more frequent in desmoplastic-type medulloblastomas.[24] However, a mutated *PTCH* gene may also be observed in occasional tumors with classic histology.[25,26] Most mutations appear to cause truncated proteins. It is believed that inactivation of *PTCH* results in activation of the growth-related *hedgehog/patched* pathway and may lead to inappropriate proliferation of cerebellar progenitor cells.[27,28] These data raise the intriguing possibility that developmental control genes play an essential role in the pathogenesis of medulloblastoma.

Medulloblastomas and colorectal neoplasms are among the major manifestations in patients with the Turcot syndrome. Germ-line mutations of the *APC* gene are responsible for this condition. Mutations of the *APC* and *beta-catenin* genes, both of which activate the Wnt pathway, have been shown to be present in approximately 13 per cent of sporadic medulloblastomas.[29–31]

Cell-biological studies have provided evidence that the two major subtypes of medulloblastoma, i.e. classical and desmoplastic/nodular medulloblastoma, originate from distinct cerebellar precursors. A periventricular progenitor cell appears to give rise to the classic form, whereas the desmoplastic/nodular form arises from external granular cells.[32,33]

Medulloepithelioma

Medulloepithelioma is a very rare embryonal tumor of the CNS. Most reported cases occur in children within the first five years of life in both supra- and infratentorial compartments. The histologic hallmark of this neoplasm is a mitotically active, pseudostratified columnar epithelium arranged in ribbons and tubules with invariable interposition of stromal elements.[34,35] These structures recapitulate the primitive epithelium of the neural tube (Plate 2). Immunohistochemical studies have shown abundant vimentin-like, nestin-like, insulin-like, and fibroblast growth factors. Glial fibrillary acid protein (GFAP), beta-III-tubulin, and neurofilaments are not usually expressed.[35]

Atypical teratoid/rhaboid tumor

AT/RT constitutes a highly malignant neoplasm with a complex and variable histology occurring predominantly in children under three years of age. It is composed of rhabdoid cells with undifferentiated, epithelial-like, and mesenchymal components, and with immunoreactivity for GFAP, cytokeratins, synaptophysin, chromogranin, and smooth-muscle actin (Plate 3). AT/RTs can occur at any location along the neuroaxis, but they occur most frequently in the cerebellum, cerebral hemisphere, and cerebellopontine angle.[36,37] When involving the cerebellum, this neoplasm has to be differentiated from medulloblastoma.[37] In previous studies, many of these neoplasms have been classified as medulloblastoma or PNET. Their distinction is, however, of great importance, since AT/RT carries a poor prognosis compared with medulloblastoma. Ninety per cent of AT/RTs demonstrate monosomy or deletion of chromosome 22. The gene involved in AT/RTs, *hSNF5/INI1*, maps to chromosome band 22q11.2. The INI1 protein is a component of the mammalian SWI/SNF complex, which functions in an ATP-dependent manner to alter chromatin structure. Somatic mutations or intragenic deletions have been documented in the majority of cases, most of which create a novel stop codon.[38,39] Germ-line INI1 mutations have been detected in patients with a combination of AT/RT of the brain and renal rhabdoid tumor.[38]

GLIAL NEOPLASMS

Astrocytoma

A useful distinction for this group of neoplasms is to differentiate diffuse astrocytomas (fibrillary astrocytoma, anaplastic astrocytoma, glioblastoma) from other astrocytic tumors (pilocytic astrocytoma, pleomorphic xanthoastrocytoma, subependymal giant-cell astrocytoma).[40,41]

Diffuse astrocytomas represent a continuous morphologic spectrum of differentiation and tumor grades. They are graded according to the WHO classification as well-differentiated astrocytoma (WHO grade II), anaplastic astrocytoma (WHO grade III), and glioblastoma multiforme (GBM; WHO grade IV). The WHO grading system is based on the presence of atypia, hypercellularity, mitoses, vascular proliferation, and necrosis.[41] Compared with astrocytomas occurring in adults, diffuse astrocytic neoplasms in children tend to be of high grade and are located more frequently in the brainstem (Plate 4). Moreover, histological grading of malignant variants (WHO grade III versus WHO grade IV) may not be as significant in terms of survival in children as in adults. Malignant astrocytomas in children appear to differ from adult glioblastomas in a number of ways, the most significant being the general absence of a preceding low-grade astrocytoma. Indeed, most low-grade astrocytomas in children do not progress to high-grade tumors, unlike in adults.[42]

High-grade pediatric astrocytomas also show different molecular genetics alterations compared with adult counterparts. Molecular genetic studies have defined at least three different subtypes among adult glioblastomas.[43] One subtype carries mutations of the *TP53* gene associated with immunohistochemically detectable p53 protein but lacks amplification and overexpression of the *EGFR* gene. This type can develop as secondary GBM, which derives from a preceding low-grade astrocytoma. A second subtype lacks mutations in the *TP53* gene but shows amplification and overexpression of the *EGFR* gene and often exhibits homologous deletions of the *p16^{INK4a}* gene and mutations of the *PTEN/MMAC1* gene on chromosome 10. This genetic profile characterizes the primary or de novo GBM. A third subtype is recognized that contains both *TP53* mutations and amplification and overexpression of the *EGFR* gene. This molecular variant may display the histologic appearance of giant-cell GBM.[44]

Molecular genetic studies in pediatric high-grade astrocytomas have shown that although glioblastomas in children usually arise de novo, their genetic profile is more similar to secondary GBM, with a high rate of *TP53* mutations (40–90 per cent of cases), very low incidence of amplification of the *EGFR* gene (zero to six per cent of cases), and low frequency of *p16^{INK4a}* deletions (13 per cent of cases).[45–47] Malignant astrocytomas in young children (under three years old) show a significant lower frequency of *TP53* mutations compared with older children.[48]

Pilocytic astrocytomas represent the most common glioma entity in children. They occur in the cerebellum, optic pathway, hypothalamus, brainstem, and basal ganglia. i.e. in midline structures. Radiographically, they often present as contrast-enhancing, solid, or cystic lesions. It is very important to distinguish this lesion from diffuse astrocytoma, because the two entities differ greatly in their clinical behavior. Histologically, pilocytic astrocytomas are composed of fusiform, piloid astrocytes disposed in both compact and loosely structured areas. Rosenthal fibers and eosinophilic granular bodies are histological hallmarks (Plate 5).

Pilomyxoid astrocytoma, a newly described entity of uncertain relationship to the pilocytic group, develops as a suprasellar neoplasm, mostly in infants under three years of age.[49] The term "pilomyxoid astrocytoma" indicates the presence of a mucinous background and piloid features. These tumors lack a biphasic architecture, Rosenthal fibers, and granular bodies, but they may show prominent angiocentric architectures (Plate 6). Mitoses are more frequent than in classic pilocytic astrocytoma. Additional studies are required to demonstrate whether the pilomyxoid variant really constitutes a distinct clinicopathological entity with a less favorable outcome.

In general, pilocytic astrocytomas are associated with a benign clinical course and carry a favorable prognosis. However, there is increasing evidence for more aggressive variants.[50–52] Criteria for atypical subtypes need to be defined. Rare disseminated forms are observed in infants carrying large hypothalamochiasmatic tumors.[53] Regression has been reported in neurofibromatosis type 1 (NF-1) patients.[54,55]

Cytogenetic studies of pilocytic astrocytomas have revealed either a normal karyotype or a variety of aberrations. No distinct pattern suggesting loss of a particular tumor suppressor gene has been identified.[56] However, CGH analyses in a large number of cases have shown various chromosomal imbalances, with gains and deletions on chromosome 19 and gains on chromosome 22 being the most common change observed.[57]

In contrast to the diffuse astrocytomas, mutations of the *TP53* gene, *CDKN2A* deletion, *EGFR* amplification, and *PTEN* mutations are absent or very rare in pilocytic astrocytoma.[58] About 20 per cent of sporadic pilocytic astrocytomas may show a loss of chromosome 17q, which includes the region encoding the *NF-1* gene.[59] However, screening of the *NF-1* gene in sporadic tumors has failed to detect mutations. Its role in pilocytic astrocytomas remains uncertain.[60]

Pleomorphic xanthoastrocytoma is a superficial lesion occurring in children and young adults. Histopathologically, it is characterized by the presence of large, bizarre cells with multiple nuclei and abundant, often foamy cytoplasm (Plate 7). A prominent intercellular reticulin network can be observed particularly in superficial, subarachnoid parts of the tumor. It reflects the presence of basal lamina material at the ultrastructural level. Mitoses are absent or rare and the MIB1 labeling index is usually below two per cent. In contrast to their pleomorphic histological appearance, pleomorphic xanthoastrocytomas are frequently associated with a benign clinical course. For lesions with high mitotic activity (five or more mitoses per ten high-power fields (HPFs)) and/or with foci of necrosis, the designation "pleomorphic xanthoastrocytoma with anaplastic features" has been proposed.[61] It is not yet established completely whether such tumors with anaplastic features display a more aggressive behavior. *TP53* mutation appears to be an uncommon genetic event and does not appear to be involved in tumor progression. This suggests that the genetic pathways in pleomorphic xanthoastrocytomas are different from those observed in diffuse astrocytomas.[62]

Subependymal giant-cell astrocytoma represents a well-demarcated, intraventricular tumor composed of large, epithelioid cells with features ranging from gemistocytes to ganglion cells. Such cells may show immunohistochemical features of both glial and neuronal lineages, with expression of S-100, beta-III tubulin, and neurofilaments. This benign neoplasm usually occurs in the setting of tuberous sclerosis.[63]

Oligodendroglioma

Oligodendrogliomas are well-differentiated tumors that develop predominantly in the cerebral hemispheres in adults. Histologically, they are composed of tumor cells with round nuclei and clear cytoplasm, which tend to form honeycomb architectures. Additional features include calcifications, mucoid degeneration, and a dense network (chicken wire) of branching capillaries. Marked nuclear atypia and occasional mitoses are compatible with the diagnosis of WHO grade II, but significant mitotic activity, prominent microvascular proliferation, or necrosis indicates a progression to anaplastic oligodendroglioma WHO grade III.[64] In contrast to most other gliomas, specific immunohistochemical markers for oligodendrogliomas are not available.

Molecular genetic alterations in oligodendrogliomas are quite distinct form those accompanying the development of astrocytomas. Losses of chromosome 1p and 19q are the aberrations observed most commonly in oligodendrogliomas, occurring in approximately 40–75 per cent of these tumors.[65] Despite the apparently different molecular genetic events that accompany early oligodendroglial transformation as compared with astrocytic tumors, malignant progression in oligodendroglioma may be associated with 9p and 10 deletions, similar to anaplastic astrocytomas and glioblastomas. An important relationship between the molecular genetic profile and chemotherapeutic response has been established in oligodendrogliomas. High-grade oligodendrogliomas with 1p allelic deletions show chemosensitivity and carry a better prognosis, whereas homozygous deletions of the *CDKN2A* gene on chromosome 9p (p16) appear to predict an unfavorable outcome.[66] Mutations of *TP53* may occur in oligodendrogliomas but are much less frequent compared with astrocytic neoplasms.[58]

Only a few pediatric series of oligodendrogliomas have been reported, and none of these included a molecular characterization.[67,68] Taking into account that oligodendroglioma-like features can be observed in various tumor entities, such as clear-cell ependymoma, pilocytic astrocytoma, neurocytoma, ganglioglioneurocytoma (extraventricular neurocytoma), and dysembryoplastic neuroepithelial tumor (DNT), and that most of these entities occur primarily in children, it cannot be ruled out that oligodendroglioma tends to be overdiagnosed in the pediatric population. The true incidence in the pediatric age group remains to be determined.

Ependymomas

Ependymomas represent eight to ten per cent of intracranial tumors in childhood. They are classified histologically into four major subtypes: myxopapillary, subependymomas, ependymomas, and anaplastic ependymomas. Myxopapillary ependymomas and subependymomas are rare in children.[69] Myxopapillary ependymomas occur primarily in the region of the filum terminale, while subependymomas are intraventricular lesions. Most subependymomas are incidental tumors discovered at autopsy, but occasionally they can become symptomatic. After surgical resection, long-term prognosis is excellent. Anaplastic progression does not usually develop in these entities. Myxopapillary ependymomas and subependymomas are considered to be WHO grade I.[70]

Ependymomas may occur at any site of the ventricular system and in the spinal canal. In children, the most frequent localization is the fourth ventricle. Histologically, the classic ependymoma manifests as a moderately cellular neoplasm with distinct perivascular pseudorosettes (Plate 8). Additional, less common features include ependymal rosettes and tubular structures termed "ependymal canals." Histological variants have been defined as cellular, papillary, tanycytic, and clear-cells ependymomas.

According to the WHO grading system, ependymomas can be separated into ependymoma WHO grade II and anaplastic ependymoma WHO grade III.[70,71] In several studies, only a loose correlation has been reported between histological appearance and clinical outcome. The exact definition of anaplastic ependymoma is controversial. In the current WHO classification, anaplastic ependymomas are characterized by high mitotic activity and the presence of a highly cellular, poorly differentiated component.[71] Vascular proliferation and necrosis are of uncertain significance. The validity of this novel grading system has to be confirmed in future clinicopathological studies.

The most frequent cytogenetic change, observed in 30 per cent of ependymomas, is monosomy 22. Less frequent are abnormalities of chromosomes 9q, 10, 17, and 13.[72,73]

An analysis of 62 ependymomas for LOH 22q and LOH 10q and for mutations of the *NF-2* and *PTEN* tumor suppressor genes revealed six cases with mutant neurofibromatosis type 2 (NF-2), all of which were located in the spinal cord.[72] This suggests that spinal ependymomas constitute a distinct molecular variant. Genes involved in cerebral ependymomas remain largely unknown.

Choroid plexus neoplasms

These neoplasms are derived from the choroid plexus and display a morphologic spectrum from very well differentiated papillomas to frankly anaplastic tumors with minimal epithelial differentiation. Tumors with intermediate or atypical appearance can occur de novo or during anaplastic transformation.[74]

Choroid plexus neoplasms in children usually arise within the lateral ventricle; less frequently, they may occur in the third ventricle. Papillomas may produce hydrocephalus by secreting cerebrospinal fluid (CSF) and through obstruction of the ventricular system.[75]

The vast majority of choroid plexus tumors are papillomas and correspond to WHO grade I. They exhibit papillae composed of a single layer of columnar epithelium resting on a fibrovascular stalk. These tumors usually show a well-formed continuous basement membrane. Mitotic figures are absent or very rare. Occasionally, the epithelial cells may contain a large number of mitochondria, which results in an oncocytic phenotype. Bone and cartilaginous metaplasia may be present in rare cases.

Lesions exhibiting significant cytologic atypia, scattered mitoses, and nests of cells that have broken through the basement membrane into the stroma have been designated as atypical choroid plexus papilloma.[75]

Anaplastic choroid plexus papillomas or choroid plexus carcinomas (both synonymous and WHO grade III) display unequivocal signs of cytologic and histological malignancy. These neoplasms present as highly cellular lesions with multilayered epithelia, complex glandular structures, and cribriform arrangements. Papillae are usually poorly formed or completely absent. Large necrotic areas and invasion of the adjacent brain are often observed.

Immunohistochemically, choroid plexus neoplasms express cytokeratins, S-100, protein and occasionally GFAP. Transthyretin (pre-albumin) has been evaluated as a marker for normal and neoplastic choroid plexus epithelia. However, as many as 20 per cent of choroid plexus papillomas are negative, and other brain tumors as well as metastatic carcinomas may be positive.

Benign choroid plexus papillomas may seed along the CSF compartment. Usually, such foci are detectable only at the microscopic level and are clinically asymptomatic. In contrast, choroid plexus carcinoma may produce frank metastases along CSF pathways.

Choroid plexus neoplasms occasionally occur in the setting of Li–Fraumeni syndrome, which is caused by a *TP53* germ-line mutation.[76] However, no *TP53* mutations have been detected in sporadic choroid plexus tumors.

Classical cytogenetics and FISH analysis have demonstrated hyperdiploidy, with gains particularly on chromosomes 7, 9, 12, 15, 17, and 18.[77] INI1 mutations have been reported in cases of choroid plexus carcinoma.[78,79]

NEURONAL AND GLIONEURONAL TUMORS

Ganglioglioma

These are benign neoplasms (WHO grade I) composed of dysplastic ganglion cells and a variable astrocytoma component. They may occur throughout the CNS. The majority are supratentorial and involve the temporal lobe. Affected patients frequently have a history of long-standing temporal lobe epilepsy.[80,81] Rare cases with anaplastic changes of the glial component have been reported.[82]

A variant of ganglioglioma is the papillary glioneuronal tumor. This is characterized by the formation of pseudopapillary architectures with a single layer of pseudostratified, small, cuboidal cells arranged around hyalinized blood vessels. A second component of this tumor contains sheets of neurocytes and ganglion cells. It remains to be demonstrated whether the papillary glioneuronal tumor constitutes a separate entity.[83–85]

Central neurocytoma

Central neurocytoma occurs predominantly in the lateral ventricle in the region of the foramen of Monro.

It develops mostly in young adults, but cases in the pediatric age group have been reported. Histologically, neurocytoma is composed of a uniform population of cells with round to oval nuclei and a finely speckled chromatin. The cytoplasm is usually clear, conferring an oligodendroglioma-like appearance. The cells are embedded in a conspicuously fibrillated neuropil matrix. Microcalcification and perivascular rosettes can be seen. The latter led to the original classification as "foramen Monroi ependymoma." Rarely, brisk mitotic activity, necrosis, and endothelial proliferation can be observed. The neuronal nature of the tumor is confirmed by immunohistochemistry for synaptophysin and other neuronal proteins. Ultrastructural features, such as clear and dense-core granules, cellular processes with microtubular arrays, and synapses, document the neuronal origin of the neoplastic cells.[86,87] In general, central neurocytoma carries a very favorable prognosis. It corresponds to WHO grade II. Occasional neurocytomas with a higher Ki-67/Mib1 labeling index (greater than two per cent) show a higher recurrence rate.[88] Extraventricular location of neurocytic neoplasms has also been reported.[89]

Desmoplastic infantile ganglioglioma and astrocytoma

Both neoplasms are related closely and may represent a spectrum of a single entity.[90] They occur in children under two years of age, with a mean age of seven months. Both tumors involve superficial cortex and leptomeninges and are often attached to the dura. The radiological appearance is that of a large cyst with an overlying solid, contrast-enhancing component. Histopathological features include neuroepithelial and fibroblastic elements intermingled with reticulin fibers and collagen deposits. The neuroepithelial component shows a variable proportion of astrocytes and neuronal cells. In desmoplastic infantile astrocytomas, this component is limited to the glial cell population. The neuronal elements range from atypical ganglioid cells to small polygonal cell types. Immunohistochemical detection of synaptophysin and/or neurofilaments facilitates the identification of the neuronal cell population. In addition, these tumors may contain a population of more primitive cells. Such an undifferentiated cell component is present in both tumor types and may predominate in some areas. In such areas, mitoses and microscopic necroses can be observed. Despite the ambiguous histology, the prognosis of desmoplastic infantile ganglioglioma/astrocytoma is very good; therefore, it corresponds to WHO grade I. Molecular genetic studies have demonstrated that in contrast to diffuse astrocytomas, desmoplastic infantile astrocytomas do not display allelic loss on chromosomes 17p and 10 and do not carry *TP53* gene mutations.[91]

Dysembryoplastic neuroepithelial tumor

DNT is a benign glioneuronal neoplasm characterized by a multinodular architecture and a predominant intracortical location. It usually occurs in the first two decades of life. Seizures of the partial or complex type are the most important symptom. DNTs are usually supratentorial and located most frequently in the temporal lobe. Rare cases involving the basal ganglia have been described. Magnetic resonance imaging (MRI) shows the cortical location of the lesion better than CT scanning. These tumors are hypointense in T1-weighted images and hyperintense on T2. Peritumoral edema and mass effect are absent. Histologically, DNT exhibits a multinodular architecture; the nodules are composed of oligodendrocyte-like cells with abundant intercellular mucin mixed with astrocytes and small neurons, which typically appear to "float" in a mucoid matrix (Plate 9). Tumor cells tend to be arranged in a columnar fashion. The cortex surrounding DNT displays disorganization of the histoarchitecture and loss of normal lamination (cortical dysplasia). A glioneuronal nature of this lesion is not only confirmed by the presence of mature neurons as an essential component; immunohistochemical and ultrastructural studies suggest that the oligodendrocyte-like elements are capable of divergent glial/neuronal differentiation.[92] Significant cellular atypia is absent in DNT, but occasionally mitoses can be observed. Proliferative indexes evaluated with Ki67/Mib1 are generally low (less than one per cent). Patients with NF-1 may rarely develop DNT.[93,94]

According to the WHO classification, a classical and a complex variant of DNT can be distinguished. The complex form exhibits a glioma-like component in addition to the characteristic DNT element. A definitive diagnosis of DNT based only on histological criteria can be very difficult on non-representative or fragmented minute specimens, where it may mimic low-grade gliomas, particularly oligodendrogliomas. The diagnosis of DNT should be taken into consideration when the following clinicoradiological criteria are present: (i) partial seizures beginning before age 20 years; (ii) absence of a progressive neurological deficit; (iii) predominant cortical topography on MRI; and (iv) no mass effect, except if related to a cyst, and no peritumoral edema. DNTs are associated with a very favorable prognosis, even after subtotal resection, and correspond histologically to WHO grade I.

PINEAL PARENCHYMAL TUMORS

Tumors deriving from pineocytes account for 11–28 per cent of pineal-region tumors in children. The current WHO classification distinguishes three entities, ranging from the highly malignant *pineoblastoma* (WHO grade IV) composed of primitive immature cells to the well-differentiated *pineocytoma* (WHO grade II). The third group, *pineal parenchymal tumors of intermediate differentiation*, comprises tumors with intermediate morphological and clinical properties.[94]

Other neoplasms located in the pineal area but not originating from pineocytes or their precursors include astrocytomas, in particular pilocytic astrocytomas and germ-cell tumors.

Pineoblastoma

Pineoblastomas account for approximately 3–17 per cent of pineal region tumors in children. They may develop at any age, but they occur predominantly in the first decade of life, with a male/female ratio of two to one. Pineoblastomas are highly cellular neoplasms composed of small, poorly differentiated, and pleomorphic cells arranged in patternless sheets. Formation of Homer–Wright or Flexner–Wintersteiner rosettes can be observed in some cases. The latter indicate an ontogenetic origin from the human pineal gland as a photoreceptor organ.[94,95] Rarely, a papillary pattern may be seen. The immunophenotype of pineoblastoma reflects the neuronal and photoreceptor differentiation with immunoreactivity for synaptophysin, neurofilaments, and retinal S-antigen. Compared with other PNETs, synaptophysin expression is usually prominent. Pineoblastomas are highly aggressive neoplasms and correspond histologically to WHO grade IV.

Occasionally, pineoblastomas may be encountered in patients with familial (bilateral) retinoblastoma, a condition termed trilateral retinoblastoma syndrome. A single case of pineoblastoma has also been reported in a patient with familiar adenomatous polyposis. Molecular genetic studies have, so far, not shown any specific alterations.

Pineocytoma

Pineocytomas are generally more common in adults than children; however, there is a wide variation of age at presentation (11–78 years). These neoplasms present as well-demarcated masses compressing adjacent structures.[94–96] Histologically, they are composed of small, uniform cells surrounding delicately fibrillated anuclear areas termed pineocytomatous rosettes, which probably represent pineocytic maturation of neoplastic cells. Such structures are readily apparent with synaptophysin immunostaining. The prognosis of pineocytomas is usually favorable following successful gross surgical removal. Pineocytomas correspond histologically to WHO grade II. In small surgical specimens, the distinction of pineocytoma and pineal parenchyma with reactive changes may pose considerable problems.

Pineal parenchymal tumor of intermediate differentiation

The morphologic features of this entity are intermediate between those of pineocytoma and pineoblastoma, i.e. high cellularity with mild nuclear atypia, rare mitoses, and absence of pineocytomatous rosettes. Such neoplasms constitute approximately ten per cent of all pineal parenchymal tumors. They occur at all ages, from young children to adults, with a higher prevalence in adults. The clinical behavior of these tumors is variable.[95,96] Few cases have been associated with CSF dissemination. Although not assigned specifically in the WHO classification, the biological behavior corresponds to that of a WHO grade III tumor.

MENINGIOMAS

Although common in adults, meningiomas are rare in children. The reported incidence in pediatric brain tumor series is less than two per cent. Most meningiomas are benign and can be graded as WHO grade I. Certain subtypes are associated with a greater likelihood of recurrence and/or aggressive behavior and correspond to WHO grades II and III. In children, there is a tendency towards more aggressive forms of meningiomas.[97–100]

Several variants of meningiomas have been described, reflecting the mesenchymal and epithelial histogenetic potential of arachnoid cells.[99] Meningothelial and transitional meningiomas constitute the most typical phenotype of these tumors, characterized by groups of cells with poorly defined cell borders forming characteristic whorls and by psammoma bodies. The cells contain nuclei with finely distributed chromatin and inconspicuous nucleoli. A mesenchymal appearance of arachnoid cells can be seen in fibrous (fibroblastic), angiomatous, and metaplastic meningiomas, whereas epithelial features predominate in the microcystic, secretory, clear-cell, chordoid, and papillary variants. Clear-cell and chordoid meningiomas behave more aggressively. Clear-cell meningiomas are composed of polygonal cells with a clear cytoplasm filled with glycogen. These meningiomas may occur at a very young age in the lumbar region. Familial occurrence in a mother and child with spinal location has been reported. Chordoid meningiomas display histological features similar to those observed in chordomas, with ribbons of eosinophilic, vacuolated cells in a mucoid background.[101] This variant must be distinguished from chordoma and chordoid glioma. Immunohistochemical features of meningiomas are consistent with the dual mesenchymal and epithelial nature of arachnoid cells. Vimentin is expressed consistently. Immunoreactivity for S-100 protein is variable and present in about 50 per cent of cases. Epithelial membrane antigen (EMA) is usually expressed. Its pattern of immunoreactivity can be focal or diffuse.

The WHO classification includes atypical meningioma (WHO grade II) as variant, with a biological behavior intermediate between the classical benign (WHO grade I) and the anaplastic meningioma (WHO grade III). Histologic criteria for atypical meningiomas include increased mitotic activity (four or more mitoses per ten HPFs) or three of the following features: hypercellularity, diffuse or sheet-like growth, prominent nucleoli, and foci of necrosis.[99,102]

Brain invasion may occur in histologically benign, atypical, or malignant meningiomas. The presence of brain invasion is associated with a greater likelihood of recurrence. Brain-invasive, histologically benign meningiomas have a clinical course similar to atypical meningiomas. In children, meningioangiomatosis can occur in association with a meningioma and may mimic brain invasion. Meningioangiomatosis represents a malformative lesion composed of superficial and intracortical, often perivascular, aggregates of meningothelial cells and vascular channels. This entity presents sporadically or in a hereditary setting, such as NF-2. It has been suggested that the relative high frequency of brain invasion observed in pediatric series of meningiomas may be attributed to the presence of this unrecognized association.[103]

Anaplastic (malignant) meningiomas (WHO grade III) differ from atypical meningioma by the presence of advanced histological features of malignancy, such as very high mitotic index (20 or more mitoses per ten HPFs) or morphological patterns reminiscent of sarcoma, carcinoma, or melanoma.[104] In addition, WHO grade III has been assigned to the two meningioma subtypes papillary meningioma and rhabdoid meningioma.

Papillary meningioma is a rare variant that occurs more frequently in children than in adults and has a high propensity for recurrence and for the development of distant metastases.[105,106] Accordingly, papillary meningiomas correspond to WHO grade III. Histologically, this tumor appears highly cellular and composed of epithelial-like cells with well-defined cellular borders. Tumor cells are frequently arranged in papillary structures around blood vessels (Plate 10). High mitotic activity and brain invasion are common. Although the papillary pattern may be predominant, areas with a classic meningothelial appearance can usually be found.

Rhabdoid meningiomas constitute rare neoplasms that contain a significant proportion of rhabdoid cells, i.e. cells with abundant eosinophilic cytoplasm, eccentric nuclei, and hyaline paranuclear inclusions. The presence of this component indicates a highly aggressive biologic behavior and results in the grading as WHO grade III meningioma. In the largest reported series (15 cases), there was only a single case of rhabdoid meningioma in a child, who experienced multiple recurrences for a period of 17 years.[107]

The most consistent cytogenetic change in meningiomas involves allelic imbalance or losses of chromosome 22, indicating that this chromosome harbors a meningioma-associated gene. In general, karyotypic and molecular genetic abnormalities are more extensive in atypical and malignant meningiomas. LOH for loci on chromosome 22q has been demonstrated in 40–80 per cent of sporadic meningiomas, and this correlates with mutations of the *NF-2* gene in more than 60 per cent of sporadic cases.[108] *NF-2* mutations are significantly less common in the meningothelial subtype compared with fibrous meningiomas. Allelic losses on chromosomes 1, 10, and 14 appear to be associated with atypical features and malignant progression.[109]

GERM-CELL TUMORS

Germ-cell tumors of the CNS comprise a group of rare neoplasms that occur primarily during childhood and adolescence. They tend to arise in midline structures, including pineal and sellar regions, the third ventricle, and the hypothalamus, but only rarely in the spinal cord. The histogenesis and classification of germ-cell tumors in the CNS are considered analogous to those of their gonadal and extragonadal counterparts.[110] *Germinomas* are the prevalent entity in the suprasellar compartment and basal ganglionic/thalamic regions. Non-germinomatous germ-cell tumors appear to predominate at other sites. Multifocal germ-cell tumors usually involve the pineal region and suprasellar compartment simultaneously or sequentially. Bilateral basal ganglia and thalamic lesions have also been reported.[111]

Germinomas

Germinomas constitute the most frequent germ-cell tumor of the CNS. They are composed of polygonal cells with large, vesicular nuclei and prominent nucleoli. Tumor cells can be separated by a fibrovascular stroma infiltrated by small lymphocytes, principally of T-cell origin (Plate 11). Some tumors show a very prominent lymphoid reaction, which may mask neoplastic elements in the biopsy material. Some germinomas exhibit a striking granulomatous reaction, which should not be misinterpreted as sarcoidosis or tuberculosis. Immunostaining for placental alkaline phosphatase (PLAP) identifies the neoplastic germ cells. Otherwise, typical germinomas may contain syncytiotrophoblastic giant cells that display cytoplasmic immunolabeling for beta-human chorionic gonadotrophin (β-HCG). The presence of such cells does not modify the biologic behavior and radiosensitivity of germinomas.

In contrast, mixed germ-cell tumors with a prominent germinoma component and additional elements of yolk-sac tumor or embryonal carcinoma carry a significantly less favorable prognosis. Immunohistochemical reactions for alpha-fetoprotein and cytokeratin can be helpful to identify minor non-germinomatous portions.

Embryonal carcinoma and yolk–sac tumors (endodermal sinus tumors)

Embryonal carcinomas and yolk-sac tumors are among the most primitive germ-cell neoplasms. The *yolk-sac tumor* is composed of cuboidal/columnar epithelial cells arranged in tubules and papillary structures, and exhibits a delicate connective stroma with capillary-sized vessels. Schiller–Duval bodies and periodic acid–Schiff (PAS)-positive hyaline globules are usually present. Cytoplasmic immunoreactivity for alpha-fetoprotein in the epithelial component can be useful in distinguishing this neoplasm from germinoma and embryonal carcinoma. The hyaline globules also stain positively for this developmental antigen.

Embryonal carcinoma presents as a less differentiated tumor. It displays patternless sheets of cells with large, vesicular nuclei and prominent nucleoli. Embryoid-body-like aggregates may occur. The neoplastic cells show dense and diffuse cytoplasmic labeling for cytokeratins, distinguishing these neoplasms from germinomas.

Choriocarcinomas

Pure choriocarcinomas develop in the CNS only rarely. However, syncytiotrophoblastic and cytotrophoblastic elements may be observed as components of other germ-cell tumors. Histologically, choriocarcinoma is characterized by a combination of syncytiotrophoblastic and cytotrophoblastic elements surrounded by sinusoidal vessels. Syncytiotrophoblastic giant cells show strong immunoreactivity for β-HCG.

Teratomas

Teratomas are tumors composed of a mixture of tissues derived from all three germinal layers. They account for approximately 0.5 per cent of all intracranial neoplasms and occur more frequently in males, preferentially involving the pineal region. As in the gonadal and extragonadal examples, three variants can be distinguished. *Mature teratomas* exclusively show fully differentiated, adult-type tissue of ectodermal, mesodermal, and endodermal origin. The more common ectodermal components encountered in such tumors include skin, brain, and choroid plexus. Mesodermal tissues include cartilage, bone, fat, and muscle. Cysts lined by epithelia of respiratory or enteric type constitute typical endodermal features.

Immature teratomas are characterized by incompletely differentiated components resembling fetal tissues. Hypercellular and mitotically active stroma, reminiscent of embryonic mesenchyme, and primitive neuroectodermal elements that resemble the developing neural tube, such as neuroepithelial rosettes and tubular structures, often predominate. Melanin-pigmented neuroepithelium indicates retinal differentiation. Immature intracranial teratomas may undergo spontaneous differentiation into fully mature tissue. Complete maturation can also be observed in specimens from patients whose immature teratomas or mixed germ-cell tumors have been subject to radio- and/or chemotherapy.[112] Such maturation presumably reflects the selective treatment sensitivity of the more actively proliferating immature components. Occasionally, teratomas may harbor an additional malignant element with features of a distinct malignant neoplasm. Such tumors are termed *teratoma with malignant transformation*. The most frequent malignant somatic components are rhabdomyosarcoma or undifferentiated sarcoma, and less frequently squamous cell carcinoma and enteric-type adenocarcinoma.[111]

Intracranial germ-cell tumors have been observed in patients with Klinefelter syndrome, which is characterized by a 47 XXY genotype. Such patients also carry an increased risk for mediastinal germ-cell tumors as well as for mammary carcinoma. Germ-cell tumors frequently exhibit additional X chromosomes. The susceptibility of Klinefelter syndrome patients to such tumors could result from the increased dosage of an X-chromosome-associated gene. Individuals with Down syndrome, which show a higher incidence of testicular germ-cell tumors, have also been reported to develop intracranial germ-cell tumors more frequently. Few case reports have documented germ-cell tumors in the setting of NF-1. Rarely, patients with germ-cell tumors of the CNS have been reported to develop secondary gonadal germ-cell tumors, suggesting that some individuals bear an increased general risk for the development of germ-cell neoplasms.[113]

Cytogenetic abnormalities in CNS germ-cell tumors appear similar to those reported in morphologically homologous tumors of the testis and other extracranial sites. Such abnormalities involve the X chromosome, alterations of chromosome 1 resulting in additional copies of the 1q21-1qter region, and a high incidence of numerical and structural anomalies affecting chromosome 12 such as chromosome 12p duplication (isochromosome 12p), a specific marker found in approximately 80 per cent of testicular and mediastinal germ-cell tumors.[114]

Molecular genetic analyses performed in a few cases have reported a low incidence of *TP53* gene mutations.[115]

Craniopharyngioma

Craniopharyngiomas are epithelial tumors of the sellar region, presumably derived from Rathke pouch epithelium. Two clinicopathological forms have to be differentiated: the *adamantinomatous* and the *papillary craniopharyngioma* forms. The latter occurs almost exclusively in adults at a mean age of 40–45 years, while the adamantinomatous form can be observed in children aged 5–14 years as well as in adults. The most frequent location is suprasellar with an intrasellar component.[116] Craniopharyngiomas manifest as solid tumors with a variable, sometimes prevalently cystic, component and frequent calcifications. The cysts of the adamantinomatous type contain brownish, machine-oil-like fluid rich in cholesterol. Adamantinomatous craniopharyngiomas are composed histologically of strands and cords of a multistratified squamous epithelium, with peripheral palisading of nuclei with nodules of compact keratin and dystrophic calcifications. The adjacent brain tissue displays an intense reactive gliosis, with abundant Rosenthal fibers, and may contain small tumor islets. No genetic susceptibility has been reported. Cytogenetic analyses in few cases have demonstrated abnormalities involving chromosomes 2 and 12.[117] Mutations of the *TP53* gene do not appear to play a role.

GLIAL TUMORS OF UNCERTAIN HISTOGENESIS

Three neoplasms of presumably glial origin have been assigned to this group: astroblastoma, gliomatosis cerebri, and chordoid glioma of the third ventricle.

Astroblastoma is a rare glial tumor characterized by a perivascular pattern of GFAP-positive cells with broad, non-tapering processes radiating towards a central blood vessel. Because such a perivascular pattern may be observed in high-grade gliomas, the designation of astroblastoma should be limited to those rare neoplasms in which this architecture is predominating and that lack prominent features of diffuse astrocytomas or ependymomas. On neuroimaging, astroblastomas appear as well-circumscribed, solid, and occasionally cystic masses. The cerebral hemispheres are most often affected, but the entity can also occur at other sites in the CNS. Astroblastomas develop more frequently in young adults, but pediatric cases have been reported. Histologically, low-grade and high-grade astroblastomas may be distinguished based on the presence of marked cellular atypia, vascular proliferation, and necrosis. Gross total resection of these tumors can result in long-term survival, even in histologically malignant lesions.[118]

Gliomatosis cerebri represents a diffuse glial tumor infiltrating extensively into both cerebral hemispheres,

Table 5.2 *Brain tumors in hereditary tumor syndromes*

Syndrome	Gene	Chromosome	Brain tumors
Neurofibromatosis 1	*NF-1*	17q11	Pilocytic astrocytoma of the optic pathway Astrocytoma DNT
Neurofibromatosis 2	*NF-1*	22q12	Bilateral acoustic schwannomas Meningioma Meningioangiomatosis, spinal ependymomas, astrocytomas
Von Hippel–Lindau	*VHL*	3p26–p25	Hemangioblastoma
Tuberous sclerosis	*TSC1* *TSC2*	9q34 16p13	SEGA
Li–Fraumeni	*TP53*	17p13	Astrocytoma, PNET
Turcot	*APC* *hMLH1* *hPSM2*	5q21 3p21 7p22	Medulloblastoma Glioblastoma
Cowden	*PTEN* (MMAC)	10q23	Dysplastic gangliocytoma of the cerebellum
NBCCS	*PTCH*	9q31	Medulloblastoma

DNT, dysembryoplastic neuroepithelial tumor; NBCCS, nevoid basal cell carcinoma syndrome; SEGA, subependymal giant cell astrocytoma.

with frequent extension into infratentorial structures. Three lobes of the brain must be affected by definition. Microscopically, gliomatosis cerebri features elongated glial cells that resemble astrocytes. A solid portion may be present in some cases but absent in others. When infiltrating myelinated tracts, the cells often display an elongated shape. Usually, mitotic activity is low and vascular proliferation is absent. Mitotically active, anaplastic variants may, however, be encountered. In few reported cases, the morphology of neoplastic cells resembles oligodendrogliomas. Few cases have been reported in children, with the majority of these tumors occurring in adults.[119]

Chordoid glioma of the third ventricle has been described recently as a new entity. This low-grade lesion occurs exclusively within the third ventricle of adult patients. Histologically, it is composed of epithelioid GFAP-positive glial cell embedded in a mucoid stroma. No cases have been reported in children. The differential diagnosis includes chordoma and chordoid meningioma.[120]

BRAIN TUMORS IN THE CONTEXT OF HEREDITARY TUMOR SYNDROMES

Various brain tumors in children can occur in the setting of familial tumor syndromes. Most of these syndromes have been characterized genetically, and genes responsible for the disease have been identified. Some of the affected tumor suppressor genes have been demonstrated to play an important role in the formation of sporadic neoplasms. It is beyond the scope of this chapter to review the phenotypic and molecular genetic alterations of these syndromes, and we refer the reader to specialized reviews on the subject. Table 5.2 summarizes the frequently observed brain tumor entities in these hereditary disorders.

BRAIN TUMORS AS SECONDARY MALIGNANCIES

Treatment for acute leukemia and other malignancies in children frequently includes irradiation of the CNS. A tragic consequence of this aggressive therapy has been the rare occurrence of radiation-induced malignant brain tumors. Histologically, these neoplasms resemble either spontaneous supratentorial PNET[121] or malignant astrocytomas.[122] Molecular characterization has revealed an activating point mutation of the *K-ras* proto-oncogene in a radiation-induced PNET. Radiotherapy-associated astrocytomas lack *K-ras* mutations and show *TP53* mutations and *EGFR* amplification in a manner similar to that described in sporadic high-grade astrocytomas.[122] Additional entities to be observed in irradiated patients include meningiomas and sarcomas.

REFERENCES

1 Kleihues P, Cavanee WK. *Pathology and Genetics of Tumours of the Nervous System.* Lyon: IARC Press, 2000.

2 Rorke LB, Hart MN, Mc Lendon RE. Supratentorial primitive neuroectodermal tumour (PNET). In: Kleihues P, Cavanee WK (eds) *Pathology and Genetics of Tumours of the Nervous System*. Lyon: IARC Press, 2000; pp. 141–4.

3 Burnett ME, White EC, Sih S, von Haken MS, Cogen PH. Chromosome arm 17p deletion analysis reveals molecular genetic heterogeneity in supratentorial and infratentorial primitive neuroectodermal tumors of the central nervous system. *Cancer Genet Cytogenet* 1997; **97**:25–31.

4 Biegel JA. Cytogenetics and molecular genetics of childhood brain tumors. *Neuro-Oncol* 1999; **1**:139–51.

5 Reifemberger J, Janssen G, Weber RG, *et al.* Primitive neuroectodermal tumors of the cerebral hemispheres in two siblings with TP53 germline mutations. *J Neuropathol Exp Neurol* 1998; **57**:179–87.

6 Cruz-Sanchez FF, Rossi ML, Hughes JT, Moss TH. Differentiation in embryonal neuroepithelial tumors of the central nervous system. *Cancer* 1991; **67**:965–76.

7 Eberhart CG, Brat DJ, Cohen KJ, Burger PC. Pediatric neuroblastic brain tumors containing abundant neuropil and true rosettes. *Pediatr Dev Pathol* 2000; **3**:346–52.

8 Giangaspero F, Bigner SH, Kleihues P, Pietsch T, Trojanowski JQ. Medulloblastoma. In: Kleihues P, Cavanee WK (eds) *Pathology and Genetics of Tumours of the Nervous System*. Lyon: IARC Press, 2000; pp. 129–37.

9 Giangaspero F, Perilongo G, Fondelli MP, *et al.* Medulloblastoma with extensive nodularity: a variant with favorable prognosis. *J Neurosurg* 1999; **91**:971–7.

10 Giangaspero F, Rigobello L, Badiali M, *et al.* Large-cell medulloblastomas. A distinct variant with highly aggressive behavior. *Am J Surg Pathol* 1992; **16**:687–93.

11 Brown HG, Kepner JL, Perlman EJ, *et al.* "Large cell/anaplastic" medulloblastoma: a Pediatric Oncology Group Study. *J Neuropathol Exp Neurol* 2000; **59**:857–65.

12 Leonard JR, Cai DX, Rivet DJ, Kaufman BA, Park TS, Levy BK, Perry A. Large cell/anaplastic medulloblastoma and medullomyoblastoma: clinicopathological and genetic features. *J Neurosurg* 2001; **95**:82–8.

13 Smith TW, Davidson RI. Medullomyoblastoma. A histologic, immunohistochemical and ultrastructural study. *Cancer* 1984; **54**:323–32.

14 Baylac F, Martinoli A, Marie B, *et al.* Une variété exceptionelle de medulloblastome: le medulloblastome mélanotique. *Ann Pathol* 1997; **17**:403–5.

15 Vagner C, Zattara C, Gambarelli D, *et al.* Detection of i(17q) chromosome by fluorescent *in situ* hybridization (FISH) with interphase nuclei in medulloblastoma. *Cancer Genet Cytogenet* 1994; **78**:1–6.

16 Reardon DA, Michalkiewicz E, Boyett JM, *et al.* Extensive genomic abnormalities in childhood medulloblastoma by comparative genomic hybridization. *Cancer Res* 1997; **57**:4042–7.

17 Cogen PH, McDonald JD. Tumor suppressor genes and medulloblastoma. *J Neuro-Oncol* 1996; **29**:103–12.

18 Adesina AM, Nalbantoglu J, Cavanee WK. *p53* gene mutation and *mdm2* gene amplification are uncommon in medulloblastoma. *Cancer Res* 1994; **54**:5649–51.

19 Badiali M, Iolascon A, Loda M, *et al.* p53 gene mutations in medulloblastoma. Immunohistochemistry, gel shift analysis and sequencing. *Diagn Mol Pathol* 1993; **2**:23–8.

20 Ohgaki H, Eibl RH, Wiestler OD, Yasargil MG, Newcomb EW, Kleihues P. *p53* mutations in nonastrocytic human brain tumors. *Cancer Res* 1991; **51**:6202–5.

21 Albrecht S, von Deimling A, Pietsch T, *et al.* Microsatellite analysis of loss of heterozygosity on chromosomes 9q, 11p, and 17p in medulloblastomas. *Neuropathol Appl Neurobiol* 1994; **20**:74–81.

22 Shofield DE, West DC, Anthony DC, Marshal R, Sklar J. Correlation of loss of heterozygosity at chromosome 9q with histologic subtype in medulloblastomas. *Am J Pathol* 1995; **146**:472–80.

23 Hahn H, Wiching C, Zaphiropoulos PG, *et al.* Mutations of the human homolog of *Drosophila* patched in the nevoid basal cell carcinoma syndrome. *Cell* 1996; **85**:841–51.

24 Pietsch T, Waha A, Koch A, *et al.* Medulloblastoma of the desmoplastic variant carry mutations of the human homologue of *Drosophila* patched. *Cancer Res* 1997; **57**:2085–8.

25 Wolter M, Reifenberger J, Sommer C, Ruzicka T, Reifenberger G. Mutations in the human homologue of the *Drosophila* segment polarity gene patched (PTCH) in sporadic basal cell carcinomas of the skin and primitive neuroectodermal tumors of the central nervous system. *Cancer Res* 1997; **57**:2581–5.

26 Raffel C, Jenkins RB, Frederick L, *et al.* Sporadic medulloblastomas contain PTCH mutations. *Cancer Res* 1997; **57**:842–5.

27 Zurawel RH, Allen C, Chiappa S, *et al.* Analysis of PATCH/SMO/SHH pathway genes in medulloblastoma. *Genes Chromosomes Cancer* 2000; **27**:44–51.

28 Goodrich LV, Milenkovic L, Higgins KM, Scott MP. Altered neural cell fates and medulloblastoma in mouse patched mutants. *Science* 1997; **277**:1109–13.

29 Eberhart CG, Tihan T, Burger PC. Nuclear localization and mutation of beta-catenin in medulloblastomas. *J Neuropathol Exp Neurol* 2000; **59**:333–7.

30 Huang H, Mahler-Araujo BM, Sankila A, *et al.* APC mutations in sporadic medulloblastoma. *Am J Pathol* 2000; **156**:433–7.

31 Koch A, Waha A, Tonn JC, *et al.* Somatic mutations of WNT/wingless signaling pathway components in primitive neuroectodermal tumors. *Int J Cancer* 2001; **93**:445–9.

32 Buhren J, Christoph AHA, Buslei R, Albrecht S, Wiestler OD, Pietsch T. Expression of the neurotrophin receptor p75ntr in medulloblastomas is correlated with distinct histological and clinical features: evidence for a medulloblastoma subtype derived from the external granule cell layer. *J Neuropathol Exp Neurol* 2000; **59**:229–40.

33 Eberhart CG, Kaufman WE, Tihan T, Burger PC. Apoptosis neuronal maturation, and neurotrophin expression within medulloblastoma nodules. *J Neuropathol Exp Neurol* 2001; **60**:462–9.

34 Molloy PT, Yachnis AT, Rorke LB, *et al.* Central nervous system medulloepithelioma: a series of eight cases including two arising in the pons. *J Neurosurg* 1996; **84**:430–6.

35 Becker LE, Sharma MC, Rorke LB. Medulloepithelioma. In: Kleihues P, Cavanee WK (eds) *Pathology and Genetics of Tumours of the Nervous System*. Lyon: IARC Press, 2000; pp. 124–6.

36 Rorke LB, Packer RJ, Biegel JA. Central nervous system atypical teratoid/rhabdoid tumors of infancy and childhood: definition of an entity. *J Neurosurg* 1996; **85**:56–65.

37 Burger PC, Yu IT, Tihan T, *et al.* Atypical teratoid/rhabdoid tumor of the central nervous system: a highly malignant tumor of infancy and childhood frequently mistaken for medulloblastoma: a Pediatric Oncology Group study. *Am J Surg Pathol* 1998; **22**:1083–92.

38 Biegel JA, Zhou JY, Rorke LB, Stenstrom C, Wainwright LM, Fogelgren B. Germ-line and acquired mutations of INI1 in atypical teratoid and rhabdoid tumors. *Cancer Res* 1999; **59**:74–9.

39 Rousseau-Merck M-F, Versteege I, Legrand I, *et al.* hSNF5/INI1 inactivation is mainly associated with homozygous deletions and mitotic recombinations in rhabdoid tumors. *Cancer Res* 1999; **59**:3152–6.

40 Burger PC, Sheithauer BW. Atlas of tumor pathology. In: *Tumors of the Central Nervous System.* Washington: AFIP, 1994; pp. 25–106.

41 Cavanee WK, Furnari FB, Nagane M, *et al.* Diffusely infiltrating astrocytomas. In: Kleihues P, Cavanee WK (eds) *Pathology and Genetics of Tumours of the Nervous System.* Lyon: IARC Press, 2000; pp. 10–21.

42 Packer RJ. Brain tumors in children. *Arch Neurol* 1999; **56**:421–5.

43 Kleihues P, Ohgaki H. Primary and secondary glioblastoma: from concept to clinical diagnosis. *Neuro-Oncol* 1999; **1**:44–51.

44 Peraud A, Watanabe K, Schwechheimer K, Yonekawa Y, Kleihues P, Ohgaki H. Genetic profile of the giant cell glioblastoma. *Lab Invest* 1999; **79**:123–9.

45 Cheng Y, Ng Hk, Zhang SF, *et al.* Genetic alterations in pediatric high-grade astrocytomas. *Hum Pathol* 1999; **30**:1284–90.

46 Sung T, Miller DC, Hayes RL, Alonso M, Yee H, Newcombo EW. Preferential inactivation of the p53 tumor suppressor pathway and lack of EGFR amplification distinguish de novo high grade pediatric astrocytomas from de novo adult astrocytomas. *Brain Pathol* 2000; **10**:249–59.

47 Raffel C, Frederick L, O'Fallon JR, *et al.* Analysis of oncogene and tumor suppressor gene alterations in pediatric malignant astrocytomas reveals reduced survival for patients with PTEN mutations. *Clin Cancer Res* 1999; **5**:4085–90.

48 Pollack IF, Finkelstein SD, Burnham J, *et al.* Age and TP53 mutation frequency in childhood malignant gliomas: results in a multi-institutional cohort. *Cancer Res* 2001; **61**:7404–7.

49 Tihan T, Fisher PG, Kepner JL, *et al.* Pediatric astrocytomas with monomorphous pilomyxoid features and less favorable outcome. *J Neuropathol Exp Neurol* 1999; **58**:1061–8.

50 Dirks PB, Jay V, Becker LE, *et al.* Development of anaplastic changes in low-grade astrocytomas of childhood. *Neurosurgery* 1994; **34**:68–78.

51 Tomlinson FH, Scheithauer BW, Hayostek CJ, *et al.* The significance of atypia and histologic malignancy in pilocytic astrocytoma of the cerebellum: a clinicopathologic and flow cytometry study. *J Child Neurol* 1994; **9**:301–10.

52 Krieger MD, Gonzalez-Gomez I, Levy ML, McComb JG. Recurrence patterns and anaplastic change in a long-term study of pilocytic astrocytomas. *Pediatr Neurosurg* 1997; **27**:1–11.

53 Perilongo G, Carollo C, Salviati L, *et al.* Diencephalic syndrome and disseminated juvenile pilocytic astrocytomas of the hypothalamic-optic chiasm region. *Cancer* 1997; **80**:142–6.

54 Gottschalk S, Tavakolian R, Buske A, Tinshert S, Lehmann R. Spontaneous remission of chiasmatic/hypothalamic masses in neurofibromatosis type 1: report of two cases. *Neuroradiology* 1999; **41**:199–201.

55 Perilongo G, Moras P, Carollo C, *et al.* Spontaneous partial regression of low-grade glioma in children with neurofibromatosis-1: a real possibility. *J Child Neurol* 1999; **14**:352–6.

56 Ransom DT, Ritland SR, Kimmel DW, *et al.* Cytogenetic and loss of heterozygosity studies in ependymomas, pilocytic astrocytomas and oligodendrogliomas. *Genes Chromosomes Cancer* 1992; **5**:348–56.

57 Szymas J, Wolf G, Petersen S, Schluens K, Nowak S, Petersen I. Comparative genomic hybridisation indicates two distinct subgroups of pilocytic astrocytoma. *Neurosurg Focus* 2000; **8**:1–6.

58 Ohgaki H, Eibl RH, Schwab M, *et al.* Mutations of the p53 tumor suppressor gene in neoplasms of the human nervous system. *Mol Carcinog* 1993; **8**:74–80.

59 Von Deimling A, Louis DN, Menon AG, *et al.* Deletions on the long arm of chromosome 17 in pilocytic atrocytoma. *Acta Neuropathol (Berl)* 1993; **86**:81–5.

60 Platten M, Giordano MJ, Dirven CM, Gutmann DH, Louis DN. Up-regulation of specific NF1 gene transcripts in sporadic pilocytic astrocytoma. *Am J Pathol* 1996; **149**:621–7.

61 Giannini C, Scheithauer BW, Burger PC, *et al.* Pleomorphic xanthoastrocytoma. What do we really know about it? *Cancer* 1999; **85**:2033–45.

62 Giannini C, Hebrink D, Scheithauer BW, Dei Tos AP, James CD. Analysis of p53 mutation and expression in pleomorphic xanthoastrocytoma. *Neurogenetics* 2001; **3**:159–62.

63 Wiestler OD, Lopes BS, Green AJ, Vinters HV. Tuberous sclerosis complex and subependymal giant cell astrocytoma. In: Kleihues P, Cavanee WK (eds) *Pathology and Genetics of Tumours of the Nervous System.* Lyon: IARC Press, 2000; pp. 227–30.

64 Reifenberger G, Kros JM, Burger PC, Louis DN, Collins VP. Oligodendroglioma. In: Kleihues P, Cavanee WK (eds) *Pathology and Genetics of Tumours of the Nervous System.* Lyon: IARC Press, 2000; pp. 56–61.

65 Reifenberger J, Reifenberger G, Liu L, James CD, Wechsler W, Collins VP. Molecular genetic analysis of oligodendroglial tumors shows preferential allelic deletions on 19q and 1p. *Am J Pathol* 1994; **145**:1175–90.

66 Ino Y, Betensky RA, Zlatescu MC, *et al.* Molecular subtypes of anaplastic oligodendroglioma: implications for patient management at diagnosis. *Clin Cancer Res* 2001; **7**:839–45.

67 Rizk T, Mottolese C, Bouffet E, *et al.* Cerebral oligodendrogliomas in children: an analysis of 15 cases. *Childs Nerv Syst* 1996; **12**:527–9.

68 Razack N, Baumgartner J, Bruner J. Pediatric oligodendrogliomas. *Pediatr Neurosurg* 1998; **28**:121–9.

69 Prayson RA. Myxopapillary ependymomas: a clinicopathologic study of 14 cases including MIB-1 and p53 immunoreactivity. *Mod Pathol* 1997; **10**:304–10.

70 Wiestler OD, Schiffer D, Coons SW, Prayson RA, Rosenblum MK. Ependymoma. In: Kleihues P, Cavanee WK (eds) *Pathology*

and Genetics of Tumours of the Nervous System. Lyon: IARC Press, 2000; pp. 72–6.

71 Wiestler OD, Schiffer D, Coons SW, Prayson RA, Rosenblum MK. Anaplastic ependymoma. In: Kleihues P, Cavanee WK (eds) *Pathology and Genetics of Tumours of the Nervous System.* Lyon: IARC Press, 2000; pp. 76–7.

72 Ebert C, von Haken M, Meyer-Puttilitz B, *et al.* Molecular genetic analysis of ependymal tumors. NF2 mutations and chromosome 22q loss occur preferentially in intramedullary spinal ependymomas. *Am J Pathol* 1999; **155**:627–32.

73 Hirose Y, Adalpe KA, Bollen A, *et al.* Chromosomal abnormalities subdivide ependymal tumors into clinically relevant groups. *Am J Pathol* 2001; **158**:1137–43.

74 Chow E, Jenkins JJ, Burger PC, *et al.* Malignant evolution of choroids plexus papilloma. *Pediatr Neurosurg* 1999; **31**:127–30.

75 Pencalet P, Sainte-Rose C, Lellouch-Tubiana A, *et al.* Papillomas and carcinomas of the choroids plexus in children. *J Neurosurg* 1998; **88**:521–8.

76 Vital A, Bringuier PP, Huang H, *et al.* Astrocytomas and choroids plexus tumors in two families with identical *p53* germline mutations. *J Neuropathol Exp Neurol* 1998; **57**:1061–9.

77 Donovan MJ, Yunis EJ, De Girolami U, Fletcher JA, Schofield DE. Chromosome aberrations in choroid plexus papillomas. *Genes Chromosomes Cancer* 1994; **11**:267–70.

78 Sevenet N, Sheridan E, Amram D, Scheneider P, Hangretinger R, Delattre O. Constitutional mutations of the hSNF/INI1 gene predispose to a variety of cancers. *Am J Hum Genet* 1999; **65**:1342–8.

79 Weber M, Stockhammer F, Schmitz U, von Deimiling A. Mutational analysis of INI1 in sporadic human brain tumors. *Acta Neuropathol* 2001; **101**:479–82.

80 Prayson RA, Khajavi K, Comair YG. Cortical architectural abnormalities and MIB1 immunoreactivity in gangliogliomas: a study of 60 patients with intracranial forms. *J Neuropathol Exp Neurol* 1995; **54**:513–20.

81 Hirose T, Scheithauer BW, Lopes MB, *et al.* Ganglioglioma: an ultrastructural and immunohistochemical study. *Cancer* 1997; **79**:989–1003.

82 Hayashi Y, Iwato M, Hasegawa M, Tachibana O, von Deimling A, Yamashita J. Malignant transformation of a gangliocytoma/ ganglioglioma into a glioblastoma multiforme: a molecular genetic analysis. Case report. *J Neurosurg* 2001; **95**:138–42.

83 Komori T, Scheithauer BW, Anthony DC, *et al.* Papillary glioneuronal tumor: a new variant of mixed neuronal-glial neoplasm. *Am J Surg Pathol* 1998; **22**:1171–83.

84 Prayson RA. Papillary glioneuronal tumor. *Arch Pathol Lab Med* 2000; **124**:1820–3.

85 Bouvier-Labit C, Daniel L, Dufour H, Grisoli F, Figarella-Branger D. Papillary glioneuronal tumor: clinicopathological and biochemical study of one case with 7-year follow up. *Acta Neuropathol (Berl)* 2000; **99**:321–6.

86 Hassoun J, Soylemezoglu F, Gambarelli D, Figarella-Branger D, von Ammon K, Kleihues P. Central neurocytoma: a synopsis of clinical and histological features. *Brain Pathol* 1993; **3**:297–306.

87 Jay V, Edwards V, Hoving E, Rutka J, Becker L, Zielenska M, Teshima I. Central neurocytoma: morphological, flow cytometric, polymerase chain reaction, fluorescence *in situ* hybridization, and karyotypic analysis, Case report. *J Neurosurg* 1999; **90**:348–54.

88 Mackenzie IR. Central neurocytoma: histologic atypia, proliferation potential and clinical outcome. *Cancer* 1999; **85**:1606–10.

89 Giangaspero F, Cenacchi G, Losi L, Cerasoli S, Bisceglia M, Burger PC. Extraventricular neoplasms with neurocytoma features. A clinicopathological study of 11 cases. *Am J Surg Pathol* 1997; **21**:206–12.

90 VandenBerg SR. Desmoplastic infantile ganglioglioma and desmoplastic cerebral astrocytoma of infancy. *Brain Pathol* 1993; **3**:255–68.

91 Taratuto AL, Sevlever G, Schultz M, Gutierrez M, Monges J, Sanchez M. Demoplastic cerebral astrocytoma of infancy (DCAI). Survival data of the original series and report of two additional cases, DNA, kinetic and molecular genetic studies. *Brain Pathol* 1994; **4**:423.

92 Daumas-Duport C. Dysembryoplastic neuroepithelial tumours. *Brain Pathol* 1993; **3**:283–95.

93 Lellouch-Tubiana A, Bourgeois M, Vekemans M, Robain O. Dysembryoplastic neuroepithelial tumors in two children with neurofibromatosis type 1. *Acta Neuropatol (Berl)* 1995; **90**:319–22.

94 Mena H, Nakazato Y, Jouvet A, Scheithauer BW. Pineal parenchymal tumours. In: Kleihues P, Cavanee WK (eds) *Pathology and Genetics of Tumours of the Nervous System.* Lyon: IARC Press, 2000; pp. 116–21.

95 Juovet A, Saint-Pierre G, Fauchon F, *et al.* Pineal parenchymal tumors: a correlation of histological features with prognosis in 66 cases. *Brain Pathol* 2000; **10**:49–60.

96 Schild SE, Scheithauer BW, Schomberg PJ, *et al.* Pineal parenchymal tumors. Clinical, pathologic, and therapeutic aspects. *Cancer* 1993; **72**:870–80.

97 Davidson GS, Hope JK. Meningeal tumors of childhood. *Cancer* 1989; **63**:1205–10.

98 Germano IM, Edwards MS, Davis RL, Schiffer D. Intracranial meningiomas of the first two decades of life. *J Neurosurg* 1994; **80**:447–53.

99 Louis DN, Budka H, von Deimling A. Meningiomas. In: Kleihues P, Cavanee WK (eds) *Pathology and Genetics of Tumours of the Nervous System.* Lyon: IARC Press, 2000; pp. 176–84.

100 Perilongo G, Sutton L, D'Angio JG, *et al.* Childhood meningiomas. Experience in the modern imaging era. *Pediatr Neurosurg* 1992; **128**:12–19.

101 Zorludemir S, Scheithauer BW, Hirose T, *et al.* Clear cell meningiomas. A clinicopathologic study of a potentially aggressive variant of meningioma. *Am J Surg Pathol* 1995; **19**:493–505.

102 Perry A, Stafford SL, Scheithauer BW, Suman VJ, Lohse CM. Meningioma grading: an analysis of histologic paramenters. *Am J Surg Pathol* 1997; **21**:1455–65.

103 Giangaspero F, Guiducci A, Lenz FA, Mastronardi L, Burger PC. Meningioma with meningiomatosis: a condition mimicking invasive meningiomas in children and young adults. Report of two cases and review of the literature. *Am J Surg Pathol* 1999; **23**:872–5.

104 Perry A, Scheithauer BW, Stafford SL, Abell-Aleff PC, Meyer FB. "Rhabdoid" meningioma: an aggressive variant. *Am J Surg Pathol* 1998; **22**:1482–90.

105 Ludwin SK, Rubinstein LJ, Russel DS. Papillary meningiomas a malignant variant of meningioma. *Cancer* 1975; **36**:1363–73.

106 Bouvier C, Zattara-Canoni H, Daniel L, Gentet JC, Lena G, Figarella-Branger D. Cerebellar papillary meningioma in a 3-year-old boy: the usefulness of electron microscopy for diagnosis. *Am J Surg Pathol* 1999; **23**:844–8.

107 Perry A, Scheithauer BW, Stafford SL, Lohse CM, Wollan PC. "Malignancy" in meningiomas: a clinicopathologic study of 116 patients, with grading implications. *Cancer* 1999; **85**:2046–56.

108 Leone PE, Bello MJ, de Campos JM, *et al.* NF2 gene mutations and allelic status of 1p,14q, 22q in sporadic meningiomas. *Oncogene* 199; **18**:2231–39.

109 Cai DX, Banerjee R, Scheithauer BW, Lohse CM, Kleinschmidt-Demasters BK, Perry A. Chromosome 1p and 14q FISH analysis in clinicopathologic subsets of meningiomas: diagnostic and prognostic implications. *J Neuropathol Exp Neurol* 2001; **60**:628–36.

110 Bjornsson J, Scheithauer BW, Okazaki H, *et al.* Intracranial germ cell tumors: pathological and immunohistochemical aspects of 70 cases. *J Neuropathol Exp Neurol* 1985; **44**:32–46.

111 Rosenblum MK, Matsutani M, Van Meir EG. CNS germ cell tumours. In: Kleihues P, Cavanee WK (eds) *Pathology and Genetics of Tumours of the Nervous System*. Lyon: IARC Press, 2000, pp. 208–14.

112 Shaffrey ME, Lanzino G, Lopes MBS, *et al.* Maturation of intracranial immature teratomas. Report of two cases. *J Neurosurg* 1996; **85**:672–6.

113 Watanabe T, Makiyama Y, Nishimoto H, Matsumoto M, Kikuchi A, Tsubokawa T. Metacronous ovarian dysgerminoma after a suprasellar germ-cell tumor treated by radiation therapy. Case report. *J Neurosurg* 1995; **83**:149–53.

114 Losi L, Polito P, Hagemeijer A, Buonamici L, Van den Berghe H, Dal Cin P. Intracranial germ cell tumour (embryonal carcinoma with teratoma) with complex karyotype including isochromosome 12p. *Virchows Arch* 1998; **433**:571–4.

115 Kim SK, Cho BK, Paek SH, *et al.* The detection of *p53* gene mutation using a microdissection technique in primary intracranial germ cell tumors. *Int J Oncol* 2001; **18**:111–16.

116 Thapar K, Kovacs K. Neoplasms of the sellar region. In: Bigner DD, McLendon RE, Bruner J (eds) *Russell and Rubinstein's Pathology of Tumours of the Nervous System*, 6th edition. London: Arnold, 1989; pp. 629–40.

117 Gorski GK, McMorrow LE, Donaldson MH, Freed M. Multiple chromosomal abnormalities in a case of craniopharyngioma. *Cancer Genet Cytogenet* 1992; **60**:212–13.

118 Brat DJ, Hirose Y, Cohen KJ, Feuerstein BG, Burger PC. Astroblastoma: clinicopathologic features and chromosomal abnormalities defined by comparative genomic hybridization. *Brain Pathol* 2000; **10**:342–52.

119 Cummings TJ, Hulette CM, Longee DC, Bottom KS, McLendon RE, Chu CT. Gliomatosis cerebri: cytologic and autopsy findings in a case involving the entire neuraxis. *Clin Neuropathol* 1999; **18**:190–7.

120 Brat DJ, Scheithauer BW, Staugaitis SM, Cortez SC, Brecher K, Burger PC. Third ventricular chordoid glioma: a distinct clinico-pathologic entity. *J Neuropathol Exp Neurol* 1998; **57**:283–90.

121 Brustle O, Ohgaki H, Schmitt HP, Walter GF, Ostertag H, Kleihues P. Primitive neuroectodermal tumors after prophylactic central nervous system irradiation in children. Association with an activated K-ras gene. *Cancer* 1992; **69**:2385–9.

122 Brat DJ, James CD, Jedlicka AE, *et al.* Molecular genetic alterations in radiation-induced astrocytomas. *Am J Pathol* 1999; **154**:1431–8.

PART III

Diagnosis and treatment planning

6

Clinical syndromes

JONATHAN A. G. PUNT

INTRODUCTION

Until 25 years ago, there were many barriers to the timely diagnosis of brain and spinal tumors in children. Few family doctors or pediatricians had a good grasp of clinical neurology. The radiological modalities available were concentrated in specialist centers, and in general access to them was only through sometimes less than accessible colleagues in the form of neurosurgeons or neurologists, often at institutions some way from the child's home. Before the advent of computed tomography (CT) scanning in the late 1970s, and magnetic resonance imaging (MRI) in the mid-1980s, investigation of a child suspected of harboring a brain or spinal tumor was a truly frightening experience for all concerned. Investigations were invasive, painful, and even dangerous. The most frequently used modalities of imaging were ventriculography, for suspected intracranial mass lesions, and myelography, for suspected intraspinal tumors. Textbooks often painted pictures of late stages in disease processes, emphasizing the importance of rather gross physical signs. Pediatricians were reluctant to refer children until clinical features were relatively far advanced, with the consequence that the neurosurgeon was faced all too often with the prospect of a child in poor condition and with advanced neurological disease.

In countries enjoying a level of technology appropriate to the third millennium, these problems should now be a matter of historical curiosity. Whereas it has often been suggested over the past decade that the only indication for performing a neurological examination is a negative CT or MRI scan, such an approach is far from the truth.

It is precisely because there is the real possibility of making diagnoses early that proper attention to symptoms is all the more important. This chapter will draw heavily on the experiences of personal clinical and medicolegal practice to emphasize the possibilities and the pitfalls.

SYNDROMES OF RAISED INTRACRANIAL PRESSURE

In children, the predilection for tumor location in or adjacent to the cerebral midline makes raised intracranial pressure through the mechanism of hydrocephalus a frequent feature. Solid or cystic tumors can attain considerable size, the effects of which may be exaggerated by cerebral edema and ventricular dilatation. The younger child in particular may hide a sizable mass in a non-dominant frontal or temporal location, producing only features of intracranial hypertension rather than focal neurology. In infancy, the initial features will be of rather non-specific irritability and vomiting. The latter may be mistaken for the much more commonly encountered gastrointestinal upsets of infancy. Persistent or regularly recurrent vomiting, without other concomitants of gastrointestinal disturbance, should raise the suspicion of intracranial pathology. With more slowly progressive intracranial hypertension, infants may show a disproportionately accelerating rate of growth in head circumference. Babies will display a tense anterior fontanelle and distended scalp veins. Downward, divergent deviation of the eyes may occur with severely raised intracranial pressure in babies and infants, regardless of whether there is hydrocephalus.

It is important to understand that the features of raised intracranial pressure in infancy are not synonymous with a diagnosis of "simple" infantile hydrocephalus, and other possibilities must always be considered. Cranial ultrasound scanning, frequently used by pediatricians as a screening test in babies and infants, may easily overlook a posterior fossa mass, especially if the radiologist is asked simply whether there is hydrocephalus.

The infant with a rapidly enlarging head and who is clearly unwell is more likely to have a neoplasm than the other causes of infantile hydrocephalus. Occasionally, an older child with tumoral hydrocephalus is encountered with an abnormally large head circumference; such a finding indicates that there has been intracranial hypertension since before the child was around five years of age. Such a long evolution may augur benign histology. The child who has reached speech age will usually complain of headaches, although the much-hallowed history of early-morning headaches, with or without vomiting, is relatively unusual. The only characteristic feature of the headaches of raised intracranial pressure is, in fact, their novelty for that patient. Many attempts have been made to create algorithms for the investigation of headaches in childhood. Although it must be acknowledged that tumor is a rare cause compared with more benign and banal conditions, such as migraine and scalp tension, it cannot be denied that it must be among the most serious. Given the relative lack of hazard accompanying CT and MRI compared with the risks involved in missing raised intracranial pressure, whether tumoral or otherwise, it is difficult to accept that there is any logical or reasonable basis for failing to obtain cranial imaging in children of any age who present with novel or recurrent headaches.

The absence of papilledema can never be taken as an indication that headaches are not due to raised intracranial pressure, especially if the observer is less than skilled at examining the fundi. The presence of raised intracranial pressure is suspected on the history, and hence

definitive imaging is obligatory as the only sure method of excluding the presence of an intracranial mass.

Later features of raised intracranial pressure (see box above) include:

- diplopia due to sixth cranial nerve dysfunction;
- visual failure due to papilloedema;
- neck stiffness and disturbed neck posture;
- deteriorating consciousness.

FOCAL NEUROLOGICAL DISTURBANCES

With midline lesions, whether above or below the tentorium cerebelli, the features of raised intracranial pressure tend to predominate. Lateralized cerebral hemisphere lesions may produce focal features appropriate to their location. Thus, frontoparietal lesions may cause contralateral motor weakness, frontal lesions may cause altered mood and behavior, and occipital lesions may cause hemianopic visual loss. Lesions in the posterior frontal and superior temporal parts of the dominant (usually the left) cerebral hemisphere will produce dysphasia in children of speech age. With respect to disturbance of speech and language, the importance of inquiring after handedness is very frequently forgotten in the pediatric setting.

Deeply placed lesions in the thalamus and basal ganglia produce profound contralateral hemiparesis and, occasionally, disturbances of posture. Occasionally, a tumor in the thalamus or basal ganglia produces a movement disorder, such as a tremor.

Below the tentorium cerebelli, lesions in the cerebellar vermis frequently show no focal features but may produce truncal ataxia, and lesions in the cerebellar hemispheres may show relatively mild ipsilateral limb ataxia. The relative paucity of focal neurological disturbance, and the predominance of features of raised intracranial pressure, may be factors in any failure to recognize the real significance of headaches. The absence of neurological features does not diminish the need for imaging in cases of novel headache.

By contrast, intrinsic lesions in the pons and medulla oblongata produce marked neurological disturbance in terms of eye movement disturbance, impairment of swallowing, changes in voice, and both weakness and clumsiness of the limbs, while being relatively free of features of raised intracranial pressure. One unusual but characteristic presentation of an intrinsic medullary tumor in infancy is poor feeding and vomiting, producing unexplained failure to thrive. The rare extra-axial masses in the posterior cranial fossa, such as acoustic nerve tumors and chordomas, may also produce dysfunction of one or more of the lower cranial nerves. The extra-axial component of an exophytic brainstem tumor may also impact on the lower cranial nerves.

Urgent symptoms of intracranial tumors

The features that signal imminent danger and that dictate *immediate* action are:

- severe headaches;
- neck pain and stiffness, especially when associated with extension of the head and neck;
- visual failure, whether progressive or intermittent;
- altered consciousness;
- episodes of decerebrate posturing;
- status epilepticus;
- altered cardiorespiratory function.

It is important to note that cerebellar ataxia may be a false localizing sign produced either by hydrocephalus or by a large frontal or temporal mass, especially in the non-dominant cerebral hemisphere. Thus, the features of raised intracranial pressure accompanied by ataxia may indicate a supratentorial rather than an infratentorial mass.

Epilepsy and brain tumors

Unlike in adults, epilepsy is a relatively unusual presenting feature of childhood brain tumors, probably due to the relative rareness of intrinsic primary and secondary cerebral-hemisphere tumors and extrinsic meningeal tumors in childhood. Epilepsy is very unusual in midline supratentorial, cerebellar, and brainstem tumors. Very few children who present with a seizure disorder will have a brain tumor. That notwithstanding, it is difficult to understand the logical basis for not investigating by MRI all new cases of childhood seizure disorder to look for a structural cause of some sort. It has to be in the best interest of the child to establish a cause for epilepsy if this is possible. This is especially the case for children whose seizures include focal features. Oligodendrogliomas seem to have a particular tendency to present with seizures. Status epilepticus may be a presentation of an intrinsic frontal lobe tumor.

A number of children undergoing investigation with a view to surgical treatment for medically intractable epilepsy, especially those with complex partial seizures of temporal lobe origin, will have brain tumors of low histological grade, usually astrocytomas, gangliogliomas, or dysembryoplastic neuroepithelial tumors (DNTs).

In patients with an established seizure disorder, a change in the seizure pattern or increasing difficulty with seizure control may mark the progression of a causative tumor. This is particularly the case in children with partial epilepsy that becomes difficult to control. Children with epilepsy in relation to tuberous sclerosis may display deteriorating seizure control if they develop subependymal giant-cell astrocytomas around the interventricular foramina. It should also be remembered that neurofibromatosis type 1 (NF-1) and tuberous sclerosis predispose to the development of both intracranial tumors in childhood and seizure disorders.

A very rare, but highly specific, seizure disorder is that of gelastic epilepsy, which can be symptomatic of a hypothalamic hamartoma.

Epilepsy can also arise in the course of treatment of brain tumors, either as a manifestation of disease progression or as the result of local irritation from surgical interventions, including ventricular shunts, or secondary to metabolic derangements such as hyponatremia and hypomagnesemia.

It is crucially important not to mistake the paroxysmal, opisthotonic, extensor spasms of severely raised intracranial pressure for epileptic seizures. Too ready, and erroneous, acceptance of "fitting" as a diagnosis in a child who is displaying the posturing of raised intracranial pressure takes the child one step nearer to death or severe permanent disability.

OPHTHALMIC MANIFESTATIONS

Disturbance of some aspect of visual function is very common in children with intracranial tumors. The range of abnormalities encountered is shown in the box below. Each abnormality can occur as a result of direct compression or invasion of neural tissue, or as an indirect effect of raised intracranial pressure.

Ophthalmic features of childhood brain tumors

Ophthalmic features include:

- failing visual acuity;
- disorders of eye movement and ocular posture;
- reduction in visual field;
- fundal abnormalities;
- loss of pupillary reflexes;
- ocular features of phakomatoses.

Visual acuity

Visual acuity may fail from direct invasion of the optic nerves, the optic chiasm, or, less frequently, the optic tracts by low-grade astrocytomas of the chiasmatic-hypothalamic region, and from direct compression from craniopharyngiomas. The aforementioned are two of the most frequently encountered supratentorial neoplasms in childhood. Lesions seen less frequently include germ-cell tumors of the anterior third ventricle, pituitary adenomas, and tumors of the skull base, such as chordomas and metastatic neuroblastoma. Malignant histiocytoses, metastatic retinoblastoma, and malignant lymphomas may all, rarely, involve the optic nerves and chiasm. Loss of color vision is seen early in compressive lesions of the optic nerves and chiasm, but this will be detected only in children of appropriate age and development.

More common than any of these is indirect loss of visual acuity as a consequence of severe papilledema due to unrelieved raised intracranial pressure. Visual acuity secondary to intracranial hypertension may fail progressively, or the child may display intermittent obscurations of vision, during which vision becomes blurred, gray, or black or is even lost completely. Such obscurations may affect either eye or both eyes, together or separately.

The true significance of papilledema is the very real propensity for it to progress to optic atrophy and permanent visual loss. Any child who is found to have papilledema is at risk of blindness and should have the visual acuity monitored carefully. Once vision starts to fail, there may be progressive loss even when the pressure is relieved. This danger continues after surgical decompression. Extreme vigilance is required postoperatively, especially following removal of posterior fossa tumors, lest persistent or recurrent hydrocephalus threatens vision. This is particularly important in the case of children whose care is transferred from the neuroscience service to the oncology service, perhaps in a different institution.

The assessment of visual acuity, and the recognition of visual loss, is difficult in childhood, and children of pre-speech age can only be assessed by careful observation of behavior. Children in the first decade of life frequently do not report visual loss. Direct inquiry should always be made regarding visual symptoms. The author recalls one child in whom severe visual loss due to a chiasmatic glioma was discovered only when it was found that she was relying on her Labrador to fulfil her newspaper deliveries. Sadly, children may show features of failing vision that are ignored by the carer or by the physician, and visual loss may be regarded by the ophthalmologist simply as "amblyopia" secondary to squint or even attributed to behavioral disturbance. The error may be compounded by regarding associated headaches as being due to "eyestrain."

Any child who shows progressive loss of visual acuity, whether unilateral or bilateral, and whose acuity can not be improved to 6/9 or better by refraction, must be assumed to have a compressive or infiltrative lesion of the anterior visual pathways until proved otherwise by high-quality, dedicated MRI. Reliance on plain skull radiographs for this purpose is not adequate; in addition, axial CT may miss lesions near the skull base.

Disorders of eye movement and ocular posture

Such disorders are common, the most frequent being the unilateral or bilateral convergent strabismus resulting from weakness or paralysis of the sixth cranial nerves secondary to raised intracranial pressure. Loss of visual acuity and restriction of visual field may lead to a failure to develop, or a loss of, conjugate gaze.

Direct involvement of the neural pathways controlling eye movement is a major feature of intrinsic tumors of the brainstem. It is also seen in children with focal lesions in the pineal region due to disturbance of the tectal plate of the midbrain, resulting in a combination of loss of upgaze, impaired accommodation, and abnormal pupillary reflexes, often referred to as Parinaud's syndrome, although the features are frequently incomplete. Children with lesions in this region may show recrudescence of eye movement disturbance, even following successful control

of disease, if they develop hyponatremia due to postoperative metabolic imbalance. Hydrocephalus per se can produce failure of upgaze or downward divergent gaze due to distortion of pathways in the rostral midbrain.

In its most extreme form, this constitutes the "sunsetting" more often encountered in babies with non-tumoral hydrocephalus. Sunsetting can also be observed in babies and infants with severely raised intracranial pressure from any cause, including massive solid tumors that are not producing hydrocephalus. It is important to remember that the most frequent ophthalmic manifestation of a blocked ventricular shunt is loss of previously present upgaze; this is a more reliable sign than papilledema. In the follow-up of children with hydrocephalus shunts or third ventriculostomies, it is a wise precaution to check and record whether upgaze is full in health, as this can be referred to at times of recurrent symptoms. A rarely seen, but highly characteristic, disorder of eye posture is the rhythmic 2–3-Hz oscillatory movements of the head produced by lesions in or around the anterior third ventricle or by dilation of the third ventricle by hydrocephalus – the bobble-head doll syndrome. Rarer still are the paroxysmal, rapid, chaotic eye movements associated with jerking of the limbs seen as a non-metastatic manifestation of neuroblastoma – opsoclonus-myoclonus encephalopathy.

Visual field loss

This can involve central or peripheral fields of vision as a consequence of direct invasion or compression. Exceptionally, a chronically enlarged third ventricle can produce chiasmal compression. The blind spot can enlarge secondary to peripapillary edema in severe papilledema. Severe hydrocephalic crises can cause cortical visual loss due to occipital ischemia secondary to central transtentorial herniation and distortion of the posterior cerebral arteries. Severe unilateral uncal herniation can produce ipsilateral occipital infarction and a resultant contralateral hemianopia.

Formal evaluation of visual fields requires a degree of sophistication, but even in very young children an impression can be gained from the child's spontaneous behavior and responses to appropriate stimuli. Loss of visual field can produce eye movement disturbance; if severe, there will be frank breakdown of conjugate gaze. Children with bitemporal hemianopia due to chiasmatic lesions may display a divergent pattern of squint.

Fundal abnormalities

Fundal abnormalities that may be seen are papilledema, occasionally with peripapillary hemorrhages, and optic atrophy. The latter may result from the direct effects of invasion or compression, such as from craniopharyngioma or anterior visual pathway astrocytoma. After the insults of prematurity, the most common cause of optic atrophy in infancy is intracranial tumor. As has been already indicated, the overriding importance of papilledema is that its presence may herald visual loss. Some children with long-standing neoplasms in and around the optic nerves and chiasm may have very small optic discs.

Pupillary abnormalities

These include loss of the light reflex, which can result from severe loss of acuity due to optic nerve dysfunction from direct destruction or may be secondary to raised intracranial pressure. With relative impairment of optic nerve conduction, there may be an afferent pupillary defect, whereby the pupil in the affected eye dilates rather than constricts when subjected to a bright light. The pupillary light reflex may be lost if there is severe uncal herniation, but this will almost invariably have been heralded and preceded by reduction in conscious level.

Impairment of the pupillary light reflex in association with disturbance of upgaze is seen with pineal-region masses and lesions in the dorsal part of the rostral midbrain.

General examination of the eye

A general eye examination may show the abnormalities associated with the phakomatoses, namely iris hamartomas (Lisch nodules) in NF-1 and peripapillary retinal hamartomas in tuberous sclerosis.

NEUROENDOCRINE, GROWTH, AND NUTRITIONAL DISTURBANCES

Most children with malignant intracranial tumors will have lost some weight, often in excess of that which might be expected from the amount of vomiting. This seems to be a particular feature in infants, and may in itself require attention before embarking upon major intracranial surgery. Young children with hypothalamic tumors may present with failure to thrive; older children may present with delayed puberty and hypothalamic wasting disorders (the diencephalic syndrome). The author has seen a number of children with craniopharyngiomas and extreme inanition who were diagnosed erroneously as having anorexia nervosa. Children with slowly progressive intrinsic lesions of the medulla oblongata can present in infancy as failure to thrive, usually associated with repeated vomiting. On occasion, many years can elapse before neurological features develop. The author has encountered a number of children with holocord spinal tumors and who have developed severe weight loss and anorexia, often associated with depression.

Tumors in and around the hypothalamus often cause neuroendocrine disturbances. The most frequently encountered lesions are craniopharyngiomas and astrocytomas, and the function that is most often impaired is growth hormone secretion. It is therefore important to include inquiries and measurement of growth in any clinical evaluation. The finding of clinical features of slowing down of growth velocity should increase the clinical suspicion of the presence of a structural lesion of the hypothalamus.

Once the diagnosis of a craniopharyngioma or hypothalamic glioma is established by imaging, it is important to involve a pediatric endocrinologist in the formal assessments of corticosteroid and thyroid function, as failure to identify and correct these before any surgical intervention may prove dangerous or even fatal. Diabetes insipidus is unusual preoperatively in craniopharyngiomas, but it is a common presenting feature in germ-cell tumors involving the anterior third ventricle and in malignant histiocytoses, sometimes preceding any other symptoms by many months. Pituitary adenomas are rare in childhood, but the hypersecretory endocrine syndromes of pituitary-driven Cushing's disease and of gigantism are encountered occasionally.

Children with pineal-region tumors may develop precocious puberty.

Children with NF-1 may display systemic symptoms due to pheochromocytoma. Children with neuroblastoma may exhibit diarrhea due to production of gastrointestinal peptide hormones. The importance of examining the whole patient, especially the skin, merits reiteration. The cutaneous manifestations of NF-1 and tuberous sclerosis (see box below) should be sought in the patient and, if relevant, also in the parents.

Cutaneous manifestations of the phakomatoses

Neurofibromatosis type 1
- café-au-lait spots (six or more lesions of diameter >5 mm in prepubertal children and >15 mm in postpubertal patients);
- axillary freckles;
- cutaneous neurofibromas (more than two);
- plexiform neurofibromas.

Tuberous sclerosis
- ash-leaf macules;
- shagreen patches;
- adenoma sebaceum;
- periungual fibromas;
- gingival fibromas;
- fibrous plaque on scalp.

BEHAVIORAL AND DEVELOPMENTAL DISTURBANCES

In general terms, frank behavioral disturbances are very rarely due to brain tumor. However, more subtle psychological symptoms are seen quite frequently in certain circumstances. Parents regularly report that children with brainstem glioma become withdrawn before the appearance of symptoms of focal neurological dysfunction. Children with intrinsic frontal and temporal lobe tumors may display changes in mood. The most frequent observation from the carer is the identification that their child has changed, often in an indefinable fashion. Schoolteachers may report a decline in aptitude and concentration.

Babies and infants with hypothalamic tumors may show developmental delay out of proportion to any disturbance of vision, nutrition, or neuroendocrine function.

The unwelcome incursion of any severe, frightening, and debilitating disease at a time of life that is characteristically associated with good health can be associated with depression, especially in adolescence, and there is probably a tendency for secondary mood disturbance to be under-recognized. This is particularly the case in those services that do not make age-appropriate arrangements for the management of adolescents.

SPINAL TUMORS

The first symptom of an intraspinal tumor is frequently midline or paraspinal pain that is characteristically worse at night and wakes the child from sleep. With tumors in the upper spinal canal, neck stiffness is common; a head tilt may be adopted, or the head and neck may be extended as if to relieve dural tension. In the lower spinal canal, a loss of the usual childhood fluidity of movement is seen, and gait appears stiff. There may be a posture of exaggerated lumbar lordosis, and the older patient may observe, if asked, that the adoption of such a posture relieves pain. Progressive spinal deformity leading to severe kyphoscoliosis may be seen. The absence of neurological signs does not exclude the possibility of tumor, which is often intrinsic and extensive. Back pain in childhood should not be attributed to mechanical or psychogenic causes without very careful consideration, including positive exclusion of spinal tumor by MRI. Radicular pain may occur with nerve-sheath tumors and, occasionally, with very focal intrinsic tumors. The organic nature of such pains may also be misinterpreted, especially if they occur in unusual or emotionally sensitive areas, such as the genitalia or rectum. The onset and progression of neurological symptoms is usually insidious, although hemorrhage or cystic change may occasionally lead to an abrupt presentation. Rarely, a neurofibroma or ependymoma may present with subarachnoid hemorrhage. Motor symptoms predominate over sensory features, the most common presentation being gait disturbance. Sphincter disturbance is usually gradual in onset and may also be mistaken for delay in maturation or psychological in origin. Recurrent urinary and vaginal infections may develop.

Intradural spinal tumors can be associated with hydrocephalus, attributable to very high levels of protein in the cerebrospinal fluid (CSF); hydrocephalus can even be the presenting feature, the tumor coming to light only when there is neurological deterioration following insertion of a ventricular shunt.

Tumors of paraspinal origin and location, notably neuroblastoma and ganglioneuroblastoma, and also the occasional Ewing's tumor, may invade the spinal canal and produce symptoms of spinal cord or nerve-root compression. The occasional baby with a congenital neuroblastoma may be paraplegic at birth. As well as the local symptomatology, there may be other features if there is metastatic disease. Malignant lymphomas can present as extradural spinal tumors.

It is difficult to comprehend how the combination of back pain and neurological symptoms in the limbs in a child or young person could ever fail to register the very real probability of serious disease. All children with scoliosis should undergo MRI to exclude an intraspinal tumor.

SYMPTOMATOLOGY OF EXTENSIVE DISEASE AND OF RECURRENCE

Through the use of whole-neuraxis MRI in standardized imaging protocols, it is now appreciated that extensive neuraxial and leptomeningeal spread of primary central nervous system (CNS) tumors at diagnosis, and later in their course, is more common than was thought previously. This applies not only to those tumors such as the primitive neuroectodermal tumors (PNETs) that have a marked predilection to show neuraxial metastasis, but also to tumors of histologically lower grades, such as astrocytomas and oligodendrogliomas. The child who looks systemically ill but who has a relatively small tumor with minimal features of raised intracranial pressure probably has a tumor that has already metastasized through the neuraxis. Spinal-nerve root pain or sphincter disturbance in a child with an intracranial tumor usually signals subarachnoid metastases. The child with a spinal tumor, usually an ependymoma, and who presents with subarachnoid hemorrhage should be assumed to be at risk of having developed disseminated disease as a result of the hemorrhage. Children with raised intracranial pressure and apparently negative imaging may not have benign intracranial hypertension (BIH), and this diagnosis should be viewed with skepticism in children in whom there is no apparent reason for having BIH; this is especially the case in prepubertal males. The diagnosis should not be made without whole-neuraxis MRI and cytological and biochemical examination of the CSF to exclude diffuse subarachnoid malignancy. Repeat imaging after an interval is an advisable precautionary measure, along with regular clinical reviews.

Similarly, unexplained communicating hydrocephalus outside the infant period requires whole-neuraxis MRI to exclude extensive malignancy and spinal tumor.

Recurrence of a brain or spinal tumor is usually heralded by a return of the original symptoms or appearance of new features, such as epilepsy. Whenever a child with a hydrocephalus shunt inserted as part of the management of an intracranial tumor returns with symptoms, it is vital to consider whether those symptoms are consistent with shunt malfunction or whether they are really those of recurrent or metastatic disease. Unexplained subdural effusions and recurrent mysterious shunt malfunctions may herald extensive subarachnoid spread of disease. Children with occult leptomeningeal spread may develop an unexpected encephalopathy when given chemotherapy. This may relate to an effect of the chemotherapy itself, possibly through release of excitotoxic amines, or it may simply be due to fluid loading in relation to platinum-based chemotherapy. The condition is usually associated with seizures progressing to status epilepticus, and it is often fatal. Occasionally, children with PNETs or intracranial germ-cell tumors may develop symptoms of systemic spread to bone, bone marrow, lymph nodes, or the peritoneal cavity; the latter usually occurs in the presence of a ventricular shunt. The accurate evaluation of children undergoing adjuvant therapy and surveillance following completion of therapy can only be accomplished through good multidisciplinary team working in combined ward units and clinics.

SOURCES OF DIAGNOSTIC ERROR

The author is sadly in a position to attest, not only from his own clinical experiences but also from a considerable clinical negligence practice, that after alleged breaches of duty of care relating to the diagnosis and management of hydrocephalus, the failure to make an appropriately rapid diagnosis of an intracranial or intraspinal tumor features very large. There is generally a tendency to believe, erroneously, that intermittent symptoms cannot be the result of progressive disease. This applies particularly to headache and to visual disturbance. Children may be seen by physicians by virtue of their regional or system specialty but who do not have special knowledge of childhood illness or the skills required to listen to children and their carers. In the experience of the author, this applies particularly to adult neurologists, ophthalmic surgeons, orthopedic surgeons, and rheumatologists.

Teenagers who are seen in adult services are at particular hazard. Apart from ignorance of the conditions, the most common source of error is the failure to listen to the child or the carer and to discard too readily the sense of the parent that the child is somehow different. The next most common mistake is an obsession with the necessity of finding physical signs, the absence of which must never be regarded as being a reliable indicator of the absence of serious disease. There is a regrettable tendency to attribute symptoms that are not accompanied by signs to psychological causes; this applies not only to headache and backache but also to disorders of vision, sphincter control, and nutrition.

To ascribe a child's symptoms erroneously to a psychological response to life events is to ignore the fact that the inherent nature of childhood is one of an ever-changing and evolving environment.

Whereas there is a perception that neoplastic disease may be far down the list of differential diagnoses, the consequences of delayed recognition are so great, and the diagnostic tools so safe and applied so easily, that there is no competent excuse for failing to employ them. The risk/benefit analysis makes it only logical and reasonable that children with symptoms such as headache and backache are investigated by imaging on the basis of the history and the observations of the carer.

Another source of error relates to imaging, and to the interpretation of imaging. It is clearly important that the clinician shares with the radiologist the relevant clinical data, rather than simply submitting a perfunctory request that states, for example, "Headaches" or "Fits." It is important that the correct modality of imaging is employed; although most intracranial tumors in childhood will be found on an unenhanced CT scan, lesions near the skull base, small lesions in and around the midbrain and pineal region, and diffuse lesions in the brainstem may be overlooked, especially by the non-specialist radiologist working on minimal clinical information.

Failure to review, reconsider, refer to a specialist colleague, or to otherwise make any, or any adequate, attempt to address persistent symptoms are further causes for delay. The non-specialist clinician relying too heavily on the opinion of the non-specialist radiologist is the technology era's version of the blind leading the blind.

It must be remembered that failure to make a timely diagnosis may not only prejudice the outcome in terms of survival but may also lead to avoidable disability, and it will inevitably have serious adverse effects on the psychological well-being of the carer, and perhaps also the child, such that the management of the illness becomes much more difficult. The neuro-oncology team embarking on a lengthy and complicated course of management for a patient whose family has lost confidence has an additional hurdle to confront.

CONCLUSIONS AND DIRECTIONS FOR FUTURE RESEARCH

Early diagnosis of neuraxial tumors in children can now be achieved in the vast majority of cases by application and correct interpretation of appropriate imaging. Although it needs to be demonstrated that there is a relationship between lag time from onset of symptoms to diagnosis and the ability to gain durable control of disease, there is little doubt that rapid diagnosis has an impact on avoidable neurological disability, as well as on the psychological state of the carer, and possibly also the child. If early diagnosis is to be achieved and improved upon, then education of doctors and the population is required. This should be coupled to improved access to diagnostic imaging and to appropriate specialist medical care. Those public healthcare systems, such as the UK's National Health Service, that introduce "gatekeepers" must examine and reconsider whether this is really in the best interest of patients. Research is required to explore and to develop the optimal models.

It may be that a relatively simple algorithm could be developed for use by paramedical staff involved in child health programs. The role of the carer in identifying changes in the health status of the child must never be forgotten.

A personal tale of two cities

The year 1983, and a child of 2.5 years is brought to the emergency room of a large Canadian children's hospital by his mother, who is concerned that the child has woken uncharacteristically early for several consecutive mornings on account of severe headaches, which settle by breakfast time. She asks to see a neurosurgeon. The child is seen in the emergency room by the then chief of service. CT is performed the same day, revealing a benign cerebellar astrocytoma, which is removed the next day. Recovery is uneventful.

Move on 18 years. The year 2001, and a child of similar age, with very similar symptomatology, is brought to the emergency room of a large UK teaching hospital. Despite there being a pediatric neurosurgeon on site, and available to be consulted, it takes three attendances and two admissions over a number of weeks before imaging is considered and a specialist opinion is sought, by which time there are severe neurological deficits, a very ill child, and distraught parents. Some healthcare systems clearly have to serve children better.

7

Diagnostic imaging

TIMOTHY JASPAN, with contribution from PAUL D. GRIFFITHS

INTRODUCTION

Central nervous system (CNS) tumors are now the commonest group of tumors in childhood, accounting for 25–30 per cent of all pediatric cancers. Primary tumors account for over 99 per cent of CNS tumors at this age. This chapter deals with issues related to imaging of tumors of the brain and spine. Particular emphasis will be given to the appropriate imaging modalities, techniques, protocols, and pitfalls of imaging encountered.

Radiological imaging of infants and children with suspected CNS tumors is often complex and requires close interaction with the other specialties involved in their management. As such, the imaging should be undertaken in tertiary centers or in close conjunction with referring institutions, according to specified protocols and guidelines for reporting. It is increasingly evident that radiological imaging of childhood CNS tumors should be undertaken as part of a multidisciplinary team, working in close conjunction with a range of specialties, including neurosurgeons, oncologists, radiotherapists, and pathologists. Imaging must cater for the specific requirements of the diagnostic, treatment-planning, and monitoring phases of the management of these children.

AIMS OF IMAGING

Imaging should be directed at:
- diagnosing the lesion, its origin, local extent, and presence of metastatic spread;

- differentiating tumors from granulomatous and infectious processes, hamartomas, vascular malformations, and heterotopias;
- directing appropriate management, including surgical planning, biopsy site selection, and radiation therapy planning;
- diagnosing tumor-related secondary complications, such as hydrocephalus, edema, intratumoral hemorrhage, and compressive cysts and brain herniation;
- diagnosing treatment-related complications;
- monitoring tumor progress or response to therapy.

IMAGING MODALITIES

The primary imaging modalities employed are computed tomography (CT) and magnetic resonance imaging (MRI). Ultrasound, single-photon-emission computed tomography (SPECT), positron-emission tomography (PET), and catheter angiography are used in selected cases and as research tools. The radiological modalities available for the evaluation of pediatric neuraxial tumors are discussed below.

Skull radiography

Plain skull radiography has no role in the investigation of suspected CNS tumors other than for specific issues related to the skull, such as evaluating the need for restorative cranial surgery and infection of surgical bone flaps.

Computed tomography

Children will often present to a community or district hospital staffed by general pediatricians for the investigation of suspected neurological disorders or with an acute neurological crisis. In many institutions, CT will be undertaken as the first line of investigation. This is because of its ubiquity, tolerance of life-support equipment, speed of scanning (often less than five to ten minutes of scanning time), and the relative simplicity of the diagnostic information provided.

Magnetic resonance imaging

The evaluation of neuraxial tumors is undertaken most completely and accurately by MRI. MRI is more sensitive than CT and demonstrates more fully and accurately the extent of the disease.[1] Preoperative evaluation by MRI provides the best platform for treatment decision-making and planning as well as for assessing the outcome of therapeutic interventions, and now forms the basis for all childhood CNS tumor treatment and investigative protocols.

Ultrasound

The value of ultrasound in the evaluation of neuraxial tumors is governed by the presence of an acoustic window. Patency of the anterior fontanelle provides access to the intracranial compartment, providing diagnostic information up to the first six to nine months of life. The quality of information provided is limited, however, and follow-up monitoring of the disease is curtailed by progressive closure of the fontanelle. Spinal imaging is dependent upon an even more limited temporal window. Progressive ossification of the posterior neural arches during the second to third months of life results in diminishing visualization of the thecal sac and cord. Paraspinal structures and tumors located at these sites may, however, be assessed, coupled with an examination of the abdominal contents. Sacrococcygeal lesions are also amenable to ultrasonic examination. The need to examine the entire neuraxis, however, limits the overall value of this modality.

Intraoperative ultrasound

The ability to guide and monitor tumor biopsies or resection interactively has secured some enthusiastic proponents of this technique. Ill-defined infiltrative tumors may be difficult to identify surgically but are often clearly apparent sonographically due to the differential echotexture of the tumor compared with normal adjacent brain. Future development of neuronavigational techniques and real-time intraoperative MRI may, however, supersede ultrasound in this capacity.

Intraoperative spinal ultrasound scanning can be very useful in delineating tumor margins and clearly defines tumoral and non-tumoral cysts. The ability to image the cord before opening the dura is an added advantage and may help surgical planning and selection of a biopsy site.

Catheter angiography

Modern imaging techniques have replaced angiography in the diagnosis of pediatric craniospinal tumors. There remains a limited role in the management of selected tumors, when superselective catheterization of vessels supplying a tumor and subsequent embolization may be beneficial in the perioperative management, diminishing tumor vascularity to improve intraoperative conditions. Local chemotherapy may also be undertaken in selected circumstances.[2]

Magnetic resonance spectroscopy

Magnetic resonance spectroscopy (MRS) is employed increasingly in the evaluation of pediatric brain tumors. Tissue function may be inferred by measuring the composition of selected metabolites within a region(s) of interest in the brain. The hydrogen proton is employed most widely in view of its abundance. Modern magnetic resonance scanners now permit MRS and conventional MRI to be undertaken using the same radiofrequency surface coil, with increasingly automated analysis of the spectroscopic data. Consequently, MRS may now be undertaken as an additional sequence at the end of a routine magnetic resonance examination with relatively little additional imaging time.

Single-voxel MRS, the analysis of a small volume ($\sim 8\,cm^3$) of tissue using a stimulated echo sequence point-resolved spectroscopy (PRESS) or stimulated-echo acquisition mode (STEAM) is commonly undertaken in view of the relatively short scan time (five to six minutes). However, this technique requires additional measurement of a selected control area of the brain for comparison. The recent introduction of multi-voxel two-dimensional (single-slice) and three-dimensional (multi-slice) real-time chemical shift imaging (CSI), employing 16 small voxels per slice, permits evaluation of larger areas of the brain that incorporate tumor and normal brain, the technique being termed "magnetic resonance spectroscopic imaging" (MRSI).

The major metabolites are N-acetyl aspartate (NAA; a marker for neuronal viability and density), creatine (Cr; a marker for energy metabolism and used as an internal reference), choline (Cho; involved in cell-membrane function and integrity), glutamate (Gl), and myoinositol (mI; an astrocytic marker). The major abnormal metabolites encountered are lactate (La; a marker of cell necrosis) and lipid (Li). The relative levels for the metabolite peaks

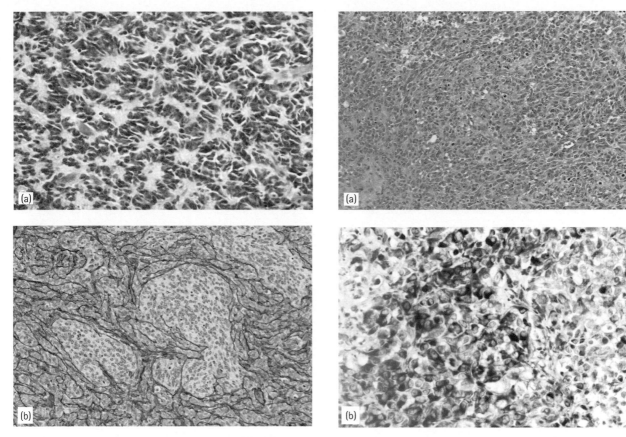

Plate 1 *Medulloblastoma and desmoplastic medulloblastoma (World Health Organization grade IV). (a) Poorly differentiated, blue-cell neoplasm with formation of neuroblastic (Homer–Wright) rosettes. (b) The desmoplastic medulloblastoma features differentiating tumor-cell islands surrounded by reticulin fibers.*

Plate 3 *Atypical teratoid/rhabdoid tumor (AT/RT) (World Health Organization grade IV). Highly cellular neoplasm composed of rhaboid, neuroepithelial, ectodermal, and mesodermal elements. Immunohistochemical reactions are helpful in identifying these components. (a) Hematoxylin and eosin staining; (b) immunohistochemical reaction with an antibody to vimentin yields a characteristic perinuclear staining pattern.*

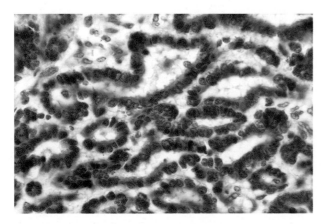

Plate 2 *Medulloepithelioma (World Health Organization grade IV). This primitive neuroepithelial neoplasm exhibits prominent neural tube-like structures.*

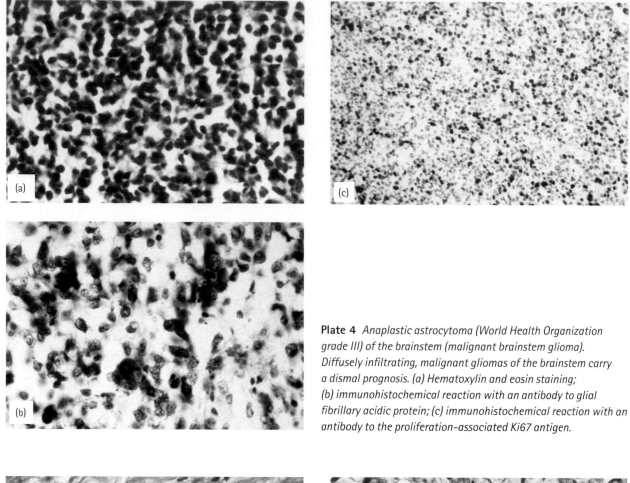

Plate 4 *Anaplastic astrocytoma (World Health Organization grade III) of the brainstem (malignant brainstem glioma). Diffusely infiltrating, malignant gliomas of the brainstem carry a dismal prognosis. (a) Hematoxylin and eosin staining; (b) immunohistochemical reaction with an antibody to glial fibrillary acidic protein; (c) immunohistochemical reaction with an antibody to the proliferation-associated Ki67 antigen.*

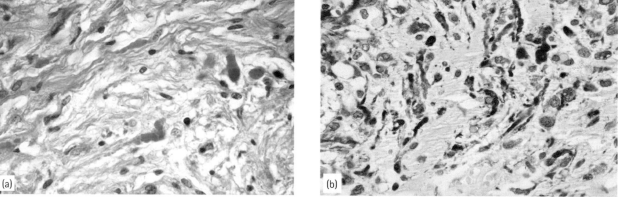

Plate 5 *Pilocytic astrocytoma (World Health Organization grade I). Microscopic hallmarks of this neoplasm include elongated, bipolar tumor cells, Rosenthal fibers, and protein droplets. (a) Hematoxylin and eosin staining; (b) immunohistochemical reaction with an antibody to glial fibrillary acidic protein.*

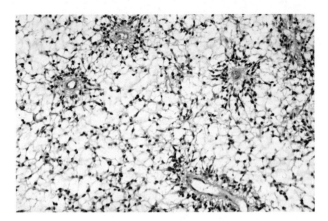

Plate 6 *Pilomyxoid astrocytoma. Such a variant shows a mucinous background and a prominent angiocentric pattern.*

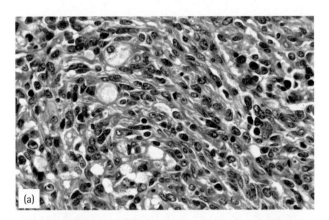

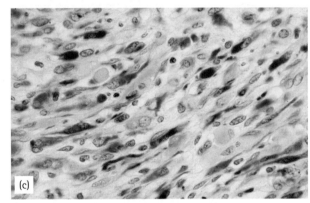

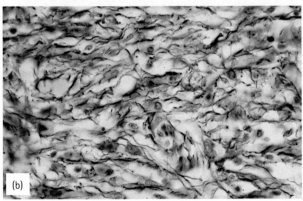

Plate 7 *Pleomorphic xanthoastrocytoma (World Health Organization grade II). Polymorphic astrocytic neoplasm (a) with fascicular growth, foamy cells, and a superficial component with production of reticulin fibers (b) and expression of glial fibrillary acidic protein (c). In contrast to their pleomorphic phenotype, many of these gliomas show a rather benign course.*

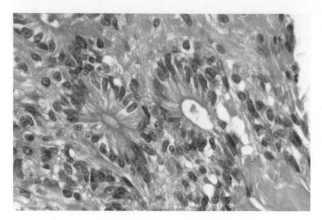

Plate 8 *Ependymoma (World Health Organization grade II). Glial neoplasms characterized by the formation of ependymal and perivascular rosettes. Anaplastic variants exhibit hypercellular, poorly differentiated components with marked mitotic activity.*

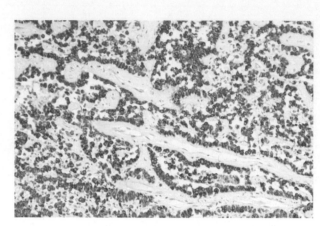

Plate 10 *Papillary meningioma (World Health Organization grade III). This anaplastic meningeal tumor features prominent papillary architectures (immunohistochemical reaction with an antibody to vimentin).*

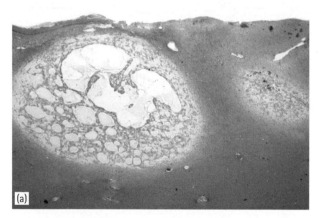

(a)

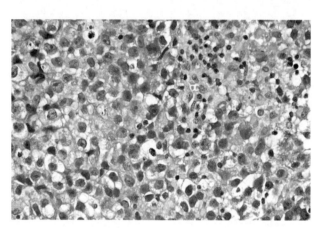

Plate 11 *Germinoma. Malignant germ-cell tumor, showing a combination of epithelioid neoplastic cells and prominent lymphocytic infiltrates. The histopathological appearance is indistinguishable from seminomas of the testis. Other germ-cell components, such as yolk sac or teratoma elements, must be excluded.*

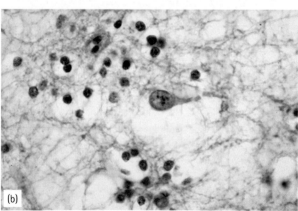

(b)

Plate 9 *Dysembryoplastic neuroepithelial tumor (DNT). Multinodular, cortical neoplasm (a) characterized by islands of clear cells in a mucoid matrix, floating neurons (b), and formation of columnar patterns. The adjacent cortex may show dysplastic change. Complex DNTs contain areas of pilocytic astrocytoma in addition.*

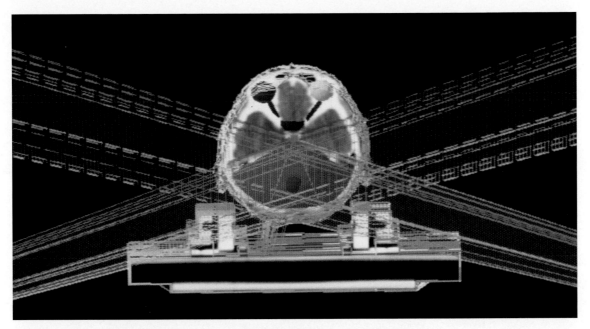

Plate 12 *Beam's-eye view of three-dimensional treatment planning of posterior fossa fields.*

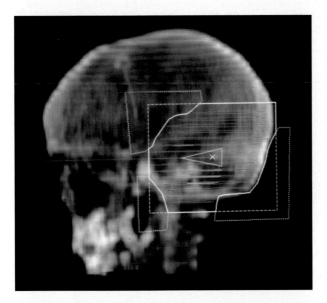

Plate 13 *Digitally reconstructed radiograph displaying oblique portal for posterior fossa boost.*

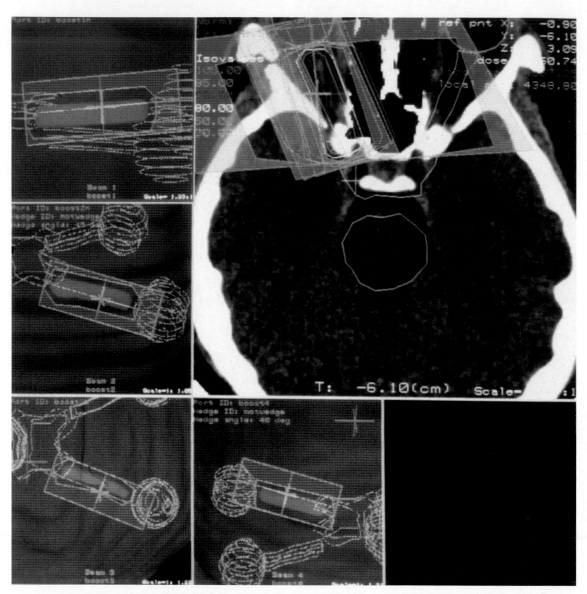

Plate 14 *Conformal radiation therapy of an optic nerve sheath meningioma in a 15-year-old boy. Treatment plan in three-dimensional conformal therapy. Radiotherapy is focused on the tumor site. The contralateral eye is spared completely, and the doses to the pituitary gland and the optic chiasm are minimized.*

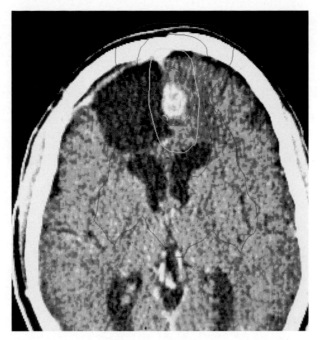

Plate 15 *Hypofractionated convergent beam radiotherapy in recurrent malignant glioma. Isodose distribution on transversal plane (three moving arcs).*

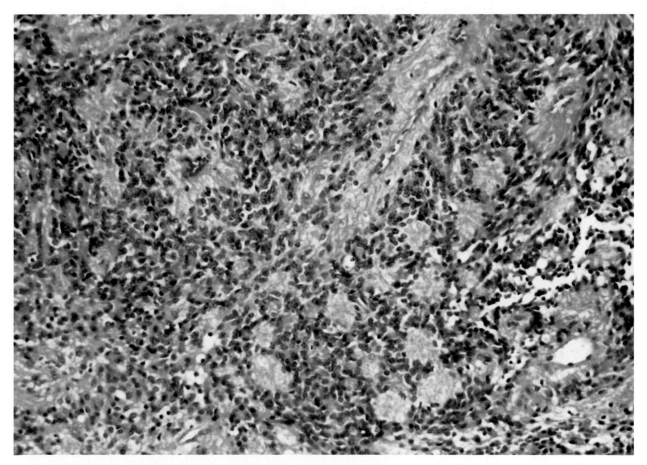

Plate 16 *Photomicrograph demonstrating perivascular pseudorosettes, created by the cytoplasmic processes of tumor cells around blood vessels. (Courtesy of Dr L. E. Becker, Hospital for Sick Children, Toronto, Canada.)*

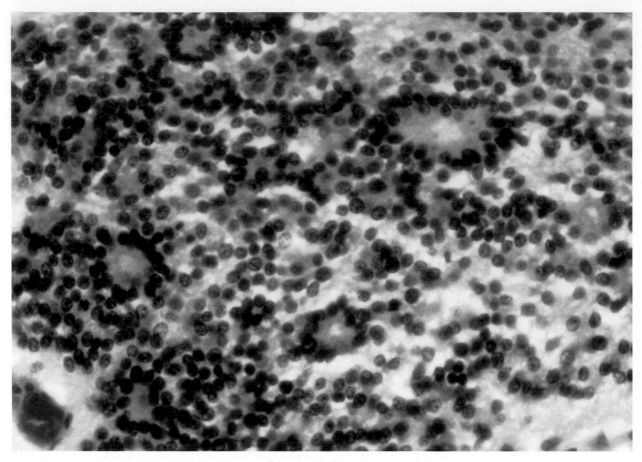

Plate 17 *Photomicrograph demonstrating true ependymal rosettes, in which the central lumen is created by the surface of the tumor cells themselves. (Courtesy of Dr L. E. Becker, Hospital for Sick Children, Toronto, Canada.)*

and metabolite ratios (NAA/Cho, NAA/Cr, Cho/Cr) may be derived.

In general, abnormal NAA serves as a non-specific marker of diseased tissue. Tumors generally display decreased NAA levels, increased choline levels, and variable lipid, lactate, and creatine levels. The level of choline correlates with the proportion of tumor in the measured volume. MRSI is not predictive of histology, but it may be helpful in evaluating tumor grade and behavior, in the selection of a stereotactic site to better target parts of a tumor expressing more aggressive features, and in the differentiation between radionecrosis and recurrent tumor.[3,4]

Perfusion magnetic resonance imaging

Dynamic, first-pass, contrast-enhanced, fast-gradient echo sequences, either T1- or T2-weighted, are employed for perfusion imaging and enable quantitative analysis of the regional cerebral blood flow (CBF) in normal brain and diseased tissue. The imaging is undertaken following a bolus injection of a contrast agent; the need for suitable intravenous access may thus prove problematic in very young infants. The relative cerebral blood volume (CBV), a function of tissue perfusion, is derived, which in the context of oncological investigations reflects tumor angiogenesis.

Tumor angiogenesis underpins the processes of tumor growth, progression, and spread. Whereas T1-weighted contrast images depict areas of breakdown or absence of the blood–brain barrier as enhancement, perfusion magnetic resonance imaging (pMRI) identifies overall tumor vascularity and intratumoral variations and may indicate the proliferative potential and malignancy of a tumor. Low-grade tumors exhibit low CBV in contradistinction to higher-grade tumors, which are more vascular.[3] Differentiation of tumor from radionecrosis, which has very low CBF, is possible. As with MRS, pMRI may enable better targeting of stereotactic biopsy sites, selecting regions of a tumor exhibiting the highest regional CBV and thus greater malignant and proliferative potential. Similarly, evaluating response to therapy may be enhanced by employing pMRI techniques. Restrictions of pMRI relate largely to inherent susceptibility artifacts associated with osseous structures (particularly around the skull base), metallic fragments and implants, calcification, and hemorrhage.

Single–photon–emission computed tomography and positron–emission tomography

SPECT with ^{201}Tl is being used increasingly to evaluate residual and recurrent brain tumors with a high level of specificity.[5] In patients who have undergone radiation therapy, high uptake of ^{201}Tl is associated with locally recurrent tumor, while low uptake is conversely seen in radiation necrosis. The ability to differentiate high-grade from low-grade tumors, tumor types, and biological activity is of unproven value in children,[6] except in the context of brainstem gliomas.[7]

PET allows quantitative assessment of brain tumor pathophysiology and biochemistry, providing an index for the metabolic activity of the lesion. Parameters that may be evaluated include blood flow, blood volume, oxygen, amino acid and glucose uptake, protein and nucleic acid synthesis, cerebral pH, and blood–brain barrier integrity. Unlike SPECT imaging, which is available widely in most well-equipped centers, PET is, at present, restricted to a relatively few centers. ^{18}F-Fluorodeoxyglucose (FDG) is used as a tracer for tumor imaging, being taken up by cells by mechanisms similar to cellular glucose utilization.

FDG-PET has been used to monitor the response of tumors to treatment, particularly radiation therapy, and to assess radiation necrosis. Identification of the metabolically most active parts of a tumor may enable better targeting for biopsy and differentiation of viable tumor from necrosis.[8] PET has also been used to differentiate high-grade from low-grade tumors – the higher the grade, the more hypermetabolic the tumor. Subtle metabolic changes may be measured with relatively high spatial resolution (3–4 mm); however, in terms of differentiating between high- and low-grade tumors, the sensitivity and specificity is probably less than with Tl SPECT.[9]

For both SPECT and PET, computer-assisted co-registration with anatomical studies such as CT or MRI adds to the power of these techniques greatly, as does close clinical correlation.

Meta–iodobenzylguanidine scintigraphy

Neuroblastomas are some of the commonest solid malignant tumors of childhood; they are metastatic at presentation in 80 per cent of cases. Neuroectodermally derived tumors, including neuroblastomas and paraganglionomas, have been shown to take up meta-iodobenzylguanidine (MIBG), an aralkylguanidine noradrenaline analog, which is iodinated with I-131 or I-123. The sensitivity of MIBG for detecting primary and secondary neuroblastomas approaches 100 per cent. The sensitivity in detecting sites on a lesion-by-lesion basis is about 80 per cent, with a 90–95 per cent sensitivity in terms of staging.[10] As the detection and the staging of the disease have a major impact on the treatment and prognosis, MIBG scanning has become integral to the management of these tumors.

SEDATION AND ANESTHESIA FOR IMAGING

The decision to image an infant or child needs to be made in close conjunction with the referring clinician and, where necessary, an experienced pediatric anesthetist. The child needs to keep still for the duration of the examination, both for CT and, especially, MRI. Children presenting acutely, particularly with clinical features indicative of raised intracranial pressure, should be imaged under general anesthesia. Imaging of the entire neuraxis requires the use of different surface coils to cover both the head and the spine, extending the length of the procedure. The sedation must therefore be sufficient to ensure immobility and handling of the child between imaging of different body parts, and the administration of contrast agent and sedation must be sufficiently long-lasting to enable the examination to be completed safely.

Infants under three months of age may be scanned following a feed; however, sedation is usually required. Oral chloral hydrate is used widely in both infants and older children up to the age of three to four years (dose 50–100 mg/kg), supplemented by rectal paraldehyde for top-up sedation. Between the ages of three and seven years, quinalbarbitone (dose 5–10 mg/kg), rectal thiopentone, or oral, buccal, intranasal, or rectal midazolam are used, the latter with high rates of success. Close monitoring is required before, during, and after administration of the sedative/anesthetic. Physiological monitoring must include pulse oximetry and trained nursing or medical staff supervising the procedure. More comprehensive magnetic-resonance-compatible monitoring equipment, including capnography and electrocardiography (ECG), must be available. The presence of a dedicated sedation nurse is strongly recommended to ensure optimal coordination with the radiographic staff and correct timing and administration of the sedation.

Training and parental involvement in the scanner room may enable the older child (over seven years of age) to undergo the examination without sedation, particularly for children undergoing frequent repeat scanning. While the above sedative agents may be used, there should be a low threshold for resorting to general anesthesia or controlled sedation undertaken by an appropriately trained anesthetist.

VENOUS ACCESS

Venous access should be secured before the child has been sedated and transferred to the imaging suite. Use of a local anesthetic Emla® cream patch is highly recommended before attempted vein cannulation. In-dwelling intravenous central lines must be used with an appropriate aseptic technique.

IMAGING PROTOCOLS

The wide range of institutions receiving and investigating childhood CNS tumors has resulted in a heterogeneous imaging methodology.[11] Because of the relatively small numbers of cases in each center, it is essential that multicenter trials be conducted to facilitate research-based therapeutic intervention and overall management of these children. There is thus a strong need for conformity in the image acquisition and presentation. An adapted "cookbook" of MRI is provided in Tables 7.1–7.3, based on the consensus document produced by the UK Children's Cancer Study Group (UKCCSG) and the Société Française d'Oncologie Pédiatrique (SFOP).[12,13]

IMAGE PRESENTATION

Conformity in the way images are acquired and presented is essential for continuity of monitoring tumor evolution and the efficient analysis of the imaging for diagnostic and research purposes. All images should be acquired using the same anatomical landmarks, the scan pilot displaying the slice orientation being recorded on each occasion such that all subsequent follow-up imaging employs the same technique. Axial imaging should be oriented to a plane parallel to a line drawn from the

Table 7.1 *Supratentorial tumors*

Sequence	Presentation	Immediately postoperative	Follow–up
Axial T2 SE or FSE	+	+	+
Coronal T1 SE	+	+	+
Post-contrast T1 SE in two orthogonal planes	+	+	+
Sagittal T1 SE whole spine	+	Spinal imaging not performed preoperatively	Protocol-driven or tumors with high risk of leptomeningeal spread
Axial T1 SE spine if equivocal area(s)	+	Spinal imaging not performed preoperatively	Protocol-driven or tumors with high risk of leptomeningeal spread

FSE, fast spin echo; SE, spin echo.

anterior commissure to posterior commissure (AC–PC axis). Imaging should be undertaken from inferior to superior in the axial plane, and from right to left in the coronal and sagittal planes.

TUMOR EVALUATION

Tumor measurement should be based on the enhancing component of the lesion, where present, recording the maximal dimensions in at least two and preferably all three orthogonal planes. There has been recent discussion about the modes of tumor measurement, including use of a single maximal dimension[14] and three-dimensional volumes.[15] Ultimately, three-dimensional volumetric evaluations employing automatic MRI multispectral segmentation techniques (including eigen-image filter and other semi-automated computer methods) may allow a more complete assessment of tumors and their response to therapy and reduce the significant element of intra- and interobserver errors in manual visual metric methods.[15–17] However, most neuro-oncology protocols are currently based on the use of two or three orthogonal tumor dimension measurements (visual metric assessment).

In the standard approach, tumor response is based on a percentage change in the dimensions and categorized into cure (complete response), partial response (which may be subdivided further into improvement), stable disease, and progression.

Follow-up imaging should be evaluated on the basis of the previous examination. All previous imaging must be available to assess the magnetic resonance characteristics and enhancement pattern of the lesion at diagnosis and any morphological evolution, which may aid in the evaluation of abnormal tissue at the primary or distant sites. Tumor cysts should not be included in the tumor volume, as there is no associated proliferative potential. The cysts, may, however result in the symptomatic presentation of the child and dictate the need for and timing of surgery.

Presence of distant disease and a qualitative evaluation of the tumor should be recorded. For non-enhancing tumors, such as brainstem fibrillary astrocytomas, tumor measurements are evaluated on the dimensions of the T2 signal abnormality obtained from two orthogonal planes of imaging.

Tumor response should be by independently verified measurements obtained not less than four weeks apart, and are evaluated as follows:

- *Complete response*: no measurable tumor.
- *Partial response*: greater than 50 per cent reduction in tumor volume.

Table 7.2 *Infratentorial tumors*

Sequence	Presentation	Immediately postoperative	Follow–up
Axial T2 SE or FSE	+	+	+
Sagittal T1 SE	+	+	+
Sagittal T2 FSE (for BSG)	+	−	+(for BSG)
Post-contrast T1 SE in two orthogonal planes	+	+	+
Sagittal T1 SE whole spine	+	Spinal imaging not performed preoperatively	Protocol-driven or tumors with high risk of leptomeningeal spread
Axial T1 SE spine if equivocal area(s)	+	Spinal imaging not performed preoperatively	Protocol-driven or tumors with high risk of leptomeningeal spread

BSG, brainstem glioma; FSE, fast spin echo; SE, spin echo.

Table 7.3. *Spinal tumors*

Sequence	Presentation	Immediately postoperative	Follow–up
Sagittal T2 FSE	+	+	+
Sagittal T1 SE	+	+	+
Axial T1 SE through lesion	+	+	+
Sagittal T1 SE post-contrast	+	+	+
Axial T1 SE post-contrast	+	+	+
Cranial post-contrast in two orthogonal planes	+	Cranial imaging not undertaken preoperatively	Protocol-driven or tumors with high risk of leptomeningeal spread

FSE, fast spin echo; SE, spin echo.

- *Improvement*: 25–50 per cent reduction in tumor volume.
- *Stable disease*: less than 25 per change in volume, or tumor growth of less than 25 per cent.
- *Disease progression*: greater than 25 per cent increase in tumor volume, or appearance of a new tumor.

Leptomeningeal disease is recorded as linear or nodular enhancement. Thin pial enhancement following surgery should be regarded as reactive if not present on the preoperative scan. Pachymeningeal enhancement in the intracranial compartment is commonly encountered postoperatively and may persist for several months or even years.[18]

Staging of the extent of surgical resection

The extent of surgical resection may be evaluated by the following criteria:

- *S0*: no residual tumor visible.
- *S1*: residual tumor less than 1.5 cm in diameter.
- *S2*: residual tumor 1.5 cm or more in largest diameter.
- *S3*: residual tumor infiltrating the brainstem (for posterior fossa) or the ventricles (for supratentorial).
- *S4*: residual tumor extending outside of its natural compartment e.g. from infra- to supratentorial or into the spinal canal.

Staging of leptomeningeal tumor

Leptomeningeal tumors are classified as follows:

- *M0*: no leptomeningeal abnormality.
- *M1*: tumor cells in the cerebrospinal fluid (CSF) (more than 14 days after surgery) but no leptomeningeal disease seen on neuroimaging.
- *M2*: intracranial leptomeningeal abnormality defined by:
  - thin laminar layers;
  - discrete nodular lesions or thick laminar layers.
- *M3*: intraspinal leptomeningeal disease defined by:
  - thin laminar layers;
  - discrete nodular lesions or thick laminar layers.
- *M4*: metastases outside the CNS.

TUMOR PATTERNS

Approximately one-third of intracranial solid tumors in children occur in the supratentorial compartment. Radiological evaluation of CNS tumors may be analyzed in terms of anatomical localization in conjunction with the pathological classification of lesions at each specific site.

Supratentorial tumors

HEMISPHERIC TUMORS

Neuroepithelial tumors

Astrocytomas Almost 50 per cent of cerebral hemispheric tumors are astrocytic in origin,[19,20] of which the astrocytomas are by far the most common. The World Health Organization (WHO) uses a three-category classification, with low-grade astrocytoma, anaplastic astrocytoma, and glioblastoma multiforme (GBM). The imaging characteristics and enhancement pattern provide helpful and often diagnostic information with regard to tumor grading. However, tumor histological heterogeneity and biological evolution are such that surgical biopsy is essential if treatment planning and evaluation are to have a rational basis. Approximately 70 per cent of astrocytomas are infiltrative in nature. Tumor extension is invariably beyond the confines of the lesion as defined by CT or MRI.[21]

Pilocytic astrocytomas Less common than diffuse fibrillary astrocytomas (vide infra), these tumors are typically located in the hypothalamus, optic nerves, and optic chiasm (vide infra), and, to a lesser extent, the thalami and basal ganglia. Hemispheric locations, particularly the frontal lobes, are less common. The tumors are well demarcated, appearing iso- or hypodense on CT scanning. Calcification is uncommon (less than 10 per cent). Tumor-related cysts are frequently present. On MRI, the solid components are isointense on T1- and hyperintense on T2-weighted images. Cystic elements follow CSF signal characteristics. Contrast enhancement is usually moderate to marked. Whilst frequently benign and insidious, the location of the tumor may result in a more aggressive presentation. Leptomeningeal metastatic spread is seen occasionally.

Fibrillary astrocytomas Of the diffuse astrocytic tumors, the low-grade diffuse fibrillary astrocytomas are the most common in childhood, most being hemispheric in location. These lesions are often poorly defined and infiltrative; however, in a minority of cases, they may appear well circumscribed. The temporal lobes are involved most frequently, followed by the frontal, parietal, and occipital lobes.[22] The CT characteristics are of an ill-defined mildly hypo- or isodense lesion that may evade detection on initial scanning. Calcification occurs in approximately 20 per cent of cases. Cystic change is uncommon. On MRI, the tumors are hypo- to isointense with respect to normal brain and hyperintense on T2-weighted images. Cortical involvement is identified by thickening as well as signal changes. Cystic change is unusual, and enhancement is characteristically absent or minimal. Perilesional edema is notable by its absence, and mass effect, if present, is seldom significant.

Anaplastic astrocytoma These tumors share similar locations with the fibrillary astrocytomas. They are unusual in childhood, but if present they occur in the second decade of life. They are more common in the fourth and fifth decades. On CT scanning, there is greater heterogeneity with foci of calcification or hemorrhage, edema, and mass effect. Enhancement is variable. Necrosis should not be present. Magnetic resonance characteristics mirror these different elements. Patchy hyperintensity on T1-weighted images, related to microcalcifications and hemorrhage, is superimposed on hypo- or isointense tumor. The tumor margins are defined poorly, and the T2 signal abnormality of the tumor merges imperceptibly with surrounding vasogenic edema. Enhancement is seen more frequently than in fibrillary astrocytomas but is patchy and variable.

Glioblastoma multiforme   These tumors, being the most aggressive astrocytic lesions, are uncommon in children. There is a biphasic age distribution with peaks at four to five and 11–12 years of age.[23] Like adult GBM, tumor necrosis is the index histological and imaging feature. On CT scanning, the tumor is iso- to mildly hyperdense, with surrounding edema. Intralesional hemorrhage is common. T1-weighted MRI demonstrates an ill-defined, irregular, iso- to mildly hyperintense lesion with irregular hypointense necrotic foci centrally. Enhancement is strong, with a thick irregular rim often highlighting a necrotic center (Figure 7.1). On T2-weighted images, solid tumor is hyperintense, the necrotic foci being of particularly high signal. Commissural extension, particularly via the corpus callosum, is a typical feature. Metastatic leptomeningeal spread is seen in 20 per cent of cases.[24]

Pleomorphic xanthoastrocytoma   This relatively rare entity, representing approximately one per cent of all gliomas in early life, has been added to the WHO list of astrocytic tumors only recently. The tumors occur most commonly in the temporal lobes and less commonly in the parietal, occipital, and frontal lobes.[25] Their derivation from subpial astrocytes underlies their typical superficial cortical location with a meningeal attachment.[24] Although classified as low-grade tumors, as implied by the name, there is often marked cellular pleomorphism and a subset of more aggressive lesions that are associated with a poor three-year survival rate.[26]

The lesion is often large at presentation, is usually well circumscribed, and may be predominantly cystic, with a mural nodule. When present, the mural nodule frequently abuts the leptomeninges. In some cases, the tumor is largely solid. Scalloping and thinning of the overlying calvarium may be seen and reflects the slow-growing nature of the tumor. Enhancement of the tumor nodule is strong on both CT scanning and MRI. On MRI, the solid tumor is hypo- to isointense and hyperintense on T2-weighted images, with typical signal characteristics for the cyst (Figure 7.2). In addition to the nodular component, gyral and/or meningeal enhancement may be seen[27] and may presage local recurrence following

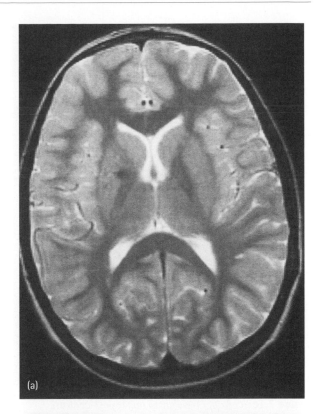

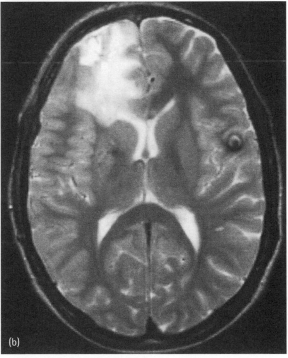

Figure 7.1a,b *Glioblastoma multiforme occurring in a boy treated previously with craniospinal radiotherapy for central nervous system lymphoma. (a) Axial T2 image post-radiotherapy showing a small cavernous malformation in the right globus pallidus. (b) Axial T2 image four years later. Ill-defined hyperintensity in the right frontal lobe has developed in addition to a second cavernous malformation in the left frontal operculum.*

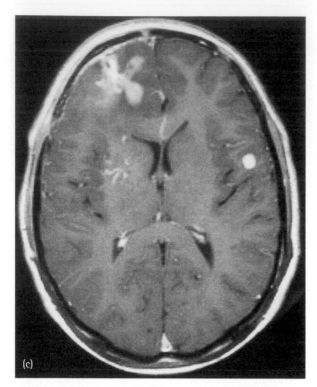

Figure 7.1c *(c) Axial T1-weighted image post-contrast demonstrates strong, irregular enhancement, highlighting a small peripheral necrotic focus. Dural enhancement is associated with a burr-hole biopsy site and dural extension of tumor. There is incidental enhancement of a venous angioma adjacent to the right pallidal cavernoma and enhancement of the left frontal opercular cavernoma.*

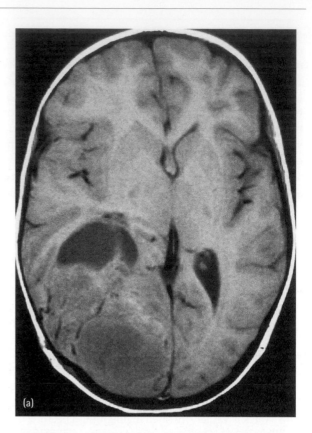

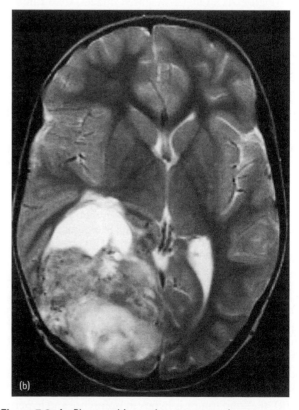

Figure 7.2a,b *Pleomorphic xanthoastrocytoma in a ten-year-old girl. (a) Axial T1 image. Large right occipitotemporal tumor with variable elements, including a small eccentric cyst and cortical involvement. (b) Axial T2-weighted image showing the heterogeneous nature of the lesion and highlighting the cyst.*

surgery. Catheter angiography reveals the tumor to be highly vascular, often deriving a dural supply from meningeal arteries.

Gliomatosis cerebri This is a rare tumor in childhood. The diffuse infiltrating nature of the lesion is often accompanied by relatively little neurological evidence of disease due to late preservation of neuronal function. CT demonstrates very subtle and widespread parenchymal abnormality, with mild hypo- to isodensity. The superiority of MRI is well exemplified by such a tumor, which defines more clearly the presence of ill-defined diffuse T2 hyperintensity involving the white matter. T1-weighted imaging may show little apparent abnormality other than expansion of the brain, particularly the gyri. Despite the presence of extensive tumor, relatively normal structure of the brain may be preserved until late in the disease process, which carries a poor prognosis. Enhancement is uncommon. The diagnosis may remain elusive for some time, being dependent on stereotactic biopsy, or it may become apparent only at autopsy. MRS may provide useful additional information in the detection of this lesion and monitoring progress.[28]

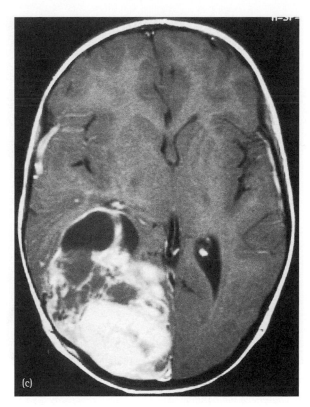

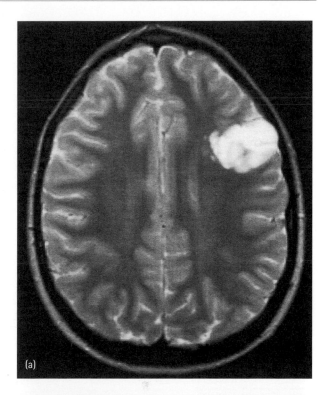

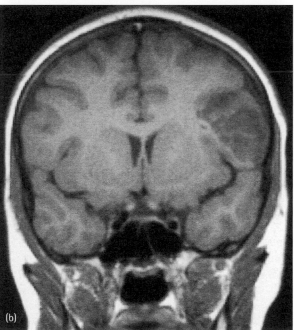

Figure 7.2c *(c) Post-contrast axial T1-weighted image. The tumor enhances avidly but irregularly.*

Oligodendroglial tumors

Oligodendrogliomas Approximately five to ten per cent of oligodendrogliomas occur in childhood,[29,30] with a peak age of 6–12 years.[31] The frontal lobes are involved most frequently, followed by the parietal and temporal lobes.[30,32] Histological heterogeneity, with astrocytic elements within the tumor, is present in approximately 50 per cent of cases. Oligoastrocytomas share similar imaging characteristics with the histologically purer oligodendrogliomas. The tumors frequently occur in the cortex or subcortical region and may exhibit local subpial or wider leptomeningeal extension.

CT optimally identifies intralesional calcifications (50 per cent) and hemorrhage (20 per cent). The tumors are, however, often iso- to hypodense on CT and less well defined on CT than by MRI. Tumor cysts are common. Enhancement is variable but often mild.

MRI demonstrates a hypointense tumor on T1-weighted images with more conspicuous margins and enhancement (Figure 7.3). Greater intensity of enhancement probably reflects more aggressive histological features.[33] On T2 imaging, the lesion, in particular any cystic elements, is hyperintense; hypointensities reflect the presence of calcifications or hemosiderin from previous hemorrhages.

The more aggressive anaplastic oligodendrogliomas are seen less frequently in children. When present, local tumor recurrence following surgery is not uncommon.

Figure 7.3a,b *Oligodendroglioma in a six-year-old boy. (a) Axial T2 image showing a well-delineated hyperintense left frontal lobe lesion involving and expanding the cortex. (b) Coronal T1 image. The heterogeneously hypointense lesion extends inferiorly to the frontal operculum, clearly having a cortical base.*

Ependymomas Approximately 30–40 per cent of ependymomas are supratentorial, arising most commonly in the third and lateral ventricles. The lesions may also be entirely parenchymal, being derived from ependymal cell

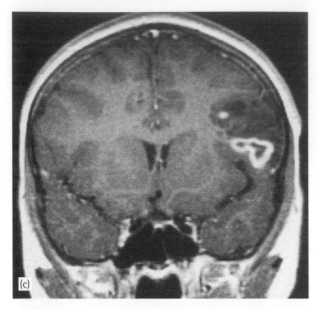

Figure 7.3c *(c) Post-contrast coronal T1 image. There is strong ring-like and nodular enhancement deep within the tumor and in the cortex.*

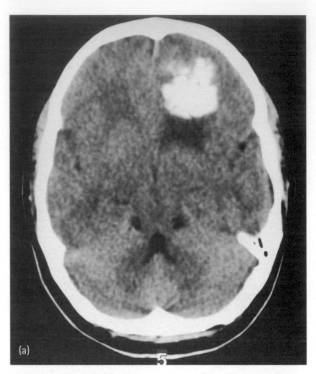

Figure 7.4a *Cerebral ependymoma. (a) Unenhanced axial computerized tomography scan, demonstrating craggy calcification in a left frontobasal tumor.*

rests in the white matter. Unlike the commoner posterior fossa tumors, the age of presentation of patients with supratentorial ependymomas is older, peaking in the latter half of the second decade; the tumors are larger and more often malignant.

Calcification is present in approximately 50 per cent of cases. Unlike posterior fossa ependymomas, cyst formation is common. On CT, the tumors tend to be heterogeneous in nature, with large cysts, amorphous calcifications, and patchy enhancement. MRI demonstrates a well-defined mass of mild hypo- to isointensity on T1-weighted images and hyperintensity on T2-weighted images. Enhancement is usually heterogeneous (Figure 7.4).

Neuronal and mixed neuronal-glial tumors

Gangliocytomas and gangliogliomas   These tumors are defined histologically by the presence of neuronal and glial cells. Gangliocytomas contain mature neoplastic ganglionic cells, while gangliogliomas have varying degrees of glial tissue interspersed between the ganglionic elements. There is a predilection for the temporal lobes for both. Gangliocytomas may also involve the hypothalamus. Gangliogliomas occur less frequently elsewhere in the cerebral hemispheres. Gangliocytomas are rare and may occur anywhere in the cerebral hemispheres and sellar region.

The imaging characteristics of both types of tumors are similar, the lesions being peripheral in location, rounded, well-defined, and hypodense on CT. There is variable presence of cysts (30–50 per cent), the incidence being higher in children than adults. Calcification, which

may be craggy and prominent, occurs in 30–40 per cent of cases. Tumoral hemorrhage is seen occasionally. A mural nodule may be seen with largely cystic tumors. On MRI, there is a heterogeneous appearance on T1-weighted imaging, while on T2 imaging the lesions are generally hyperintense, although they may be modified by the presence of calcification or blood products. There is little or no perilesional edema (Figure 7.5). Enhancement occurs in approximately 50 per cent of cases (Figure 7.6).[34,35] Gangliogliomas may infiltrate the leptomeninges, although this does not necessarily connote malignancy. Distant leptomeningeal spread may, however, occur in a small proportion of cases, identified most readily if the primary lesion enhances.

Dysembryoplastic neuroepithelial tumors   These lesions are of low grade; debate persists over whether they are true neoplasms or rather hamartomatous overgrowth of glioneuronal tissue. The clinical presentation of children with dysembryoplastic neuroepithelial tumors (DNTs) is typically with seizures, usually commencing in the second decade of life. The tumors are characteristically intracortical and multinodular, the thickened cortex around the margins of the lesion being due to a combination of tumor and cortical dysplasia. The slow-growing nature of the tumor explains the occasional finding of calvarial scalloping or thinning. Whilst typically located in the temporal lobes medially, they may

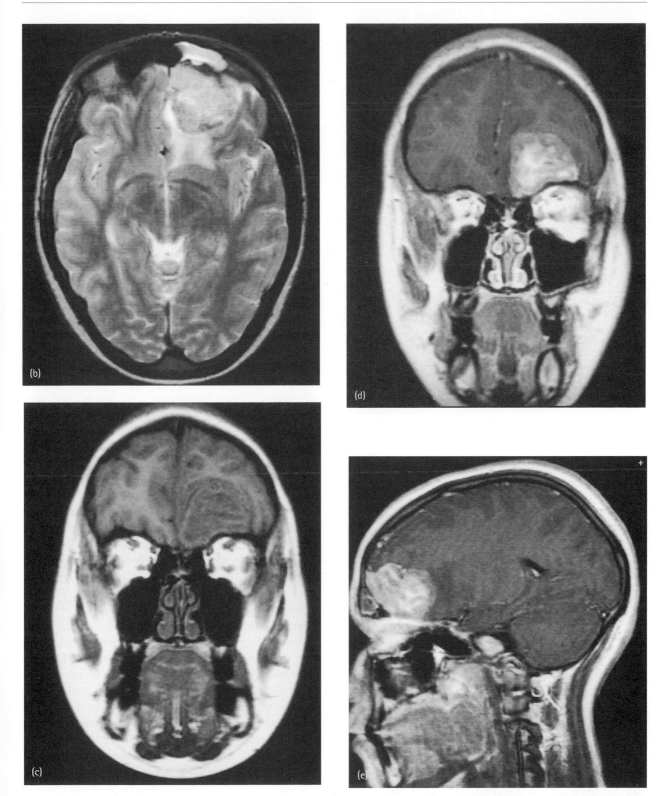

Figure 7.4b–e *(b) Axial T2 image. The lesion is heterogeneously mildly hyperintense, with some surrounding edema. (c) Pre-contrast coronal T1 image. The lesion is mildly hypointense. (d) Coronal and (e) Sagittal T1 images, demonstrating patchy moderately strong lesion enhancement.*

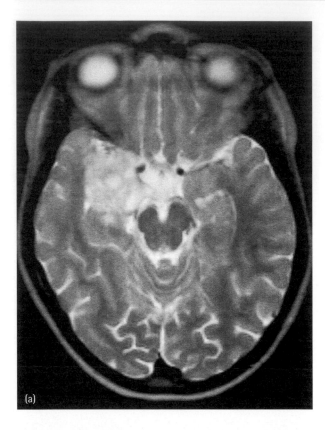

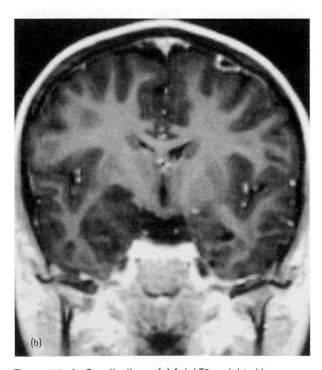

Figure 7.5a,b *Ganglioglioma. (a) Axial T2-weighted image.*
A discrete hyperintense lesion is present based on the mesial right
temporal lobe. Note the absence of edema. (b) Post-contrast
coronal T1-weighted image, showing a cortically based
non-enhancing lesion, isointense in comparison to the adjacent
cortex.

be found elsewhere in the cerebral hemispheres in a cortical location.

The CT appearance is of a hypodense peripheral mass, possibly with cystic foci and occasionally calcification and enhancement following contrast administration. On MRI, the mass is usually well circumscribed, appearing as a ribbon-like intracortical hypointensity on T1-weighted images and is hyperintense on T2-weighted images (Figure 7.7). The cortex may appear multinodular, distorted, and thickened, and there may be abnormal signals in the underlying whiter matter. Three-dimensional T1-weighted gradient echo techniques are especially useful in defining the associated cortical dysplasia associated with more complex forms of DNT because of the improved anatomical resolution. Punctate foci of enhancement may occur, but this is not typically a feature.

Desmoplastic infantile gangliogliomas Desmoplastic infantile ganglioglioma (DIG) is a rare, relatively recently described, benign tumor usually occurring in the first year of life. Unlike its variant, ganglioglioma, the typical sites of involvement are the frontal, parietal, and temporal lobes.[36,37] The tumors are typically large and cystic at presentation, often measuring over 10 cm, and have a superficial location. Leptomeningeal involvement is common. The prognosis is good following surgical resection. Imaging typically reveals a large hypodense cyst and a hyperdense peripherally located solid component that enhances avidly following contrast administration. MRI demonstrates corresponding appearances with signal intensities consistent with cyst fluid. The solid component of the tumor may be hypo-, iso-, or hyperdense on T2-weighted images (Figure 7.8) and enhances strongly on T1 images, highlighting a broad base upon the leptomeninges.

Embryonal tumors

Primitive neuroectodermal tumors PNETs are characterized by the presence of small, undifferentiated, round cells with variable cellular differentiation. The term "primitive neuroectodermal tumor" (PNET) now encompasses histological entities such as cerebral neuroblastoma, medulloepithelioma, ependymoblastoma, medulloblastoma, retinoblastoma, and pineoblastoma. Approximately five to ten per cent of PNETs occur in the cerebral hemispheres, where they are typically large at presentation. Supratentorial PNETs, along with atypical teratoid/rhabdoid tumors (vide infra), may occur in the neonatal period and in the first year of life.[38] The small number of tumors occurring in the second and third decades of life are more often a desmoplastic variant of PNET. The frontal lobes are involved most often, followed by the parietal, temporal, and occipital lobes. Calcification is a dominant feature, occurring in 50–70 per cent of cases; hydrocephalus is also frequently present.

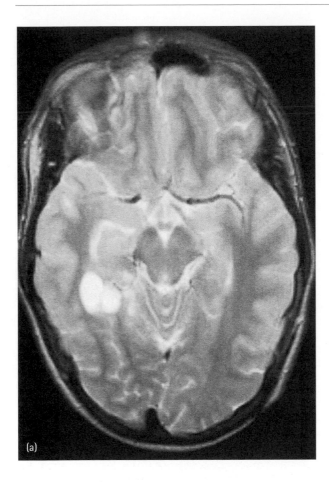

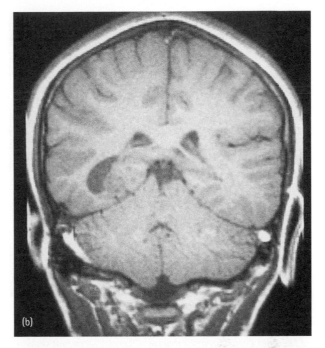

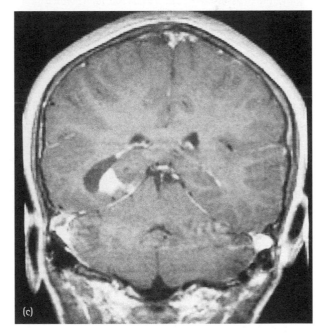

Figure 7.6a–c *Gangliocytoma. (a) Axial T2-weighted image, showing a discrete hyperintensity in the deep right temporal lobe. (b) Coronal T1 image. The lesion, based on the occipitotemporal gyrus, has a peripheral solid component isointense in comparison with the adjacent cortex and a deeper cystic element. (c). Post-contrast coronal T1 image, showing strong enhancement of the solid cortically based component.*

The tumors are well defined and are markedly heterogeneous in appearance on both CT and MRI due to the presence of calcification, hemorrhage, necrosis, and the highly cellular nature of the tumor. There is usually little or no edema. Patchy contrast enhancement is seen, particularly with MRI, in the solid components of the tumor. MRI also optimally demonstrates leptomeningeal spread, which occurs in 40 per cent of cases.[39]

Atypical teratoid/rhabdoid tumors These tumors occur at a younger age (often within the first year of life)

than parenchymal ependymomas and PNETs, with which they share similar imaging characteristics and which they are frequently mistaken for.[40] The tumors are usually large at presentation and appear of heterogeneous mild hyperdensity on CT. Cysts, foci of necrosis, and calcification may be seen. Enhancement is variable. On MRI, the solid components of the tumor appear isointense on T1-weighted images and heterogeneous mild hyperintensity on T2 imaging, reflecting the presence of necrosis cellular atypia. Enhancement is similarly heterogeneous.

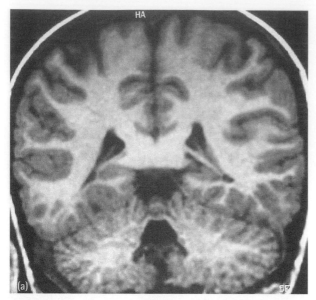

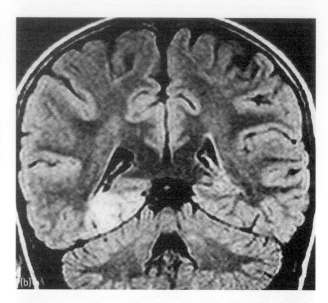

Figure 7.7a,b *Dysembryoplastic neuroepithelial tumor. (a) Coronal T1-weighted image, showing irregular thickening of the right occipitotemporal gyrus. Adjacent slices (not shown) demonstrated associated cortical dysplasia. (b) A coronal fluid-attenuated inversion recovery (FLAIR) image defines the lesion more clearly.*

Germ–cell tumors

Teratomas Parenchymal teratomas are rare but important causes of tumors in the first year of life. These tumors are often huge at the time of presentation, which may be at birth. The characteristic imaging finding on both CT and MRI is of an extremely heterogeneous mass reflecting the various cellular elements, cysts, and necrosis. Coarse calcification is a constant feature.[38] Enhancement is variable. The prognosis for both atypical teratoid/rhabdoid tumors and teratomas is poor.

Lymphomas and hematopoietic tumors Primary cerebral involvement with lymphoma is uncommon in childhood; secondary involvement is rare. Primary non-Hodgkin's cerebral lymphoma occurs as a discrete hemispheric mass associated with cerebral edema and mass effect. CT typically demonstrates a mildly hyperdense mass on pre-contrast images. On T1-weighted images, the tumor is mildly hypointense and correspondingly iso- to mildly hyperintense on T2-weighted images. Contrast enhancement is characteristically strong on both CT and MRI (Figure 7.9).

Metastatic spread of acute leukemia to the brain or leptomeninges may be manifest only by mild non-specific ventricular dilation and cerebral sulcal widening. This may reflect concurrent chemotherapy or impaired CSF absorption. Enhancing tumor is uncommon, but when

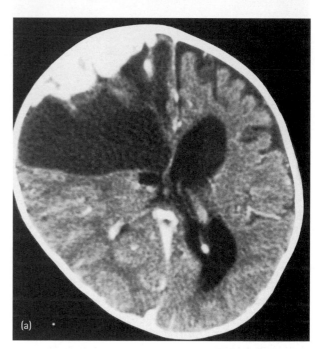

Figure 7.8a *Desmoplastic infantile ganglioglioma. (a) Post-contrast axial computerized tomography scan. Solid superficial tumor enhances strongly, overlying a large hypodense tumor cyst.*

present it typically involves the leptomeninges with extensive nodular or sheet-like enhancement better defined by MRI (Figure 7.10).

SELLAR AND PERISELLAR TUMORS

Craniopharyngiomas

Accounting for approximately 50 per cent of all suprasellar tumors, craniopharyngiomas are the most common

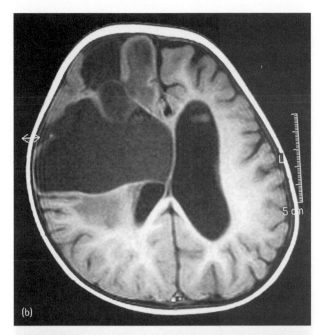

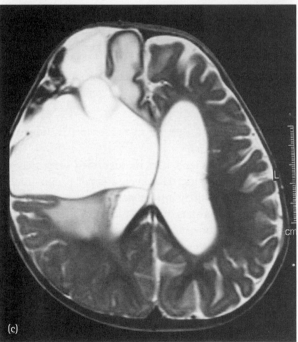

Figure 7.8b,c *(b) Axial T1 and (c) T2 images, showing the heterogeneous appearances of the peripheral solid component of the tumor with hypointensity on the T2 images. Note edema anteromedial and posterior to the tumor.*

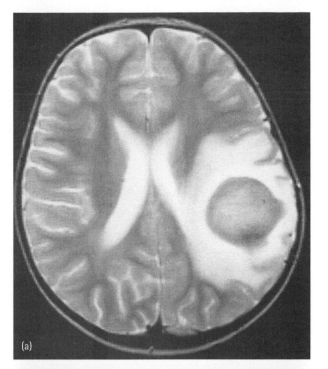

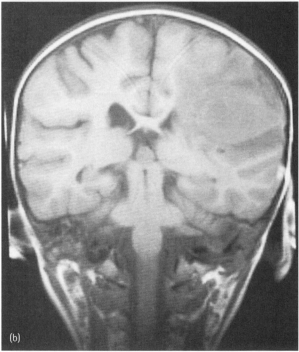

Figure 7.9a,b *Non-Hodgkin's lymphoma. (a) Axial T2-weighted image, demonstrating a left parietal well-circumscribed lesion with intense surrounding edema and localized mass effect. (b) Coronal T1-weighted image. The lesion is mildly hypointense.*

non-neuroepithelial tumor of childhood.[41] The large majority are suprasellar, but a small proportion may be found within the sellar or third ventricle. Childhood tumors tend to be histologically adamantinous and occur usually in the second decade. These tumors are histologically benign, but they behave aggressively by

invading adjacent structures. Although they may have well-defined and encapsulated components, other parts of the lesion are often adherent to the base of the brain, optic chiasm, hypothalamus, and circle of Willis vessels,

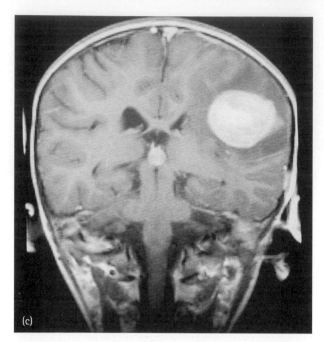

Figure 7.9c *(c) Post-contrast T1-weighted image, showing strong homogeneous enhancement of the parietal tumor and a smaller pineal mass.*

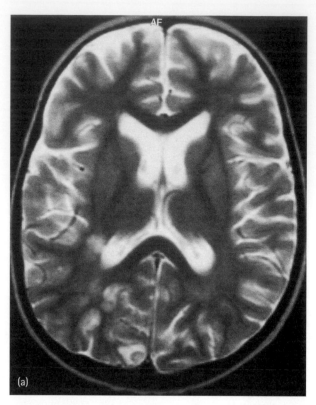

Figure 7.10a *Acute lymphoblastic leukemia. (a) Axial T2 image. Right-sided periventricular and occipital cortical hyperintensities are present.*

and they may extend to fill the third ventricle and project into the anterior and middle cranial fossae.

On imaging, adamantinous tumors frequently exhibit calcification, which can be demonstrated by CT in approximately 90 per cent of cases, with a similar frequency of cystic change and enhancement.[42] The calcification may be delicate, lining a cyst wall, patchy, or large and craggy. The tumors are often lobulated and may encase the internal carotid arteries. The cystic elements tend to be low in density but higher than CSF and may enlarge rapidly following intracyst hemorrhage. Enhancement is patchy but tends to be strong.

MRI reflects the heterogeneous histological nature of the lesion. Highly proteinaceous fluid, cholesterol crystals, keratin, and/or blood products accounts for the mixed appearance of the cysts on T1-weighted imaging. The cyst fluid may thus appear hypo-, iso-, or, frequently, hyperintense corresponding with the "engine-oil" nature of the fluid identified at surgery.[43] There is similar heterogeneity on T2 imaging, with calcification and methemoglobin producing hypointense foci. Enhancement clearly identifies the solid elements of the tumor and helps to define the extent of local involvement. High-resolution heavily T2-weighted sequences may also be helpful in delineating clearly the tumor margins and cystic elements before surgical intervention (Figure 7.11). The tumor typically has a lobulated appearance and may extend down into the sella, with a dumbbell configuration due to the restricting nature of the diaphragma sella.

The pituitary gland may be identified separately on good-quality imaging. However, a small proportion of tumors may be entirely intrasellar. The presence of epithelial rests in the margins of the tumor accounts for the frequent invagination of tumor into surrounding structures, such as the hypothalamus, thalamus, optic chiasm, and adjacent temporal and frontal lobes. Tumor extirpation is thus frequently impossible, and recurrence, which may be very late, is common.

Disruption of the cystic elements either before or following surgery can produce a chemical meningitis and local T2 hyperintensity. Superior extension of the tumor may result in hydrocephalus, which occurs in approximately 50 per cent of cases.[44]

Differentiation from a Rathke's cleft cyst may be difficult. However, these lesions are found more commonly incidentally in adults during MRI examinations. The cysts are usually intrasellar and non-calcified and do not enhance. On CT, the cysts are mildly hypodense and may show a rim of enhancement. The cysts may have cerebrospinal-fluid-like characteristics on MRI. The presence of cholesterol crystals or blood products may, however, result in T1 hyperintensity and iso- to hypointensity on T2-weighted images.[45] The typical origination of the Rathke's cleft cysts from the pars

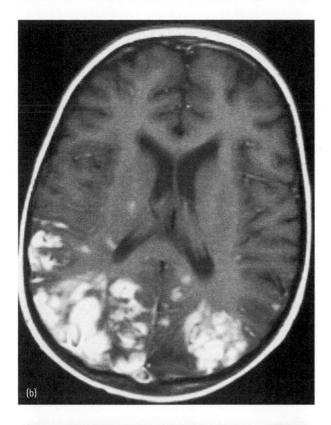

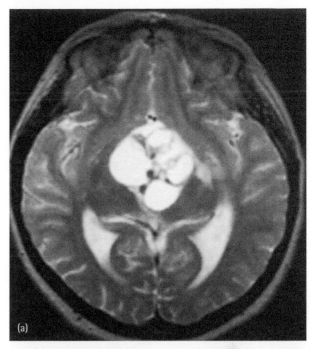

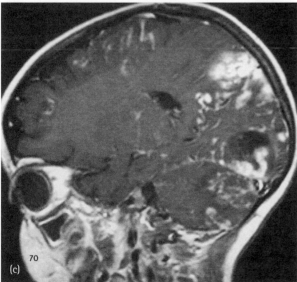

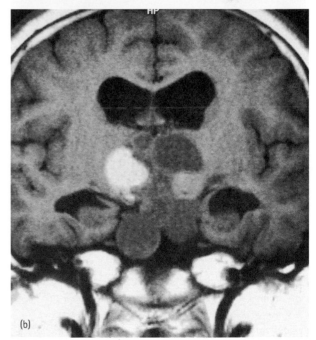

Figure 7.10b,c *(b) Axial and (c) Sagittal T1-weighted post-contrast images, demonstrating extensive leptomeningeal enhancing tumor.*

Figure 7.11a,b *Craniopharyngioma. (a) Axial T2 image, showing a well-defined suprasellar mass of mixed hyperintense cystic and more heterogeneously hypointense tissue. Note edema extending into the left optic tract. (b) Coronal T1 image, showing hyper- and hypointense elements of the tumor.*

intermedia of the pituitary gland results in the anterior displacement of the pituitary stalk, a helpful diagnostic feature.[46]

Germinomas

Germinomas are the most common germ-cell tumors in the suprasellar region. They may occur as isolated lesions or secondary to CSF spread from a pineal primary. Synchronous pineal and suprasellar germinomas occur in 6–12 per cent of cases.[47] Approximately 20–30 per cent of all intracranial germinomas occur in the suprasellar

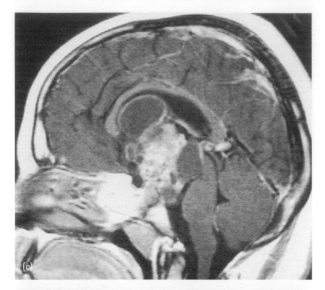

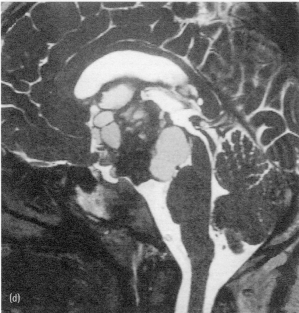

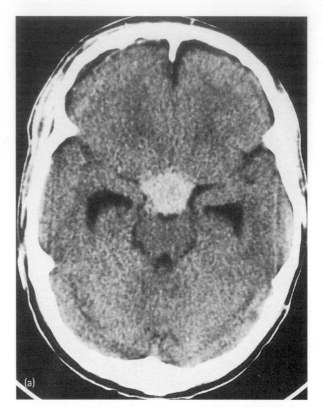

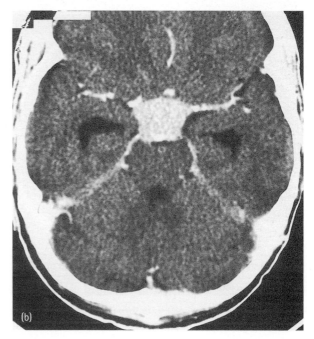

Figure 7.11c,d *(c) Sagittal post-contrast image. There is patchy strong enhancement centrally, with non-enhancing cystic components superiorly and posteriorly. (d) Sagittal constructive interference in the steady state sequence, demonstrating more clearly the morphology of the tumor and relation to adjacent structures, such as the pituitary gland and the third ventricular floor.*

Figure 7.12a,b *Suprasellar germinoma. (a) Axial pre-contrast computerized tomography (CT) scan. The hyperdense tumor fills the suprasellar cistern. (b) Axial post-contrast CT, demonstrating moderate homogeneous enhancement of the tumor.*

region, being the second most common site of these germ-cell tumors after a pineal location. Unlike the pineal-region tumors, suprasellar germinomas are more common in girls.[19] CT scanning is very helpful in evaluating germinomas in the suprasellar region. Mild to moderate hyperdensity is characteristic, reflecting the highly cellular nature of the lesion (Figure 7.12). In contrast, suprasellar astrocytomas, which may be otherwise not dissimilar in

appearance, are hypodense before contrast administration. The mass is well circumscribed, round or lobulated, and homogeneous in appearance; however, hyperdensity due to hemorrhage may be seen. Enhancement is generally

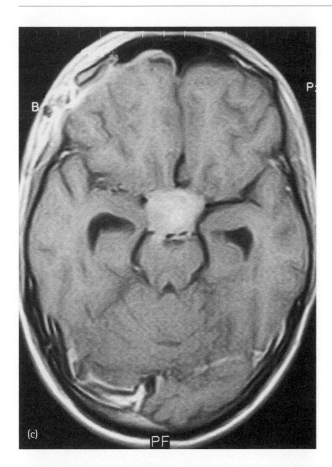

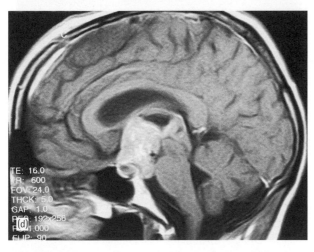

Figure 7.12c,d *(c) Axial and (d) Sagittal post-contrast T1-weighted images, showing a moderately enhancing mass in the suprasellar region and within the posterior part of the third ventricle.*

uniform and strong. T1-weighted magnetic resonance demonstrates a mildly hypointense lesion and intermediate signal intensity on T2 images. There is generally strong enhancement following gadolinium administration (Figure 7.12). CSF extension with diffuse leptomeningeal spread is not uncommon.

Opticochiasmatic and hypothalamic astrocytomas

These tumors occur predominantly in the first decade of life and account for 25–30 per cent of all suprasellar tumors. They are associated with neurofibromatosis type 1 (NF-1) in 50 per cent of pediatric cases.[48] Optic-nerve gliomas (ONGs) are the most common neoplastic intracranial manifestation of NF-1. These tumors may occur as entirely intraorbital lesions. There may be variable extension into the cisternal segment of the optic nerve (Figure 7.13) or into the optic chiasm. The diagnosis is usually made between the ages of one and seven years. Most of these tumors are slow-growing, but approximately 20 per cent take an aggressive course.

Both hypothalamic and opticochiasmatic astrocytomas share histological characteristics, being typically pilocytic in type. Hypothalamic astrocytomas often grow upwards into the third ventricle, where they tend to obstruct the foramina of Monro, while opticochiasmatic tumors usually extend into the cisternal and intraorbital segments of the optic nerves. There is, however, considerable overlap between the two, as both the hypothalamus and the chiasm are involved, irrespective of the site of origin of the lesion. While there are no particular distinguishing differences between NF-1- and non-NF-1-related tumors, there is a lesser degree of involvement of the optic nerves in non-NF-1 cases. In addition, a useful discriminating factor is the frequent occurrence of the characteristic non-tumoral hyperintense lesions of NF-1 seen in the optic radiations, thalami, basal ganglia, brainstem cerebellar peduncles, and cerebellar hemispheres on MRI.[49]

On CT, the tumors are generally mildly hypodense. Calcification is uncommon, as are cysts and intratumoral hemorrhages. Expansion of one or both optic nerve canals may be identified along with dysplasia of the sphenoid bone and orbital contents in NF-1 cases. Enhancement is strong but may be focal. Magnetic resonance is optimal for defining the extent of intraorbital and intracranial involvement and the accompanying hyperintense NF-1 lesions. T1-weighted images show a mildly hypointense mass, which is of intermediate to marked hyperintensity on T2 imaging. Enhancement is often strong (Figure 7.14). In those lesions extending into the optic nerves, enhancement within the intraorbital segments of the tumor may be less pronounced or absent. Tumors extending posteriorly into the optic radiations may be differentiated from non-tumoral NF-1-related T2-hyperintense lesions by the presence of enhancement. CSF-borne metastases may occur occasionally (Figure 7.14).

Hypothalamic hamartomas

These lesions arise from the region of the tuber cinereum and project inferiorly into the suprasellar cisterns. Being composed of disorganized heterotopic neural tissue, they are not true neoplasms, but they may enlarge slowly. The bland appearance, similar to brain tissue, and often small

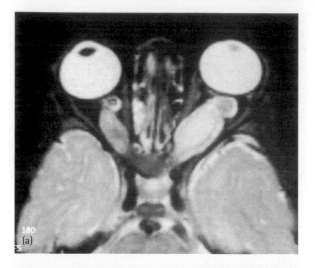

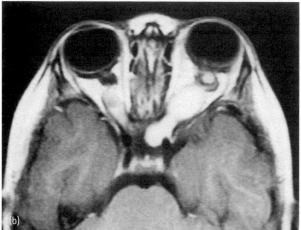

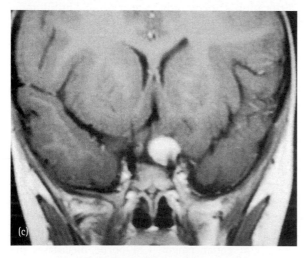

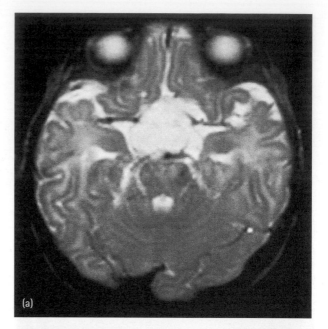

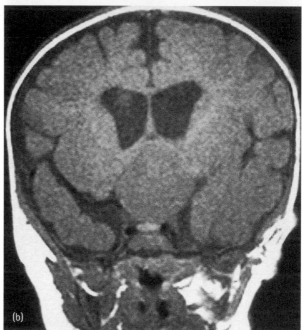

Figure 7.14a,b *Optico-hypothalamic astrocytoma. (a) Axial T2 image, showing a hyperintense lesion filling the suprasellar cistern. (b) Coronal T1-weighted image. The tumor is mildly hypointense in comparison with the adjacent brain tissue and extends superiorly to obstruct the foramina of Monro. Note the normal slightly hyperintense pituitary gland underlying the lesion.*

Figure 7.13a–c *Optic-nerve gliomas. (a) Axial T2-weighted fat-saturated image, showing bilaterally expanded and hyperintense optic nerves. (b) Axial T1-weighted image following contrast administration. There is extension of tumor to involve the intracanalicular segment of the optic nerve on the left. (c) Coronal T1-weighted image. The tumor extends posteriorly to involve the cisternal segment of the left optic nerve.*

size may lead to a lack of appreciation of these lesions on CT scanning. MRI elegantly defines a sessile or pedunculated mass below the third ventricular floor as an isointense mass surrounded by CSF on T1-weighted images.[50]

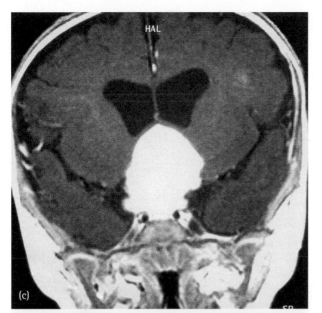

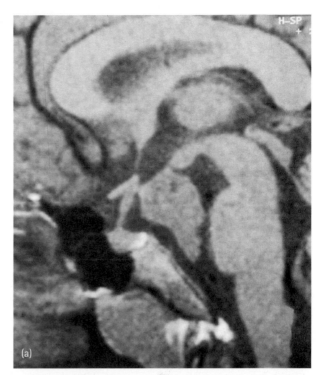

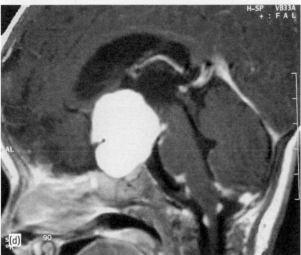

Figure 7.14c,d *(c) Post-contrast coronal T1-weighted image. The tumor enhances intensely and homogeneously. (d). Sagittal T1-weighted image, demonstrating the suprasellar tumor and distant enhancing tumor coating the surface of the brainstem and cerebellum, indicative of leptomeningeal tumor spread.*

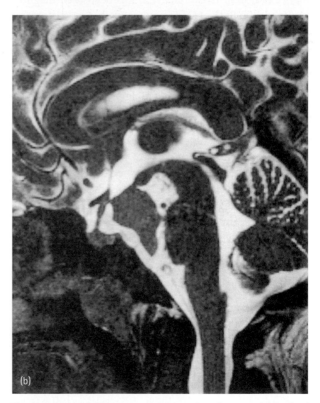

Enhancement is notable by its absence (Figure 7.15). T2 imaging may demonstrate mild hyperintensity, which may be more prominent on fluid-attenuated inversion recovery (FLAIR) images. Ultra-high-resolution, heavily T2-weighted sequences are particularly useful in defining the smaller lesions (Figure 7.15).

Meningiomas

Meningiomas are rarely encountered in childhood, accounting for less than three per cent of all childhood intracranial neoplasms. Cystic change is more common than in the adult variant. The imaging characteristics are

Figure 7.15a,b *(a) Hamartoma of the tuber cinereum. (a) Sagittal T1-weighted image. The tumor, which is isointense with respect to the adjacent brain, extends inferiorly from the floor of the third ventricle. There was no enhancement following contrast administration (not shown). (b) Sagittal constructive interference in the steady state defines more clearly the tumor's origin from the floor of the third ventricle.*

otherwise similar, being iso- or mildly hyperdense on CT.[51] Calcification may be seen. Focal hyperostosis may be seen on bone window settings. Enhancement is generally prominent. On MRI, the iso- to mildly hyperintense mass generally exhibits strong enhancement, while T2-weighted images may show mild hyperintensity. Edema may occur in the adjacent white matter and in the optic chiasm.

PINEAL–REGION TUMORS

Tumors in the pineal region account for approximately ten per cent of all intracranial brain tumors.[52] Histological classification is broken down into germ-cell tumors, pineal-cell tumors, and parapineal tumors.

Germ-cell tumors

These tumors are derived from pluripotential primordial germ cells and account for 50–70 per cent of all pineal-region tumors. Of the pineal germ-cell tumors, 65 per cent are germinomas, 25 per cent are non-germinomas, and ten per cent are mature teratomas.[53] Germinomas are highly radiosensitive, a fact that has been used diagnostically, although the trend is increasingly towards obtaining definitive histological confirmation by stereotactic biopsy.[54] Non-germinomatous tumors do not respond favorably to radiotherapy, in contradistinction to the highly radiosensitive germinomas. Unlike the suprasellar germinomas, there is a strong male predominance.[52,53]

Germinomas The majority (approximately 60 per cent) of intracranial germinomas occur in the pineal region. The high nuclear-to-cytoplasm ratio of germinomas accounts for the typical mild to moderately hyperdense appearance on CT scanning. The tumors are well defined but may be craggy. Calcification may be seen in up to 50 per cent of cases but may also represent incorporation of normal calcified pineal tissue into the tumor. Enhancement is strong to intense.

On MRI, the lesion appears morphologically homogeneous, being slightly hypo- to isointense on T1 imaging and iso- to hyperintense on T2-weighted images. Cysts and hemorrhage are variably present. Enhancement is strong and homogeneous (Figure 7.16). Infiltration of structures around the pineal gland may occur. Local mass effect and invasion results in third ventricular obstruction and hydrocephalus. MRI is mandatory in the evaluation of intracranial or intraspinal metastases. Intracranial metastases occur particularly within the ventricles, notably in the anterior recesses of the third ventricle.

Teratomas These tumors have a strong male preponderance and a peak incidence around puberty, although they may occur throughout the first two decades.[55] Imaging of these tumors reflects their derivation from

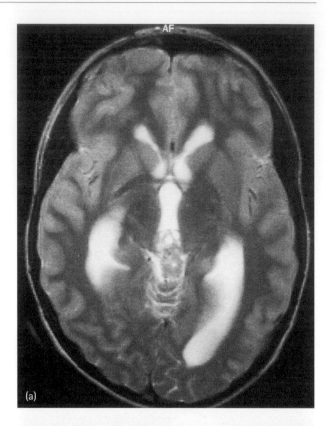

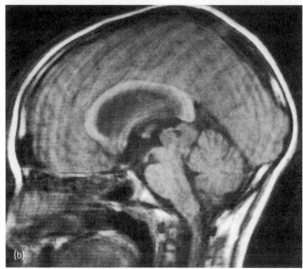

Figure 7.16a,b *Pineal germinoma. (a) Axial T2 image. There is a small, irregular lesion protruding into the posterior third ventricle. Note mild hydrocephalus. (b) Sagittal T1-weighted image. The pineal region tumor is isointense with respect to adjacent brain tissue. The upper tectum and aqueduct are compressed by the tumor.*

all three germ-cell layers and their variable maturity and malignancy. The more benign mature teratomas are characterized by fully differentiated tissue, while the malignant immature tumors contain primitive cellular

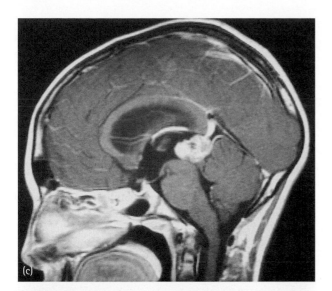

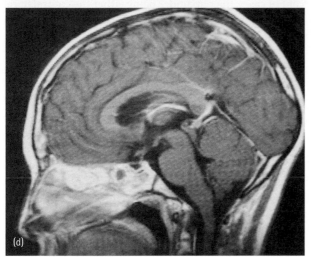

Figure 7.16c,d *(c) Sagittal T1 post-contrast image. The tumor enhances strongly, highlighting small central cystic foci. (d) Sagittal T1 post-contrast image six weeks following radiotherapy. The tumor has regressed fully.*

tissue. The lesions appear characteristically heterogeneous on both CT and MRI. Calcification, fat, bone, hemorrhage, and cysts may be variously identified. Enhancement may be ring-like.[56]

Non-germinomatous germ-cell tumors   These tumors are rare and share similar imaging characteristics with other pineal germ-cell tumors. Features that may be helpful include a greater propensity to invade the tectum and thalamus, a higher incidence of hemorrhage, and more intense enhancement.[57]

Pineal–cell tumors

Pineal parenchymal tumors are rare in childhood. There are three primary types: pineocytoma (presenting in the third and fourth decades of life), pineoblastomas (peak incidence in the latter half of the second decade of life), and intermediately differentiated pineal tumors. There is no significant sex difference. Calcification occurs in approximately 50 per cent of cases and tends to occur peripherally. The pineal-cell tumors tend to produce a sharply marginated convex mass bulging into the third ventricle.

Pineocytomas   Pineocytomas are generally well defined and have a lobulated appearance resembling the normal pineal gland. They occur slightly more often in males than females. They are very uncommon below the age of 18 years. On T1-weighted images the lesions are hypo- or isointense, and on T2 imaging they tend to be moderately hyperintense. Contrast enhancement tends to be strong but heterogeneous.

Pineoblastomas   The imaging features of pineoblastomas are indistinguishable from PNETs elsewhere in the neuraxis. There is greater heterogeneity due to the increased incidence of hemorrhage, necrosis, and cyst formation, being reflected in the appearances on MRI, although they tend to be less hyperintense than pineocytomas. Enhancement is strong, and distant CSF spread at the time of presentation is present in approximately ten per cent of cases.[58] Children under two years of age with bilateral retinoblastoma may occasionally have an accompanying pineoblastoma, the so-called "trilateral retinoblastoma syndrome."

Parapineal tumors

Astrocytomas   Gliomas of the tectum or tegmentum of the midbrain are fibrillary or pilocytic astrocytomas. The presentation is with hydrocephalus, the cause of which may evade detection, particularly if CT is the only diagnostic modality employed. Ill-defined tumors of the subthalamic or thalamic region may similarly obstruct the posterior third ventricle and there may also be subtle abnormalities on CT. The tectal tumors tend to be isodense with respect to gray matter; enhancement is typically absent. Sagittal plane imaging, particularly using heavily T2*-weighted three-dimensional Fourier transform sequences, is helpful in defining the often subtle distortion of the tectal anatomy.[59] The lesions are usually isointense on T1-weighted images and mild to moderately hyperintense on T2-weighted images, and typically do not enhance (Figure 7.17). Astrocytomas in the tegmentum or thalamic regions may exhibit greater heterogeneity on both pulse sequences, cysts, and patchy or more focal strong enhancement.

Meningiomas   Meningiomas in the parapineal region are rare in childhood. The imaging characteristics are similar to those of meningiomas located elsewhere in the intracranial compartment.

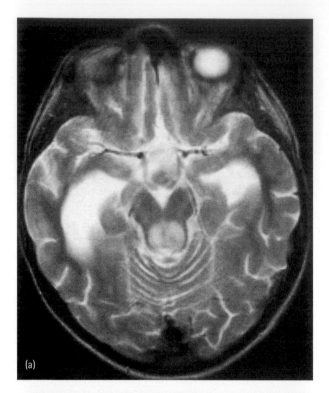

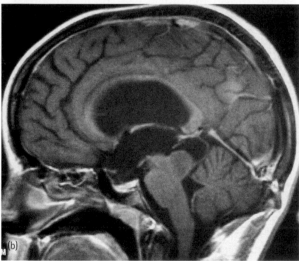

Figure 7.17a,b *Tectal glioma. (a) Axial T2 image, showing a hyperintense lesion expanding the tectum of the midbrain. The temporal horns of the lateral ventricles are dilated. (b) Sagittal post-contrast T1 image. The mildly hypointense tumor shows no enhancement. The aqueduct is occluded. There is a small diverticulum arising from the posterior third ventricle overlying the tumor.*

Pineal cysts Simple pineal cysts need to be considered in view of their frequency as a normal finding in childhood. The cysts are usually small but may grow to up to 2 cm in diameter.[60] On imaging, rim calcification is often identified by CT. MRI is particularly sensitive in the detection of these lesions, which are now identified frequently during investigation of non-tumoral conditions in both adults and children. The cysts generally follow CSF in the signal characteristics and may demonstrate peripheral enhancement.

PERIVENTRICULAR TUMORS

Choroid plexus papillomas and carcinomas

Choroid plexus tumors represent approximately three per cent of all pediatric brain tumors, of which 70 per cent are benign choroid plexus papillomas (CPPs), 20 per cent are choroid plexus carcinomas (CPCs), and the remainder are atypical choroid plexus tumors.[61] The lateral ventricles are most commonly involved, often centered on the atrium. The peak age of incidence is under two years. The tumors are contained at one site in 86 per cent of cases, the remainder being either the contralateral lateral ventricle or elsewhere in the third or fourth ventricle.[62]

Ultrasound scanning is particularly well suited for detecting tumors in early infancy, when the presentation is with hydrocephalus. The lesion appears as a multilobulated hyperechogenic mass typically within a lateral ventricle and especially in the region of the trigone. On CT, both CPPs and CPCs appear hyperdense and lobulated. Amorphous or punctate calcification is often present. Enhancement is frequently very strong. On MRI, the lesions are usually hypo- to isointense on T1-weighted images and hyperintense on T2-weighted images and show intense enhancement. Parenchymal enhancement, edema, and nodular intraventricular and/or intraspinal metastases are more suggestive of a CPC.

Ependymomas

Most supratentorial ependymomas lie within the brain parenchyma; however, 15–25 per cent may occur within the third or lateral ventricles.[63] The tumor is often large, lobulated, and well-defined. Intratumoral calcification and cysts may be found on pre-contrast CT, the mass usually being isodense. Enhancement is strong. MRI demonstrates a mildly hypointense mass on T1 imaging and hyperintensity on T2-weighted images. Enhancement, like CT, is strong and heterogeneous and may also identify adjacent ependymal enhancement. In general, there are no diagnostic features to clearly differentiate ependymomas from other gliomas. The location of a lesion with such characteristics is, however, of significant diagnostic importance.[64]

Subependymal giant-cell astrocytomas

These tumors occur almost uniquely in association with tuberous sclerosis. Any subependymal nodular lesion in excess of 1 cm and located in a lateral ventricle at or near the foramen of Monro should be regarded as being such

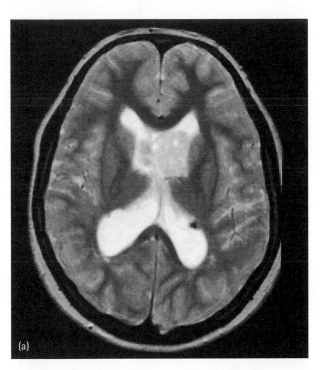

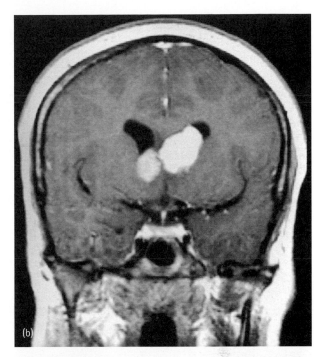

Figure 7.18a *Subependymal giant-cell astrocytoma. (a) Axial T2 image. A lobulated, slightly hyperintense lesion is present in the anterior horns of the lateral ventricles, with mild ventricular enlargement. Note the calcified subependymal tuber in the left lateral ventricle.*

a tumor. Obstruction of the foramen of Monro results in either ipsilateral or bilateral ventricular dilatation.

CT scanning is helpful in identifying the presence of calcified subependymal and/or subcortical tubers elsewhere, as well as calcification within the tumor itself. The lesion is hypo- to isodense and well-circumscribed, and shows strong enhancement following contrast administration. Progressive growth helps to distinguish the lesion from tubers, which may also show some enhancement. Magnetic resonance reflects the CT appearances, with hypo- to isointensity on T1 imaging, variable T2 hyperintensity, and strong enhancement following intravenous gadolinium (Figure 7.18). MRI is also best suited to display the associated features of tuberous sclerosis, particularly the subcortical tubers and cortical dysplasia.

Neurocytomas

These are uncommon, slow-growing, low-grade tumors, which typically occur in late adolescence or early adulthood. They arise in close association with the septum pellucidum. The entity of central neurocytoma has been recognized only relatively recently, having been classified as tumors such as oligodendrogliomas in the past. Calcification is frequently identified on CT. The tumors occur within the lateral and/or third ventricles and are

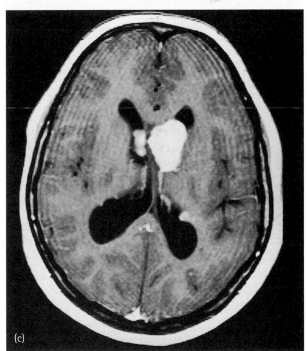

Figure 7.18b,c *(b) Coronal and (c) axial post-contrast T1-weighted images. There are strongly enhancing lesions based on the region of the foramina of Monro (blandly hypointense on pre-contrast images, not shown). In addition, enhancement is seen at the site of the calcified subependymal tuber on the left and subtle smaller subependymal lesions in the right lateral ventricle.*

often large at the time of presentation. The magnetic resonance characteristics are of a lesion exhibiting mixed signal intensities on both T1- and T2-weighted images. Enhancement is often only mild and patchy, although it may be more focally prominent, as best appreciated on MRI (Figure 7.19).

Meningiomas

Intraventricular meningioma is an uncommon entity in childhood but should be considered in a child presenting with a large ventricular-based lesion associated with hydrocephalus. On CT scanning, the tumor is typically iso- to mildly hyperdense and enhances strongly. MRI characterizes more clearly and localizes the lesion, which is mildly hyperintense with respect to brain tissue on T1-weighted images and of heterogeneous signal characteristics on T2 imaging, reflecting the variable presence of calcification. As with CT, strong enhancement is the norm (Figure 7.20).

Infratentorial tumors

Approximately 50–55 per cent of pediatric intracranial tumors are located in the posterior fossa.[65] Supratentorial tumors predominate in the first two years of life, while infratentorial tumors are more common between the ages of three and 11 years. Most posterior fossa tumors in childhood occur in the brainstem and cerebellar hemispheres, with astrocytic tumors such as gliomas and ependymomas being most prevalent, followed by PNETs.

MRI of posterior fossa tumors is particularly important in view of the inherent problems associated with CT in this compartment, particularly the beam-hardening artifact associated with the juxtaposition of the large bony masses of the petrous bones adjacent to the cisterns, brainstem, and cerebellar hemispheres.

BRAINSTEM TUMORS

Brainstem gliomas

Brainstem gliomas (BSGs) account for 25–30 per cent of all infratentorial pediatric tumors. They occur particularly in the first decade of life, with a mean age of seven years at diagnosis.[66,67] Most are low-grade diffuse fibrillary astrocytomas. A minority are higher-grade astrocytomas (including GBM, which have a propensity to metastasize in the CSF) or, least commonly, pilocytic astrocytomas. Irrespective of histological grade or appearance, 80 per cent of patients with BSG present with a rapidly progressive clinical syndrome characterized by cerebellar, cranial nerve, or long tract signs and a diffuse expanding lesion based on the pons. The combination of this clinical syndrome combined with the radiological features is sufficiently specific such that biopsy is now no longer undertaken routinely, particularly as there is poor concordance between histological grade and outcome.[68] The prognosis is uniformly poor, with survival beyond one to two years being rare.

CT characteristics of BSG are of a hypodense expansile brainstem mass. Calcification and hemorrhage are

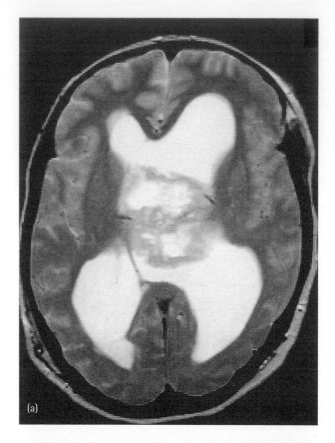

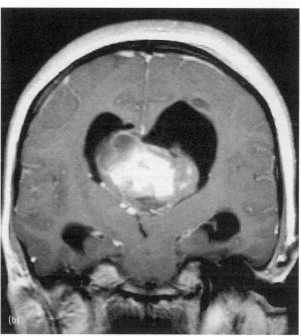

Figure 7.19a,b *Neurocytoma. (a) Axial T2-weighted image, demonstrating a heterogeneously hyperintense intraventricular mass obstructing the foramina of Monro. There is asymmetrical ventricular dilation. (b) Coronal T1-weighted image following contrast administration. There is central strong enhancement (the pre-contrast image, not shown, showed a mildly hypointense lesion).*

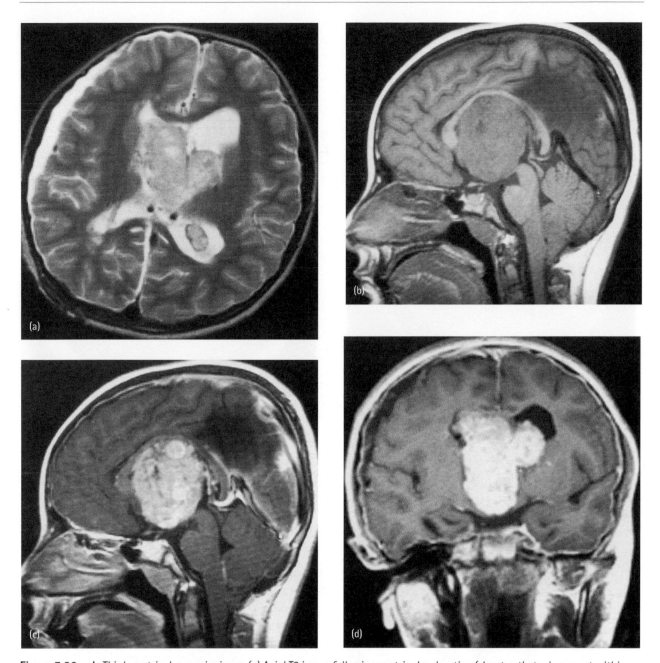

Figure 7.20a–d *Third-ventricular meningioma. (a) Axial T2 image following ventricular shunting (shunt catheter is present within the right lateral ventricle, with a post-shunting, right-sided subdural hygroma). There is a mildly heterogeneously hyperintense intraventricular mass. (b) Sagittal T1-weighted image. The third ventricular mass is isointense with respect to the adjacent gray matter, filling the ventricle and splaying the corpus callosum. (c) Sagittal and (d) Coronal post-contrast T1 images, showing strong tumor enhancement. The lesion extends through the foramina of Monro into the lateral ventricles.*

relatively rare.[67] There is little or no enhancement, although patchy enhancement may be seen in some cases. On MRI, the lesions are hypointense on T1- and hyperintense on T2-weighted images. As with CT, enhancement is generally absent (Figure 7.21). Tumor evaluation is thus heavily dependent upon the hyperintense abnormality identified on at least two orthogonal T2-weighted images. Freeman and Farmer described

four types of BSG: diffuse, focal, dorsal exophytic, and cervicomedullary.[66]

Diffuse BSGs are commonest (80 per cent), occurring particularly in the pons, and are histologically more aggressive. Growth may be caudocephalad. Exophytic growth is most commonly ventral into the prepontine cistern, with variable encasement of the basilar artery,[69] or dorsally into the cerebellar peduncles or fourth ventricle. The pons is

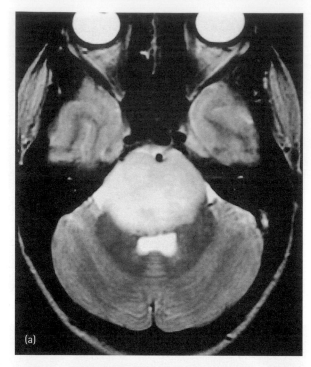

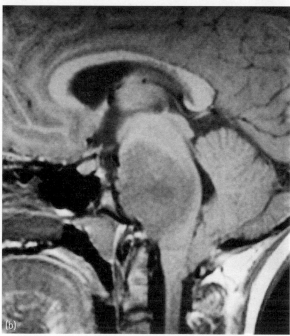

Figure 7.21a,b *Diffuse brainstem glioma. (a) Axial T2-weighted image, showing a diffusely expanded and hyperintense pons, the tumor surrounding the basilar artery anteriorly. (b) Sagittal T1 image. The tumor is mildly hypointense. There are small nodular projections of the tumor anteriorly. There is accompanying cerebellar tonsillar ectopia.*

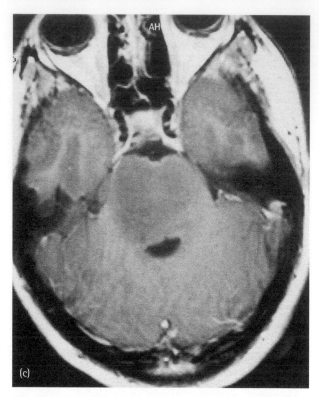

Figure 7.21c *(c) Axial post-contrast T1-weighted image. The tumor shows no enhancement.*

long tract signs, and ataxia. Enhancement is usually absent or minimal, except following radiotherapy. Progression tends to be rapid and CSF spread may occur. The prognosis is poor, with an overall five-year survival of 10–15 per cent.

Five to ten per cent of BSGs are *focal*, well-defined, generally smaller, and usually limited to part of the brainstem.[66] Such tumors may have significant cystic components, but edema is usually absent in keeping with the low-grade nature. Exophytic growth into adjacent cisterns or the fourth ventricle of variable size may be present. Sagittal and axial plane imaging is required to demonstrate resectability of tumors that extend to the surface of the brainstem. Enhancement is variable but may be strong.

Dorsal exophytic tumors arise from the subependymal region of the floor of the fourth ventricle, into which they grow. These tumors are generally pilocytic astrocytomas and characteristically may enhance strongly. The tumors involve adjacent cranial nerve nuclei within the dorsal part of the brainstem, but they tend to spare the more ventrally located long tracts.

Cervicomedullary tumors expand the upper cervical cord and extend into the dorsal medulla. Lower-grade tumors typically exhibit posterior exophytic extension into the cisterna magna, whereas more aggressive lesions infiltrate more extensively into the adjacent brainstem.

typically expanded, with diffuse infiltration along fiber tracts of the brainstem. The fourth ventricle is often flattened; however, hydrocephalus is generally absent, presentation being typically with multiple lower cranial palsies,

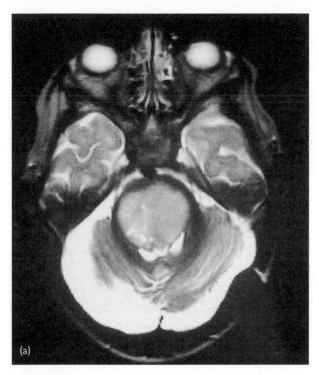

Figure 7.22a *Brainstem primitive neuroectodermal tumor.*
(a) Axial T2-weighted image, showing a heterogeneously
hyperintense central pontine lesion.

Focal, exophytic, and cystic tumors, as well as those
located at the midbrain or cervicomedullary junction,
generally carry a better prognosis.[70,71]

Primitive neuroectodermal tumors

Although uncommon, PNETs may occur entirely within
the brainstem, usually the pons.[72] The imaging aspects are
variable, but edema, patchy or more solid enhancement,
and an aggressive course is the norm (Figure 7.22).

CEREBELLAR TUMORS

Medulloblastomas (primitive neuroectodermal tumors of the posterior fossa)

These are the commonest posterior fossa tumors in
childhood, accounting for 30–40 per cent of tumors at
this site. The peak incidence is between the ages of five and
eight years, with a second peak in adolescents and young
adults. There is a male predominance in the order of two
or three to one. In children the tumors are characteristically undifferentiated and highly malignant, arising from
the anterior aspect of the inferior vermis and inferior
medullary velum.

Tumors may extend anteriorly through the fourth
ventricle to invade the brainstem, inferiorly and laterally
into the cisterna magna, perimedullary and cerebellopontine cisterns via the fourth ventricular foramina, and diffusely within the neuraxis by CSF dissemination. In older
children, in whom desmoplastic PNETs are more common,

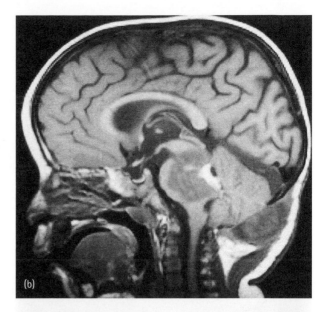

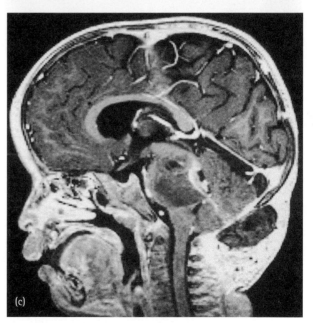

Figure 7.22b,c *(b) Sagittal T1 image (post-biopsy). The*
hypointense tumor is well defined. Hemorrhage is present
posteriorly at the biopsy site. The fourth ventricle is effaced.
(c). Post-contrast T1-weighted three-dimensional volume image,
showing no intralesional enhancement.

the tumors occur more frequently in the cerebellar hemispheres laterally and often abut the tentorium or extend
to the surface of the cerebellum.

The typical aspect of a medulloblastoma on CT is a
midline well-defined isodense to mildly hyperdense mass
lying posterior to the fourth ventricle. Extension superiorly to obstruct the fourth ventricle results in the frequent occurrence of hydrocephalus. Calcification may be
apparent in up to 20 per cent of cases. A more heterogeneous pattern of medulloblastoma is associated with

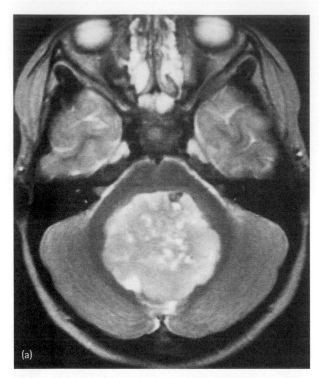

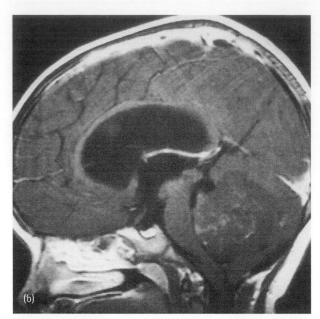

Figure 7.23b *(b) Post-contrast T1 image, showing patchy enhancement centrally within the tumor (pre-contrast image, not shown, showed a blandly hypointense lesion).*

Figure 7.23a *Medulloblastoma. (a) Axial T2 image. A large heterogeneously hyperintense tumor fills the fourth ventricle, compressing the pons.*

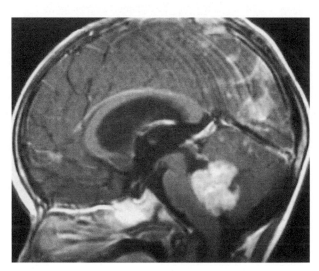

Figure 7.24 *Medulloblastoma. Post-contrast sagittal T1 weighted image, demonstrating a strongly enhancing tumor filling the fourth ventricle. Note delicate subependymal spread within the dilated rostral fourth ventricle and supratentorial leptomeningeal spread posteriorly and in the subfrontal region.*

cysts and necrotic foci, which may lead to diagnostic confusion with cerebellar astrocytomas. The mild hypodensity of the latter is an important discriminating factor. Enhancement tends to be strong, particularly in the more homogeneous tumors.

As with the majority of posterior fossa tumors, MRI is optimal, particularly in the sagittal plane. The origin of the tumor from the inferior medullary velum is often apparent, with an ill-defined zone of transition from the vermis to the tumor. The tumor projecting into the fourth ventricle is sharply delineated, with the fourth ventricle draped over the superior and posterior surfaces of the lesion. The signal characteristics are non-specific. On T1 images the tumor tends to be mildly hypointense, while on T2-weighted images it is usually of mild to moderate hyperintensity. Perilesional edema may be present but is not a prominent feature. The presence of calcifications and cysts results in considerable heterogeneity on T2-weighted images.[73] Enhancement is variable and may be mild, patchy, and heterogeneous (Figure 7.23) or strong (Figure 7.24).

Demonstration of leptomeningeal spread, which is of great importance in defining treatment strategies and prognosis, typically occurs in the subfrontal regions, sylvian fissures, basal cisterns, posterior fossa cisterns, and thoracic and lumbosacral regions, requires post-contrast

T1-weighted imaging of the entire neuraxis before surgery. The incidence of leptomeningeal spread at the time of diagnosis probably approaches 40 per cent.[74] The deposits usually enhance and may be nodular (Figure 7.25) or drop-like or appear as sheets of tumor producing a "sugar-candy" coating of the spinal cord or brainstem. Postoperative artifacts, blood clot, and possible contrast leakage into the CSF may lead to considerable diagnostic difficulties (see below).

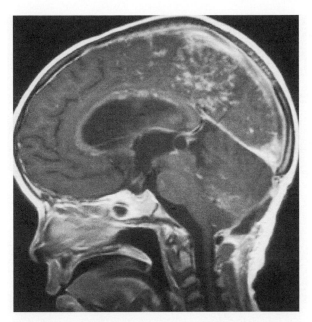

Figure 7.25 *Metastatic medulloblastoma. Post-contrast T1 image, showing multiple small deposits related to the cerebral falx and corpus callosum.*

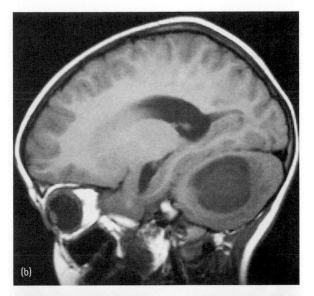

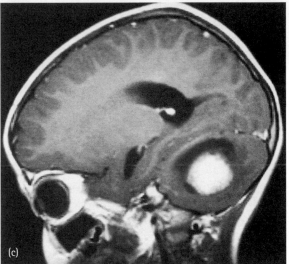

Figure 7.26b,c *(b) Pre- and (c) post-contrast sagittal T1 images. The solid nodule is hypointense and shows strong uniform enhancement.*

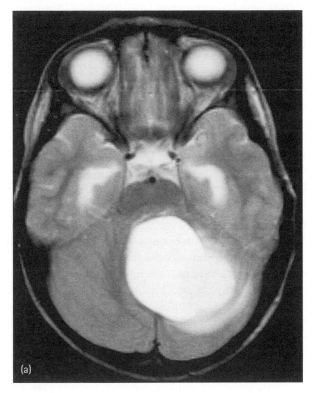

Figure 7.26a *Cerebellar pilocytic astrocytoma. (a) Axial T2-weighted image. The predominantly cystic tumor is strongly hyperintense, with a smaller solid mural element of slightly reduced intensity posterolaterally.*

Astrocytomas

These tumors are characteristically juvenile pilocytic astrocytomas. However, fibrillary astrocytomas as well as more malignant histological types (anaplastic astrocytoma, GBM) may be encountered.[75] Most tumors are large at presentation and may appear as cystic with a mural nodule of tumor (50 per cent), solid with cystic/necrotic foci (40 per cent), or purely solid. Solid tumors tend to arise from the vermis, occur in younger children, and are histologically more aggressive, while cystic tumors tend to occur in older children. Calcification is seen in 10–20 per cent. Intratumoral hemorrhage is rare.

On imaging, pilocytic astrocytomas are characterized by a cystic mass with an iso- or mildly hypodense nodule or solid component on CT. The midline vermian tumors have a tendency to be hyperdense. Characteristic of pilocytic astrocytomas is the presence of open fenestrations and tight junctions within the endothelial cells of these tumors, which exhibit abundant vascular proliferation.

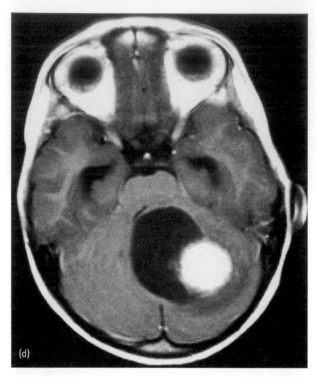

Figure 7.26d *(d) Axial post-contrast T1 image, demonstrating the smaller enhancing mural nodule. There is no enhancement related to the wall of the larger cystic element.*

The consequence is that the solid component(s) of the tumor tends to show intense enhancement. Necrotic tumors demonstrate irregular craggy enhancement. Non-pilocytic astrocytomas tend to show less or even no enhancement of the solid parts of the tumor. Of the cystic tumors, demonstration of enhancement of the wall of the cyst indicates that the wall is tumor-lined and requires resection. Non-enhancing cyst walls are consistent with compressed non-neoplastic glial tissue.[65] However, tumor cannot be excluded in all cases, probably due to the insensitivity of CT in particular to detect subtle enhancement or the presence of a thin layer of non-enhancing tumor.

Evaluation of the tumor is more complete with MRI. The imaging characteristics of pilocytic astrocytomas are of a mildly hypointense mass on T1-weighted images, cystic elements being more prominently hypointense. T2 imaging shows a combination of moderate hyperintensity of the solid element of the lesion and intense T2 shortening of the cyst. Enhancement tends to be strong and homogeneous (Figure 7.26). Non-pilocytic astrocytomas present as diffuse and often ill-defined hyperintense lesions on T2 imaging and with corresponding mild hypointensity on T1-weighted images. Enhancement is variable and patchy and may be absent. In the context of NF-1, differentiation from the non-glial hamartomatous hyperintense signal lesions can be difficult (Figure 7.27). These lesions may be extensive in both the pons and the cerebellar hemispheres; they are also encountered frequently in the

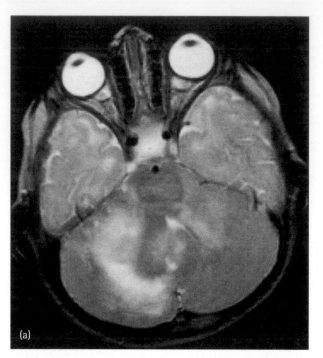

Figure 7.27a *Diffuse cerebellar astrocytoma in a 13-year-old girl with neurofibromatosis type 1 (NF-1). (a) Axial T2 image at presentation, showing prominent ill-defined hyperintensity in the deep right cerebellar hemisphere, with compression of the fourth ventricle. There are further abnormalities in the vermis, left cerebellar hemisphere, and pons, which may represent NF-1-related hyperintense signal change or tumor. Similar lesions are also present in the subcortical white matter of temporal lobes.*

internal capsules, lentiform nuclei, and splenium of the corpus callosum. Mass effect, edema, and contrast enhancement are not features of these lesions. However, the astrocytomas associated with NF-1 may occasionally undergo spontaneous involution (Figure 7.27).

Ependymomas

Ependymomas constitute approximately ten per cent of posterior fossa tumors in childhood. These tumors are derived from ependymal cells lining the ventricles or in ependymal cell rests, which may sometimes occur quite distant from the ventricles, giving rise to hemispheric tumors. The floor of the fourth ventricle is the most common site, and the tumor typically fills the fourth ventricle. The more desmoplastic ependymomas have a tendency to extend out through the foramina of Magendie or Luschka in a toothpaste-like fashion; however, tumors may also originate in the lateral recesses or cerebellopontine angle cisterns.

In contradistinction to medulloblastomas, there is often an ill-defined interface between the brainstem and the tumor, whereas a distinct plane of cleavage is usually preserved between the lesion and the vermis. In addition, the tumors tend to grow outside the ventricular walls to locally invade adjacent structures, such as the brainstem and

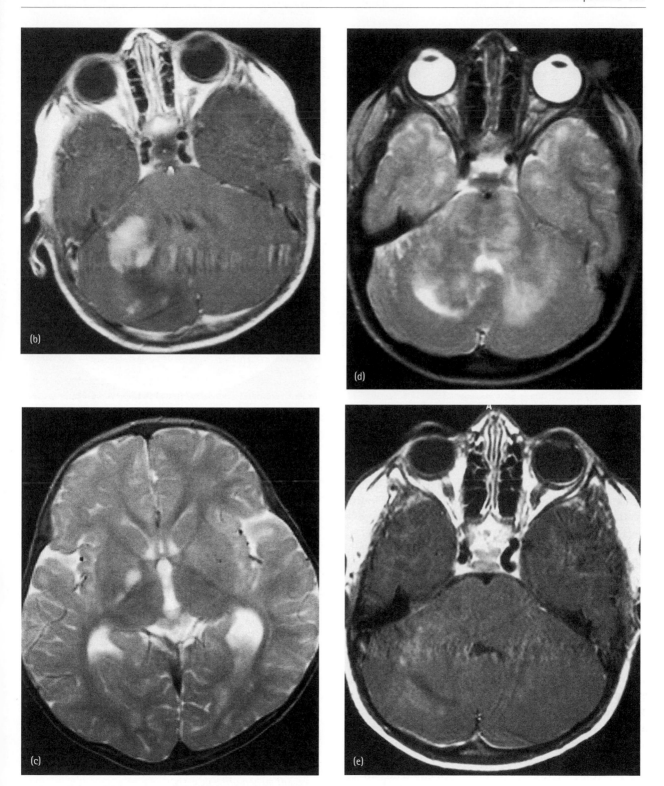

Figure 7.27b–e *(b) Axial T1-weighted image following contrast administration at the same level, demonstrating strong enhancement within the right-sided cerebellar lesion, indicative of tumor. The other pontine and cerebellar lesions do not enhance. (c) Axial T2 image through basal ganglia. There are small NF-1-related hyperintense signal lesions in the globus pallidi and posterior capsule on the right. (d) Axial T2 image four years later. There had been no treatment in the intervening period. The right cerebellar abnormality has regressed, but there is increased prominence of the pontine and left cerebellar hyperintensities. There is slight mass effect associated with the posterior pontine lesion. (e) Axial post-contrast image. The enhancement associated with the left cerebellar lesion has almost disappeared.*

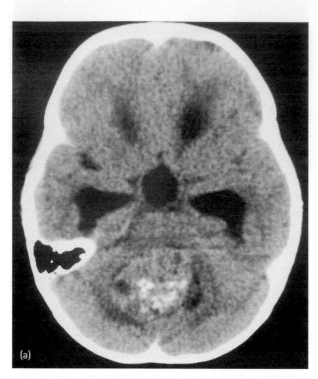

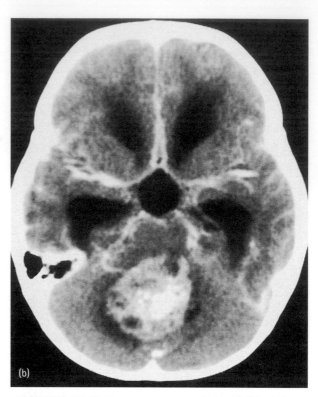

Figure 7.28a,b *Ependymoma. (a) Axial computerized tomography scan. There is an isodense lesion filling the fourth ventricle, containing small hypodense cysts and punctate calcifications. (b) Following contrast administration, there is heterogeneous enhancement. Supratentorial hydrocephalus is present.*

cerebellar hemispheres. This makes total resection difficult and accounts for the frequent local recurrence. The fourth ventricle is frequently draped over the superior surface of the tumor. Hydrocephalus is commonly present.[76]

On CT scanning, the tumor appears iso- to mildly hyperdense. Punctate or amorphous calcification is present in approximately 50 per cent of cases (Figure 7.28). Intratumoral hemorrhage, which may produce rapid enlargement of the lesion and precipitate symptomatic presentation, and small cysts may be seen.[76] Following contrast administration, there is often only mild to moderate heterogeneous enhancement. MRI tends to reflect the cellular heterogeneity of these tumors, the solid components being hypo- to isointense to brain tissue on T1-weighted images and iso- to hyperintense on T2-weighted images. Patchy hemorrhage may be identified by the presence of hyperintense foci within the lesion on T1-weighted images, being correspondingly hypointense on T2 imaging (Figure 7.29). Enhancement tends to be more striking than appreciated on CT, and may be patchy in nature, but it may be absent or homogeneous in some cases. Tumor demarcation tends to be poor, reflecting local infiltration of adjacent tissues; however, unlike medulloblastomas, vermian infiltration is not a feature (Figure 7.29). Local extension within the posterior fossa and into the upper cervical spine is not uncommon at the time of diagnosis (Figure 7.30).

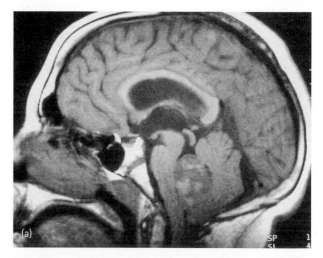

Figure 7.29a *Ependymoma. (a) Sagittal T1 magnetic resonance image. The mildly hypointense tumor filling the fourth ventricle contains several small hyperintense foci, most probably representing hemorrhagic cysts.*

Recurrence following surgery is most often local at the tumor bed. However, extension into the upper cervical spine or laterally into the cerebellopontine angle cisterns and more distant CSF spread is not uncommon. Completeness of the primary tumor excision reflects the greatest potential for long-term disease-free survival.

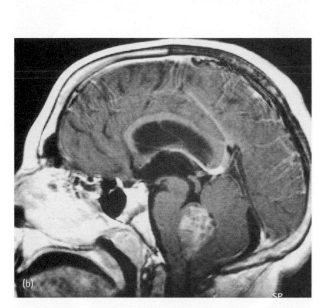

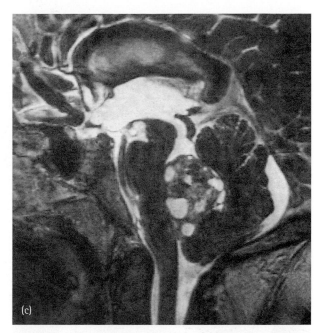

Figure 7.29b,c *(b) Post-contrast sagittal T1 image, showing patchy strong enhancement, the tumor being seen to protrude into the foramen of Luschka. (c) Sagittal constructive interference in the steady state image demonstrates clearly the topographical anatomy of the tumor and the lack of involvement of the vermis. Note the clear demonstration of the cystic nature of the small hemorrhagic foci.*

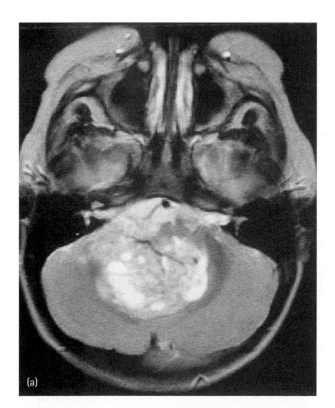

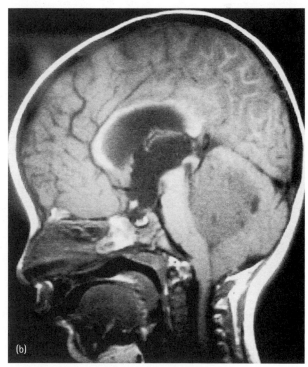

Figure 7.30a,b *Ependymoma. (a) Axial T2-weighted image, showing a heterogeneously hyperintense midline posterior fossa lesion containing cysts, a prominent vessel, and small hypointensities indicative of calcification. (b) Sagittal T1 image. The lesion is mildly hypointense, with several small hypointense cystic foci.*

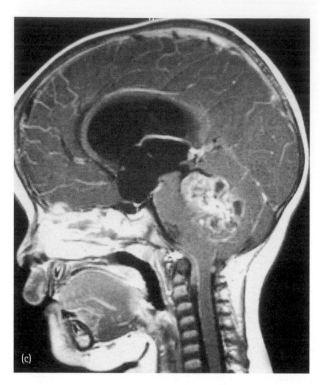

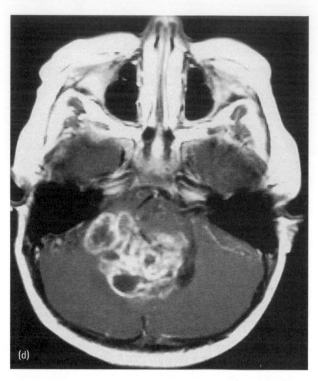

Figure 7.30c,d *(c) Sagittal post-contrast image. The tumor enhances strongly, highlighting the cystic foci. There is contiguous tumor lying anterior to the craniocervical junction, with delicate linear enhancement extending caudally on the ventral surface of the cord. (d) Axial T1-weighted image, showing tumor extending out of the fourth ventricle via the foramen of Luschka.*

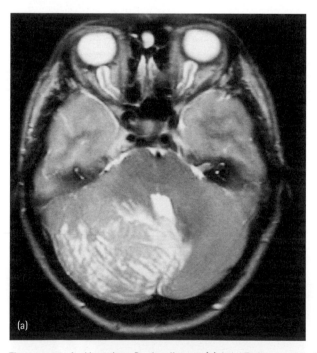

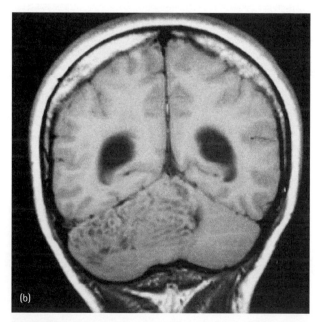

Figure 7.31a,b *Lhermitte–Duclos disease. (a) Axial T2 image, showing a mass-like lesion expanding the right cerebellar hemisphere and compressing the fourth ventricle. Note the characteristic parallel linear striations within the lesion. (b) Coronal T1 image. The hypointense striations appear prominently within the minimally hypointense tumor. Note the expansion of the posterior fossa on the right.*

Atypical teratoid/rhabdoid tumors

These tumors, which represent a newly recognized entity among malignant pediatric brain tumors,[40] share similar imaging characteristics to medulloblastomas and ependymomas. However, they tend to occur in children under the age of two years and are commoner in boys than girls. The prognosis is poor, with CSF dissemination frequently present at the time of presentation.

Dysplastic gangliocytomas (Lhermitte–Duclos disease)

These uncommon lesions occur in older children and young adults. They may be associated with neurofibromatosis or Cowden's disease (multiple hamartoma syndrome).[77] The lesion appears as a large cerebellar mass with thickened cerebellar folia, giving the mass a striate aspect. On CT scanning, the lesion appears hypodense with mild to moderate mass effect, which may result in supratentorial mass effect. MRI demonstrates a hypointense mass on T1-weighted images and heterogeneous hyperintensity on T2 imaging. Linear relatively parallel striations on the surface of the lesion are a striking feature on both pulse sequences (Figure 7.31). Expansion of the ipsilateral cerebellar hemisphere with thinning and bulging of the overlying skull is indicative of the longstanding nature of this lesion, which shares neoplastic and hamartomatous features. Contrast enhancement is not a feature, although it has been reported,[78] and pial vessels may appear particularly prominent.

FOURTH-VENTRICULAR TUMORS

Choroid plexus papillomas and carcinomas

The fourth ventricle is an uncommon site for choroid plexus tumors in childhood. The benign CPPs and more aggressive CPCs share similar appearances histologically and on imaging. The choroid plexus is located at the roof of the fourth ventricle and extends out through the foramina of Luschka (the lateral fourth ventricular outlet foramina) into the cerebellopontine angle cisterns. Thus, the tumors may be located in an extraventricular location. The tumors are often large, frond-like, friable, and hypervascular. Calcification is present in approximately 25 per cent of cases. The imaging characteristics are as those described for the supratentorial tumors.

Astrocytomas

Cerebellar astrocytomas usually originate from the vermis and extend anteriorly into the fourth ventricle. However, occasionally, these tumors may be entirely intraventricular in location. The imaging characteristics are typically those of a pilocytic astrocytoma, with a hypointense mass on T1-weighted images filling the fourth ventricle and showing strong enhancement following contrast administration.

EXTRA-AXIAL TUMORS

Nerve–sheath tumors

Schwannomas, benign neoplasms consisting of Schwann cells arising from the nerve sheath, occur most commonly in association with the vestibulocochlear nerve. They are rare in childhood. Particularly when bilateral, they occur in association with the central, type 2 form of neurofibromatosis (NF-2). Less commonly, schwannomas may arise from the fifth or ninth cranial nerves,

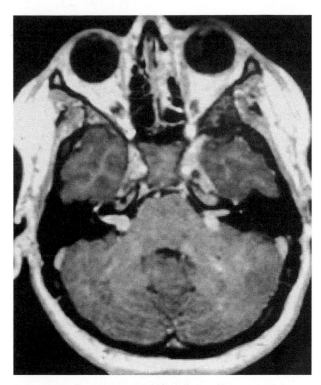

Figure 7.32 *Neurofibromatosis type 2 in a 13-year-old girl. Axial post-contrast image, showing small, bilateral acoustic schwannomas. A left convexity meningioma, spinal-cord ependymomas, and multiple neurinomas of the cauda equina were also present.*

the cardinal features being that of an extra-axial posterior fossa lesion. Imaging by magnetic resonance is optimal, particularly for identifying the small intracanalicular lesions (Figure 7.32). Schwannomas generally appear hypointense on T1 images and homogeneously or heterogeneously hyperintense on T2-weighted images (Figure 7.33). Cysts may be identified within the lesion, or there may be entrapped pouches of CSF forming capping cysts. Enhancement of the solid portions of the tumor is strong.

Neurofibromas, nerve-sheath tumors of the peripheral nervous system, are similarly uncommon in childhood but may occur at the skull base, typically in children with NF-1.

Meningiomas

Meningiomas are uncommon within the posterior fossa in childhood. Atypical histological features are not uncommon. The imaging characteristics are similar to the supratentorial lesions and those seen in adulthood. The masses may attain a large size before presentation (Figure 7.34).

Chordomas

These tumors, derived from notochordal remnants, are very unusual in children. Typically, they occur in

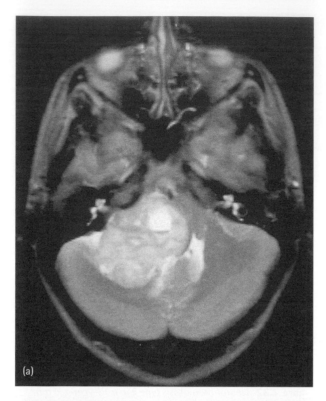

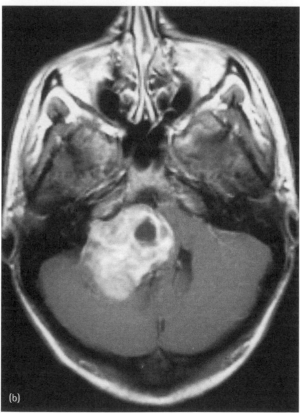

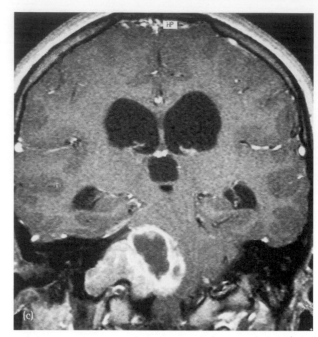

Figure 7.33c *(c) Post-contrast coronal T1 image, demonstrating clearly the tumor extending into the jugular foramen. The cyst is demarcated clearly.*

Figure 7.33a,b *Glossopharyngeal schwannoma in an 11-year-old girl. (a) Axial T2 image, showing a large, discrete, heterogeneously hyperintense extra-axial mass and a hemorrhagic cyst containing a fluid–fluid layer. (b) Post-contrast axial T1-weighted image, demonstrating strong patchy enhancement.*

middle age. Their location is usually in association with the spheno-occipital synchondrosis.[79] The mass is focally destructive and may extend into the nasopharynx, sphenoid sinus, or upper cervical region. CT scanning is helpful, identifying spicular or more complex calcifications. On CT, the mass is hypodense. T1-weighted MRI demonstrates a hypointense mass, with corresponding mixed but essentially hyperintense signal on T2-weighted images. Unlike in adults, enhancement in children tends to be less marked.

Metastases

Metastatic tumors in the posterior fossa are rare in childhood outside of primary intracranial tumors. A range of supratentorial, infratentorial, and spinal tumors may spread to the posterior fossa, reflecting widely differing histological phenotypes and proliferative/malignant features. The deposits may be discrete and linear, or they may occur as larger nodular masses in the posterior fossa (Figure 7.35).

Primitive round–cell tumors

Ewing's sarcoma and neuroblastoma arise in the skull base in a small proportion of childhood CNS tumors and share similar imaging characteristics.[80] The tumors may be primary or secondary. There may be variable expansion into the extra-axial spaces within the posterior fossa. The affected part of the skull base is typically expanded. There is typically both intra- and extracranial disease,

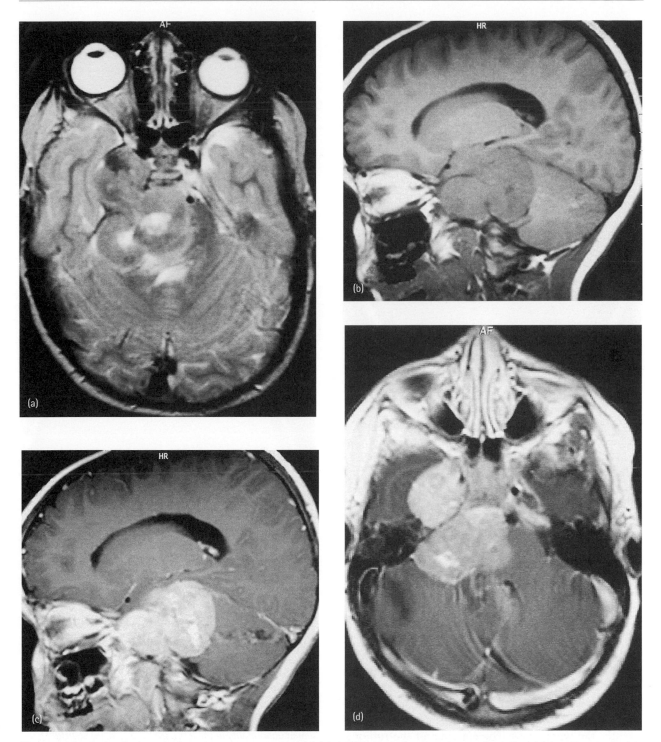

Figure 7.34a–d *Atypical meningioma in a nine-year-old girl. (a) Axial T2 image, showing a large, mixed-signal-intensity extra-axial lesion compressing the brainstem and fourth ventricle and extending into the right parasellar region. (b) Sagittal T1-weighted image. The tumor is slightly hypointense and well-defined. (c) Post-contrast sagittal and (d) axial T1-weighted images, showing strong heterogeneous enhancement.*

with focal infiltration of bone and soft tissues (Figure 7.36). MRI is most useful in evaluating the extent of the disease. Post-contrast fat-suppressed T1-weighted sequences are particularly useful, the tumor enhancing strongly. Elevation of the periosteum helps to differentiate these tumors from the normal but prominent enhancement that may be seen in association with the normal enhancing hematopoietic marrow of childhood.

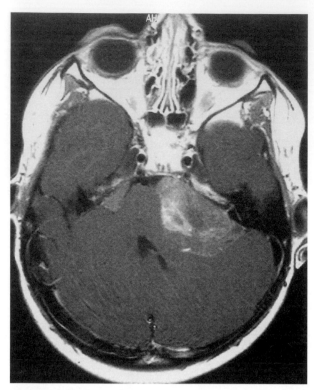

Figure 7.35 *Metastatic glioblastoma multiforme. Post-contrast axial T1-weighted image, demonstrating variably enhancing lesions in the cerebellopontine angle cisterns. The primary cerebral tumor (not shown) exhibited similar enhancing characteristics.*

Spinal tumors

INTRADURAL INTRAMEDULLARY TUMORS

Astrocytomas

Intramedullary spinal tumors account for approximately five per cent of childhood CNS neoplasms, of which astrocytomas are the commonest, accounting for approximately 60 per cent of tumors in this location. Most occur in the first five years of life and, unlike in adults, tend to preponderantly involve the rostral spinal cord.[81] The majority of tumors are low-grade lesions, but there is a significant minority of grade 3 and 4 gliomas.

MRI typically demonstrates fusiform expansion of the cord, usually involving several segments or, not infrequently, the whole cord. The epicenter of the tumor is usually iso- to slightly hypointense on T1-weighted images and heterogeneously hyperintense on T2 imaging. Exophytic growth of the tumor is not uncommon and is best evaluated on axial images. There are frequently abnormal glial-lined cysts or necrotic foci within the solid part of the tumor, the cyst fluid being highly proteinaceous, resulting in higher signal intensity on T1 imaging. Peritumoral cysts, probably representing syringohydromyelic cavities, may also accompany the diffuse cord expansion occurring both rostral and caudal to the solid portion of the tumor.

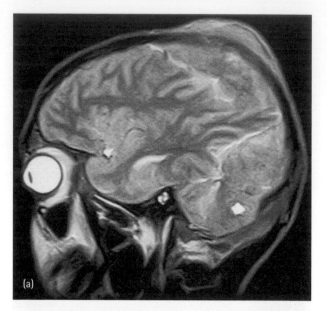

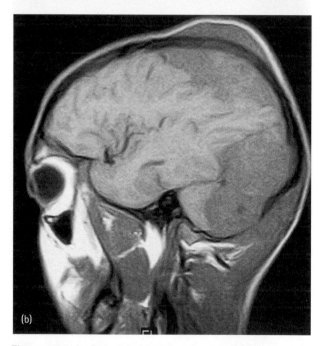

Figure 7.36a,b *Ewing's sarcoma in a 12-year-old boy. (a) Sagittal T2-weighted image, demonstrating a heterogeneously mildly hypointense posterior fossa extra-axial mass involving the occipital bone and extracranial soft tissues. There is further similar abnormality in the left parietal region. (b) Sagittal T1 image. The lesion is correspondingly hypointense.*

Enhancement is variable, and in some astrocytomas there may be little or none. Overall, the enhancement tends to be less prominent and less well-defined than in ependymomas.[82] Definition of the margins of associated cystic lesions is better appreciated following contrast administration. As with intracranial astrocytomas, tumor infiltration should be regarded as extending beyond the

Ependymomas

Ependymomas represent approximately 30 per cent of intrinsic cord tumors, most occurring in the conus region. Myxopapillary ependymomas of the filum terminale, characteristically seen in adults, are uncommon in children. The cervical cord is affected in older children and young adults, particularly in association with NF-2.

These tumors are usually well-defined and exhibit heterogeneous signal characteristics on both T1- and T2-weighted sequences, corresponding to the presence of cysts, hemorrhage, and microcalcifications. Edema invariably accompanies the intramedullary tumors, expanding the cord caudocephalad to the solid tumor. Enhancement is typically moderate to strong, defining a well-marginated mass (Figure 7.38). This pattern of enhancement is not, however, uniform and may be heterogeneous or even minimal.[83] Multiple spinal-cord ependymomas may occur, particularly in association with NF-2, where there may also be accompanying meningiomas (Figure 7.38). Cranial imaging should be undertaken at the end of the examination in view of the propensity for these tumors to seed in the CSF.

Miscellaneous tumors

Other primary cord tumors are rare. Gangliogliomas, gangliocytomas, PNETs, and intramedullary metastases from intracranial primary CNS tumors may be encountered. Spinal gangliogliomas are uncommon cord tumors with a heterogeneous appearance on T1-weighted imaging[84] and enhancement frequently extending over eight vertebral body segments.[82] Hemangioblastomas occur occasionally as isolated tumors in childhood, typically in the cervical spine. There is typically a cyst, a strongly enhancing mural nodule, and a leash of prominent vessels surrounding the lesion in the cord or perimedullary region. In general, the imaging characteristics of these lesions tend to be non-specific, requiring biopsy or resection for a definitive diagnosis.

INTRADURAL EXTRAMEDULLARY TUMORS

The commonest tumors in this compartment are leptomeningeal metastatic deposits and nerve-sheath tumors.

Leptomeningeal metastatic disease

CSF-borne metastases are particularly characteristic of pediatric primary CNS tumors, of which medulloblastomas are the foremost source. Other tumors associated with spinal CSF dissemination include other PNETs, pineocytomas, ependymoma, malignant gliomas, germinomas, gangliogliomas, and even occasionally low-grade gliomas. MRI has a greater diagnostic accuracy than CSF cytological analysis for the early detection of disseminated medulloblastoma.[85]

Leptomeningeal deposits occur typically in the mid- and lower thoracic region, cauda equina, and sacral thecal sac.

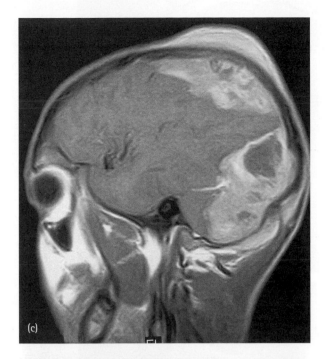

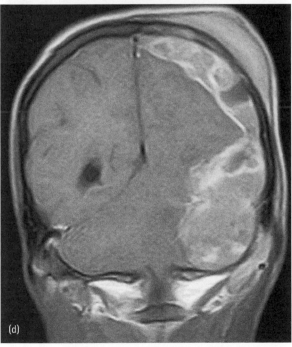

Figure 7.36c,d *(c) Post-contrast sagittal T1 image. There is strong heterogeneous enhancement, highlighting cystic/necrotic foci and adjacent dural enhancement. (d) Post-contrast coronal T1 image, demonstrating more clearly the contiguous nature of the tumor and the extracranial spread.*

enhancing tumor, being present within the typically extensive cord edema. Aggressive tumors may be encountered, with intratumoral hemorrhage, necrosis, and diffuse leptomeningeal spread throughout the neuraxis (Figure 7.37).

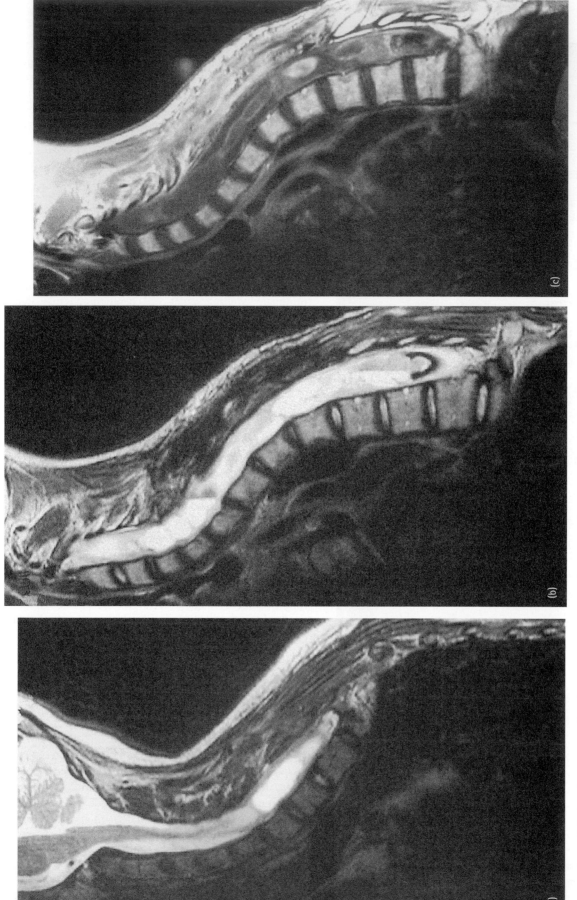

Figure 7.37a–c Spinal cord astrocytoma in a nine-year-old girl with a progressive scoliotic deformity. (a) Sagittal T2-weighted image, demonstrating cord expansion and a hyperintense cord cyst at the cervicothoracic junction. (b) Sagittal T2-weighted image eight months later, following acute neurological deterioration. The cord expansion has increased greatly, with fluid levels in the cervicothoracic junction and mid-thoracic cysts indicative of hemorrhage into the tumor. (c) Post-contrast sagittal T1-weighted image, showing patchy foci of mixed/strong enhancement throughout the thoracic and cervical cord (also seen on adjacent images).

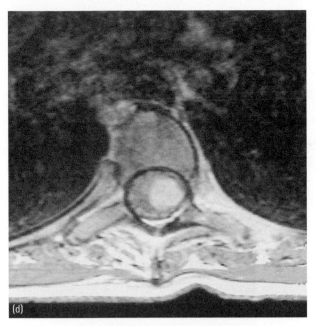
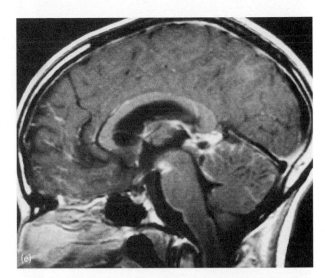

Figure 7.37d,e *(d) Axial post-contrast T1-weighted image. A strongly enhancing lesion is present eccentrically within the left side of the expanded cord. (e) Post-contrast sagittal T1 image through the brain, demonstrating delicate linear enhancing tumor over the surface of the brainstem, cerebellar hemispheres, and further leptomeningeal metastatic disease in the supratentorial compartment.*

Contrast-enhanced T1-weighted imaging is optimal for identifying these lesions, which appear as enhancing nodular lesions (Figure 7.39), thickening of nerve roots, or diffuse enhancement over the surface of the cord. Normal vessels, particularly on the dorsal surface of the lower thoracic cord, may simulate metastatic deposits. However, the curvilinear nature of the enhancement should help to differentiate between the two. Caution should also be exercised in patients in whom the primary tumor shows little or no enhancement. In addition, the spinal metastases of some children with enhancing medulloblastomas do not exhibit enhancement and could thus be overlooked.[73] In these patients, a heavily T2-weighted sequence may be more helpful in detecting their presence. Imaging following a recent craniectomy is associated frequently with the presence of blood products and confusing patterns of enhancement that may simulate metastases. Pre-contrast T1 imaging should be undertaken to identify any hyperintense methemoglobin. Delaying postoperative imaging by more than two weeks can reduce false-positive results when a preoperative spinal study was not undertaken.[85]

Nerve-sheath tumors

The two principal types of nerve-sheath tumors are neurofibromas, which typically occur in patients with NF-1, and schwannomas, which are rare in childhood outside of the context of NF-2. Neurofibromas in NF-1 are typically multiple, being associated with the spinal nerves or nerve sheaths. They appear as nodular or more confluent lesions thickening the nerve roots, particularly in the lumbosacral spine, being mildly hypointense on T1-weighted images. On T2-weighted images, there is typically an outer zone of hyperintensity surrounding a central core that is relatively hypointense, probably representing dense collagenous stroma.[86] These lesions are best identified following contrast administration, with mild to moderate enhancement of the tumors. Multiple small intrathecal schwannomas, particularly in the lumbosacral region, are a characteristic feature of spinal involvement in NF-2 (Figure 7.40). There may be accompanying small meningiomata or cord tumors.

Solitary neurofibromas are rare in childhood. When present, they may be identified as an intraspinal mass that may be associated with cord compression, vertebral body scalloping, expansion of an adjacent neuroforaminal canal, laminar thinning, or a mass extending in a so-called dumbbell fashion into the paraspinal soft tissues. Plexiform neurofibromas are large, confluent masses that occur typically in the paraspinal or pelvic soft tissues.

Meningiomas

These lesions, which are primarily intradural, are rare in childhood, accounting for less then five per cent of pediatric spinal tumors. MRI demonstrates a sharply delineated dural-based mass with signal characteristics similar to spinal cord tissue or slightly less intense than the spinal cord itself on both T1- and T2-weighted images. Enhancement is generally strong.

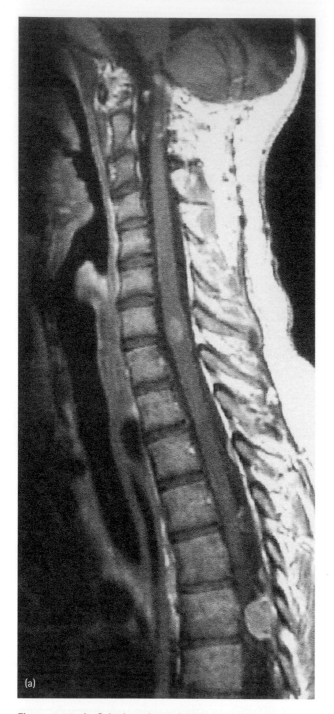
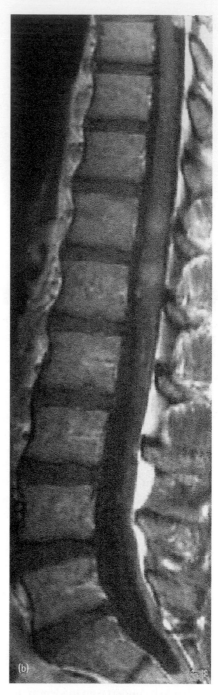

Figure 7.38a,b *Spinal-cord ependymomas in a 12-year-old girl with neurofibromatosis type 2. (a) and (b) Post-contrast sagittal T1-weighted images of the spine, demonstrating intermediately enhancing intramedullary lesions at the cervicothoracic junction and at T12 and L1. T2 images (not shown) demonstrated extensive associated cord edema and expansion. Note the extramedullary lesion at T6, most probably a meningioma, and small neurinomas at the C2 level.*

EXTRADURAL TUMORS

Tumors involving the extradural compartment of the spine in childhood are derived mainly from extraspinal masses invading the spinal canal via the neuroforaminal canal. Primarily osseous tumors will not be reviewed here, with a limited discussion of soft-tissue-derived lesions with direct CNS involvement.

Teratomas

These tumors are derived from tissues arising from germinal pluripotential cells occurring at ectopic sites.

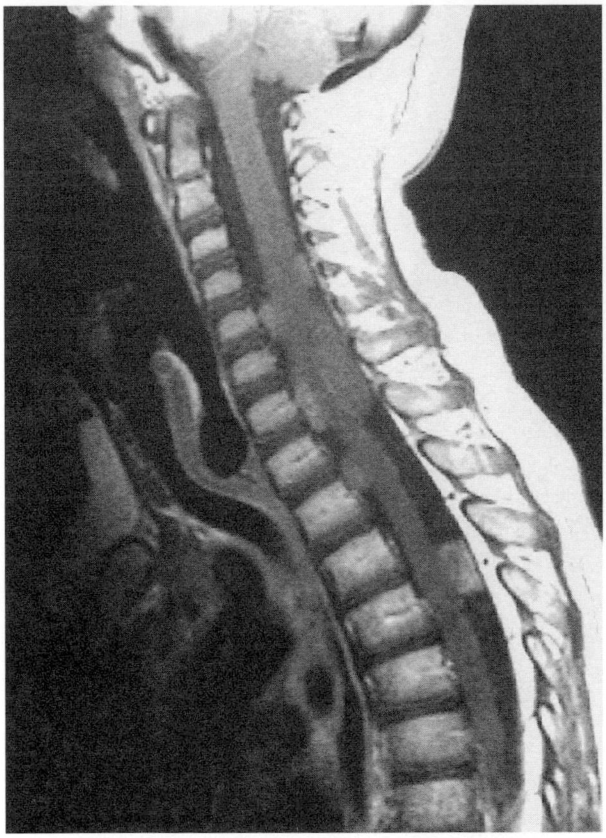

Figure 7.39 *Metastases from a glioblastoma multiforme in a four-year-old boy (same case as in Figure 7.35). Post-contrast sagittal T1 image, showing large mild to moderately enhancing nodular deposits on the dorsal and ventral aspects of the cervical and thoracic cord.*

Sacrococcygeal teratomas are congenital tumors that are more frequent in girls than boys and usually present as large posterior masses, with variable degrees of anterior pelvic extension. A small minority exist as purely presacral lesions. Teratomas may arise predominantly within the thoracolumbar spinal canal in a small proportion of cases in childhood, with a more even sex distribution and wider age spectrum.

The spinal canal is generally markedly expanded. Sacrococcygeal tumors may present as largely cystic masses. The imaging characteristics reflect the existence of tissues derived from ectoderm, mesoderm, and endoderm, with fatty tissue, calcifications, bone, teeth, solid tissue, and cysts containing fluid of diverse contents. The tumors are consequently typically heterogeneous on all pulse sequences. Magnetic resonance is particularly helpful in identifying the presence of intramedullary tumors (Figure 7.41). Enhancement is variable but usually present. Fat-suppression techniques may be helpful in defining the full extent of the tumor, particularly in the pelvis, and in confirming the lipomatous nature of the tumor.

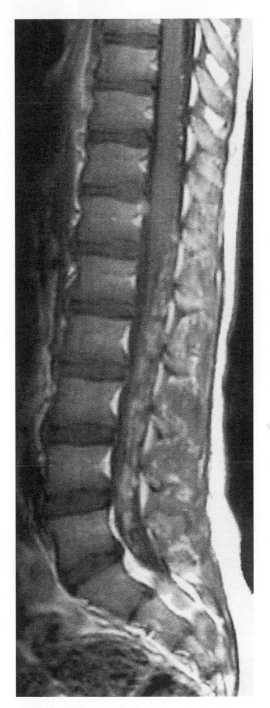

Figure 7.40 *Neurinomas of the cauda equina in a ten-year-old girl with neurofibromatosis type 2. Sagittal post-contrast T1 image, showing multiple, small, enhancing lesions throughout the lumbar thecal sac.*

Tumors of the autonomic nervous system

Neuroblastomas (and rarely ganglioneuromas and ganglioneuroblastomas) involving the spine arise from neuroblasts derived from the autonomic nervous system. The paraspinal sympathetic chain at the thoracolumbar and posterior mediastinal regions are most commonly

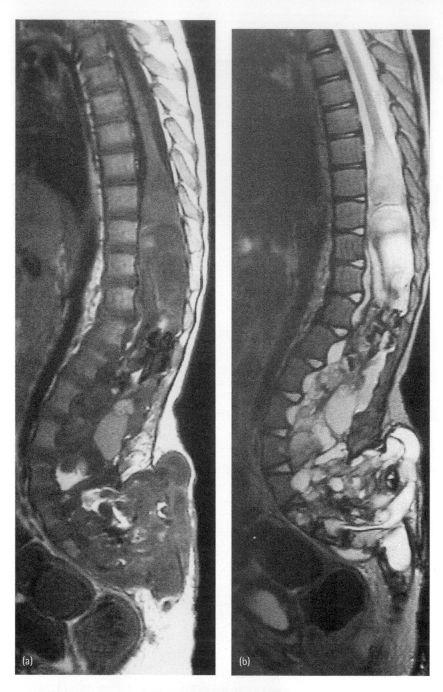

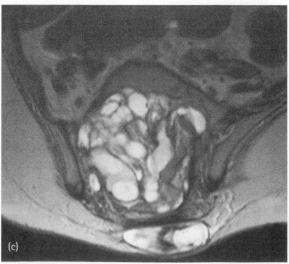

Figure 7.41a–c *Lumbosacral malignant teratoma in a one-year-old girl. Sagittal (a) T1- and (b) T2-weighted images and (c) axial T2-weighted images, showing a large heterogeneous mixed cystic-solid tumor filling and expanding the spinal canal. Tumor extends confluently into the spinal cord.*

involved, with a large paraspinal mass extending over several vertebral body segments. Extension into the spinal canal via the neuroforaminal canal leads to tumor within the extradural compartment, occasionally breaching the dura to lie within the subdural compartment. Asymptomatic cord compression is a not uncommon presentation.[87]

The imaging characteristics of these tumors are very similar, with a large paraspinal soft-tissue mass extending in a dumbbell fashion into the spinal canal or, particularly in the case of neuroblastomas, infiltrative metastatic disease affecting one or several vertebral bodies with contiguous extradural tumor. The tumor appears generally as a homogeneous isointense mass on T1 images and moderately to markedly hyperintense on T2-weighted images. Foci of hemorrhage, necrosis, or calcification may be present, resulting in focal alterations in the signal characteristics (Figure 7.42). Enhancement following contrast administration tends to be strong. Fat-suppression techniques may be helpful in identifying the degree of any vertebral body infiltration.

Peripheral primitive neuroectodermal tumors

These tumors, previously known as extraosseous Ewing's sarcoma, arise from small round cells within the paraspinal soft tissues, meninges or the calvarium.[88] Intraspinal extradural lesions frequently result in cord compression and presentation with a progressive spastic paraparesis or tetraparesis. MRI demonstrates a smoothly expansile mass, which is generally mildly hypo- or isointense on T1-weighted images and iso- to mildly hyperintense on T2-weighted images, with variable enhancement following contrast administration. Cystic or necrotic foci may be identified.

CLINICAL TRIALS

The incidence of specific childhood tumors is such that unless collaborative multinational multicenter trials are undertaken, then therapeutic interventions are difficult if not impossible to evaluate. Radiological imaging plays an integral part in these trials and studies. Imaging panels derived from accredited experts in pediatric neuroradiology are required to undertake this activity. Generally, this involves a tumor panel of two neuroradiologists, with a third neuroradiologist providing a casting vote in cases of disagreement or equivocation. Such a model has been developed in the UK and France, with close collaboration between the UKCCSG and the SFOP.

Significant intra- and interobserver error is inherent in the evaluation of response to anti-tumor therapy. In a French study, major disagreements occurred in 40 per cent and minor disagreements in 10.5 per cent of all tumor

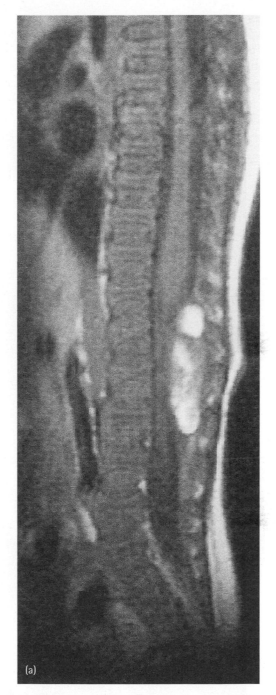

(a)

Figure 7.42a *Lumbar neuroblastoma in a three-year-old boy. (a) Sagittal T1-weighted image, showing a dorsally located heterogeneously hyperintense extradural mass compressing the conus and cauda equina.*

response evaluations in a multicenter oncological trial assessed subsequently by an evaluation committee.[11] The percentage of significant tumor response consequently fell by 23.2 per cent. Reasons for disagreement included errors in tumor measurement, errors in selection of measurable targets, intercurrent diseases, and radiological technical factors. The conclusions were that all therapeutic trials requiring neuroradiological response criteria and that are to be published in peer-reviewed journals should be undertaken by an evaluation committee.

Future developments will include the increased use of advanced MRI techniques, such as perfusion imaging and two-dimensional and three-dimensional MRS techniques in tumor evaluation, both for management and for clinical trials. Issues such as lesional boundaries for tumor volume measurements will remain problematic in the near future, particularly in the context of ill-defined or

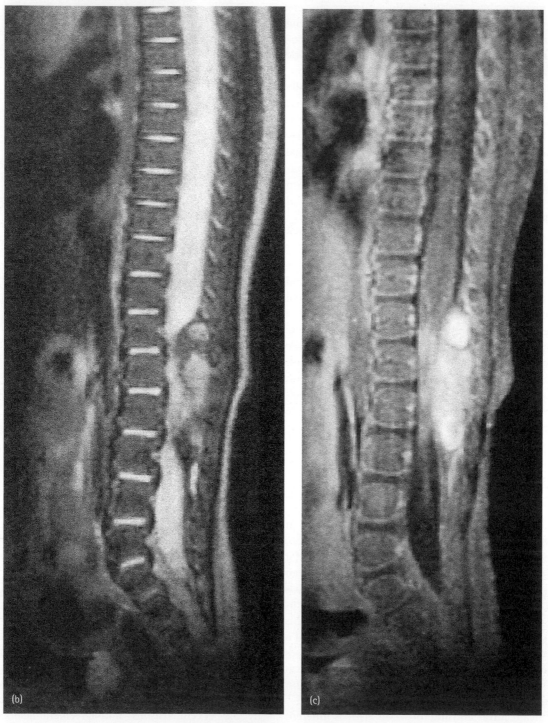

Figure 7.42b,c *(b) Sagittal short tau inversion recovery, showing the mass to be of mixed signal characteristics. (c) Post-contrast sagittal T1-weighted fat-saturated sequence. The lesion enhances strongly. Apparent enhancement of the cauda equina is artifactual, being due to partial volume averaging related to the tumor wrapping itself around the thecal sac posteriorly.*

poorly enhancing tumors, where these advanced techniques may demonstrate more extensive tumor than that defined by the contrast enhancing component of a lesion (Figure 7.43).

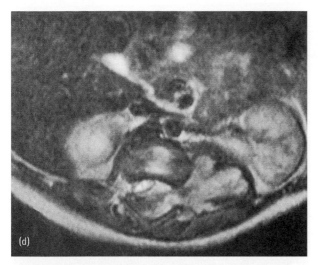

Figure 7.42d *(d) Axial T2 image, showing the dorsal location of the mass, particularly on the left and extending outwards through the related neuroforaminal canal into the paraspinal region.*

PITFALLS OF IMAGING

Postsurgical enhancement

Evaluation of the extent of tumor resection should be undertaken within 48–72 hours. This timeframe is a compromise between pragmatic considerations (patient compliance, surgical paraphernalia) and the onset of reactive enhancement, generally assumed to commence after 48 hours (Figure 7.44). There are traps and pitfalls to consider, however. Very early non-tumoral enhancement probably occurs to a greater or lesser extent in the majority of cases, which needs to be borne in mind constantly. To complicate the issue further, residual tumor may show diminished enhancement within the first 24 hours following surgery,[89] and concurrent steroid medication can significantly reduce the degree of tumoral enhancement. Whilst macroscopic tumor residuum is generally detected readily on early postoperative imaging, smaller tumor remnants can represent a significant diagnostic challenge (Figure 7.45). In general, residual tumor appears as nodular enhancement, whereas postoperative non-tumoral enhancement tends to be linear or curvilinear, conforming to resection margins or punctate.[90,91]

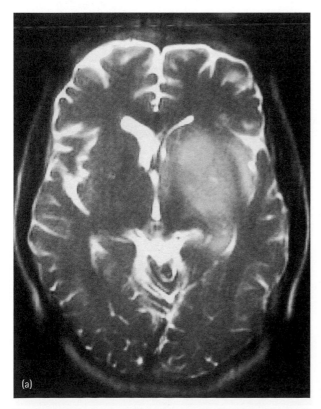

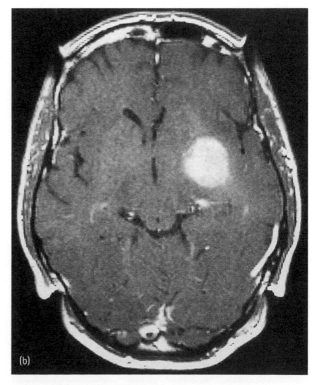

Figure 7.43a,b *Grade 3 left basal-ganglia-based tumor in a 17-year-old male. (a) Axial T2-weighted image, demonstrating an ill-defined hyperintense lesion with localized mass effect. (b) Post-contrast axial T1 image, showing a clear-cut central area of enhancement within the T2 abnormality.*

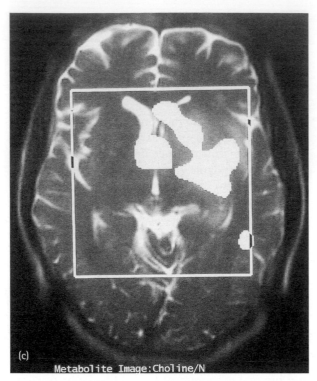

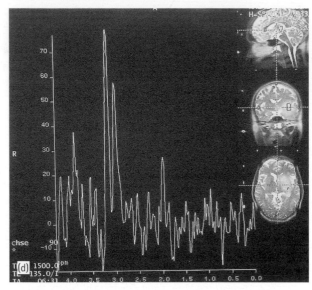

Figure 7.43c,d *(c) Magnetic resonance spectroscopy metabolite map, showing abnormally increased choline/N-acetyl aspartate (NAA) ratios extending beyond the confines of the T1-enhancing abnormality. (d) Magnetic resonance spectrum, demonstrating an abnormally elevated choline peak and depressed NAA peak measured at the posterior margin of the T2 abnormality, indicative of tumor.*

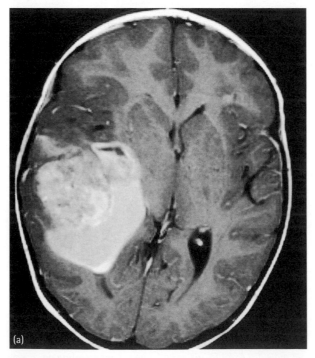

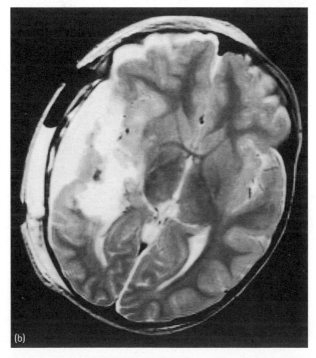

Figure 7.44a,b *Temporal lobe ganglioglioma in an 11-year-old girl. (a) Preoperative axial T1-weighted image, demonstrating a large, heterogeneously right-temporal-lobe-based enhancing mass. (b) Imaging undertaken 24 hours postoperatively, demonstrating macroscopic resection and postoperative changes.*

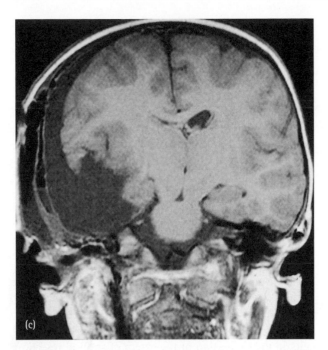

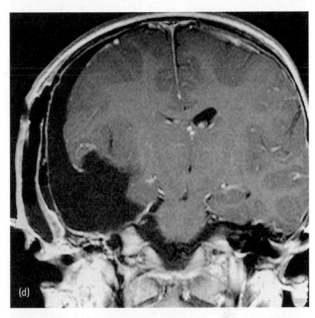

Figure 7.44c,d *(c) Pre-contrast coronal T1-weighted image, demonstrating a clear plane of resection with an overlying subdural hygroma. (d) Following contrast administration, note that the only enhancement seen is in relation to surface vessels.*

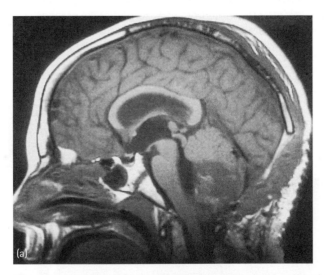

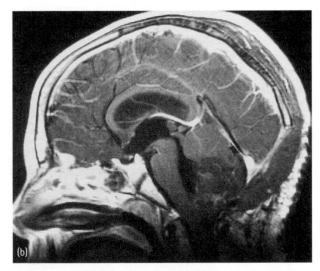

Figure 7.45a,b *Postoperative imaging in a 15-year-old male 24 hours following resection of an ependymoma (preoperative imaging demonstrated a large heterogeneously enhancing tumor). (a) Sagittal T1 image. There is some ill-defined hyperintensity within the bed of the resected tumor, representing hematoma (hyperintense despite being only 24 hours old). Tumor bed hemostatic material was not used, and there was no intralesional hemorrhage on the preoperative imaging. (b) Post-contrast sagittal T1-weighted image, showing no related enhancement in the midline.*

Non-tumoral enhancement related to the surgical procedure occurs as a consequence of four major factors:[13]

- focal breakdown of the blood–brain barrier, with leakage of contrast, which may occur as early as the first few hours following surgery[92] and probably occurs in 50–60 per cent of MRI studies;[91,93]
- local tissue trauma, resulting in hyperemia and contrast extravasation, which commences after the third postoperative day and has a peak effect in the fifth to fourteenth days postsurgery;[89]
- neovascularization due to angiogenesis within the tumor bed, commencing within the first postoperative week and persisting for several weeks. This manifests itself initially as delicate linear enhancement but becomes progressively thicker and more problematic in terms of differentiation from tumor residuum;

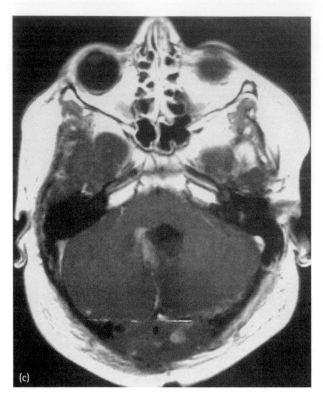

Figure 7.45c *(c) Axial post-contrast T1 image. There is enhancing tumor in the right side of the resection cavity, extending confluently into the dorsal pons. Invasion of the brainstem precluded complete excision of the tumor. There is no enhancement elsewhere within the surgical bed. Later interval scanning (not shown) showed progression of the tumor at this site.*

- chronic gliosis and disruption of the blood–brain barrier, which may manifest as persisting enhancement for many months postsurgery.

Surgical intervention, particularly burr holes and craniotomies, produces an immediate alteration in the status of the dura due to an inflammatory reaction and probable hyperemia. The dura may enhance within the first few hours following surgery, and the enhancement may persist for months or even years.[18]

Tumor bed material

The commonest non-tumoral abnormalities encountered in the postoperative tumor bed are blood and hemostatic material, particularly hemostatic gauze. Degradation of blood clot to methemoglobin occurs within the first two to three days following surgery, and may be even earlier (Figure 7.45). The hyperintensity of extracellular methemoglobin on T1-weighed images presents potential difficulty in the evaluation of the extent of surgical resection and tumor residuum.[92] Blood tracking down into the spinal thecal sac will similarly provide potential pitfalls in the assessment of the presence of CSF tumor spread. Thus, every attempt should be made to undertake preoperative whole-neuraxial imaging. If preoperative spinal imaging cannot be undertaken, then the spine should be examined at least three weeks after surgery.

Hemostatic gauze within the operative bed will appear mild to moderately hyperintense on T1-weighted images immediately following surgery and may persist as such for weeks or even months (Figure 7.46). Blood clot adherent to and enmeshed within the hemostatic gauze

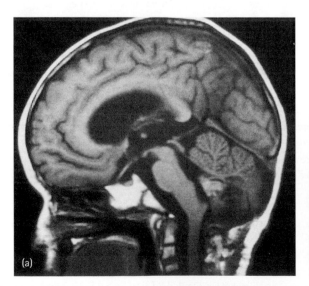
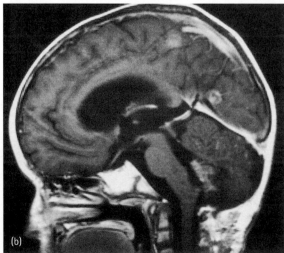

Figure 7.46a,b *Images in a six-year-old girl imaged four weeks following resection of a medulloblastoma. (a) Sagittal T1-weighted image, showing hyperintensity in the inferior vermian region. Hemostatic gauze had been placed in the tumor bed to assist hemostasis. (b) Post-contrast T1 image, demonstrating a little enhancement around the T1 hyperintensity in keeping with postsurgical reactive enhancement. Discrete enhancing lesions are present in the midline in the supratentorial compartment, consistent with metastases (more identified on adjacent slices).*

probably accounts for the more prominently hyperintense appearance seen in some cases.

CONCLUSION

The radiological evaluation of childhood CNS cancer has become an integral part of the management of these tumors. As many of these tumors are individually uncommon, epidemiological studies and evaluation of treatment protocols will necessarily involve multicenter multinational collaborative studies. The recent development of imaging protocols will help to standardize and systematize the imaging strategy, which is of fundamental importance for neuro-oncological therapeutic trials.

The continual evolution of imaging techniques offers the potential for increasingly sensitive and targeted diagnostic information. In the meantime, adherence to the imaging principles described above and increased implementation of neuroradiological tumor panels will provide an important platform for these future developments.

REFERENCES

1 Lee BC, Kneeland JB, Cahill PT, Deck MD. MR recognition of supratentorial tumors. *Am J Neuroradiol* 1985; **6**:871–8.
2 Dahlborg SA, Petrillo A, Crossen JR, *et al.* The potential for complete and durable response in nonglial primary brain tumors in children and young adults with enhanced chemotherapy delivery. *Cancer J Sci Am* 1998; **4**:110–24.
3 Tzika AA, Vajapeyam S, Barnes PD. Multivoxel proton MR spectroscopy and hemodynamic MR imaging of childhood brain tumors. Preliminary observations. *Am J Neuroradiol* 1997; **18**:203–18.
4 Girard N, Wang ZJ, Erbetta A, *et al.* Prognostic value of proton MR spectroscopy of cerebral hemisphere tumors in children. *Neuroradiology* 1998; **40**:121–5.
5 Hustinx R, Alavi A. SPECT and PET imaging of brain tumors. *Neuroimaging Clin N Am* 1999; **9**:751–66.
6 Rollins NA, Lowry PA, Shapiro KN. Comparison of gadolinium-enhanced MR and thallium-201 single photon emission computed tomography in pediatric tumors. *Pediatr Neurosurg* 1995; **22**:8–14.
7 Maria BL, Drane WB, Quisiling RJ, Hoang KB. Correlation between gadolinium-diethylenetriaminepentaacetic acid contrast enhancement and thallium-201 chloride uptake in pediatric brainstem glioma. *J Child Neurol* 1997; **12**:341–8.
8 Roelcke U, Leenders KL. PET in neuro-oncology. *J Cancer Res Clin Oncol* 2001; **127**:2–8.
9 Tamura M, Shibaski T, Zama A, *et al.* Assessment of malignancy of glioma by positron emission tomography with ^{18}F-fluorodeoxyglucose and single photon emission computed tomography with thalium-201 chloride. *Neuroradiology* 1998; **40**:210–15.
10 Perel Y, Conway J, Kletzel M, *et al.* Clinical impact and prognostic value of metaiodobenzylguanidine imaging in children with metastatic neuroblastoma. *J Pediatr Hematol Oncol* 1999; **21**:13–18.
11 Thiesse P, Ollivier L, Di Stefano-Louineau D, *et al.* Response rate accuracy in oncology trials:reasons for interobserver variability. *J Clin Oncol* 1997; **15**:3507–14.
12 Griffiths PD. A protocol for imaging paediatric brain tumours. *Clin Radiol* 1999; **54**:558–62.
13 Thiesse P, Jaspan T, Couanet D, Bracard S, Neuenschwander S, Griffiths PD. Un protocol d'imagerie des tumeurs cerebrales de l'enfant. *J Radiol* 2001; **82**:11–16.
14 Therasse P, Arbuck SG, Eisenhauer EA, *et al.* New guidelines to evaluate the response to treatment in solid tumors. *J Natl Cancer Inst* 2000; **92**:205–16.
15 Shi W-M, Wildrick, Sawaya R. Volumetric measurement of brain tumors from MR imaging. *J Neuro Oncol* 1998; **37**:87–9.
16 Peck DJ, Windham JP, Emery LL, *et al.* Cerebral tumor volume calculations using planimetric and eigen image analysis. *Med Phys* 1996; **23**:2035–42.
17 Joe BN, Fukui MB, Meltzer CC, *et al.* Brain tumor volume measurement: comparison of manual and semiautomated methods. *Radiology* 1999; **212**:811–16.
18 Hudgins PA, Davies PC, Hoffman JC. Gadopentetate dimeglumine-enhanced MR imaging in children following surgery for brain tumor: spectrum of meningeal findings. *Am J Neuroradiol* 1991; **12**:301–7.
19 Becker LE, Halliday WC. Central nervous system tumors of childhood. *Perspect Pediatr Pathol* 1987; **10**:86–134.
20 Zimmerman RA. Pediatric supratentorial tumors. *Semin Roentgenol* 1990; **25**:225–48.
21 Earnest F, Kelly PJ, Scheithauer BW, *et al.* Cerebral astrocytomas: histopathologic correlation of MR and CT contrast enhancement with stereotactic biopsy. *Radiology* 1988; **166**:823–7.
22 Naidich TP, Zimmerman RA. Primary brain tumors in children. *Semin Roentgenol* 1984; **19**:100–114.
23 Dohrmann GJ, Farwell JR, Flannery JT. Glioblastoma multiforme in children. *J Neurosurg* 1976; **44**:442–8.
24 Wisoff JH, Boyett JM, Berger MS, *et al.* Current neurosurgical management and the impact of the extent of resection in the treatment of malignant gliomas of childhood: a report of the Children's Cancer Group trial no. CCG-945. *J Neurosurg* 1998; **89**:52–9.
25 Giannini C, Scheithauer BW. Classification and grading of low-grade astrocytic tumors in children. *Brain Pathol* 1997; **7**:785–98.
26 Bucciero A, De Caro M, De Stefano V, *et al.* Pleomorphic xanthoastrocytoma: clinical, imaging and pathological features of four cases. *Clin Neurol Neurosurg* 1997; **99**:40–5.
27 Tonn JC, Paulus W, Warmuth-Metz, *et al.* Pleomorphic xanthoastrocytoma: report of six cases with special consideration of diagnostic and therapeutic pitfalls. *Surg Neurol* 1997; **47**:162–9.
28 Bendszus M, Warmuth-Metz M, Klein R *et al.* MR spectroscopy in gliomatosis cerebri. *Am J Neuroradiol* 2000; **21**:375–80.
29 Razack N, Baumgartner J, Bruner J. Pediatric oligodendrogliomas. *Pediatr Neurosurg* 1998; **28**:121–9.
30 Shaw EG, Scheithauer BW, O'Fallon JR, Tazelaar HD, Davis DH. Oligodendrogliomas: the Mayo Clinic experience. *J Neurosurg* 1992; **76**:428–34.

31 Tice H, Barnes PD, Goumnerova L, Scott RM, Tarbell NJ. Pediatric and adolescent oligodendrogliomas. *Am J Neuroradiol* 1993; **14**:1293–300.

32 Ludwig CL, Smith MT, Godfrey AD, Armbrustmacher VW. A clinicopathological study of 323 patients with oligodendrogliomas. *Ann Neurol* 1986; **19**:15–21.

33 Lee YY, Van Tassel P. Intracranial oligodendrogliomas: imaging findings in 35 untreated cases. *Am J Roentgenol* 1989; **152**:361–9.

34 Castillo M. Gangliogliomas: ubiquitous or not? *Am J Neuroradiol* 1998; **19**:807–9.

35 Zentner J, Wolf HK, Ostertun B, *et al.* Gangliogliomas: clinical, radiological, and histopathological findings in 51 patients. *J Neurol Neurosurg Psychiatry* 1994; **57**:1497–502.

36 Martin DS, Levy B, Awwad EE, Pittman T. Desmoplastic infantile ganglioglioma: CT and MR features. *Am J Neuroradiol* 1991; **12**:1195–7.

37 Tenreiro-Picon OR, Kamath SV, Knorr JR, *et al.* Desmoplastic infantile ganglioglioma: CT and MRI features. *Pediatr Radiol* 1995; **25**:540–3.

38 Buetow PC, Smirniotopoulos JG, Done S. Congenital brain tumors: a review of 45 cases. *Am J Neuroradiol* 1990; **11**:793–9.

39 Davis PC, Wichman RD, Takei Y, Hoffman JC. Primary cerebral neuroblastoma: CT and MRI findings in 12 cases. *Am J Neuroradiol* 1990; **11**:115–20.

40 Oka H, Scheithauer BW, Tanaka R, Yamada K. Clinicopathological characteristics of atypical teratoid/rhabdoid tumor. *Neurol Med Chir* 1999; **39**:510–18.

41 Miller DC. Pathology of craniopharyngiomas: clinical import of pathological findings. *Pediatr Neurosurg* 1994; **21**:11–17.

42 Maroldo TV, Barkovich AJ. Pediatric brain tumors. *Semin Ultrasound CT MR* 1992; **13**:412–48.

43 Sartoretti-Schefer S, Wichmann W, Aguzzi A, Valavanis A. MR differentiation of adamantinous and squamous-papillary craniopharyngiomas. *Am J Neuroradiol* 1997; **18**:77–87.

44 Villani RM, Tomei G, Bello L, *et al.* Long-term results of treatment for craniopharyngioma in children. *Childs Nerv Syst* 1997; **13**:397–405.

45 Crenshaw WB, Chew FS. Rathke's cleft cyst. *Am J Roentgenol* 1992; **158**:1312.

46 Donovan JL, Nesbit GM. Distinction of masses involving the sella and suprasellar space: specificity of imaging features. *Am J Roentgenol* 1996; **167**:597–603.

47 Sugiyama K, Uozumi T, Kiya K, *et al.* Intracranial germ-cell tumor with synchronous lesions in the pineal and suprasellar regions: report of six cases and review of the literature. *Surg Neurol* 1992; **38**:114–20.

48 Pont MS, Elster AD. Lesions of skin and brain: modern imaging of the neurocutaneous syndromes. *Am J Roentgenol* 1992; **158**:1193–203.

49 Hurst RW, Newman SA, Cail WS. Multifocal intracranial MR abnormalities in neurofibromatosis. *Am J Neuroradiol* 1988; **9**:293–6.

50 Boyko OB, Curnes JT, Oakes WJ, Burger PC. Hamartomas of the tuber cinereum: CT, MR, and pathologic findings. *Am J Neuroradiol* 1991; **12**:309–14.

51 Darling CF, Byrd SE, Reyes-Mugica, *et al.* MR of pediatric intracranial meningiomas. *Am J Neuroradiol* 1994; **15**:435–44.

52 Kang JK, Jeun SS, Hong YK, *et al.* Experience with pineal region tumors. *Childs Nerv Syst* 1998; **14**:63–8.

53 Choi JU, Kim DS, Chung SS, Kim SS. Treatment of germ cell tumors in the pineal region. *Childs Nerv Syst* 1998; **14**:41–8.

54 Popovic EA, Kelly PJ. Stereotactic procedures for lesions of the pineal region. *Mayo Clin Proc* 1993; **68**:965–70.

55 Prahlow JA, Challa VR. Neoplasms of the pineal region. *South Med J* 1996; **89**:1081–7.

56 Zee CS, Segall H, Apuzzo M, *et al.* MR imaging of pineal region neoplasms. *J Comput Assist Tomogr* 1991; **15**:56–63.

57 Smirniotopoulos JG, Rushing EJ, Mena H. Pineal region masses: differential diagnosis. *Radiographics* 1992; **12**:577–96.

58 Schild SE, Scheithauer BW, Schomberg PJ, *et al.* Pineal parenchymal tumors. Clinical, pathologic, and therapeutic aspects. *Cancer* 1993; **72**:870–80.

59 Laitt RD, Malluci CL, Jaspan T, *et al.* Constructive interference in steady-state 3D Fourier-transform MRI in management of hydrocephalus and third ventriculostomy. *Neuroradiology* 1999; **41**:117–23.

60 Fetell MR, Bruce JN, Burke AM, *et al.* Non-neoplastic pineal cysts. *Neurology* 1991; **41**:1034–40.

61 Laurence KM. The biology of choroid plexus papilloma in infancy and childhood. *Acta Neurochir (Wien)* 1979; **50**:79–90.

62 Berger C, Thiesse P, Lellouch-Tubiana A, *et al.* Choroid plexus carcinomas in childhood: clinical features and prognostic factors. *Neurosurgery* 1998; **42**:470–5.

63 Armington WG, Osborn AG, Cubberley DA, *et al.* Supratentorial ependymoma: CT appearance. *Radiology* 1985; **157**:367–72.

64 Spoto GP, Press GA, Hesselink JR, Solomon M. Intracranial ependymoma and subependymoma: MR manifestations. *Am J Neuroradiol* 1990; **11**:83–91.

65 Naidich TP, Zimmermann RA. Primary brain tumors in children. *Semin Roentgenol* 1984; **19**:100–14.

66 Freeman CR, Farmer JP. Pediatric brain stem gliomas: a review. *Int J Radiat Oncol Biol Phys* 1998; **40**:265–71.

67 Kaplan AM, Albright AL, Zimmerman RA, *et al.* Brainstem gliomas in children. A Children's Cancer Group review of 119 cases. *Pediatr Neurosurg* 1996; **24**:185–92.

68 Albright AL, Packer AL, Zimmerman R, *et al.* Magnetic resonance scans should replace biopsies for diagnosis of diffuse brainstem gliomas. A report from the Children's Cancer Study Group. *Neurosurgery* 1993; **33**:1026–9.

69 Khatib ZA, Heideman RL, Kovnar EH, *et al.* Predominance of pilocytic histology in dorsally exophytic brain stem tumors. *Pediatr Neurosurg* 1994; **20**:2–10.

70 Robertson PL, Muraszko KM, Brunberg JA, *et al.* Pediatric midbrain tumors: a benign subgroup of brain stem gliomas. *Pediatr Neurosurg* 1995; **22**:65–73.

71 Barkovich AJ, Krischer J, Kun LE, *et al.* Brain stem gliomas: a classification system based on magnetic resonance imaging. *Pediatr Neurosurg* 1990–1991; **16**:73–83.

72 Behnke J, Mursch K, Bruck W, Christen HJ, Markakis E. Intra-axial endophytic primitive neuroectodermal tumors in the pons: clinical, radiological and immunohistochemical aspects in four children. *Childs Nerv Syst* 1996; **12**:125–9.

73 Meyers SP, Kemp SS, Tarr RW. MR imaging features of medulloblastomas. *Am J Roentgenol* 1992; **158**:859–65.

74 Rorke LB, Trojanowski JQ, Lee VM, *et al.* Primitive neuroectodermal tumors of the central nervous system. *Brain Pathol* 1997; **7**:765–84.

75 Kuroiwa T, Numaguchi Y, Rothman MI, *et al.* Posterior fossa glioblastoma multiforme: MR findings. *Am J Neuroradiol* 1995; **16**:583–9.

76 Tortori-Donati P, Fondelli MP, Cama A, *et al.* Ependymomas of the posterior cranial fossa: CT and MRI findings. *Neuroradiology* 1995; **37**:238–43.

77 Kulkantrakorn K, Awwad EE, Levy B, *et al.* MRI in Lhermitte–Duclos disease. *Neurology* 1997; **48**:725–31.

78 Awwad EE, Levy E, Martin DS, Merenda GO. Atypical MR appearance of Lhermitte–Duclos disease with contrast enhancement. *Am J Neuroradiol* 1995; **16**:1719–20.

79 Matsumoto J, Towbin RB, Ball WS. Cranial chordomas in infancy and childhood. A report of two cases and review of the literature. *Pediatr Radiol* 1989; **20**:28–32.

80 Hadfield MG, Luo VY, Williams RL, Ward JD, Russo CP. Ewing sarcoma of the skull in an infant. A case report and review. *Pediatr Neurosurg* 1996; **25**:100–104.

81 Steinbok P, Cochrane DD, Poskitt K. Intramedullary spinal cord tumors in children. In: Berger MS (ed.) *Pediatric Neuro-oncology.* Philadelphia: Saunders, 1992, pp. 931–45.

82 Koeller KK, Rosenblum RS, Morrison AL. Neoplasms of the spinal cord and filum terminale: radiologic-pathologic correlation. *Radiographics* 2000; **20**:1721–49.

83 Kahan H, Sklar EM, Post MJ, Bruce. MR characteristics of histopathologic subtypes of spinal ependymoma. *Am J Neuroradiol* 1996; **17**:143–50.

84 Patel U, Pinto RS, Miller DC, *et al.* MR of spinal cord gangliogliomas. *Am J Neuroradiol* 1998; **19**:879–87.

85 Meyers SP, Wildenhain SL, Chang JA, *et al.* Postoperative evaluation for disseminated medulloblastoma involving the spine: contrast-enhanced MR findings, CSF cytologic analysis, timing of disease occurrence, and patient outcomes. *Am J Neuroradiol* 2000; **21**:1757–65.

86 Burk DL, Brunberg JA, Kanal E, *et al.* Spinal and paraspinal neurofibromatosis: surface coil imaging at 1.5T. *Radiology* 1987; **162**:797–801.

87 Punt J, Pritchard J, Pincott JR, Till K. Neuroblastoma: a review of 21 cases presenting with spinal cord compression. *Cancer* 1980; **45**:3095–101.

88 Kimber C, Michalski A, Spitz L, Pierro A. Primitive neuro-ectodermal tumors: anatomic location, extent of surgery, and outcome. *J Pediatr Surg* 1998; **33**:39–41.

89 Forsyth PA, Petrov E, Mahallati H, *et al.* Prospective study of postoperative magnetic resonance imaging in patients with malignant gliomas. *J Clin Oncol* 1997; **15**:2076–81.

90 Albert FK, Forsting M, Sartor K, Adams HP, Kunze S. Early postoperative magnetic resonance imaging after resection of malignant glioma: objective evaluation of residual tumour and its influence on regrowth and prognosis. *Neurosurgery* 1994; **34**:45–60.

91 Henegar MM, Moran CJ, Silbergeld DL. Early postoperative magnetic resonance imaging following nonneoplastic cortical resection. *J Neurosurg* 1996; **84**:174–9.

92 Spetzger U, Thron A, Gilsbach JM. Immediate postoperative CT contrast enhancement following surgery of cerebral tumoral lesions. *J Comput Assist Tomogr* 1998; **22**:120–5.

93 Oser AB, Moran CJ, Kaufman BA, Park TS. Intracranial tumor in children: MR imaging findings within 24 hours of craniotomy. *Radiology* 1997; **205**:807–12.

8

Clinical trials

RICHARD SPOSTO

INTRODUCTION AND OVERVIEW

A clinical trial is "any form of planned experiment which involves patients and is designed to elucidate the most appropriate treatment of future patients with a given medical condition."[1] This definition describes concisely the structured clinical investigation necessary to acquire a clear understanding of the prognosis and treatment of pediatric central nervous system (CNS) tumors. The definition encompasses a spectrum of types of clinical trials, which differ in their objectives, complexity, target population, duration, and the numbers of patients involved.

In clinical oncology research, it is convenient, although not always completely accurate, to categorize clinical trials as phase I, phase II, or phase III. In the conventional and idealized sequence, phase I trials are preliminary studies of new single agents or combination treatments to establish a *maximum tolerated dose* (MTD). These are followed by phase II trials, which obtain preliminary evidence of efficacy of the drug or combination at the MTD using short-term or surrogate efficacy endpoints. Finally, phase III trials provide evidence of (lack of) efficacy compared with a control or standard treatment based on definitive, long-term endpoints. Many clinical trials cannot be categorized so easily, and designing trials to fit into only one of these categories can be counterproductive. However, it is useful to frame the discussion of clinical trials within this simplest classification scheme.

There is a large literature on the design and analysis of phase I, phase II, and phase III oncology clinical trials.

These methods were developed first in the context of adult cancer, and they may not address adequately the additional challenges presented by the design of clinical trials in childhood CNS tumors. Most pediatric CNS tumors are rarer than many adult cancers and other pediatric cancers, which limits the numbers of patients available to clinical trials. CNS tumors are biologically diverse, so this small patient resource must be divided further into smaller homogeneous groups within which meaningful phase II and phase III trials can be performed. In addition, entities such as medulloblastoma and primitive neuroectodermal tumor (PNET) occur primarily in children, which means that investigations will not have the benefit of information provided by studies already conducted in adults with similar tumors.

In this chapter, we will discuss clinical trials with emphasis on their application to research in pediatric CNS tumors. Each topic could easily be the subject of a chapter itself. Hence, our objective is to highlight important aspects of clinical trials and to provide references that will assist the interested reader in further examination of subtler issues.

PHASE I TRIALS

Phase I clinical trials are used to establish, as rapidly as possible, the highest (maximum) tolerated dose of treatment, and to determine the type and frequency of toxicity that will occur with the treatment.[2] Phase I trials would ideally lead to phase II trials of treatment efficacy, which in most cases is best done at the highest dose that can be administered safely.[2]

In a typical phase I trial, successive cohorts of patients are treated with a sequence of higher and higher doses until unacceptable levels of toxicity are encountered. One presumes with these designs that increases in dose will result in an increase in toxicity rate, an increase in efficacy, or both. Dose can be thought of not only literally as the dose of a chemotherapeutic agent, but any successive change in dose, schedule, infusion rate, etc., of a drug or other treatment modality that is thought potentially to increase efficacy but also potentially to increase rates of unacceptable toxicity. A dose-escalation algorithm with well-understood statistical properties ensures that a minimum number of patients are treated at inappropriately low levels or at unacceptably high dose levels.

In phase I trials in children, the MTD in adults often has been determined already, so that problems associated with underdosing early patients is less of a concern.[2] In cases where the MTD has not been determined, because pediatric CNS tumors are rare, accelerated escalation designs may provide added efficiency in terms of the numbers of patients and the time required to reach the MTD, while still minimizing the number of patients treated at presumably subtherapeutic doses and without compromising the precision of MTD estimates or placing more patients at risk for excess toxicity.[3]

Given the small sample sizes inherent in phase I trials, determination of the MTD is very imprecise.[4] Hence, the evaluation of toxicity at the MTD will continue past phase I into phase II, with the possibility of subsequent increases or decreases of the dose, depending on the additional toxicity and pharmacokinetics data that will become available during the phase II trial.

Eligible patient population

The eligible population for a phase I trial comprises patients who have adequate physiological status, so that toxicities that are observed can be attributed primarily to the agent being administered, rather than to a patient's poor status.[2] Since the aim of phase I trials is to establish a safe dose of a drug or treatment modality in advance of subsequent treatment-efficacy studies, it is neither critical nor necessarily desirable to limit the trial to patients with a specific histological diagnosis or tumor location, unless the toxicity of the treatment is likely to be affected by these considerations. Because phase I trials are sometimes performed without prior human data on toxicity and efficacy, they are typically restricted to patients for whom all known available treatments have been attempted and failed, or in newly diagnosed patients whose prognosis is known to be extremely grave, even with the best available treatment (e.g. intrinsic brainstem glioma).

Definitions of dose–limiting toxicity and maximum tolerated dose

Dose-limiting toxicities (DLTs) are toxicities whose occurrence in a sufficiently large fraction of patients will cause one to consider treatment infeasible. There is no one definition of DLT that is applicable to all situations, so it is important to define precisely what will be considered as a DLT. For example, with myelosuppressive chemotherapy, expected hematological toxicities would typically not be considered DLTs unless they resulted in death or unacceptable delays in therapy administration. Serious non-hematological toxicities would be included. The definition of DLT as the occurrence of any of the following may be applicable to many situations:

- toxic death, which is death primarily attributable to treatment;
- any grade 4 non-hematological toxicity;
- any grade 3 non-hematological toxicity that does not resolve within seven days after appropriate intervention (grade 3 nausea and vomiting is not included in this definition);
- failure to recover to absolute neutrophil count (ANC) >500/μl and platelets >25 000/μl within seven days of the last dose of therapy in any cycle.

There is some confusion in the literature and textbooks about the definition of MTD, or at least inconsistency in the use of terminology (e.g. see Smith *et al.*[2] and Arbuck[5]). The MTD is a population quantity that represents the dose above which the rate of occurrence of any DLT will exceed the tolerable rate. For example, given the above definition of DLT, we may define the MTD as the maximum dose at which 20 per cent of patients of the type in the study would experience the DLT. The purpose of a phase I trial is to estimate the MTD based on data. Because of statistical variation, it is entirely possible (and, in fact, expected) that the estimate of the MTD will differ from the true population value of the MTD.

Standard cohort design

The "standard" phase I design treats cohorts of three to six patients at each dose in a predetermined sequence of escalating doses, as follows:[6]

1 Treat up to six patients at each dose level, but only three at a time, starting with the lowest dose level.
2 If none of the first three patients at the dose level experiences a DLT, then go up a dose level and treat three patients. If exactly one experiences a DLT, then treat three more at this level; if at most one of six has experienced a DLT, then go up a dose level and treat three patients. However, if two or more patients experience DLTs at the dose level, then go down a

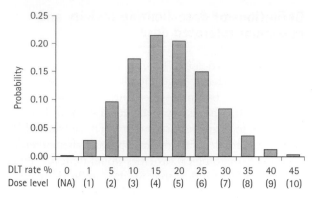

Figure 8.1 *Probability of dose-limiting toxicity (DLT) at the selected maximum tolerated dose (MTD).*

dose level (if a lower dose exists) and treat three more patients (to a maximum of six).

3 The estimated MTD is the highest dose level at which six patients are treated and no more than one patient experiences a DLT.

When defining DLT, it is important to understand that the MTD selected by the standard design is not likely to be a dose at which DLTs would occur rarely in the treated population. Rather, this statistical rule will, on average, settle on MTDs that cause DLTs in 15–20 per cent of treated patients. This level of toxicity at the MTD may be appropriate for serious but manageable toxicities, but it is unlikely to be appropriate for toxicities resulting in death or permanent organ damage. This is illustrated in Figure 8.1, which is based on a simulation of 1000 identical phase I trials using the standard design. The figure shows dose levels used in the trials (starting dose 1), the true DLT rates in the target population of patients at each dose level, and the probability that different dose levels are selected as the MTD.

Note that the modal estimate of MTD is dose level 4, which has a population DLT rate of 15 per cent. The average DLT rate of the selected MTD in these 1000 trials is 18 ± 9 (mean ± standard deviation (SD)) per cent, with DLT rates of 25 per cent and above selected with probability 0.29, and those with rates of 35 per cent and above selected with probably 0.051. Hence, if 20 per cent is the acceptable rate for the DLT, then this rule will significantly underdose (DLT rate ≤ 10 per cent) with probability 0.30 and significantly overdose (DLT rate ≥ 30 per cent) with probability 0.14. On the other hand, if ten per cent was the highest acceptable DLT rate, then this rule will significantly overdose (≥20 per cent) with probability 0.49.

Other phase I designs

This points out one of the deficiencies in the standard phase I design. Although this design is ubiquitous, simple,

and intuitive, its statistical rationale is weak.[7,8] The design does not allow one to target a different DLT rate when this is dictated by considerations of the type and severity of toxicities likely to be encountered. The MTD determination also largely ignores the considerable information available about toxicity from patients treated around the selected dose.[9] The design can also result in the treatment of many patients at therapeutically suboptimal doses when low starting doses are mandated. This creates an ethical concern, since many patients go into these trials with at least some expectation of deriving therapeutic benefit from the treatment.[8] In recent years, phase I trial designs have been proposed to address many of these perceived deficiencies, including multistage designs[3,6,8] and continual reassessment method (CRM).[10–16] A very good comparison of the properties of a number of proposed designs is provided by Ahn.[17] Designs in which the starting dose and escalation scheme are guided by pharmacokinetic parameters have been used,[7,18–20] which is important when one considers interpatient variability in drug metabolism and distribution, especially in the context of variable doses of steroid or other supportive care agents.

Procedural aspects and patient safety monitoring

The purpose of the staged designs used in phase I trials is to ensure that patients are not treated at a higher dose level before the current level can reasonably be certified as safe. If a DLT can occur at any time during, say, an eight-week course of treatment, then additional enrollment should not occur into the study during the eight-week evaluation period for the last patient entered from the current stage. A deliberate effort should be made after each stage to collect all relevant toxicity data, to review these data within a small committee of coordinating investigators, and to make a formal judgment of which patients DLTs have occurred in. Procedures should be in place in the study coordinating office to automatically halt enrollment when enrollment of a stage has been completed, and to restart enrollment only when the reviewing committee has authorized it.

PHASE II TRIALS

The objective of phase II trials is to assess rapidly the efficacy of a treatment. Most phase II studies are "group-sequential," enrolling and treating first an initial small cohort of patients, with enrollment of additional cohorts if adequate treatment response is observed. Designs that utilize this philosophy are described by Chang *et al.*[21] and Simon.[22]

Eligibility

The eligibility criteria for phase II studies are often similar to those of phase I studies, but with two key refinements. While phase I studies can be conducted in histologically heterogeneous groups of tumors, phase II studies will often necessarily target (histologically, biologically, stage) similar groups of tumors to establish the efficacy within each type. Secondly, patients enrolled on phase II studies must have disease that is assessable for documenting response to treatment. In the case of pediatric CNS tumors, this almost always means that patients must have radiologically identifiable tumors that can be measured serially during therapy.

Definition of response

The primary endpoint for most phase II trials is tumor response, which for CNS tumors has typically been defined in terms of the reduction in maximum cross-sectional area by computed tomography (CT) or magnetic resonance imaging (MRI). More recently, however, the so-called response evaluation criteria in solid tumors (RECIST) criteria have been devised, whereby response assessments are based on the maximum tumor diameter. This simple measurement is ostensibly easier to assess, is more reproducible, and results in equivalent conclusions about treatment efficacy compared with definitions that depend on cross-sectional area or tumor volume.[23–25] Although there continues to be discussion about the appropriateness of RECIST,[26] it is useful to describe response endpoints in this context, since it illustrates the essential features of the problem and is easily adapted to include measurements based on tumor area.

In RECIST criteria, lesions are classified as measurable (i.e. can be measured in at least one dimension) or non-measurable (e.g. positive cerebrospinal fluid (CSF) cytology, diffuse seeding of tumor in the leptomeninges, or other lesions that cannot be quantified but for which a qualitative assessment of "positive" or "negative" can be made). Some or all measurable lesions are identified as "target lesions" and are used to define the reference (baseline) measurement, which is the sum of the largest diameter (SLD) of all the identified target lesions. All other lesions are identified as non-target lesions and are not measured, although their presence or absence is noted. The response to treatment of target lesions is classified as follows:

- *Complete response (CR)*: complete disappearance.
- *Partial response (PR)*: 30 per cent reduction in the SLD.
- *Progressive disease (PD)*: 20 per cent increase in SLD compared with its smallest value during treatment, or appearance of new lesions.
- *Stable disease (SD)*: all other situations.

Non-target lesions are classified as follows:

- *CR*: complete disappearance.
- *Incomplete response/SD*: less than complete disappearance, but no new lesions.
- *PD*: appearance of new lesions.

The overall response to treatment is a synthesis of response in target lesions, response in non-target lesions, and the appearance of new lesions. For example, CR in both target and non-target lesions without any new lesions would be considered an overall CR, whereas CR in target lesions but incomplete response/SD in non-target lesions without new lesions would be considered overall PR. Complete details of the RECIST criteria can be found in Therasse *et al.*[23]

Standard two-stage design

The standard two-stage phase II study design involves enrolling a small number of patients, evaluating the response in this cohort, and then recruiting a second cohort or halting the study, depending on the response in the first cohort. In order to design a phase II trial, one first selects a minimum acceptable response rate (p_0) for the treatment under study and also a higher response rate (p_1) that is high enough to definitely be of interest. Typically, CR and PR are combined to compute overall response rate. One then devises a simple statistical rule that limits the chance of accepting a treatment that has poor efficacy (i.e. its response rate p is less than p_0), while having a good chance of accepting a treatment with good efficacy (i.e. its response rate p is at least p_1). This is usually expressed in terms of a statistical hypothesis test:[27]

$$H_0: p \leq p_0 \quad v. \quad H_A: p > p_0$$

where appropriate values are chosen for the α-error rate (type I error, false-positive rate) and β-error rate (type II error, false-negative rate) corresponding to p_0 and p_1, respectively. It is typical to set $\alpha = 0.05$ and $\beta = 0.80$. However, it is best to judge a rule by considering the entire characteristic function (i.e. power curve).

Figure 8.2 shows the characteristic function for three different two-stage rules, as described by Simon.[22] These designs were selected with the aid of a computer program, OPT.[28] All three rules have $\alpha \leq 0.05$ when $p_0 = 0.20$, which implies that treatments that produce a response in less than 20 per cent of patients should be accepted only rarely. Rules 1 and 2 were set so that $\beta \leq 0.20$ when $p_1 = 0.35$; in other words, these rules will accept, with probability 0.80, treatments that have a 35 per cent response rate. Note that these two rules will accept nearly 100 per cent of treatments that have a response rate of 0.45 or more, but will accept only 50 per cent of treatments that have a response rate of 0.30. Hence, even though a treatment that produces a response rate of 0.30

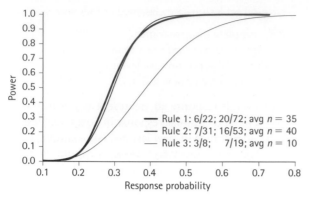

Figure 8.2 *Operating characteristic for two-stage phase II designs.*

may be of some interest, the chosen design has only a 50/50 chance of identifying these treatments as promising. Rules 1 and 2 are different in the average number of patients that will be treated. Rule 1 minimizes the average number of patients that would be treated if the true response rate were $p_0 = 0.20$. One treats 22 patients in the first stage and recruits 50 more patients if at least six of 22 show response. Ultimately, at least 20 of 72 responses are required to accept the treatment as effective. Rule 2 minimizes the maximum number of patients treated and requires at least seven of 31 responses in the first stage and 16 of 53 responses ultimately to declare the treatment effective. Rule 3 was devised with $\beta = 0.20$ when $p_1 = 0.50$ and hence is less likely to detect a very large response rate. Whereas rules 1 and 2 will identify a treatment with a 0.30 response rate 80 per cent of the time, rule 3 will identify such a treatment 40 per cent of the time.

Other phase II designs and combined phase I/phase II designs

While the study design described above is appropriate when the intent is to identify drugs or treatments that are cytotoxic, neither the RECIST criteria nor the design is necessarily appropriate when the drug or modality is cytostatic (e.g. anti-angiogenesis agents, differentiation agents).[29,30] Phase II trials in this context will rely on longer-term endpoints, such as time to tumor progression, and hence will resemble single-arm screening trials that compare, for example, one-year progression-free survival percentage with a historical or hypothetical baseline.

One issue that is of certain relevance to pediatric CNS tumor trials is that of resource allocation. Since the number of available patients is limited, it is important to allocate patients to trials optimally.[31] Randomized phase II trials[32] have been proposed as a strategy to conduct concurrent phase II evaluations of several therapies. In situations where there are more therapeutic options concurrently available than there are patients to evaluate them,

randomized phase II designs that compare efficacy can be used to screen efficiently for the most effective treatments.[33,34] These strategies are predicated to some extent on synchronous development of competing therapies through phase I development. Hybrid phase I/II studies,[35] possibly with intrapatient dose escalation[36] to enhance dose intensity, and designs that evaluate simultaneously both toxicity and efficacy endpoints,[37,38] are also possible.

PHASE III TRIALS

Phase III, or confirmatory, trials are prospective trials in which a large number of patients are assigned randomly to two or more different treatments, and then followed for outcome. Randomized trials minimize or eliminate bias that occurs with non-randomized, historically controlled trials or reports of case series. Since patients who are assigned to different treatments are treated and followed in contemporary time, improvements in imaging technology, surgical technique, and supportive care measures, changes in definitions of pathological entities, and other factors that affect outcome are represented equally in all treatment groups. Random allocation also ensures that inadvertent preferential selection of patients with better or worse prognosis for a particular treatment does not occur.

There is continued discussion on the need for performing randomized trials to demonstrate the efficacy of new treatments.[39–41] Non-randomized, historically controlled trials may sometimes be attractive in research in pediatric CNS tumors because these diseases are rare, and traditionally sized (by adult cancer standards) phase III randomized trials may take many years to complete, even in multi-institutional settings. Ironically, it is the fact that pediatric CNS tumors are rare that makes historical controls less attractive, because a sufficiently sized historical cohort accumulated over many years will not likely be comparable with a similarly sized cohort treated prospectively over a similar number of years. Hence, well-designed, randomized clinical trials provide the most convincing evidence of which of several alternative treatments is best. Nevertheless, when outcome with standard or available treatments is predictably grave, such as for pediatric brainstem tumors[42] or high-grade glioma,[43] then a randomized trial, although perhaps scientifically desirable, may be less ethically justifiable or practically feasible since randomization to a known ineffective treatment is unattractive to patients and physicians.[44]

Eligible patient population

Patients who are included in a phase III trial should be those to whom the scientific question will apply and for whom the proposed therapy or therapies are appropriate and safe. The patient cohort should otherwise mimic clinical practice as closely as possible by allowing entry of any patients for whom the treatments in the study would be appropriate.[45]

Patients should never be excluded from analysis – i.e. described as "not eligible" or censored (see below) – based on events that occur after the patient has been enrolled and the treatment has started. Especially in randomized trials, one assumes that any and all events that occur after the start of treatment are possibly related to the treatment. Excluding patients based on post-entry events distorts the patient population and reduces the generalizability of the study, since it defines the population based on information that will not be available to a physician who is deciding on what treatment course to take for a new patient. For example, patients who cannot tolerate an assigned treatment and hence must receive a significantly modified treatment or alternative treatment must be included because they inform about the practical efficacy of the treatment in the general population. The outcome in only the patients who can complete the therapy is irrelevant to a physician who must decide whether to use the treatment.

Endpoints for phase III trials

Phase III trials in pediatric CNS tumors are almost always designed to decide which treatment can most effectively control and, ideally, eliminate the tumors, while causing the least possible morbidity. Whereas the primary endpoints for analysis of phase I and phase II studies are the short-term endpoints of toxicity and tumor response, the endpoints for phase III trials measure disease control and patient cure and morbidity in the long term. Typical primary endpoints for phase III trials are:

- *overall survival (OS)*: the time from the start of treatment (or other appropriate time) to death from any cause;
- *event-free survival (EFS)*: the time from start of treatment to radiologically confirmed disease progression or recurrence, death from any cause, or occurrence of a second malignant neoplasm (SMN), whichever comes first.

Notice that the definition of EFS includes all possible events that can be considered treatment failures, whether they are related directly to disease recurrence or related indirectly to the side effects of the treatment. Although including non-cancer related events may seem counterintuitive, the alternative will lead to biased comparisons. If one were to compare a "mild" treatment that cures 50 per cent of patients with an "aggressive" treatment that results in toxic death in 16 per cent of patients but cures 60 per cent of the patients who survive the treatment, the latter treatment would look superior if only disease recurrence or progression were counted, but would be nearly identical in terms of EFS, and would overall be inferior when one considers also the toxicity of the treatment.

In some trials, other endpoints can be used. For example, neuroaxis dissemination may be an important endpoint for the study of reduced-dose neuroaxis radiation therapy in non-disseminated medulloblastoma. It is important, however, to analyze these specific endpoints as components of more general, primary endpoints, such as EFS, which reflect overall treatment success.[46]

Randomization and stratification

Randomization is a process by which one of several alternative treatments is assigned to patients independently of influence from the patient, the treating physician, and the study investigators. Clearly, a randomized trial cannot be promoted ethically to a patient who prefers a treatment that is available without study participation, or participated in by a physician who cannot recommend any of the study treatments to the patient with clinical equipoise or substantial uncertainty as to which, if any, of the treatments is better (although there is considerable ongoing debate, beyond the scope of this chapter, on what comprises an acceptable degree of equipoise or uncertainty[47–50]). Given that this hurdle has been surmounted, there are a number of ways to generate randomized treatment assignments.

The simplest method is simple random allocation. For a two-treatment randomized trial, this is equivalent to flipping a coin and assigning "heads" to one treatment and "tails" to another. Today, one would use computer-generated pseudo-random numbers. For example, to randomize between one of three treatments, one could generate a random number between 1 and 999 inclusive, and allocate treatment 1 if number 1–333 occurred, treatment 2 if number 334–666 occurred, and treatment 3 if number 667–999 occurred. In most randomized trials, however, blocked randomization or stratified/blocked randomization is employed. Stratified/blocked randomization guarantees that similar numbers of patients are treated with each treatment, and that important patient characteristics are approximately balanced in all treatment groups. These methods also simplify presentation of data and can increase statistical precision in analysis, although with some increased organizational overhead.[28,51]

There are a number of rules that should be followed in randomization. First, randomization should occur only for patients who can be treated appropriately with any of the possible treatments in the study. Patients who are not eligible in this sense should be screened out before randomization.

Second, treatment assignments are final and irrevocable. For example, if a patient is randomized within the wrong stratum (e.g. in the age under ten years stratum versus the age 11 years or over stratum), there is no option to re-randomize the patient within the "correct" stratum, nor is there any need to make this correction, since stratum mistakes are generally inconsequential to the analysis. Allowing re-randomization opens the process to manipulation that can introduce bias.

Third, in order to assure that the required eligibility screening and unbiased treatment assignment are performed, randomization should be made by a central coordinating office. The practice of distributing envelopes to individual centers or allowing centers to perform their own randomization is unacceptable, since such systems can be manipulated.

Fourth, randomization should occur as closely as possible to the point at which the experimental treatments differ. For treatments that differ early, the randomization can occur at the time of study entry – patients eligible for the randomization are the same as those eligible for the study. However, for treatments that differ late in treatment, the randomization should also occur late in treatment, and hence a separate screening for randomization eligibility should be undertaken.[52]

METHODS FOR SURVIVAL ANALYSIS

The most commonly used methods of analysis of phase III trials in oncology are based on the product limit (Kaplan–Meier) estimate, which is used to estimate the percentage of patients who survive or survive event-free (e.g. five-year OS, three-year EFS, etc.), and the log-rank test and Cox regression analysis, which are used to compare OS and EFS among treatment or prognostic groups.[53,54] These methods account correctly for patient censoring, which is a unique feature of survival data. Censoring occurs because many patients in clinical trials do not experience the treatment failure endpoint during the trial period, either because they have essentially been cured of the disease or because they have not been followed long enough at the time of analysis. As noted above, patients should not be censored in survival analysis for reasons that can possibly be related to the treatment or the disease.

The log-rank test is based on the notion that a treatment that results in a higher long-term OS or EFS exhibits at all times a lower failure (or hazard) rate (i.e. the number of events that occur per unit time). This test is most sensitive to these so-called proportional-hazards (PH) differences. Although there is no biological reason to believe that the PH assumption will hold absolutely, and in fact there are examples where it clearly does not hold,[55,56] in most circumstances the PH assumption provides a reasonable description of the difference in outcome between treatment or prognostic groups.

The quantity that reflects PH differences is the relative failure rate (RFR), which equals one when two treatments result in the same EFS, and equals 0.5 when one treatment results in a failure rate that is half the failure rate of another treatment.

How big should a phase III trial be?

In statistical hypothesis testing, one asks whether the data from a clinical trial provide compelling evidence that the true value of a parameter (in this case, RFR) are different from a hypothesized value. Since one wants to make positive assertions based on the data, the null hypothesis (H_0) usually represents the state of nature that is not of interest, and the alternative hypothesis (H_A) represents that which is of interest. For the log-rank test, the null and alternative hypotheses would be stated as:

$$H_0: RFR = 1 \quad v. \quad H_A: RFR \, 1$$

One first adjusts the test's critical value (the log-rank value above which one would declare a difference) to achieve an acceptable α-error (type I error, false-positive) rate and recruits sufficient numbers of patients to achieve a low β-error (type II error, false-negative) rate for the smallest difference of practical clinical interest. Commonly accepted values are $\alpha = 0.05$ and $\beta = 0.20$; $1 - \beta$ is called the power of the test.

An important feature of the log-rank test is that the effective sample size is not the number of patients that are randomized but rather the average number of treatment failure events that will be observed during the trial. Hence, a trial with 43 patients in each of two treatments, one with long-term EFS of 0.25 and the other with long-term EFS of 0.50, will have about the same power to detect this twofold difference as a study of 185 patients in each of two treatments, where the long-term EFS is 0.81 and 0.90, respectively. Note that even though RFR is 0.5 in both situations, in absolute terms the first study detects a 0.25 difference in long-term EFS (0.50 versus 0.25) whereas the second detects a difference of 0.09 (0.90 versus 0.81). In other words, the same RFR difference between two treatments will correspond to different absolute difference in EFS or OS, depending on the average prognosis of the patients being studied. (An algebraic consequence of the PH assumption is that $EFS_B = EFS_A^{RFR}$, where EFS_B and EFS_A are the EFS percentages for treatments B and A, respectively, and RFR is the relative failure rate in group B compared with group A.)

As a rule of thumb, one has to observe 70 failures in the course of the trial to detect RFR = 0.5 with power of 0.80, using a two-sided 0.05 log-rank test, 100 events to detect RFR = 0.56, 200 events to detect RFR = 0.67, and 350 events to detect RFR = 0.75. A method for computing sample size that is appropriate for pediatric cancer, where it is expected that a non-negligible fraction of patients will be cured of disease, is described by Sposto and Krailo.[57]

A dilemma that sometimes occurs in conducting randomized studies in rare pediatric CNS tumors is that even with large, multi-institutional collaborations, it may be impossible to design a trial that can be accomplished in a reasonable time (e.g. less than ten years) and that is sufficiently large to achieve traditionally small α- and β-errors to detect the smallest difference that is really of clinical interest. In this case, the only available options are (i) to conduct a very large, long, randomized study, the results from which may be irrelevant when they become available; (ii) to conduct a smaller, randomized trial that is well-controlled but has higher-than-traditional error rates; (iii) to conduct a single-treatment, historically controlled study that is somewhat more precise but may be subject to bias; and (iv) to conclude that the proposed study question can never be feasibly answered. There is no uniformly best option to choose, although conducting a smaller, randomized trial is a reasonable approach in some situations.[58]

Intent–to–treat analysis

In randomized clinical trials, there is an accepted convention of intent-to-treat analysis. Although there are several, distinct issues of intent-to-treat, the most important for randomized trials is concerned with how one handles deviations from assigned treatment. Sometimes a patient will agree to be randomized, but after randomization will switch or be switched to another of the available treatments on the study, or the patient or physician may opt for an entirely different treatment, either because of preference or because the treatment cannot be tolerated. The principle of intent-to-treat says that patients who switch or otherwise deviate from the assigned treatment may not be excluded from the randomized trial, and nor should they be censored at the time of deviation from treatment. Rather, they should be included in the primary analysis according to the randomly assigned treatment. This may seem counterintuitive, but there are sound reasons to adhere to this philosophy, since decisions to change treatment are often influenced by factors that also influence prognosis, and excluding such patients potentially renders the randomized groups incomparable.[59] It is best to think of a randomized trial as a comparison of groups of patients treated by different initial intents but who may unavoidably deviate from the intended treatment, rather than thinking of it as a comparison of artificially constructed, "pure" groups of patients who receive only the experimental treatment, when such groups of patients do not exist in practice.

Interim safety monitoring and criteria for early stopping

As in phase I and phase II trials, phase III trials will include scheduled, interim analyses of the data in order to discover early, compelling evidence that one treatment is superior or inferior to the others. Depending on the length of the study and the rapidity with which events are observed, these interim analyses may be scheduled semi-annually, annually, or perhaps at one or two key times during the study. The motivation for performing interim analyses is to avoid the unacceptable situation wherein one discovers at the end of a long, randomized trial that an extremely large benefit for one treatment exists and that this would have been abundantly clear early on in the study. Sophisticated statistical methods have been developed to conduct these analyses in a way that does not compromise the statistical design of the study by inflating the false-positive (α) error rate.[60,61]

Reduction in treatment (equivalence) trials

As treatments for pediatric CNS tumors improve, or as homogeneous subsets of patients with better long-term prognosis are identified, the objectives of randomized trials shift from improving EFS with minimal increase in morbidity to decreasing morbidity with minimal decrease in efficacy. Consider, for example, the treatment of average-risk medulloblastoma.[62,63] These so-called reduction-in-therapy or equivalence trials will include primary endpoints that reflect both efficacy (e.g. EFS) and morbidity (e.g. quality of life, cognitive function). These studies will be designed to protect against clear reductions in efficacy while simultaneously detecting important improvements in long-term morbidity.[64-67]

SOME GENERAL ISSUES IN CLINICAL TRIALS

The study protocol document

All clinical trials should be described in a protocol document, which is a comprehensive description of all aspects of the study. The protocol should describe the objectives of the research, the rationale and background for performing the research, the details of treatment and patient management, guidelines for surgery, radiology, radiation therapy, chemotherapy, pathology, and any other medical disciplines in the study. The protocol should also describe which patients are eligible for the study, the study design, including the number of patients required, the duration of the study, the primary and secondary endpoints, planned statistical analyses, interim safety monitoring rules, the data that are to be collected, and enrollment and randomization procedures. This is by no means a comprehensive list. The protocol document should contain any information that is required by physicians involved in treating or managing patients on the study, or staff involved in coordinating or administering the study, or reviewers charged with scientific, methodological, patient safety, or ethical review of the study. An excellent discussion of the required contents of protocol documents can be found in Piantadosi.[28]

Data acquisition, quality assurance, and security

The data that will be required to analyze and administer a clinical trial should be planned in advance. This will naturally include data to establish eligibility, any other pretreatment data that will be of research interest, and follow-up data that comprise toxicity, details of treatment administration, tumor response, disease recurrence, and follow-up and life status. The amount of detail that is necessary in each of these broad categories depends on whether the primary focus of the study is toxicity (phase I), short-term response (phase II), or long-term outcome (phase III). For any study, the research data collection should be parsimonious. The goal is to include only those data necessary to answer the research questions and to coordinate the study. The goal is not to computerize the medical record.

One should maintain a regular schedule for reviewing and updating the trial data. For small, single-institution studies, a weekly or monthly review of patient charts should be conducted, and the new data entered in the database. For larger, multi-institutional studies, paper forms or computer/web-based data entry mechanisms should be provided by which data can be submitted at will by participating institutions. As part of every review and update cycle, computerized data reports should be produced that identify missing or contradictory data items and delinquencies in follow-up, so that these can be corrected. Ensuring that data are kept accurate and up-to-date is essential, since an important part of the coordination of a clinical trial is the protection of patient safety through periodic monitoring and analysis. Safety monitoring procedures will be ineffective if current, accurate data are not available.

Data from a clinical trial should be backed up routinely and securely. Most large institutions have centrally administered computer networks with sophisticated procedures for backing up network volumes. These institutions also maintain firewalls and anti-virus software to protect the network from external snooping, vandalism, and computer viruses. In this kind of environment, one should avoid storing computerized research data on individual computer workstations, instead making sure that they are stored on network volumes. If a centrally administered computer environment is not available, then procedures for routine back-up, anti-virus protection, and security will have to be provided on the computer or computers where the data are stored.

Guidelines for reporting the results of clinical trials

Careful, thorough, and concise reporting of the results of clinical trials is important in getting the result of the trials accepted and in allowing others to compare the results of the trial with other research and with their own experience. Recently, detailed guidelines for the reporting of randomized clinical trials have been described (the CONSORT statement[68,69]). In addition, an excellent, detailed discussion of reporting of all types of clinical trials is given by Piantadosi.[28]

ETHICAL ISSUES IN THE CONDUCT OF CLINICAL TRIALS

The important difference between clinical trials and other types of experimental science is the involvement of humans, and the resulting requisite care on the part of the investigators to ensure that patients are informed fully of their participation in an experiment and that there are risks as well as possible benefits that derive from their participation.

Declaration of Helsinki

Virtually all countries that perform clinical trials adhere to the Declaration of Helsinki, the international agreement that outlines ethical principles in the conduct of medical research.[49,70] This agreement reaffirms the duty of physicians to safeguard the welfare of patients, and to participate only in research that is scientifically sound, sufficiently important that benefits to society can outweigh risks to subjects, conducted with the full knowledge and voluntary participation of the subjects, and reviewed independently for adherence to accepted ethical and safety conventions. The most recent version of the Declaration of Helsinki includes revisions designed to address the issue of randomized trials conducted in developing nations, and adds a statement that the results of the medical research must have a reasonable likelihood of benefiting the population in which the research was conducted.[70]

Institutional review board or research ethics committee

Study protocols should be reviewed by special ethical review committees that are independent of the investigators or sponsors of the research. The composition of these committees will differ, depending on the laws and regulations of the country where the research is performed. The charge of this committee is to ensure that the research adheres to accepted ethical and patient safety practices. Most major institutions participating in clinical research have a standing research ethics committee that reviews all research conducted at the institutions, regardless of whether the institution has originated the research or is simply participating in it.

Informed consent

All patients should be aware that they will be participating in scientific research, that there may be risks as well as benefits to participating in this research, and that they can decline to participate in the research or withdraw from participation in the research at any time without compromising the care that they will receive. These rights should be explained to patients and their parents or responsible carers in person, either by the treating physician or another member of the medical team who is familiar with the research. In addition, the parents (or responsible carers) and patients should be provided with an "informed consent" document that describes in detail, but in understandable language, the risks and benefits of participating in the research, and their rights and expectations as patients. An informed consent document should be signed by the patient or the patient's guardian *before* enrollment into the study and *before* the start of any part of the treatment that can be considered experimental.[71]

Patient confidentiality

Patient confidentiality with respect to the data collected in clinical trials must be maintained as stringently (or more so) as would be the case for patients' medical records. Since clinical trials data will be reviewed and analyzed by non-medical personnel (e.g. statisticians, study coordinators) who are not primarily responsible for the patient's care, the research charts should be available only to those people who need to see them. In addition, the computerized research data should be stored without patient names, instead being identified with a unique patient-identification number. There will be a need to link this at times to the patient's name, but the correspondence between the identifier and the named patient should be kept in a separate, secure computer file with restricted access.

Data and safety monitoring board

In randomized, phase III clinical trials, it is an accepted practice that a data and safety monitoring board (DSMB) or data monitoring committee (DMC) be constituted.[72–74] The rationale for these committees is that investigators who are involved directly in the trial are probably not in the best position to evaluate impartially the accumulating evidence about whether treatments differ, and to weigh this information against the risks and benefits to future patients of continuing the trial. The membership of the DSMB should include, at least, several physicians who are expert in research in the treatment of CNS tumors, and a non-affiliated biostatistician; the board may also include an expert on ethics and a lay patient advocate. The DSMB will usually meet every six months or yearly, depending on the study and the details of the interim statistical monitoring. The board will be provided with a detailed report of treatment toxicities and other side effects, deaths, and treatment failures that have occurred, and a formal interim statistical analysis of the result to date. These will be provided in a report produced by the study biostatistician. They will also include a discussion of problems with occurrence and management of toxicities provided by the physician coordinator of the study. In most instances, the physician coordinator will be blinded to any of the interim statistical analysis. It should be said that there is no uniform agreement about the need for an independent monitoring committee.[75]

MULTIDISCIPLINARY COLLABORATION IN THE DESIGN OF CLINICAL TRIALS

As this chapter has highlighted, there are many important aspects of clinical trials that can affect the ability of the trial to answer the scientific question that is being posed. It is important, therefore, that the design of clinical trials be developed with close collaboration between representatives of all medical (e.g. surgery, pathology, radiology) and non-medical (e.g. biostatistics, pharmacy, nursing) disciplines that will be instrumental to the conduct of the trial, care of patients enrolled on the trial, and the analysis and publication of results. Multidisciplinary collaboration ensures that studies address well-defined hypotheses and objectives, that endpoints for achieving these objectives are defined clearly, that the data necessary to evaluate the objectives will be collected, that patients are treated and managed according to the treatment as described in the protocol, that the study design is efficient, that statistical analyses provide a clear answer, and that statistically valid patient safety monitoring rules are in place.

REFERENCES

1 Pocock SJ. *Clinical Trials: A Practical Approach*. New York: John Wiley and Sons, 1983.

2 Smith M, Bernstein M, Bleyer WA, *et al.* Conduct of phase I trials in children with cancer. *J Clin Oncol* 1998; **16**:966–78.

3   Simon R, Freidlin B, Rubinstein L, Arbuck SG, Collins J, Christian MC. Accelerated titration designs for phase I clinical trials in oncology. *J Natl Cancer Inst* 1997; **89**:1138–47.

4   Christian MC, Korn EL. The limited precision of phase I trials. *J Natl Cancer Inst* 1994; **86**:1662–3.

5   Arbuck SG. Workshop on phase I study design. Ninth NCI/EORTC New Drug Development Symposium, Amsterdam, March 12, 1996. *Ann Oncol* 1996; **7**:567–73.

6   Korn EL, Midthune D, Chen TT, Rubinstein LV, Christian MC, Simon RM. A comparison of two phase I trial designs. *Stat Med* 1994; **13**:1799–806.

7   Mick R, Ratain MJ. Model-guided determination of maximum tolerated dose in Phase I clinical trials: evidence for increased precision. *J Natl Cancer Inst* 1993; **85**:217–23.

8   Ratain MJ, Mick R, Schilsky RL, Siegler M. Statistical and ethical issues in the design and conduct of phase I and II clinical trials of new anticancer agents. *J Natl Cancer Inst* 1993; **85**:1637–43.

9   Storer BE. Design and analysis of phase I clinical trials. *Biometrics* 1989; **45**:925–37.

10 Miller S. An extension of the continual reassessment methods using a preliminary up-and-down design in a dose finding study in cancer patients, in order to investigate a greater range of doses. *Stat Med* 1995; **14**:911–22, 923.

11 O'Quigley J, Pepe M, Fisher L. Continual reassessment method: a practical design for phase 1 clinical trials in cancer. *Biometrics* 1990; **46**:33–48.

12 O'Quigley J, Chevret S. Methods for dose finding studies in cancer clinical trials: a review and results of a Monte Carlo study. *Stat Med* 1991; **10**:1647–64.

13 Goodman SN, Zahurak ML, Piantadosi S. Some practical improvements in the continual reassessment method for phase I studies. *Stat Med* 1995; **14**:1149–61.

14 Chevret S. The continual reassessment method in cancer phase I clinical trials: a simulation study. *Stat Med* 1993; **12**:1093–108.

15 Piantadosi S, Fisher JD, Grossman S. Practical implementation of a modified continual reassessment method for dose-finding trials. *Cancer Chemother Pharmacol* 1998; **41**:429–36.

16 Rinaldi DA, Burris HA, Dorr FA, *et al*. Initial phase I evaluation of the novel thymidylate synthase inhibitor, LY231514, using the modified continual reassessment method for dose escalation. *J Clin Oncol* 1995; **13**:2842–50.

17 Ahn C. An evaluation of phase I cancer clinical trial designs. *Stat Med* 1998; **17**:1537–49.

18 Gianni L, Vigano L, Surbone A, *et al*. Pharmacology and clinical toxicity of 4′-iodo-4′-deoxydoxorubicin: an example of successful application of pharmacokinetics to dose escalation in phase I trials. *J Natl Cancer Inst* 1990; **82**:469–77.

19 Collins JM, Grieshaber CK, Chabner BA. Pharmacologically guided phase I clinical trials based upon preclinical drug development. *J Natl Cancer Inst* 1990; **82**:1321–6.

20 Berlin J, Stewart JA, Storer B, *et al*. Phase I clinical and pharmacokinetic trial of penclomedine using a novel, two-stage trial design for patients with advanced malignancy. *J Clin Oncol* 1998; **16**:1142–9.

21 Chang MN, Therneau TM, Wieand HS, Cha SS. Designs for group sequential phase II clinical trials. *Biometrics* 1987; **43**:865–74.

22 Simon R. Optimal two-stage designs for phase II clinical trials. *Control Clin Trials* 1989; **10**:1–10.

23 Therasse P, Arbuck SG, Eisenhauer EA, *et al*. New guidelines to evaluate the response to treatment in solid tumors. European Organization for Research and Treatment of Cancer, National Cancer Institute of the United States, National Cancer Institute of Canada. *J Natl Cancer Inst* 2000; **92**:205–16.

24 James K, Eisenhauer E, Christian M, *et al*. Measuring response in solid tumors: unidimensional versus bidimensional measurement. *J Natl Cancer Inst* 1999; **91**:523–8.

25 Hilsenbeck SG, Von Hoff DD. Measure once or twice – does it really matter? *J Natl Cancer Inst* 1999; **91**:494–5.

26 Gehan EA, Tefft MC. Will there be resistance to the RECIST (Response Evaluation Criteria in Solid Tumors)? *J Natl Cancer Inst* 2000; **92**:179–81.

27 Dixon WJ, Massey FJ. *Introduction to Statistical Analysis*, 3rd edn. New York: McGraw-Hill, 1969.

28 Piantadosi S. *Clinical Trials: A Methodologic Perspective*. New York: John Wiley & Sons, 1997.

29 Mick R, Crowley JJ, Carroll RJ. Phase II clinical trial design for noncytotoxic anticancer agents for which time to disease progression is the primary endpoint. *Control Clin Trials* 2000; **21**:343–59.

30 Korn EL, Arbuck SG, Pluda JM, Simon R, Kaplan RS, Christian MC. Clinical trial designs for cytostatic agents: are new approaches needed? *J Clin Oncol* 2001; **19**:265–72.

31 Whitehead J. Designing phase II studies in the context of a programme of clinical research. *Biometrics* 1985; **41**: 373–83.

32 Simon R, Wittes RE, Ellenberg SS. Randomized phase II clinical trials. *Cancer Treat Rep* 1985; **69**:1375–81.

33 Strauss N, Simon R. Investigating a sequence of randomized Phase II trials to discover promising treatments. *Stat Med* 1995; **14**:1479–89.

34 Thall PF, Estey EH. A Bayesian strategy for screening cancer treatments prior to phase II clinical evaluation. *Stat Med* 1993; **12**:1197–211.

35 Thall PF, Russell KE. A strategy for dose-finding and safety monitoring based on efficacy and adverse outcomes in phase I/II clinical trials. *Biometrics* 1998; **54**:251–64.

36 Blaney SM, Needle MN, Gillespie A, *et al*. Phase II trial of topotecan administered as 72-hour continuous infusion in children with refractory solid tumors: a collaborative Pediatric Branch, National Cancer Institute, and Children's Cancer Group Study. *Clin Cancer Res* 1998; **4**:357–60.

37 Conaway MR, Petroni GR. Bivariate sequential designs for phase II trials. *Biometrics* 1995; **51**:656–64.

38 Conaway MR, Petroni GR. Designs for phase II trials allowing for a trade-off between response and toxicity. *Biometrics* 1996; **52**:1375–86.

39 Pocock SJ, Elbourne DR. Randomized trials or observational tribulations? *N Engl J Med* 2000; **342**:1907–1909.

40 Concato J, Shah N, Horwitz RI. Randomized, controlled trials, observational studies, and the hierarchy of research designs. *N Engl J Med* 2000; **342**:1887–92.

41 Benson K and Hartz AJ. A comparison of observational studies and randomized, controlled trials. *N Engl J Med* 2000; **342**:1878–86.

42 Mandell LR, Kadota R, Freeman C, *et al*. There is no role for hyperfractionated radiotherapy in the management of children with newly diagnosed diffuse intrinsic brainstem tumors: results of a Pediatric Oncology Group phase III trial comparing

conventional vs. hyperfractionated radiotherapy. *Int J Radiat Oncol Biol Phys* 1999; **43**:959–64.

43 Finlay JL, Boyett JM, Yates AJ, *et al.* Randomized phase III trial in childhood high-grade astrocytoma comparing vincristine, lomustine, and prednisone with the eight-drugs-in-1-day regimen. Childrens Cancer Group. *J Clin Oncol* 1995; **13**:112–23.

44 Emanuel EJ, Patterson WB. Ethics of randomized clinical trials. *J Clin Oncol* 1998; **16**:365–6, 366–71.

45 George SL. Reducing patient eligibility criteria in cancer clinical trials. *J Clin Oncol* 1996; **14**:1364–70.

46 Prentice RL, Kalbfleisch JD, Peterson AV, Jr, Flournoy N, Farewell VT, Breslow NE. The analysis of failure times in the presence of competing risks. *Biometrics* 1978; **34**:541–54.

47 Sackett DL. Uncertainty about clinical equipoise. There is another exchange on equipoise and uncertainty. *Br Med J* 2001; **322**:795–6.

48 Lilford RJ. Uncertainty about clinical equipoise. Clinical equipoise and the uncertainty principles both require further scrutiny. *Br Med J* 2001; **322**:795.

49 Lilford RJ, Djulbegovic B. Declaration of Helsinki should be strengthened. Equipoise is essential principle of human experimentation. *Br Med J* 2001; **322**:299–300.

50 Weijer C, Shapiro SH, Cranley Glass K. For and against: clinical equipoise and not the uncertainty principle is the moral underpinning of the randomised controlled trial. *Br Med J* 2000; **321**:756–8.

51 Peto R, Pike MC, Armitage P, *et al.* Design and analysis of randomized clinical trials requiring prolonged observation of each patient. I. Introduction and design. *Br J Cancer* 1976; **34**:585–612.

52 Durrleman S, Simon R. When to randomize? *J Clin Oncol* 1991: **9**:116–22.

53 Kalbfleisch J, Prentice R. *The Statistical Analysis of Failure Time Data*. New York: John Wiley and Sons, 1980.

54 Peto R, Pike MC, Armitage P, *et al.* Design and analysis of randomized clinical trials requiring prolonged observation of each patient. II. analysis and examples. *Br J Cancer* 1977; **35**:1–39.

55 Matthay KK, Villablanca JG, Seeger RC, *et al.* Improved outcome for high risk neuroblastoma with high dose therapy and purged autologous bone marrow transplantation and with subsequent 13-cis-retinoic acid. *N Engl J Med* 1999; **341**:1165–73.

56 Nesbit ME, Buckley JD, Feig SA, *et al.* Chemotherapy for induction of remission of childhood acute myeloid leukemia followed by marrow transplantation or multiagent chemotherapy: a report from the Children's Cancer Group. *J Clin Oncol* 1994; **12**:127–35.

57 Sposto R, Sather HN. Determining the duration of comparative clinical trials while allowing for cure. *J Chronic Dis* 1985; **38**:683–90.

58 Sposto R, Stram DO. A strategic view of randomized trial design in low-incidence cancer. *Stat Med* 1999; **18**:1183–97.

59 Lee YJ, Ellenberg JH, Hirtz DG, Nelson KB. Analysis of clinical trials by treatment actually received: is it really an option? *Stat Med* 1991; **10**:1595–605.

60 Lan KK, Rosenberger WF, Lachin JM. Use of spending functions for occasional or continuous monitoring of data in clinical trials. *Stat Med* 1993; **12**:2219–31.

61 Betensky RA. Conditional power calculations for early acceptance of H0 embedded in sequential tests. *Stat Med* 1997; **16**:465–77.

62 Packer RJ, Goldwein J, Nicholson HS, *et al.* Treatment of children with medulloblastomas with reduced-dose craniospinal radiation therapy and adjuvant chemotherapy: a Children's Cancer Group Study. *J Clin Oncol* 1999; **17**:2127–36.

63 Bailey CC, Gnekow A, Wellek S, *et al.* Prospective randomised trial of chemotherapy given before radiotherapy in childhood medulloblastoma. International Society of Paediatric Oncology (SIOP) and the (German) Society of Paediatric Oncology (GPO): SIOP II. *Med Pediatr Oncol* 1995; **25**:166–78.

64 Durrleman S, Simon R. Planning and monitoring of equivalence studies. *Biometrics* 1990; **46**:329–36.

65 Fleming TR. Design and interpretation of equivalence trials. *Am Heart J* 2000; **139**:S171–6.

66 Com-Nougue C, Rodary C, Patte C. How to establish equivalence when data are censored: a randomized trial of treatments for B non-Hodgkin's lymphoma. *Stat Med* 1993; **12**:1353–64.

67 Whitehead J. Sequential designs for equivalence studies. *Stat Med* 1996; **15**:2703–15.

68 Altman DG, Begg C, Cho M, *et al.* Better reporting of randomised controlled trials: the CONSORT statement. *Br Med J* 1996; **313**:570–1.

69 Begg C, Cho M, Eastwood S, *et al.* Improving the quality of reporting of randomized controlled trials. The CONSORT statement. *J Am Med Assoc* 1996; **276**:637–9.

70 Reynolds T. Declaration of Helsinki revised. *J Natl Cancer Inst* 2000; **92**:1801–3.

71 Grossman SA, Piantadosi S, Covahey C. Are informed consent forms that describe clinical oncology research protocols readable by most patients and their families? *J Clin Oncol* 1994; **12**:2211–15.

72 Wittes J. Behind closed doors: the data monitoring board in randomized clinical trials. *Stat Med* 1993; **12**:419–24.

73 Whitehead J. On being the statistician on a Data and Safety Monitoring Board. *Stat Med* 1999; **18**:3425–34.

74 DeMets DL, Pocock SJ, Julian DG. The agonising negative trend in monitoring of clinical trials. *Lancet* 1999; **354**:1983–8.

75 Harrington D, Crowley J, George SL, Pajak T, Redmond C, Wieand S. The case against independent monitoring committees. *Stat Med* 1994; **13**:1411–14.

Treatment techniques and neurotoxicities

9

Neurosurgical techniques

PAUL D. CHUMAS AND ATUL TYAGI

INTRODUCTION

Neurosurgery has changed more than most other surgical specialties over the past 30 years. The most fundamental change has been in the availability of new diagnostic techniques, with the advent of computed tomography (CT) scanning in the 1970s and of magnetic resonance imaging (MRI) in the 1980s. For the first time, the brain and spinal cord could be visualized directly. More recently, functional imaging with positron-emission tomography (PET), single-photon-emission computed tomography (SPECT), magnetic resonance spectroscopy (MRS), and functional magnetic resonance imaging (fMRI) have allowed direct examination of brain metabolism.

The use of the operating microscope has been another significant step, giving the surgeon both illumination and magnification. Other important improvements in instrumentation include safe forms of rigid fixation of the head, self-retaining retractor systems, dissecting instruments, high-speed drills and craniotomes, and the ultrasonic aspirator. The latter device is of especial importance in the removal of tumors; it works by fragmenting the tumor ultrasonically and then removing the tumor by aspiration. Obviously, accurate localization of the tumor is paramount. With large tumors and tumors near specific internal landmarks, assistance may not be required. However, for small tumors and tumors in eloquent areas, a stereotactic system may be necessary. These systems integrate fixed external landmarks with the imaging (CT or MRI) and are highly accurate. In the past few years, attempts have

been made to combine all these advances by giving the surgeon real-time imaging by operating within the MRI environment. The various forms of stereotactic surgery will be discussed in more detail later in this chapter.

It is important to recognize the role that anesthesia has had in making neurosurgery safer. A better understanding of the pathophysiology of raised intracranial pressure and how best to counter this has been aided by various monitoring techniques and by various new anaesthetic agents. The anesthetist's task is often made more difficult by the position in which the surgeon places the patient (e.g. the sitting position, with the attendant risk of air embolism and the problems of venous stasis, or the "park-bench" or lateral position, with concerns about pressure sores and brachial plexus injury).

The care offered by the neuroanesthetist does not stop in the operating suite but continues in the intensive-care and high-dependency units. This allows for further careful neurological monitoring of the patient, with particular emphasis on detecting postoperative complications (e.g. intracranial hematoma or the development of hydrocephalus and the control of seizures). Blood loss is of particular importance in small children. Fluid balance in general needs careful monitoring, as patients are susceptible to diabetes insipidus, inappropriate antidiuretic hormone (ADH) secretion, and cerebral salt wasting.

Anesthetic techniques are not limited purely to general anesthesia. Perhaps the most challenging (for patient and anesthetist alike) is the awake craniotomy. This technique allows eloquent areas (speech, motor cortex, etc.)

to be mapped and hence avoided. The child must be old enough to cooperate. The method consists of initially administering a general anesthetic (using a laryngeal rather than an endotracheal tube), during which time the craniotomy is performed. The child is then allowed to wake up, so that eloquent areas may be mapped before putting the child back to sleep for the remainder of the procedure.

Pediatric neurosurgery is a relatively new field and is still not recognized as a subspecialty in many countries. More than most areas of neurosurgery, pediatric neurosurgery relies on a multidisciplinary team approach. This includes both medical (neuroradiologists, neuro-oncologists, neurologists, radiotherapists, endocrinologists) and non-medical (nurses, physiotherapists, occupational therapists, speech therapists, social workers, health visitors, psychologists, school teachers) staff. While the management strategy at the initial presentation is often fairly straightforward, the treatment of recurrent or residual disease requires far more discussion. In particular, the role of second-look surgery needs to be defined more clearly. Certainly, chemotherapy and/or radiotherapy can alter the residual tumor (e.g. secreting germ-cell tumors can be left as mature dermoid tumors) and salvage an inoperable case (e.g. decrease the vascularity of a choroid-plexus carcinoma).

Depending on the site of the tumor, it is not infrequent for combined procedures to be undertaken with other surgical disciplines. This is particularly the case with skull-base tumors, where ear/nose/throat (ENT), maxillofacial, and plastic surgery may all be involved. Likewise, combined procedures with orthopedic surgeons may be necessary when rigid spinal fixation or instrumentation is required. Conversely, neurosurgery may offer access to the orbit via the cranium for ophthalmic surgeons.

This chapter aims to give an overview of the most common surgical approaches used to reach pediatric brain tumors. As the majority of patients present initially with hydrocephalus, it seems appropriate to start with the management of this condition before discussing the surgical techniques used to remove the tumor itself.

TREATMENT OF HYDROCEPHALUS

Raised intracranial pressure is by far the most common presentation for children with brain tumors. This is usually secondary to hydrocephalus rather than a primary effect of the size of the tumor itself. The majority of pediatric tumors occur in the midline and obstruct the fourth ventricle, the aqueduct of Sylvius, or the third ventricle. This type of hydrocephalus is therefore termed "obstructive." In contrast, blood or infection in the cerebrospinal fluid (CSF) pathways can interfere with the absorption of the CSF; this type of hydrocephalus is termed "communicating."

Before the advent of modern imaging, it was not uncommon for children to present late with a long history of headache and vomiting and to be dehydrated on admission. When shunts became available in the 1950s, it became routine practice to treat the hydrocephalus with a shunt before tumor surgery. This practice is no longer necessary as, in general, tumors are diagnosed much earlier and the child is therefore usually in a better clinical state. Overall, only about one-third of posterior fossa tumors now require a permanent shunt, almost always receiving this at some point in the postoperative period.

Modern management consists of commencing the child on steroids and early surgery. At the time of tumor surgery, many surgeons will either place an external ventricular drain (a silastic catheter passing through the brain into the lateral ventricle) or place a burr hole, so that if there is an urgent requirement in the postoperative period to drain CSF, access is available. Occasionally, children still present with marked hydrocephalus and are drowsy and require external ventricular drain (EVD) before tumor surgery. The main risk associated with EVD insertion is infection. By ten days, virtually all EVDs will have been colonized. The other risk (albeit very rare) of treating the hydrocephalus before removal of a posterior fossa tumor is that of upward herniation.

Shunts

A shunt usually consists of a ventricular catheter connected to a valve and reservoir, which allows CSF to be tapped through the skin. On to this is attached a catheter, which is tunneled subcutaneously to a distal site. Although most cavities in the body have been tried, the abdomen, the atrium, and the pleura are used most widely. Atrial shunts were commonplace in the 1960s and 1970s, but problems with endocarditis and glomerulonephritis have resulted in the abdominal cavity becoming the site of preference.

Before the advent of shunts in the 1950s, hydrocephalus was frequently fatal. While shunts were therefore considered a huge advance, it quickly became apparent that shunts had problems of their own. In particularly, virtually all studies to date have shown that approximately 40 per cent of shunts will malfunction within the first year of implantation[1–3] and that the exponential decline in shunt function then continues at approximately five per cent per year (Figure 9.1). This malfunction may be the result of one of the following:

- *Mechanical failure*: complete, partial, or intermittent obstruction, fracture, migration, or disconnection of the shunt system. Obstruction is the cause of 50 per cent of primary shunt malfunctions, and the vast majority of these are blockages of the ventricular catheter.[1]

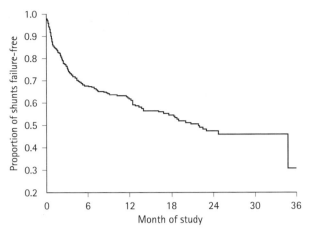

Figure 9.1 *Kaplan–Meier curve, showing the proportion of shunts that are failure-free. (From Drake JM, Kestle JRW, Milner R, et al. Randomized trial of cerebrospinal fluid shunt valve design in pediatric hydrocephalus.* Neurosurgery *1998; **43**:294–305.)*

- *Functional failure*: most commonly overdrainage, causing symptoms of low-pressure headaches, slit-ventricle syndrome, and subdural hematomas.
- *Infection*: the most common infecting organisms are *Staphylococcus epidermidis* (40 per cent) and *Staphylococcus aureus* (20 per cent).

Although some single-institution studies have quoted infection rates of less than one per cent, the generally accepted rate is of the order of ten per cent (with far higher figures being seen in the neonatal period).[2,3] Furthermore, concurrent surgical procedures and hydrocephalus secondary to obstruction of the CSF pathways by tumor have been shown to be independent risk factors for shunt failure.[4] It is not, therefore, surprising that much time and research have been invested in trying to improve shunt function (flow-regulated valves, anti-siphon devices, programmable valves). However, the fundamental problem is how to design a shunt that functions adequately in the horizontal position but that does not then overdrain (due to siphoning) in the vertical position. Despite the advertising propaganda pedaled by shunt manufacturers, there is no evidence to suggest that any one shunt is superior.[3]

Third ventriculostomy

With obstructive hydrocephalus, it is assumed that the CSF absorption pathways are normal. This means that it should be theoretically possible to internally bypass the obstruction and relieve the hydrocephalus. The operation of third ventriculostomy consists of making a hole in the floor of the third ventricle, thus allowing the CSF to pass into the prepontine cistern and hence avoiding any distal obstruction (i.e. posterior thalamic, pineal region, posterior fossa). Although this technique has come into favor only

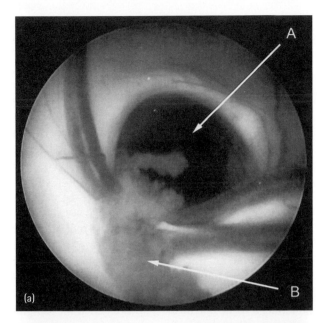

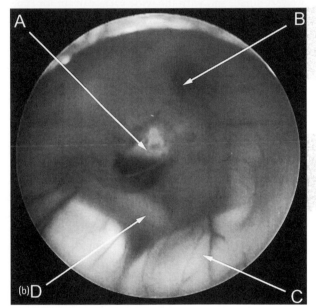

Figure 9.2a,b *(a) Endoscopic view of the foramen of Monroe (A); the choroid plexus (B) is seen passing into the third ventricle. (b) The floor of the third ventricle is shown with the hole (A) into the prepontine system. The landmarks are also clearly visible: the infundibular recess (B), the right mammillary body (C), and the basilar artery (D). Note the thinness of the floor of the ventricle.*

in recent years, it was first described in the 1920s by Walter Dandy, and the first endoscopic procedure was undertaken by Mixter in 1922.[1,2] The resurgence in third ventriculostomy can be put down to a combination of improved instrumentation (in particular, the optics) and an attempt to avoid the complications associated with shunting.

Endoscopic third ventriculostomy consists of placing a burr hole just anterior to the coronal suture, passage of the endoscope through the brain into the lateral ventricle, and navigation through the foramen of Monroe into the third ventricle (Figure 9.2). Once in the third ventricle, the landmarks are the mammillary bodies posteriorly and the infundibular recess (a small red dot) anteriorly. Usually, the floor of the third ventricle in patients with triventricular hydrocephalus is very thin. A small hole is made in the floor of the third ventricle anterior to the mammillary bodies and just in front of the basilar artery (which bifurcates just beneath the floor of the third ventricle).

The success rate for endoscopic third ventriculostomy in patients with tumoral obstructive hydrocephalus is reported to be of the order of 70 per cent.[2] The majority of failures occur in the first few weeks, but delayed failures have been reported. Perhaps the clearest indication for third ventriculostomy is in those patients with pineal region tumors. In this scenario, the endoscopic third ventriculostomy fulfils many functions, allowing the CSF to be sampled, treating the hydrocephalus, and possibly obtaining a tissue diagnosis. (However, often the samples are very small, and with the wide variety of tumor types found in this region, diagnosis may be difficult.)

While endoscopic third ventriculostomy is esthetically pleasing to surgeon and patient alike, it is inherently more dangerous than shunt insertion (with particular risk to vascular structures). Perhaps the most important issue to stress (irrespective of the type of treatment the patient has received) is the need to have a low threshold to immediately reinvestigate any patient with hydrocephalus and who presents with symptoms suggestive of raised intracranial pressure. A CT scan should be performed and the neurosurgical team informed as soon as possible. Unfortunately, avoidable deaths due to undiagnosed shunt malfunction or failure of third ventriculostomy occur each year. It can be difficult to differentiate the symptoms of a shunt malfunction from the drowsiness and vomiting associated with the hydration required with high-dose chemotherapy or with the somnolence seen after radiotherapy. Nonetheless, it is better to err on the side of caution and arrange a scan to determine the cause of the patient's symptoms rather than miss the diagnosis of acute hydrocephalus.

Third ventriculostomy is not the only role for neuroendoscopy. Traditionally, patients with obstruction around the foramen of Monroe (e.g. due to a craniopharyngioma) have been treated by insertion of bilateral shunts. With an endoscope, it is possible to make a hole through the interventricular septum and thus communicate the two lateral ventricles and then insert a single shunt. Endoscopy can also be utilized to biopsy tumors located within the ventricular system.

Finally, the role of intrathecal drug administration must be discussed. Most commonly, this consists of inserting an access device in the frontal region so that intrathecal chemotherapy may be administered (e.g. in patients with central nervous system (CNS) involvement with leukemia). An access device consists of a subcutaneous silastic dome connected to a ventricular catheter. It is then possible, using a sterile technique, to place a needle through the skin and into the dome and thus connect directly into the ventricular system. Other methods of drug delivery have been developed for the administration of morphine and baclofen (to decrease spasticity). These consist of motorized pumps that are placed into the subcutaneous tissue of the abdominal wall. A tube leads from the pump, passes around the flank, and is then inserted into the lumbar theca. It is possible that these continuous infusion systems will become important aids for the delivery of chemo- and immunotherapies over the next few years.

TECHNIQUES FOR TUMOR BIOPSY

Certain tumors are extremely responsive to adjuvant therapy, and once a histological diagnosis is made definitive treatment with chemotherapy or radiotherapy can be started without the need for surgical debulking. Likewise, with tumors in eloquent areas, surgical resection might not be feasible but histological diagnosis may still be required. Tissue for histology short of an open operation can be obtained by the following means.

Stereotactic biopsy

This is carried out using a rigid frame screwed firmly into the skull. The patient is then imaged using either CT or MRI, and the *xyz* coordinates of the tumor are obtained. A biopsy is then performed by passing a needle through an appropriately sited burr hole. A histological diagnosis can almost always be achieved by this technique, and biopsies have been obtained of tumors in virtually all locations. In pediatric oncological practice, the indications for stereotactic biopsy are mainly for diencephalic, cerebral hemispheric, and pineal tumors. While stereotactic biopsies can be done relatively safely in the diencephalic and hemispheric location, hemorrhage is the main potential problem with pineal tumors, as they are surrounded by the deep venous system. A further problem with pineal region tumors is that associated with sampling errors. However, two large series looking at stereotactic biopsy of pineal region tumors have shown this technique to be safe and accurate.[5,6]

Neuronavigation

In effect this is "frameless" stereotaxy. This technology aims to use the detail of neuroimaging to help direct the surgeon during the operation. This neuronavigation relies on infrared cameras to track the patient's head and to track surgical instruments with light-emitting diodes (LEDs) attached and to relay this information to a workstation on

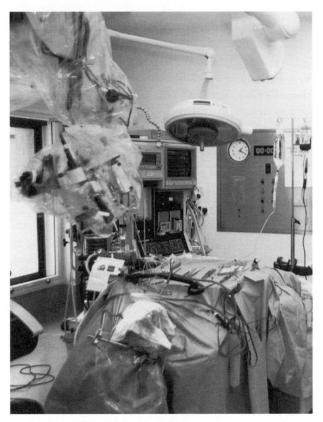

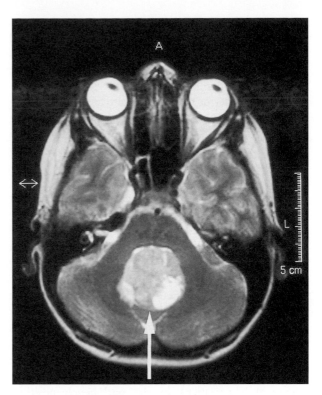

Figure 9.4 *Midline suboccipital craniotomy for midline posterior fossa lesions.*

Figure 9.3 *Neuronavigational system, with infrared cameras and a computer terminal. This figure also shows the limited access to the patient that the anesthetist has once the patient has been draped.*

which the preoperative imaging studies are held (Figure 9.3). Thus, as the surgeon brings an instrument into the operative field, the appropriate slice on the CT or MRI scan is displayed on the computer terminal. Most of the systems available have a biopsy program, but although they are very accurate they do not have the degree of accuracy associated with a rigid frame. However, the fact that the imaging data can be collected before surgery is obviously very important with children. The placement of a rigid frame in children usually requires a general anesthetic.

Endoscopy

With tumors that are visible within the ventricular system, tumor tissue can be obtained via an endoscope. The biopsy can be combined with a third ventriculostomy for the treatment of hydrocephalus.[7] The tumor specimen obtained using this technique is generally small, and expert neuropathological support is necessary. Another problem with endoscopic biopsy is bleeding, which may obscure vision.

The ability to sample CSF (for markers and cytology), treat the hydrocephalus, and biopsy the tumor under direct vision makes endoscopy the favored option in the management of pineal tumors when only a tissue diagnosis is planned.

Surgical resection of tumors in most locations intracranially can be carried out thanks largely to the advances outlined above. However, the actual approach used will vary according to the location and the tumor type. The following section describes the common operative approaches used in dealing with pediatric brain and spinal tumors.

POSTERIOR FOSSA

The posterior fossa is the most common site for both malignant and low-grade tumors in children. Most of these tumors are midline and are best approached suboccipitally via a midline incision (Figure 9.4). The patient may be placed prone (the most commonly used position), in the "Concorde position," or in the sitting position. The advantages of the sitting position include the fact that there is no pooling of blood and that it gives a good view to tumors that extend high up towards the tentorium. The disadvantages of this position include the risks of air embolism and the fact that the surgeon is left in an uncomfortable position with their hands outstretched. By monitoring cardiac Doppler and end tidal carbon dioxide, it is possible to detect the consequences of air embolism early and to take steps to seal the source of the embolism.

The degree of tonsillar herniation and the inferior extent of the tumor will determine the number of cervical laminae that are exposed. As mentioned earlier, many surgeons place an occipital burr hole and insert an external ventricular drain as the initial step in the operation. The actual bone removal can be undertaken piecemeal (craniectomy) or, more commonly, en bloc (craniotomy). With the latter approach, the bone is replaced at the end of the procedure. Most posterior fossa tumors are located within the fourth ventricle, and the approach consists of dividing the vermis to expose the tumor. Although the mechanism is not understood, it is generally accepted that the cerebellar mutism seen occasionally after posterior fossa surgery is related to the splitting of the vermis.

Although the surgeon will usually claim a "watertight closure" of the dura in the operation notes, CSF leakage and pseudomeningocele formation (collection of CSF under the skin) are relatively common. This is an indication of ongoing abnormal CSF dynamics, which may take many days or even weeks to settle. A mixture of suturing, pressure bandages, and lumbar puncture/lumbar drain insertion are usually sufficient to tide the patient over until a new equilibrium between CSF production and absorption is reached.

Laterally placed tumors, in particular cerebellar pontine angle (CPA) tumors, are best approached directly (Figure 9.5), with the patient in the park-bench position. The patient is placed on their side with a sandbag under the axilla to avoid brachial plexus injury, and with the

dependant arm either hanging in a sling or strapped across the chest. The incision is placed just medial to the mastoid process and continues down into the neck. The main risks of this approach include damage to the vertebral artery, problems with CSF rhinorrhea if entry into the air cells is not dealt with, and damage to the lower cranial nerves that run through the CPA.

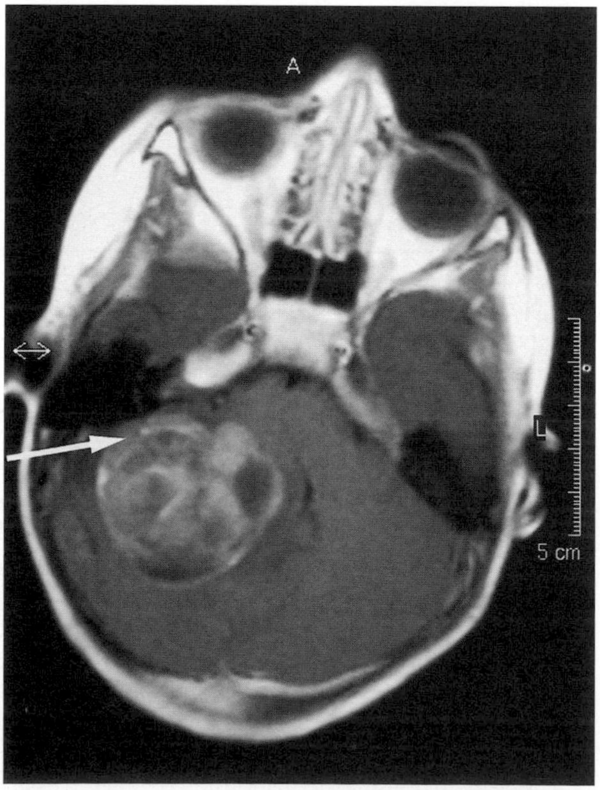

PINEAL REGION

The role of endoscopy in pineal region tumors has been stressed, as has the possibility of stereotactic biopsy. An alternative strategy is to perform an open biopsy with the option of proceeding to definitive surgery depending on the results of the intraoperative pathological assessment. Open operation may also be indicated following adjuvant therapy as a second-look procedure to resect residual tumor. The two main approaches to a tumor in this location are the supracerebellar and the occipital transtentorial.

Supracerebellar infratentorial approach

The tumor is approached through a midline posterior fossa craniotomy (Figure 9.6).[8] The route taken is between the superior aspect of the cerebellum and the tentorium. This approach is useful for essentially midline pineal region tumors. The tumor is resected from between the deep veins,

Figure 9.5 *Lateral (retro sigmoid) approach to cerebellopontine region tumors.*

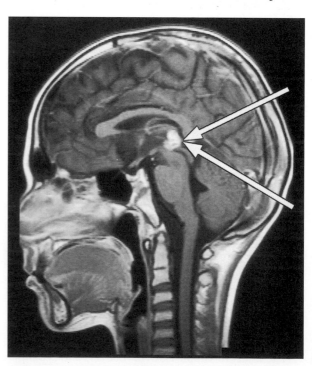

Figure 9.6 *Approaches to the pineal region. The upper arrow shows the route taken in the occipital transtentorial approach. The lower arrow demonstrates the supracerebellar infratentorial approach.*

the splenium of the corpus callosum, and the colliculi inferiorly. Injury to the deep veins, hemorrhage, and impairment of upward gaze can occur. The other complications of this approach relate to positioning, with many surgeons utilizing the sitting position. The mortality rate in one large series of pineal region tumors operated using this approach was 3.5 per cent (7/196).[8]

Occipital transtentorial approach

The tumor is approached between the occipital lobe and the falx cerebri (Figure 9.6). The tentorium cerebelli is divided to one side of the straight sinus, and the tumor is exposed in the quadrigeminal cistern. The tumor is then resected from under the deep veins. The occipital lobe can be injured by retraction in this approach, leading to a hemianopia, which is generally transient.[9]

THIRD VENTRICULAR TUMORS

A variety of tumors can present as masses within the third ventricle. These may arise primarily within the third ventricle or extend from one of the walls of the third ventricle. The common pathologies seen in this location are astrocytomas, pineal region tumors bulging forward, craniopharyngiomas, epidermoids/dermoids, and colloid cysts. Again, hydrocephalus is a common cause of presentation and endoscopy may be useful to biopsy the tumor, to perform a third ventriculostomy, or to fenestrate the interventricular septum and hence avoid the need for bilateral shunts.

The surgical routes available for tumors in this location are the transcortical and the interhemispheric. Additionally, tumors located posteriorly in the third ventricle can be resected using the approaches described for pineal region tumors.

Transcortical approach

The third ventricle is approached through the frontal cortex. The lateral ventricle is entered and the third ventricular tumor approached either through a dilated foramen of Monro or between the choroid plexus of the lateral ventricle and the thalamus. Dilated ventricles are a prerequisite for this approach. The exposure is also essentially unilateral. The need to make a cortical incision may increase the risk of epilepsy in the long term.

Interhemispheric approach

The tumor is approached from the midline (Figure 9.7). The space between the falx cerebri medially and the medial aspect of the cerebral hemisphere laterally is developed. An anterior corpus callosotomy, usually 2–2.5 cm in length, is made. The third ventricle is then entered between the bodies of the fornices leading to the roof of the third ventricle, via the lateral ventricle and then through the foramen of Monro between the choroid plexus and the thalamus.

Any of these approaches can be used to resect tumors within the third ventricle, but the working space is narrow, which prohibits the use of many of the instruments detailed previously. Cognitive deficits can occur following this approach. These deficits tend to be transient, but permanent changes are seen in five to ten per cent of patients. Other effects, such as altered consciousness, transient mutism, impairment of memory, and contralateral limb weakness, may also occur, but these tend to resolve spontaneously within a few weeks. Despite resection of the tumor, hydrocephalus may persist in up to 30 per cent of patients. The reported mortality rate for resection of third ventricular tumors is 5–12 per cent.

SUPRASELLAR TUMORS

Various tumors can present as masses in the suprasellar area, e.g. craniopharyngiomas, optic chiasm/hypothalamic glioma, and pituitary adenomas. Biopsy and partial

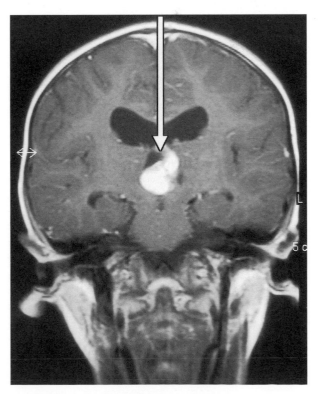

Figure 9.7 *Interhemispheric approach to third ventricular tumors.*

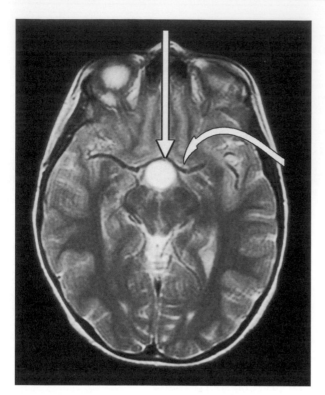

Figure 9.8 *Approaches to suprasellar lesions. The curved arrow shows the pterional route. The straight arrow indicates the subfrontal route.*

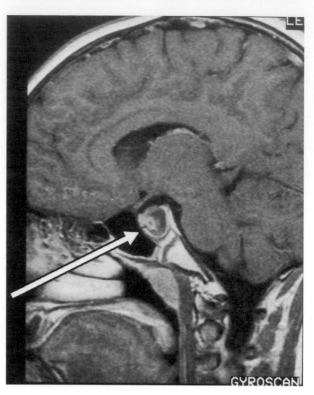

Figure 9.9 *The trans-sphenoidal route to sellar lesions.*

or total resection of tumors in this location can be achieved by various routes:

Pterional route

The pterional route is essentially an anterolateral approach to the suprasellar region (Figure 9.8). The approach can be used for virtually all suprasellar tumors, but tumor resection may have to be done between the structures in the suprasellar cisterns, i.e. the internal carotid artery and its branches, and the optic nerve. A certain degree of frontal and temporal lobe retraction is required in this approach. The pterional route is frequently adapted to allow access from more than one direction. Thus, the frontal aspect of the craniotomy may be extended to allow a subfrontal approach. Additionally, the supraorbital bar and the zygomatic process may be removed to widen the exposure and decrease the need for retraction of the brain. It is also possible to extend the temporal aspect of the approach to allow for subtemporal access.

Subfrontal approach

A midline frontal approach can be used, which allows good visualization of the optic nerves and the internal carotid arteries bilaterally (Figure 9.8). The tumor is resected from between the optic nerves. The frontal lobes may suffer retraction injury during this approach, and the olfactory nerves may be damaged, resulting in anosmia. Tumors extending laterally or posteriorly into the interpeduncular fossa can be difficult to resect using this approach.

Trans-sphenoidal route

The trans-sphenoidal route is used mainly for tumors in the sellar region (Figure 9.9). The base of the skull and the sphenoid bone is approached through the nasal cavity in the midline. The sphenoid sinus is entered and the sella turcica is visualized. The pituitary fossa can then be entered by opening the basal dura. Pneumatization of the sphenoid sinus increases the ease of the operation. In children under five years of age, the sphenoid bone may have to be drilled out in order to access the pituitary fossa.[10] This route is used mainly for pituitary adenomas and intrasellar craniopharyngiomas with or without suprasellar extension. Total excision of craniopharyngiomas has been achieved by this route.[11,12] The main problems of this approach are with CSF leakage. Rarely injury to the internal carotid artery in the cavernous sinus may occur. The main advantage of this approach is the avoidance of a craniotomy and the associated risk of epilepsy.

HEMISPHERIC TUMORS

The most common tumors seen in this location in children tend to be gliomas.[13] Total or near-total resection of the tumor, without major neurological deficit if feasible, is the goal of surgical intervention. This may be possible only in superficially located tumors and those that are well demarcated from the surrounding brain substance. For diffuse tumors located in the basal ganglionic and thalamic region, stereotactic biopsy of the tumor to establish the histological diagnosis followed by adjuvant therapy may be the best option.

Resection of these tumors has been helped by the advent of neuronavigation, which allows precise localization of the tumor and maximizes resection of these tumors.[14] Preoperative investigations such as fMRI can help to localize eloquent cortical and subcortical areas and their relation to the tumor, allowing planning of the extent of surgical resection.[15]

Various neurophysiological intraoperative techniques allow the surgeon to localize areas such as the motor and sensory cortices. Cortical stimulation techniques are useful in identifying speech and motor areas intraoperatively.[16] Motor mapping can be achieved in an anesthetized patient, but speech localization requires an awake patient, which can only be carried out in older children.[17,18]

Intraoperative MRI has been used in some centers to allow real-time imaging of the extent of tumor resection and thus maximize tumor resection.[19]

SKULL–BASE APPROACHES

These approaches involve a more extensive removal of bone from the cranium. This allows the tumor to be approached along the skull base, thus decreasing the amount of brain retraction required. Commonly used techniques are the removal of the orbital bar for resection of craniopharyngiomas, and removal of the orbital roof and lateral wall, including the zygomatic arch for access to parasellar tumors. Lateral approaches through the petrous bone can be used to expose the anterior and anterolateral portions of the posterior fossa. These involve extensive petrous temporal bone drilling and are often carried out by an ENT surgeon.

SPINAL TUMORS

Spinal tumors are divided into extradural and intradural tumors. The latter are subdivided further into those that are intrinsic to the spinal cord (intramedullary) and those that are not arising from the spinal cord but are pressing on it (extramedullary). Extradural tumors (34.5 per cent) comprise the largest group of spinal tumors in children, followed by the intramedullary tumors (29.7 per cent), and intradural extramedullary tumors (24.6 per cent).[20]

Extramedullary tumors

Intradural extramedullary tumors are generally benign tumors (nerve-sheath tumors, dermoid/epidermoid), and the treatment is predominantly surgical excision. Some tumors, such as nerve-sheath tumors, may extend extradurally and into the paraspinal tissues through the neural foramen. These tumors require resection of the intraspinal component followed by resection of the paraspinal component, which may need the involvement of other surgical disciplines, depending on whether access to the chest, abdomen, or pelvis is required. Dermoid tumors can be adherent to the spinal cord, in which case only debulking may be carried out safely. These tumors are approached posteriorly. Laminectomy, in which the laminar arch and the spinous process are removed, or laminotomy, in which the lamina and the spinous process are removed en bloc and replaced following tumor resection, are used to provide surgical access. Preoperative localization of the intraspinal lesion is usually carried out. Intraoperative tools such as ultrasound are helpful in localizing the tumor extent before the dura is opened. It can also help to locate a syrinx associated with the tumor.[21]

Most extradural tumors in children are extensions of malignant paraspinal neoplasms, e.g. neuroblastomas, sarcomas that invade the spinal canal through the neural foramen. Surgery may be required in order to make a tissue diagnosis or as an emergency procedure if there is evidence of sudden neurological deterioration secondary to cord compression at the time of presentation or during medical therapy.

Surgery can be carried out with minimal morbidity and no mortality.[22] Multilevel laminectomy, however, can lead to progressive spinal deformity, depending on the level at which it is performed, the highest risk being in the cervical region. Laminotomy is being performed more often to reduce the incidence of postoperative spinal deformity, although this has not been proven.

Intramedullary tumors

The predominant intramedullary tumors in children tend to be low-grade tumors. Two-thirds of intramedullary tumors are low-grade astrocytomas or gangliogliomas. In one study, ependymomas constituted 11.6 per cent of the tumors.[23] The aim of surgery in these tumors remains total/near-total resection if safely and technically possible. A laminotomy – i.e. en bloc removal of multiple lamina and the spinous processes with the attached ligamentum flavum and interspinous ligaments – is carried out if multiple levels need to be exposed. The tumor margins can then be defined using intraoperative ultrasound. Following dural opening, a myelotomy is made in the midline and the tumor margins are identified. The tumor can then be debulked using an ultrasonic aspirator. The tumor, if well-defined, can be separated from the surrounding cord and resected. If there is an associated syrinx, then that is also drained. The laminae are then replaced and held in place with suture material or plates.

Major postoperative morbidity tends to be a new neurological deficit or worsening of existing deficits. For a patient who has no preoperative motor deficit, the likelihood of this complication is less than five per cent.[23] Progressive spinal deformity can occur, especially in the cervical and thoracic spine. Although unproven, it is hoped that laminoplasty will reduce this spinal deformity.

RECENT ADVANCES IN TUMOR SURGERY

In an attempt to make surgical resection safer, some new technological advances have been made, including intraoperative spinal cord monitoring, fMRI, and intraoperative MRI.

Spinal cord monitoring

Somatosensory evoked potentials (SSEPs) have been used widely in spinal scoliosis surgery. SSEPs are signal-averaged data and are not real-time measurements. The data are collected at frequent intervals to maximize sensitivity to operative events.[24] While false-negative outcomes do occur, the true-negative rate has been reported to be as high as 99.93 per cent.[25] In patients with intramedullary tumors, SSEPs can be difficult to obtain if proprioception is impaired. Motor-evoked potentials (MEPs) are being used for motor tract assessment. The experience of one group showed that epidural MEPs are reliable predictors of postoperative neurological status: a less than 50 per cent reduction of intraoperative epidural MEPs amplitude signified a transient paresis, while a greater than 50 per cent reduction in MEPs was associated with a more profound postoperative neurological deficit.[23]

Intraoperative magnetic resonance imaging

This is a new application of MRI. The patient is operated on in a modified operating room containing an MRI scanner, and magnetic-resonance-compatible instruments and anesthetic equipment are used. The operating field is within the scanner gantry, allowing observation of the surgical resection of the brain tumor. The advantages are accurate localization of the tumor and of the extent of surgical resection. In one study, intraoperative imaging showed residual tumor when resection appeared complete on the basis of surgical observation alone in more than one-third of cases.[19] Intraoperative complications could also be identified and dealt with immediately. The drawbacks are the confined space available, the fact that much equipment is still not magnetic-resonance-compatible, and the enormous expense. There is certainly no evidence that these systems are cost-effective.

Functional magnetic resonance imaging

This can be used to map cerebral functions in patients with frontal and parietal tumors preoperatively. It can be used to locate eloquent areas, i.e. motor, sensory, and language, in relation to the tumor. fMRI helps to determine the risk of postoperative neurological deficit from surgical resection of tumors located near eloquent areas.[26]

REFERENCES

1   Drake JM, Sainte-Rose C. *The Shunt Book*. New York: Blackwell Scientific, 1995.
2   Chumas P, Tyagi A, Livingston J. Hydrocephalus – what's new? *Arch Dis Child Fetal Neonatal Ed* 2001; **85**:F149–54.
3   Drake JM, Kestle JRW, Milner R, *et al*. Randomized trial of cerebrospinal fluid shunt valve design in pediatric hydrocephalus. *Neurosurgery* 1998; **43**:294–305.
4   Tuli S, Drake JM, Lawless J, *et al*. Risk factors for repeated cerebrospinal shunt failures in pediatric patients with hydrocephalus. *J Neurosurg* 2000; **92**:31–8.
5   Regis J, Bouillot P, Rouby-Volot F, Figarella-Branger D, Dufor H, Peragut JC. Pineal region tumors and the role of stereotactic biopsy: review of the mortality, morbidity and diagnostic rates in 370 cases. *Neurosurgery* 1996; **39**:907–14.
6   Kreth F, Schatz CR, Pagenstecher A, Faist M, Volk B, Ostertag, Christoph B. Stereotactic management of lesions of the pineal region. *Neurosurgery* 1996; **39**:280–91.
7   Oi S, Shibata M, Tominaga J, *et al*. Efficacy of neuroendoscopic procedures in minimally invasive preferential management of pineal region tumors: a prospective study. *J Neurosurg* 2000; **93**:245–53.
8   Bruce JN, Stein BM. Supracerebellar approach to pineal region neoplasms. In Schmidek HH and Sweet WH (eds) *Operative Neurosurgical Techniques. Indications, Methods and Results*, Second edition. Philadelphia: WB Saunders Co., 1988, pp. 405–9.
9   Nazzaro JM, Shults WT, Neuwelt EA. Neuro-ophthalmological function of patients with pineal region tumors approached transtentorially in the semisitting position. *J Neurosurg* 1992; **76**:746–51.
10 Partington MD, Davis DH, Laws ER, Scheithauer BW. Pituitary adenomas in childhood and adolescence. Results of transphenoidal surgery. *J Neurosurg* 1994; **80**:209–16.
11 Takumi A, Ludecke DK. Transnasal surgery for infradiaphragmatic craniopharyngiomas in paediatric patients. *Neurosurgery* 1998; **44**:957–66.

12 Landolt AM, Zachmann M. Results of transphenoidal extirpation of craniopharyngiomas and Rathke's cysts. *Neurosurgery* 1991; **28**:410–15.

13 Pollack IF. Brain tumors in children. *N Engl J Med* 1994; **331**:1500–7.

14 Drake JM, Prudencio J, Holowka S, *et al.* Frameless stereotaxy in children. *Paediatr Neurosurg* 1994; **20**:152–9.

15 Puce A, Constable T, Luby ML, *et al.* Functional magnetic resonance imaging of sensory and motor cortex: comparison with electrophysiological localization. *J Neurosurg* 1995; **83**:262–70.

16 Berger MS, Ojemann GA, Lettich E. Neurophysiological monitoring during astrocytoma surgery. *Neurosurg Clin North Am* 1990; **1**:65–80.

17 Berger MS. The impact of technical adjuncts in the surgical management of cerebral hemispheric low-grade gliomas of childhood. *J Neuro-Oncol* 1996; **28**:129–55.

18 Taylor MD, Bernstein M. Awake craniotomy with brain mapping as the routine surgical approach to treating patients with supratentorial intra-axial tumors: a prospective trial of 200 cases. *J Neurosurg* 1999; **90**:35–41.

19 Black PM, Alexander E, 3rd, Martin C, *et al.* Craniotomy for tumor treatment in an intraoperative magnetic resonance imaging. *Neurosurgery* 1999; **45**:423–31.

20 Yamamoto Y, Raffel C. Spinal extradural neoplasms and intradural extramedullary neoplasms. In: Albright L, Pollack I, Adelson D (eds) *Principles and Practice of Pediatric Neurosurgery.* New York: Thieme Medical Publishers, 1999, p. 686.

21 Epstein F, Rhagavendra NB, John RE, Pritchett L. Spinal cord astrocytomas of childhood: surgical adjuncts and pitfalls. *Concepts Paediatr Neurosurg* 1985; **5**:224–37.

22 Raffel C, Neave VCD, Lavine S, McComb JG. Treatment of spinal cord compression by epidural malignancy in childhood. *Neurosurgery* 1991; **28**:349–52.

23 Muszynski CA, Constantini S, Epstein FJ. Intraspinal Intramedullary neoplasms. In: Albright L, Pollock I, Adelson D (eds) *Principles and Practice of Pediatric Neurosurgery.* New York: Thieme Medical Publishers, 1999, p. 699.

24 Padberg AM, Bridwell KH. Spinal cord monitoring. Current state of art. Disorders of pediatric and adolescent spine. *Orthop Clin North Am* 1999; **30**:407–33.

25 Schwartz DM, Sestokas AK, Turner LA, *et al.* Neurophysiological identification of iatrogenic neural injury during complex spinal surgery. *Semin Spine Surg* 1998; **10**:242–51.

26 Mueller WM, Yetkin FZ, Hammeke TA, *et al.* Functional magnetic resonance imaging mapping of the motor cortex in patients with cerebral tumors. *Neurosurgery* 1996; **39**:515–20.

10

Radiotherapy techniques

ROLF D. KORTMANN, CAROLYN R. FREEMAN AND ROGER E. TAYLOR with CHRISTINE ABERCROMBIE (ANESTHESIA) AND ANNE INGLE (PLAY THERAPY)

INTRODUCTION

For the majority of children with tumors of the central nervous system (CNS), surgery is the most important treatment modality. However, radiotherapy has also been accepted as having a major role for many patients, since Cushing first reported its essential role in the curative therapy of medulloblastoma in 1919.[1] With the recognition of the different patterns of biological behavior of CNS tumors, techniques and dose fractionation regimens specific to the various tumor types were developed. In 1953, Paterson and Farr noted the need for precise coverage of the craniospinal target volume and an appropriate radiation dose to achieve optimal results for children with medulloblastoma.[2] Over the past 40 years, there has been progressive improvement in the outcome of treatment of children with CNS tumors. Bloom and colleagues observed an increase in ten-year survival from 38 to 58 per cent when comparing patients treated between 1950 and 1970 with a cohort treated between 1970 and 1981.[3] Recent advances in radiotherapy techniques have the potential to better the outcome by improving tumor control and reducing radiation toxicity. These high-precision treatment techniques, as well as fractionation schedules, exploit the radiobiological properties of tumor and normal tissue. Quality-control programs ensure precise and reproducible treatments.

Physical properties of ionizing irradiation

In clinical practice, photons are predominantly used in radiation therapy. They are generated by hitting a dense metal target with a focused beam of electrons accelerated to very high energy. The acceleration of electrons can be achieved by a high-frequency electromagnetic field in a linear tube (linear accelerator). They can also be produced by radioisotopes emitting high-energy photons in their decay process, such as cobalt-60 used in telecobalt units and in the "gamma knife." Other isotopes, such as iodine-125, are generally used in brachytherapy. Electrons from an accelerator can be used directly to form a therapeutic field. Photon beams of various energies differ in their ability to penetrate the tissue. The curves show a build-up region between the point of entry and the depth of the dose maximum, where the dose gradually grows from a low superficial value to a maximum. These properties provide a skin-sparing effect. The high-penetration ability of photons is the basis for computer-assisted treatment planning in which different fields from different angles can be applied and superimposed, leading to a homogeneous maximum dose distribution around their points of intersection (the isocenter). Electrons, however, display a sharp dose fall-off beyond their dose maximum, which ranges energy-dependently between 0.5 and 6 cm. This makes crossing electron fields impractical. Therefore, they are used as simple static fields for superficial targets, such as in irradiation of the spinal canal.

Biological properties of ionizing irradiation

The underlying principle of cell death caused by ionizing irradiation is focused essentially on the production of hydroxyl radicals leading to DNA double-strand breaks.

Radiation-induced cell death, however, is a complex issue comprising many molecular genetic mechanisms leading to apoptosis. Tumor and normal cells can repair sublethal cell damage. The capacity of tumor tissue, however, is limited compared with normal tissue, leading to a progressive reduction of tumor cells without compromising normal tissue.

RADIOBIOLOGICAL CONSIDERATIONS

Total dose and fractionation

The time/dose pattern and its effect on tumor and normal tissue cells impacts significantly on tumor control and acute side effects as well as late sequelae. Single high-dose irradiation (radiosurgery) causes frank necrosis and, if administered focally within tumor, effectively controls localized disease. Fractionation exploits the differences in response to radiation between normal and tumor tissue, taking advantage of the well-established radiobiological fact that normal tissue can tolerate many small doses of irradiation much better than a single larger fraction. Fractionated radiation therapy administers a higher cumulative dose to the target volume with multiple treatments extending over several weeks.

The tolerance of normal brain parenchyma and its vascular and supporting structures becomes the limiting factor in external beam therapy, and the risk of particularly long-term sequelae is the dose-limiting factor. White matter tends to be more sensitive than gray matter in young children (under two years of age), in whom myelinization is incomplete. Late effects appear in a predictable manner in relation to volume, dose, and fractionation. Frank radiation necrosis is seen with threshold doses of approximately 45 Gy in ten fractions, 60 Gy in 35 fractions, and 70 Gy in 60 fractions. Small target volumes, low daily doses, and multiple fractions all decrease the incidence of late effects associated with conventional external beam therapy. With conventional fractionation schedules of 1.8–2.0 Gy/day, total doses of up to 54 Gy are tolerated well for limited intracranial fields.

HYPERFRACTIONATION

The rationale for hyperfractionation is to try to reduce the delayed effects of radiation injury and to prevent tumor repopulation by giving more than one radiation fraction per day in smaller doses per fraction. Small doses given more than once a day, usually six to eight hours apart, produce a redistribution of proliferating tumor cells, with some cells entering a radiosensitive stage. Other non-proliferating or dose-limiting tissue, such as normal brain, will potentially be spared this effect of redistribution. There are also important differences in repair

capacity between tumor and late-responding normal tissue. In CNS irradiation, hyperfractionated radiotherapy may therefore allow a higher total dose and result in increased tumor cell kill without increasing normal tissue toxicity.

The results of two phase II studies in the treatment of medulloblastoma using hyperfractionation were promising, achieving long-term survival rates up to 93 per cent in low- and high-risk medulloblastoma and supratentorial primitive neuroectodermal tumor (PNET).[4–9] In the study of Prados and colleagues, 33 of 39 patients received hyperfractionated radiotherapy of 30 Gy to the neuraxis followed by a boost to the posterior fossa to 72 Gy.[4] There were only three treatment failures at the primary tumor site exposed to a total dose of 72 Gy. In a series of 23 patients who were classified as poor-risk by a high T- or M-stage, hyperfractionation was given with a dose to the craniospinal axis of 36 Gy followed by a boost to the posterior fossa up to 54 Gy and to the tumor site up to 72 Gy.[6] Fifteen patients had a high T-stage without evidence of metastases. Of these patients, 14 (93 per cent) have remained in continuous complete remission for a median of 68 months, and none has died. This treatment strategy was subsequently investigated by the Children's Cancer Group (CCG) in high-stage medulloblastoma and supratentorial PNET, including those with metastatic disease.

In ependymoma, the use of local dose escalation with hyperfractionation is also promising. Preliminary data show an increased progression-free survival of 74 per cent at five years.[10] In the Paediatric Oncology Group POG-8132 study, a three year progression-free survival of 53 per cent in incompletely resected tumors was achieved.[11] The approach of hyperfractionation is currently under investigation in European and American working groups. In brainstem glioma, this approach was, however, unsuccessful.[12–14] Hyperfractionated schedules from 1.0 to 1.26 Gy twice daily were applied up to 75.6 Gy, tested prospectively by the Children's Cancer Study Group (CCSG) and the POG, and compared in a randomized phase III trial with conventional fractionation. The median progression-free survival ranged between six and eight months, but no survival advantage was seen.

DOSE PRESCRIPTIONS

Adequate dose prescriptions are necessary to meet the radiobiological requirements to achieve maximal tumor cell kill and to allow recovery of normal tissue from the effects of ionizing irradiation. Although novel fractionation schemes such as hyperfractionation have given disappointing results in brainstem glioma, fast proliferating embryonal tumors such as medulloblastoma seem to be responsive, which is leading to better tumor control while sparing normal tissue.

ROLE OF PLAY SPECIALISTS IN PREPARATION FOR CRANIOSPINAL RADIOTHERAPY

The role of hospital play specialists is to look at the psychological and emotional needs of sick children in hospital. Part of this role is to prepare children for their treatment, enabling them to understand their treatment and to cooperate with it, without any psychological distress. Using play tools such as dolls, photographs, videos, and information booklets, play specialists can explain exactly what is going to happen, using play as a medium all children understand. Play specialists can alleviate any fears, anxieties, or misconceptions that the child may have. This process gives the child the opportunity to ask questions and receive answers.

Antony Oakhill states:

> Research has shown significant stress reduction in play preparation programmes that combine giving information, demonstrating procedures and having the child play with equipment for the medicosurgical procedure he is to undergo. This cognitive, psychological approach helps the child acknowledge and play through his fantasies and misconceptions.[15]

For a child undergoing craniospinal radiotherapy, play preparation is very important if they are to be able to accept the treatment without distress. While the actual treatment itself does not hurt (it cannot be seen, felt, or heard), the process of preparation for and delivery of the treatment that the child undergoes is very invasive and upsetting. The preparation can be the most distressing part.

Planning

MAKING THE MOULD

In order to deliver radiation therapy accurately and safely, the child must lie still in exactly the same position every day for the whole course of daily or twice-daily treatments. In order to achieve the same position, a mould of the head must be made, which is subsequently fixed to the treatment table. The preparation of the mould is the first stage of planning.

This starts with an impression being taken of the child's face and head. The child has to lie still while their hair is covered with a swimming cap. Aqueous cream is then applied to the face and ears, and small strips of plaster-of-Paris bandage are dipped in warm water and applied to the face. The eyes, nostrils, and mouth are left uncovered. The child has to lie still until the plaster cast has set. The mould is removed and is used by the technicians to make a see-through Perspex mask.

The child returns later for the back of the mask to be made. This is made with the child lying face down in the front half of the Perspex mask. The back of the head is covered in cling film, and plaster-of-Paris bandage is applied. When the back mask is completed, the child returns for the fitting, in which the front and back masks are joined together with four plastic poppers that connect them together.

SIMULATION/COMPUTED TOMOGRAPHY SCAN PLANNING

The next stage is simulation. This uses a simulated radiotherapy machine with a gantry that rotates around a bed. The child lies face down in the mask, keeping very still on the bed while the machine rotates around them taking a series of X-ray pictures. The child has to be in the room alone while the pictures are being taken; this can take between 15 and 45 minutes. The parents can see their child and talk to them via an audiovisual link when they are excluded from the room, and they can rejoin the child during periods when the machine is being adjusted.

Sometimes for the planning, the child may need to have a computed tomography (CT) scan in their mask before they have their simulation. After all the X-rays have been taken, the child can go home. They will be contacted when they have a date to start the treatment.

Treatment

If spinal radiotherapy is required, the child will need to have a small tattoo/dot put on the skin at the base of the spine. A local anesthetic cream can be used so the child does not feel the needle as it is dipped in dye and then inserted just underneath the skin. The process of the delivery of treatment is a repeat of the simulation process. The child has to be on their own when the radiotherapy is given, but the parents can watch their child on a TV monitor and talk to them.

Play therapy preparation

The key to successful play preparation is for the play specialist to start play preparation in plenty of time, sometimes weeks before the event. Using dolls, the child can experience making a mask themselves. This is very beneficial as the child is able to handle the medical equipment and experience what it feels like. The child can put cream on the doll's face and then use plaster bandage to make an impression of the doll's face. Other techniques that may be used, according to the child's individual needs, include making masks using bandages and balloons, and making casts of hands and feet.

Information

The author (CA) and her colleagues have written information booklets about radiotherapy that give information and show photographs of the radiotherapy department and machines. At the author's hospital, a video film has been made that shows children undergoing treatment.

For continuity of care, the play specialist accompanies the child and family to the consultation with the radiotherapy consultant, takes them on a visit around the radiotherapy department, then follows them through the planning, simulation, and treatment stages. All the play equipment can go home with the child and family, so they are able to carry on the preparation work at home. There are huge benefits to this, as the child is in their own familiar environment. The play can then be done as part of their daily activities, without any undue pressure. Parents can actively help their child to feel involved and therefore have some control over the situation when treatment begins.

The author, during her 12 years in this line of work, has learnt to expect the unexpected and never to assume one knows what the child is frightened of. This is very clear in the following case study:

A three-year-old boy needed craniospinal radiotherapy. He had spent most of his life in hospital since he was nine months old. He was getting fed up with coming to hospital, becoming distressed on occasions. After spending some time with the family, we decided to make the mask impressions under general anesthetic and to carry out the treatment while the child was awake.

We made an extra mask, which I took out to the boy's home, where we carried out the play preparation. The mask stayed at the boy's home, where he practiced wearing it and then lying still it in it, with his parents helping him. We visited the radiotherapy department on several occasions, choosing quiet times so the boy could go in the rooms, play on the beds, and operate the machinery without anything happening to him.

This continued for several weeks, until we all thought the boy was ready to begin. The boy was fine until he was asked to take off his vest, at which point he became very distraught. When asked what had upset him, he replied that he did not want to take his vest off or people to look at his back.

The solution was simple: we created a special radiotherapy vest with a window cut out of the back. This worked well, as the child kept his vest on and the radiographers could get to the area they needed to visualize. Of all the things that had happened to the child – the machinery in the room, strange people, strange surroundings – the most traumatic thing for him was the removal of his vest. It is important to always listen to the child. This boy sailed through the rest of his treatment without any problems.

Conclusion

Sometimes the preparation process is brief and straightforward, but sometimes it can involve considerable time. This commitment to achieving radiotherapy with cooperation of the child is not always compatible with commencing treatment in a short timeframe. Inclusion of the play therapist in multidisciplinary discussions surrounding scheduling of treatments is essential to achieving a happy and cooperative child in the first day of treatment.

By using these methods of preparation techniques tailored to the individual's needs, the play specialist reduces the anxiety, fears, and misconceptions, not only for the child but also for the family. This enables the child to cooperate with the treatment with a reduced risk of long-term psychological trauma. It makes life easier for all concerned and frequently saves the need for general anesthesia with all its clinical and financial consequences.

Using play specialists would result in a huge saving in cost and a reduction in risk because every general anesthetic (GA) involves risk. Often radiotherapy lasts 30 days which means 30 + GAs, but most of all it benefits the child in terms of self confidence and self esteem because they learn how to cope. The cost of two children's GAs for 30 days will pay for one hospital's play specialist's salary.[16]

ANESTHESIA FOR RADIOTHERAPY: A PEDIATRIC ANESTHETIST'S VIEW

Introduction

When there is no prospect of a child remaining motionless for cranial radiotherapy for whatever reason, anesthesia is used to immobilize the child in order to make the application of radiotherapy safe and controllable. This situation happens most frequently in preschool children (under five to six years) and in children with developmental delay. In our practice, we have rejected restraint (straps) as a method for immobilizing children during non-anesthetized radiotherapy.

Craniospinal radiotherapy is the most complex radiation field delivered. New techniques of hyperfractionated radiotherapy and conformal treatments mean that the risks of radiotherapy on long-term neurological damage versus its benefit in tumor cure are being reconsidered for younger children. It is likely, therefore, that radiotherapy under anesthesia will continue to be a regular feature of the pediatric radiotherapy department as anesthetic techniques have developed considerably in the past decade, making anesthesia safer. Careful consideration needs to be given to the specialist environment, staffing, and planning that modern anesthetic techniques require for their safe application for this indication.

This section has been written as a personal view of anesthetizing children for radiotherapy over a number of years. Some of the discussion will center upon the physical environment that exists in our hospital, which, of course, will be different in other institutions. However, consideration of the physical environment is central to planning anesthesia for this subgroup of children.

The problems

THE CHILD

The young or handicapped child who requires craniospinal radiotherapy has commonly been treated intensively with other cancer treatments, including surgery and chemotherapy. The child may have physical or neurological disability, and they may come with a family that is concerned about the chances of success of the treatment and is unsure about the consequences of the radiotherapy being offered.

The delivery of radiotherapy is commonly in a hospital distant from the child's cancer unit. The radiotherapy machines are accommodated in concrete-lined rooms with no windows, often in the basement of the hospital. The child's previous experience of going to theater, having chemotherapy, and undergoing physiotherapy and rehabilitation will have colored their view of whether they can trust the adults delivering their treatment.

The child needs to be starved for general anesthetic, thus the timing of general anesthesia is crucial. An early start means that three meals a day can be achieved. A 2 p.m. start means no lunch, which leads to a malnourished child.

THE PARENTS

The parents are frequently extremely anxious about the process of anesthesia on one occasion, but to undergo it repeatedly on a daily basis for several weeks is a dimension of commitment with which they are unfamiliar. Clear explanations are required of the methods of anesthetic used, the feasibility of repeated intravenous or inhaled inductions, the safety of the child during the anesthetic, the time taken for the child to recover, and the accommodation of the child and the family during this prolonged period, whether it be in hospital or at home. Traveling to the hospital on a daily basis for treatment is often problematic but avoids the dislocation of the child, plus a parent, from the rest of the family for a period of several weeks. For some patients, "night care" has proven popular, i.e. the child arrives at bedtime and departs mid-morning after recovery from the general anesthetic.

THE ANESTHETIC TEAM

The majority of centers offer anesthetics for radiotherapy as an exceptional service rather than a routine service. Therefore, unless the child is being cared for in a very large treatment center, there will not be a regular anesthetic list to cover radiotherapy anesthetics on a daily basis throughout the year. This means that each child's treatment must be arranged in a specific way, using anesthetically trained medical, nursing, and theatre staff at a non-theatre location and ensuring continuity of availability of these staff on a daily basis for the four to five weeks of treatment.

The radiotherapy environment in which the anesthetic is delivered is often designed primarily not for anesthesia but for delivery of radiotherapy. The availability of piped oxygen, anesthetic-scavenging equipment, sufficient space, and recovery equipment is highly variable between centers. More recently designed units are increasingly having radiotherapy rooms installed with anesthetic facilities.

Finally, the radiotherapy department may be in a hospital without regular pediatric medical services. This poses a particular difficulty for providing suitable resources to support cardiac arrest and transfer to a children's intensive care area if an unexpected severe anesthetic incident occurs. These matters are the subjects of a variety of safety standards, which vary from country to country, but clearly awareness of these standards is a critical part of planning such a service.

The radiotherapy technique

Listening carefully to the special needs of the child and their family, providing clear explanations of the procedure and risks, giving the child and the family opportunities to get to know the anesthetic team, and a personal and professional strategy by the anesthetist that is child-friendly and cooperative are all important for the planning of any individual child's treatment program involving anesthesia. Play preparation of the child (see above) is critical for trying to gain the child's cooperation for anesthesia, and indeed for full radiotherapy treatments; it is preferable that cooperation be gained for the former even if it cannot be gained for the latter. If the anesthetic personnel are to change through the treatment period, then clear explanations to the child and family that this will occur may well help them conquer their natural suspicion of new faces.

The anesthetic

Careful assessment of the radiotherapy area for delivery of anesthetics is critical to safe practice. A selection of suitable equipment that can be transported to the area safely with built-in safeguards to cover against unexpected eventualities is critical. The installation or availability of piped oxygen and anesthetic-scavenging equipment is a standard that should be available. Use of a very large "J" oxygen cylinder may be a substitute for pipeline oxygen. If no scavenging is available, then engineers may be asked to increase the airflow to the radiotherapy suite, and the consultant may select a circuit with lower flow requirements and use an oxygen/air/vapor mixture rather than oxygen/nitrous oxide/vapor. Careful selection of anesthetic agents for induction and maintenance of anesthesia to provide rapid "street fitness" is desirable, e.g. propofol for induction and sevoflurane or isoflurane for maintenance. The selection of methods for anesthetic monitoring is important, whether it be by having monitoring devices within the radiotherapy suite monitored by a television camera, or by having bespoke monitoring equipment within the radiotherapy suite console into which monitoring devices can be plugged. Television monitors, if used, should be color-sensitive so that the patient's condition can be monitored, and the television system must have high resolution so that detail can be seen appropriately. Access to a central venous catheter for repeated intravenous induction is the preferred method of anesthesia because of its speed of action and lack of discomfort. Routine use of antiemetics to minimize the risk of radiotherapy-induced nausea and vomiting should be used in order to optimize the recovery on each day. Finally, recovery after anesthesia needs to be a specific task for the anesthetic team and is not easy to delegate routinely to non-anesthetic-trained nurses, since they are unfamiliar with the stages of recovery and may miss changes indicative of unexpected difficulty.

Patient selection for anesthesia

- *Preschool (under five to six years)*: optional.
- *Under three years old*: all children.

Positioning

Most radiation oncologists prefer the prone position for delivering of radiotherapy to the back of the head, the cranium, and the spinal column. However, the prone position is probably unsuitable for regular anesthetics without intubation. Repeated intubations over four to five weeks on a daily basis are potentially hazardous because of the local trauma to the vocal cords and the possibility of laryngospasm during periods of recovery. In our practice, we have insisted, as anesthetists, on a supine position; the radiotherapists have responded to

this in the interests of patient safety by redesigning their system for delivery (Figure 10.1).[17] It does put the radiotherapy technicians at greater inconvenience in monitoring their fields to the spine, as these need to be delivered from below rather than above the table, and the marks for positioning fields therefore must be directed through the table. However, we have found that by adopting a supine position, we have been able to induce anesthesia using intravenous agents and maintain an airway with a laryngeal mask, thereby avoiding the need for repetitive intubation. This, in turn, allows the child to breathe spontaneously during the anesthetic. We use a fast-acting inhalational anesthetic (sevoflurane) using an oxygen/air mixture. The avoidance of the prone position precludes the need for regular intubation, avoids the need to provide appropriate position support under the shoulders and hips to allow for unimpeded diaphragmatic movement, and in obese patients avoids the risk of compression of the chest by the abdominal contents due to obesity.

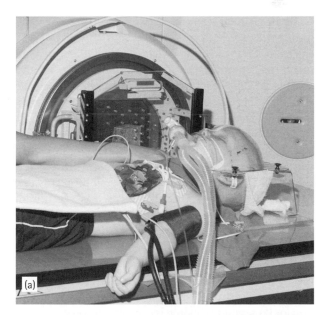

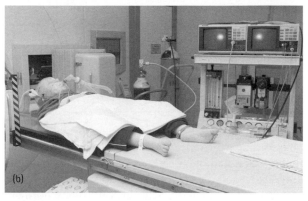

Figure 10.1 *Supine positioning for craniospinal radiotherapy under general anesthesia.*

Editorial comment

Although some pediatric anesthesiologists may prefer or even insist on the supine position for radiotherapy, this is not a universally held view. Many others are prepared to anesthetize children in the prone position for craniospinal irradiation. Where there is a choice between prone and supine positions, it is reasonable to choose the latter for children requiring anesthesia. For craniospinal irradiation, many radiation technologists prefer to be able to visualize the junction between the head and spine fields, and also to check alignment of the spinal fields. However, with the development of newer technologies for positioning and verification (such as real-time electronic portal imaging), this view may change.

Completing the course

Once the radiotherapy course has started, there is a commitment to see it through to the end on a daily basis, since there is evidence that delays in radiotherapy treatments can compromise the anti-tumor effect. For the anesthetist, this means that giving an anesthetic to a child with an upper respiratory tract infection or other anesthetic risk factor must be considered an acceptable risk by adopting appropriate techniques. The potential for laryngospasm, coughing, and breath-holding in a child with an upper respiratory tract infection with possible consequent desaturation episodes are all problems that have to be overcome rather than be used as a reason for delaying or omitting anesthesia.

Delivery of radiotherapy under anesthesia by the anesthetic team is one of the more rewarding aspects of our work. The regular appointments for these anesthetics mean that the team, the child, and the family form a sustained relationship. There is a feeling that immobilization for these young children is contributing very positively to the possibility of them being cured of their tumor, and the technical challenge of delivering safe anesthesia on a daily basis for several weeks is personally and professionally satisfying.

Supportive care

The acute side effects of irradiation are normally acceptable, leading to a grade I or II erythema within the treatment portals and other early reactions such as radiation esophagitis and diarrhea from the spinal component of craniospinal irradiation. Neurological toxicity normally does not exceed World Health Organization (WHO) grade I or II toxicity, requiring steroids only in rare cases.[18]

A child- and family-centered approach is an integral part of supportive care during radiotherapy. This should be delivered by a dedicated multiprofessional team. Play therapists can play a pivotal role in the preparation of the child for radiotherapy. Information given to the family by the clinicians should be reinforced by other professionals, particularly nurses. High-quality, multiprofessional care requires close and compassionate cooperation between the radiotherapy and pediatric oncology departments.

TECHNICAL CONSIDERATIONS

Treatment planning/definition of target volumes

Radiotherapy is a local treatment; therefore, the target volumes are defined according to the pathological and biological behavior of the tumor to be treated, specifically its tendency to infiltrate and recur locally or to spread within the brain or entire CNS (Table 10.1). The improvements in radiotherapy treatment and delivery techniques allow better coverage of target volume in order to ensure maximal tumor control while sparing as much normal tissue as possible to reduce the risk of toxicity secondary to treatment.

TARGET VOLUME

Treatment planning comprises the exact definition of the volumes to be treated according to internationally formalized standards, i.e. those of the International Commission for Radiation Units (ICRU).[19] Important developments have been the production of the ICRU-50 and ICRU-62 documents. These define how tumor, patient, and treatment parameters are taken into account when defining radiotherapy target volumes. These volumes are essentially based on gross tumor volume (GTV), clinical target volume (CTV), and planning target

Table 10.1 *Clinical target volume according to areas at risk defined by tendency of the tumor to spread within the central nervous system (CNS)*

Primary tumor site "limited volume irradiation"	Whole-brain technique	CNS "neuraxis"
Low-grade glioma	Leukemia	Medulloblastoma/PNET
High-grade glioma	Germinoma	Anaplastic ependymoma*
Ependymoma	Lymphoma	Germinoma*
Craniopharyngioma		Secreting germ-cell
Teratoma		tumor*

PNET, primitive neuroectodermal tumor.
*Advised in some clinical situations.

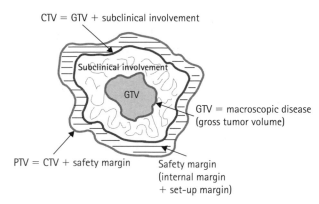

Figure 10.2 *Definition of target volumes in treatment planning according to the International Commission for Radiation Units ICRU 50/62 rules.*[19] (CTV, clinical target volume; GTV, gross tumor volume; PTV planning target volume.)

volume (PTV); they also take into account precision of imaging, geometric precision of treatment technique, and organs at risk (Figure 10.2).

Definitions of target volumes (ICRU-50)

- *GTV*: gross visible/demonstrable extent and location of malignant tumor.
- *CTV*: volume that contains subclinical tumor that is required to be eradicated.
- *PTV*: a geometrical concept defined to select appropriate beam sizes and arrangements, taking into account the net effect of all the possible geometrical variations.

DOSE PRESCRIPTION AND SPECIFICATION

The radiotherapy dose prescription is given according to internationally accepted recommendations such as the ICRU-50 and ICRU-62 rules.[19] Total dose, fractionation, and the definition and tolerance levels of dose homogeneity within the target volumes should be standardized, including reference points within the target volumes and corresponding reference doses (dose specification). In addition, the dose to critical organs (organs at risk, OARs) should be recorded. In whole-brain irradiation, the dose is specified at the midplane of the central axis of the two parallel opposed fields. In irradiation of the spinal canal, the depth of the maximum dose is determined using a CT or a lateral simulation film in the treatment position. It is necessary to calculate the minimum and maximum depth of the target volume at the posterior border of the vertebral bodies. The points of maximum depth are usually at C7 and L5. The spinal dose must be recorded as a maximum and minimum

corresponding to the minimum and maximum depths of the posterior vertebral bodies, and the doses should be prescribed to the minimum. If the calculated dose to these points varies by more than ten per cent, then a compensator should be designed to improve the uniformity of dose. In the case of electrons, the energy should be chosen such that the 90 per cent isodose line encompasses the deepest part of the target volume; the dose specification is made at the 90 per cent isodose. Radiation dose specification in irradiation of the tumor region is done with the ICRU reference point in the center of the target volume (100 per cent). The ICRU-50/62 document recommends that dose inhomogeneity within the target volume should not exceed the tolerance limits of minus five per cent to plus seven per cent.

DOSE HOMOGENEITY

The goal is to achieve a homogeneous dose distribution throughout the planning target volume within a range of minus five per cent and plus seven per cent. Dose homogeneity within the planning target volume is affected by a number of factors, including the shape of the patient's surface and position parallel to the central axis of the beam. Previously, wedge filters were used to achieve a homogeneous dose distribution. The beam intensity is decreased more along that part of the beam rays travelling through the thicker part of the wedge. Intensity is absorbed according to the different angles of the wedges. Alternatively, a standardized wedge moves into the field (dynamic wedge) when the beam is on, and a computer controls the speed of blade moving in and out of the beam. In recent years, however, multileaf collimators have been used to achieve an intensity-modified beam by superimposing differently shaped portals.

FIELD–SHAPING

The planning target volume is often irregularly shaped, mandating individualized field-shaping and alignments in order to shield normal tissue and OARs, such as the eyes, in the whole-brain technique. Traditionally, blocking was achieved by manually cutting a cast to the shape and pouring hot cerrobend (an alloy of bismuth, lead, tin, and cadmium) into the cast with a thickness of three to five half-value layers (one half-value layer attenuates the beam by 50 per cent). These blocks were attached to a tray, which was mounted in the head of the treatment machine. With recent computer technologies and rapid advances in imaging software, virtual three-dimensional reconstruction of the anatomy can be made from CT or magnetic resonance imaging (MRI) scans. For multiple non-coplanar beams, accurate shielding can now be achieved by introducing multileaf collimators, thereby avoiding the labor-intensive manufacture of cerrobend blocks.

INTENSITY MODULATED RADIOTHERAPY

Intensity-modulated radiotherapy (IMRT) is an important development that is likely to be used increasingly. Using multileaf collimators, it is possible to develop systems to vary the intensity within the radiation beam during a radiation exposure. IMRT uses either the "step-and-shoot" technique or dynamic IMRT, which is provided by moving multileaf collimator leaves ("sliding window"). IMRT relies on an inverse planning system, whereby dose and dose-distribution limits are predetermined, and the computer planning system calculates multiple beam weights and profiles. Several radiotherapy planning studies examining radiotherapy planning for brain tumors have confirmed the potential for IMRT to offer an improved radiotherapy dose distribution in patients with brain tumors when compared with other conformal planning techniques.[20–22] Using a micro-multileaf collimation system, intensity-modulated stereotactic radiosurgery[23] can provide an improved dose distribution compared with static fields. IMRT allows a better coverage of clinical target volume and a better sparing of surrounding normal tissue, particularly for irregularly shaped or concave radiotherapy target volumes. However, IMRT is a complex system requiring an optimal software system combined with three-dimensional treatment planning. Additionally, a precise reproducibility of field alignment is a prerequisite to meet the advantages of this new technique. Optimization of field arrangements and dose calculations go hand in hand with automated procedures to evaluate the technique. The present developments are aiming at an automatic mathematical optimization of treatment technique and dose distribution.

There are several potential roles for IMRT in the management of pediatric brain tumors. IMRT allows for improved dose distribution within the target volume compared with surrounding normal tissue. It may be used to reduce the dose to surrounding normal brain as in conformal treatment of the tumor bed in medulloblastoma. It can be used to compensate for changing

---

Treatment planning

Computer-assisted treatment planning, including modern imaging techniques, has become standard in radio-oncology in recent years. A precise three-dimensional delineation of the tumor in conjunction with a corresponding three-dimensional treatment planning allows precise and reproducible coverage of target volumes while sparing normal surrounding tissue. Local high-dose delivery and a reduced dose to healthy tissue lead to better tumor control and a reduction in side effects.

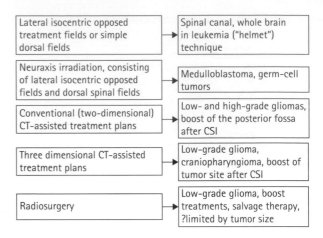

Figure 10.3 *Corresponding treatment techniques after definition of target volumes.* (CSI, craniospinal irradiation; CT, computed tomography.)

patient contour, as an alternative to fixed tissue compensators, e.g. in radiotherapy of the spinal axis.

Treatment techniques

The treatment technique is selected based on clinical requirements. Treatment techniques include simple treatment portals and complex treatment techniques, such as irradiation of the craniospinal axis and irradiation of the primary tumor site by using computer-assisted treatment planning (Figure 10.3).

WHOLE-BRAIN IRRADIATION

Whole-brain irradiation is an integral part of the treatment of acute leukemia, medulloblastoma, and intracranial germ-cell tumors. Parallel-opposed isocentric lateral treatment portals are used to encompass the entire intracranial contents. Head immobilization is necessary to achieve a reproducible treatment (Figure 10.4). The appropriate beam energy for irradiation of the entire intracranial contents is usually below 10 MV to avoid underdosing brain tissue and meninges close to the surface, which is within the dose built-up region. Anatomical landmarks (generally bone) visible on simulation or portal localization radiographs are used to define the field borders. The inferior border should be inferior to the cribriform plate, the middle cranial and posterior fossae, and the foramen magnum. The safety margins critically depend on the geometric precision of field alignments, the width of the penumbra, and individual anatomic factors. Even under optimal conditions, the safety margins should be at least 1 cm (Table 10.2). To achieve a homogeneous dose distribution, especially at the subfrontal region, the isocenter should be placed in the area of the cribriform plate. This will also reduce the risk of damage to the contralateral lens from the divergent beam. Individualized blocks along the base of the skull usually allow sufficient sparing of the lenses. However, since the cribriform plate can be projected over the upper third of the orbit in a considerable proportion of children,[24] it may not be possible to shield the lenses, since a miss of the clinical target volume at the cribriform plate may account for CNS relapses found in the subfrontal region.[25] It is now thought preferable to achieve coverage of this region even at the risk of cataract development.

IRRADIATION OF THE CRANIOSPINAL AXIS

The aim is to achieve a homogeneous dose distribution throughout the entire intracranial contents and the spinal axis. Craniospinal axis irradiation basically consists

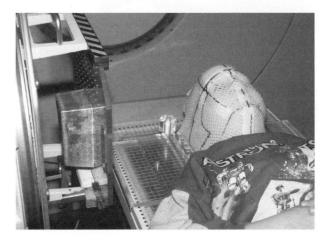

Figure 10.4 *Head fixation with thermoplastic facemask in irradiation of the entire intracranial contents in supine position on the treatment machine (thermoplastic facemask). Cerrobend blocks are attached to a tray mounted on the gantry, in order to shield the face (whole-brain technique).*

of the whole brain volume plus an adjacent dorsal field for the spinal canal (Figure 10.5). The quality of craniospinal irradiation considerably impacts the risk for relapse, especially in the management of medulloblastoma (Table 10.3). In the prospective study of Packer and colleagues,[26,27] inadequate radiotherapy was associated with a worse survival. The French working group for the treatment of medulloblastoma in childhood reviewed the radiation therapy protocol of the multicenter study M7 and assessed the contribution of radiotherapy techniques to tumor relapse.[28] Of 82 patients treated for medulloblastoma, 22 had recurrent disease. In ten (45.4 per cent) cases, the relapses could be attributed to an inadequate treatment technique. In a subsequent analysis, Carrie and colleagues assessed the frequency of failures and survival with respect to quality of radiation therapy in medulloblastoma and noted a dramatic reduction in survival with increasing frequency of protocol violations.[29] In contrast, the prospective quality-assurance program of the Hirntumoren (HIT) studies for the treatment of malignant brain tumors in childhood resulted in radiotherapy performed according to protocol guidelines in 95 per cent of children, and it is reasonable to postulate that high quality of radiotherapy may have contributed to the good outcome of patients treated in these studies.[8,18]

In recent years, treatment techniques have been introduced that ensure reliable administration of radiotherapy. These new developments have in common the fact that the traditional treatment technique of using lateral isocentric opposed fields to irradiate the whole brain and the irradiation of the spinal canal by using a dorsal field remains unchanged. CT simulation of craniospinal fields is able to improve treatment accuracy and patient comfort.[30] A volumetric dataset acquired by sequential CT scans allows a computer-assisted virtual simulation of field alignments. Comparison of digitally reconstructed

Table 10.2 *Geometric precision of current treatment techniques in irradiation of primary tumor site. Geometric precision is defined as random linear deviations of field alignment between simulation and first session and between each subsequent session (with the exception of radiosurgery measurements with a phantom)*

Ref.	Technique	Immobilization system	Geometric (mean, mm)	Precision (maximal, mm)
41	Craniospinal axis	Vacuum pillow, cast	5.0	13.0
24	Lateral, isocentric opposed fields (whole-brain technique)	Thermoplastic facemask	4.0	10
47	Conventional CT-assisted radiotherapy (two-dimensional)	Thermoplastic facemask	2.5	5.0
8	Conformal radiotherapy (three-dimensional)	Rigid facemask (bandage/cast), bite block	0.9	3.0
75	Fractionated convergence therapy	Gill–Thomas–Cosman ring (relocatable)	1.0	2.3
54	"Radiosurgery" (high single dose)	Invasive, stereotactic frame	0.3	1.0

CT, computed tomography.

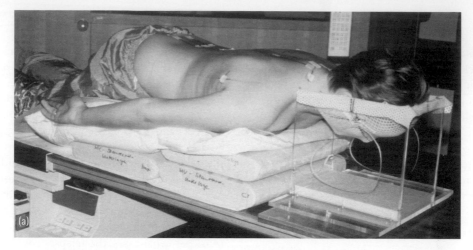

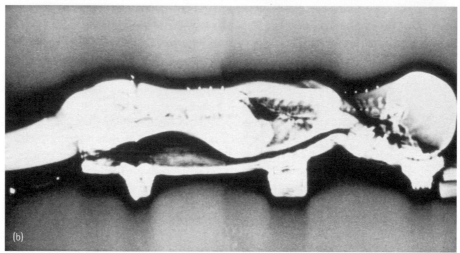

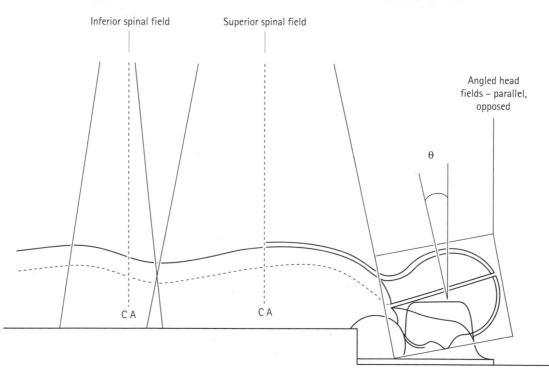

Inferior spinal field   Superior spinal field

Angled head
fields – parallel,
opposed

θ

C A   C A

Figure 10.5a,b,c *(a) Conventional craniospinal irradiation. The patient is in prone position. Cast for fixation to assure reproducibility of field alignment. The whole brain is treated by two lateral isocentric opposed fields. The spinal canal is treated by a dorsal treatment portal. (b) Computed tomography scan, displaying patient positioning for treatment planning. (c) Schematic display of field alignment.*

Table 10.3 *Impact of quality of radiotherapy on outcome in radiotherapy of medulloblastoma*

Ref.	Patients (*n*)	"High quality"	"Low quality"	Survival	Differences
27	108	Radiotherapy 1983–89, *n* = 41	Radiotherapy 1975–82, *n* = 67	Five-year survival 49% v. 82% five-year-PFS	Significant, *P* = 0.004
28	88	CSA + e⁻	CSA + X	4 v. 0 relapse	Not stated
76	40	Radiotherapy before 1980	Radiotherapy after 1980	Five-year survival 64% v. 80%	Significant, *P* = 0.02
67	77	41 adequate whole-brain fields	36 inadequate whole-brain fields	Five-year PFS 94% v. 72%	Significant, *P* = 0.016
29	169	49 (29%)	Minor deviations = 67 (40%); major deviations (md) = 53 (31%), of these 36 = one md, 11 = two md, six = three md	Three-year relapse rate after treatment: 33% for all patients, 23% for correct treatment, 17% for one md, 67% for two md, 78% for three md	Significant, *P* = 0.04
26	63	No deviations = 43	Deviations = 20	Five-year PFS 81% v. 70%	Not significant, *P* = 0.42

CSA + e⁻, craniospinal axis irradiation with electrons; CSA + X, craniospinal axis irradiation with photons; PFS, progression-free survival.

radiographs of the virtually simulated fields with verification films taken during treatment set-up confirms a high degree of accuracy.

WHOLE-BRAIN TECHNIQUE

This technique is described above, with modifications to meet the requirements for a homogeneous dose distribution of the field junction. The field extends to the C3–C4 interspace, where it adjoins the spinal volume. Collimator rotation is required to match the whole-brain portals to the divergent edge of the adjacent spine field. Care has to be taken for the abutting borders of the whole brain and spinal portals. The depth of the dose maximum has to be determined using a CT scan in the treatment position. As an alternative, lateral simulator films with metal skin markers can be used.

SPINAL FIELD

The spinal canal is irradiated using a single, direct, dorsal portal. In adolescents, the field length may not be sufficient, making necessary the use of two dorsal portals. The occurrence of metastases from medulloblastoma by way of seeding along cerebrospinal fluid (CSF) pathways to the spinal canal is well recognized. It is therefore indispensable to provide a reliable coverage of the entire dural sac. MRI (normally done for staging) should be used whenever possible to determine the lower field border and width in the sacral region. The width of the field should cover the lateral borders of the pedicles and allow for scoliosis or rotation of the vertebral column.

Individualized field-shaping in the upper region of the spinal fields using multileaf collimators will help to reduce irradiation of normal tissue and OARs, such as the heart and lungs. The design of the inferior portion of the spinal field of craniospinal irradiation is a matter of custom but not consensus. There are no data in the literature evaluating the frequency of recurrent disease with respect to field alignment. Many radiotherapists widen the inferior aspect of field to encompass the sacroiliac joints in order to safely cover the sacral nerve roots. The field design is commonly referred to as a "spade field" by virtue of its resemblance to a spade. However, gross anatomy, myelography, and spinal CT and MRI scanning show that the spinal canal extends laterally no further than the point of exit of the spinal nerves through the intervertebral foramina, suggesting that the widening of the treatment portal in the sacral region is not necessary.[31,32] MRI can be used to determine the thecal sac in order to adjust the caudal border of the spinal field. In one analysis, it was demonstrated that the thecal sac terminated below the S2–S3 interspace in only two (8.7 per cent) of 23 children. MRI can be used to individualize the lower border of the spinal field to minimize scattered radiation to the gonads.[32]

ELECTRON BEAMS FOR SPINAL FIELDS

Electron fields may be utilized if the depth of the target volume is within the therapeutic range of electrons. Precise selection of energy is necessary to avoid underdosage in some cases. Electron beams offer a potential advantage in limiting exit dose to the vertebral bodies, thus reducing the risk for growth retardation and myelosuppression. In one study, the thyroid dose was decreased from 73 to seven per cent, the heart dose from 59 to six per cent, and the kidney dose from 76 to 31 per cent. However, lateral scatter of electrons increased the dose to the lungs from ten to 35 per cent.[33] Using tertiary collimation close to the skin of electron beams at extended source-to-surface distance may reduce the penumbra width.[34] However, the clinical significance of these dosimetric findings remains to be demonstrated. Gaspar and colleagues followed 32 patients who received electron irradiation to the spinal field.[35] Complications following treatment were compared with reported complications following treatment with photons to the spinal field. The authors found no differences in late complications, suggesting that the dose reduction to OARs has little clinical impact.

FIELD-MATCHING

Devising a treatment technique that prevents overdosage and underdosage at the junction between the whole brain and cranial spinal field requires complex three-dimensional matching of adjacent fields. There are several ways to achieve a homogeneous dose distribution: by rotating the collimator of the whole-brain technique according to the beam divergence of the upper spinal field, by moving junctions, and by using penumbra modifiers.[35–38] Most commonly, the collimator is rotated to produce a smooth variation of dose between the adjacent portals. This results in an exact match of cranial and spinal doses without the need for a gap. The divergence of the cranial fields can be compensated by rotating the treatment couch such that the inferior edges of the cranial fields become coplanar with the upper edges of the spinal fields. This technique, however, increases the divergence of the beams at the subfrontal region, with resulting dose inhomogeneities in this area.

Dose profiles across the junction have shown an underdosage of 60 per cent with a gap of 1 cm and an overdosage of up to 40 per cent in an overlap of 5 mm when using 4-MV photons.[38] The optimal dose distribution is a tight junction.[36,38] Isocentric half-field techniques using an penumbra modifier at the field junction achieve dose variations of less than ten per cent across the match zone.[37] To minimize cumulative local dose irregularities and underdosage, a practice of changing the location of the junction one or more times during the course of treatment ("feathering") has been generally adopted. The increment of movement should be 1–2 cm. When moving the junction by 1 cm, underdosage can be reduced to 20–30 per cent and overdosage to 10–20 per cent. Tinkler and colleagues, however, noted that moving junctions appeared not to be necessary in terms of clinical significance.[39] In a series of 34 patients with a constant

junction, no morbidity or relapses were observed, indicating that the necessity for feathering is questionable. Another technique to provide sufficient dose homogeneity is computer-assisted dynamic radiotherapy achieved by using interactive movement of the couch for treating the spinal fields.[40] Additionally, random set-up errors will tend to eliminate hot or cold spots at the junction.[41]

Field-matching between two spinal fields is usually done with a tight junction at the level of the dorsal border of the vertebral body, thereby leaving a small gap in the spinal canal and a skin gap of at least 1 cm. Under these circumstances, a moving junction is indispensable to avoid cold and hot spots along the spinal canal and vertebral bodies. Three-dimensional treatment planning allows optimized dose distribution across the junction. By using this technique, neither increased relapse rates nor cases of myelopathy have been observed.

PATIENT POSITIONING

Manufacture of a fixation device for the head and trunk is indispensable for providing a stable and reproducible treatment delivery. The spine should be made as straight as possible to achieve a constant-depth dose distribution along the spinal canal. Normally, the child is treated in the prone position. In recent years, the supine position has also been used, but this requires precise computer-assisted treatment planning to avoid dose irregularities across the matching zone of treatment portals.[41,42]

Posterior fossa/primary tumor site

Craniospinal irradiation is normally followed by a boost to the posterior fossa in medulloblastoma or to the tumor site in supratentorial PNETs and germ-cell tumors. Computer-assisted treatment planning should be performed to achieve reliable coverage of the treatment volume and to allow optimal sparing of normal tissue (Plates 12 and 13). The posterior fossa can be treated using lateral opposed fields. Lateral fields can be angled in order to spare the inner ears. The anterior field border should encompass the clinoid process, the posterior field border should encompass the occipital bone, and the inferior border should encompass the first cervical segment. Conformal radiotherapy is under investigation for posterior fossa boost irradiation because of better sparing of other structures. Paulino and colleagues analyzed different conformal treatment techniques with the conventional lateral isocentric opposed field technique and found an advantage of conformal therapy in terms of coverage of the planning target volume and dose reduction to the cochlea, pituitary gland, and non-posterior fossa brain, albeit at the expense of increased dose exposure to the thyroid gland and other tissues in the neck.[43] Although there is ongoing discussion as to whether to treat the entire posterior fossa in medulloblastoma, the entire posterior fossa is at risk for recurrent disease according to intraoperative pathological findings in five craniotomies that demonstrated extensive tumor spread within the entire posterior fossa.[44,45] Increased recurrence rates were observed in patients with protocol violations and who were treated with reduced field sizes in the large prospective trial Société International d'Oncologie Pédiatrique (SIOP) II.[46] This issue is still unsolved, and standard treatment techniques should therefore encompass the entire posterior fossa. In the treatment of the primary tumor site in supratentorial PNETs and germ-cell tumors, the techniques of irradiating limited volumes are the standard of care (see below and Chapter 16).

Treatment techniques

Whole-brain fields and irradiation of the craniospinal axis are the classical techniques for treating macroscopic tumor and areas of possible tumor spread within the brain or entire CNS. The treatment fields cover larger areas of normal tissue requiring an adequate dose prescription, which is able to control disease in adjuvant areas and which considers normal tissue tolerance. As a rule, the total doses are therefore limited and smaller doses per fraction are normally applied to allow optimal recovery of normal cells.

Irradiation of the primary tumor

Usually, computer-assisted treatment planning is used. It is recommended that an individualized facemask be used to guarantee reproducibility of head positioning. A headrest should be chosen in order to provide sufficient head inclination so that anterior–posterior beams will not traverse the lenses of the eyes. Devices for head fixation are indispensable for providing a reproducible field alignment. They usually include thermoplastic facemasks with individually made mouthpieces or bite frames attached to the table. Field alignment achieved by using fixation systems can be reproduced reliably in clinical practice with deviations of 2.5 mm.[47] Reproducibility is significantly less accurate if no fixation system is applied (Table 10.2).

The CTV encompasses visible tumor as seen on CT or MRI (T1 contrast enhanced or T2-weighted plain images) and areas of possible tumor infiltration. When defining the CTV, anatomical borders must be considered, i.e. in tumors of the frontal region, tumor spread normally does not cross the falx to the contralateral side. The PTV encompasses the CTV with an additional margin according to the precision of treatment technique (0.2–0.5 cm

if rigid head fixation, 0.5–1.0 cm if a conventional facemask/head shell is used).[48]

In tumors of the spinal canal, a simple dorsal field is normally sufficient to meet the requirements of homogeneous dose distribution. Definition of the CTV should be done using MRI. Safety margins of one vertebral segment are recommended.[49]

Two-dimensional (conventional) treatment planning and delivery techniques

The introduction of computer-assisted treatment planning systems led to two-dimensional radiation therapy. Beam angles can be modified to avoid direct beams to especially sensitive organs, such as the eye, optic nerves, and chiasm. Targets near the surface can be treated by using two orthogonal fields (such as an anterior or posterior and lateral field), using wedges to provide a homogeneous dose distribution across the planning target volume. In more central tumors, three or four field techniques are usually applied; simple lateral opposed portals should be avoided whenever possible in order to reduce normal tissue irradiation. Non-coplanar treatments can be performed by using beams that are not in an axial plane, by rotating the treatment couch, and by moving the gantry to the decided position. Straightforward noncoplanar beams, such as an anterior, lateral, or vertex field, can be used for lateral lesions, especially in the area of the temporal lobes. A pair of parallel opposed fields augmented by a vertex field can be administered for lesions along the midline.

Current two-dimensional radiation therapy techniques are usually based on a single-axial CT scan of the patient. The major shortcomings of two-dimensional treatment planning systems are the lack of a realistic display of GTV and CTV. Correspondingly, the real volume of normal tissue or OARs included in the 95 per cent isodose is not appreciated sufficiently, resulting in a failure to compute the dose prescriptions throughout the target volumes and normal tissue.

THREE-DIMENSIONAL (FRACTIONATED) CONFORMAL RADIOTHERAPY

Current radiation techniques of limited volume irradiation of brain tumors using modern three-dimensional conformal treatment planning systems are essentially based on quantitative data acquired during the CT planning examination (Plate 14). The major advantages of CT planning in conjunction with registration of MRI scans are the exact localization of target volumes with respect to the surrounding tissue, body outline, and internal and external landmarks, and more accurate delineation of critical organs such as the brainstem and optic chiasm.

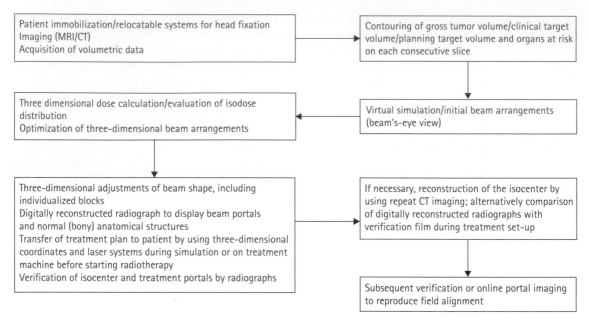

Figure 10.6 *Process of treatment planning and delivery in fractionated conformal radiotherapy.*

With these data, optimal three-dimensional beam modeling and dose distribution calculation can be performed.

Three-dimensional treatment planning and conformal radiation therapy promises high precision in dose delivery to a defined target volume and represents a major improvement over conventional two-dimensional radiation therapy. The process of three-dimensional conformal irradiation comprises several steps. An adequate acquisition of volumetric data by imaging is a prerequisite to precisely delineate anatomical structures, i.e. the tumor and OARs. According to the ICRU-50/62 rules, GTV, CTV, and PTV are contoured on each consecutive CT or MRI slice. The data are then transferred to the three-dimensional treatment planning system, which reconstructs all target volumes and normal tissue structures (Figure 10.6).

When the treatment plan is evaluated, additional tools such as dose–volume histograms, dose–surface displays, and dose statistics can be used to optimize the treatment plan (Figure 10.7). In order to improve delineation of tumor and normal tissue, image fusion of MRI with the corresponding CT imaging is being used increasingly.[50] The advantages, however, can gain clinical importance only if they are combined with a rigid head fixation system. By using this technique, the accuracy of field alignment can be improved to 1.0–2.0 mm (Table 10.2).[8]

CLINICAL APPLICATIONS

Circumscribed brain tumors such as glioma of the optic pathway are often irregularly shaped and localized in close proximity to OARs, such as the eye, pituitary gland,

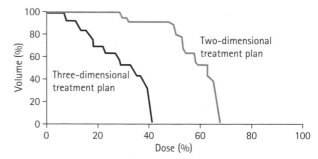

Figure 10.7 *Dose–volume histograms in fractionated conventional two-dimensional and three-dimensional conformal radiotherapy of irregularly shaped tumors. The dose–volume histogram displays the relative contribution of the total dose administered with respect to the volume irradiated. In three-dimensional treatment planning, the dose to the optic chiasm and the pituitary gland has been reduced significantly (40 per cent) as compared with the conventional two-dimensional treatment plan.*

and brainstem. Multiple static fields that conform to the irregular shape of the tumor achieve a maximum dose within the lesion while sparing normal surrounding structures (Figure 10.3). In contrast to convergence therapy, tumors of almost all sizes and shapes can be treated with identical geometric accuracy (Table 10.2).[8,48] Three-dimensional treatment planning with conformal techniques allows a 30–40 per cent reduction in the volume of normal brain tissue exposed to high-dose irradiation as compared with conventional two-dimensional treatment.[48] At present, however, clinical data are scarce for childhood brain tumors. Debus and colleagues treated ten patients with optic gliomas and favored a conformal fractionated approach because of the possibility of minimizing the amount of normal tissue within the high-dose volume.[51] Although not investigated in their series, the risk for therapy-induced endocrinological disorders can be reduced substantially by decreasing the dose to the pituitary gland and hypothalamus. Consequently, in optic-pathway tumors as well as other tumor types, there is increasing interest in early treatment with fractionated conformal radiotherapy to avoid tumor-related morbidity.

STEREOTACTIC IRRADIATION TECHNIQUES

The direct correlation between radiation dose and tumor control suggests the desirability of increasing dose levels for many malignant CNS tumors. Concerns regarding the potential toxicity of higher doses of irradiation demand restriction of the volume of brain tissue exposed to high doses. Combined with innovations in sophisticated three-dimensional stereotactic and imaging procedures, the dose–response–volume interactions have heightened interest in potentially idealized physical delivery of radiation therapy. Fractionated or conformal or convergent therapy proton therapy, brachytherapy, and high-single-dose radiotherapy ("radiosurgery") are examples of techniques to achieve focal high-dose radiation delivery.

Treatment planning in stereotactic irradiation

For treatment planning, a stereotactic head frame system is used with an additional set of plastic indicators with fiducial markers for magnetic resonance and/or CT imaging. A three-dimensional Cartesian coordinate system (xyz) is used to specify the target coordinates in stereotactic space. The volumetric data obtained by MRI or CT are then entered into the treatment planning system as input data for fitting the parameters of a mathematical model for the surface of the head and for dose calculation. Reliable definition of the target volumes is achieved by superimposing CT and MRI images.

Stereotactic convergence therapy ("radiosurgery")

The direct correlation between radiation dose and tumor control suggests the strategy of increasing dose levels within macroscopic tumor. The term "radiosurgery" was coined to describe a technique of delivering a large single dose of irradiation to a well-defined target volume. The technique allows delivery of a high dose to a circumscribed volume and with a steep dose gradient to surrounding normal tissue. Necrosis within the lesion is the primary aim of treatment, and the response depends on the pathobiological properties of the tumor itself. Due to the high geometric precision of this technique, necrosis of surrounding tissue is a rare event. Adjacent neural structures, however, may exhibit a tissue reaction on

imaging displaying features of edema, which requires supportive medication in some cases. The underlying principle of radiosurgery is the use of multiple beams of radiation focused on a single volume in space, adding the numerous small doses of the incident paths through the normal brain that converge on the tumor site.

The existing systems meet the requirements for a highly precise treatment delivery and basically consist of a stereotactic frame, a treatment planning system, and adequate imaging procedures. However, they may differ in various ways relating to localization of target volumes, geometric accuracy of dose delivery, accuracy of dose calculation, treatment-verification systems, and possibilities to compare alternative treatment plans. A stereotactic frame is fixed to the patient's skull, providing highly precise fiducial landmarks that allow stereotactic localization of the intracranial target. The frame is used to identify the target on MRI or CT, with respect to a specified xyz coordinate system. The defined relationship between the stereotactic coordinate system and the radiation source ensures accurate delivery of radiation dose to the target. The process of treatment planning consequently requires acquisition of accurate stereotactic images and reliable definition of target and critical normal CNS anatomy. A computerized simulation of the treatment plan is necessary to optimize the radiation beam configuration in order to conform the isodose surface to the target volume. Quality assurance tests are essential for highly accurate treatment delivery.

Linear accelerator-based systems

Linear accelerator-based radiosurgery techniques are based on the modification of standard linear accelerators with the addition of tertiary collimation and a stereotactic frame and involve rotations of the gantry. The McGill group used additionally simultaneous couch movements such that the exit doses did not overlap with the beam entrance.[52,53] The collimators in use have circular diameters ranging from 5 to 30 mm at the linear accelerator isocenter. The isocenter is the point of intersection between the gantry rotation axis and the rotation axis of the treatment couch. Ellipsoidal isodose surfaces can be obtained by computer-controlled arc rotation combined with different fixed gantry angles. The plane of the arcs is vertical, and the arcs are of equal angular distance from each other. Usually, a set of circular secondary collimators (cones) is used to produce small circular field sizes, which are defined by the diameter of the collimator. Unlike in the gamma knife, it is not necessary to use multiple isocenters for large spherical targets. Even targets with elliptical shapes can be treated with a single isocenter by carefully adjusting the field sizes, arcs, length, and planes. Irregularly shaped targets, however, might require multiple isocenter treatments. Dose prescription is usually at the 80 per cent isodose surface relative to the maximum dose. For a multiple isocenter treatment, the dose prescription is given to the highest isodose surface covering the target. The dose distribution throughout the target volume is therefore more homogeneous than in gamma knife treatments. Film techniques allow verification of all positioning adjustments after the coordinates of the isocenters are determined. The geometric precision of mechanical field alignment is 0.1–0.5 mm. In conjunction with an invasive rigid fixation system, radiosurgery achieves a high degree of precision and reproducibility at median deviations from the isocenter of 0.3 mm (Table 10.2).[54]

Gamma knife

A similar principle underlies the gamma knife as with the moving arcs in linear accelerator based radiosurgery. The gamma knife is a unit containing more than 200 independent static cobalt-60 sources, each oriented towards a defined isocenter at which the maximum dose is achieved. The radiation beam from each individual source is collimated, and all beams converge precisely to a common focal point or isocenter at the center of the spherical radiation unit. The diameter of the maximum dose area is determined by a helmet with special collimators focusing the incident beams. Interchangeable collimator helmets provide varying beam diameters between 4 and 18 mm in order to meet the requirements of an adequate coverage of target volume with an accuracy of 0.1 mm.

Clinical application

Preliminary data in several small series reveal low acute toxicity and promising results in recurrent tumors as well as in primary treatment. In a series of 22 children with recurrent localized CNS tumors, including ependymoma, astrocytoma, and medulloblastoma, and who received radiosurgery following prior conventional irradiation, 18 were free of progression at a median interval of nine months.[55] The feasibility of this approach was subsequently investigated in 14 patients with recurrent medulloblastoma and in seven patients with residual medulloblastoma after conventional irradiation of neuraxis. All patients are alive without evidence of disease, indicating that escalating the dose to the tumor might improve local control if part of primary treatment in conjunction with conventional radiation.[56,57] In contrast, six of 11 patients who were treated for recurrent disease have died of progressive tumor.[56] The predominant site of failure was distant within the CNS, and no child failed locally.

Grabb and colleagues investigated the role of radiosurgery in a series of 25 children with astrocytomas, ependymomas, and malignant gliomas.[58] Eleven children had received fractionated irradiation before stereotactic radiosurgery. With a median follow-up of 21

months, 11 of the 13 children with benign glial neoplasms had tumor control with stereotactic radiosurgery alone, and all of them have remained alive. In the series of Ganz and colleagues, eight tumors in seven patients were treated with gamma-knife radiosurgery.[59] A complete remission on imaging could be obtained in one child, four showed a reduction in size, and three were stable at a mean follow-up of 21 months. No acute toxicity was reported. These results could be confirmed in nine patients treated by Somaza and colleauges.[60] The dose was 15 Gy, and the progression-free survival was 100 per cent at a median follow-up of 19 months. When deciding on radiosurgery, it should be considered that the tissue around the tumor might bear microscopic disease due to infiltrating tumor. This area at risk receives an inadequate dosage, and a relevant incidence of short-term recurrent disease arising from undertreated tumor cells cannot be excluded. Whether stereotactic radiation therapy with either of the latter techniques will add substantially to disease control and preserve neurologic function remains to be established and should be part of future investigations.

Fractionated stereotactic convergence therapy

Fractionated stereotactic convergence radiotherapy is a new modality that combines the accurate focal dose delivery of stereotactic radiosurgery with the biological advantages of conventional radiation therapy (Figure 10.8 and Plate 15). The modality requires sophisticated treatment planning, a dedicated high-energy linear accelerator, and a relocatable immobilization device assuring precise treatment (Table 10.2). However, this technique is limited to tumors of less than 5 cm in diameter of spheroid configuration. Dunbar and colleagues treated 33 children with different tumors comprising craniopharyngiomas, meningiomas, pilocytic astrocytomas, and retinoblastomas.[61] In 25 per cent of patients, a reduction of tumor volume of more than 50 per cent could be obtained; the other 75 per cent of cases showed stable disease. A multiple-fraction program of linear accelerator radiosurgery using 6.3–7.5-Gy fractions on alternate days, adding up to 37.8 or 45.5 Gy in two weeks, was reported from the McGill group in 15 patients, including several children, who were treated at recurrence or primary presentation of astrocytoma, craniopharyngioma, or chordoma.[60] Early results have been excellent. Freeman and colleagues reported on ten patients with previously untreated primary brain tumors and who were managed with stereotactic hypofractionated convergence radiotherapy.[53] Five of them had grade 1 or grade 2 astrocytoma. The total dose ranged between 36.0 and 43 Gy at a median dose of 42 Gy, given in six or seven fractions. Clinical and radiological improvement was achieved in all patients, and an almost complete remission was achieved in two patients at a follow-up of between five and 47 months. In the subsequent series

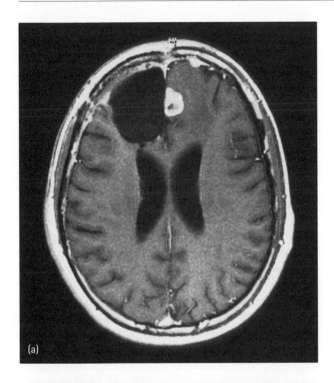

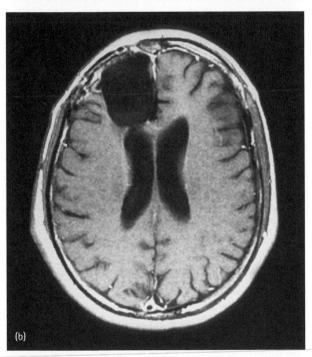

Figure 10.8a,b *Hypofractionated convergent beam radiotherapy in recurrent malignant glioma. (a) In a 17-year old boy, a localized glioblastoma recurrent in the left frontal region one year after conventional fractionated irradiation (total dose 60 Gy) is displayed on a gadolinium-enhanced T1-weighted magnetic resonance image. Hypofractionated radiotherapy (4 × 5 Gy, total dose 20 Gy) using a convergence technique was applied using a relocatable base plate. (b) One year later, the tumor was in continuous complete remission. However, disease recurred in the spinal canal.*

of Benk and colleagues from the same institution, the outcome in 14 children was evaluated.[62] The median total dose given to the 90 per cent isodose line around the visible tumor was 39 Gy, with a range between 18 and 24 Gy given in 3–10-Gy fractions once every other day. The mean biological effective dose was 57.6 Gy (given in 2-Gy fractions). The actuarial five-year overall survival rate was 100 per cent and the progression-free survival was 60 per cent at a median follow-up of 42 months. The investigators concluded that hypofractionated stereotactic radiotherapy is a valid option for non-resectable tumors in children, and it is becoming standard treatment for exploiting differences in the response to irradiation between tumor and normal tissue. As in radiosurgery, further investigations are warranted to assess the role of this approach.

Frameless stereotactic radiosurgery

The frameless stereotactic technique comprises an image-guided robotic system, including computer-assisted treatment planning, real-time imaging, and delivery components, all integrated by a powerful computer system. This system avoids the shortcomings of external frame fixation, which often limits the application of arcs. Moreover, fixation to the skull causes discomfort in children and can be problematic if fractionated radiotherapy is intended. In frameless stereotactic radiosurgery, two X-ray imaging devices are positioned on either side of the patient's head and acquire real-time radiographs of the skull at repeated intervals during treatment. These images are compared automatically with the digitally reconstructed radiographs obtained from the treatment planning system. This process allows a precise comparison of treatment position and adjustment of the coordinate system. In case of patient movement, changes in field positioning are detected automatically, and the beam arrangement is realigned with the target. However, no clinical experience has been reported using this system for childhood brain tumors.

Proton therapy

Proton therapy has been used for more than 40 years but only in very few institutions worldwide. It is now being used increasingly, and it has entered routine practice for some tumor types. The major advantage of proton therapy over conventional radiation techniques is the high degree of dose conformity around the tumor that can be achieved, since protons have no exit dose beyond the target. The incident monoenergetic beam of charged particles provides a dose distribution characterized by a precise range and a dose built-up effect called the Bragg peak near the end of the range. The range and distance of the particles depend on the energy and the physical characteristics of the absorbing tissue. These two factors allow a modification of the length of travel path and the distance of the maximum dose relative to surface. Proton radiation dose is normally expressed as cobalt Gray equivalent, which employs a relative biologic effectiveness factor of 1.1 for protons versus cobalt-60. Therefore, the distal edge of the Bragg peak can be placed in any given position in tissue by a specific range-modulation process. The energy of the emerging particles from the accelerator can be changed, or material can be inserted into the path of the beam before entering the patient; the energy of some of the particles will be absorbed by this material, reducing their range in tissue. An additional modification of the range is the spreading out of the Bragg peak. The dose distribution can be lengthened by an addition of different successive beams with Bragg peaks of progressively shorter ranges, thereby adding the peaks to a plateau. Additionally, collimators and multiple intersecting beams are able to create an individualized dose distribution. Combining collimators and proton beams with decreasing energy, the incident portal can be scanned throughout the target volume to achieve a homogeneous dose distribution from the proximal to the distal tumor edges.

This physical dose distribution has been used to treat adult patients with chordomas of the base of the skull. These tumors are generally difficult to irradiate because of their close proximity to the brainstem. In a report from the Massachusetts General Hospital, actuarial local control rates for 115 adult patients with base-of-skull chordomas treated between 1978 and 1993 with doses around 70 cobalt Gray equivalent (CGE; calculation to a biologically equivalent dose factor using cobalt-60) were 59 per cent at five years and 44 per cent at ten years.[63]

Treatment of base-of-skull and cervical spine chordomas in children has also been shown to be safe and effective.[64] Eighteen children aged between four and 18 years were treated at the Massachusetts General Hospital and Harvard Medical School with a mixed-photon/160-MeV proton (80 per cent proton contribution) 69 CGE. With a median follow-up of 72 months, the five-year actuarial survival was 68 per cent and disease-free survival was 63 per cent. Long-term effects were acceptable. Two children developed growth hormone deficiency, three children developed impaired hearing, and one required surgical excision of an area of temporal necrosis that had resulted in epilepsy.

Additionally charged particle beams have minimal lateral scatter, producing markedly more sharp edges compared with photon beams. An advantage of proton therapy over photon therapy in irradiation of the spinal canal has been suggested by Miralbell and colleagues.[65] Dosimetric studies revealed that the proportions of the vertebral body volume receiving more than 50 per cent of the prescribed dose were 100 per cent in 6-MV photons and only 20 per cent in protons. For 6-MV photons, more than 60 per cent of the dose prescribed to the target was delivered to 44 per cent of the heart volume, while proton beams were able to completely avoid the heart. When comparing the dose distribution with electrons, however, no definitive advantage can be seen.

McAllister and colleagues suggested that proton therapy can significantly reduce treatment-related morbidity.[66] The cohort of 28 children, however, was very heterogeneous, and although treatment-related morbidity was found to be low, the results were not convincing. Miralbell and colleagues performed dosimetric studies in whole-brain irradiation for protons and photons.[67] In their analysis, proton beams succeeded better in reducing the dose to the brain hemispheres. In a model to predict normal tissue complication probabilities for IQ deficits, proton therapy revealed only a slight advantage over photon beams (2.5 per cent as calculated to the normal healthy population IQ values). Children between the ages of four and eight years benefited most from the dose reduction, suggesting that modulated proton beams may help to reduce the irradiation of normal brain while optimally treating all meningeal sites.

Brachytherapy

Interstitial brachytherapy, although a new method in the management of childhood brain tumors, has gained importance, particularly for low-grade glioma. Brachytherapy represents a different treatment modality for a selected patient population. It is suited for children with unifocal, circumscribed tumors, with a diameter of less than 4 cm, in any location. As in external stereotactic radiotherapy, the main advantage of brachytherapy is the ability to give a high dose to a well-circumscribed tumor volume with minimal dose to neighboring normal tissue.

The ionizing irradiation is most commonly produced by iodine-125 seeds. Image-guided stereotactic implantation of the seeds and a three-dimensional calculation of isodose distribution is a prerequisite to obtaining a precise and reproducible treatment. Normal brain tissue and tumor display characteristic morphological changes when exposed to irradiation with respect to the typical dose distributions. Due to the high local dose, a circumscribed area of radionecrosis is a constant feature that spreads from the center of the implant to the periphery within weeks. Beyond the necrotic area, normal tissue potentially infiltrated by tumor cells receives a non-necrotizing dose. It is hypothesized that programmed cell arrest or death is induced. The volume of the area of necrosis and response to irradiation depends on the total dose, the dose rate, and the energy of the radioactive source. Treatment outcome is therefore a combination of tumor cell death, including necrotic changes and stable tumor or shrinkage in the periphery. The radioactive source may disturb the capillary physiology of the normal surrounding tissue, leading to acute and late effects. A temporary increase in capillary permeability may occur possibly causing extensive oedema accompanied by a reduced regional cerebral blood flow.[68] Increased intracranial pressure may occur, and steroid medication may be necessary to control symptoms.

The largest series of interstitial radiosurgery in childhood and adult low-grade glioma was published by Kreth and colleagues.[69] A total of 455 patients with low-grade glioma were treated using I-125 either as permanent or temporary implants. The seeds had a low activity, emitting X-rays at an energy of 27–35 keV. A reference dose of 60–100 Gy calculated at the outer rim of the tumor was applied. The specific dose rate factor was 1.32 Gy/hour/mCi at 1 cm. Permanent implants were performed in 261 (57.4 per cent) patients; temporary implants were performed in 194 patients (42.6 per cent). A complete to major response was obtained in 135 of 455 patients, while a partial to minor response was observed in 96 patients, 1.5 years after initial radiosurgery. The five- and ten-year survival rates in 97 patients with pilocytic astrocytoma were 85 and 83 per cent, respectively; in patients with WHO grade II astrocytomas (250 patients), the rates were 61 and 51 per cent, respectively. Of 455 patients, 124 were children and adolescents, 54 had a WHO grade II glioma, and 70 had a pilocytic astrocytoma. A five-year survival of 84 per cent was obtained in astrocytoma WHO II, while that for pilocytic astrocytoma was 90 per cent.

Scerrati and colleagues also used either 192-Ir or 125-I sources as permanent or temporary implant.[70] A mean peripheral dose of 89.7 Gy for permanent implants and 42.8 Gy for the temporary implants was administered in 36 patients (two pilocytic astrocytoma, 23 astrocytoma, 11 oligodendroglioma). The survival estimates were 83 per cent at five years and 39 per cent at ten years.

In the absence of properly controlled clinical trials, it is impossible to define the best treatment concept for every patient. Whether large but circumscribed tumors should be treated preferably with surgery, conventional radiotherapy, or stereotactic radiotherapy remains unclear. There is a necessity for a more detailed analysis of retrospective data for better evaluation of currently available treatment modalities, especially in the absence of prospective randomized studies. No studies have concentrated on survival time after therapy in relation to quality of life, complications, and invasiveness of therapy. In high-grade glioma, the results are dismal. In one series, all patients died between five and 36 months after implantation.[71]

Limited volume radiotherapy

Modern treatment techniques using rigid head fixations and three-dimensional treatment-planning open up the possibility to improve local tumor control in limited volume irradiation. It is a fast developing area in radiation therapy and comprises high local doses ("radiosurgery" and brachytherapy) and fractionated dose prescriptions, including various techniques:

- *Radiosurgery*: high local single dose (linear accelerator-based systems/ "gamma knife").
- *Fractionated convergence therapy*: linear, accelerator-based systems using a relocatable frame for head-fixation.
- *Fractionated conformal radiotherapy*: multiple, static, non-coplanar fields using a rigid, relocatable, head-fixation.
- *Proton therapy*: fractionated radiotherapy with a high degree of dose conformity to target (few institutions worldwide).
- *Brachytherapy*: stereotactically implanted radioactive sources (iodine-125 seeds).

Fractionated conformal radiotherapy in conjunction with modern dose calculations such as IMRT will further improve local tumor control and reduce the risk of side effects.

Quality assurance

Recent advances in radiation therapy have opened up new possibilities for integration of radiotherapy in the therapeutic plan for tumors of the CNS, but the superior performance of modern equipment cannot be exploited fully unless a high degree of accuracy and reliability in dose delivery is achieved. This in turn leads to strong demands on quality assurance and quality control for all of the steps between treatment planning and end of treatment delivery. Quality assurance in radiotherapy of tumors of the CNS is required to guarantee an optimal and adequate treatment by means of quality-control procedures and is becoming an integral component of prospective controlled trials.[72,73]

DEFINITION

Quality assurance in radiotherapy has been defined by the WHO and comprises all those procedures that ensure consistency of the medical prescription and the safe fulfillment of that prescription as regards dose to the target volume, dose to normal tissue, minimal exposure of personnel, and adequate patient monitoring aimed at determining the end result of treatment. Quality control comprises the regulatory process through which the actual quality performance is measured, compared with existing standards and finally the actions necessary to keep or regain conformance with the standards. In general, radiation therapy of CNS tumors includes additional specific safeguards.

RECOMMENDATIONS FOR QUALITY ASSURANCE AND QUALITY CONTROL

Quality assurance and quality control programs should be based on both radiation physics and clinical assessment. There are already some recommendations on general quality standards for radiotherapy, including the irradiation of CNS tumors.[74] It is necessary that these recommendations should be considered for future cooperative trials. In addition, quality control procedures should meet the appropriate standards agreed and adopted by all centers treating children with brain tumors.

ACCURACY OF TREATMENT

The process of treatment planning and delivery can be subdivided into many steps that are closely interrelated. The application of a specific treatment technique comprises specially designed treatment-planning systems, designing individualized treatment portals and field alignments in the majority of patients. The definition of target volumes (GTV, CTV, PTV) should be done according to the ICRU 50/62 rules. Dose prescription/specification should be according to the ICRU 50/62 rules.[19]

Immobilization devices

The reproducibility and geometric precision of field alignment depend strongly on the immobilization obtained by individual facemasks or other fixation systems.

The geometric precision that can be achieved for different treatment techniques and immobilization devices is summarized in Table 10.2 and must be considered when selecting the adequate treatment technique and

---

Immobilization devices

Immobilization devices include:

- stereotactic frame for radiosurgery;
- relocatable bite-block systems attached to a stereotactic frame;
- rigid facemask (cast material) for three-dimensional fractionated conformal radiation therapy;
- thermoplastic facemask for whole-brain irradiation;
- cast material and vacuum pillows for craniospinal irradiation.

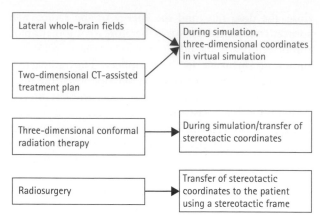

Figure 10.9 *Transfer of treatment plan. The process to transfer the intended plan to the patient is chosen according to the treatment technique applied.*

when deciding on the safety margins for the definition of the planning target volume.

Transfer of treatment plan

The transfer of a treatment plan requires an adequate technique to avoid localization errors that might potentially lead to a systematic miss of the target volume, which in turn might cause an underdosage of the tumor and an overdosage to normal tissue (Figure 10.9).

Treatment delivery

The accuracy of field alignment during treatment delivery is determined by the immobilization device, treatment technique, mechanical inaccuracies of treatment machine and couch, movement of the patient, and the technician positioning the portals before delivery of treatment. It is reflected by random, statistical fluctuations of treatment portals within a limited range.

Quality control procedures

For all steps between treatment planning and delivery, it is necessary to use control procedures to ensure a reliable treatment regarding the geometric precision and dosimetry. It is necessary to record the corresponding data.

Methods for reproducing geometric precision

Methods for reproducing geometric precision include:

- verification films;
- repeated CT examinations;
- newer techniques;
- repeated simulations;
- online (portal) imaging.

The factors shown in Figure 10.10 have an impact on geometric precision and are interrelated closely.

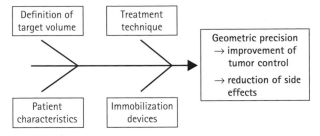

Figure 10.10 *Schema for the radiotherapy planning process.*

REPRODUCIBILITY OF TREATMENT/RECORDING OF DATA

Parameters specific for each patient as well as data regarding radiation therapy should be recorded to achieve a reproducible treatment. With these data, it must be possible to reconstruct the whole process of treatment planning and delivery by an external institution.

Minimal requirements for recording data

The minimal requirements for recording data are:

- definition of target volume;
- radiation protocols;
- dose prescription/specification;
- immobilization devices;
- treatment technique (i.e. computer-assisted treatment plans);
- control procedures/documentation.

That is, imaging should include simulation films of treatment portals, repeated CT examinations, verification films, instant pictures of patient positioning, and field alignment.

The increasing complexity of irradiation techniques in the treatment of CNS malignancies mandates the use of formalized systems and comprehensive quality assurance programs that cover the complete radiotherapy process. As all steps in the process of treatment planning and delivery are interlinked closely, possible errors introduced at one step impact on the quality of the radiotherapy and on the outcome in terms of tumor control and possible side effects.

Quality assurance

This is a comprehensive system to guarantee a precise, reliable, and reproducible treatment not only for one particular patient but for all treatments performed in the radiotherapy institution. It aims to achieve a high-quality level of radiation therapy for all institutions worldwide.

THE FUTURE

In the past five to ten years, there have been important developments in the planning and delivery of radiotherapy. These have come about as a consequence of the rapid development of computing technology. However, it is important that advances in radiotherapy planning should be accompanied by concurrent improvements in treatment accuracy and immobilization. New therapeutic modalities such as IMRT are likely to further improve the conformity of the treated volume to the clinical target volume, which should hopefully lead to reduced normal tissue morbidity. It is important that the benefits from the introduction of these technologies should be assessed critically. Proton therapy has potential advantages, but the relative lack of access in most countries will remain a challenge. There has been a trend towards the automatic delay or attempted avoidance of radiotherapy for children with CNS tumors, often leading to a poor outcome. It is likely that in the twenty-first century we will see a reappraisal of the role of radiotherapy in the management of children with brain tumors, with rational use of this important modality, with the aim of achieving the maximum therapeutic ratio.

REFERENCES

1 Cushing H. Experiences with cerebellar astrocytoma. A critical review. *Acta Pathol Microbiol Scand* 1930; **7**:1–86.

2 Paterson E, Farr RF. Cerebellar medulloblastoma: treatment by radiation of the whole central nervous system. *Acta Radiol* 1953; **39**:323–336.

3 Bloom HJ, Glees J, Bell J, Ashley SE, Gorman C. The treatment and long-term prognosis of children with intracranial tumors: a study of 610 cases, 1950–1981. [Published erratum appears in *Int J Radiat Oncol Biol Phys* 1990; **19**:829.] *Int J Radiat Oncol Biol Phys* 1990; **18**:723–45.

4 Prados MD, Wara WM, Edwards MHB, Cogen PH. Hyperfractioned craniospinal radiation for primitive neuroectodermal tumors; early results of a pilot study. *Int J Radiat Oncol Biol Phys* 1993; **28**:431–8.

5 Prados MD, Edwards MSB, Chang SM, *et al.* Hyperfractionated craniospinal radiation therapy for primitive neuroectodermal tumors: results of a phase II study. *Int J Radiat Oncol Biol Phys* 1999; **43**:279–85.

6 Allen JC, Donahue B, DaRosso R, Nierenberg A. Hyperfractionated craniospinal radiotherapy and adjuvant chemotherapy for children with newly diagnosed medulloblastoma and other primitive neuroectodermal tumors. *Int J Radiat Oncol Biol Phys* 1996; **30**:1155–61.

7 Marymont MH, Geohas J, Tomita T, Strauss L, Brand WN, Mittal BB. Hyperfractionated craniospinal radiation in medulloblastoma. *Pediatr Neurosurg* 1996; **24**:178–84.

8 Halperin EC, Friedman HS, Schold SC, Jr, *et al.* Surgery, hyperfractionated craniospinal irradiation, and adjuvant chemotherapy in the management of supratentorial

embryonal neuroepithelial neoplasms in children. *Surg Neurol* 1993; **40**:278–83.

9   Ricardi U, Besenzon L, Cordero di Montezomolo L, *et al.* Low dose hyperfractionated craniospinal radiation therapy for childhood cerebellar medulloblastoma: early results of a phase I/II study. *Eur J Cancer* 1997; **33**:911.

10 Needle MN, Goldwein JW, Grass J, *et al.* Adjuvant chemotherapy for the treatment of intracranial ependymoma of childhood. *Cancer* 1997; **80**:341–7.

11 Kovnar E, Curran W, Tomita T, *et al.* Hyperfractionated irradiation for childhood ependymoma: early results of a phase III Pediatric Oncology Group study. *VIIth Symposium. Pediatr Neurooncol* 1997; **33**:268.

12 Freeman CR, Krischer JP, Sanford RA, *et al.* Final results of a study of escalating doses of hyperfractionated radiotherapy in brain stem tumors in children: a Pediatric Oncology Group Study. *Int J Radiat Oncol Biol Phys* 1993; **27**:197–206.

13 Packer RJ, Boyett JM, Zimmerman RA, *et al.* Outcome of children with brain stem gliomas after treatment with 7800 cGy of hyperfractionated radiotherapy. A Children's Cancer Group phase I/II trial. *Cancer* 1994; **74**:1827–34.

14 Mandell LR, Kadota R, Freeman C, *et al.* There is no role for hyperfractionated radiotherapy in the management of children with newly diagnosed diffuse intrinsic brainstem tumors: results of a Pediatric Oncology Group phase III trial comparing conventional vs. hyperfractionated radiotherapy. *Int J Radiat Oncol Biol Phys* 1999; **43**:959–64.

15 Oakhill A (ed), *The Supportive Care of the Child with Cancer.* Bristol: IOP Publishing, 1988.

16 Tweed J, NHS for children to see major shake up. *Nursery World* July 2001; 4.

17 Rades D, Munte S, Baumann R, Karstens JH, Piepenbrock S, Leuwer M. Avoiding tracheal intubation in children during craniospinal irradiation. *Paediatr Anaesth* 2001; **11**:629–32.

18 Kortmann RD, Kuhl J, Timmermann B, *et al.* Postoperative neoadjuvant chemotherapy before radiotherapy as compared to immediate radiotherapy followed by maintenance chemotherapy in the treatment of medulloblastoma in childhood: results of the German prospective randomized trial HIT '91. *Int J Radiat Oncol Biol Phys* 2000; **46**:269–79.

19 International Commission on Radiation Units and Measurements. Report 50/62. Dose specification for reporting external beam therapy with photons and electrons. Bethesda, MD: International Commission on Radiation Units and Measurements, 1993.

20 Cardinale RM, Benedict SH, Wu Q, Zwicker RD, Gaballa HE, Mohan R. A comparison of three stereotactic radiotherapy techniques: ARCS vs. noncoplanar fixed fields vs. intensity modulation. *Int J Radiat Oncol Biol Phys* 1998; **42**:431–6.

21 Fraass BA, Kessler ML, McShan DL, *et al.* Optimization and clinical use of multisegment intensity-modulated radiation therapy for high-dose conformal therapy. *Semin Radiat Oncol* 1999; **9**:60–77.

22 Khoo VS, Oldham M, Adams EJ, Bedford JL, Webb S, Brada M. Comparison of intensity-modulated tomotherapy with stereotactically guided conformal radiotherapy for brain tumors. *Int J Radiat Oncol Biol Phys* 1999; **45**:415–25.

23 Benedict SH, Cardinale RM, Wu Q, Zwicker RD, Broaddus WC, Mohan R. Intensity-modulated stereotactic radiosurgery using dynamic micro-multileaf collimation. *Int J Radiat Oncol Biol Phys* 2001; **50**:751–8.

24 Kortmann RD, Hess CF, Hoffmann W, Jany R, Bamberg M. Is the standardized helmet technique adequate for irradiation of the brain and the cranial meninges? *Int J Radiat Oncol Biol Phys* 1995; **32**:241–4.

25 Jereb B, Krishnaswami S, Reid A, Rajender KA. Radiation for medulloblastoma adjusted to prevent recurrence to the cribriform plate region. *Cancer* 1984; **54**:602–4.

26 Packer RJ, Goldwein HS, Nicholson LG, Vezina JC, Allen MD, Ris K. Treatment of children with medulloblastomas with reduced-dose craniospinal radiation therapy and adjuvant chemotherapy: a Children's Cancer Group study. *J Clin Oncol* 1999; **17**:2127–36.

27 Packer RJ, Sutton LN, Goldwein JW, *et al.* Improved survival with the use of adjuvant chemotherapy in the treatment of medulloblastoma. *J Neurosurg* 1991; **74**:433–40.

28 Carrie C, Alapetite C, Mere P, Aimard L. Quality control of radiotherapeutic treatment of medulloblastoma in a multicentric study. The contribution of radiotherapy technique to tumour relapse. The Fench Medulloblastoma Group. *Radiother Oncol* 1992; **24**:77–81.

29 Carrie C, Hoffstetter S, Gomez F, *et al.* Impact of targeting deviations on outcome in medulloblastoma: study of the French Society of Pediatric Oncology (SFOP). *Int J Radiat Oncol Biol Phys* 1999; **45**:435–9.

30 Mah K, Danjoux CE, Manship S, Makhani N, Cardoso M, Sixel KE. Computed tomographic simulation of craniospinal fields in pediatric patients: improved treatment accuracy and patient comfort. *Int J Radiat Oncol Biol Phys* 1998; **41**:997–1003.

31 Halperin EC. Concerning the inferior portion of the spinal radiotherapy field for malignancies that disseminate via the cerebrospinal fluid. *Int J Radiat Oncol Biol Phys* 1993; **26**:357–62.

32 Scharf CB, Paulino AC, Goldberg KN. Determination of the inferior border of the thecal sac using magnetic resonance imaging: implications on radiation therapy treatment planning. *Int J Radiat Oncol Biol Phys* 1998; **41**:621–4.

33 Li C, Muller Runkel R, Vijayakumar S, Myrianthopoulos LC, Kuchnir FT. Craniospinal axis irradiation: an improved electron technique for irradiation of the spinal axis. *Br J Radiol* 1994; **67**:186–93.

34 Roback DM, Johnson JM, Khan FM, Engeler GP, McGuire WA. The use of tertiary collimation for spinal irradiation with extended SSD electron fields. *Int J Radiat Oncol Biol Phys* 1997; **37**:1187–92.

35 Gaspar LE, Dawson DJ, Tilley Gulliford SA, Banerjee P. Medulloblastoma: long-term follow-up of patients treated with electron irradiation of the spinal field. *Radiology* 1991; **180**:867–70.

36 Bamberg M, Schmitt G, Quast U. Therapie und Prognose des Medulloblastoms, Fortschritte durch neuartige Bestrahlungstechniken. *Strahlentherapie* 1980; **156**:1–17.

37 Sohn JW, Schell MC, Dass KK, Suh JH, Tefft M. Uniform irradiation of the craniospinal axis with a penumbra modifier and an asymmetric collimator. *Int J Radiat Oncol Biol Phys* 1994; **29**:187–90.

38 Tatcher M, Glicksman AS. Field matching considerations in craniospinal irradiation. *Int J Radiat Oncol Biol Phys* 1989; **17**:865–9.

39 Tinkler SD, Lucraft HH. Are moving junctions in craniospinal irradiation for medulloblastoma really necessary? *Br J Radiol* 1995; **68**:736–9.

40 Verellen D, Van den Heuvel F, De Neve W, De Beukeleer M, Storme G. Dynamic radiotherapy: interactive movement of patient couch for treatment of craniospinal axis. *Int J Radiat Oncol Biol Phys* 1996; **35**:771–7.

41 Kortmann RD, Timmermann B, Kuhl J, *et al*. HIT '91 (prospective, co-operative study for the treatment of malignant brain tumors in childhood): accuracy and acute toxicity of the irradiation of the craniospinal axis – results of the quality assurance program. *Strahlentherapie und Onkologie* 1999; **175**:162–9.

42 Tenhunen M, Usenius T, Lahtinen T. Irradiation of the whole neuraxis. A method for field positioning. *Acta Oncol* 1994; **33**:661–5.

43 Paulino AC, Narayana A, Mohideen MN, Jeswani S. Posterior fossa boost in medulloblastoma: an analysis of dose to surrounding structures using 3-dimensional (conformal) radiotherapy. *Int J Radiat Oncol Biol Phys* 2000; **46**:281–6.

44 Tomita T, McLone DG. Spontaneous seeding of medulloblastoma: results of cerebrospinal fluid cytology and arachnoid biopsy from the cisterna magna. *Neurosurgery* 1983; **12**:265–7.

45 Fukunaga Johnson N, Lee JH, Sandler HM, Robertson P, McNeil E, Goldwein JW. Patterns of failure following treatment for medulloblastoma: is it necessary to treat the entire posterior fossa? *Int J Radiat Oncol Biol Phys* 1998; **42**:143–6.

46 Rottinger EM, Bailey CC, Bamberg M. Treatment of medulloblastoma – dependence of outcome on quality of radiotherapy. *Radiother Oncol* 1994; **32**:138.

47 Kortmann RD, Hess CF, Jany R, Bamberg M. Repeated CT examinations in limited volume irradiation of brain tumors: quantitative analysis of individualized (CT-based) treatment plans. *Radiother Oncol* 1994; **30**:171–4.

48 Kortmann RD, Timmermann B, Becker G, Kuhl J, Bamberg M. Advances in treatment techniques and time/dose schedules in external radiation therapy of brain tumours in childhood. *Klin Padiatr* 1998; **210**:220–6.

49 Linstadt DE, Wara WM, Leibel SA, Gutin PH, Wilson CB, Sheline GE. Postoperative radiotherapy of primary spinal cord tumors. *Int J Radiat Oncol Biol Phys* 1989; **16**:1397–403.

50 Thornton AF, Jr, Sandler HM, Ten Haken RK, *et al*. The clinical utility of magnetic resonance imaging in 3-dimensional treatment planning of brain neoplasms. *Int J Radiat Oncol Biol Phys* 1992; **24**:767–75.

51 Debus J, Kocagoncu KO, Hoss A, Wenz F, Wannenmacher M. Fractionated stereotactic radiotherapy (FSRT) for optic glioma. *Int J Radiat Oncol Biol Phys* 1999; **44**:243–8.

52 Podgorsak EB, Olivier A, Pla M, Lefebvre PY, Hazel J. Dynamic stereotactic radiosurgery. *Int J Radiat Oncol Biol Phys* 1988; **14**:115–26.

53 Freeman CR, Souhami L, Caron JL, *et al*. Stereotactic external beam irradiation in previously untreated brain tumors in children and adolescents. *Med Pediatr Oncol* 1994; **22**:173–80.

54 Becker G, Major J, Christ G, Duffner F, Bamberg M. Stereotaxic convergent-beam irradiation. Initial experiences with the SRS 200 system. *Strahlenther Onkol* 1996; **172**:9–18.

55 Loeffler JS, Neozi L, Kooy HM. Results of radiosurgery in the management of recurrent pediatric brain tumors. *Harvard Medical School Continuing Education Course* 1990; Boston.

56 Patrice SJ, Tarbell NJ, Goumnerova LC, Shrieve DC, Black PM, Loeffler JS. Results of radiosurgery in the management of recurrent and residual medulloblastoma. *Pediatr Neurosurg* 1995; **22**:197–203.

57 Woo C, Stea B, Lulu B, Hamilton A, Cassady JR. The use of stereotactic radiosurgical boost in the treatment of medulloblastomas. *Int J Radiat Oncol Biol Phys* 1997; **37**:761–4.

58 Grabb PA, Lunsford LD, Albright AL, Kondziolka D, Flickinger JC. Stereotactic radiosurgery for glial neoplasms of childhood. *Neurosurgery* 1996; **38**:696–701.

59 Ganz JC, Smievoll AI, Thorsen F. Radiosurgical treatment of gliomas of the diencephalon. *Acta Neurochir Suppl (Wien)* 1994; **62**:62–6.

60 Souhami L, Olivier A, Podgorsak EB, Villemure JG, Pla M, Sadikot AF. Fractionated stereotactic radiation therapy for intracranial tumors. *Cancer* 1991; **68**:2101–8.

61 Dunbar SF, Tarbell NJ, Kooy HM, *et al*. Stereotactic radiotherapy for pediatric and adult brain tumors: preliminary report. *Int J Radiat Oncol Biol Phys* 1994; **30**:531–9.

62 Benk V, Bouhnik H, Raquin MA, Kalifa C, Habrand JL. Quality control of low dose craniospinal irradiation for low risk medulloblastoma. *Br J Radiol* 1995; **68**:1009–13.

63 Terahara A, Niemierko A, Goitein M, *et al*. Analysis of the relationship between tumor dose inhomogeneity and local control in patients with skull base chordoma. *Int J Radiat Oncol Biol Phys* 1999; **45**:351–8.

64 Benk V, Liebsch NJ, Munzenrider JE, Efird J, McManus P, Suit H. Base of skull and cervical spine chordomas in children treated by high-dose irradiation. *Int J Radiat Oncol Biol Phys* 1995; **31**:577–81.

65 Miralbell R, Lomax A, Russo M. Potential role of proton therapy in the treatment of pediatric medulloblastoma/primitive neuro-ectodermal tumors: spinal theca irradiation. *Int J Radiat Oncol Biol Phys* 1997; **38**:805–11.

66 McAllister B, Archambeau JO, Nguyen MC, *et al*. Proton therapy for pediatric cranial tumors: preliminary report on treatment and disease-related morbidities. *Int J Radiat Oncol Biol Phys* 1997; **39**:455–60.

67 Miralbell R, Bleher A, Huguenin P, *et al*. Pediatric medulloblastoma: radiation treatment technique and patterns of failure. *Int J Radiat Oncol Biol Phys* 1997; **37**:523–9.

68 Kreth FW, Faist M, Rossner R, Birg W, Volk B, Ostertag CB. The risk of interstitial radiotherapy of low-grade gliomas. *Radiother Oncol* 1997; **43**:253–60.

69 Kreth FW, Faist M, Warnke PC, Rossner R, Volk B, Ostertag CB. Interstitial radiosurgery of low-grade gliomas. *J Neurosurg* 1995; **82**:418–29.

70 Scerrati M, Montemaggi P, Iacoangeli M, *et al*. Interstitial brachytherapy for low-grade cerebral gliomas: analysis of results in a series of 36 cases. *Acta Neurochir* 1994; **131**: 97–105.

71 25. Healey EA, Shamberger RC, Grier HE, Loeffler JS, Tarbell NJ. A 10-year experience of pediatric brachytherapy. *Int J Radiat Oncol Biol Phys* 1995; **32**:451–5.

72 Kortmann RD, Kuhl J, Timmermann B, *et al.* Postoperative neoadjuvant chemotherapy before radiotherapy as compared to immediate radiotherapy followed by maintenance chemotherapy in the treatment of medulloblastoma in childhood: results of the German prospective randomized trial HIT '91. *Int J Radiat Oncol Biol Phys* 2000; **46**:269–79.

73 EORTC Brain Tumor Group, Guidelines for Quality Assurance. www.eortc.be

74 Thwaites D, Scalliet P, Leer JW, Overgaard J. Quality assurance in radiotherapy. European Society for Therapeutic Radiology and Oncology Advisory Report to the Commission of the European Union for the "Europe Against Cancer Programme". *Radiother Oncol* 1995; **35**:61–73.

75 Warrington AP, Laing RW, Brada M. Quality assurance in fractionated stereotactic radiotherapy. *Radiother Oncol* 1994; **30**:239–46.

76 Grabenbauer GG, Beck JD, Erhardt J, *et al.* Postoperative radiotherapy of medulloblastoma: impact of radiation quality on treatment outcome. *Am J Clin Oncol* 1996; **19**:73–7.

11

Neuropsychological outcome

MAUREEN DENNIS, BRENDA J. SPIEGLER, DARIA RIVA AND DAUNE L. MACGREGOR

INTRODUCTION

Injury to the immature brain alters neurocognitive outcome by affecting the level of intellectual, academic, neuropsychological, and psychosocial function. Brain injury affects the entire trajectory of development. Some skills are lost, and the rate of new development is altered. Understanding the outcome of children who have been treated for a brain tumor involves four questions: (i) What are the important outcome domains? (ii) What are the factors that shape or predict outcome? (iii) When should outcome be evaluated within the trajectory of development? (iv) Can pharmacologic or behavioral interventions ameliorate the long-term cognitive effects of brain tumors and their treatment?

In this chapter, we will use these questions to focus a review of neurocognitive outcome after childhood brain tumors, and we will explore their implications for predicting outcome. We will consider how biological, developmental, and reserve factors influence outcome in cognitive, academic, neuropsychological, and psychosocial domains, and how these relations are expressed at different time points after diagnosis (Figure 11.1).

OUTCOME DOMAINS

Outcome after childhood brain tumors involves multiple domains of function. *Physical* outcome refers to whether the child's height, weight, fatigue tolerance, endurance, and motor performance are normal for age. *Cognitive-academic* outcome is usually measured by a standard intelligence test and by assessment of academic skill attainments. *Neuropsychological* outcome refers to capacities such as psychomotor speed, attention, and memory, as well as to functions such as language and visual perception. *Psychosocial* outcome refers to an individual's ability to function in the social world of family, school, and community. *Quality-of-life* outcome, incorporating all these factors, focuses on the individual's life satisfaction. Measures of quality of life may involve global indices[1] and measures relevant specifically to pediatric cancer.[2,3]

Intelligence

Intelligence, the most frequent outcome measure in the pediatric oncology literature, has been related to age at treatment[4–7] and time since treatment.[4,6] It has also been related to treatment with cranial radiation[5,7–10] and/or chemotherapy.[11]

In the study of IQ in children with brain tumors, two measurement issues are important. First, changes in the form of the IQ test to accommodate a child's increasing age affect the analyses of data in longitudinal outcome studies.[12] Second, short-form IQ tests are sometimes used to estimate IQ;[13,14] while their suitability in normal populations has been established,[15] it is unclear how well short-form IQ tests estimate cognitive ability in children with brain tumors.

Academic and vocational outcomes

Children treated for brain tumors often have less than favorable academic and vocational outcomes. Two-thirds

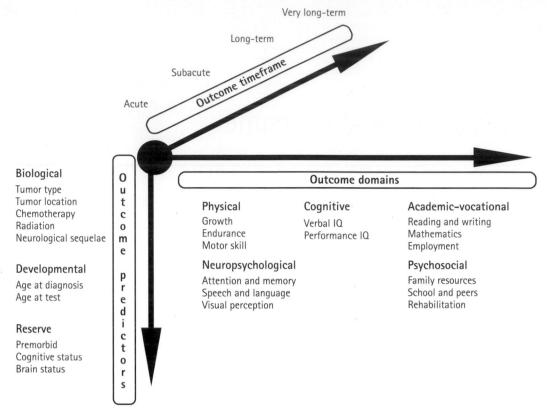

Figure 11.1 *Outcome algorithm for childhood brain tumors.*

of children with diverse types of brain tumor require special education for learning disability.[16] Reading and spelling achievement in medulloblastoma survivors is lower than that of their siblings.[17]

Vocational outcome after childhood brain tumors is often limited. Only one-quarter of adult survivors of childhood brain tumors radiated before the age of four years have post-secondary education, and one-third have never been employed.[18]

Neuropsychological outcome

MEMORY AND ATTENTION

Memory and attention deficits are often described as part of the cognitive morbidity of childhood brain tumors.[19] Children with diverse tumor types show problems in memory[20,21] and attention.[22] Impairment in several forms of memory and attention has been described in children with treated brain tumors:

- *Explicit memory*, which requires the conscious retrospective recall of previously stored information.[5,20,23]
- *Implicit memory*, in which past experiences and exposures to events influence present memory without awareness or voluntary control.[19]

- *Working memory*, in which information is maintained online while new, incoming information is processed.[19]

Memory and attention deficits are functionally significant. Explicit memory is important for the short- and long-term recall of information and for the new learning required for successful academic and vocational function. Implicit memory is a mechanism for learning without conscious attention. Working memory is important for the successful performance of many cognitive and academic tasks, including reading comprehension and mathematics. Deficits in the memory and attention domain limit the ability to learn new information and prevent the effective utilization and activation of previous learning. Attention and memory deficits limit the amount of available knowledge; a limited information base, in turn, makes it more difficult to accrue new knowledge, and thus the rate of new learning is impaired further.

SPEECH AND LANGUAGE

Brain tumors in children may produce speech and language disturbances[24] that can range from difficulties with speech production, articulation, and phonation, to problems with word-finding and difficulty in understanding language at the level of text and discourse. These deficits may involve oral language, written language, or both.

Language deficits disrupt not only academic function in language-based skills such as reading, writing, and spelling, but also social communication involving the pragmatic understanding of literal, inferential, and non-literal language.

PREDICTORS OF OUTCOME

At least three factors predict neurocognitive outcome after childhood brain tumors. One set of factors is *biological*, which concern the tumor type and location, the physiological effects of adjuvant treatment such as chemotherapy and cranial radiation, and the short- and long-term neurological sequelae associated with tumor location or treatment. A second set of factors is *developmental*, which concern the chronological age and developmental stage of the child, referenced both to the age at diagnosis and treatment and to the age at outcome evaluation. A third set of factors involves *reserve*, including prediagnosis cognitive and psychosocial resources, as well as post-diagnosis resources in the child, family, school, and community.

Because children with brain tumors are not a homogeneous group, variability in outcome is not random and can be related to aspects of biology, development, and reserve. Outcome is often determined multiply. For example, a biologically aggressive tumor treated with radiation (biological factor) in a very young child (developmental factor) will certainly have a notably adverse outcome in multiple domains.

Biological factors

Biological factors include tumor localization and lateralization (Table 11.1), tumor treatment, and neurological sequelae such as hydrocephalus and epilepsy.

Table 11.1 *Anatomical factors predicting outcome*

Site and interactions	Key impairment
Cortical v. subcortical damage	Greater IQ loss with cortical damage
White matter damage	Cognitive, processing speed and other deficits
Frontal lobes	Motor speech, articulation, and executive dysfunction
Posterior cortical	
Lateralization	Limited information available
Temporal lobe	Memory
Midline tumors	Memory and behavior
Infratentorial tumors	Memory, attention, cognition, language, timing and behavior

TUMOR LOCALIZATION AND LATERALIZATION

Cortical versus subcortical tumors

In the absence of adjuvant treatments, which add to the cognitive morbidities of childhood brain tumors, cortical tumors are generally associated with lower IQs compared with subcortical and posterior fossa tumors.[7,8] Language deficits vary by tumor localization and lateralization. For tumors above the tentorium, the relations between language symptoms and side and site of tumor are sometimes similar to those reported for adults. Right-handed children with tumors localized in the left hemisphere show two different types of aphasia: those with lesions in the pre- or peri-rolandic areas exhibit a non-fluent type of aphasia, while those with temporal-parietal tumors have a fluent type of aphasia.[25]

White–matter tumors

Tumor localization in the white matter (whether the primary lesion site or a secondary result of radiation or chemotherapy therapy) disturbs complex information transmission between different brain regions, with functional deficits in response consistency and processing speed. Damage to the white matter is associated with impairments of non-verbal intelligence, fluency, and executive function.[26]

Frontal lobe tumors

Frontal lobe tumors produce patterns of deficits related to intra-regional localization.[25] Childhood tumors involving Broca's area cause a syndrome characterized by phonetic-articulatory deficits and agrammatism, whereas tumors of the prefrontal areas produce deficits, including executive dysfunction, and problems in motor programming. These impairments are also associated with changes in personality and self-awareness.

Posterior cortical tumors

Evidence for a relation between tumor lateralization and related neuropsychological functions is scant for posterior cortical tumors. In one study, a girl with a left occipital tumor showed difficulty recognizing details of figures; in another, children with right posterior tumors showed difficulties recognizing the global pattern of visual stimuli.[27]

Temporal lobe tumors

Children with temporal lobe tumors demonstrate memory deficits.[28] The modality of the memory disorder is not always related to the lateralization of the tumor,[29,30] as it tends to be in adults. A broader pattern of neuropsychological dysfunction may be seen in children with temporal lobe tumors, a pattern associated with inadequate seizure control, postoperative complications, tumor recurrence, and younger age at diagnosis.[30]

Midline tumors

Children with tumors in the sellar or suprasellar regions, or in the chiasmatic or hypothalamic regions, often show significant neurocognitive problems at diagnosis[31] and postoperatively. Memory impairment is common, even in the absence of generalized intellectual impairment.[32] Half of a group of children treated surgically for craniopharyngioma had memory impairment.[23] Changes in social-emotional behavior can be quite prominent,[33] and may include perseveration and aggressive behavior.[34,35] The reported behavioral changes may reflect altered reciprocal connections between the frontal lobes and the limbic system and hypothalamus.[36,37]

Infratentorial tumors

Neurobehavioral outcome after cerebellar tumors varies with lateralization. Children with left cerebellar hemisphere tumors have been reported to show impairment in nonverbal functions, while children with tumors in the right cerebellar hemisphere show a decline in verbal skills.[38,39] In contrast, a recent study of 100 children treated surgically for cerebellar astrocytomas reported no differences in intellectual, academic, and adaptive outcome as a function of tumor location or lateralization within the cerebellum.[40]

Memory and attention deficits are common after tumors of the posterior fossa. Significant deficits in auditory verbal memory were evident in half of a sample of children treated with radiotherapy for posterior fossa or third ventricle tumors.[5] Children with posterior fossa tumors have attention deficits,[41] which may arise because of the proximity of the cerebellum to the brainstem ascending activating system, which, together with thalamic and cortical mechanisms, modulates arousal, alertness, and attention.[36]

Posterior fossa tumors are associated with language deficits,[24] including impairments in oral expression and auditory comprehension.[42,43]

Recent evidence has implicated the cerebellum, in particular the lateral cerebellum, in the perception of durations in the hundreds of milliseconds range, and in the cognitive timing of motor output,[44–48] which also includes speech. Survivors of childhood posterior fossa tumors have difficulties with timing; specifically, they show deficits in short-duration (about 400 ms) perception, regardless of the pathology or treatment of the tumor.[49]

Intellectual, neuropsychological, and academic difficulties have been identified in children with posterior fossa tumors, in both the short and the long term.[50,51] Academic failure occurs frequently in survivors of posterior fossa tumors, and the rate is higher in survivors of medulloblastoma than in survivors of cerebellar astrocytomas.[52,53]

TUMOR TREATMENT (Table 11.2)

Surgery

Factors related to surgical intervention apply to all types of operable tumors, benign and malignant. New

Table 11.2 *Treatment-related injury*

Treatment	Nature of injury
Surgery	Removal, section, or traction of nerve tissue
Radiation	Damage to vascular endothelium, demyelination. Effects are progressive, dose-related, and related to fields of treatment
Chemotherapy	
IV	Limited evidence of functional toxicity
RT + IV	Cerebral calcification, vascular damage, demyelination, multifocal white matter
RT + IT ± IV	Further enhanced neurotoxicity

IT, intrathecal; IV, intravenous; RT, radiotherapy.

microsurgical techniques facilitate the selective removal of tumor tissue, as do computer-guided techniques (neuronavigation).[54] Longitudinal studies of patients undergoing initial surgery show that cognitive and neuropsychological performances remain stable and may even improve slightly after surgery, before further interventions.[8]

Particular surgical approaches may be associated with selective neuropsychological deficits. Approaches involving the prolonged retraction of the frontal lobes to reach tumors of the optic chiasm, hypothalamus, or third ventricle may cause complex behavioral and mental deficits consistent with damage to the orbital frontal area. Partial sectioning of the corpus callosum to remove tumors of the third ventricle causes minor disconnection syndromes,[55] in keeping with the reported functional effects of callosal agenesis.[56]

Radiotherapy

External conventional radiotherapy is known to be associated with severe neuropsychological and intellectual deterioration. The mechanism is thought to involve a progressive vascular and demyelinating neuropathology, beginning after the end of treatment, reaching a peak over the next few years, and then maintaining a persisting but less steep decline.[57] Disordered hippocampal neurogenesis may also be involved[58]. The concomitant cognitive impairment is related inversely to age of treatment[5,59] and related directly to the dose and field of cerebral radiation.[60,61] Attempts to adjust radiation dose on the basis of age or tumor recurrence risk have not fully eliminated the cognitive deficits;[57,62] hyperfractionation of the radiation dose reduces but does not eliminate them.[25]

New radiotherapeutic techniques hold promise for improved long-term neurocognitive outcome. *Stereotactic radiotherapy* techniques can now deliver a precise dose of radiation to a predetermined target volume. *Brachytherapy* involves stereotactic implantation of a radioactive seed-containing isotope designed to deliver a radiation dose to a very localized field around the tumor bed.[63] Some preliminary evidence exists about the effects of these new, focused techniques on neurocognitive outcome. Children treated with stereotactic radiotherapy or brachytherapy for low-grade glioma have shown no deterioration in intelligence, attention, memory, language, or visuospatial functions over a five-year follow-up period; deficits are limited to those present before treatment and are related to tumor site.[25] Further study of the long-term outcome of these treatments is required, especially as they have not been in widespread use until very recently.

Chemotherapy

The role of intravenous chemotherapy in intellectual loss and neurocognitive impairment in children treated for brain tumors is still a matter of active investigation, in part because few children can be treated with chemotherapy without concomitant cranial radiation. Because of the known neurotoxicity associated with cranial radiation in young children, efforts have been made to delay the use of cranial radiation in infants with brain tumors, at least until their third birthday. A positive developmental outcome has been reported in very young children treated with chemotherapy only;[64,65] here, cognitive declines over time were minimal on a range of cognitive, academic, and neuropsychological outcomes, and scores tended to remain within normal limits.

The use of intrathecal chemotherapy, particularly methotrexate, can be associated with significant cognitive morbidity,[66] and the risk is greater when intrathecal methotrexate is used in association with radiotherapy.[67] Studies in children treated for medulloblastoma are rare but support the finding that using radiotherapy in association with intrathecal methotrexate may have particularly severe effects on cognitive development.[68] Recent studies have suggested that in very young children treated for leukemia, intrathecal methotrexate might affect the structure and function of the neocerebellar-frontal subsystem.[69]

Some studies have compared treatments across different types of cancer diagnoses. In a comparison of children with a variety of diagnoses and who received intrathecal methotrexate plus radiotherapy, or intrathecal methotrexate only, or intravenous methotrexate only, significant neuropsychological deficits were documented in the group who received radiotherapy, most of whom also had intrathecal methotrexate.[70] A recent study of children with medulloblastoma compared treatment with intraventricular methotrexate plus radiotherapy versus intraventricular methotrexate alone, radiotherapy alone, and neither treatment. Neurocognitive deficits were associated with either form of treatment used alone, but the most impaired children were those who received the combined treatments.[71]

STRUCTURAL BRAIN DAMAGE

Both radiotherapy and intravenous chemotherapy induce vascular changes, cerebral calcifications, and demyelination.[72] The white matter areas involved most frequently are the centrum semiovale and periventricular areas, in which abnormalities tend to be multifocal and symmetrical.[73] More rarely, morphological changes are visible in cortical regions. At least in the treatment of leukemia, radiotherapy and intravenous chemotherapy seem to have synergistic effects when used in combination.[74] The most extreme form of central nervous system (CNS) neurotoxicity is radiation necrosis.[75] Progressive necrotizing leukoencephalopathy can occur when radiation and chemotherapy are used in combination. These forms of brain injury occur late and may be associated with progressive neurological deterioration, including focal signs, dementia, ataxia, spasticity, seizures, coma, and even death.

Some time-related cognitive deficits in children with brain tumors are related to progressive structural brain damage that is of a less extreme nature than radiation necrosis. Brain scans of children treated with cranial radiation for primary brain or skull-based tumors show generalized brain atrophy, calcifications in brain matter distant from the site of the primary tumor, and white matter abnormalities.[76] Abnormalities are more frequent in children under the age of three years at treatment. Serial neuroimaging has demonstrated an increasing number and size of lacunae within the white matter in a proportion of children whose brain tumors were treated with radiation, and children treated before five years of age were at higher risk for this neuropathology.[77] Although the IQs of the radiated patients as a group declined over time, there was no significant difference between the rate of IQ decline in the groups with and without lacunae on neuroimaging.

Progressive white matter damage has also been documented after cranial radiation for medulloblastoma.[14,78,79] The volume of normal-appearing white matter declines over time in children treated with craniospinal radiation for medulloblastoma. The rate of loss of normal-appearing white matter does not differ in younger versus older children, but the rate of loss is faster in children receiving a higher dose of craniospinal radiation.[14,78] Neurocognitive outcome after radiation treatment for a range of childhood cancers is related to white matter integrity.[80]

NEUROLOGICAL SEQUELAE

A full understanding of the neurocognitive outcome of the child treated for a brain tumor requires consideration of both the unique and the common neurological complications of treatment. In addition to the changes in motor and cognitive skills that may be related directly to tumor location and surgery, treatment with cranial radiation and/or chemotherapy may produce medical and neurocognitive late effects,[81] even extending into adult life.[82]

Somnolence

The somnolence syndrome, occurring in up to 60 per cent of children radiated for childhood brain tumors, involves symptoms of lethargy, anorexia, apathy, and headache, which may occur six to eight weeks after radiation and may last for 4–14 days.[57] The symptoms are transient and respond to increasing doses of prednisone or the use of daily steroids.

Hydrocephalus

Hydrocephalus is a significant complication of infratentorial brain tumors.[83] Up to one-third of children with posterior fossa tumors require shunts.[83] Hydrocephalus at the time of tumor treatment does not appear to affect outcome, in that there is no relation between IQ and either postoperative ventricular dilation[52] or non-emergent shunt placement.[84] The evidence for a relation between shunt history and outcome is mixed. One study reported that non-shunted tumor patients had higher IQ scores;[85] another reported that motor function, intelligence, and academic achievement were higher in shunted medulloblastoma survivors;[53] a third study reported that IQ was unaffected by treated hydrocephalus.[8] In studying the effect of hydrocephalus on outcome, age at tumor treatment should be considered: hydrocephalus appears to be more prevalent in children with an earlier age at tumor diagnosis; these also comprise the group with elevated rates of neurological and neuropsychological difficulties.[86]

Seizures

Seizures are a complication for as many as 25 per cent of children treated for brain tumors.[82] Mechanisms of epileptogenesis in brain tumors[87] are not understood fully, but they may involve either enhanced excitatory or attenuated inhibitory influences. Brain tumors may cause "denervation hypersensitivity." Concentrations of glutamate, an excitatory neurotransmitter associated with epilepsy, are known to be increased in gliomas.

Seizures associated with brain tumors[88] are more likely to be partial (simple or complex), but there is a recognized association with absence and generalized tonic clonic seizure types. Resection of the epileptogenic zone may be an appropriate initial treatment. Delays in cerebral tumor diagnosis in children presenting with intractable epilepsy – particularly in children who have non-focal neurological examinations – can be avoided by early investigation with magnetic resonance imaging (MRI).

Syndromes

Two syndromes (cerebellar mutism with subsequent dysarthria, cerebellar cognitive-affective syndrome) associated with childhood brain tumors have been studied in some detail, with respect to both clinical features and clinicopathological correlation. Both syndromes occur after posterior fossa tumors.

Cerebellar mutism with subsequent dysarthria

- A form of acquired aphasia, mutism with subsequent dysarthria (MSD), has been identified in children with posterior fossa tumors, who acutely or progressively lose previously acquired language skills.[89–94]
- Nearly all MSD patients are under ten years of age. The condition has been described in children as young as two years.[94]
- The syndrome is characterized by a complete but transient loss of speech resolving into a dysarthria that shares some of the features of adult dysarthria: imprecise consonants, articulatory breakdowns, prolonged phonemes, prolonged intervals, slow rate of speech, lack of volume control, harsh voice, pitch breaks, variable pitch, and explosive onset.[43,95] Improvement of the dysarthria to normal speech seems to be related to the recovery of complex movements of the mouth and tongue.[94]
- Mutism has been associated with posterior fossa tumors located in the midline or vermis of the cerebellum, and with tumors that invade both cerebellar hemispheres or the deep nuclei of the cerebellum.[92,93] However, incision of the vermis does not always produce MSD,[91] and some patients with MSD have had surgery that avoided the vermis.[96]
- Brainstem involvement is common in cases of MSD.[91] It has been proposed that isolated lesions in cerebellar structures are not sufficient to produce MSD, and that an additional ventricular location of the tumor and adherence to the dorsal brainstem are necessary, an idea supported by the frequent occurrence of pyramidal and eye-movement signs in children with MSD.[94] Localization of the brainstem dysfunction in MSD appears to be rostral to the medulla oblongata and caudal to the mesencephalon.[94] It has been proposed that the mutism of MSD is related to bilateral involvement of the dentate nuclei, and also that the subsequent dysarthric speech represents a recovering cerebellar mechanism.[97]
- Risk factors for MSD include midline location of the tumor combined with postoperative complications that involve destruction of the midline roof structures and penetration of the peduncles and/or lateral wall or ventricular floor parenchyma.[92] Other risk factors include

hydrocephalus at the time of tumor presentation, ventricular localization of the tumor, and postsurgical edema of the pontine tegmentum.[94]

- Long-term recovery of the dysarthria is incomplete. Very long-term survivors of childhood cerebellar tumors continue to show ataxic dysarthric features in their spontaneous speech.[98] Furthermore, tumor survivors with a history of MSD show more ataxic dysarthria than those without MSD at the time of tumor treatment.[99]

Cerebellar cognitive–affective syndrome

- In recent years, our understanding of the role of the cerebellum has been broadened from one of motor control to one of an essential node in the neural circuitry controlling higher-order cognitive processes.[100]
- In adults, cerebellar lesions produce cognitive and behavioral changes, termed the "cerebellar cognitive-affective syndrome," including executive dysfunction in planning, mental flexibility, and working memory, as well as personality changes, including affective blunting and disinhibition.[100]
- Aspects of the cerebellar cognitive-affective syndrome have been reported in children.[51,101,102] Childhood tumors of the cerebellar vermis are associated with affective dysregulation and complex alterations in social and communicative behavior involving autistic-like symptomatology.[38] Of interest, deficits in the regulation of affect are sometimes evident in children with cerebellar tumors treated with surgery but neither radiotherapy nor chemotherapy.[101]
- Cognitive-affective changes are more evident after lesions of the posterior lobe and vermis than after anterior lobe lesions; their putative neural substrate is a disruption of the cerebellar modulation of prefrontal, posterior parietal, superior temporal, and limbic regions.[100,103] The fact that a similar neuroanatomical basis exists in children is of interest, and it has been proposed that early lesions to the cerebellum produce a wide range of cognitive deficits, both immediately and later in development,[101] which is in keeping with the persistence of other functional cerebellar deficits in long-term survivors of posterior fossa tumors of childhood.[49,103]

Developmental factors

AGE AT DIAGNOSIS AND TREATMENT

An earlier age at diagnosis and treatment entails a greater risk than an older age for later neurocognitive impairment, especially for children with brain tumors that require adjuvant treatment.[6,105,106] Intellectual impairment is more frequent and more severe in younger radiated children compared with older radiated children.[5,17,107–110]

The effects of lesions to the developing brain are often studied through the analysis of age at diagnosis and treatment effects. Age at diagnosis and treatment is a marker, albeit imperfect, for both brain development (e.g. synaptic, myelogenic, neurogenic) and cognitive development (skills already mastered, skills yet to be mastered). While biological and cognitive aspects of development occur concurrently, their separate impact on outcome in children treated for brain tumors can be studied.

BRAIN DEVELOPMENT

In humans, fundamental cycles of brain development occur prenatally, although aspects of CNS development that are important for organizing and processing sensory input and for higher-level cognition continue through childhood and into adult life. For example, synaptic development, including synaptogenesis and pruning, occurs largely in the postnatal period.[111] As with many aspects of nervous system development, synaptogenesis begins in the sensory regions of the brain and progresses to the association areas or higher cortical regions. Myelogenesis, the coating of axons in a lipid and protein sheath, also occurs in a specific sequence or cycle over the course of pre- and postnatal development.[112] Glial cells, which continue to proliferate throughout the lifespan, produce myelin in a pattern of progressive encephalization, starting in the spinal cord prenatally and ending in the higher cortical association areas in mid-life.[111]

Cycles of brain development

Synaptic development:
- synaptogenesis
- synaptic pruning.

Myelogenesis:
- glial cell proliferation
- myelinization.

The protracted development of the brain has several implications for the outcome of childhood brain tumors. Because actively dividing cells are targeted by adjuvant treatments such as cranial radiation therapy, the most actively dividing cells at time of treatment are at greatest risk for damage. More generally, white matter is especially vulnerable to the late effects of cranial radiation because the glial cells that support the formation of myelin continue to grow and divide throughout life. If cells in the hippocampus continue to divide during childhood and adolescence, then deficits in new learning will be a common neurocognitive complaint, even in older children treated with cranial radiation.[58]

COGNITIVE DEVELOPMENT

See also Chapter 26.

The typical course of cognitive development is not linear, although new skills emerge in a predictable sequence and timeframe. Just as actively dividing cells are at greatest risk for damage by cranial radiation, skills and abilities in the most active stage of development are at greatest risk for impairment as a result of brain damage in childhood.

Cognitive deficits will vary according to the level of skill development, because emerging, developing, and established skills are differentially vulnerable to the effects of childhood brain damage.

Acquired brain injuries may disrupt the development of skills that are yet to be acquired or skills emerging at the time of injury. The infant or preschooler has few well-established cognitive skills. Brain damage early in life, when most skills are either emergent or developing, and few are firmly established, puts a child at highest risk for impairment in a wide range of cognitive skills and, indeed, for generalized cognitive impairment. Consistent with this model, a young age at diagnosis and treatment for brain tumors is especially debilitating in a broad range of cognitive functions.[105]

An insult to the brain before or during a particular time window in development may change the normal developmental trajectory of a skill that is meant to emerge at that time.[113] Different patterns of outcome for a skill domain have been related to the developmental time window within which skills develop. For example, children with acquired brain injury in the preschool years develop poorer reading decoding than do children with later injuries.[114] Recent research has begun to address these skill development questions and to study how age at diagnosis and treatment for childhood brain tumors is associated with specific deficit patterns in emerging skills.

AGE AT TEST

Cognitive outcome will vary depending on the age at which outcome is assessed. Some cognitive deficits are evident only at the point in development at which the requisite skills emerge and the brain actively begins to contribute to the development of a new behavior or strategy for solving a problem, a point that may be several years removed from tumor diagnosis. For example, deficient executive and organizational skills after early frontal lobe injury

may be a latent deficit, a late-emerging impairment that becomes fully apparent only in adolescent or adult life.

Cognitive reserve

The term "cognitive reserve" refers to the capacity for adaptive, efficient, and flexible problem-solving. It has been suggested that cognitive reserve may account for the variability in outcome that occurs despite similarities in disease states, type of treatment, and time since treatment.[114,115] The cognitive reserve hypothesis proposes that factors such as premorbid intelligence and/or educational attainment may buffer or exacerbate the effects of an acquired brain injury.

The cognitive reserve hypothesis finds considerable support in the adult aging literature. Increased cognitive reserve slows the emergence of mental deficits in neurodegenerative diseases.[116] In Alzheimer's disease, the presentation of dementing symptoms varies with the degree of cognitive reserve. Individuals with a high degree of cognitive reserve exhibit signs of dementing illness at a later stage in the disease process than do those with lesser cognitive reserve; however, a prior head injury depletes cognitive reserve, so that individuals with a history of head injury begin to show signs of dementia earlier, regardless of their premorbid intelligence.[116]

Individuals with childhood brain insults reach adulthood with diminished cognitive reserve, and it has been proposed that they may be vulnerable to accelerated cognitive decline in mid- to late adulthood.[117] Our understanding of the late neurocognitive effects of childhood brain tumors will be incomplete until we can follow the natural history of survivors into middle and old age. Studies of long-term survivors of childhood brain tumors are important not only in describing the natural history of the condition but also in identifying whether the tumor and its treatment are associated with an accelerated pattern of aging.

Genetic substrate

Within the overall pattern of impairments that are observed following treatment for brain tumors in childhood, there remains a range of severity that is not accounted for easily by the tumor factors of site, histological tumor type, etc., or the therapy given. On basic principles, it would seem probable that this range of responses has a genetic basis. There is thus a need for programs of laboratory and clinical research designed to investigate what genetic mechanisms drive this observation, the purpose being to identify individuals who are at greater or lesser risk of suffering more severe adverse sequelae from therapy, especially radiation therapy, and to explore possible interventions that might modify these responses. As one example, studies are needed of outcome in children treated for brain tumors who have pre-existing diagnoses of learning disability, attention deficit hyperactivity disorder, or family histories of these disorders. To date, such children have generally been excluded from group studies, but their pre-existing disorders, or underlying predisposition to such, may in fact put them at greater risk for poor outcome.

Psychosocial and environmental factors

Extrinsic influences modify how the damaged or undamaged CNS develops and help to shape how the child will respond to brain injury. Factors such as family adaptation, individual and family coping style, personality/temperament, and environmental demands can affect a child's recovery and behavioral status after brain injury.

Because the influence of psychosocial and environmental factors on outcome is difficult to assess, these factors have often been ignored. To some extent, however, they are more easily molded, adjusted, and changed than biological factors. Recent research suggests that psychosocial and environmental factors are important moderators that act to buffer or exacerbate the effects of biological factors in producing better or poorer outcome.

Behavioral and cognitive outcomes in children treated for brain tumors depend on both illness-related variables (e.g. neurological symptoms at presentation, treatment modalities) and family-related variables (e.g. coping, family stress, family cohesiveness). In a longitudinal study, the combination of family and illness variables best predicted cognitive outcomes, and inclusion of contextual factors (e.g. family stress, maternal coping) enhanced the prediction of behavioral, adaptive, and cognitive outcome in children with brain tumors.[118]

Longitudinal models have been developed that consider direct and secondary factors affecting outcome, mediators, and moderators of recovery. These methods have been applied with considerable effect to children with closed head injury.[119] Taylor and colleagues have demonstrated that a brain injury in childhood affects a child's post-injury behavior and adjustment both directly (via neuropathological mechanisms and emotional reactions to the injury and its aftermath) and indirectly (via effects on the family's response to the child post-injury). The influence of child and family is bidirectional. Brain injury in a child can have *direct* effects on family function via post-traumatic stress reactions and changes in family roles and routines, and *indirect* effects through changes in the child's behavior or adjustment that cause further disruption to family function. These effects are interrelated, i.e. there is a relation between a child's behavioral dysfunction at one point in time and subsequent suboptimal family function.

Cultural factors

Cultural variables also influence the outcome of childhood brain tumors. In some cultures, childhood cancer is not discussed openly, even within the family, with the result that children may be unaware of their own diagnosis and treatment history or may fail to receive the encouragement, extra support, or tutoring required to become literate and numerate members of society. In other families, survival alone may be considered sufficient success, and so minimal expectations may be placed on the child with a brain tumor. Such families may feel that it is unfair to push their child beyond the bare minimum, and they may be satisfied for their child to live at home, supported by other family members or by society.

Socioeconomic factors

Socioeconomic status has implications for family stress and coping, as well as direct financial implications for rehabilitation opportunities in many countries. Private schooling, individual tutoring, and special vocational programs may be precluded in some societies for families with insufficient resources. This factor may also be tied to the ability to access services and to negotiate a path though a complex health system.

OUTCOME TIMEFRAME

Outcome is the end result of the altered developmental trajectory. As such, it is important to measure it at a number of time points. Different conclusions may be reached if "outcome" is evaluated soon after diagnosis, in the subacute phase, in the long term, or in the very long term in mid- to late adulthood. An initial primary deficit may have effects over time on the development of higher level abilities so that, in the long term, the pattern of impairment may be broader or more diffuse than was earlier appreciated. Different conclusions will be reached depending on the point of reference in relation to time since diagnosis.

Time since diagnosis and treatment

In adults, a longer time since brain injury is usually related to enhanced recovery. In children, the positive association between time since injury and recovery may not hold.[117,120] An opposite relation may hold in some instances. With some forms of brain damage in childhood, a longer time since injury can be associated with declines in level of performance, e.g. verbal intelligence declines with time since diagnosis in survivors of childhood medulloblastoma, which suggests progressive failure to assimilate new knowledge at a developmentally appropriate rate.[50]

There are two explanations for the effect by which the magnitude of a developmental cognitive deficit increases with time since diagnosis. One has to do with structural changes to the brain (as discussed earlier) and the other is concerned with rate of development and new learning.

New skill acquisition

Following treatment for a brain tumor, the child's challenge is not only to regain lost motor and cognitive skills but also to maintain an age-appropriate rate of acquisition of new skills. When one or both of these tasks cannot be achieved, as is common in children with brain tumors, cognitive deficits become increasingly apparent over time.

Children treated with cranial radiation for brain tumors exhibit a slower than normal rate of new learning. While they continue to acquire new skills and knowledge over time, their rate of gain is slower than for age peers, with the result that age-related standard scores decline over time at a rate moderated by both age at treatment and dose of craniospinal radiaton.[13] The implication is that survivors of childhood brain tumor treated with cranial radiation show smaller deficits in relation to age peers in the first few years after diagnosis but become increasingly discrepant from peers over the course of development. As yet, it is unclear how long this progressive discrepancy continues to grow. These children may be limited, not only in their rate of cognitive development, but also in the final level attained.

Persisting deficits

Thus far, we have considered changes in the upward slope of growth and development during childhood and its relation to progressive brain damage and a slowed rate of development. Some deficits emerge at diagnosis or immediately after surgery and improve in the subacute phase. Even in the very long term, however, these deficits may not recover to age-expected levels. Huber-Okrainic and colleagues demonstrated that very long-term survivors (average survival time 11 years) of posterior fossa tumors, and who had transient cerebellar mutism in the postoperative period, continued to exhibit more ataxic dysarthric speech and a slower speech rate compared with tumor survivors without a history of transient cerebellar mutism and compared with healthy controls.[99] Furthermore, adult survivors of childhood posterior fossa tumors had not made the normal developmental advances from a childhood speech rate.[98]

Psychosocial factors

When psychosocial adaptation is studied in survivors of childhood cancer, children with the diagnosis of brain tumor are often excluded.[121–124] This is due in part to the fact that problems associated with the diagnosis and treatment of brain tumors directly affect social cognition and social adaptation. Children diagnosed recently with brain tumors exhibit problems in social competence and behavior.[125] Although behavior problems settle in the long term, problems with social competence persist.[126] Children treated previously for brain tumors are perceived as more socially isolated by teachers, peers, and self-report; furthermore, classmates perceive these children as sick, fatigued, and often absent from school.[127] In the long term, the quality of life of brain tumor survivors appears to be compromised.[128]

INTERVENTIONS

Until recently, the main goal of treatment-related research for childhood brain tumors has been to increase the rates of survival and ultimate cure. Drawing from research in the rehabilitation of another major form of acquired brain damage, traumatic brain injury, recent efforts have addressed long-term deficits either through pharmacological interventions or through behaviorally-based cognitive rehabilitation programs. Little is known about whether and how intervention can ameliorate the cognitive morbidity of brain tumors and their treatment.

Pharmacological interventions

Children with brain tumors have attention problems. Medication that has proven effective in children with primary attention deficit disorder has been studied in groups of childhood cancer survivors, including those with brain tumors. The stimulant medication methylphenidate (e.g. Ritalin™) has been reported to improve attention, behavior, and academic function in a mixed group of children, including some with brain tumors.[129] In another report, however, methylphenidate did not improve attention or memory.[130] A double-blind, placebo-controlled trial of methylphenidate in survivors of childhood leukemia or brain tumors documented significant drug-related improvements in attention but not impulsivity.[131]

Cognitive/behavioral rehabilitation

Only a few investigators have designed and implemented behavioral intervention or treatment programs to ameliorate the late neurocognitive deficits associated with childhood brain tumors and their treatment. Butler and colleagues[132,133] have designed a cognitive remediation program adapted from the Attention Process Training of Sohlberg and Mateer,[134] in which hierarchically graded materials were designed to address attention, perceptual, and non-verbal cognitive processes. In work with an individual therapist, each patient learned strategies for completely scanning materials, checking his or her own work, refraining from self-distracting activities, setting personal goals, and trying out new problem-solving strategies. The results, although currently only preliminary, are encouraging: 21 children who completed the program, but not waiting-list controls, showed statistically significant gains on measures of attention and concentration.

Conclusions

- The neurocognitive outcome of childhood brain tumors is determined by four broad categories of factors: biological, developmental, reserve, and intervention.
- Different outcome levels within a given outcome domain may be related to a variety of variables in distinct ways, e.g. age at tumor diagnosis and time since tumor treatment may each make distinct contributions to intellectual morbidity.[50]
- Outcome must also be referenced to the child's age and developmental stage at the times of diagnosis and/or treatment.
- More research is required to clarify how particular biological and tumor features shape outcome. Further information is needed about the natural history of particular tumor types and their treatments.
- Childhood brain tumors are associated with a range of neurological symptoms and conditions. Some of these have negative implications for neurocognitive outcome, although the specific contribution to outcome is often imperfectly understood.
- After treatment for a brain tumor, the child has the dual tasks of regaining lost skills at the same time as attempting to master new skills, which may explain in part why a younger age is commonly associated with a greater risk for neurocognitive deficits.

FUTURE DIRECTIONS

Toxicity of surgery

National and international therapeutic trials have characteristically collected extensive acute toxicity data regarding chemotherapy and radiation therapy, but there has been little or no attempt to collect prospective surgical toxicity data. This constitutes important missing information given the emerging prognostic importance of the extent of surgical resection in many intracranial tumors and the impact of early surgical toxicity on the delivery of adjuvant therapies. High-technology approaches are being employed increasingly and even routinely, but there are scant data to enable evaluation of their benefits. Furthermore, there is the possibility of exploiting interactions between chemotherapy and surgery in some situations to facilitate surgical resection. Future clinical studies should therefore include collection of datasets that will enable the analysis of the extent and causation of surgical toxicity.

Novel therapeutic approaches

The study of novel therapeutic approaches, whether they be methods of drug delivery (e.g. intracavitary chemotherapy), different radiation therapy schedules (e.g. hyperfractionation), or new physical agents (e.g. laser-induced hyperthermia), should include standardized assessments of the neurodevelopmental and neuropsychological sequelae.

- The study of neurocognitive outcomes in children with brain tumors can profitably use models of cognitive development in the design of outcome studies, and a developmental cognitive approach to the study of childhood brain tumors might enhance the ability to predict outcome in specific ways.
- The exploration of syndromes, such as the cerebellar cognitive affective syndrome, is likely to increase our understanding of some of the long-term effects of brain tumors unique to childhood.
- With respect to models of long-term follow-up, accurate evaluation of outcome after childhood brain tumors must involve multidisciplinary expertise to measure not only physical and cognitive late effects but also psychosocial and neuropsychological sequelae.
- In the long term, many children treated for brain tumors will reach adulthood, at which point they face a number of challenges. On a practical level, they will require follow-up from professionals who must be aware of their complex neurodevelopmental history in order to design complete and appropriate outcome evaluations.
- Models of long-term follow-up may require new categories of professional expertise as more children treated for brain tumors survive and age.[117]

- In the very long term, some survivors of childhood brain tumors may face unusual challenges, such as a head injury, as well as the normal challenges of aging. How they will meet these challenges in the face of diminished reserve is a question of both theoretical and practical significance. At present, little is known about treatments that might enhance biological resilience in the face of new brain insults, such as the abnormal one of a closed head injury or the normal one of aging. We also know little about the rate of cognitive changes with aging. In view of the diminished reserve that results from a treated childhood brain tumor, this issue is of considerable importance.
- The fact that neurocognitive outcome studies are beginning to ask these questions and to draw on a range of developmental methods bodes well for a fuller understanding and appreciation of the lifespan experience of children treated for brain tumors.

REFERENCES

1 Bradlyn AS, Harris CV, Warner JE, Ritchey AK, Zaboy K. An investigation of the validity of the Quality of Well-Being Scale with pediatric oncology patients. *Health Psychol* 1993; **12**:246–50.

2 Varni JW, Katz ER, Seid M, Quiggins DJL, Friedman-Bender A. The Pediatric Cancer Quality of Life Inventory-32 (PCQL-32). *Cancer* 1998; **82**:1184–96.

3 Goodwin DAJ, Boggs SR, Graham-Pole J. Development and validation of the Pediatric Oncology Quality of Life Scale. *Psychol Assess* 1994; **6**:321–8.

4 Duffner PK, Cohen ME, Parker MS. Prospective intellectual testing in children with brain tumors. *Ann Neurol* 1988; **23**:575–579.

5 Packer JR, Sutton LN, Atkins TE, *et al.* A prospective study of cognitive function in children receiving whole-brain radiotherapy and chemotherapy: 2-year results. *J Neurosurg* 1989; **70**:707–13.

6 Hoppe-Hirsch E, Renier D, Lellouch-Tubiana A, Sainte-Rose C, Pierre-Kahn A, Hirsch JF. Medulloblastoma in childhood: progressive intellectual deterioration. *Childs Nerv Syst* 1990; **6**:60–5.

7 Jannoun L, Bloom HJG. Long-term psychological effects in children treated for intracranial tumors. *Int J Radiat Oncol Biol Phys* 1990; **18**:747–53.

8 Ellenberg L, McComb JG, Siegel SE, Stowe S. Factors affecting intellectual outcome in pediatric brain tumor patients. *Neurosurgery* 1987; **21**:638–44.

9 LeBaron S, Zeltzer PM, Zeltzer LK, Scott SE, Marlin AE. Assessment of quality of survival in children with medulloblastoma and cerebellar astrocytoma. *Cancer* 1988; **62**:1215–22.

10 Reimers TS, Ehrenfels S, Mortensen EL, *et al.* Cognitive deficits in long-term survivors of childhood brain tumors: Identification of predictive factors. *Med Pediatr Oncol* 2003; **40**:26–34.

11 Copeland DR, Moore III BD, Francis DJ, Jaffe N, Culbert SJ. Neuropsychologic effects of chemotherapy on children with cancer: a longitudinal study. *J Clin Oncol* 1996; **14**:2826–35.

12 Mulhern RK, Ochs J, Fairclough D. Deterioration of intellect among children surviving leukemia: IQ test changes modify estimates of treatment toxicity. *J Consult Clin Psychol* 1992; **60**:477–80.

13 Palmer SL, Goloubeva O, Reddick WE, *et al.* Patterns of intellectual development among survivors of pediatric medulloblastoma: a longitudinal analysis. *J Clin Oncol* 2001; **19**:2302–8.

14 Mulhern RK, Palmer SL, Reddick WE, *et al.* Risks of young age for selected neurocognitive deficits in medulloblastoma are associated with white matter loss. *J Clin Oncol* 2001; **19**:472–9.

15 Sattler JM. *Assessment of Children. WISC-III and WPPSI-R Supplement.* San Diego: Sattler, 1992.

16 Kun LE, Mulhern RK. Neuropsychological function in children with brain tumors: II. Serial studies of intellect and time after treatment. *Am J Clin Oncol* 1983; **6**:651–6.

17 Silverman CL, Palkes H, Talent B, Kovnar E, Clouse JW, Thomas RM. Late effects of radiotherapy on patients with cerebellar medulloblastoma. *Cancer* 1984; **54**:825–9.

18 Jenkin D, Danjoux C, Greenberg M. Subsequent quality of life for children irradiated for a brain tumor before age four years. *Med Pediatr Oncol* 1998; **31**:506–11.

19 Dennis M, Hetherington CR, Spiegler BJ. Memory and attention after childhood brain tumors. *Med Pediatr Oncol Suppl* 1998; **1**:25–33.

20 Kun LE, Mulhern RK, Crisco JJ. Quality of life in children treated for brain tumors. Intellectual, emotional and academic function. *J Neurosurg* 1983; **58**:1–6.

21 George AP, Kuehn SM, Vassilyadi M, *et al.* Cognitive sequelae in children with posterior fossa tumors. *Pediatr Neurol* 2003; **28**:42–7.

22 Moore BD, Copeland DR, Ried H, Levy B. Neurophysiological basis of cognitive deficits in long-term survivors of childhood cancer. *Arch Neurol* 1992; **49**:809–17.

23 Hoffman HJ, De Silva M, Humphreys RP, Drake JM, Smith ML, Blaser SI. Aggressive surgical management of craniopharyngiomas in children. *J Neurosurg* 1992; **76**:47–52.

24 Hudson LJ. Speech and language disorders in childhood brain tumours. In: Murdoch BE (ed.). *Acquired Neurological Speech/ Language Disorders in Childhood.* London: Taylor & Francis, 1990, pp. 245–68.

25 Riva D. Criteri prognostici neuropsicologici per la scelta del trattamento dei tumori cerebrali infantili. Technical report of the Italian Ministry of Health. Milan: Italian Ministry of Health, 1995.

26 Filley CM. The behavioral neurology of cerebral white matter. *Neurology* 1998; **50**:1535–40.

27 Riva D, Milani N, Pantaleoni C. Defective analytical and synthetic visual perception in children with posterior lesions. Paper given at XI European Conference of the International Neuropsychological Society; Lathi, 1988.

28 Cavazzuti V, Winston K, Baker R, Welch K. Psychological changes following surgery for tumors in the temporal lobe. *J Neurosurg* 1980; **53**:618–26.

29 Carpentieri SC, Mulhern RK. Patterns of memory dysfunction among children surviving temporal lobe tumors. *Arch Clin Neuropsychol* 1993; **8**:345–57.

30 Mulhern RK, Kovnar EH, Kun LE, Crisco JJ, Williams JM. Psychologic and neurologic function following treatment for childhood temporal lobe astrocytoma. *J Child Neurol* 1988; **3**:47–52.

31 Fouladi M, Wallace D, Langston JW, *et al.* Survival and functional outcome of children with hypothalamic/chiasmatic tumors. *Cancer* 2003; **97**:1084–92.

32 Carpentieri SC, Waber DP, Scott RM, *et al.* Memory deficits among children with craniopharyngiomas. *Neurosurgery* 2001; **49**:1053–8.

33 Spiegler BJ, Williams S. Benign tumors in malignant locations: Behavioral and social/emotional morbidity associated with craniopharyngioma in children. *J Int Neuropsychol Soc* 2000; **6**:201.

34 Cavazzuti V, Fischer EG, Welch K, Belli JA, Winston KR. Neurological and psychophysiological sequelae following different treatments of cranopharyngioma in children. *J Neurosurg* 1983; **59**:409–17.

35 Riva D, Pantaleoni C, Devoti M, Saletti V, Nichelli F, Giorgi C. Late neuropsychological and behavioral outcome of children surgically treated for craniopharyngioma. *Childs Nerv Syst* 1998; **14**:179–84.

36 Brodal A. *Neurological Anatomy in Relation to Clinical Medicine*, 3rd edition. Oxford: Oxford University Press, 1969.

37 Kupferman I. Hypothalamus and limbic system and cerebral cortex: homeostasis and arousal. In: Kandel E, Schwartz JH (eds). *Principles of Neural Sciences.* Amsterdam: Elsevier, 1985, pp. 110–23.

38 Riva D, Giorgi C. The cerebellum contributes to higher functions during development. Evidence from a series of children surgically treated for posterior fossa tumours. *Brain* 2000; **123**:1051–61.

39 Scott RB, Stoodley CJ, Anslow P, *et al.* Lateralized cognitive deficits in children following cerebellar lesions. *Dev Med Child Neurol* 2001; **43**:685–91.

40 Beebe D, Ris M, Holmes E. Location may not affect IQ and adaptive outcome in pediatric cerebellar tumors. *J Int Neuropsychol Soc* 2002; **8**:293–4.

41 Riva D, Pantaleoni C, Milani N, Belani FF. Impairment of neuropsychological functions in children with medulloblastomas and astrocytomas in the posterior fossa. *Childs Nerv Syst* 1989; **5**:107–10.

42 Hudson LJ, Murdoch BE. Chronic language deficits in children treated for posterior fossa tumour. *Aphasiology* 1992; **6**:135–50.

43 Hudson LJ, Burdoch BE, Ozanne AE. Posterior fossa tumours in childhood: associated speech and language disorders post-surgery. *Aphasiology* 1989; **3**:1–18.

44 Ivry R. Cerebellar timing systems. *Int Rev Neurobiol* 1997; **41**:555–73.

45 Ivry RB, Keele SW. Timing functions of the cerebellum. *J Cogn Neurosci* 1988; **1**:136–50.

46 Ivry R, Keele S. Timing functions of the cerebellum. *J Cogn Neurosci* 1989; **1**:136–52.

47 Nichelli P, Alway D, Grafman J. Perceptual timing in cerebellar degeneration. *Neuropsychologia* 1996; **34**:863–71.

48 Penhune VB, Zattore RJ, Evans AC. Cerebellar contributions to motor timing: a PET study of auditory and visual rhythm reproduction. *J Cogn Neurosci* 1998; **10**:752–65.

49 Hetherington R, Dennis M, Spiegler B. Perception and estimation of time in long-term survivors of childhood posterior fossa tumors. *J Int Neuropsychol Soc* 2000; **6**:682–92.

50 Dennis M, Spiegler BJ, Hetherington CR, Greenberg ML. Neuropsychological sequelae of the treatment of children with medulloblastoma. *J Neuro-Oncol* 1996; **29**:91–101.

51 Steinlin M, Imfeld S, Zulauf P, *et al.* Neuropsychological long-term sequelae after posterior fossa tumour resection during childhood. *Brain* 2003; **126**:1998–2008.

52 Hirsch JF, Renier D, Czernichow P, Benveniste L, Pierre-Kahn A. Medulloblastoma in childhood. Survival and functional results. *Acta Neurochir* 1979; **48**:1–15.

53 Johnson DL, McCabe MA, Nicholson HS, *et al.* Quality of long-term survival in young children with medulloblastoma. *J Neurosurg* 1994; **80**:1004–10.

54 Giorgi C, Casolino SD, Franzini A, *et al.* Computer-assisted planning of stereotactic neurosurgical procedures. *Childs Nerv Syst* 1989; **5**:299–302.

55 Giorgi C, Riva D. Stereotactically guided transfrontal removal of intraventricular midline tumors in children. Neurosurgical and neuropsychological considerations. *J Neurosurg* 1994; **81**:374–80.

56 Aglioti S, Beltramello A, Tassinari G, Berlucchi G. Paradoxically greater interhemispheric transfer deficits in partial than complete callosal agenesis. *Neuropsychologia* 1998; **36**:1015–24.

57 Cohen ME, Duffner PK. *Brain Tumors in Children*, 2nd edition. New York: Raven Press, 1994.

58 Monje ML, Palmer T. Radiation injury and neurogenesis. *Curr Opin Neurol* 2003; **16**:129–34.

59 Eiser C. Intellectual abilities among survivors of childhood leukaemia as a function of CNS irradiation. *Arch Dis Child* 1978; **53**:391–5.

60 Mulhern RK, Horowitz ME, Kovnar EH, Langston J, Sanford RA, Kun LE. Neurodevelopmental status of infants and young children treated for brain tumors with preirradiation chemotherapy. *J Clin Oncol* 1989; **7**:1660–66.

61 Kieffer-Renaux V, Bulteau C, Grill J, *et al.* Patterns of neuropsychological deficits in children with medulloblastoma according to craniospatial irradiation doses. *Dev Med Child Neurol* 2000; **42**:741–5.

62 Ris D, Packer R, Goldwin J, *et al.* Intellectual outcome after reduced-dose radiation therapy plus adjuvant chemotherapy for medulloblastoma: a Children's Cancer Group Study. *J Clin Oncol* 2001; **19**:3470–6.

63 Bernstein M, Laperriere N, Leung P, McKenzie S. Interstitial brachytherapy for malignant brain tumors: preliminary results. *Neurosurgery* 1990; **26**:371–9, 379–80.

64 Copeland DR, deMoor C, Moore BDI, Ater JL. Neurocognitive development of children after cerebellar tumor in infancy: a longitudinal study. *J Clin Oncol* 1999; **17**:3476–86.

65 Moore BD, Ater JL, Copeland DR. Improved neuropsychological outcome in children with brain tumors diagnosed during infancy and treated without cranial radiation. *J Child Neurol* 1992; **7**:281–90.

66 Maria BL, Dennis M, Obonsawin M. Severe permanent encephalopathy in acute lymphoblastic leukemia. *Can J Neurol Sci* 1993; **20**:199–205.

67 Bleyer WA, Poplack DG. Prophylaxis and treatment of leukemia in the central nervous system and other sanctuaries. *Semin Oncol* 1985; **12**:131–48.

68 Riva D, Giorgi C, Nichelli F, *et al.* Intrathecal methotrexate affects higher functions in children with medulloblastoma. *Neurology* 2002; **59**:48–53.

69 Lesnik PG, Ciesielski KT, Hart BL, Benzel EC, Sanders JA. Evidence for cerebellar-frontal system changes in children treated with intrathecal chemotherapy for leukemia. *Arch Neurol* 1998; **55**:1561–8.

70 Butler RW, Hill JM, Steinherz PG, Meyers PA, Finlay JL. Neuropsychologic effects of cranial irradiation, intrathecal methotrexate, and systemic methotrexate in childhood cancer. *J Clin Oncol* 1994; **12**:2621–9.

71 Ottensmeier H, Kuhl J. Pilot Trial HIT-SKK'87/HIT-SKK'92: a retrospective neuropsychological study in children less than 3 years of age with medulloblastoma. Paper given at IX International Symposium of Pediatric Neuro-Oncology; San Francisco; 2000.

72 De Reuck J, vander Eecken H. The anatomy of the late radiation encephalopathy. *Eur Neurol* 1975; **13**:481–94.

73 Lee YY, Nauert C, Glass JP. Treatment-related white matter changes in cancer patients. *Cancer* 1986; **57**:1473–82.

74 Waber DP, Tarbell NJ, Fairclough D, *et al.* Cognitive sequelae of treatment in childhood acute lymphoblastic leukemia: cranial radiation requires an accomplice. *J Clin Oncol* 1995; **13**:2490–96.

75 Maria BL, Menkes JH. Tumors of the nervous system. In: Menkes JH, Sarnat HB (eds). *Child Neurology*, 6th edition. Philadelphia: Lippincott, Williams & Wilkins, 2000, pp. 787–858.

76 Davis PC, Hoffman JC, Pearl GS, Braun IF. CT evaluation of effects of cranial radiation therapy in children. *Am J Neuroradiol* 1986; **7**:639–44.

77 Fouladi M, Langston J, Mulhern R, *et al.* Silent lacunar lesions detected by magnetic resonance imaging of children with brain tumors: a late sequelae of therapy. *J Clin Oncol* 2000; **18**:824–31.

78 Mulhern RK, Reddick WE, Palmer SL, *et al.* Neurocognitive deficits in medulloblastoma survivors and white matter loss. *Ann Neurol* 1999; **46**:834–41.

79 Reddick WE, Russell JM, Glass JO, *et al.* Subtle white matter volume differences in children treated for medulloblastoma with conventional or reduced dose craniospinal irradiation. *Magn Reson Imaging* 2000; **18**:787–93.

80 Reddick WE, White HA, Glass JO, *et al.* Developmental model relating white matter volume to neurocognitive deficits in pediatric brain tumor survivors. *Cancer* 2003; **97**: 2512–9.

81 Anderson DM, Rennie KM, Ziegler RS, *et al.* Medical and neurocognitive late effects among survivors of childhood central nervous system tumors. *Cancer* 2001; **92**:2709–19.

82 Packer RJ, Gurney JG, Punyko JA, *et al.* Long-term neurologic and neurosensory sequelae in adult survivors of a childhood brain tumor: childhood cancer survivor study. *J Clin Oncol* 2003; **21**:3255–61.

83 Raimondi AJ, Tomita T. Hydrocephalus and infratentorial tumors. Incidence, clinical picture, and treatment. *J Neurosurg* 1981; **55**:174–82.

84 Kao GD, Goldwein JW, Schultz DJ, Radcliffe J, Sutton L, Lange B. The impact of perioperative factors on subsequent intelligence quotient deficits in children treated for medulloblastoma/posterior fossa primitive neuroectodermal tumors. *Cancer* 1994; **74**:965–71.

85 Packer RJ, Sposto R, Atkins TE, *et al.* Quality of life in children with primitive neuroectodermal tumors (medulloblastoma) of the posterior fossa. *Pediatr Neurosci* 1987; **13**:169–75.

86 Chapman CA, Waber DP, Bernstein JH, *et al.* Neurobehavioral and neurologic outcome in long-term survivors of posterior fossa brain tumors: role of age and perioperative factors. *J Clin Oncol* 1995; **10**:209–12.

87 Patel H, Garg BP, Salanova V. Tumor-related epilepsy in children. *J Child Neurol* 2001; **16**:141–5.

88 Kim SK, Wang KC, Cho BK. Intractable seizures associated with brain tumor in childhood: lesionectomy and seizure outcome. *Childs Nerv Syst* 1995; **11**:634–8.

89 Di Cataldo A, Dollo C, Astuto M, *et al.* Mutism after surgical removal of a cerebellar tumor: two case reports. *Pediatr Hematol Oncol* 2001; **18**:117–21.

90 Dailey AT, McKhann GM, 2nd, Berger MS. The pathophysiology of oral pharyngeal apraxia and mutism following posterior fossa tumor resection in children. *J Neurosurg* 1995; **83**:467–75.

91 Doxey D, Bruce D, Sklar F, Swift D, Shapiro K. Posterior fossa syndrome: identifiable risk factors and irreversible complications. *Pediatr Neurosurg* 1999; **31**:131–6.

92 Humphreys RP. Mutism after posterior fossa surgery. *Concepts Pediatr Neurosurg* 1989; **9**:57–64.

93 Rekate HL, Grubb RL, Aram DM, Hahn JF, Ratcheson RA. Muteness of cerebellar origin. *Arch Neurol* 1985; **42**:697–8.

94 Van Dongen HR, Catsman-Berrevoets CE, van Mourik M. The syndrome of 'cerebellar' mutism and subsequent dysarthria. *Neurology* 1994; **44**:2040–6.

95 Van Mourik M, Catsman-Berrevoets CE, Yousef-Bak E, Paquier PF, van Dongen HR. Dysarthria in children with cerebellar or brainstem tumors. *Pediatr Neurol* 1998; **18**:411–14.

96 Siffert J, Allen JC. Late effects of therapy of thalamic and hypothalamic tumors in childhood: Vascular, neurobehavioral and neoplastic. *Pediatr Neurosurg* 2000; **33**:105–11.

97 Ammirati M, Mirzai S, Samii M. Transient mutism following removal of a cerebellar tumor. A case report and review of the literature. *Childs Nerv Syst* 1989; **5**:12–14.

98 Huber-Okrainec J, Dennis M, Bradley K, Spiegler BJ. Motor speech deficits in long-term survivors of childhood cerebellar tumors: effects of tumor type, radiation, age at diagnosis, and survival years. *Neurooncology* 2001; **3**:371.

99 Huber-Okrainec J, Dennis M, Bradley K, Spiegler BJ. Cerebellar tumor resection in childhood followed by transient cerebellar mutism: an investigation of residual speech deficits in long-term survivors. American Association of Neurological Surgeons and Congress of Neurological Surgeons Section on Pediatric Neurological Surgery, 30th Annual Meeting, New York, 2001; **3**:371.

100 Schmahmann JD, Sherman JC. The cerebellar cognitive affective syndrome. *Brain* 1998; **121**:561–79.

101 Levisohn L, Cronin-Golomb A, Schmahmann JD. Neuropsychological consequences of cerebellar tumour resection in children: cerebellar cognitive affective syndrome in a paediatric population. *Brain* 2000; **123**:1041–50.

102 Sadeh M, Cohen I. Transient loss of speech after removal of posterior fossa tumors – one aspect of a larger neuropsychological entity: the cerebellar cognitive affective syndrome. *Pediatr Hematol Oncol* 2001; **18**:423–6.

103 Marien P, Engelborghs S, Michiels E, *et al.* Cognitive and linguistic disturbances in the posterior fossa syndrome in children: A diaschisis phenomenon? *Brain Lang* 2003; **87**:162.

104 Dennis M, Hetherington CR, Spiegler BJ, Barnes MA. Functional consequences of congenital cerebellar dysmorphologies and acquired cerebellar lesions of childhood. In: Brohman SH, Fletcher JM (eds). *The Changing Nervous System: Neurobehavioral Consequences of Early Brain Disorders*. New York: Oxford University Press, 1999, pp. 172–98.

105 Radcliffe J, Bunin GR, Sutton LN, Goldwein JW, Phillips PC. Cognitive deficits in long-term survivors of childhood medulloblastoma and other noncortical tumors: age-dependent effects of whole brain radiation. *Int J Dev Neurosci* 1994; **12**:327–34.

106 Silber JH, Radcliffe J, Peckham V, *et al.* Whole-brain irradiation and decline in intelligence: the influence of dose and age on IQ score. *J Clin Oncol* 1992; **10**:1390–96.

107 Chin HW, Maruyama Y. Age at treatment and long-term performance results in medulloblastoma. *Cancer* 1984; **53**:1952–8.

108 Danoff BF, Cowchock S, Marquette C, Mulgrew L, Kramer S. Assessment of the long-term effects of primary radiation therapy for brain tumors in children. *Cancer* 1982; **49**:1580–6.

109 Mulhern RK, Hancock J, Fairclough D, Kun L. Neuro-psychological status of children treated for brain tumors: a critical review and integrative analysis. *Med Pediatr Oncol* 1992; **20**:181–91.

110 Spunberg JJ, Chang CH, Goldman M, Auricchio E, Bell JJ. Quality of long-term survival following irradiation for intracranial tumors in children under the age of two. *Int J Radiat Oncol* 1981; **7**:727–36.

111 Spreen O, Tupper D, Risser A, Tuokko H, Edgell D. *Human Developmental Neuropsychology*. New York: Oxford University Press, 1984.

112 Pfefferbaum A, Mathalon DH, Sullivan EV, Rawles JM, Zipursky RB, Lim KO. A quantitative magnetic resonance imaging study of changes in brain morphology from infancy to late adulthood. *Arch Neurol* 1994; **51**:874–87.

113 Dennis M. Language and the young damaged brain. In: Boll T, Bryant BK (eds). *Clinical Neuropsychology and Brain Function: Research, Measurement and Practice*. Washington, DC: American Psychological Association, 1988, pp. 85–123.

114 Barnes MA, Dennis M. Reading after closed head injury in childhood: effects on accuracy, fluency and comprehension. *Dev Neuropsychol* 1999; **15**:1–24.

115 Satz P. Brain reserve capacity on symptom onset after brain injury: a formulation and review of evidence for threshold theory. *Neuropsychology* 1993; **7**:273–95.

116 Stern Y, Gurland B, Tatemichi TK, Tang MX, Wilder D, Mayeux R. Influence of education and occupation on the incidence of Alzheimer's disease. *J Am Med Assoc* 1994; **271**:1004–10.

117 Dennis M, Spiegler BJ, Hetherington R. New survivors for the new millennium: cognitive risk and reserve in adults with childhood brain insults. *Brain Cogn* 2000; **42**:102–5.

118 Carlson-Green B, Morris RD, Krawiecki N. Family and illness predictors of outcome in pediatric brain tumors. *J Pediatr Psychol* 1995; **20**:769–84.

119 Taylor HG, Yeates KO, Wade SL, Drotar D, Stancin T, Burant C. Bidirectional child-family influences on outcomes of traumatic brain injury in children. *J Int Neuropsychol Soc* 2001; **7**:755–67.

120 Taylor HG, Alden J. Age-related differences in outcomes following childhood brain insults: an introduction and overview. *J Int Neuropsychol Soc* 1997; **3**:555–67.

121 Mulhern RK, Wasserman AL, Friedman AG, Fairclough D. Social competence and behavioral adjustment of children who are long-term survivors of cancer. *Pediatrics* 1989; **83**:18–25.

122 Moore IM, Glasser ME, Ablin AR. The late psychosocial consequences of childhood cancer. *J Pediatr Nurs* 1987; **3**:150–58.

123 Sloper T, Larcombe IJ, Charlton A. Psychosocial adjustment of five-year survivors of childhood cancer. *J Can Ed* 1994; **9**:163–9.

124 Fritz GK, Williams JR. Issues of adolescent development for survivors of childhood cancer. *J Am Acad Child Adolesc Psychiatry* 1988; **27**:712–15.

125 Mulhern RK, Carpentieri S, Shema S, Stone P, Fairclough D. Factors associated with social and behavioral problems among children recently diagnosed with brain tumor. *J Pediatr Psychol* 1993; **18**:339–50.

126 Carpentieri SC, Mulhern RK, Douglas S, Hanna S, Fairclough DL. Behavioral resiliency among children surviving brain tumors: a longitudinal study. *J Clin Child Psychol* 1993; **22**:236–46.

127 Vannatta K, Gartstein MA, Short A, Noll RB. A controlled study of peer relationships of children surviving brain tumors: teacher, peer and self-ratings. *J Pediatr Psychol* 1998; **23**:279–87.

128 Spiegler BJ, Glaser A, Hetherington CR, Dennis M, Greenberg M. Health-related quality of life (HRQL) in long-term survivors of childhood posterior fossa tumors. Paper given at the 5th International Conference on Long-term Complications of Children and Adolescents with Cancer, Niagara-On-the-Lake, 1998.

129 DeLong R, Friedman H, Friedman N, Gustafson K, Oakes J. Methylphenidate in neuropsychological sequelae of radiotherapy and chemotherapy of childhood brain tumors and leukemia. Letter to the Editor, *J Child Neurol* 1992; **7**:462–3.

130 Torres CF, Korones DN, Palumbo DR, Wissler KH, Vadasz E, Cox C. Effect of methylphenidate in the post-radiation attention and memory deficits in children. *Ann Neurol* 1996; **40**:331.

131 Thompson SJ, Leigh L, Christensen R, *et al.* Immediate neurocognitive effects of methylphenidate on learning-impaired survivors of childhood cancer. *J Clin Oncol* 2001; **19**:1802–8.

132 Butler RW. Attentional processes and their remediation in childhood cancer. *Med Pediatr Oncol Suppl* 1998; **1**:75–8.

133 Butler RW, Copeland DR. Attentional processes and their remediation in children treated for cancer: a literature review and the development of a therapeutic approach. *J Int Neuropsychol Soc* 2002; **8**:115–24.

134 Sohlberg MM, Mateer CA. Attention Process Training (APT). Puyallup, WA: Washington Association for Neuropsychological Research and Development, 1986.

12

Drug delivery

SUSAN M. BLANEY, STACEY L. BERG AND ALAN V. BODDY

INTRODUCTION

The successful treatment of malignant central nervous system (CNS) tumors in infants and children remains a formidable challenge. Overall progress in the development of successful treatment approaches for these tumors has been modest despite advances in neurosurgical and radiation therapy techniques and the availability of new chemotherapeutic agents. Each of these treatment modalities has certain inherent limitations: for surgical treatment, the difficulties created by tumor location and extent; for radiation therapy, the intolerance of the developing CNS to radiation; and for chemotherapy, the limited drug access imposed by the blood–brain barrier. Nevertheless, as with other childhood tumors, a multimodality treatment approach combining surgical resection (when feasible) with radiation therapy or chemotherapy, or both, has led to progress in the treatment of some childhood CNS tumors. In this chapter, we will review the role of chemotherapeutic agents and other treatment strategies that have a potential role in the treatment of primary CNS tumors or the prevention and treatment of tumors with a predilection for CNS dissemination.

BLOOD–BRAIN, BLOOD–CEREBROSPINAL FLUID, AND BLOOD–TUMOR BARRIERS

The anatomic location of the blood–brain barrier is the endothelial lining of brain capillaries. Endothelial cells in brain capillaries differ from non-CNS capillaries in several ways (Figure 12.1): (i) brain capillaries have epithelial-like, high-resistance, tight junctions that fuse brain capillary endothelia together into a continuous cellular layer separating blood and interstitial space; (ii) brain capillaries have a paucity of fenestrations and pinocytic vesicles, thereby restricting transcellular transport; (iii) brain capillaries have a greater number of mitochondria; and (iv) brain capillaries have a number of metabolic enzymes and transporters, e.g. p-glycoprotein (PGP), multidrug resistance-associated proteins (MRP1 and 3), and organic acid transporters (OATs), which are not normally found in endothelial cells.[1–7] Thus, access to the interstitial space of the brain requires agents to pass through two membranes (luminal and abluminal plasma membranes) and the endothelial cell cytoplasm, which is accomplished by either passive diffusion or facilitated transport.[4] As a result, the blood–brain barrier is selectively permeable to lipophilic compounds, which can diffuse readily through lipid plasma membranes, and to nutrients, including glucose and amino acids, for which there are specific transporters to facilitate passage across plasma membranes.[4,8,9]

The blood–cerebrospinal fluid (CSF) barrier serves as the other major natural membrane barrier in the CNS.[9] Drug concentrations in the CSF are often used as a surrogate for concentrations in the brain interstitial space because of the relative availability of CSF versus brain tissue. However, it is important to remember that the blood–CSF and blood–brain barriers are not equivalent.[4] The blood–CSF barrier, which has a surface area approximately 5000-fold less than that of the blood–brain barrier, is located in the epithelium of the tiny organs that surround the ventricles (e.g. choroid plexus, median eminence, area postrema). Capillaries in the region of the blood–CSF barrier are porous, allowing small molecules to penetrate the interstitial space of the circumventricular, organs including the surface of the ependymal-lined ventricles. The ependyma are fused together by low-resistance tight junctions. Therefore, the composition of the CSF is determined by secretory processes in the choroid plexus ependymal epithelial cells rather than the capillary endothelial cells. As a result, for some agents, the concentration in the CSF may be substantially different from that in the brain interstitium.[4,9] Similar to the blood–brain barrier, some drug transporters such as PGP, MRP, and OAT have been postulated to play a drug-transporting role in the blood–CSF barrier at the level of the choroid plexus.[6,10,11]

The blood–tumor barrier is another important variable that plays a role in restricting the delivery of systemically administered chemotherapy to the tumor tissue relative to plasma. As discussed previously, simple diffusion is the primary route by which drugs cross the blood–brain barrier. However, in brain tumors, permeability is an even more complex issue, since within a given tumor there may be more than one microvessel population, each with its own permeability characteristics.[12,13] Another complicating factor involves the spatial distribution of the target capillaries. Although the capillaries within the tumor may have increased permeability, the permeability in the brain adjacent to tumor rapidly returns to normal brain values within just a few millimeters of the tumor margin. Since individual tumor cells may be located centimeters away from the tumor edge, the spatial variability in capillary permeability will also impact drug delivery.[12–14]

Physiochemical properties affecting the blood–brain barrier

Factors that influence the penetration of a drug across the blood–brain barrier include the physiochemical properties of the agent, the degree of protein binding,

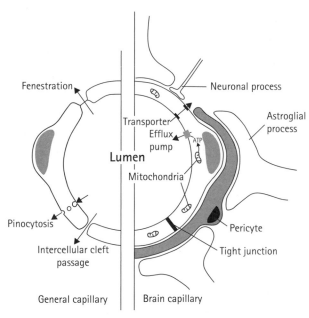

Figure 12.1 *Differences between brain capillary endothelial cells and endothelial cells in other organs. Brain capillary endothelial cells have tight intercellular junctions and lack fenestrations and pinocytic vesicles. The cytoplasm of the brain capillary endothelial cells are rich in mitochondria, which supply energy to the various transport systems for passage of nutrients into the brain and to pump out potentially toxic compounds. Processes from astrocytes, pericytes, and neurons are associated closely with brain capillaries and trophically influence the specialized functions of brain capillary endothelial cells. Reproduced with permission from Patel et al.[4]*

Table 12.1 *Central nervous penetration of commonly used anticancer drugs (adapted from Balis and Poplack[163])*

Drug	CSF/plasma ratio (%)
Alkylating agents	
Cyclophosphamide	50/15[a]
Ifosfamide	30/15[a]
Thiotepa	>95
Carmustine (BCNU)	>90
Platinum analogs	
Cisplatin	40/<5[b]
Carboplatin	30/<5
Antimetabolites	
Methotrexate	3
6-Mercaptopurine	25
Cytarabine	15
5-Fluorouracil	50/15[c]
Anti-tumor antibiotics	
Anthracyclines	ND
Dactinomycin	ND
Plant alkaloids	
Vinca alkaloids	5
Epipodophyllotoxins	<5
Topoisomerase I inhibitors	
Topotecan	30
Irinotecan	14
SN-38	≤8[d]
Miscellaneous	
Prednisolone	<10
Dexamethasone	15
L-asparaginase	ND[e]

CSF, cerebrospinal fluid; ND, drug not detectable in cerebrospinal fluid. [a]Includes parent compound/active metabolite. [b]Includes free (ultrafilterable)/total platinum. [c]Includes bolus dose/infusion. [d]Active metabolite of irinotecan. [e]Although drug is not detectable in cerebrospinal fluid, cerebrospinal fluid L-asparagine is depleted by systemic administration of L-asparaginase.

and the affinity of the agent for carriers that facilitate transport of endogenous compounds into the CNS. Characteristics that adversely affect drug penetration across the blood–brain barrier include poor lipid solubility, significant ionization, and high protein or tissue binding.[15–17] For most anticancer agents that have been studied, penetration across the blood–brain barrier is limited (Table 12.1). Nevertheless, because of the observations that there are several agents that penetrate the blood–brain barrier poorly yet have activity against CNS tumors, and the concentration of chemotherapy in the majority of the tumor is higher than that in the adjacent normal brain,[4,18] there is still controversy over the magnitude of the blood–brain barrier's role in the resistance of CNS tumors to chemotherapy.[19]

STRATEGIES FOR INCREASING CENTRAL NERVOUS SYSTEM DRUG DELIVERY

Many therapeutic strategies have been developed in an attempt to either disrupt or circumvent the blood–brain barrier in order to enhance drug delivery to the target tumor site within the CNS, including: (i) blood–brain barrier disruption with agents such as mannitol and vasoactive compounds; (ii) administration of very high-dose systemic chemotherapy; and (iii) regional chemotherapy administration using the intrathecal, intra-arterial, and intratumoral routes. These approaches and their potential advantages and/or disadvantages are outlined in Table 12.2.

Disruption of the blood–brain and blood–tumor barriers

A number of mechanisms have been employed to disrupt the blood–brain and blood–tumor barriers. The most common approach involves the use of agents such as mannitol to increase the osmotic potential of plasma. Newer approaches include strategies to chemically modify the blood–brain barrier, using vasoactive compounds and attempts to prevent drug efflux from tumor tissue through inhibition of transport pumps such as PGP. Although objective evidence of anti-tumor response has been observed with each of these approaches, the use of such approaches outside the context of a clinical trial cannot be recommended, since their role in the treatment of children with CNS tumors has not been defined.

Table 12.2 *Comparison of different methods drug delivery to brain tumors (adapted from Groothuis[12])*

Approach	Primary advantages	Primary disadvantages	Limiting factors
BBB disruption	First-pass increase in AUC, increased permeability	Invasive, differential effect on brain and tumor, short-lived, potential for unpredictable neurotoxicity	BBB/BTB permeability, systemic toxicity
Chemical modification with vasoactive compounds	First-pass increase in AUC, increased permeability (theoretically selective to BTB)	Invasive, short-lived	BBB/BTB permeability, systemic toxicity
Radiation therapy	Greater selectivity for BBB	Long-term neurological sequelae in developing CNS	Patient age, potential systemic/neurologic toxicity
Inhibiting drug efflux	Decreased efflux	Not selective for BTB, therefore potential for increased neurotoxicity	
New drug formulations	Potential for BTB selectivity	Must be evaluated for each agent	BBB/BTB permeability, systemic toxicity
Intrathecal (intralumbar or intraventricular)	Easy access, ideal for leptomeningeal disease	Not useful for parenchymal disease or bulky leptomeningeal disease, non-uniform distribution in CNS	Bulk flow rate of CSF
Intratumoral therapy (biodegradable polymers, convection-enhanced delivery)	Bypasses BBB, 100% drug delivered to target	Invasive, distribution is diffusional	Unpredictable distribution, increased potential for local neurotoxicity
Intra-arterial therapy	First-pass increase in AUC	Invasive, small increase in AUC	BBB/BTB permeability, systemic toxicity
High-dose systemic chemotherapy	Higher concentrations at target site, uniform drug delivery		Systemic toxicity

AUC, area under curve; BBB, blood–brain barrier; BTB, blood–tumor barrier; CNS, central nervous system; CSF, cerebrospinal fluid.

Randomized clinical trials to assess the impact of such interventions on either response or progression-free survival have not yet been performed.

OSMOTIC DISRUPTION

This approach involves intra-arterial infusion, via an intracerebral or vertebral artery, of a hyperosmolar solution to induce blood–brain barrier disruption. Exposure of the capillary endothelial cells to the hyperosmolar solution leads to cell shrinkage and stress on the tight junctions.[20] As a result, the junctions are pulled apart, allowing increased capillary permeability. Hypertonic mannitol (25 per cent) is the most commonly used agent for blood–brain barrier disruption, although hypertonic arabinose has also been utilized.[4,21] The intra-arterial infusion of the hypertonic solution is frequently preceded by intravenous administration of chemotherapeutic agents that require systemic activation, e.g. cyclophosphamide, and is generally followed by intra-arterial administration of another chemotherapeutic agent such as methotrexate or carboplatin.[20]

Considerable controversy has been generated by the use of osmotic blood–brain barrier disruption, for a variety of reasons. First, the actual effectiveness of blood –brain barrier disruption in increasing drug delivery to tumors is uncertain. The enhancement of drug uptake into tumors is variable because blood–tumor barrier permeability is not homogeneous.[22,23] As a result, the relative increase in exposure within the tumor may be less than that within normal brain or brain adjacent to tumor. This was demonstrated elegantly by Zunkeler and colleagues,[24] who evaluated the pharmacokinetics of methotrexate, an agent with low CNS permeability, after blood–brain barrier disruption with mannitol. They found that the peak absolute percentage increases in the permeability of tumor and normal blood brain vessels were 60 per cent and 1000 per cent, respectively. In addition, there is little rationale for using this approach to administer a cell-cycle-specific agent, such as methotrexate, because the duration of exposure above a threshold concentration is a much more important determinant of response than is exposure to high concentrations for a brief period of time.[4]

Although blood–brain barrier disruption has been shown to be feasible in a limited multicenter setting, it has many drawbacks, including the need for general anesthesia and intra- blood–brain barrier (BBB) catheterization.[25] Despite the overall low risk of neurological complications after osmotic BBB disruption, there may be profound or unpredictable toxicities, including pulmonary embolus, stroke, visual deterioration, hearing loss, and seizures.[4,25] In addition, osmotic disruption of the blood–brain barrier is non-specific (i.e. not limited to the tumor) and therefore may be associated with increased neurotoxicity. Indeed, unexpected high-frequency hearing loss occurred in almost 80 per cent of patients receiving carboplatin after osmotic blood–brain barrier disruption, necessitating a change in treatment plan and investigation of chemoprotecant strategies.[20,26,27] Unpredictable neurological toxicities associated with combinations of certain anticancer agents and anesthetics, as demonstrated in preclinical studies with etoposide phosphate, may also occur.[28]

CHEMICAL MODIFICATION USING VASOACTIVE COMPOUNDS

A variety of chemical agents that are derivatives of normal vasoactive compounds, including labradimil, the synthetic analog of bradykinin,[29–31] interleukin-2,[32] leukotriene C4,[33] and others,[34] have been investigated, either preclinically or clinically, for their ability to disrupt the blood–brain barrier.

Bradykinin, a naturally occurring nonapeptide, and its synthetic analog labradimil (Cereport, RMP-7) bind specifically to B2 receptors expressed on the luminal and abluminal surfaces of brain and brain tumor capillaries. This results in transient relaxation of the tight junctions and increased permeability to a variety of agents.[30,35] Recent studies have demonstrated that bradykinin and labradimil can increase the permeability of the blood–tumor barrier at doses lower than those required for disruption of the blood–brain barrier.[30,36] The obvious appeal of this strategy, which in theory selectively increases the permeability of the blood–tumor barrier, is that it avoids the potential for unpredictable neurotoxicity associated with high drug concentrations in normal brain. Labradimil has the advantage of having a longer half-life than bradykinin.[37] Thus, strategies using labradimil to selectively increase the permeability of the blood–tumor barrier are currently being evaluated in clinical trials.[31,38] Early results indicate that labradimil administered in combination with carboplatin is tolerated well.[38] There are currently two ongoing studies within the Children's Oncology Group (COG) of labradimil in children with CNS tumors, one a study of concurrent labradimil and carboplatin with radiation therapy for patients with newly diagnosed brainstem gliomas, and the other a phase II trial of labradimil and carboplatin in patients with recurrent or refractory CNS tumors.

RADIATION

Ionizing radiation can impair the integrity of the blood–brain barrier at doses exceeding 10–15 Gy.[39] Although the mechanism of this response is not understood entirely, it may be due to the activation of vesicular transport. A pilot study evaluating the effects of radiation on the blood–brain barrier using ^{99M}Tc-glucoheptonate in patients with localized brain tumors revealed that the blood–brain barrier in the irradiated normal brain was disrupted and that the degree of disruption was directly proportional to the radiation dose. In addition, an evaluation of one patient in this study demonstrated that there was partial disruption of the blood–brain barrier (~22 per cent) within the tumor pre-radiation, and that the permeability increased post-radiation (~75 per cent) and then decreased (to <20 per cent) over the ensuing eight months.[40] The impact of radiation on the disposition of chemotherapy within the CNS has not been well studied. However, based on these observations, it has been proposed that radiotherapy (to doses of 20–30 Gy) should precede chemotherapy in order to disrupt the blood–brain barrier and facilitate the delivery of drugs to the tumor.[40]

INHIBITION OF DRUG EFFLUX

Access of many drugs to the brain is limited by active efflux, mediated by PGP and related transporters that confer resistance to cancer cells by allowing them to move a variety of chemotherapeutic agents against a concentration gradient.[6,7,41] PGP, an ATP-dependent transport protein, and the *mdr-1* gene that encodes for it are normally expressed in the apical membranes of a number of epithelial cell types in the body (e.g. the biliary canaliculi, the proximal tubules in the kidney, the mucosal lining of the jejunum and colon, and the adrenal gland), including the blood luminal membrane of the brain endothelial cells that make up the blood–brain barrier. In addition, PGP is expressed in a variety of human tumors, including CNS tumors such as gliomas.[12,42,43] Extensive preclinical experiments in knockout mice that lack an *mdr-1* gene demonstrate highly increased CNS concentrations following systemic administration of drugs such as vinblastine and cyclosporin, known substrates for PGP.[44] Similarly, a role for MRP in excluding etoposide from CSF has been demonstrated from experiments utilizing knockout mice.[11] As a result, it has been postulated that highly effective inhibitors of PGP may be effective in blocking PGP in the blood–brain barrier. However, this strategy has not been successful in preclinical studies in non-human primates, where PGP-inhibitory concentrations of cyclosporin A failed to increase the CSF penetration of doxorubicin.[45] More potent PGP inhibitors that may be more effective are being developed.

An obvious potential drawback to this strategy is that, like osmotic blood–brain barrier disruption, it is not selective for the blood–tumor barrier and therefore it has the potential to increase toxicity to normal brain. In addition, the recent identification of functional polymorphisms of the *mdr-1* gene suggests that there may be interpatient variability in PGP modulation of CNS drug penetration.[46]

NOVEL METHODS OF INTRAVASCULAR DRUG DELIVERY

The use of liposomal drug formulations that selectively accumulate in brain tumors is another approach that is being explored in an attempt to overcome the blood–brain barrier. Relatively selective delivery to tumor has been reported for liposomal formulations of daunorubicin and doxorubicin in patients with glioblastoma multiforme.[47,48] Results from a recent study indicate that accumulation of radiolabeled "stealth" liposomal doxorubicin was 13–19 times higher in glioblastomas and 7–13 times higher in metastatic lesions, as compared with normal brain. The effectiveness of liposomal delivery of drugs to brain tumors is not yet proven.

Regional drug delivery

INTRATHECAL THERAPY

Intrathecal administration of chemotherapy, one of the earliest approaches used to circumvent the blood–brain barrier, is utilized routinely in the treatment and prevention of CNS leukemias and lymphomas. Intrathecal drug delivery can be accomplished via lumbar puncture or via the use of an in-dwelling ventricular access device (e.g. Ommaya reservoir) or an in-dwelling lumbar reservoir. The primary advantage of this form of regional therapy is that very high drug concentrations can be achieved in the CSF using relatively small doses because the initial volume of distribution in the CSF is small compared with that in plasma (150 ml for CSF, 3500 ml for plasma).[49–51] As a result of the lower total drug dose, the potential for systemic toxicity is minimized.

Despite the significant pharmacologic advantages resulting from intrathecal drug administration, there are several inherent limitations to this approach: (i) the penetration of drug into the brain parenchyma after intrathecal dosing is only a few millimeters,[52] thereby limiting the utility of this approach in patients with parenchymal or bulky leptomeningeal tumors; (ii) drug distribution throughout the neuraxis is not uniform, as has been demonstrated in non-human primates following intralumbar methotrexate;[53] and (iii) the presence of alterations in CSF flow due to hydrocephalus, a ventriculoperitoneal shunt, or the leptomeningeal disease itself may significantly alter drug distribution and elimination from the CSF.[54] Other potential disadvantages of intrathecal therapy include pain and inconvenience if the intralumbar route is used for drug delivery, and technical problems with drug delivery to the intended target site, as evidenced by radioisotope studies demonstrating that in approximately ten per cent of intralumbar injections, drug is injected or leaks into the subdural or epidural space instead of the subarachnoid space.[55] Some of these limitations can be overcome by direct delivery of drug into the ventricle using a ventricular access device, which ensures drug delivery into the CSF and results in more uniform drug distribution. Although the pharmacokinetic advantages of intraventricular drug delivery are substantial, this approach requires a neurosurgical procedure and is therefore most often reserved for patients with overt leptomeningeal disease.

Standard agents for intrathecal administration

Methotrexate and cytarabine administered alone or in combination with hydrocortisone are the cornerstones of both the treatment and the prevention of CNS disease in children with acute leukemia or lymphoma. Important pharmacological principles have been derived from their routine use in childhood leukemias that have widespread applicability to other intrathecal agents. For example, unlike systemically administered chemotherapy, in which dosing is based on body surface area, intrathecal chemotherapy is generally administered at a fixed dose in all patients over three years of age. This practice is based on the observation that the CNS, including the CSF volume, approaches adult size in children at this age.[56] Bleyer and colleagues demonstrated that age-based dosing both improved response to and decreased toxicity of intrathecally administered methotrexate.[57] Virtually all intrathecal drug administration in children now follows this approach.

Unfortunately, neither methotrexate nor cytarabine is particularly useful for the treatment of brain tumors. Thiotepa, which has modest activity against pediatric brain tumors when administered systemically,[58] has also been administered intrathecally. In a retrospective review, five of 14 patients with leptomeningeal gliomatosis responded radiographically to intraventricular administration of thiotepa.[59] However, in a prospective, randomized study of thiotepa compared with methotrexate in patients with leptomeningeal spread of solid tumors, no patient in either arm had significant clinical improvement, and the median survival time for patients treated with thiotepa was 14 weeks.[60] There is no current standard intrathecal therapy for leptomeningeal malignancy.

Investigational agents

A number of other agents have been studied in clinical trials of intrathecal administration. These include diaziquone,[61] 6-mercaptopurine,[62] mafosfamide,[63,64] and topotecan.[65] In addition, a liposomally encapsulated form of cytarabine, DepoCyt™, which provides pharmacokinetic advantages compared with free cytarabine, is also being studied for both leukemia/lymphomas and solid tumors that have spread to the leptomeninges.[66–68] Although some of these agents have shown anti-tumor activity in the phase I setting, it is too early to recommend their use outside the investigational setting.

Ongoing studies in children to evaluate new agents for intrathecal administration include a COG phase II trial of intrathecal topotecan, a Pediatric Brain Tumor Consortium (PBTC) phase I study of a form of intrathecal busulfan (Spartaject®-Busulfan), and a PBTC pilot study of intrathecal mafosfamide in infants with newly diagnosed embryonal tumors.

INTRATUMORAL THERAPY

Biodegradable polymers

Microencapsulated, drug-loaded, biodegradable polymers implanted into brain or tumor tissue at the time of surgery provide a mechanism for timed release of cytotoxic therapy.[69] Gliadel, a 3.85 per cent carmustine-impregnated polymer, is the first biodegradable polymer approved for use by the US Food and Drug Administration (FDA) in adults with high-grade recurrent gliomas. A phase III randomized, placebo-controlled study of gliadel demonstrated an increase in median survival from 23 weeks to 31 weeks in the patients who received surgically implanted carmustine-loaded polymers.[70] The primary advantage of this approach is that it bypasses the blood–brain barrier, allowing direct delivery of high concentrations of drug to the tumor tissue or tumor bed with a small total drug dose, thereby minimizing potential for systemic toxicity.[71] However, some clinical studies have demonstrated the potential for increased local toxicities, including wound infection, CSF leak, sepsis, and cerebral edema.[72,73]

The primary limitation to the use of biodegradable polymers is the poor diffusion of the drug through tumor and brain interstitium. As a result, only a small volume of tissue surrounding the drug source is treated.[74] In addition, there may be limitations or resistance that are inherent to the agent utilized within the polymer.[73] For example, carmustine resistance may be due, in part, to the presence in tumor of high levels of the DNA repair protein alkylguanyl-DNA alkyltransferase (AGT).[75,76] O^6-benzylguanine (O^6BG) is an inhibitor of AGT that may provide a strategy for overcoming this resistance mechanism (see below). In theory, systemic administration of O^6BG in conjunction with use of the carmustine-loaded polymers may potentially increase the efficacy of the polymer. This treatment strategy is, at the time of writing, being evaluated in a clinical trial sponsored by the National Cancer Institute for adults with CNS tumors.[71] Ongoing studies are also evaluating carmustine-loaded polymers containing higher doses of carmustine (20 per cent and 32 per cent) in an attempt to take advantage of the steep dose–response curve for alkylating agents. Preliminary results of these studies suggest that polymers loaded with up to 20 per cent carmustine are tolerated well.[77]

Other agents are also being evaluated using biodegradable polymers as a vehicle for drug delivery. The feasibility of administering intratumoral 5-fluorouracil (5-FU) using poly(D,L, lactide-co-glycolide) (PLAGA) microspheres in patients with newly diagnosed glioblastoma multiforme has recently been confirmed in a pilot study. 5-FU-loaded PLAGA microspheres were surgically implanted into the surgical resection cavity. Radiation therapy commenced within seven days of surgery. Sustained concentrations of 5-FU were present in the CSF for at least one month postoperatively. Overall tolerance to the treatment was good, and median survival in this small study increased from 51 weeks to 98 weeks.[78] The role of biodegradable polymers in the treatment of childhood CNS tumors has not yet been evaluated.

Convection–enhanced delivery

Convection-enhanced delivery, also referred to as intracerebral clysis,[79] is a method of delivering drug to CNS tumors directly using a catheter that has been implanted into the tumor or tumor cavity to directly infuse drug solutions. A subcutaneously implanted Ommaya reservoir facilitates administration of intermittent bolus injections or continuous infusion of the solution over prolonged periods of time. This drug delivery technique can be used to deliver drugs or large macromolecules (e.g. immunotoxin, cytokines) efficiently and homogeneously to a large volume of brain over a short period of time, since unlike diffusion, convection (bulk flow) results from a pressure gradient.[71,74,80,81] The volume of distribution with convection delivery is linearly proportional to the volume of the infusion and the type of tissue being infused.[12,82,83] The maximum concentration of drug in the infusate will be limited by toxicity to normal brain within the central part of the convective component of the infusion.[12] The feasibility of convection-enhanced delivery has been evaluated preclinically in a variety of experimental brain tumor models[79,84,85] and in non-human primates.[82] Clinical trials using this approach are ongoing in adults with supratentorial CNS tumors, but the approach has not been evaluated in children.

INTRA–ARTERIAL THERAPY

In theory, intra-arterial delivery of chemotherapy to CNS tumors, as to tumors elsewhere in the body, offers a potential pharmacokinetic advantage over intravenous infusions because higher blood concentrations of drug are achieved during the first pass through the brain. This advantage is most pronounced for agents that have a high total body clearance and for agents that are metabolized or inactivated after the first pass through the liver.[4,86] In contrast, if a drug is not cleared rapidly from the systemic circulation, or if high local concentrations result in undue toxicity, then the intra-arterial approach is not advantageous. The delivery of drugs to brain tumors by intra-arterial infusion is particularly complex because of streaming and non-uniform mixing of drug administered in this fashion. In addition, cannulation of different arteries and different infusion techniques may

result in unexpected differences in the properties of drug distribution. For example, Saris and colleagues studied the effects of various infusion techniques on the distribution of infusate using a labeled tracer and positron-emission spectroscopy imaging.[86] Supraophthalmic artery drug infusions resulted in pronounced vascular streaming and heterogeneity of tracer distribution in the brain. In contrast, after infraophthalmic infusions into the cervical carotid artery there was little or no intravascular streaming, probably because increased turbulence in this area resulted in more uniform drug mixing in the blood near the site of administration. In addition, the use of diastole-phased pulse infusions substantially reduced drug streaming following supraophthalmic administration.[86] Thus fluid mechanics, in addition to pharmacokinetics, have a major impact on the potential advantages of intra-arterial drug administration.

Intra-arterial therapy has not yet been demonstrated to provide a clinically meaningful advantage for patients with CNS tumors.[4] Furthermore, it has been associated with significant morbidity, including irreversible encephalopathy and visual loss, in addition to the inherent potential risks associated with carotid artery catheterization.[86,87] There is not currently a role for intra-arterial infusions in the treatment of children with CNS tumors.

High–dose systemic chemotherapy

Systemic administration of high doses of chemotherapy is another strategy that has been utilized to overcome the limited blood–brain barrier penetration of most systemically administered anticancer agents. The primary theoretic advantage of high-dose systemic therapy over regional therapy is that while both approaches produce high drug concentrations in the target site, systemic therapy results in more uniform delivery and more sustained exposure in the brain and CSF.[4] This approach has been used successfully with agents such as methotrexate and cytarabine in the treatment of childhood leukemias. A primary limitation to this approach is the potential for severe systemic toxicity,[88,89] although this can be ameliorated in part by the use of hematological support, such as stem-cell or bone-marrow transplant.

High-dose chemotherapy approaches in children and adults with primary or recurrent CNS tumors using stem-cell or bone-marrow rescue have demonstrated minimal to modest anti-tumor activity in a variety of adult and pediatric CNS tumors.[89–93] In general, embryonal tumors appear to be most responsive, while gliomas appear to be relatively unresponsive. In addition, this therapy has sometimes been associated with early toxic deaths and neurologic complications.[90,91] Unfortunately, the interpretation of clinical trials utilizing this approach is confounded by the various treatment regimens selected, the heterogeneity of previous or subsequent radiotherapy, and the assorted tumor types and locations studied. The role of high-dose chemotherapy in the treatment of children with CNS tumors has not yet been defined.

STANDARD CHEMOTHERAPY APPROACHES

Alkylating agents

Alkylating agents are highly active in the treatment of a variety of malignant childhood tumors, including those of the CNS. These agents exert their cytotoxic effect by producing alkylation of DNA through the formation of reactive intermediates that attack nucleophilic sites.[94] Since alkylating agents demonstrate a steep dose–response curve in experimental tumor model systems, they are frequently incorporated into high-dose chemotherapy regimens that employ either bone-marrow or peripheral stem-cell rescue, as discussed above.[95]

Alkylating agents may differ greatly in their toxicity profiles and anti-tumor activity as a result of differences in pharmacokinetic profiles, lipid solubility, membrane transport properties, ability to penetrate the CNS, and detoxification reactions.[94] Myelosuppression is the primary acute toxicity associated with alkylating agent therapy. However, it may be delayed and/or cumulative following treatment with some agents, e.g. the nitrosoureas. Other common acute toxicities of alkylating agents include nausea, vomiting, alopecia, and allergic reactions. Gastrointestinal and neurological toxicities may be observed at high doses. Delayed toxicities include pulmonary fibrosis, gonadal atrophy, and impaired renal function. In addition, these agents are carcinogenic, mutagenic, and teratogenic.[96–98]

The alkylating agents used most widely in the treatment of CNS tumors include cyclophosphamide, procarbazine, and the nitrosoureas (carmustine, lomustine).

CYCLOPHOSPHAMIDE

Cyclophosphamide, an inactive prodrug that requires activation by hepatic microsomal enzymes in order to exert a cytotoxic effect, is one of the most widely utilized anticancer agents for the treatment of embryonal tumors of the CNS as well as for a variety of other childhood tumors. Cyclophosphamide is usually administered as either a single bolus dose or a fractionated dose over two to three days. This agent is usually administered in combination chemotherapy regimens, but it has also demonstrated single-agent activity in patients with recurrent medulloblastoma and gliomas.[99–101] In addition, cyclophosphamide is used widely in preparative regimens for autologous bone-marrow transplant and in regimens that utilize high-dose chemotherapy with peripheral blood stem-cell rescue.

PROCARBAZINE

In the earliest phase II study of procarbazine in patients with brain tumors, the response rate was 48 per cent.[102] It is worth noting, however, that the initial estimates of response to procarbazine, as to many of the older agents generally considered active against brain tumors, came before the advent of computed tomography (CT) and magnetic resonance imaging (MRI). Thus, it is difficult to compare the single-agent activity of these drugs with that of drugs developed more recently. In a recent phase II study in previously untreated children with high-grade glioma, procarbazine was inactive.[103] Procarbazine is now used most commonly in combination with lomustine, or with lomustine and vincristine, although the activity of these combinations is limited.[104]

NITROSOUREAS

The nitrosoureas have been used for the treatment of brain tumors for more than 40 years. Early single-agent response rates ranged from 30 to 70 per cent.[105] However, in a more recent study comparing procarbazine with carmustine in adults with gliomas, the response rate was 35 per cent for procarbazine and 23 per cent for carmustine.[106] As discussed above, the DNA repair enzyme AGT may be at least partly responsible for nitrosourea resistance. O^6BG acts as a fraudulent substrate for AGT, depleting AGT and interfering with DNA repair. Thus, this agent increases tumor cell sensitivity to alkylating agents such as carmustine and lomustine.[76] Recent studies have demonstrated that AGT inhibition in tumor tissue is feasible.[107] However, normal tissue, particularly bone marrow, is also sensitized and the dose of nitrosoureas must be reduced when given with O^6BG.[108] The ultimate utility of this approach is unproven.

Non–classical alkylating agents

TEMOZOLOMIDE

Temozolomide is an oral imidazotetrazine derivative that was developed as an alternative for dacarbazine. Both agents are prodrugs for the active moiety MTIC (methyltriazenyl imidazole carboximide). However, unlike dacarbazine, which requires hepatic activation, temozolomide decomposes spontaneously at physiological pH to its active metabolite. Temozolomide is distributed widely in tissues and penetrates well across the blood–brain barrier.[109] Preclinical models suggested that the anti-tumor activity of temozolomide was schedule-dependent, leading to initial evaluation of single daily dosing for five consecutive days. Temozolomide has shown activity in a number of studies,[110,111] and it is approved as second-line treatment for anaplastic astrocytoma in adults.[112] Results of a CCG phase II trial of temozolomide in children have not yet been published.

Tumor levels of AGT (see above) and of DNA mismatch repair proteins are important in determining response to temozolomide and other alkylating agents.[107] Therefore, a pediatric phase I study of temozolomide in combination with O[6]BG is currently under way.

Platinum analogs

Along with the nitrosoureas and other alkylating agents, cisplatin and carboplatin are among the most widely used agents in the treatment of brain tumors. Cisplatin is highly protein-bound and penetrates poorly into the CSF,[113] although tumor concentrations of cisplatin have been reported to be much higher than those in normal brain tissue.[114] The dose-limiting toxicities of cisplatin are nephrotoxicity and ototoxicity, which are not always reversible.[115] Single-agent studies of cisplatin have demonstrated a response rate of 30–80 per cent, depending on tumor histology, with medulloblastomas being particularly sensitive.[116–119]

Carboplatin is less protein-bound than cisplatin and penetrates much better into the CSF.[113] It achieves cytotoxic concentrations in brain tumors following intravenous administration.[120] In contrast to cisplatin, the dose-limiting toxicity of carboplatin is myelosuppression, especially thrombocytopenia. Because thrombocytopenia is correlated closely with total systemic exposure to carboplatin, which in turn may be predicted based on an individual patient's glomerular filtration rate, several equations have been developed that permit selection of a carboplatin dose that will produce a tolerable platelet nadir on an individualized basis.[115] A somewhat unusual toxicity of carboplatin is hypersensitivity reactions, which appear to occur more commonly in patients who receive a higher number of carboplatin infusions.[121] Carboplatin has demonstrated single-agent activity against childhood brain tumors in a number of phase II trials, although the response rates vary.[122–125] It is also active against low-grade gliomas and optic pathway tumors, including those that arise in patients with neurofibromatosis type 1 (NF-1).[126–128]

Topoisomerase inhibitors

EPIPODOPHYLLOTOXINS

The epipodophyllotoxins etoposide and teniposide are used widely in the treatment of various childhood malignancies. Etoposide is particularly active against many solid tumors. Its activity against brain tumors, however, is uncertain. A phase II study in children with recurrent or refractory brain tumors showed only a low level of activity, with a response rate of less than 20 per cent.[129] Because there is some evidence that a protracted schedule may be

more active, etoposide has also been studied following daily oral dosing for a prolonged period, usually of 21 consecutive days or longer. Results of these studies have been mixed, but the activity of etoposide administered in this fashion appears to be modest at best.[130–134] Similarly, there appears to be little role for teniposide in the treatment of childhood brain tumors.[135,136]

TOPOISOMERASE I POISONS

Topoisomerase I poisons produce DNA strand breaks by forming a ternary complex with DNA and the topoisomerase I enzyme. Optimal binding of these agents to topoisomerase I requires the presence of an intact alpha-hydroxylactone moiety (E-ring). This lactone ring is labile in aqueous solutions, undergoing reversible hydrolysis to a relatively inactive open-ring carboxylate form that predominates at physiologic pH. Modifications of the A and B rings of the pentacyclic backbone affect the water solubility and protein binding of the various camptothecin analogs. Topotecan and irinotecan are the most extensively studied topoisomerase I poisons.

Topotecan

In preclinical studies, topotecan penetrated well into the CSF of non-human primates[137,138] and demonstrated significant anti-tumor activity against human brain tumor xenografts (glioma and medulloblastoma).[139] These characteristics provided a strong rationale to study the activity of topotecan against childhood brain tumors. Two phase II studies of topotecan in children with refractory or high-risk CNS tumors were thus performed, one evaluating a 24-hour infusion and the other evaluating a 72-hour infusion. Topotecan was inactive in patients with glioblastoma multiforme, brainstem glioma, and medulloblastoma in both studies. However, in each study, there were several children who experienced prolonged periods of stable disease, including patients with low-grade gliomas, malignant neuroepithelial tumor, ependymoma, and optic glioma.[140,141]

The relative inactivity of topotecan in phase II clinical trials may be related, in part, to the metabolic disposition of this agent. The primary route of topotecan elimination is renal,[142–144] although a small fraction of topotecan is eliminated following oxidative metabolism to an N-desmethyl metabolite.[145] The latter pathway becomes clinically important in patients receiving concomitant medications that induce oxidative metabolism, e.g. anticonvulsants such as phenytoin, because there is a subsequent marked increase in topotecan clearance and an overall decrease in exposure that may affect drug efficacy.[146] Thus, higher doses of topotecan may be required for patients receiving such medications. The interaction between topotecan and enzyme-inducing anticonvulsants was not recognized until after the completion of the phase II studies. Therefore, it is possible that some of the patients enrolled in the phase II studies were relatively underdosed compared with patients who were not receiving anticonvulsants. As a result of this uncertainty, a study is under way to evaluate the efficacy of topotecan in children with newly diagnosed medulloblastoma, and who receive a four-hour infusion of topotecan daily for five days, with the dose adjusted based on real-time pharmacokinetic studies to achieve targeted topotecan plasma concentrations. Results of this study should clarify the activity of topotecan against medulloblastoma.

Irinotecan

Irinotecan is a prodrug that is converted by carboxylesterase in the liver, intestinal tract, and some tumors to an active metabolite, SN-38, which is 100- to 1000-fold more potent than the parent irinotecan.[147] Irinotecan has shown promising activity against recurrent or progressive glioma in adults.[148] There is currently a COG phase II study of irinotecan in children with CNS tumors. As with topotecan, however, concomitant administration of enzyme-inducing anticonvulsants can increase drug clearance, thus decreasing drug exposure and compromising activity.[148,149] As a result, there are ongoing studies in both children and adults to define the maximum tolerated dose of irinotecan in patients who are receiving these drugs, so that an adequate evaluation of the activity of irinotecan in these patients can be made.

Vinca alkaloids

In an early study of vincristine in children with recurrent brain tumors, eight of 17 children showed neurologic responses after treatment with weekly vincristine.[150] Vincristine is currently a part of many first-line combination chemotherapy regimens for children with brain tumors, although part of this widespread use may be attributed to vincristine's lack of overlapping toxicities, particularly myelosuppression, when administered with other cytotoxic agents.

Antimetabolites

Antimetabolites are not used widely in the treatment of pediatric brain tumors. Methotrexate in high doses administered with leucovorin rescue may have some activity in limited tumor types.[151] Low-dose, orally administered methotrexate is not active.[152]

Corticosteroids

Corticosteroids are commonly administered in high doses to patients with brain tumors in an attempt to decrease tumor-related edema and therefore ameliorate symptoms. This activity is believed to related to steroid-induced decreases in blood–brain barrier permeability (reviewed by Koehler[153]). However, some evidence suggests that these same mechanisms of action may have a negative impact on the anti-tumor efficacy of chemotherapy. In preclinical studies, administration of dexamethasone to rats with experimental brain tumors reduced uptake of cisplatin into areas of the brain surrounding the tumor, although uptake into the tumor itself was not affected.[154] Although clinical data are limited, MRI studies suggest that dexamethasone may reduce vascular permeability across the blood–tumor barrier in patients with brain tumors.[155] Currently, there is insufficient evidence to indicate that corticosteroid therapy has a negative effect on anticancer therapy; however, it is generally recommended that corticosteroids not be used as antiemetics in the treatment of patients with CNS tumors.

Novel agents

ANTI–ANGIOGENIC AGENTS

Abnormal angiogenesis has been implicated in the development of many tumor types, including brain tumors. It presents an attractive strategy for the targeted development of new anticancer agents. Among the anticancer agents investigated recently, or being studied currently, in brain tumors are SU5416, a small molecule inhibitor of vascular endothelial growth factor, TNP-470, a fumagillin analog, and thalidomide. A comprehensive review of this topic has been published by Kirsch and colleagues.[156] Although anti-angiogenesis represents an exciting area of new drug development, it is too early to know whether any of these anti-angiogenic agents will have a place in the treatment of childhood brain tumors.

STI–571

The tyrosine kinase inhibitor Gleevec (STI-571) competitively inhibits the bcr-abl tyrosine kinase that results from the Philadelphia (9,22) chromosome translocation in chronic myelogenous leukemia.[157,158] In addition, Gleevec also inhibits platelet-derived growth factor (PDGF) receptor, stem cell factor (SCF) receptor, and c-kit-mediated signaling.[159–161] Since PDGF may play a role in brain tumors, particularly gliomas,[162] early studies of Gleevec for the treatment of pediatric brain tumors are under way in children with newly diagnosed brainstem gliomas and in children with refractory or progressive high-grade gliomas.

CONCLUSIONS AND DIRECTIONS FOR FUTURE RESEARCH

Multimodality therapy has improved the outcome of some childhood brain tumors. Some CNS tumors types, however, remain refractory to current therapeutic modalities.

Future research must be directed towards identifying the reasons for intrinsic resistance to therapy and for disease recurrence after initially successful therapy. New chemotherapeutic agents must be identified that can overcome drug resistance. As our understanding of the molecular pathogenesis of pediatric brain tumors improves, the use of specifically targeted agents to treat these tumors must be investigated. In addition, we must actively evaluate new drug-delivery strategies for the treatment of childhood CNS tumors.

REFERENCES

1 Bradbury M. The blood–brain barrier. *Exp Physiol* 1993; **78**:53–72.

2 De Boer A, Breimer D. The blood–brain barrier: clinical implications for drug delivery to the brain. *J R Coll Phys Lond* 1994; **28**:502–6.

3 Johansson B. The physiology of the blood–brain barrier. *Adv Exp Med Biol* 1990; **27**:25–39.

4 Patel M, Blaney S, Balis F. Pharmacokinetics of drug delivery to the central nervous system. In: Grochow L, Ames M (eds). *A Clinician's Guide to Chemotherapy Pharmacokinetics and Pharmacodynamics*. Baltimore: Williams & Wilkins, 1998, pp. 67–90.

5 Bart J, Groen HJ, Hendrikse N, van der Graaf W, Vaalburg W, de Vries EG. The blood–brain barrier and oncology: new insights into function and modulation. *Cancer Treat Rev* 2000; **26**:449–62.

6 Rao VV, Dahlheimer JL, Bardgett ME, *et al.* Choroid plexus epithelial expression of MDR1 P glycoprotein and multidrug resistance-associated protein contribute to the blood-cerebrospinal-fluid drug-permeability barrier. *Proc Natl Acad Sci U S A* 1999; **96**:3900–5.

7 Schinkel AH. P-Glycoprotein, a gatekeeper in the blood–brain barrier. *Adv Drug Deliv Rev* 1999; **36**:179–94.

8 Betz A. An overview of the multiple functions of the blood–brain barrier. *NIDA Res Monogr* 1992; **120**:5–72.

9 Pardridge W, Oldendorf W, Cancilla P, *et al.* Blood–brain barrier: interface between internal medicine and the brain. *Ann Intern Med* 1986; **105**:82–95.

10 Angeletti RH, Novikoff PM, Juvvadi SR, Fritschy JM, Meier PJ, Wolkoff AW. The choroid plexus epithelium is the site of the organic anion transport protein in the brain. *Proc Natl Acad Sci USA* 1997; **94**:283–6.

11 Wijnholds J, deLange EC, Scheffer GL, *et al.* Multidrug resistance protein 1 protects the choroid plexus epithelium and contributes to the blood–cerebrospinal fluid barrier. *J Clin Invest* 2000; **105**:279–85.

12 Groothuis D. The blood–brain and blood–tumor barriers: a review of strategies for increasing drug delivery. *Neuro-Oncol* 2000; **2**:45–59.

13 Blasberg R, Kobayashi T, Horowitz M, *et al.* Regional blood-to-tissue transport in ethylnitrosourea-induced brain tumors. *Ann Neurol* 1983; **14**:202–15.

14 Burger P. The anatomy of astrocytomas. *Mayo Clin Proc* 1987; **62**:527–9.

15 Poplack D, Bleyer W, Horowitz M. *Pharmacology of Antineoplastic Agents in Cerebrospinal Fluid*. New York: Plenum Press, 1980.

16 Mellet L. Physiochemical considerations and pharmacokinetic behavior in delivery of drugs to the central nervous system. *Cancer Treat Rep* 1977; **61**:527–31.

17 Koch-Weser J, Sellers E. Binding of drugs to serum albumin. *N Engl J Med* 1976; **294**:311–16.

18 Stewart D. A critique of the role of the blood–brain barrier in the chemotherapy of human brain tumors. *J Neuro-Oncol* 1994; **20**:121–39.

19 Vick NA, Khandekar J. Chemotherapy of brain tumors: the "blood–brain" barrier is not a factor. *Arch Neurol* 1977; **34**:523–6.

20 Doolittle N, Petrillo A, Bell S, Cummings P, Eriksen S. Blood–brain barrier disruption for the treatment of malignant brain tumors: the National Program. *J Neuroscience Nurs* **30**:81–90.

21 Neuwelt E, Rapoport S. Modification of the blood–brain barrier in the chemotherapy of malignant brain tumors. *Fed Proc* 1984; **43**:214–19.

22 Shapiro WR, Voorhies RM, Hiesiger EM, Sher PB, Basler GA, Lipschutz LE. Pharmacokinetics of tumor cell exposure to [14C]methotrexate after intracarotid administration without and with hyperosmotic opening of the blood–brain and blood–tumor barriers in rat brain tumors: a quantitative autoradiographic study. *Cancer Res* 1988; **48**:694–701.

23 Hiesiger EM, Voorhies RM, Basler GA, Lipschutz LE, Posner JB, Shapiro WR. Opening the blood–brain and blood–tumor barriers in experimental rat brain tumors: the effect of intracarotid hyperosmolar mannitol on capillary permeability and blood flow. *Ann Neurol* 1986; **19**:50–9.

24 Zunkeler B, Carson RE, Olson J, *et al.* Quantification and pharmacokinetics of blood–brain barrier disruption in humans. *J Neurosurg* 1996; **85**:1056–65.

25 Doolittle ND, Miner ME, Hall WA, *et al.* Safety and efficacy of a multicenter study using intraarterial chemotherapy in conjunction with osmotic opening of the blood–brain barrier for the treatment of patients with malignant brain tumors. *Cancer* 2000; **88**:637–47.

26 Williams PC, Henner WD, Roman-Goldstein S, *et al.* Toxicity and efficacy of carboplatin and etoposide in conjunction with disruption of the blood–brain tumor barrier in the treatment of intracranial neoplasms. *Neurosurgery* 1995; **37**:17–27, 27–8.

27 Doolittle ND, Muldoon LL, Brummett RE, *et al.* Delayed sodium thiosulfate as an otoprotectant against carboplatin-induced hearing loss in patients with malignant brain tumors. *Clin Cancer Res* 2001; **7**:493–500.

28 Fortin D, McCormick CI, Remsen LG, Nixon R, Neuwelt EA. Unexpected neurotoxicity of etoposide phosphate administered in combination with other chemotherapeutic agents after blood–brain barrier modification to enhance delivery, using propofol for general anesthesia, in a rat model. *Neurosurgery* 2000; **47**:199–207.

29 Elliott PJ, Hayward NJ, Huff MR, Nagle TL, Black KL, Bartus RT. Unlocking the blood–brain barrier: a role for RMP-7 in brain tumor therapy. *Exp Neurol* 1996; **141**:214–24.

30 Liu Y, Hashizume K, Chen Z, *et al.* Correlation between bradykinin-induced blood–tumor barrier permeability and B2 receptor expression in experimental brain tumors. *Neurol Res* 2001; **23**:379–87.

31 Cloughesy TF, Black KL, Gobin YP, *et al*. Intra-arterial Cereport (RMP-7) and carboplatin: a dose escalation study for recurrent malignant gliomas. *Neurosurgery* 1999; **44**:270–8, 278–9.

32 Gutman M, Laufer R, Eisenthal A, *et al*. Increased microvascular permeability induced by prolonged interleukin-2 administration is attenuated by the oxygen-free-radical scavenger dimethylthiourea. *Cancer Immunol Immunother* 1996; **43**:240–4.

33 Black KL, Chio CC. Increased opening of blood–tumour barrier by leukotriene C4 is dependent on size of molecules. *Neurol Res* 1992; **14**:402–4.

34 De Vries H, Blom-Roosemalen M, van Oosten M, *et al*. The influence of cytokines on the integrity of the blood–brain barrier in vitro. *J Neuroimmunol* 1996; **64**:37–43.

35 Raymond J, Robertson D, Dinsdale H. Pharmacological modification of bradykinin induced breakdown of the blood–brain barrier. *Can J Neurol Sci* 1986; **13**:214–20.

36 Inamura T, Black K. Bradykinin selectively opens blood–tumor barrier in experimental brain tumors. *J Cereb Blood Flow Metab* 1984; **14**:862–70.

37 Emerich DF, Dean RL, Osborn C, Bartus RT. The development of the bradykinin agonist labradimil as a means to increase the permeability of the blood–brain barrier: from concept to clinical evaluation. *Clin Pharmacokinet* 2001; **40**:105–23.

38 Thomas J, Lind M, Ford J, Bleehen N, Calvert A, Boddy A. Pharmacokinetics of carboplatin administered in combination with the bradykinin agonist Cereport (RMP-7) for the treatment of brain tumors. *Cancer Chem Pharmacol* 2000; **45**:284–90.

39 Trnovec T, Kallay Z, Bezek S. Effects of ionizing radiation on the blood–brain barrier permeability to pharmacologically active substances. *Int J Radiat Oncol Biol Phys* 1990; **19**:1581–7.

40 Qin DX, Zheng R, Tang J, Li JX, Hu YH. Influence of radiation on the blood–brain barrier and optimum time of chemotherapy. *Int J Radiat Oncol Biol Phys* 1990; **19**:1507–10.

41 Schinkel A. P-glycoprotein, a gatekeeper in the blood–brain barrier. *Adv Drug Deliv Rev* 1999; **36**:179–94.

42 Balis FM, Holcenberg JS, Blaney SM. General principles of chemotherapy. In: Pizzo P, Poplack D (eds). *Principles and Practice of Pediatric Oncology*, 4th edition. Philadelphia: Lippincott-Raven, 2002, pp. 237–309.

43 Chaudhary PM, Roninson IB. Expression and activity of P-glycoprotein, a multidrug efflux pump in human hematopoietic stem cell. *Cell* 1991; **66**:85–94.

44 Schinkel AH, Wagenaar E, Mol CA, van Deemter L. P-glycoprotein in the blood-brain barrier of mice influences the brain penetration and pharmacological activity of many drugs. *J Clin Invest* 1996; **97**:2517–24.

45 Warren KE, Patel MC, McCully CM, Montuenga LM, Balis FM. Effect of P-glycoprotein modulation with cyclosporin A on cerebrospinal fluid penetration of doxorubicin in non-human primates. *Cancer Chemother Pharmacol* 2000; **45**:207–12.

46 Hoffmeyer S, Burk O, von Richter O, *et al*. Functional polymorphisms of the human multidrug-resistance gene: multiple sequence variations and correlation of one allele with P-glycoprotein expression and activity in vivo. *Proc Natl Acad Sci USA* 2000; **97**:3473–8.

47 Zucchetti M, Boiardi A, Silvani A, Parisi I, Piccolrovazzi S, D'Incalci M. Distribution of daunorubicin and daunorubicinol in human glioma tumors after administration of liposomal daunorubicin. *Cancer Chemother Pharmacol* 1999; **44**:173–6.

48 Koukourakis MI, Koukouraki S, Fezoulidis I, *et al*. High intratumoural accumulation of stealth liposomal doxorubicin (Caelyx) in glioblastomas and in metastatic brain tumours. *Br J Cancer* 2000; **83**:1281–6.

49 Poplack D, Riccardi R. Pharmacologic approaches to the treatment of central nervous system malignancy. In: Poplack D, Massimo L, Cornaglia-Ferraris P (eds). *The Role of Pharmacology in Pediatric Oncology*. Boston: Martinus Nijhoff, 1987, pp. 137–56.

50 Chabner B. The role of drugs in cancer treatment. In: Chabner B (ed.). *Pharmacologic Principles of Cancer Treatment*. Philadelphia: WB Saunders, 1982, pp. 3–14.

51 Collins J. Regional therapy: an overview. In: Poplack D, Massimo L, Cornaglia-Ferraris P (eds). *The Role of Pharmacology in Pediatric Oncology*. Boston: Martinus Nijhoff, 1987, pp. 125–35.

52 Blasberg R, Patlak C, Fernstermacher J. Intrathecal chemotherapy. Brain tissue profiles after ventriculo-cisternal perfusion. *J Pharmacol Exp Ther* 1975; **195**:73–83.

53 Blaney S, Poplack D, Godwin K, McCully C, Murphy R, Balis F. The effect of body position on ventricular cerebrospinal fluid methotrexate concentration following intralumbar administration. *J Clin Oncol* 1995; **13**:177–9.

54 Bomgaars L, Chamberlain M, Poplack D, Blaney S. Leptomeningeal metastases. In: Levin VA (ed.): *Cancer in the Nervous System*, 2nd edition. New York: Oxford University Press, 2002, pp. 375–93.

55 Larson S, Johnson G, Ommaya A, Jones A, Chiro GD. The radionuclide ventriculogram. *J Am Med Assoc* 1973; **224**:853–7.

56 Bleyer W. Clinicalpharmacology of intrathecal methotrexate. II. An improved dosage regimen derived from age-related pharmacokinetics. *Cancer Treat Rep* 1977; **61**:1419–25.

57 Bleyer W, Coccia PF, Sather HN, *et al*. Reduction in central nervous system leukemia with a pharmacokinetically derived intrathecal methotrexate dosage regimen. *J Clin Oncol* 1983; **1**:317–25.

58 Heideman R, Packer R, Reaman G, *et al*. A Phase II evaluation of thiotepa in central nervous system malignancies. *Cancer* 1992; **72**:271–5.

59 Witham T, Fukui M, Meltzer C, Burns R, Konziolka D, Bozik M. Survival of patients with high grade glioma treated with intrathecal thiotriethylenephosphoramide for ependymal or leptomeningeal gliomatosis. *Cancer* 1999; **86**:1347–53.

60 Grossman SA, Finkelstein DM, Ruckdeschel JC, Trump DL, Moynihan T, Ettinger DS. Randomized prospective comparison of intraventricular methotrexate and thiotepa in patients with previously untreated neoplastic meningitis. Eastern Cooperative Oncology Group. *J Clin Oncol* 1993; **11**:561–9.

61 Berg S, Balis F, Zimm S, *et al*. Phase I/II trial and pharma-cokinetics of intrathecal diaziquone in refractory meningeal malignancies. *J Clin Oncol* 1992; **10**:143–8.

62 Adamson P, Balis F, Arndt C, *et al*. Intrathecal 6-mercaptopurine: preclinical pharmacology, phase I/II trial, and pharmacokinetic study. *Cancer Res* 1991; **51**:6079–83.

63 Blaney S, Balis F, Arndt *et al*. A phase I study of intrathecal mafosfamide (MF) in patients wtih refractory meningeal malignancies. *Proc Am Soc Clin Oncol* 1992; **11**:113.

64 Slavc I, Schuller E, Czech T, Hainfellner J, Seidl R, Dieckmann K. Intrathecal mafosfamide therapy for pediatric brain tumors with meningeal dissemination. *J Neuro-Oncol* 1998; **38**:213–18.

65 Blaney S, Heideman R, Cole D, *et al.* A phase I study of intrathecal topotecan. *Proc Am Soc Cancer Res* 1998; **39**:2198.

66 Glantz M, Jaekle K, Chamberlain M, *et al.* A randomized controlled trial comparing intrathecal sustained-release cytarabine (DepoCyt) to intrathecal methotrexate in patients with neoplastic meningitis from solid tumors. *Clin Cancer Res* 1999; **5**:2294–402.

67 Bomgaars L, Geyer J, Franklin J, *et al.* A phase I dose escalation study of intrathecal DepoFoam™ encapsulated cytarabine (DTC101) in pediatric patients with advanced malignancies. *Am Soc Ped Hem Oncol* 1998; **30**:683.

68 Jaeckle K, Phuphanich S, Bent M, *et al.* Intrathecal treatment of neoplastic meningitis due to breast cancer with a slow-release formulation of cytarabine. *Br J Cancer* 2001; **84**:157–63.

69 Menei P, Benoit JP, Boisdron-Celle M, Fournier D, Mercier P, Guy G. Drug targeting into the central nervous system by stereotactic implantation of biodegradable microspheres. *Neurosurgery* 1994; **34**:1058–64.

70 Brem H, Piantadosi S, Burger PC, *et al.* Placebo-controlled trial of safety and efficacy of intraoperative controlled delivery by biodegradable polymers of chemotherapy for recurrent gliomas. The Polymer-brain Tumor Treatment Group. *Lancet* 1995; **345**:1008–12.

71 Haroun RI, Brem H. Local drug delivery. *Curr Opin Oncol* 2000; **12**:187–93.

72 Subach B, Witham T, Kondziokla D, Lunsford L, Bozik M, Schiff D. Morbidity and survival after 1,3-bis (2-chloroethyl)-1-nitrosourea water implantation for recurrent glioblastoma: a retrospective case-matched cohort series. *Neurosurgery* 1999; **45**:17–23.

73 Engelhard HH. The role of interstitial BCNU chemotherapy in the treatment of malignant glioma. *Surg Neurol* 2000; **53**:458–64.

74 Bobo R, Laske DW, Akbasak A, Morrison P, Dedrick R, Oldfield EH. Convection-enhanced delivery of macromolecules in the brain. *Proc Natl Acad Sci USA* 1994; **91**:2076–80.

75 Friedman HS, Dolan ME, Moschel RC, *et al.* Enhancement of nitrosourea activity in medulloblastoma and glioblastoma multiforme. *J Natl Cancer Inst* 1992; **84**:1926–31.

76 Dolan ME, Mitchell RB, Mummert C, Moschel RC, Pegg AE. Effect of O6-benzylguanine analogues on sensitivity of human tumor cells to the cytotoxic effects of alkylating agents. *Cancer Res* 1991; **51**:3367–72.

77 Olivi A, Bruce J, Saris S, *et al.* Phase I study of escalating doses of interstitial BCNU administered via wafer in patients with recurrent malignant glioma. *Proc Am Soc Clin Oncol* 1998; **17**:A1490.

78 Menei P, Venier MC, Gamelin E, *et al.* Local and sustained delivery of 5-fluorouracil from biodegradable microspheres for the radiosensitization of glioblastoma: a pilot study. *Cancer* 1999; **86**:325–30.

79 Kaiser MG, Parsa AT, Fine RL, Hall JS, Chakrabarti I, Bruce JN. Tissue distribution and antitumor activity of topotecan delivered by intracerebral clysis in a rat glioma model. *Neurosurgery* 2000; **47**:1391–8, 1398–9.

80 Fernstermacher J, Kaye T. Drug "diffusion" within the brain. *Ann N Y Acad Sci* 1988; **531**:29–39.

81 Rosenberg G, Kyner W, Estrada E. Bulk flow of brain interstitial fluid under normal and hyperosmolar conditions. *Am J Physiol* 1980; **238**:F42–9.

82 Laske DW, Morrison PF, Lieberman DM, *et al.* Chronic interstitial infusion of protein to primate brain: determination of drug distribution and clearance with single-photon emission computerized tomography imaging. *J Neurosurg* 1997; **87**:586–94.

83 Lieberman D, Laske DW, Morrison PF, Bankiewicz K, Oldfield EH. Convection-enhanced distribution of large molecules in gray matter during interstitial drug infusion. *J Neurosurg* 1995; **82**:1021–9.

84 Viola JJ, Agbaria R, Walbridge S, *et al.* In situ cyclopentenyl cytosine infusion for the treatment of experimental brain tumors. *Cancer Res* 1995; **55**:1306–9.

85 Heimberger A, Archer G, McLendon RE, *et al.* Temozolomide delivered by intracerebral microinfusion is safe and efficacious against malignant gliomas in rats. *Clin Cancer Res* 2000; **6**:4148–53.

86 Saris SC, Blasberg RG, Carson RE, *et al.* Intravascular streaming during carotid artery infusions. Demonstration in humans and reduction using diastole-phased pulsatile administration. *J Neurosurg* 1991; **74**:763–72.

87 Shapiro WR. Chemotherapy of malignant gliomas: studies of the BTCG. *Rev Neurol (Paris)* 1992; **148**:428–34.

88 Berg S, Poplack D. Advances in the treatment of meningeal cancers. *Crit Rev Oncol Hematol* 1995; **20**:87–98.

89 Abrey LE, Rosenblum MK, Papadopoulos E, Childs BH, Finlay JL. High dose chemotherapy with autologous stem cell rescue in adults with malignant primary brain tumors. *J Neuro-Oncol* 1999; **44**:147–53.

90 Papadakis V, Dunkel IJ, Cramer LD, *et al.* High-dose carmustine, thiotepa and etoposide followed by autologous bone marrow rescue for the treatment of high risk central nervous system tumors. *Bone Marrow Transplant* 2000; **26**:153–60.

91 Kochi M, Ushio Y. High-dose chemotherapy with autologous hematopoietic stem-cell rescue for patients with malignant brain tumors. *Crit Rev Neurosurg* 1999; **9**:295–302.

92 Finlay J, Stewart S, Wong M, *et al.* Pilot study of high-dose thiotepa and etoposide with autologous bone marrow rescue in children and young adults with recurrent CNS tumors. *J Clin Oncol* 1996; **14**:2495–503.

93 Guruangan S, Dunkel IJ, Goldman S, *et al.* Myeloablative chemotherapy with autologous bone marrow rescue in young children with recurrent malignant brain tumors. *J Clin Oncol* 1998; **16**:2486–93.

94 Colvin M, Chabner B. Alkylating agents. In: Chabner B, Collins JM (eds). *Cancer Chemotherapy: Principles and Practice.* Philadelphia: JB Lippincott, 1990, pp. 276–313.

95 Frei E, Teicher B, Holden S, Cathcar K, Wang Y. Preclinical studies and clinical correlation of the effect of alkylating dose. *Cancer Res* 1988; **48**:6417–23.

96 Connors T. Alkylating drugs, nitrosoureas and dimethyl-triazenes. In: Pinedo HM (ed.). *Cancer Chemotherapy.* New York: Elsevier, 1981, pp. 32–47.

97 Mirkes P. Cyclophosphamide teratogenesis: a review. *Teratog Carcinog Mutagen* 1985; **5**:75–88.

98 Balis FM, Holcenberg JS, Blaney SM. General principles of chemotherapy. In: Pizzo P, Poplack D (eds). *Principles and*

Practice of Pediatric Oncology, 4th edition. Philadelphia: Lippincott-Raven, 2002, pp. 237–309.

99 Abrahamsen TG, Lange BJ, Packer RJ, *et al.* A phase I and II trial of dose-intensified cyclophosphamide and GM-CSF in pediatric malignant brain tumors. *J Pediatr Hematol Oncol* 1995; **17**:134–9.

100 Yule SM, Foreman NK, Mitchell C, Gouldon N, May P, McDowell HP. High-dose cyclophosphamide for poor-prognosis and recurrent pediatric brain tumors: a dose-escalation study. *J Clin Oncol* 1997; **15**:3258–65.

101 Allen JC, Helson L. High-dose cyclophosphamide chemotherapy for recurrent CNS tumors in children. *J Neurosurg* 1981; **55**:749–56.

102 Kumar A, Renaudin J, Wilson C, Boldrey E, Enot K, Levin V. Procarbazine hydrochloride in the treatment of brain tumors. *J Neurosurg* 1974; **40**:365–71.

103 Chintagumpala M, Burger P, McCluggage C, *et al.* Response to procarbazine in newly diagnosed patients with high-grade glioma: a Pediatric Oncology Group (POG) study. *Proc Annu Meet Am Soc Clin Oncol* 1999; **18**:A2153.

104 Galanis E, Buckner JC, Burch PA, *et al.* Phase II trial of nitrogen mustard, vincristine, and procarbazine in patients with recurrent glioma: North Central Cancer Treatment Group results. *J Clin Oncol* 1998; **16**:2953–8.

105 Edwards M, Levin V, Wilson C. Brain tumor chemotherapy: an evaluation of agents in current use for phase II and III trials. *Cancer Treat Rep* 1980; **64**:1179–205.

106 Newton H, Bromberg J, Junck L, Page M, Greenberg H. Comparison between BCNU and procarbazine chemotherapy for treatment of gliomas. *J Neuro-Oncol* 1993; **15**:257–63.

107 Friedman H, Kokkinakis D, Pluda J, *et al.* Phase I trial of O6-benzylguanine for patients undergoing surgery for malignant glioma. *J Clin Oncol* 1998; **16**:3570–5.

108 Schilsky R, Dolan M, Bertucci D, *et al.* Phase I clinical and pharmacological study of O6-benzylguanine followed by carmustine in patients with advanced cancer. *Clin Cancer Res* 2000; **6**:3025–31.

109 Agarwala S, Kirkwood J. Temozolomide, a novel alkylating agent with activity in the central nervous system, may improve the treatment of advanced metastatic melanoma. *Oncologist* 2000; **5**:144–51.

110 Newlands ES, O'Reilly SM, Glaser MG, *et al.* The Charing Cross Hospital experience with temozolomide in patients with gliomas. *Eur J Cancer* 1996; **32A**:2236–41.

111 Bower M, Newlands ES, Bleehen NM, *et al.* Multicentre CRC phase II trial of temozolomide in recurrent or progressive high-grade glioma. *Cancer Chemother Pharmacol* 1997; **40**:484–8.

112 Friedman H, Pluda J, Quinn J, *et al.* Phase I trial of carmustine plus O6-benzylguanine for patients with recurrent or progressive malignant glioma. *J Clin Oncol* 2000; **18**:3522–8.

113 Patel M, Godwin K, McCully C, Adamson P, Balis F. Plasma and cerebrospinal fluid pharmacokinetics of carboplatin and cisplatin. *Proc Am Assoc Cancer Res* 1996; **37**:A2753.

114 Van den Bent M, Schellens J, Vecht C, *et al.* Phase II study on cisplatin and ifosfamide in recurrent high grade gliomas. *Eur J Cancer* 1998; **34**:1570–4.

115 Murry D. Comparative clinical pharmacology of cisplatin and carboplatin. *Pharmacotherapy* 1997; **17**:140–455.

116 Bertolone SJ, Baum ES, Krivit W, Hammond GD. A phase II study of cisplatin therapy in recurrent childhood brain tumors. A report from the Childrens Cancer Study Group. *J Neuro-Oncol* 1989; **7**:5–11.

117 Khan A, D'Souza B, Wharam M, *et al.* Cisplatin therapy in recurrent childhood brain tumors. *Cancer Treat Rep* 1982; **66**:2013–20.

118 Sexauer C, Khan A, Burger P, *et al.* Cisplatin in recurrent pediatric brain tumors: a POG phase II study. *Cancer* 1985; **56**:1497–501.

119 Walker RW, Allen JC. Cisplatin in the treatment of recurrent childhood primary brain tumors. *J Clin Oncol* 1988; **6**:62–6.

120 Whittle I, Malcolm G, DI DJ, Reid M. Platinum distribution in malignant glioma following intraoperative intravenous infusion of carboplatin. *Br J Neurosurg* 1999; **13**:132–7.

121 Markman M, Kennedy A, Webster K, *et al.* Clinical features of hypersensitivity reactions to carboplatin. *J Clin Oncol* 1999; **17**:1141–5.

122 Allen JC, Walker R, Luks E, Jennings M, Barfoot S, Tan C. Carboplatin and recurrent childhood brain tumors. *J Clin Oncol* 1987; **5**:459–63.

123 Gaynon PS, Ettinger LJ, Moel D, *et al.* Pediatric phase I trial of carboplatin: a Children's Cancer Study Group report. *Cancer Treat Rep* 1987; **71**:1039–42.

124 Gaynon PS, Ettinger LJ, Baum ES, Siegel SE, Krailo MD, Hammond GD. Carboplatin in childhood brain tumors. A Children's Cancer Study Group phase II trial. *Cancer* 1990; **66**:2465–9.

125 Friedman HS, Krischer JP, Burger P, *et al.* Treatment of children with progressive or recurrent brain tumors with carboplatin or iproplatin: a Pediatric Oncology Group randomized phase II study. *J Clin Oncol* 1992; **10**:249–56.

126 Packer RJ, Lange B, Ater J, *et al.* Carboplatin and vincristine for recurrent and newly diagnosed low-grade gliomas of childhood. *J Clin Oncol* 1993; **11**:850–6.

127 Packer RJ, Goldwein J, Nicholson HS, *et al.* Treatment of children with medulloblastomas with reduced-dose craniospinal radiation therapy and adjuvant chemotherapy: a Children's Cancer Group Study. *J Clin Oncol* 1999; **17**:2127–36.

128 Mahoney DH, Jr., Cohen ME, Friedman HS, *et al.* Carboplatin is effective therapy for young children with progressive optic pathway tumors: a Pediatric Oncology Group phase II study. *Neuro-Oncol* 2000; **2**:213–20.

129 Kobrinsky NL, Packer RJ, Boyett JM, *et al.* Etoposide with or without mannitol for the treatment of recurrent or primarily unresponsive brain tumors: a Children's Cancer Group Study, CCG-9881. *J Neuro-Oncol* 1999; **45**:47–54.

130 Ashley DM, Meier L, Kerby T, *et al.* Response of recurrent medulloblastoma to low-dose oral etoposide. *J Clin Oncol* 1996; **14**:1922–7.

131 Chamberlain MC. Recurrent cerebellar gliomas: salvage therapy with oral etoposide. *J Child Neurol* 1997; **12**:200–4.

132 Chamberlain MC. Recurrent intracranial ependymoma in children: salvage therapy with oral etoposide. *Pediatr Neurol* 2001; **24**:117–21.

133 Korones DN, Fisher PG, Cohen KJ, Dubowy RL. No responses to oral etoposide in 15 patients with recurrent brain tumors. *Med Pediatr Oncol* 2000; **35**:80–2.

134 Needle MN, Molloy PT, Geyer JR, *et al.* Phase II study of daily oral etoposide in children with recurrent brain tumors and other solid tumors. *Med Pediatr Oncol* 1997; **29**:28–32.

135 Sullivan MP, van Eys J, Herson J, Starling KA, Ragab A, Sexhauer C. Nonresponsiveness of brain tumors to VM-26 therapy in children. *Cancer Treat Rep* 1979; **63**:155–6.

136 Seiler RW. Combination chemotherapy with VM 26 and CCNU in primary malignant brain tumors of children. *Helv Paediatr Acta* 1980; **35**:51–6.

137 Blaney S, Cole D, Balis F, Godwin K, McCully C, Poplack D. Plasma and CSF pharmacokinetic study of topotecan in nonhuman primates. *Cancer Res* 1992; **53**:725–7.

138 Sung C, Blaney S, Cole D, Balis F, Dedrick R. A pharmacokinetic model of topotecan clearance from plasma and cerebrospinal fluid. *Cancer Res* 1994; **54**:5118–22.

139 Friedman H, Houghton P, Schold S, Keir S, Bigner D. Activity of 9-dimethylamiomethyl-10-hydroxycamptothecin against pediatric and adult central nervous system tumor xenografts. *Cancer Chem Pharmacol* 1994; **34**:171–4.

140 Blaney S, Phillips P, Packer R, *et al.* Phase II evaluation of topotecan for pediatric central nervous system tumors. *Cancer* 1996; **78**:527–31.

141 Kadota R, Stewart C, Horn M, *et al.* Topotecan for the treatment of recurrent or progressive central nervous system tumors: a Pediatric Oncology Group phase II study. *J Neuro-Oncol* 1999; **43**:43–7.

142 Blaney S, Balis F, Cole D, *et al.* Pediatric phase I trial and pharmacokinetic study of topotecan administered as a 24-hour continuous infusion. *Cancer Res* 1993; **53**:1032–6.

143 Furman W, Baker S, Pratt CB, Rivera G, Evans WE, Stewart C. Escalating systemic exposure to topotecan following a 120-hour continuous infusion in children with relapsed acute leukemia. *J Clin Oncol* 1996; **14**:1504–11.

144 Stewart C, Baker S, Heideman R, Jones D, Crom W, Pratt C. Clincal pharmacodynamics of continuous infusion topotecan in children: systemic exposure predicts hematologic toxicity. *J Clin Oncol* 1994; **12**:1946–54.

145 Rosing H, Herben V, van Gortel-van Zomeren D, *et al.* Isolation and structural confirmation of *N*-desmethyl topotecan, a metabolite of topotecan. *Cancer Chemother Pharmacol* 1997; **39**:498–504.

146 Zamboni W, Gajjar A, Heideman R, *et al.* Phenytoin alters the disposition of topotecan and *N*-desmethyl topotecan in a patient with medulloblastoma. *Clin Cancer Res* 1998; **4**:783–9.

147 Kunimoto T, Nitta K, Tanaka T, *et al.* Antitumor activity of 7-ethyl-10-[4-(1-piperidino)-1-piperidino]carbonyloxy-camptothecin, a novel water-soluble derivative of camptothecin. *Cancer Res* 1987; **47**:5944–7.

148 Friedman H, Petrow W, Friedman A, *et al.* Irinotecan therapy in adults with recurrent or progressive malignant glioma. *J Clin Oncol* 1999; **17**:1516–25.

149 Murry D, Cherrick I, Salama V, *et al.* Influence of phenytoin on the disposition of irinotecan: a case report. *J Pediatr Hematol Oncol* 2002; **24**:130–3.

150 Rosenstock J, Evans A, Schut L. Response to vincristine of recurrent brain tumors in children. *J Neurosurg* 1976; **45**:135–9.

151 Rosen G, Ghavimi F, Nirenberg A, Mosende C, Mehta BM. High-dose methotrexate with citrovorum factor rescue for the treatment of central nervous system tumors in children. *Cancer Treat Rep* 1977; **61**:681–90.

152 Mulne AF, Ducore JM, Elterman RD, *et al.* Oral methotrexate for recurrent brain tumors in children: a Pediatric Oncology Group study. *J Pediatr Hematol Oncol* 2000; **22**:41–4.

153 Koehler PJ. Use of corticosteroids in neuro-oncology. *Anticancer Drugs* 1995; **6**:19–33.

154 Straathof CS, van den Bent MJ, Ma J, *et al.* The effect of dexamethasone on the uptake of cisplatin in 9L glioma and the area of brain around tumor. *J Neuro-Oncol* 1998; **37**:1–8.

155 Ostergaard L, Hochberg FH, Rabinov JD, *et al.* Early changes measured by magnetic resonance imaging in cerebral blood flow, blood volume, and blood–brain barrier permeability following dexamethasone treatment in patients with brain tumors. *J Neurosurg* 1999; **90**:300–5.

156 Kirsch M, Schacker G, Black P. Anti-angiogenic treatment strategies for malignant brain tumors. *J Neuro-Oncol* 2000; **50**:149–63.

157 Deininger M, Goldman J, Lydon N, Melo J. The tryosine kinase inhibitor CGP57148B selectively inhibits the growth of BCR-ABL positive cells. *Blood* 1997; **90**:3691–8.

158 Druker B, Tamura S, Buchdunger E, *et al.* Effects of a selective inhibitor of the Abl tyrosine kinase on the growth of Bcr-Abl positive cells. *Nat Med* 1996; **2**:561–6.

159 Buchdunger E, Cioffi C, Law N, *et al.* Abl protein-tyrosine kinase inhibitor STI571 inhibits in vitro signal transduction mediated by c-kit and platelet-derived growth factor receptors. *J Pharmacol Exp Ther* 2000; **295**:139–45.

160 Carroll M, Ohno-Jones S, Tamura S, *et al.* CGP 57148, a tyrosine kinase inhibitor, inhibits the growth of cells expressing BCR-ABL, TEL-ABL, and TEL-PDGFR fusion proteins. *Blood* 1997; **90**:4947–52.

161 Heinrich M, Griffith D, Druker B, Wait C, Ott K, Ziggler A. Inhibition of c-kit receptor tyrosine kinase activity by STI 571, a selective tyrosine kinase inhibitor. *Blood* 2000; **96**:925–32.

162 Nistér M, Claesson-Welch L, Eriksson A, Heldin C-H, Westermark B. Differential expression of platelet-derived growth factor receptors in human malignant glioma cell lines. *J Biol Chem* 1991; **266**:16755–63.

163 Balis FM, Poplack DG. Cancer Chemotherapy. In: Nathan DG, Oski FA (eds). *Hematology of Infancy and Childhood.* Philadelphia: W.B. Saunders, 1993, pp. 1207–38.

Disease-specific multidisciplinary management

PART

V

Disease-specific multidisciplinary

Astrocytic tumors, low-grade: general considerations

ASTRID K. GNEKOW, ROGER J. PACKER AND ROLF D. KORTMANN

INTRODUCTION

Due to the misconception that the low-grade astrocytic tumors are uniformly benign neoplasms curable by surgery alone, there has been widespread and long-lasting underestimation of the diagnostic and therapeutic challenges posed by these tumors. This chapter and Chapter 13b will detail the broad spectrum of presentation, biologic behavior, and basic management strategies for the group of histopathologically variable tumors categorized as low-grade glioma.

EPIDEMIOLOGY

Low-grade gliomas comprise approximately 30–40 per cent of all primary brain tumors of childhood. Their annual incidence varies between 10 and 12 per million children under the age of 15 years in Western countries (France, USA, Scandinavia) and between three and five per million children under the age of 15 years in China and Japan.[1]

Low-grade gliomas may occur at any age. The mean age of diagnosis varies but ranges between six and 11 years. Some subgroups of low-grade glioma, such as desmoplastic infantile ganglioglioma/astrocytoma (DIG/DIA), peak at a different age. There is no general consensus concerning the impact of age on the risk of disease progression. The male/female overall ratio is 1.2 to one.[1] However, some diagnoses, such as DIG/DIA, show a more marked male preponderance.

Familial and heritable disease associations

There is a striking association of specific variants of low-grade glioma and heritable diseases, which, in part, may serve as a model for cancer development.

NEUROFIBROMATOSIS TYPE 1

Neurofibromatosis type 1 (NF-1) in both its familial and sporadic forms is caused by mutations within the *Neurofibromin* gene located on the long arm of chromosome 17 (17q11.2). This evolutionary, highly conserved gene spanning 350 kb of genomic DNA is organized in more than 50 exons. Transcripts have been found to be tissue- and cell-type-specific and to be expressed differentially in neurons and glia.[2,3] Highest levels of the gene product, neurofibromin, have been detected within the central and peripheral nervous systems and in the adrenal glands.

The NF-1 gene can be regarded primarily as a histogenesis control gene, which also functions as a tumor suppressor gene.[4] While the occurrence of two independent mutations for the rise of malignant tumors seems to be the case for malignant neurofibrosarcoma, it is doubtful that this model also explains the development of low-grade astrocytic lesions in NF-1.

Low-grade gliomas, primarily of the optic nerves and diencephalon, but also of other regions of brain, arise in 5–15 per cent of patients with NF-1.[5–9] Up to 50 per cent of patients with visual pathway gliomas will have NF-1; an even higher proportion of those with isolated optic nerve gliomas will have this condition.[10–13] Since the presence of an optic pathway glioma puts NF-1 patients at risk for later development of other, even more malignant, brain tumors, there may exist a subset of NF-1 patients with increased vulnerability for glial tumors. It is unresolved as to whether specific genetic mutations of the NF-1 gene, or the effects of modifying genes or other modifying factors, predispose to the evolution of visual pathway gliomas in NF-1.[9,14]

TUBEROUS SCLEROSIS

Tuberous sclerosis complex is an autosomal dominantly inherited multisystem disorder characterized by widespread hamartomas in almost every organ, but predominantly brain, kidneys, liver, heart, skin, and eyes. Molecular studies have shown mutations on chromosomes 16p13 and 9q34. The presence of subependymal giant-cell astrocytoma is one of the major diagnostic criteria.[15] The tumors appear with increasing frequency throughout childhood, reaching an incidence of 15 per cent in adolescence.[16]

LI–FRAUMENI SYNDROME

Low-grade astrocytomas occur with increased incidence in Li–Fraumeni syndrome, a genetic condition characterized by an excessive aggregation of tumors in more than two generations or in siblings, by the occurrence of tumors at an unusual age for the tumor type or in an atypical gender, and by the sequential appearance of other cancers in the same individual, associated with genetic disorders and birth defects.[17–19] A germ-line mutation in the *p53* locus on chromosome 17p13 triggers the susceptibility to develop multiple tumors, among which brain tumors are frequently encountered. Children present mainly with medulloblastoma/primitive neuroectodermal tumor (PNET) or choroid plexus tumors, but astrocytic tumors associated with the Li–Fraumeni syndrome occur mainly in the third and fourth decades of life.[20]

Other associations

Although radiation-induced brain tumors are mostly meningioma or high-grade glioma, low-grade gliomas may also occur.[21] Even among children irradiated for tinea capitis, long-term follow-up has disclosed the development of intracranial tumors, including low-grade glioma, after long latency periods.[22]

DETERMINANTS OF BIOLOGIC BEHAVIOR

Despite repeated attempts of conventional karyotyping and comparative genomic hybridization, specific gene loci with frequent alterations have not been characterized in childhood low-grade glioma, unlike in adult glioma, where progressive DNA alterations within one given tumor representing progressive degrees of malignancy have been found.[23,24]

The World Health Organization (WHO) suggests a role for the (altered) NF-1 gene or its signal transduction pathway in the development of sporadic juvenile pilocytic astrocytoma (JPA), although this has not been proven by specific gene deletions or changes of gene expression. Occasionally in cases of sporadic pilocytic astrocytoma, there is loss of chromosome 17q, including the region of the NF-1 gene, without a specific mutation.[25,26] Even the differential expression of some NF-1 transcripts does not separate reactive and neoplastic astrocytes.

Unlike the adult experience, in children the DNA index possesses no independent prognostic significance when survival is stratified by tumor grade.[27] All types of low-grade glioma are characterized by a biologically indolent growth pattern that is not explained well by histological features. However, even after incomplete surgical resections, some tumors do not exhibit growth for extended periods of time. Alterations in blood supply, decelerating growth kinetics within the tumor over time due to a change in the ability of the tumor to maintain an adequate level of autocrine growth factors (e.g. epidermal growth factor receptor (EGFR), c-erbB-2 oncoprotein, transforming growth factor alpha (TGF-α)), and an increase in the spontaneous rate of apoptosis could contribute to this erratic pattern of growth.[28–30]

There are other speculations about factors responsible for tumor growth. In adults, the presence of a higher proliferation rate, as identified by Ki-67/MIB-1-staining, elevated levels of vascular endothelial growth factor (VEGF), and downregulation of neural cell adhesion molecule (N-CAM) correlate with a higher rate of tumor progression.[31–33]

For childhood low-grade glioma, no unequivocal findings have been established. In general, non-aggressive behavior has been correlated with a low rate of DNA synthesis, as reflected by the bromodeoxyuridine labeling index.[34] However, the proliferation associated marker Ki 67 and its equivalent, MIB-1, for formalin-fixed, paraffin-embedded tissue, present in G1, S, G2, and M phases, but not in G0,[35] has shown marked variability without clear-cut correlation with natural behavior. Studies have correlated the MIB-1 staining index with recurrence in low-grade glioma.[32,36,37] A cut-off value of more than one per cent could be established for progressive pilocytic astrocytoma of the visual pathways by some authors,[38] but it was not confirmed as a predictive value.[39] Malignant progression and unfavorable prognosis might follow the additional clonal expansion of *p53*-mutated tumor cells,[40,41] whereas *p53* mutation by itself does not seem to predict aggressive tumor behavior.[42]

CLASSIFICATION

See Chapter 5.

GENERAL PRINCIPLES OF TREATMENT STRATEGY

Diagnosis

Reflecting the generally low proliferative potential of low-grade astrocytic tumors, clinical signs and symptoms evolve gradually in most cases. First symptoms may be traced back for years, but rapidly progressive signs can be noted as well.

Focal neurological signs and symptoms of increased intracranial pressure may be present, varying according to the location of the primary tumor. Focal neurological signs are related directly to the functional brain area at the site of tumor growth and are described in the respective sections.

Neuroimaging

See Chapter 7.

Histologic confirmation

Despite considerable recent advances in neuroimaging, there still is a need for histologic confirmation of the majority of lesions suspected to be low-grade tumors. Biopsy, either by open surgery or by stereotactic techniques, confirms the presence of a neoplasm and, if specific, the tumor type. It also provides prognostic information from histologic and molecular features.

Surgery is the first therapeutic step when approaching most pediatric low-grade gliomas.[43,44] There are a few clearly defined situations that do not require surgery and/or biopsy or resection. Unresectable, dorsally extending optic pathway gliomas will be of low-grade, usually pilocytic, histology in patients with NF-1, especially if there is unequivocal, extensive, and contiguous involvement of the visual pathways. Tumors should present the typical hypodense appearance on plain computed tomography (CT) scans. If these characteristics are not met, then biopsy of the tumor should be undertaken (Figure 13a.1).

BASIC CONSIDERATIONS CONCERNING TREATMENT STRATEGY

Analyzing overall survival as outcome parameter for the success of a given treatment strategy may not be adequate in low-grade astrocytic tumors. Since long phases

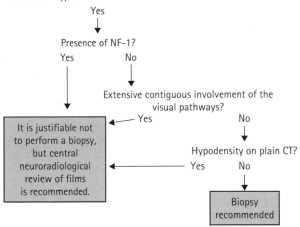

Figure 13a.1 *Decision-making process for biopsy of a chiasmatic-hypothalamic tumor.*

(10–15 years) of patient survival are common, and since survivors will experience late effects of all treatments applied, it is pertinent to evaluate the additional damage produced by any therapeutic measure.

Surgery

There is general consensus that primary surgical excision is the treatment of choice for almost all low-grade tumors at diagnosis and even at recurrences (Table 13a.1). Specialized imaging may help to trace the tumor margins and thereby permit the surgeon to spare critical functional areas.[44–46] Since these lesions are generally well demarcated with apparently minimal invasion of the surrounding brain tissue, they can be resected totally in some regions, such as the cerebellum and cerebral hemispheres. However, pathological review has shown that two-thirds of the tumors infiltrate the surrounding parenchyma, particularly the white matter.[47] Recent reports indicate that total removal is possible in up to 90 per cent of cerebral hemispheric gliomas[48] and in two-thirds of cerebellar astrocytomas.[49] Long-term follow-up shows survival rates after complete resection above 90 per cent.[48,50–55] However, even in these cohorts, a small percentage of progression occurs over time, justifying long-term follow-up, particularly after a second resection.

Many tumors, however, are not amenable to complete resection because of location or growth characteristics. In such circumstances, surgery is limited to biopsy. Stable disease for extended periods of time has been described following subtotal resection or less for tumors in almost all regions of the brain and spine. The literature would suggest a poorer long-term prognosis for such patients, as compared with those with totally resected lesions, 15–50 per cent survival at ten years being reported in all anatomical locations, with a high rate of early progression.[49,53,55–58]

Table 13a.1 *Surgery: recommendations and points of discussion*

Procedure	Known/recommended	Points of discussion
Biopsy	Indicated in all cases of LGG to obtain tissue for diagnosis and biological investigation if appropriate	Is biopsy indicated in case of unequivocal neuroradiologic evidence of optic pathway glioma or hypothalamic-chiasmatic LGG in children without NF-1?
	Not indicated in cases of unequivocal neuroradiologic evidences of optic pathway glioma in children with NF-1	
Surgical resection	Complete resection represents the cure for most childhood LGG	Are debulking procedures to be recommended in case of a non-symptomatic exophytic hypothalamic chiasmatic glioma?
	Complete surgical resection indicated if achievable "safely" (cortical/cerebellar/exophytic brainstem/spinal LGG)	
	Debulking surgical procedures may be indicated in cases of symptomatic exophytic hypothalamic chiasmatic glioma (e.g. associated with hydrocephalus)	
	Always indicated in cases of pure optic nerve glioma of an already blind and/or proptotic eye with important aesthetic consequences	

LGG, low-grade glioma; NF-1, neurofibromatosis type 1.

Table 13a.2 *Initial observation time: recommendations and points of discussion*

Known/recommended	Points of discussion
Initial observation time always recommended in cases of complete tumor resection and in cases of unresectable, non-progressive, and/or non-symptomatic LGG affecting "young" children and affecting NF-1 patients regardless of age	Does immediate treatment improve the progression-free survival and quality of life of older children with an unresectable, non-progressive, and/or non-symptomatic LGG?

LGG, low-grade glioma; NF-1, neurofibromatosis type 1.

For cerebral hemispheric and cerebellar astrocytoma, the volume of residual tumor has proved to be the best predictor of the risk of disease progression.[45,49] For hypothalamic or visual pathway tumors, however, Janss and colleagues have shown that tumor volume at diagnosis does not predict the need for subsequent treatment with surgery or adjuvant chemotherapy.[59] In their series of 46 patients, only 23 per cent and 19 per cent had avoided interventions at two and five years, respectively.

There has been debate advocating tumor management with radical rather than conservative surgery, even for children with midline supratentorial glioma, in order to reduce the rate of progression.[57,58,60] Since radical surgery cannot achieve complete resection in every case, the late consequences of such intervention need to be balanced against the chances of relieving severe symptoms or saving life.[58]

Wait-and-see approach

After complete resection of a childhood low-grade glioma, no further therapy is generally required. A period of close observation – "wait and see" – is also usually recommended for those children who did not undergo surgery and for whom macroscopic residual disease was left after surgery if there is no clinical evidence of symptomatic or progressive disease on imaging (Table 13a.2).

Since no clear-cut predictive clinical, biological, or histopathological features have been determined, it cannot be predicted with certainty which low-grade tumors will show an indolent clinical behavior and which will run an aggressive course. It is not known whether all low-grade tumors possess proliferative potential; therefore, it is unclear whether all low-grade gliomas ultimately need treatment.

Spontaneous involution has been unequivocally documented only rarely. Perilongo and colleagues reported two children with NF-1, in whom contrast-enhancing, space-occupying lesions regressed widely without any therapeutic intervention throughout observation periods of six and ten months, respectively, with stable disease thereafter.[61] Similar courses with regression occurring within two years after diagnosis have been reported for other children with NF-1,[61] whereas in patients without NF-1 the phenomenon of tumor regression of a low-grade lesion has primarily been described following previous partial resection or biopsy.[62] All of these tumors

Table 13a.3 *Radiotherapy: recommendations and points of discussion*

Known/recommended	Points of discussion
Represents the gold standard of treatment of "old" children affected by small unresectable progressive or symptomatic LGG	Does radiotherapy improve overall survival in children with unresectable progressive or symptomatic LGG?
Indicated in children with unresectable progressive or symptomatic LGG after having failed chemotherapy	What are the most effective doses?
	Do highly focused radiotherapy techniques (e.g. conformational or stereotactic fractionated radiotherapy) have the same local tumor control rates as conventional techniques?

LGG, low-grade glioma.

had been located in the chiasmatic-hypothalamic region. For lesions in children with NF-1, tumor regrowth within the extended follow-up period has been reported.[61,63] Whether massive apoptosis, as claimed by Takeuchi and colleagues for one of their cases,[64] underlies the phenomenon of spontaneous regression remains to be elucidated.

Radiotherapy

Although radiation therapy has been the standard treatment for low-grade glioma for many years, the optimal approach is a matter of debate (Tables 13a.3 and 13a.4). Radiotherapy alone is utilized primarily in tumors not amenable to surgical resection. Its role as an adjunct to surgery and its impact on progression-free and overall survival is difficult to assess. A benefit of radiotherapy on survival has been detected in selected subgroups of adult patients with subtotally resected low-grade astrocytomas, oligodendrogliomas, and oligoastrocytomas. However, a survival advantage with radiotherapy is less certain for children undergoing either total or subtotal resection.[50,65–68] Since the treatment was not randomized in the published series, selection for this treatment modality may have led to the inclusion of patients with more aggressive tumors in the radiotherapy group. In gliomas of the optic pathway, radiotherapy plays a role in the improvement or stabilization of visual function.[10]

The optimal timing of radiotherapy is an unsettled issue. In childhood low-grade glioma, routine irradiation after complete resection is not applied. In those cases in which less than a complete resection was performed, there is considerable controversy in the literature as to whether to proceed with adjuvant radiotherapy. Despite a significantly higher progression-free survival rate in some series, an advantage for overall survival was not generally observed with immediate postoperative radiotherapy.[50,65]

The effect of radiotherapy after chemotherapy has failed is largely unknown. In children under the age of five years and in whom radiotherapy has been postponed by chemotherapy, those that progress following irradiation most likely represent a cohort with poor prognostic features.[59] In older children, the subsequent progression-free survival and overall survival do not differ from patients having received radiotherapy as first-line treatment.[69]

The optimum dose for radiation therapy in childhood low-grade glioma has not been well established. The selection of dose prescriptions is influenced strongly by patient age, extent, and site of tumor, with a tendency to a lower dose in younger children with larger tumors (larger treatment portals); consequently, the reported results are conflicting (Table 13a.5). Recently recommended and generally accepted dose prescriptions range between 50.4 and 54 Gy. These dose levels are not associated with a significant risk for visual dysfunction or radionecrosis, provided that the fractionated dose does not exceed 2.0 Gy.

Although stereotactic biopsies have shown tumor cells extending beyond imaging abnormalities, accumulated data support the use of localized fields to treat low-grade gliomas.[70] In childhood low-grade glioma, local failure is the predominant feature in progressive or recurrent disease, and leptomeningeal spread is a rare event.[71] This implies that treatment fields encompassing the tumor are appropriate.[70]

In studies where there is imaging evidence of response, this may take place gradually over a period of years.[72,73] In many cases, such shrinkage is not related directly to tumor control or improvement of symptoms. Short-term treatment-related changes on magnetic resonance imaging (MRI) might be misleading and should be distinguished from tumor progression.[74]

Stereotactic irradiation techniques in conjunction with rigid head-fixation systems comprising single high-dose delivery ("radiosurgery"), fractionated convergence therapy, and fractionated three-dimensional conformal therapy are new techniques to improve the therapeutic ratio by focusing the dose to tumor while sparing surrounding normal tissue. Although these techniques are well established in adults, data for childhood central nervous system (CNS) malignancies, in particular low-grade glioma, are scarce (Table 13a.6). The direct correlation between radiation dose and tumor control suggests the strategy of

Table 13a.4 Survival after radiotherapy with and without surgery, surgery alone, or surveillance of low-grade glioma in childhood

Ref.	Period	Patients (n)	Tumor	Treatment	Survival		Follow-up
					Progression-free	Overall	
106	1977	16	Optic glioma	RT 3.5–65.0 Gy	n.m.	5/10 years 80%, 12/16 patients alive	1–14 years (mean 6.3 years)
107	1956–1977	18	Optic glioma	RT 50–60 Gy, FD 1.8–2.5 Gy	n.m.	5 years 83%, 10 years 73%	1–19 years
108	1950–1975	42	Chiasmal glioma	RT alone 35–60 Gy, FD n.m.	n.m.	Anterior chiasmal glioma: 5 years 91.7%, 10 years 72.4% Posterior chiasmal glioma: 5 years 87.7%, 10 years 40%	n.m.
109	1951–1981	29	Optic glioma	RT 45–50 Gy, FD 1.8–2.0 Gy	5 years 100%, 10 years 90%	5 years 100%, 10 years 93%	1–30 years (median 10 years)
110	1953–1984	36	Optic glioma	RT, 24 patients; RT in progressive disease, 12 patients: 35–61 Gy, FD 1.5–2.0 Gy	10 years 55%	10 years 87%	7 months–33.4 years (mean 9.4 years)
111	1961–1984	14	Optic nerve glioma	RT alone 40–56 Gy, FD n.m.	5 years 90% (3/14), 10 years 60% (5/14)	5 years 100%, 10 years 100%	1–20 years (median 8 years)
112	1965–1983	36	Glioma of optic nerve and chiasm	RT 38.0–56.86 Gy, FD 1.4–2.0 Gy	n.m.	5 years 94%, 10 years 31%, 15 years 31%	2–21 years (mean 10.3 years)
113	1956–1986	33	Glioma of optic nerve and chiasma	Surgery + RT, 22 patients; RT alone, 11 patients: 37.86–61 Gy, FD 0.76–2.0 Gy	5 years 85%, 10 years 75%, 15 years 75%	5 years 94%, 10 years 81%, 15 years 74%	2–31 years (mean 12.3 years)

Ref	Years	n	Site	Treatment	Survival	Survival	Follow-up
114	1971–1986	24	Optic glioma	RT alone 45–56.6 Gy, FD 1.8–2.0 Gy	6 years 88%	6 years 100%	24 months–17 years (median 6 years)
72	1970–1986	57	Chiasm glioma	RT alone 40–60 Gy, FD 1.45–2.15 Gy	5 years 89.05%, 10 years 82.0%	5 years 83.5%, 10 years 83.5%	2.5–16.5 years (mean 7.5 years)
66	1958–1990	87	Optic glioma	RT 36–55.12 Gy, FD 1.8–2.0 Gy; RT (a) 38 patients, surveillance (b) 49 patients	5 J (a/b): 80%/64%; 10 J (a/b): 73%/64%; 15 J (a/b): 65%/64%	5 J (a/b): 94%/95%; 10 J (a/b): 79%/92%; 15 J (a/b): 69%/80%	n.m.
50	1956–1991	71	Hemispheric glioma	RT dose n.m., (a) postoperative RT (35 patients), (b) surveillance (35 patients), (c) postoperative RT after incomplete resection (33 patients), (d) surveillance after incomplete resection (16 patients)	10 years (a/b/c/d), 83%/75%/82%/40%	10 years (a/b/c/d), 90%/97%/89%/94%	1–420 months (median 99 months)
115	1973–1994	33	Optic and hypothalamic glioma	RT 40–60 Gy, FD 1.8–2.0 Gy	5 years 82%, 10 years 77%	5 years 93%, 10 years 79%	0.5–16 years (mean 13.6 years)
116	1984–1994	142	All sites	Patients with progressive tumors: 13 surgery, 30 RT 38–72 Gy (median 54 Gy)	n.m.	4 years 65%	n.m.
117	1963–1995	19	all sites	RT (for macroscopic tumor) median 54 Gy, FD 1.8 Gy	5 years 88%, 10 years 68%	5 years 94%, 10 years 80%	Median 5.6 years
73	1975–1997	25	Optic glioma and thalamic glioma	RT 45–60 Gy, FD 1.6–2.0 Gy	10 years 69%	10 years 94%	1.5–23.0 years (mean 9 years)
69	1992–1999	96	All sites	RT in progressive disease: 81 patients, 54 Gy, FD 1.8 Gy; brachytherapy: 15 patients, 60 Gy	3 years 87.1%	3 years 95.7%	0–96 months (mean 19.4 months)

FD, fractional dose; n.m., not mentioned; RT, radiotherapy.

Table 13a.5 *Progression-free survival (PFS) in children and adults with low-grade glioma: dose–response relationship (retrospective analyses)*

Ref.	Patients (*n*)	Total dose (Gy)	Fractionated dose (Gy)	PFS (5 years)	PFS (10 years)	*P*
118	171	45.0	1.8	47%	Not reached	NS
	172	59.4		50%		
106	7	≤42	n.m.	43%	n.m.	n.m.
	9	≥50		100%		
108	13	35–45	n.m.	Relapse rate 11/13	n.m.	n.m.
	29	50–60		Relapse rate 8/29		
119	52	>45.0	n.m.	80%	65%	n.m.
	62	<45.0		65%	55%	
112	12	>45.0	Calculation according	100%		0.045
	12	<45.0	to nominal standard dose	75%		
113	3	<40.0	n.m.	0%	0%	<0.0001
	30	>40.0		90%	79%	
66	19	>50.0	n.m.	88%	88%	0.37 (NS)
	15	<50.0		72%	57%	
73	9	44–45	1.6–2.0	87%	36%	0.04
	16	45.1–60		90%	85%	

n.m., not mentioned; NS, not significant.

Table 13a.6 *Stereotactic fractionated and high single-dose radiotherapy ("radiosurgery") in childhood low-grade gliomas*

Ref.	Technique	Patients	Outcome	Follow–up (months)
120	Fractionated convergence therapy (5 × 1.8–2.0 Gy/45–54 Gy) + dose escalation 60 Gy	11 (initial RT), 9 (recurrence)	No acute side effects, 1 CR, 19 PR/SD, overall survival 100%	16
77	High single-dose ("radiosurgery"), dose 12 Gy	7 patients, 8 tumors	No acute side effects, 1 CR, 4 PR, 3 SD, overall survival 100%	21
78	High single-dose ("radiosurgery"), dose 11–20 Gy	13	4 transient edema, 4 CR, 5 PR, 2 SD, 2 PD, overall survival 100%	21
80	High single-dose ("radiosurgery"), dose 15 Gy	9	PFS 100%, overall survival 100%	19
79	High single-dose ("radiosurgery"), dose 12–14.4 Gy	2	No side effects, decrease in tumor size and improvement of vision in both patients	24–43
74	Fractionated convergence therapy (5 × 1.8–2.0 Gy/52.2–60.0 Gy)	28	Overall survival 100%, decrease in tumor size in 15 patients, stable tumor size in 1 patient, increased tumor size (transient, 15–21 months) in 13 patients	24
75	Hypofractionated convergence therapy (median total dose 39–18.0–42.0 Gy in 6–10 fractions)	8	1 edema, 1 edema + tumor necrosis, 1 tumor necrosis, 5-year PFS 60%, overall survival 100%	42
76	Fractionated conformal radiotherapy (median total dose 52.4 Gy/1.6–2.0 Gy fractionated dose)	10	PFS at 5 years 90%, overall survival 100%, no acute toxicity	12–72

CR, complete response; PD, progressive disease; PFS, progression-free survival; PR, partial response; SD, stable disease.

increasing dose levels within macroscopic tumor. Preliminary data reveal low acute toxicity and promising results in recurrent tumors as well as in primary treatment.[74–81] Whether stereotactic radiation therapy with either of the latter techniques will add substantially to disease control and preserve neurologic function remains to be established and should be part of future investigations.

Chemotherapy

Investigation of chemotherapy treatment strategies for young children under the age of five years assumed a high priority to avoid early radiotherapy, especially for those with visual pathway gliomas (Table 13a.7). Several reports produced evidence that cytotoxic drugs are active

Table 13a.7 *Chemotherapy: recommendations and points of discussion*

Known/recommended	Points of discussion
Stabilizes tumor growth for relatively long periods of time, allowing significant tumor volume reduction in many cases	What are the long-term effects of chemotherapy?
Indicated in young children with unresectable progressive or symptomatic LGG	Does chemotherapy represent the first line of treatment for all children with unresectable progressive or symptomatic, hypothalamic-chiasmatic LGG regardless of age?
Indicated in all children with NF-1 and affected by unresectable progressive or symptomatic LGG, regardless of age	What are the most important prognostic factors in children treated with chemotherapy for progression and radiation free-survival?
	What are the most effective and "safe" drugs?
	How long should these children been treated?
	Does chemotherapy induce chemo- and radio-resistance?

LGG, low-grade glioma; NF-1, neurofibromatosis type 1.

against low-grade astrocytic tumors and that they may permit delay or obviate the need for radiation therapy. Although short-term efficacy with transient tumor control is the primary target for these approaches, no data exist to clarify the role of chemotherapy for long-term outcome.

Measuring response by conventional criteria, such as complete response or partial response (tumor volume reduction of >50 per cent) may not be appropriate for low-grade astrocytoma, as prolonged stable disease may be a better measure of success.[13]

Limited studies suggest that chemotherapy has little or no adverse effects on cognitive or endocrine function, but the inherent long-term risks concerning organ toxicity and carcinogenic and mutagenic risks have to be followed closely.

Reports on the effectiveness of chemotherapy in low-grade glioma have comprised newly diagnosed as well as relapsed patients treated with single agents or drug combinations for variable lengths of time. Table 13a.8 focuses on response only, since survival and progression-free or event-free survival data are not available for the smaller series and cannot be compared due to the diverse study conditions.

SINGLE-AGENT THERAPY

The effect of single-agent therapy has been assessed for vincristine, carboplatin, etoposide, and cyclophosphamide. Radiographic response rates, including complete and partial response as well as stable disease, range from 54 to 75 per cent, being sustained for three years in up to 83 per cent.[82–89] High-dose ifosfamide and oral low-dose methotrexate have demonstrated comparable but short lived responses.[90,91] No conclusive data have been published on the use of topotecan or temozolomide.[92,93]

COMBINATION-AGENT THERAPY

Since the first report on the delay of radiotherapy following prolonged administration of vincristine and actinomycin D

in 24 children,[94] several series have showed objective response rates of 50–65 per cent, including stable disease of 80–90 per cent, for various combinations of carboplatin and vincristine.[13,95–97] Progression rates have been around 35 per cent at three years, indicating that two-thirds of the children do not have to be irradiated within this interval.[13] Children with stable disease after treatment have the same progression-free interval as those with measurable response.[13] Carboplatin has well-known myelotoxicity but only minor nephro- and ototoxicity. Allergies have been reported in 6–30 per cent of children treated with repeat doses.[13,96,97]

Comparable results have been obtained with high-dose carboplatin in combination with etoposide.[11,98] More short-lived responses followed therapy with etoposide and vincristine.[99]

A five-drug, nitrosourea-based regimen prompted a response rate of 95 per cent, including stable disease, with median time to progression of 132 weeks.[100,101] Given the differences in patient age at diagnosis and tumor location, these data are not directly comparable with those of carboplatin/vincristine.

There are also approaches to intensify chemotherapy in an attempt to increase overall response and ultimately disease control. The French multiagent protocol, originally intended to treat medulloblastoma and PNET, has been investigated for spinal, chiasmatic-hypothalamic, and low-grade astrocytoma.[102] Response rates and progression-free survival rates are virtually identical to those obtained with carboplatin/vincristine. However, progression-free survival seems higher for children with a significant objective response than for those with a minor response or stable disease.

The first study to randomize chemotherapy in newly diagnosed chiasmatic-hypothalamic low-grade astrocytomas, using either the carboplatin and vincristine regimen or the five-drug nitrosourea-based regimen (6-thioguanine, procarbazine, dibromodulcitol, CCNY (lomustine), and

Table 13a.8 *Chemotherapy for low-grade glioma: response assessment*

Drug(s)	Ref.	Patients (n)	Dose/m²	Treatment interval	Assessment of response by	Time of assessment	CR	PR	MR	SD	PD
Carboplatin	85	R 7	560 mg	4 weeks	CT/MRI	8 weeks				5	2
	87	ND 4, R 2	560 mg	4 weeks	MRI	8 weeks				6	2
	82	ND 12	560 mg	4 weeks				4		6	
Iproplatin	85	R 15	270 mg	3 weeks	CT/MRI	6 weeks		1		10	4
Cyclophosphamide	121	4	4–5 g	4 weeks	MRI	No information		2	1	1	
	122	R 6, diss. 4	4–5 g	4 weeks				5	1	3	1
	88	ND 15	1.2 g	3 weeks	CT/MRI	12 weeks	1			9	5
Ifosfamide	90	R 6, diss. 4	3 × 3 g	3 weeks	CT/MRI	6 weeks		1		3	2
Temozolomide	CCG (unpublished)	R 20	5 × 200 mg	4 weeks	CT/MRI	8 weeks		1		8	
MTX	91	R 10	7.5 mg × 8 (every 6 h)	1 week	CT/MRI	2 months		2		5	3
Topotecan	92	R 2	5.5–7.5 mg	3 weeks	CT/MRI	6 weeks		1		1	
	88	R 11	3–3.75 mg (CI)	3 weeks	CT/MRI	6 weeks				5	6
Etoposide	83	R 14 chiasmatic-hypothalamic	50 mg × 21 days	5 weeks	CT/MRI	8 weeks	1	4		3	6
	84	R 12 cerebellar	50 mg × 21 days	5 weeks	CT/MRI	8 weeks		2		4	6
Vincristine + actinomycin D	94	ND 24	1.5 mg vincristine, 15 μg actinomycin D	12-weekly		12 weeks		3	6	14	1
Vincristine + carboplatin	95	ND 37	1.5 mg–175 mg	Weekly	CT/MRI	10 weeks	1	15	7	13	1
	95	R 23	1.5 mg–175 mg	Weekly	CT/MRI	10 weeks		7	5	5	6
	13	ND 78	1.5 mg–175 mg	Weekly	MRI	10 weeks	4	22	18	29	5
	96	ND 132	1.5 mg–550 mg	3–4 weeks	CT/MRI	10 weeks	5		56	49	22
Carboplatin + etoposide	11	ND 17, R 2	300–1000 mg carboplatin, 600 mg etoposide	3–4 weeks	CT/MRI	12–16 weeks	1	1	6	8	4
Etoposide + vincristine	99	R 14, ND 6	1.5 mg–5 × 100 mg	6 weeks	CT/MRI			1	3	11	5
TPDCV	100	ND 15	See ref.	6 weeks	CT/MRI	No information		11		2	2
	101	ND 42	See ref.	6 weeks	CT/MRI	6 weeks			15	25	2
BB SFOP	123	ND 84	See ref.		CT/MRI						

BB SFOP, Baby Société Francaise d'Oncologie Pédiatrique; CCG, Children's Cancer Group; CI, confidence interval; CR, complete response; CT, computed tomography; diss., disseminated tumors; MR, minor response (tumor volume reduction <50% but >25% of initial volume); MRI, magnetic resonance imaging; MTX, methotrexate; ND, newly diagnosed; PD, progressive disease (tumor volume increase >25%); PR, partial response (tumor volume reduction >50%); R, relapsed; SD, stable disease; TPDCV, 6-thioguanine, procarbazine, dibromodulcitol, CCNY (lomustine), and vincristine.

vincristine; TPCDV), is still open for accrual and preliminary data have not been published.

Indications for starting non-surgical therapy

In selecting the optimal strategy, the relative effectiveness of surgery, chemotherapy, and irradiation must be balanced against their potential complications. The risks of delayed non-surgical treatment include irreversible neurologic impairment and a potentially lower probability of tumor control. General rules for initiating treatment have not been universally agreed. Non-surgical therapy for unresectable or incompletely resected tumors should be considered at diagnosis for children presenting with severe neurologic symptoms, such as diencephalic syndrome, focal neurologic deficits, convulsions, and increased intracranial pressure. For children who have been observed initially, clinical or radiographic progression, even in the absence of clinical symptoms, may justify the necessity for non-surgical treatment.[13,59,81,103,104]

Current treatment recommendations offer a common strategy for all low-grade histologies (outlined in Figure 13a.2). The necessity for a tailored management of subgroups, possibly characterized perhaps by histology, location, extent of surgical resection, or any other factor, have yet to be defined.

Since older children are more likely to develop disease progression while on chemotherapy,[13] and since the rationale for delaying radiotherapy in older children, especially if only for one to two years, is less clear, most studies contain a recommended age for the choice of chemotherapy versus radiotherapy in progressive or symptomatic tumors. Preliminary data suggest that children receiving radiotherapy for tumor progression following initial chemotherapy do not fare worse than those receiving primary irradiation.[69] The groups differ, however, with respect to tumor histology and location in this study.

Since children with NF-1 are at a greater risk for developing second tumors within the brain and carry a significant risk for vasculopathy, they may be treated for visual pathway gliomas with chemotherapy even at older ages.[14,105]

In summary, the principles that underlie the management strategies for children affected by malignant CNS tumors can be applied directly to children with low-grade astrocytic tumor. Most of these patients are expected to be long-term survivors, and thus their condition should be considered as a chronic disorder rather than a life-threatening neoplastic condition. Selection of treatment approaches should involve careful consideration to the impact of the tumor and its treatment upon future health status. Furthermore, for a variety of reasons, many aspects of their biology, clinical behavior, and consequently treatment approach have still not been investigated well. Finally, there is still a great deal to be learned about the tumor biology, clinical behavior, and interaction with treatments.

REFERENCES

1   Stiller C, Nectoux J. International incidence of childhood brain and spinal tumours. *Int J Epidemiol* 1994; **23**:458–64.

2   Bernards A. Neurofibromatosis type I and ras-mediated signaling: filling in the GAP's. *Biochim Biophys Acta* 1995; **1242**:43–59.

3   Shen M, Harper P, Upadhyaya M. Molecular genetics of neurofibromatosis type 1 (NF1). *J Med Genet* 1996; **33**:2–17.

4   Riccardi V. Histogenesis control genes and neurofibromatosis 1. *Eur J Pediatr* 2000; **159**:475–6.

5   Riccardi V. Neurofibromatosis: past, present and future. *N Engl J Med* 1991; **324**:1283–5.

6   Riccardi V. Neurofibromatosis: phenotype, natural history and pathogenesis. Baltimore, MD: Johns Hopkins University Press, 1992.

7   Lewis R, Gerson L, Axelson K, Riccardi V, Whitford R. Von Recklinghausen neurofibromatosis II. Incidence of optic gliomata. *Ophthalmology* 1984; **91**:929–35.

8   Listernick R, Louis D, Packer R, Gutmann D. Optic pathway gliomas in children with neurofibromatosis 1: consensus statement from the NFA Optic Pathway Glioma Task Force. *Ann Neurol* 1997; **41**:143–9.

9   Vinchon M, Soto-Ares G, Ruchoux M, Dhellemmes P. Cerebellar gliomas in children with NF1: pathology and surgery. *Childs Nerv Syst* 2000; **16**:417–20.

10 Capelli C, Grill J, Raquin M, *et al.* Long-term follow up of 69 patients treated for optic pathway tumours before the chemotherapy era. *Arch Dis Child* 1998; **79**:334–8.

11 Castello M, Schiavetti A, Varrasso G, Clerico A, Capelli C. Chemotherapy in low-grade astrocytoma management. *Childs Nerv Syst* 1998; **14**:6–9.

12 Dutton J. Gliomas of the anterior visual pathway. *Surv Ophthalmol* 1994; **38**:427–52.

13 Packer R, Ater J, Allen J, *et al.* Carboplatin and vincristine chemotherapy for children with newly diagnosed progressive low-grade gliomas. *J Neurosurg* 1997; **86**:747–54.

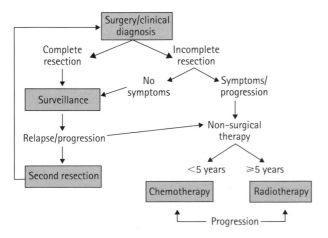

Figure 13a.2 *Treatment strategy for low-grade astrocytic tumors.*

14 Friedman J, Birch P. An association between optic glioma and other tumors of the central nervous system in neurofibromatosis type I. *Neuropediatrics* 1997; **28**:131–2.

15 Roach E, Gomez M, Northrup H. Tuberous sclerosis complex consensus conference: revised diagnostic criteria. *J Child Neurol* 1998; **13**:624–8.

16 Jozwiak S, Schwartz R, Janniger C, Bielicka-Cymerman J. Usefulness of diagnostic criteria of tuberous sclerosis complex in pediatric patients. *J Child Neurol* 2000; **15**:652–9.

17 Li F, Fraumeni JJ. Prospective study of a family cancer syndrome. *J Am Med Assoc* 1982; **247**:2692–4.

18 Lynch H, Katz D, Bogard P, Lynch J. The sarcoma, breast cancer, lung cancer and adrenocortical carcinoma syndrome revisited: childhood cancer. *Am J Dis Child* 1985; **139**:134–6.

19 Malkin D, Li F, Strong L, *et al.* Germ line p53 mutations in a familial syndrome of breast cancer, sarcomas and other neoplasms. *Science* 1990; **250**:1233–8.

20 Ohgaki K, Vital A, Kleihues P, Hainaut P. Li–Fraumeni syndrome and TP53 germline mutations. In: Kleihues P, Cavenee W (eds). *Pathology and Genetics: Tumors of the Nervous System.* Lyon: IARC Press, 2000, pp. 231–4.

21 Amirjamshidi A, Abbassioun K. Radiation-induced tumors of the central nervous system occurring in childhood and adolescence. *Childs Nerv Syst* 2000; **16**:390–7.

22 Shore R, Albert R, Pasternack B. Follow up study of patients treated by x-ray epilation for tinea capitis. *Arch Environ Health* 1976; **31**:21–8.

23 Miettinen H, Kononen J, Sallinen P, *et al.* CDKN2/p16 predicts survival in oligodendrogliomas: comparison with astrocytomas. *J Neuro-Oncol* 1999; **41**:205–11.

24 Smith J, Perry A, Borell T, *et al.* Alterations of chromosome arms 1p and 19q as predictors of survival in oligodendrogliomas, astrocytomas and mixed oligoastrocytomas. *J Clin Oncol* 2000; **18**:636–45.

25 Von Deimling A, Louis D, Menon A, Ellison D, Wiestler O, Seizinger B. Allelic loss on the long arm of chromosome 17 in pilocytic astrocytoma. *Acta Neuropathol* 1993; **86**:81–5.

26 Ohgaki K, Schauble B, zur Hausen A, von Ammon K, Kleihues P. Genetic alterations associated with the evolution and progression of astrocytic brain tumors. *Virchows Arch* 1995; **427**:113–18.

27 Mathew P, Look T, Luo X, *et al.* DNA index of glial tumors in children. Correlation with tumor grade and prognosis. *Cancer* 1996; **78**:881–6.

28 Bodey B, Bodey BJ, Siegel S, Kaiser H. Fas (Apo-1, CD95) receptor expression in childhood astrocytomas. Is it a marker of the major apoptotic pathway or a signaling receptor for immune escape of neoplastic cells? *In Vivo* 1999; **13**:357–74.

29 Von Bossanyi P, Sallaba J, Dietzmann K, Warich-Kirches M, Kirches E. Correlation of TGF-alpha and EGF-receptor expression with proliferative activity in human astrocytic glioma. *Pathol Res Pract* 1998; **194**:141–7.

30 Rhodes R. Biological evaluation of biopsies from adult cerebral astrocytomas: cell growth/cell suicide ratios and their relationship to patient survival. *J Neuropathol Exp Neurol* 1998; **57**:746–57.

31 Abdulrauf S, Edvardsen K, Ho K, Yang X, Rock J, Rosenblum M. Vascular endothelial growth factor expression and vascular density as prognostic markers of survival in patients with low-grade astrocytoma. *J Neurosurg* 1998; **88**:513–20.

32 Hoshi M, Yoshida K, Shimazaki K, Sasaki H, Otani M, Kawase T. Correlation between MIB 1-staining indices and recurrence in low-grade astrocytomas. *Brain Tumor Pathol* 1997; **14**:47–51.

33 Sasaki H, Yoshida K, Ikeda E, *et al.* Expression of the neural cell adhesion molecule in astrocytic tumors: an inverse correlation with malignancy. *Cancer* 1998; **82**:1921–31.

34 Prados M, Krouwer H, Edwards M, Cogen P, Davis R, Hoshino T. Proliferative potential and outcome in pediatric astrocytic tumors. *J Neuro-Oncol* 1992; **13**:277–82.

35 Cattoretti G, Becker M, Key G, *et al.* Monoclonal antibodies against recombinant parts of the Ki67 antigen (MIB1 and MIB3) detect proliferating cells in microwave-processed formalin-fixed paraffin sections. *J Pathol* 1992; **168**:357–63.

36 Burger P, Shibata T, Kleihues P. The use of monoclonal antibody Ki 67 in the identification of proliferating cells: application to surgical neuropathology. *Am J Surg Pathol* 1986; **10**:611–17.

37 Dirven C, Kondstaal J, Mooij J, Molenaar W. The proliferative potential of the pilocytic astrocytoma: the relation between MIB-1 labeling and clinical and neuro-radiological follow-up. *J Neuro-Oncol* 1998; **37**:9–16.

38 Cummings T, Provenzale J, Hunter S, *et al.* Gliomas of the optic nerve: histological, immunohistochemical (MIB-1 and p53) and MRI analysis. *Acta Neuropathol* 2000; **99**:563–70.

39 Czech T, Slavc I, Aichholzer M, *et al.* Proliferative activity as measured by MIB-1 labeling index and long-term outcome of visual pathway astrocytomas in children. *J Neuro-Oncol* 1999; **42**:143–50.

40 Ishii N, Tada M, Hamou M, *et al.* Cells with TP53 mutations in low grade astrocytic tumors evolve clonally to malignancy and are an unfavorable prognostic factor. *Oncogene* 1999; **18**:5870–8.

41 Sidransky D, Mikkelsen T, Schwechheimer K, Rosenblum M, Cavenee W, Vogelstein B. Clonal expansion of p53 mutant cells is associated with brain tumor progression. *Nature* 1992; **355**:846–7.

42 Hayes V, Dirven C, Dam A, *et al.* High frequency of TP43 mutations in juvenile pilocytic astrocytomas indicates role of TP53 in the development of these tumors. *Brain Pathol* 1999; **9**:463–7.

43 Albright A, Price R, Guthkelch A. Diencephalic gliomas of children. *Cancer* 1985; **55**:2789–93.

44 Pollack I. The role of surgery in pediatric gliomas. *J Neuro-Oncol* 1999; **42**:271–88.

45 Berger M, Deliganis A, Dobbins J, Keles G. The effect of extent of resection on recurrence in patients with low grade cerebral hemispheric gliomas. *Cancer* 1994; **74**:1784–91.

46 So E. Integration of EEG, MRI and SPECT in localizing the seizure focus for epilepsy surgery. *Epilepsia* 2000; 41 (suppl. 3): S48–54.

47 Coakley K, Huston JI, Scheithauer B, Forbes G, Kelly P. Pilocytic astrocytomas: well demarcated magnetic resonance appearance despite frequent infiltration histologically. *Mayo Clin Proc* 1995; **70**:747–51.

48 Hirsch J-F, Rose C, Pierre-Kah A, Pfister A, Hoppe-Hirsch E. Benign astrocytic and oligodendrocytic tumors of the cerebral hemispheres in children. *J Neurosurg* 1989; **70**:568–72.

49 Smoots D, Geyer J, Lieberman D, Berger M. Predicting disease progression in childhood cerebellar astrocytoma. *Childs Nerv Syst* 1998; **14**:636–48.

50 Pollack I, Claassen D, Al-Shboul Q, Janosky J, Deutsch M. Low-grade gliomas of the cerebral hemispheres in children: an analysis of 71 cases. *J Neurosurg* 1995; **82**:536–47.

51 West C, Gattamaneni R, Blair V. Radiotherapy in the treatment of low grade astrocytomas I. A survival analysis. *Childs Nerv Syst* 1995; **11**:438–42.

52 Wallner K, Gonzales M, Edwards M, Wara W, Sheline G. Treatment results of juvenile pilocytic astrocytoma. *J Neurosurg* 1988; **69**:171–6.

53 Campbell J, Pollack I. Cerebellar astrocytomas in children. *J Neuro-Oncol* 1996; **28**:223–31.

54 Gjerris F, Klinken L. Long term prognosis in children with benign cerebellar astrocytoma. *J Neurosurg* 1978; **49**:179–84.

55 Pencalet P, Maixner W, Sainte-Rose C, *et al.* Benign cerebellar astrocytomas in children. *J Neurosurg* 1999; **90**:265–73.

56 Garvey M, Packer R. An integrated approach to the treatment of chiasmatic-hypothalamic gliomas. *J Neuro-Oncol* 1996; **28**:167–83.

57 Hoffman H, Soloniuk D, Humphryes R, *et al.* Management and outcome of low-grade astrocytomas of the midline in children: a retrospective review. *Neurosurgery* 1993; **33**:964–71.

58 Sutton L, Molloy P, Sernyak H, *et al.* Long-term outcome of hypothalamic/chiasmatic astrocytomas in children treated with conservative surgery. *J Neurosurg* 1995; **83**:583–9.

59 Janss A, Grundy R, Cnaan A, *et al.* Optic pathway and hypothalamic/chiasmatic gliomas in children younger than age 5 years with a 6-year follow-up. *Cancer* 1995; **75**:1051–9.

60 Wisoff J, Abbott R, Epstein F. Surgical management of exophytic chiasmatic-hypothalamic tumors of childhood. *J Neurosurg* 1990; **73**:661–7.

61 Perilongo G, Moras P, Carollo C, Battistella A, Clementi M, Laverda A. Spontaneous partial regression of low-grade glioma in children with neurofibromatosis-1: a real possibility. *J Child Neurol* 1999; **14**:352–6.

62 Kernan J, Horgan M, Piatt J, D'Agostino A. Spontaneous involution of a diencephalic astrocytoma. *Pediatr Neurosurg* 1998; **29**:149–53.

63 Schmandt S, Packer R, Vezina L, Jane J. Spontaneous regression of low-grade astrocytomas in childhood. *Pediatr Neurosurg* 2000; **32**:132–6.

64 Takeuchi H, Kabuto M, Sato K, Kubota T. Chiasmal gliomas with spontaneous regression: proliferation and apoptosis. *Childs Nerv Syst* 1997; **13**:229–33.

65 Forsyth P, Shaw E, Scheithauer B, O'Fallon J, Layton DJ, Katzman J. Supratentorial pilocytic astrocytomas. A clinicopathologic, prognostic and flow cytometric study of 51 patients. *Cancer* 1993; **72**:1335–42.

66 Jenkin D, Angyalfi S, Becker L, *et al.* Optic glioma in children: surveillance, resection or irradiation? *Int J Radiat Oncol Biol Phys* 1993; **25**:215–25.

67 Shaw E, Daumas-Duport C, Scheithauer B, *et al.* Radiation therapy in the management of low-grade supratentorial astrocytomas. *J Neurosurg* 1989; **70**:853–61.

68 Shibamato Y, Kitakabu Y, Takahashi M, *et al.* Supratentorial low-grade astrocytoma. Correlation of computed tomography findings with effect of radiation therapy and prognostic variables. *Cancer* 1993; **72**:190–5.

69 Kortmann R, Zanetti I, Mueller S, *et al.* Radiotherapy in low grade glioma: an interim analysis of the SIOP low grade glioma study. In: Proceedings of the IXth Symposium Pediatric Neuro-Oncology, San Francisco, 2000.

70 Kortmann R, Timmermann B, Becker G, Kuehl J, Bamberg M. Advances in treatment techniques and time/dose schedules in external radiation therapy of brain tumours in childhood. *Klin Pediatr* 1998; **210**:220–6.

71 Pollack I, Hurtt M, Pang D, Albright A. Dissemination of low grade intracranial astrocytomas in children. *Cancer* 1994; **73**:2869–78.

72 Bataini J, Delanian S, Ponvert D. Chiasmal gliomas: results of irradiation management in 57 patients and review of the literature. *Int J Radiat Oncol Biol Phys* 1991; **21**:615–23.

73 Grabenbauer G, Schuchardt U, Buchfelder M, *et al.* Radiation therapy of optico-hypothalamic gliomas (OHG) – radiographic response, vision and toxicity. *Radiother Oncol* 2000; **54**:239–45.

74 Bakardjiev A, Barnes P, Goumnerova L, *et al.* Magnetic resonance imaging changes after stereotactic radiation therapy for childhood low grade astrocytoma. *Cancer* 1996; **78**:864–73.

75 Benk V, Clark B, Souhami L, *et al.* Stereotactic radiation in primary brain tumors in children and adolescents. *Paediatr Neurosurg* 1999; **31**:59–64.

76 Debus J, Kocagoncu K, Hoss A, Wenz F, Wannenmacher M. Fractionated stereotactic radiotherapy (FSRT) for optic glioma. *Int J Radiat Oncol Biol Phys* 1999; **44**:243–8.

77 Ganz J, Smievoll A, Thorsen F. Radiosurgical treatment of gliomas of the diencephalon. *Acta Neurochir* 1994; **62** (suppl.):62–6.

78 Grabb P, Lunsford L, Albright A, Kondziolka D, Flickinger J. Stereotactic radiosurgery for glial neoplasms of childhood. *Neurosurgery* 1996; **38**:696–702.

79 Lim Y, Leem W. Two cases of gamma knife radiosurgery for low-grade optic chiasm glioma. *Stereotact Funct Neurosurg* 1996; **66** (suppl. 1):174–83.

80 Somaza S, Kondziolka D, Lunsford L, Flickinger J, Bissonette D, Albright A. Early outcomes after stereotactic radiosurgery for growing pilocytic astrocytomas in children. *Pediatr Neurosurg* 1996; **25**:109–15.

81 Tarbell N, Loeffler J. Recent trends in the radiotherapy of pediatric gliomas. *J Neuro-Oncol* 1996; **28**:233–44.

82 Aquino V, Fort D, Kamen B. Carboplatin for the treatment of children with newly diagnosed optic chiasm gliomas: a phase II study. *J Neuro-Oncol* 1999; **41**:255–9.

83 Chamberlain M, Grafe M. Recurrent chiasmatic-hypothalamic glioma treated with oral etoposide. *J Clin Oncol* 1995; **13**:2072–6.

84 Chamberlain M. Recurrent cerebellar gliomas: Salvage therapy with oral etoposide. *J Child Neurol* 1997; **12**:200–4.

85 Friedman H, Krischer J, Burger P, *et al.* Treatment of children with progressive or recurrent brain tumors with carboplatin or iproplatin: a Pediatric Oncology Group randomized phase II study. *J Clin Oncol* 1992; **10**:249–56.

86 McCowage G, Longee D, Fuchs H, Friedman H. Treatment of high-grade gliomas and metastatic pilocytic astrocytomas with high-dose cyclophosphamide. In: *Proceedings of the Annual Meeting of the American Society of Clinical Oncologists*, 1995, p. A290.

87 Moghrabi A, Friedman H, Burger P, Tien R, Oakes W. Carboplatin treatment of progressive optic pathway gliomas to delay radiotherapy. *J Neurosurg* 1993; **79**:223–7.

88 Kadota R, Kun L, Langston J, *et al.* Cyclophosphamide for the treatment of progressive low-grade astrocytoma: a Paediatric

Oncology Group phase II study. *J Pediatr Hematol Oncol* 1999; **21**:198–202.

89 Rosenstock J, Evans A, Schut L. Response to vincristine of recurrent brain tumors in children. *J Neurosurg* 1976; **45**:135–40.

90 Heideman R, Douglass E, Langston J, *et al.* A phase II study of every other day high-dose ifosfamide in pediatric brain tumors: a Pediatric Oncology Group study. *J Neuro-Oncol* 1995; **25**:77–84.

91 Mulne A, Ducore J, Elterman R, *et al.* Oral methotrexate for recurrent brain tumors in children: a Pediatric Oncology Group study. *J Pediatr Hematol Oncol* 2000; **22**:41–4.

92 Blaney S, Phillips P, Packer R, *et al.* Phase II evaluation of topotecan for pediatric central nervous system tumors. *Cancer* 1996; **78**:527–31.

93 Kadota R, Stewart C, Horn M, *et al.* Topotecan for the treatment of progressive central nervous system tumors: a Pediatric Oncology Group phase II study. *J Neuro-Oncol* 1999; **43**:43–7.

94 Packer R, Sutton L, Bilaniuk L, *et al.* Treatment of chiasmatic/hypothalamic gliomas of childhood with chemotherapy: an update. *Ann Neurol* 1988; **23**:79–85.

95 Packer R, Lange B, Ater J, *et al.* Carboplatin and vincristine for progressive low-grade gliomas of childhood. *J Clin Oncol* 1993; **11**:850–7.

96 Perilongo G, Walker D, Taylor R, *et al.* Vincristine (VCR) carboplatin (CBDCA) in hypothalamic-chiasmatic low grade glioma (HC-LGG). SIOP-LGG study report. *Med Pediatr Oncol* 2000; **35**:190.

97 Gnekow A, Kaatsch P, Kortmann R, Wiestler O. HIT-LGG: effectiveness of carboplatin-vincristine in progressive low-grade gliomas of childhood: an interim report. *Klin Pediatr* 2000; **212**:177–84.

98 Castello M, Schiavetti A, Padula A, *et al.* Does chemotherapy have a role in low-grade glioma management? *Med Pediatr Oncol* 1995; **25**:102–8.

99 Pons M, Finlay J, Walker R, Puccetti D, Packer R, McElwain M. Chemotherapy with vincristine and etoposide in children with low-grade astrocytoma. *J Neuro-Oncol* 1992; **14**:151–8.

100 Petronio J, Edwards M, Prados M, *et al.* Management of chiasmal and hypothalamic gliomas of infancy and childhood with chemotherapy. *J Neurosurg* 1991; **74**:701–8.

101 Prados M, Edwards M, Rabbitt J, Lamborn K, Davis R, Levin V. Treatment of pediatric low-grade gliomas with a nitrosourea-based multiagent chemotherapy regimen. *J Neuro-Oncol* 1997; **32**:235–41.

102 Doireau V, Grill J, Zerah M, *et al.* Chemotherapy for unresectable and recurrent intramedullary glial tumours in children. Brain Tumours Sub-committee of the French Society of Pediatric Oncology (SFOP). *Br J Cancer* 1999; **81**:835–40.

103 Grill J, Laithier V, Rodriguez D, Raquin M, Pierre-Kahn A, Kalifa C. When do children with optic pathway tumours need treatment? An oncological perspective in 106 patients treated in a single centre. *Eur J Pediatr* 2000; **159**:692–6.

104 Souweidane M, Hoffman H. Current treatment of thalamic gliomas in children. *J Neuro-Oncol* 1996; **28**:157–66.

105 Grill J, Couanet D, Capelli C, *et al.* Radiation-induced cerebral vasculopathy in children with neurofibromatosis and optic pathway glioma. *Ann Neurol* 1999; **45**:393–6.

106 Montgomery A, Griffin T, Parker R, Gerdes A. Optic nerve glioma: the role of radiation therapy. *Cancer* 1977; **40**:2079–80.

107 Danoff B, Kramer S, Thompson N. The radiotherapeutic management of optic gliomas of children. *Int J Radiat Oncol Biol Phys* 1980; **6**:45–50.

108 Sung D. Suprasellar tumors in children: a review of clinical manifestations and managements. *Cancer* 1982; **50**:1420–5.

109 Horwich A, Bloom H. Optic gliomas: radiation therapy and prognosis. *Int J Radiat Oncol Biol Phys* 1985; **11**:1067–79.

110 Wong J, Uhl V, Wara W, Sheline G. Optic gliomas. A re-analysis of the University of California, San Francisco, experience. *Cancer* 1987; **60**:1847–55.

111 Weiss L, Sagerman R, King G, Chung C, Dubowy R. Controversy in the management of optic nerve glioma. *Cancer* 1987; **59**:1000–4.

112 Flickinger J, Torres C, Deutsch M. Management of low grade gliomas of the optic nerve and chiasm. *Cancer* 1988; **61**:635–42.

113 Kovalic J, Grigsby P, Shepard M, Fineberg B, Thomas P. Radiation therapy for gliomas of the optic nerve and chiasm. *Int J Radiat Oncol Biol Phys* 1990; **18**:927–32.

114 Pierce S, Barnes P, Loeffler J, McGinn C, Tarbell N. Definitive radiation therapy in the management of symptomatic patients with optic glioma. *Cancer* 1990; **65**:45–52.

115 Erkal H, Serin M, Cakmak A. Management of optic pathway and chiasmatic-hypothalamic gliomas in children: tumor volume response to radiation therapy. *Radiother Oncol* 1997; **45**:11–15.

116 Gajjar A, Sanford R, Heideman R, *et al.* Low-grade astrocytoma: a decade of experience at St Jude Children's Research Hospital. *J Clin Oncol* 1997; **15**:2792–9.

117 Fisher B, Bauman G, Leighton C, Stitt L, Cairncross J, Macdonald D. Low-grade gliomas in children: tumor volume response to radiation. *J Neurosurg* 1998; **88**:969–74.

118 Karim A, Maat B, Hatlevoll R, *et al.* A randomised trial of dose-response in radiation therapy of low-grade cerebral glioma: European Organisation for Research and Treatment of Cancer (EORTC) Study 22844. *Int J Radiat Oncol Biol Phys* 1996; **36**:263–70.

119 Alvord EJ, Lofton S. Gliomas of the optic nerve or chiasm. Outcome by patients' age, tumor site and treatment. *J Neurosurg* 1988; **68**:85–98.

120 Dunbar S, Tarbell N, Kooy H, *et al.* Stereotactic radiotherapy for pediatric and adult brain tumors: preliminary report. *Int J Radiat Oncol Biol Phys* 1994; **30**:531–9.

121 McCowage G, Tien R, McLendon R, *et al.* Successful treatment of childhood pilocytic astrocytomas metastatic to the leptomeninges with high-dose cyclophosphamide. *Med Pediatr Oncol* 1996; **27**:32–9.

122 Longee D, Friedman H, Albright R, *et al.* Treatment of patients with recurrent gliomas with cyclophosphamide and vincristine. *J Neurosurg* 1990; **72**:583–8.

123 Laithier V, Raquin M, Couanet D, *et al.* Chemotherapy for children with optic pathway glioma: results of a prospective study by the French Society of Pediatric Oncology (SFOP). *Med Pediatr Oncol* 2000; **35**:190.

13b

Astrocytic tumors, low grade: treatment considerations by primary site and tumor dissemination

ASTRID K. GNEKOW, ROGER J. PACKER AND ROLF D. KORTMANN

LOW-GRADE ASTROCYTIC TUMORS OF THE CEREBRAL HEMISPHERES

Management

For all hemispheric tumors, primary surgery is the most important step within the therapeutic strategy. Further steps such as radiotherapy and chemotherapy have to be considered for children with incompletely resected tumors and those with relapse according to the general lines stated for low-grade glioma.

SURGERY AT DIAGNOSIS

The aim of surgery when a low-grade tumor is suspected in this area of the brain is to remove the tumor in order to relieve/arrest symptoms, which may be neurological or epileptic.

Completeness of resection may be a function of pre-operative tumor volume,[1] irrespective of histology, and should be confirmed by modern imaging techniques. Among pediatric series, the rate of complete resections varies between 30 and 95 per cent.[2–4] Complete resection is followed by long-term survival in over 90 per cent.[2-6]

On the other hand, preliminary data of the large natural history study conducted by the Children's Cancer Group (CCG) and the Pediatric Oncology Group (POG) suggest that among 131 relapsing patients, 60 per cent had had an initial resection of more than 95 per cent; 24 per cent (31/131) of these cases had tumors located in the cerebral cortex.[7]

Incompletely resected tumors tend to progress. Time to progression relates to the size of the postoperative residue, with smaller tumors progressing for longer time intervals.[1,4] No difference for the influence of histologic subtype upon progression-free survival has been shown, but as a group patients with non-pilocytic astrocytoma are less likely to have aggressive tumor resection.[2,4] This may imply that an aggressive surgical approach is justified even in the presence of the more infiltrative fibrillary astrocytoma, despite ill-defined margins.

SURGERY AT RELAPSE/PROGRESSION

Children with recurrent/progressive low-grade glioma should be subjected to a second attempt at total tumor removal, which may be accomplished in about half of cases.[2,4]

Non-surgical treatment

After extensive resection, residual tumors might either enlarge slowly or remain quiescent, even in the absence of adjuvant therapy. Consequently, they are best managed with close follow-up, with the option of adjuvant treatment in progressive tumor growth. As for all sites of low-grade astrocytoma, there is consensus that following primary resection, non-surgical treatment is not indicated for completely removed tumors but should be reserved for children developing progression of an incompletely removed tumor not amenable to second surgery.

Radiotherapy

Since extensive surgery is possible in many cases, the role of radiotherapy must be seen in the context of resectability. Even with incomplete tumor removal, prolonged progression-free survival is commonly achieved, and little benefit of radiotherapy can be expected for patients undergoing total or incomplete resection. Radiotherapy as primary treatment is recommended only when surgery is limited to biopsy.[8] In the series of Forsyth and colleagues, 51 patients with supratentorial pilocytic astrocytoma had an overall survival of 82 per cent at 10 and 20 years, 100 per cent for 16 patients undergoing complete resection, and 74 per cent for 35 patients following subtotal removal or biopsy.

The timing of radiotherapy following incomplete resection has therefore been variable. If offered immediately following incomplete resection, a significant difference in progression-free survival has been reported (at 10 years: 82 per cent with versus 40 per cent without radiotherapy), but no difference for overall survival has been reported (at 10 years: 89 per cent with versus 94 per cent without radiotherapy). Additionally, in nine of 16 non-irradiated, incompletely resected tumors, no progression was noted during a median observation time of 68 months.[4]

Radiation doses for the treatment of childhood hemispheric tumors have not been evaluated systematically.

Doses were not specified in the reports of Pollack and colleagues[4] and Gajjar and colleagues.[2] They ranged from 40 to 59 Gy for 19 patients in the series of Wallner and colleagues.[5] Current recommendation is a tumor dose of 54 Gy with a daily fractionation of 1.8 Gy, applying modern techniques for treatment planning.[9–11] The use of hyperfractionation, although investigated for adults,[12] has not been evaluated in children.

Stereotactic radiosurgery offers benefits for well-circumscribed hemispheric lesions by either interstitial or external technique due to its potential of sparing surrounding tissue. However, the numbers of children that have been treated are small.[4,13–17]

An issue that is frequently ignored is the role of radiotherapy in improving focal neurologic deficits. In a series of 15 children, seven of nine with focal neurologic deficits improved following radiotherapy.[18]

Chemotherapy

Only occasionally have children with supratentorial hemispheric astrocytic tumors been included in chemotherapy trials in an attempt to defer radiotherapy. There is no prospective, systematic evaluation of its effectiveness, whereas the small numbers of children having received chemotherapy for hemispheric glioma cannot always be traced within the combined series. Reports are summarized in Table 13b.1.[19–27]

Taken together, 22 children were treated with a variety of chemotherapy regimens. Response was not given for six cases, but 12 of 16 with a known response achieved a partial or minor response or stable disease. There is just one report of the use of concomitant chemoradiotherapy for incompletely resected supratentorial low-grade astrocytoma in children. Seven of 15 patients had hemispheric tumors. Following non-radical resection, three received

Table 13b.1 *Chemotherapy for pediatric supratentorial hemispheric low-grade glioma*

Ref.	Drug(s)	Patients (*n*)	CR/PR/IMP	SD	PD
24	BCNU, VCR, intrathecal MTX, Dexa	6	0/3/1	Not given	Not given
20	Carboplatin	2	0	1	1
23	Etoposide/VCR	5	0	2	3
25	CCNU/PRC/AZQ	1	0/0/1	0	0
	Cyclo	1	0	1	0
26	Carboplatin	1	Not given	Not given	Not given
21, 22	Carboplatin/VCR	3	0/2/0	1	0
43	TCDPV	2	Not given	Not given	Not given
19	Carboplatin/etoposide	1	Not given	Not given	Not given
27	Cisplatin/VCR + RT	3	3/0/0	0	0

AZQ, aziridinylbenzoquinone; BCNU, carmustine; CCNU, lomustine; CR, complete response; Cyclo, cyclophosphamide; Dexa, dexamethasone; IMP, improved; MTX, methotrexate; PD, progressive disease; PR, partial response; PRC, procarbazine; RT, radiotherapy; SD, stable disease; TCDPV, 6-thioguanine, CCNU (lomustine), procarbazine, dibromodulcitol, and vincristine; VCR, vincristine.
Chemotherapy alone, *n* = 22: CR 0, PR 5, IMP 2, SD 5, PD 4, response not given 6. Chemoradiotherapy, *n* = 3: CR 3.

cisplatin and vincristine during focal irradiation with 50–54 Gy tumor dose at a daily fraction of 2 Gy, achieving complete remission.[27]

Although numbers are too small for definite conclusions, hemispheric low-grade astrocytomas seem to respond to an equivalent degree to chemotherapy as low-grade gliomas of other anatomical sites. Chemotherapy may therefore be a treatment option for progressive low-grade glioma of the cerebral hemispheres, especially in young patients.

LOW-GRADE ASTROCYTIC TUMORS OF THE SUPRATENTORIAL MIDLINE

The management of diencephalic gliomas is dependent on tumor location, clinical presentation, the presence of NF-1, and age.

Isolated optic nerve glioma

For those children with isolated optic nerve gliomas, treatment is highly dependent on the visual acuity of the patient at the time of diagnosis and the degree of symptomatology.[28] In most patients with NF-1 and isolated optic nerve gliomas, a period of observation is judicious to see whether the tumor actually is progressing, since many patients will have relatively stable disease for many years without any specific form of intervention.[29–32] In patients with progressive orbital lesions not involving the chiasm, and in those that have caused severe visual loss, especially blindness, resection of the intraorbital portion of the nerve (attempting to spare the orbit) is usually undertaken to improve the cosmetic appearance of the child and prevent spread of the tumor more posteriorly into the chiasm.[28] However, it is unclear how frequently isolated orbital lesions will actually spread into the chiasm and even whether such surgery prevents infiltration.

In patients with relatively good visual acuity at the time of diagnosis, such surgery is infrequently recommended, since in the majority of patients diagnosis can be based on typical imaging features alone.

In patients with falling visual acuity, radiation has been utilized to attempt to maintain or improve vision. In the majority of cases, such radiation, usually in the range of 4500–5500 cGy, will at least stabilize vision and result in a decrease in the amount of proptosis.[33,34] However, radiation therapy does carry with it the risk of secondary tumors in surrounding tissues and possibly long-term facial disfigurement due to the effects of radiation on the growth of bones in the orbital region. Although chemotherapy has been used on an anecdotal basis for patients with isolated optic nerve gliomas, there are no data to support its efficacy.

Chiasmatic tumors

Treatment of patients with chiasmatic tumors is also partially dependent on the presence of NF-1. In asymptomatic patients and in patients with apparently static clinical symptomatology at the time of diagnosis, a period of observation has been recommended before specific treatment is started.[30,32]

SURGICAL TREATMENT

In patients with NF-1, biopsy is rarely required for diagnosis. In patients without NF-1, biopsy or surgical resection is most commonly recommended to confirm the type of tumor present and possibly to debulk disease, especially in children without contiguous orbital involvement. At surgery, the majority of children will be found to have pilocytic astrocytomas, but fibrillary astrocytomas may also occur.

In patients with large globular, especially cystic lesions, such surgical debulking may result in a significant amount of tumor removal, but this carries with it the risk of increased visual impairment, especially visual field loss.[35] An increase in visual impairment has been reported for 43–75 per cent of children.[32,34–36]

NON-SURGICAL TREATMENT

Following biopsy, especially in children without NF-1, and also in those patients with NF-1 and progressive symptomatology or radiographic progression on sequential studies, treatment with either radiation or chemotherapy is usually required.

Radiotherapy

Although the role of radiation therapy for children with chiasmatic/hypothalamic gliomas has not been established unequivocally, non-randomized studies have suggested that doses of radiation between 5000 and 5400 cGy result in tumor shrinkage or at least stabilization of disease in the majority of patients.[34,37] Whereas post-treatment progression is not seen in tumors confined to the optic nerve, the risk for its development rises with increasing extension of the lesions into the adjacent midbrain.[37–39] Patients with neurologic signs at time of treatment are reported to have a poorer prognosis (overall survival at five and ten years: 57 per cent with neurologic signs versus 92 per cent without neurologic signs).[38] Overall progression-free survival rates of 70–90 per cent have been reported five to ten years after treatment with radiation.

The efficacy of radiation in stabilization and improvement of visual function, which can be sustained for many years, has been confirmed by numerous reports (Tables 13b.2 and 13b.3). In many studies, radiation therapy has been performed in cases of progressive loss of vision. However, due to the nature of disease, long-term secondary failure rates of up to 40 per cent may occur.[41] Five-year

Table 13b.2 *Vision after radiotherapy of gliomas of the optic pathway*

Ref.	Patients (*n*)	Total dose (TD) and fractionated dose (FD)	Improved (%)	Stable (%)	Worse (%)
121	22	8–15 Gy	Vision 11 (50)	8 (36.4)	3 (13.6)
36	12	TD 3.5–65 Gy (almost all 50 Gy), FD n.m.	Vision 3 (25)	9 (75)	0
29	28	n.m.	Acuity 4 (14.3)	18 (28.6)	6 (21.4)
122	9	TD 37–55.8 Gy, FD 1.0–2.0 Gy	Vision 1 (11.1)	8 (88.9)	0
123	39	TD 50–60 Gy, FD n.m.	Vision 7 (19.9)	30 (76.9)	2 (5.1)
124	23	TD 45–50 Gy, FD 1.8–2.0 Gy	Acuity 10 (43), visual field 4 (18)	Acuity 11 (48), visual field 19 (82)	Acuity 2 (9), visual field 0
34	18	TD 50–60 Gy, FD 1.8–2.5 Gy	Vision 6 (33)	8 (44)	4 (22)
125	12	TD 40–56 Gy, FD n.m.	Vision 3 (25)	9 (75)	0
126	22	TD 38–56.86 Gy, FD 1.4–2.0 Gy	2 (9)	14 (77)	3 (14)
127	17	TD 35–61 Gy, FD 1.5–2.0 Gy	6 (35)	9 (53)	2 (12)
128	23	TD 45–56.6 Gy, FD 1.8–2.0 Gy	23 (30)	14 (61)	2 (9)
129	15	TD 43–60 Gy, FD n.m.	Vision 3 (20)	8 (53.3)	1 (6.6)
38	44	TD 40–60 Gy, FD 1.45–2.15 Gy	Acuity 25 (57), visual field 19 (61)	Acuity 16 (36), visual field 11 (35)	Acuity 3 (7), visual field 1 (3)
130	13	TD 40–60 Gy, FD 1.8–2.0 Gy	9 (34)	14 (54)	3 (12)
131	25	TD 45–60 Gy, FD 1.6–2.0 Gy	Acuity 9/25 (36), visual field 3/20 (15)	Acuity 13 (52), visual field 16 (80)	Acuity 3 (12), visual field 1 (5)

Table 13b.3 *Impact of fractionated dose and total dose on risk of loss of visual function after radiotherapy of tumors at the base of skull (pituitary adenoma in the majority of cases). The optic chiasm was encompassed by the treatment portals*

Ref.	Patients (%)	Dose (Gy) Single	Dose (Gy) Total
132	5/55 (9.1)	2.5	45.0–50.0
133	4/122 (3.3)	2.0–2.5	50.0
134	4/23 (17.4)	3.0	42.0–45.0

survival rates are somewhat higher in patients who have undergone radiotherapy compared with those who have not.[34,40] Overall progression-free survival rates of 70–90 per cent have been reported five to ten years after treatment with radiation.

Radiation therapy, especially because of the large size of chiasmatic and hypothalamic tumors at the time of diagnosis, may result in long-term neurocognitive damage and, in the vast majority of patients, will have significant endocrinologic sequelae, especially growth hormone insufficiency.

Chemotherapy

Given the young age of children with chiasmatic tumors, chemotherapy has often been utilized in an attempt to delay, if not obviate, the need for radiotherapy. A variety of different chemotherapeutic approaches have been utilized in children with progressive chiasmatic/hypothalamic gliomas, especially in patients under five years of age at the time of diagnosis. Drugs and drug combinations that have been utilized include carboplatin alone, oral VP16 alone, a combination of actinomycin D and vincristine, a combination of carboplatin and vincristine, the five-drug combination of BCNU, vincristine, thioguanine, procarbazine, and dibromodulcitol, and other, more intensive drug regimens.[20–23,42,43] The largest published experience has been with the carboplatin and vincristine regimen. In a recent series of 68 patients, a radiographic response was documented in over 60 per cent of patients, and 90–95 per cent of patients had at least disease stabilization while on treatment.[22]

Approximately 70 per cent of children with visual pathway gliomas remained free of progressive disease three years following the initiation of treatment (for at least two years after completion of treatment). This drug regimen was not as successful in older children, and patients with NF-1 and with progressive disease benefited as well as, if not better than, patients without NF-1.

HYPOTHALAMIC-CHIASMATIC GLIOMA: CASE 1

This case is a boy born at full term after a normal pregnancy and who was diagnosed with NF-1 at three months of age based on the presence of numerous café-au-lait spots and a positive family history (his mother and his older brother also have NF-1). His personal medical history was marked by psychomotor developmental delay. At the age of 3.5 years, the physician at the NF clinic who was following the child decided to obtain a contrast-enhanced head MRI. The MRI showed that the entire optic chiasm, the intracranial tract of the left optic nerve, and the left hypothalamus were grossly enlarged, partially deforming the third ventricle. The lesion was enhancing after contrast injection; furthermore, on the T2-weighted images, hyperintense areas were visible in the splenium of the corpus callosum, which appeared slightly thin. No history of decreased visual acuity could be documented. The Teller test revealed a visual acuity in the range of 1/50 bilaterally, while visual evoked potentials demonstrated an abnormal transmission of the visual stimulation, particularly in the pre-chiasmatic level. No accurate assessment of the visual field could be obtained.

Based on the MRI findings, a diagnosis of visual pathway glioma was formulated, and a decision was taken to defer any treatment until clinical and neuroradiological evidence of progressive disease had become evident.

Subsequently, the child underwent periodic head MRI evaluations every six months for the first year and then yearly. The reasons for such a relatively frequent neuroradiological follow-up were related to: (i) the difficulties of monitoring appropriately the visual function of this young, mentally delayed child; (ii) his relatively young age at diagnosis (it is hypothesized that optic pathway gliomas in children with NF-1 have a limited time span of growth, which usually does not overcome the first decade of life, if even the first six years of life); and (iii) the extension of the tumor (pure optic gliomas seem to have a much more indolent clinical behaviour than gliomas extending posteriorly, intracranially to reach the optic chiasm).

At five years' follow-up, the visual function has improved minimally (as expected, with the increasing age) and the optic pathway lesion has not changed. No therapy has been administered so far.

Thalamic tumors

The management of children with progressive thalamic lesions is highly dependent on the histological type of the tumor.[44] Since over 50 per cent of patients with thalamic lesions will have higher-grade tumors, biopsy and/or surgical resection is indicated in almost all patients. However, the majority of these tumors are not amenable to significant tumor resections. Patients with low-grade lesions are usually managed with radiation or chemotherapy according to the principles stated for tumors of the chiasmatic–hypothalamic region. Despite low-grade histology, bithalamic glial tumors are as aggressive as high-grade glial neoplasms with a dismal outcome, requiring novel treatment approaches.[45]

BRAINSTEM LOW–GRADE GLIOMA (NOT INCLUDING INTRINSIC DIFFUSE PONTINE GLIOMA)

Focal brainstem glioma

The outcome of children with focal lesions is better than that for children with diffuse, intrinsic tumors.

Dorsally exophytic cervicomedullary tumors have been treated with biopsy followed by radiation therapy, partial resection followed by radiation therapy, and total surgical resections.[46,47] Independent of the form of treatment, 80–90 per cent of patients can be expected to be alive five years following diagnosis, the majority with stable disease. Surgical resections for tumors in such regions, however, may result in increased neurologic compromise, including the need for prolonged ventilatory support in up to 30 per cent of patients.[46] When radiotherapy is utilized, most frequently doses between 50 and 54 Gy are delivered in conventional daily fractionated regimens. For very young children, especially those under five years of age, with residual low-grade tumors after surgery, chemotherapy has been utilized; the combination of carboplatin and vincristine has demonstrated a local control rate of approximately 70 per cent at three years following diagnosis in a small series.[21]

Management of focal brainstem lesions remains unsettled. Focal lesions, which are often cystic, can be treated by surgical resection, although such resections are often incomplete and may result in increased, and often permanent, neurologic deficits.[48] Alternatively, biopsy, especially stereotactic biopsy, to prove the low-grade nature of the lesion, followed by either local radiation therapy or, in very young children, chemotherapy, may result in similar rates of disease control and less long-term neurologic morbidity.[49]

Tectal gliomas

Patients with tectal lesions usually require CSF diversion procedures at the time of diagnosis.[50,51] Subsequently, two-thirds of patients will not require any other form of intervention for four to five years after diagnosis. In children who develop progressive disease, radiation therapy is usually employed.

Patients with NF-1 may also present with apparent brainstem gliomas. Some of these lesions will be true gliomas and will show growth over a period of observation; others may be diagnosed on screening studies at the time when the patient is asymptomatic.[52,53] In patients with progressive symptoms, treatment is usually undertaken as it would be for patients without NF-1. However, for most patients with NF-1 and a possible brainstem glioma, a period of observation coupled with serial magnetic resonance studies is recommended before any form of specific treatment.

LOW-GRADE ASTROCYTIC TUMORS OF THE CEREBELLUM

Management

Surgery plays the key role within the treatment strategy for cerebellar astrocytoma. Numerous reports indicate that the extent of resection is correlated well with long-term outcome. Thus, the surgical plan is to achieve complete resection of the lesion whilst avoiding severe neurological damage. The operation will also permit sufficient material for histopathologic diagnosis to be obtained and restoration of pathways for the CSF circulation.

Surgery

If preoperative investigations confirm that the origin of the tumor is the cerebellar hemisphere, the vermis, or the fourth ventricular floor, then total removal should be the goal of surgical intervention.[54,55] To avoid postoperative mutism, no extended vermian incision should be performed.[55]

Despite the limitations of early postoperative scans,[56] there is consensus to confirm the extent of surgical resection by postoperative contrast-enhanced CT or MRI. In 20–30 per cent, this may not correlate with the surgeon's estimate of completeness.[57,58] If postoperative scans disclose resectable tumor, immediate reoperation should be considered to achieve complete tumor removal.[55]

Complete surgical resection, as judged by postoperative neuroimaging and operative notes, appears possible in 84–90 per cent of all patients.[2,54] Series preceding the modern imaging era and modern neurosurgical techniques report complete resections in 45–76 per cent.[57,59–62] Completely resected cerebellar astrocytoma has a long-term prognosis for relapse-free survival and overall survival exceeding 80 and 90 per cent, respectively. However, even after complete resection, a small percentage of relapses occur throughout the years.[2,57,58,61,63]

Incomplete removal is inevitable if the tumor extends into the brainstem, if there is leptomeningeal infiltration, and if there is involvement of cranial nerves. However, even for tumors involving the brainstem, complete resection appears possible today in up to 62.5 per cent of cases.[64] Since non-pilocytic (diffuse, fibrillary) astrocytomas are found more often in this location, the presence of fibrillary histology is an added adverse prognostic factor.[58,64,65] Technical adjuncts, such as monitoring the electromyogram of cranial nerves, may assist the surgeon in achieving more extensive resection with safety.[55]

Extended periods of stable disease, and sporadic cases of tumor regression, following partial resection are reported for small numbers of patients.[57,60,65,66] However, the majority of tumor residues tends to progress over time, mostly within four to five years after initial operation,

and progression-free survival rates range between 29–80 per cent and 0–79 per cent at five and ten years, respectively.[5,54,57,58,60,61,63–67] For residual volumes above 3 cm^3, progression-free survival drops below 50 per cent at 100 months.[58] It should be acknowledged that recurrences of cerebellar astrocytoma may occur late, well beyond the time predicted by Collins' law.[66,68]

Upon relapse or progression, reoperation is recommended to try and achieve a delayed gross total resection.[2,64,65,69] Although this appears to be successful in up to 30 per cent of patients, individual patients can be managed by multiple reinterventions.[54,61,64]

Most failures are local, yet leptomeningeal spread to brain and/or spine has been reported.[5,70–74]

Operative procedures of midline cerebellar tumors have an inherent risk of causing transient mutism following bilateral lesion of the dentate nucleus.[75,76] Complete absence of speech without associated brainstem signs may develop within several days postoperatively, lasting days to several months. When speech is regained, it passes through a state of dysarthria (see Chapter 24).

Pseudobulbar palsy may have a similarly delayed onset. Supranuclear lesions are associated with emotional lability. This has been attributed to retraction of the cerebellar hemispheres and vermian incision and extension of edema along the middle and superior cerebellar peduncles into the upper pons and midbrain. Gradual resolution of the symptoms takes several months.[76,77]

Non-surgical treatment

Due to the fact that only small numbers of patients cannot be managed by (repeat) surgical intervention, there are no prospective studies concerning non-surgical treatment.

RADIOTHERAPY

Postoperative radiotherapy has been applied to patients with residual, progressive, or recurrent cerebellar astrocytoma in a rather unsystematic pattern. Occasionally, the decision for irradiation has depended only on the preference of the referring neurosurgeon.[63] However, routine radiotherapy for incompletely excised cerebellar tumors has not been advocated.[69]

Indications for radiotherapy have been recurrent tumor after secondary or multiple operation, residual tumor at inoperable sites, tumor that had just been biopsied, and symptomatic patients following subtotal resection.[2,57,69] More recently, radiotherapy has been reserved for children over five years old.[2]

Results concerning the effectiveness of radiotherapy are conflicting and are difficult to interpret due to small numbers and extended periods of recruitment, changes in techniques, doses, and fractionation, and inconsistent indications for initiating adjuvant therapy. Some authors have not demonstrated a beneficial effect of radiotherapy.[78] Progression-free survival has been prolonged, but no survival advantage was shown for the group with incomplete resection plus radiation.[5,63,69] Griffin and colleagues demonstrated a relapse-free survival rate of 83 per cent following radiotherapy, no matter how many previous surgeries were performed, but no patient survived if the preceding surgery was less than subtotal.[61]

Current recommendations follow the general treatment strategy for low-grade glioma, with treatment being indicated for symptomatic and/or progressive tumors that are not amenable to surgical resection. Modern planning systems should be applied, especially considering adequate field size and correct margins to reduce the radiation dose to critical organs of the brain.

CHEMOTHERAPY

There have been no prospective studies of chemotherapy for low-grade cerebellar tumors. Inclusion of patients with recurrent or progressive cerebellar astrocytoma into ongoing chemotherapy studies has yielded few preliminary results. Mostly, these children were young and chemotherapy was applied to defer radiotherapy, justifying this approach.

The role of radiotherapy as well as chemotherapy for the treatment of progressive/relapsed tumors has not been established prospectively, but preliminary information suggests that progression-free survival can be prolonged.

LOW-GRADE ASTROCYTIC TUMORS OF THE SPINAL CANAL

Management

As in all other regions of the CNS, treatment strategy for spinal-cord astrocytoma has to balance functional outcome and the risks of tumor progression or relapse. Due to the rarity of these tumors, larger series have most often comprised tumors treated during extended periods of time, where not only equipment and technical possibilities, but also the general treatment philosophy, have changed.[79–84]

Surgery

Most patients will require surgical intervention to at least diagnose the type of tumor present, since other tumor histologies, such as ependymomas or intrinsic primitive neuroectodermal tumors of the spinal cord, cannot be distinguished on neuroradiographic features alone.[85,86] Furthermore, higher-grade gliomas carry a much less favorable prognosis than, and must be distinguished from, lower-grade tumors.[87]

Surgery has to provide spinal decompression and to remove safely as much tumor as possible, despite the intrinsic nature of the tumors and extent at the time of diagnosis, taking into account that attempts to remove these lesions may cause severe additional neurologic deficits.[88] Radical excision of intramedullary spinal cord tumors has been recommended as treatment of choice, provided that at least subtotal resection is possible. Multiple surgical interventions may be performed.[81,86, 88–90] The use of modern technical adjuncts, such as intraoperative ultrasound, intraoperative monitoring with spinal somatosensory evoked potentials (SEPs), and spinal cord evoked potentials (SCEPs), facilitates tumor removal.[86] In pediatric series, gross total and/or subtotal resection has been achieved in 49 per cent[91] and 76.8 per cent,[89,92] but not all patients in the latter series had low-grade tumors (131/164, 79.9 per cent).

Even when microscopic residues are present, tumors may remain quiescent for extended periods of time. However, tumor progression and worsening of the functional neurologic status will ensue in patients treated expectantly after primary biopsy only.[81]

The postoperative functional status is determined by the degree of the preoperative deficit. Patients with no or only mild deficits before surgery rarely deteriorate. In a report of 164 patients aged 21 years or younger, clinical symptomatology was said to be unchanged in 60 per cent, improved in 16 per cent, and worse in 24 per cent three months following surgery.[89,92] Five-year progression-free survival was similar for patients who had a gross total resection compared with those who had a subtotal resection (defined in this series as an 80–95 per cent resection).

A discrete postoperative increase of preoperative dysfunction is transient in nature in most cases, but patients with extensive non-cystic tumors and severe preoperative disability are likely to deteriorate from surgery.

Radiotherapy

Because of the lack of prospective trials with sufficient follow-up, treatments are based on strategies for equivalent histologies of intracranial tumors on the assumption that the tumor behavior would be comparable. Considering the advances in imaging, surgical skills, and radiation techniques, it becomes difficult to assess the value of each therapeutic intervention. The role of radiation therapy has yet to be defined with respect to preservation or improvement of neurological function, site and extent of disease, surgical resectability, age, and recently chemotherapy.

Where an intramedullary infiltrating tumor has spread, extensive surgery is not favored and radiotherapy is traditionally used. Many authors stress that radiotherapy may be postponed until signs of progression occur.[83,84,91,93,94]

After various degrees of resection with or without post-operative radiotherapy, the survival rates in patients with low-grade gliomas have ranged between 60 and 80 per cent at five years and between 55 and 70 per cent at ten years.[92,95] In earlier reports, routine postoperative radiation had been given in all tumors irrespective of the degree of resection, resulting in survival rates of between 80 and 67 per cent and relapse-free survival rates between 73 and 53 per cent at 10 and 20 years, respectively. There was a trend towards better survival for patients receiving radiotherapy in pilocytic astrocytoma (85 per cent versus 75 per cent after surgery) and a significant advantage for non-pilocytic astrocytoma in one analysis (Table 13b.4).[83] Some series could not identify a benefit of radiation following total and subtotal resection, but patients had prolonged survival when they were irradiated following incomplete surgery.[84,91,93] When deciding on treatment, it should be considered that a more aggressive surgical approach can be associated with higher neurologic morbidity. Control of neurological deficits is a major option for the selection of treatment, but there are limited data evaluating the impact of radiotherapy on neurological function. One retrospective analysis reports improvement of neurological deficits in 12/23 patients, stable status in 9/23 patients, and deterioration in only 2/23 patients at six months after radiotherapy.[96]

In the majority of cases, low-grade gliomas recur locally after initial treatment (in 30–80 per cent of patients) and metastatic spread is a rare event.

In all published series, radiotherapy to the tumor site only was performed. With the use of MRI, the gross tumor volume according to the ICRU-50 report can be delineated accurately, and a safety margin in the craniocaudal direction of one vertebral body is recommended in the literature.[84,97]

The threshold for radiation injury of tumor-containing cord is encountered at 45–50 Gy using conventional fractionation,[93,98] thus radiosensitivity of the spinal cord limits the dose that can be given to the tumor. Due to a presumed shallow dose–response curve, it appears that doses in excess of 45 Gy are sufficient for tumor control. Doses of less than 40 Gy may be associated with an increased failure rate. Beyond 50 Gy, no additional benefit in terms of progression-free survival has been observed.[83,84,91,93] With respect to the assumed dose– response relationship of their intracranial counterparts, doses between 45 and 50 Gy are currently recommended. The role of the length of the spinal cord field has not been determined.[99]

Chemotherapy

The role of chemotherapy in the treatment of spinal-cord low-grade astrocytomas remains poorly defined. Chemotherapy has been utilized especially for young infants with progressive low-grade tumors.[21] There are a few case reports, or very small series, suggesting that various chemotherapeutic regimens produce responses in either incompletely resected or inoperable tumors with marked functional improvement.[79,80,91,90,100,101] As in other sites, chemotherapy may delay the need for radiotherapy or even obviate its use,[79,80,100] although close monitoring for progression is necessary.[102]

Prognosis

The survival of patients with low-grade gliomas of the spinal cord is usually favorable, thus their functional outcome is of main concern.

Data of series including all types and grades of intramedullary pediatric tumors yield five-year survival rates between 39 and 90 per cent and event-free survival rates between 14 and 77 per cent.

Overall survival rates for low-grade tumors regardless of previous treatment are reported at 76 per cent at ten years, and including radiotherapy at 83 per cent at ten years,[91] 88 per cent at a median follow-up of 4.8 years,[80,100] and 83 per cent at ten years.[84] Five-year progression-free survival was reported to be 79 per cent following aggressive surgical intervention alone.[89] About half of the unresectable tumors being treated with chemotherapy progress.[80,90,100,102]

Table 13b.4 *Effect of radiotherapy on low-grade spinal tumors in children*

Ref.	Patient characteristics	Radiation dose (Gy)	Fractionation (Gy/fraction)	Ten-year survival (irradiated v. non-irradiated) (%)
91	21 irradiated of 49 low-grade glioma	30–50	Not given	83 v. 70, NS
94	9 irradiated of 18, 4/11 with low-grade glioma	43–50	Not given	3/4 alive v. 7/7 alive at 3–18 years
83	14 children <20 years/ 79 patients all ages	13.1–66.6 (median 49.8)	1.44–2.5 (median 1.8)	80–85 v. 55–60 (pilocytic astrocytoma, all ages, n = 43), NS
84	12 low-grade glioma/31 children	30–56	Not given	83 (all irradiated)

NS, not significant.

Factors influencing outcome have been the duration of presenting symptoms before diagnosis, specifically the development of spinal deformity, the preoperative neurologic condition, and the type of tumor,[86,91] whereas the extent of disease at diagnosis (number of vertebral segments involved) has not proved to have a significant influence.[83] Differences between histologic subtypes have not been assessed separately for children. Relapse and progression usually occur within the first five years, but they may develop after more than ten years of follow-up.

Post-tumor-related therapeutic follow-up also has to focus on spinal deformity. This may result from neurogenic defect, laminectomy/laminotomy, and, if applied, radiotherapy. Specific sequelae of radiotherapy include radionecrosis, vasculopathy, and impaired spinal growth. Depending on the age of the patient and the length of the radiation field, radiogenic growth disturbances can enhance pre-existing spinal deformities, such as kyphoscoliosis. They may be progressive, even requiring orthopedic surgery (i.e. spinal fusion).[86,99] An incidence of second tumors of 13 per cent at ten and 20 years has been reported.[84]

DISSEMINATED LOW-GRADE ASTROCYTIC TUMORS

Incidence

A small percentage of low-grade gliomas develop leptomeningeal dissemination either at presentation or during follow-up. Chiasmatic and hypothalamic lesions have especially been found to be associated with CSF seeding.

Most reports focus on the course of single patients. An estimate of the incidence of leptomeningeal spread comes from institutional retrospective analyses: about five per cent of children presented with leptomeningeal spread at diagnosis, whereas dissemination was diagnosed in 12 per cent at progression.[71,73,103,104] With improvements in neuroimaging technology, this phenomenon may be identified with increasing frequency.

Age and sex

Children diagnosed with leptomeningeal spread had a median age of eight years (five months to 20 years).[73] Those that developed dissemination, mostly within two years following initial diagnosis, were younger, with a median age of 16 months (five months to 43 years, including two adults).[71] There seems to be a marked male preponderance (male/female ratios 5:3 and 9:2).[71,103,104]

Tumor location

The majority of primary tumors are located in the chiasmatic-hypothalamic and thalamic area (37/56 cases), but primaries have also been reported in the cerebellum, brainstem, and spinal cord (Table 13b.5).

Leptomeningeal spread involves all areas of the CNS. Despite a low risk for tumor spread via shunting devices even in malignant brain tumors,[105] leptomeningeal seeding associated with spread via a ventriculoperitoneal shunt into the abdominal cavity has been reported.[73,106] On the other hand, even if it has been investigated, tumor cells have rarely been found in the CSF.

Histology

Juvenile pilocytic astrocytoma, and other categories of low-grade glioma, have been the histologies in most cases. No unique histological features have been identified, nor has malignant transformation been found on re-biopsy. Proliferation indices, if determined, correspond to those of the primary tumor.[74]

The primary lesions arising in close proximity to the ventricles and basal cisterns may show a predisposition to dissemination, but it is not clear whether they constitute a distinct entity. Patterns of adhesion molecule production, protease secretion, and growth factor pathway activation may play a part in determining the ability of free-floating tumor cells to become adherent to, and to multiply on, ependymal and leptomeningeal surfaces.[70,73,107] When dissemination is present at diagnosis, it cannot be excluded that tumors arise simultaneously at various sites.

Signs and symptoms

Leptomeningeal spread is rarely symptomatic at diagnosis. Even if seeding occurs at progression, there may be no symptoms at all, or not all sites involved may cause symptoms.[71,103,108–110] There has been one report of a sacral intradural metastasis with paraparesis, saddle-type anesthesia, diminished ankle jerk in the lower extremities, and bladder dysfunction at diagnosis without concomitant symptoms that could be attributed to the chiasmatic primary.[111]

Clinical signs related to dissemination mainly are pain, meningeal syndrome, radicular compression, raised intracranial pressure, and seizures.[71,103,109] In a report from Perilongo and colleagues, primary dissemination was diagnosed in three infant boys who had presented with diencephalic syndrome due to an extensive chiasmatic-hypothalamic pilocytic astrocytoma.[104] Only one similar observation was reported by Pollack and colleagues,[73] thus it is not clear whether this association is a

Table 13b.5 *Clinical features of metastatic low-grade astrocytoma in children*

Ref.	No. of children with dissemination	Age at diagnosis	Location of primary tumor	CSF-positivity	Location of multicentric spread	Present at diagnosis	Present at progression (interval from diagnosis to spread)	Histology of primary tumor
106	1	3.5 years	Chiasmatic-hypothalamic	1/1	Leptomeningeal	–	1/1: 10 months	Astrocytoma grade I
70	2/94	4.75 years, 8.5 years	Chiasm 1, cerebellum 1	?	Leptomeningeal 2 (cerebral and spinal)	–	2/2: 3.5 years, 6 years	2 PA
135	1	10 years	Chiasm	?	Spinal leptomeningeal 1	–	1/1: 2 years	1 PA
136	1	1.3 years	Chiasm	?	Posterior fossa + spinal leptomeningeal 1	–	1/1: 8.5 years	1 PA
25	2/11	10.8 years (both)	Primary bifocal tumors	Not given	Temporal right + cerebellar vermis 1, thalamus right + hypothalamus left 1	2/2	–	2 PA
137	1/25	12 years	Tectal region	?	Spinal leptomeningeal 1	1/1	–	1 LGG
73	3/76	6 months, 4 years, 5 years	Chiasm 1, cerebellum 2	0/3 (1 atypical cells)	Subependymal ventricular 3, leptomeningeal 3	2/3	1/3: 4.75 years	1 PA, 2 LGG
71	11/90 JPA	5 months–43 years	Hypothalamus 10, cerebellar vermis 1	2/3 with leptomeningeal spread	Cerebral hemisphere 2, posterior fossa 3, spinal cord 6, leptomeningeal 3, subependymal 4	3/11	8/11: median 12 months (4–108 months)	11 JPA

Reference(s)	N	Age	Location				Diagnosis
103	8/150 LGG	5 months–20 years	Hypothalamus 4, temporal lobe 1, spinal cord 2, pons 1	0/2	Cerebral hemisphere 5, posterior fossa 6, spinal cord 6, leptomeningeal not given, subependymal 4	8/8	–	3 JPA, 5 astrocytoma n.o.s.
110, 138	4	2.5 years, 5 years, 7 years, 8 years	Third ventricle 1, cerebellum 1, hypothalamic 1, third ventricle 1	0/3	Posterior fossa 1, spinal cord 2, leptomeningeal 2, subependymal 2	1/4	3/4: 8 months, 32 months, 44 months	3 PA
108	1	14 years	Chiasm, both optic tracts	Not given	Cerebral hemisphere, posterior fossa, spinal canal	–	1/1: 39 months	1 PA
104	3/43	6 months, 7 months, 18 months	Chiasmatic-hypothalamic 3	0/1	Leptomeningeal 3 (intraventricular, cerebral, spinal)	3/3	–	3 PA
74	2	4 years, 6 years	Chiasmatic-hypothalamic 1, cerebellum 1	Not given	Cerebral hemisphere 1, cerebellum 1, spinal cord 1, leptomeningeal 2	–	2/2: 4.66 years, 4.75 years	2 PA
109	16	5 years (5 months–12.5 years)	Chiasmatic-hypothalamic 8, thalamus 1, brainstem 2, spinal cord 3, leptomeningeal gliomatosis 2	Not given	Isolated nodules, location not given 3, diffuse leptomeningeal 7, both types 5, cystic lesion 1	6/16	10/16: median 3 years (11 months–9 years)	5 PA, 6 astrocytoma n.o.s., 2 oligodendroglioma, 2 mixed glioma, 1 clinical diagnosis
111	1	8 years	Chiasmatic-hypothalamic	Not given	Spinal cord (sacral intradural)	1/1	–	Astrocytoma grade II

CSF, cerebrospinal fluid; JPA, juvenile pilocytic astrocytoma; LGG, low-grade glioma; n.o.s, not otherwise specified; PA, pilocytic astrocytoma.

result of thorough clinical investigation or has a common pathological background.

Diagnostic procedure

MRI of brain and spine, as performed by standard techniques, may either show enhancing nodular deposits or may demonstrate lining of the leptomeninges, revealed most impressively by subtraction techniques.[103]

Routine MRI of the spinal axis probably is not needed in patients with unifocal intracranial disease and no symptoms that can be referred to the spine.[73] However, investigation of the entire neuroaxis is mandatory if leptomeningeal or periventricular deposits on the initial or follow-up cranial neuroimaging studies are noted and in cases with symptoms related to potential metastatic sites.[111]

Cytologic examination of the CSF can be negative even in cases of unequivocal spinal deposits or leptomeningeal lining. It should be performed in patients with positive neuroimaging, but it is not recommended routinely in imaging-negative children.[73]

There is no uniform policy concerning the necessity of a separate biopsy of at least one of the metastatic lesions. Where metastatic sites have been biopsied, pathological findings have mirrored the primary tumor appearances.[71,73,108,111]

Management

Treatment has been instituted in most but not all patients with multicentric disease following diagnosis of metastases. Recommended approaches take their pattern from the general treatment strategies for pediatric low-grade glioma.

SURGERY

If there are only singular lesions, then their surgical removal is recommended.[71,111] However, multiplicity of deposits or the presence of leptomeningeal "coating" limit this approach. Besides, surgery only has not been sufficient to prevent progressive disease in individual cases.[103]

The question as to whether to proceed with radiotherapy or chemotherapy remains open and must include consideration of the age of the patient, whether the patient has undergone radiotherapy for the primary tumor, and, if so, the interval since that previous irradiation.

RADIOTHERAPY

Radiotherapy for multicentric disease has been applied in a variety of prescriptions, not allowing direct comparison. Among those 56 cases shown in Table 13b.5, ten children have been treated primarily with radiation and five have received additional chemotherapy preceding or following radiotherapy. Six children received craniospinal irradiation. Doses ranged from 60 Gy in hyperfractionated technique (2×1 Gy/day) to the brain and 30 Gy to the spinal cord plus a local boost of 14.5 Gy to conventionally fractionated 40 Gy to the brain and 30 Gy to the spine. One child received cranial irradiation with 39 Gy, two were treated with spinal fields up to 48 Gy, and no details are given in five cases.

At the time the reports were published, four children had died of progressive disease and 11 are alive following multiple interventions (of those receiving radiotherapy only, two died and eight are alive). Limited information indicates that individual children retained normal endocrine function, continued their school education, and did not develop additional neurologic deficits.[72,73]

CHEMOTHERAPY

For 39 of 57 children listed in Table 13b.5, chemotherapy has been the primary approach to multicentric disease. Whereas five of 57 received additional radiotherapy, most children have been treated with individualized strategies. Thus, the success of any given approach cannot be evaluated. Protocols based on carboplatin and cisplatin were predominant (26/44), alkylating agents were given to 13 of 44 (six cyclophosphamide, one ifosfamide, six BCNU/CCNU), and multiagent chemotherapy was applied in two of 44 cases (miscellaneous three: VP16, AZQ, PCV). Although nearly all patients showed initial responses, these were often of short duration, and subsequent progression was reported in 27 of 44 patients. Thirty-two children were alive and 12 had died from further progression at the time of publication.

Recommendation

The presence of multicentric disease at diagnosis or its emergence upon progression is viewed as indication for therapy. Treatment modalities for multicentric disease must be considered individually, since an optimum strategy has not been determined. In accord with current recommendations, younger children receive initial chemotherapy following contemporary protocols to delay irradiation. Radiotherapy options include craniospinal irradiation with 35–39 Gy in conventional fractions or even 40–48 Gy hyperfractionated plus a boost to the primary tumor. Focal irradiation follows the general prescriptions.

The course of disease is extremely variable. Progression following transient response to therapeutic interventions is frequent, but prolonged disease stabilization is possible. Successful treatment of widespread seeding does not preclude good quality of life.

HYPOTHALAMIC–CHIASMATIC GLIOMA: CASE 2

This case is a Caucasian boy, referred at the age of eight months to medical attention for failure to thrive, which had become evident after the age of four months. Since then, the child's medical history was unremarkable, as was his family history. Mild irritability had been reported recently, along with occasional morning vomiting. In the previous month or so, loss of appetite was also reported. The child had no stigmata of NF-1. His physical examination was negative, except for a body weight below the tenth percentile, compatible with a growth curve that was normal up to the age of four months and had plateaued thereafter. His neurological examination was normal apart from the presence of nystagmus on lateral gaze. After an extensive gastroenterologic and metabolic work-up, it was decided to obtain a head MRI. The study showed a large contrast-enhancing, non-cystic, lobulated hypothalamic-chiasmatic lesion. Furthermore, on the head examination, enhancing nodules along the anterior aspect of the pons were also visible. Because of this finding, the MRI investigation was extended to include the entire spine, where other subarachnoidal discrete nodules were visible. Significant ventriculomegaly was also reported. Subsequently, the child was brought to surgery for a ventriculoperitoneal shunt placement and biopsy of the mass. No debulking procedures were thought to be possible. The histological diagnosis was in favour of a classical, bona fide pilocytic astrocytoma.

Due to the age of the child, the dimension of the lesion, and the presence of a diencephalic syndrome, it was decided to treat the child with chemotherapy, specifically the combination of carboplatin and vincristine. The child received the 12-month schedule of chemotherapy. The tumor mass and the subarachnoidal nodules decreased in size (and number); after the first three months of therapy, the child started to gain weight. At the end of chemotherapy, his body weight was between the twenty-fifth and fiftieth centiles. The child was followed periodically. At eight months off therapy, the hypothalamic-chiasmatic mass started to grow again, but without provoking any clinical symptoms, while the subarachnoidal nodules remained stable in number and size. The child's visual function was never monitored carefully. On a Teller test, the visual acuity was estimated to be on the 1/50 range, with some visual field defects. Because of the tumor regrowth and the child's young age (29 months),

further chemotherapy was delivered. During this entire period, the child never stopped growing in weight and height. The tumor responded temporarily, but after ten months of further therapy, the primary tumor regrew. At that time, when the child was almost 3.5 years old, after long discussion and after having excluded the possibility of a debulking procedure, it was elected to irradiate the primary lesion, sparing for the moment the treatment of the entire craniospinal axis (as the presence of disseminated disease theoretically dictated). In fact, it was thought too deleterious to irradiate the entire craniospinal axis in a child of such a young age and with doubtful efficacy. The child was then irradiated (54 Gy). Presently, at the age of six years, the child is in a good general condition. He is slightly obese despite an apparent normal food intake, and he has some cognitive problems (he is in a special education class) and multiple endocrinologic deficits (growth and thyroid hormone deficiency), but the disease is stable. Interestingly, the discrete nodules that were visible along the spine are reducing in number as well as in the degree of post-contrast enhancement.

FUTURE CONSIDERATIONS

Low-grade gliomas span a wide spectrum of biologic entities. Thus, clinical presentation, applicability of different treatments, and prognosis vary with respect to histology, anatomical location, and the age of the patient. Despite considerable efforts, optimal management policies are not available for all subgroups. The indolent nature of some of these lesions makes treatment choices difficult, especially in children with subtle clinical symptoms.

Modern surgical techniques integrating localization techniques such as frameless stereotaxy, intraoperative ultrasound, and functional MRI, as well as electrophysiological mapping of eloquent areas, permit greater degrees of resection in larger proportions of patients.[55,112] It is probable that fewer children will need postoperative, non-surgical therapy in the future.

One of the most pertinent problems concerning at least all those tumors not amenable to complete surgical resection, is the necessity to define prognostic factors that predict disease progression.

Among pilocytic astrocytomas of the hypothalamic-chiasmatic region and the cerebellum, there may be a subset with a monomorphous pilomyxoid pattern and a less favorable outcome than classical pilocytic astrocytoma.[113] Prospective evaluation of these features and other light-microscopic, immunohistochemical, and cytogenetic and molecular studies might determine a group of tumors that are likely to progress early and possibly develop CNS dissemination.

Most probably, however, defining prognostic subgroups will rely on clinical data as well. Tumor location, extent of disease, resectability, and patient age are prognostically relevant variables in many retrospective studies. Furthermore, progression patterns of optic pathway tumors in children with NF-1 differ markedly from those in other patients.[114] Current studies have to define the population, who needs treatment, and the optimal timing for non-surgical therapy in children with residual tumor.

The proven high efficacy of radiotherapy in terms of tumor control and preservation or improvement of visual or neurologic function demands further developments in treatment techniques in order to reduce the potential detrimental effects on the developing CNS. The recent introduction of stereotactic radiation techniques yielded promising results in improving local treatment while better sparing normal tissue. These techniques are being used increasingly, but the impact on tumor control and visual function and the side effects remain to be established. The new approaches should therefore be part of future investigations.

All series demonstrate that chemotherapy has an effect in the treatment of low-grade glioma. Complete responses to chemotherapy are few, but the frequency of partial responses, minor responses, and stable disease is high, and overall response rates that include stable disease range from 70 to 100 per cent. Yet, the impact of any chemotherapy treatment has to be measured by the proportion of young children in whom radiation is delayed successfully beyond five years or later. An additional aspect is the sparing of radiotherapy in patients with NF-1, who are not only prone to subsequent, often more malignant, brain tumors,[115] but who are also at risk for vasculopathy.[115,116] Many aspects of the use of chemotherapy in low-grade glioma are still defined only poorly. Factors influencing the response to chemotherapy have been age and the presence of NF-1,[22,117] but response to treatment may be modified by other factors as well.

A large number of agents have been applied in the various series, resulting in comparable response rates. It has to be defined whether there are drugs or combinations of superior effectiveness and tolerable acute and late toxicities. Previous studies have lasted for variable lengths of time; most studies were a year long, but they range from a few months to almost two years. A direct comparison is made impossible due to the inherent differences of strategies between studies. Thus, even the optimal duration of therapy remains to be assessed. Further work is needed to correlate chemosensitivity to molecular phenotype. Additionally, novel approaches to therapy have to be investigated, such as targeting tumor angiogenesis.[118]

Due to the small numbers of these tumors even in referral centers, the therapeutic questions have to be addressed in cooperative studies in the future. Adequate management strategies will probably include a combination of treatment interventions, including surgery, radiotherapy, and chemotherapy, throughout a prolonged phase of follow-up.[119] No studies exist that evaluate the impact of the different treatment strategies that have been applied throughout the years upon quality of life for long-term survivors.

As for all other pediatric brain tumors, adequate management of children with low-grade astrocytic tumors requires a dedicated multidisciplinary team,[120] where the necessity of care for extended periods of time, adjusted to the dynamics of the tumor, is acknowledged.

REFERENCES

1   Berger M, Deliganis A, Dobbins J, Keles G. The effect of extent of resection on recurrence in patients with low grade cerebral hemispheric gliomas. *Cancer* 1994; **74**:1784–91.

2   Gajjar A, Sanford R, Heideman R, *et al*. Low-grade astrocytoma: a decade of experience at St Jude Children's Research Hospital. *J Clin Oncol* 1997; **15**:2792–9.

3   Hirsch J-F, Rose C, Pierre-Kah A, Pfister A, Hoppe-Hirsch E. Benign astrocytic and oligodendrocytic tumors of the cerebral hemispheres in children. *J Neurosurg* 1989; **70**:568–72.

4   Pollack I, Claassen D, Al-Shboul Q, Janosky J, Deutsch M. Low-grade gliomas of the cerebral hemispheres in children: an analysis of 71 cases. *J Neurosurg* 1995; **82**:536–47.

5   Wallner K, Gonzales M, Edwards M, Wara W, Sheline G. Treatment results of juvenile pilocytic astrocytoma. *J Neurosurg* 1988; **69**:171–6.

6   West C, Gattamaneni R, Blair V. Radiotherapy in the treatment of low grade astrocytomas I. A survival analysis. *Childs Nerv Syst* 1995; **11**:438–42.

7   Dhodapkar K, Wisoff J, Sanford R, Holmes E, Sposto R, Finlay J. Patterns of relapse and survival for newly-diagnosed childhood low grade astrocytoma: Initial results of CCG9891/POG9130. *Med Pediatr Oncol* 1999; **33**:205.

8   Forsyth P, Shaw E, Scheithauer B, O'Fallon J, Layton DJ, Katzman J. Supratentorial pilocytic astrocytomas. A clinicopathologic, prognostic and flow cytometric study of 51 patients. *Cancer* 1993; **72**:1335–42.

9   Kortmann R, Timmermann B, Becker G, Kuehl J, Bamberg M. Advances in treatment techniques and time/dose schedules in external radiation therapy of brain tumors in childhood. *Klin Pediatr* 1998; **210**:220–6.

10 Kortmann R, Becker G, Perelmouter J, Buchgeister M, Meisner C, Bamberg M. Geometric accuracy of field alignment in fractionated stereotactic conformal radiotherapy of brain tumors. *Int J Radiat Oncol Biol Phys* 1999; **43**:921–6.

11 Mansur D, Hekmatpanah J, Wollman R, *et al*. Low grade gliomas treated with adjuvant radiation therapy in the modern imaging era. *Am J Clin Oncol* 2000; **23**:222–6.

12 Jeremic B, Shibamotu Y, Grujicic D, *et al*. Hyperfractionated radiation therapy for completely resected supratentorial

low-grade glioma. A phase II study. *Radiother Oncol* 1998; **49**:49–54.

13 Dunbar S, Tarbell N, Kooy H, *et al.* Stereotactic radiotherapy for pediatric and adult brain tumors: preliminary report. *Int J Radiat Oncol Biol Phys* 1994; **30**:531–9.

14 Grabb P, Lunsford L, Albright A, Kondziolka D, Flickinger J. Stereotactic radiosurgery for glial neoplasms of childhood. *Neurosurgery* 1996; **38**:696–702.

15 Somaza S, Kondziolka D, Lunsford L, Flickinger J, Bissonette D, Albright A. Early outcomes after stereotactic radiosurgery for growing pilocytic astrocytomas in children. *Pediatr Neurosurg* 1996; **25**:109–15.

16 Voges J, Sturm V, Berthold F, Pastyr O, Schlegel W, Lorenz W. Interstitial irradiation of cerebral gliomas in childhood by permanently implanted 125-iodine – preliminary results. *Klin Pediatr* 1990; **2020**:270–4.

17 Schaetz C, Kreth F, Faist M, Warnke P, Volk B, Ostertag C. Interstitial 125-iodine radiosurgery of low-grade gliomas of the insula of Reil. *Acta Neurochir* 1994; **130**:80–9.

18 Fisher B, Bauman G, Leighton C, Stitt L, Cairncross J, Macdonald D. Low-grade gliomas in children: tumor volume response to radiation. *J Neurosurg* 1998; **88**:969–74.

19 Castello M, Schiavetti A, Varrasso G, Clerico A, Capelli C. Chemotherapy in low-grade astrocytoma management. *Childs Nerv Syst* 1998; **14**:6–9.

20 Friedman H, Krischer J, Burger P, *et al.* Treatment of children with progressive or recurrent brain tumors with carboplatin or iproplatin: a Pediatric Oncology Group randomized phase II study. *J Clin Oncol* 1992; **10**:249–56.

21 Packer R, Lange B, Ater J, *et al.* Carboplatin and vincristine for progressive low-grade gliomas of childhood. *J Clin Oncol* 1993; **11**:850–7.

22 Packer R, Ater J, Allen J, *et al.* Carboplatin and vincristine chemotherapy for children with newly diagnosed progressive low-grade gliomas. *J Neurosurg* 1997; **86**:747–54.

23 Pons M, Finlay J, Walker R, Puccetti D, Packer R, McElwain M. Chemotherapy with vincristine and etoposide in children with low-grade astrocytoma. *J Neuro-Oncol* 1992; **14**:151–8.

24 Sumer T, Freeman A, Cohen M, Bremer A, Thomas P, Sinks L. Chemotherapy in recurrent non-cystic low grade astrocytomas of the cerebrum in children. *J Surg Oncol* 1978; **10**:45–54.

25 Brown M, Friedman H, Oakes J, Boyko O, Hockenberger B, Schold S. Chemotherapy for pilocytic astrocytoma. *Cancer* 1993; **71**:3165–72.

26 Chang S, Fryberger S, Crouse V, Tilford D, Prados M. Carboplatin hypersensitivity in children. *Cancer* 1995; **75**:1171–5.

27 Strojan P, Petric-Grabnar G, Zupancic N, Jereb B. Concomitant chemo-radiotherapy for incompletely resected supratentorial low-grade astrocytoma in children: preliminary report. *Med Pediatr Oncol* 1999; **32**:112–16.

28 Eggers H, Jokobiec F, Jones I. Optic nerve gliomas. In: Duane T, Jaeger E (eds). *Clinical Ophthalmology.* New York: Harper & Row, 1985, pp. 1–17.

29 Hoyt W, Baghdassarian S. Optic glioma of childhood. Natural history and rationale for conservative management. *Br J Ophthalmol* 1969; **53**:793–8.

30 Listernick R, Darling C, Greenwald M, Strauss L, Charrow J. Optic pathway tumors in children: the effect of neurofibromatosis type 1 on clinical manifestations and natural history. *J Pediatr* 1995; **127**:718–22.

31 Listernick R, Charrow J, Greenwald M, Mets M. Natural history of optic pathway tumors in children with neurofibromatosis type 1: a longitudinal study. *J Pediatr* 1994; **25**:63–6.

32 Sutton L, Molloy P, Sernyak H, *et al.* Long-term outcome of hypothalamic/chiasmatic astrocytomas in children treated with conservative surgery. *J Neurosurg* 1995; **83**:583–9.

33 Chutorian A, Schwartz J, Evans R, Carter S. Optic gliomas in children. *Neurology* 1964; **14**:83–95.

34 Danoff B, Kramer S, Thompson N. The radiotherapeutic management of optic gliomas of children. *Int J Radiat Oncol Biol Phys* 1980; **6**:45–50.

35 Wisoff J, Abbott R, Epstein F. Surgical management of exophytic chiasmatic-hypothalamic tumors of childhood. *J Neurosurg* 1990; **73**:661–7.

36 Montgomery A, Griffin T, Parker R, Gerdes A. Optic nerve glioma: the role of radiation therapy. *Cancer* 1977; **40**:2079–80.

37 Rush J, Young B, Campbell R, MacCarthy C. Optic glioma, long-term follow-up of 85 histopathologically verified cases. *Ophthalmology* 1982; **89**:1213–19.

38 Bataini J, Delanian S, Ponvert D. Chiasmal gliomas: results of irradiation management in 57 patients and review of the literature. *Int J Radiat Oncol Biol Phys* 1991; **21**:615–23.

39 Kovalic J, Grigsby P, Shepard M, Fineberg B, Thomas P. Radiation therapy for gliomas of the optic nerve and chiasm. *Int J Radiat Oncol Biol Phys* 1990; **18**:927–32.

40 Jenkin D, Angyalfi S, Becker L, *et al.* Optic glioma in children: surveillance, resection or irradiation? *Int J Radiat Oncol Biol Phys* 1993; **25**:215–25.

41 Dutton J. Gliomas of the anterior visual pathway. *Surv Ophthalmol* 1994; **38**:427–52.

42 Packer R, Sutton L, Bilaniuk L, *et al.* Treatment of chiasmatic/ hypothalamic gliomas of childhood with chemotherapy: an update. *Ann Neurol* 1988; **23**:79–85.

43 Prados M, Edwards M, Rabbitt J, Lamborn K, Davis R, Levin V. Treatment of pediatric low-grade gliomas with a nitrosourea-based multiagent chemotherapy regimen. *J Neuro-Oncol* 1997; **32**:235–41.

44 Allen J. Initial management of children with hypothalamic and thalamic tumors and the modifying role of neurofibromatosis-1. *Paediatr Neurosurg* 2000; **32**:154–62.

45 Reardon D, Gajjar A, Sandford R, *et al.* Bithalamic involvement predicts poor outcome among children with thalamic glial tumors. *Pediatr Neurosurg* 1998; **29**:29–35.

46 Epstein F, McCleary E. Intrinsic brain stem tumors of childhood: surgical indications. *J Neurosurg* 1986; **64**:11–14.

47 Stroink A, Hoffman J, Hendrick E, Humphreys R, Davidson G. Transependymal benign dorsally exophytic brain stem gliomas in childhood: diagnosis and treatment recommendations. *Neurosurgery* 1987; **20**:439–44.

48 Edwards M, Wara W, Ciricillo S, Barkovich A. Focal brain stem astrocytomas causing symptoms of involvement of the facial nerve nucleus: long-term survival in six pediatric cases. *J Neurosurg* 1994; **80**:20–5.

49 Coffey R, Lunsford L. Stereotactic surgery for mass lesions of the mid-brain and pons. *Neurosurgery* 1985; **17**:12–18.

50 Pollack I, Pang D, Albright A. The long term outcome in children with late onset aqueductal stenosis resulting from benign intrinsic tectal tumors. *J Neurosurg* 1994; **80**:20–5.

51 Robertson P, Muraszko K, Brunberg J, Axtell R, Dauser R, Turrisi A. Pediatric mid-brain tumors: a benign sub-group

of brain stem gliomas. *Paediatr Neurosurg* 1995; **22**:65–73.

52 Pollack I, Shultz B, Mulvihill J. The management of brain stem gliomas in patients with neurofibromatosis 1. *Neurology* 1996; **46**:1652–60.

53 Milstein J, Geyer J, Berger M, Bleyer W. Favorable prognosis for brain stem gliomas in neurofibromatosis. *J Neuro-Oncol* 1989; **7**:367–71.

54 Abdollahzadeh M, Hoffman H, Blazer S, *et al*. Benign cerebellar astrocytoma in childhood: experience at the Hospital for Sick Children 1980–1992. *Childs Nerv Syst* 1994; **10**:380–3.

55 Pollack I. The role of surgery in pediatric gliomas. *J Neuro-Oncol* 1999; **42**:271–88.

56 Rollins N, Shapiro K. The use of early post-operative MR in detecting residual juvenile cerebellar pilocytic astrocytoma. *Am J Neuroradiol* 1998; **19**:151–6.

57 Dirven C, Mooij J, Molenaar W. Cerebellar pilocytic astrocytoma: a treatment protocol based upon analysis of 73 cases and review of the literature. *Childs Nerv Syst* 1997; **13**:17–23.

58 Smoots D, Geyer J, Lieberman D, Berger M. Predicting disease progression in childhood cerebellar astrocytoma. *Childs Nerv Syst* 1998; **14**:636–48.

59 Garcia D, Latifi H, Simpson J, Picker S. Astrocytomas of the cerebellum in children. *J Neurosurg* 1989; **71**:661–4.

60 Gjerris F, Klinken L. Long term prognosis in children with benign cerebellar astrocytoma. *J Neurosurg* 1978; **49**: 179–84.

61 Griffin T, Beaufait D, Blasko J. Cystic cerebellar astrocytomas in childhood. *Cancer* 1979; **44**:276–80.

62 Hayostek C, Shaw E, Scheithauer B, *et al*. Astrocytomas of the cerebellum: a comparative clinicopathologic study of pilocytic and diffuse astrocytomas. *Cancer* 1993; **72**:856–69.

63 Garcia D, Marks J, Latifi H, Klieforth A. Childhood cerebellar astrocytomas: is there a role for post-operative irradiation? *Int J Radiat Oncol Biol Phys* 1990; **18**:815–18.

64 Pencalet P, Maixner W, Sainte-Rose C, *et al*. Benign cerebellar astrocytomas in children. *J Neurosurg* 1999; **90**:265–73.

65 Schneider J, Raffel C, McComb J. Benign cerebellar astrocytomas of childhood. *Neurosurgery* 1992; **30**:58–93.

66 Austin E, Alvord E. Recurrences of cerebellar astrocytomas: a violation of Collins' law. *J Neurosurg* 1988; **68**:41–7.

67 Sutton L, Cnaan A, Klatt L, *et al*. Post-operative surveillance imaging in children with cerebellar astrocytoma. *J Neurosurg* 1996; **84**:721–5.

68 Brown W, Tavare C, Sobel E, Gilles F. The applicability of Collin's law to childhood brain tumors and its usefulness as a predictor of survival. *Neurosurgery* 1995; **36**:1093–6.

69 Campbell J, Pollack I. Cerebellar astrocytomas in children. *J Neuro-Oncol* 1996; **28**:223–31.

70 Civitello L, Packer R, Rorke L, Siegel K, Sutton L, Schut L. Leptomeningeal dissemination of low grade gliomas in children. *Neurology* 1988; **38**:562–6.

71 Mamelak A, Prados M, Obana W, Cogan P, Edwards M. Treatment options and prognosis for multicentric juvenile pilocytic astrocytoma. *J Neurosurg* 1994; **81**:24–30.

72 Mishima K, Nakamura M, Nakamura H, Nakamura O, Funata N, Shitara N. Leptomeningeal dissemination of cerebellar pilocytic astrocytoma. *J Neurosurg* 1992; **77**:788–91.

73 Pollack I, Hurtt M, Pang D, Albright A. Dissemination of low grade intracranial astrocytomas in children. *Cancer* 1994; **73**:2869–78.

74 Tamura M, Zama A, Kurihara H, *et al*. Management of recurrent pilocytic astrocytoma with leptomeningeal dissemination in childhood. *Childs Nerv Syst* 1998; **14**: 617–22.

75 Ammirati M, Mizai S, Samii M. Transient mutism following removal of a cerebellar tumor. *Childs Nerv Syst* 1989; **5**:12–14.

76 Pollack J, Polinko P, Pang D, Albright A, Towbin R, Fitz C. Mutism and pseudobulbar symptoms after resection of posterior fossa tumors in children: incidence and pathophysiology. *Neurosurgery* 1995; **37**:885–93.

77 Wisoff J, Epstein F. Pseudobulbar palsy after posterior fossa operation in children. *Neurosurgery* 1984; **15**:707–9.

78 Undijan S, Marinov M, Georgiev K. Long-term follow-up after surgical treatment of cerebellar astrocytomas in 100 children. *Childs Nerv Syst* 1989; **5**:99–101.

79 Bouffet E, Amat D, Devaux Y, Desuzinges C. Chemotherapy for spinal cord astrocytoma. *Med Pediatr Oncol* 1997; **29**:560–2.

80 Doireau V, Grill J, Zerah M, *et al*. Chemotherapy for unresectable and recurrent intramedullary glial tumors in children. Brain Tumors Sub-committee of the French Society of Pediatric Oncology (SFOP). *B J Cancer* 1999; **81**:835–40.

81 Epstein F, Epstein N. Surgical treatment of spinal cord astrocytomas of childhood. A series of 19 patients. *J Neurosurg* 1982; **57**:685–9.

82 Epstein F. Spinal cord tumors in children. *J Neurosurg* 1995; **82**:516–17.

83 Minehan K, Shaw E, Scheithauer B, Davis D, Onofrio B. Spinal cord astrocytoma: pathological and treatment considerations. *J Neurosurg* 1995; **83**:590–5.

84 O'Sullivan C, Jenkin D, Doherty M, Hoffman H, Greenberg M. Spinal cord tumors in children: long-term results of combined surgical and radiation treatment. *J Neurosurg* 1994; **81**:507–12.

85 Constantini S, Epstein F. Intraspinal tumors in children and infants. In: Youmans J, Becker D, Dunsker C (eds). *Neurosurgical Surgery*, 4th ed. Philadelphia: WB Saunders, 1996, pp. 3123–33.

86 Epstein F, Constantini S. Spinal cord tumors of childhood. In: Pang D (ed.). *Disorders of the Pediatric Spine*. New York: Raven Press, 1995, pp. 55–76.

87 Cohen A, Wisoff J, Allen J, Epstein F. Malignant astrocytomas of the spinal cord. *J Neurosurg* 1989; **70**:50–4.

88 Nishio S, Morioka T, Fujii K, Inamura T, Fukui M. Spinal cord gliomas: management and outcome with reference to adjuvant therapy. *J Clin Neurosci* 2000; **7**:20–3.

89 Constantini S, Miller D, Allen J, Rorke L, Freed D, Epstein F. Pediatric intramedullary spinal cord tumors: surgical morbidity and long-term follow-up. *Childs Nerv Syst* 1998; **14**:484.

90 Fort D, Packer R, Kirkpatrick G, Kuttesch JJ, Ater J. Carboplatin and vincristine for pediatric primary spinal cord astrocytomas. *Childs Nerv Syst* 1998; **14**:484.

91 Bouffet E, Pierre-Kahn A, Marchal J, *et al*. Prognostic factors in pediatric spinal cord astrocytoma. *Cancer* 1998; **83**:2391–9.

92 Constantini S, Miller D, Allen J, Rorke L, Freed D, Epstein F. Radical excision of intramedullary spinal cord

tumors: surgical morbidity and long-term follow-up evaluation in 164 children and young adults. *J Neurosurg* 2000; **93**:183–93.

93   Linstadt D, Wara W, Leibel S, Gutin P, Wilson C, Sheline G. Post-operative radiotherapy of primary spinal cord tumors. *Int J Radiat Oncol Biol Phys* 1989; **16**:1397–403.

94   Przybylski G, Albright A, Martinez A. Spinal cord astrocytomas: long-term results comparing treatments in children. *Childs Nerv Syst* 1997; **13**:375–82.

95   Hardison H, Packer R, Rorke L, Schut L, Sutton L, Bruce D. Outcome of children with primary intramedullary spinal cord tumors. *Childs Nerv Syst* 1987; **3**:89–92.

96   Jyothirmayi R, Madhavan J, Nair M, Rajan B. Conservative surgery and radiotherapy in the treatment of spinal cord astrocytoma. *J Neuro-Oncol* 1997; **33**:205–11.

97   Bamberg M, Hess C, Kortmann R. Zentralnervensystem. In: Scherer E, Sack H (eds). *Strahlentherapie/Radiologische Onkologie*, 4th ed. Heidelberg: Springer-Verlag, 1998, pp. 763–808.

98   McCunniff A, Liang M. Radiation tolerance of the cervical spinal cord. *Int J Radiat Oncol Biol Phys* 1989; **16**:675–8.

99   Marcus RJ, Million R. The incidence of myelitis after irradiation of the cervical spinal cord. *Int J Radiat Oncol Biol Phys* 1990; **19**:3–8.

100 Doireau V, Grill J, Chastagner P, *et al.* Chemotherapy for intramedullary glial tumors. *Childs Nerv Syst* 1998; **14**:484–5.

101 Lowis S, Pizer B, Coakham H, Nelson R, Bouffet E. Chemotherapy for spinal cord astrocytoma: can natural history be modified? *Childs Nerv Syst* 1998; **14**:317–21.

102 Foreman N, Hay T, Handler M. Chemotherapy for spinal cord astrocytoma. *Med Pediatr Oncol* 1998; **30**:311–12.

103 Gajjar A, Bhargava R, Jenkins J, *et al.* Low-grade astrocytoma with neuroaxis dissemination at diagnosis. *J Neurosurg* 1995; **83**:67–71.

104 Perilongo G, Carollo C, Salviati L, *et al.* Diencephalic syndrome and disseminated juvenile pilocytic astrocytomas of the hypothalamic-optic chiasm region. *Cancer* 1997; **80**:142–6.

105 Berger M, Baumeister B, Geyer J, Milstein J, Kanev P, LeRoux P. The risks of metastases from shunting in children with primary central nervous system tumors. *J Neurosurg* 1991; **74**:872–7.

106 Trigg M, Swanson J, Letellier M. Metastasis of an optic glioma through a ventricular peritoneal shunt. *Cancer* 1983; **52**:599–601.

107 Russell D, Rubinstein L. *Pathology of Tumors of the Nervous System*. Baltimore: Williams & Wilkins, 1989.

108 Braun-Fischer A, Romeike B, Eymann R, Glas B, Riesinger P, Reiche W. Pilozytisches astrocytom mit subarachnoidaler dissemination. *Radiologe* 1997; **37**:899–904.

109 Lesage F, Grill J, Cinalli G, Lellouch-Tubiana A, Cuanet, Kalifa C. Metastatic low-grade glioma in 16 children: presentation, treatment and outcome. *Childs Nerv Syst* 1998; **14**:483.

110 McCowage G, Tien R, McLendon R, *et al.* Successful treatment of childhood pilocytic astrocytomas metastatic to the leptomeninges with high-dose cyclophosphamide. *Med Pediatr Oncol* 1996; **27**:32–9.

111 Akar Z, Tanriover N, Kafadar A, Gazioglu N, Oz B, Kuday C. Chiasmatic low-grade glioma presenting with sacral intradural spinal metastases. *Childs Nerv Syst* 2000; **16**:309–11.

112 Berger M. The impact of technical adjuncts in the surgical management of cerebral hemispheric low-grade gliomas of childhood. *J Neuro-Oncol* 1996; **28**:129–55.

113 Tihan T, Fisher P, Kepner J, *et al.* Pediatric astrocytomas with monomorphous pilomyxoid features and a less favourable outcome. *J Neuropathol Exp Neurol* 1999; **58**:1061–8.

114 Grill J, Laithier V, Rodriguez D, Raquin M, Pierre-Kahn A, Kalifa C. When do children with optic pathway tumors need treatment? An oncological perspective in 106 patients treated in a single centre. *Eur J Pediatr* 2000; **159**:692–6.

115 Friedman J, Birch P. An association between optic glioma and other tumors of the central nervous system in neurofibromatosis type I. *Neuropediatrics* 1997; **28**:131–2.

116 Grill J, Couanet D, Capelli C, *et al.* Radiation induced cerebral vasculopathy in children with neurofibromatosis and optic pathway glioma. *Ann Neurol* 1999; **45**:393–6.

117 Laithier V, Raquin M, Couanet D, *et al.* Chemotherapy for children with optic pathway glioma: results of a prospective study by the French Society of Pediatric Oncology (SFOP). *Med Pediatr Oncol* 2000; **35**:190.

118 Wolff J, Egeler R. Investigational approaches to the treatment of brain tumors in children. *Med Pediatr Oncol* 1999; **32**:135–8.

119 Reddy A, Packer R. Chemotherapy for low grade gliomas. *Childs Nerv Syst* 1999; **15**:506–13.

120 Packer R. An overview of pediatric oncology as a model for interdisciplinary care. *Childs Nerv Syst* 1995; **11**:13–16.

121 Taveras J, Lester A, Wood E. The value of radiation therapy in the management of glioma of the optic nerves and chiasma. *Radiology* 1956; **66**:518–28.

122 Dosoretz D, Blitzer P, Wang C, Linggood R. Management of glioma of the optic nerve and/or chiasm: an analysis of 20 cases. *Cancer* 1980; **45**:1467–71.

123 Kalifa C, Ernest C, Rodary C, *et al.* Optic glioma in children. A retrospective study of 57 cases treated by irradiation (authors' translation). *Arch Fr Pediatr* 1981; **38**:309–13.

124 Horwich A, Bloom H. Optic gliomas: radiation therapy and prognosis. *Int J Radiat Oncol Biol Phys* 1985; **11**:1067–79.

125 Weiss L, Sagerman R, King G, Chung C, Dubowy R. Controversy in the management of optic nerve glioma. *Cancer* 1987; **59**:1000–4.

126 Flickinger J, Torres C, Deutsch M. Management of low grade gliomas of the optic nerve and chiasm. *Cancer* 1988; **61**:635–42.

127 Wong J, Uhl V, Wara W, Sheline G. Optic gliomas. A re-analysis of the University of California, San Francisco, experience. *Cancer* 1987; **60**:1847–55.

128 Pierce S, Barnes P, Loeffler J, McGinn C, Tarbell N. Definitive radiation therapy in the management of symptomatic patients with optic glioma. *Cancer* 1990; **65**:45–52.

129 Rodriguez L, Edwards M, Levin V. Management of hypothalamic gliomas in children: an analysis of 33 cases. *Neurosurgery* 1990; **26**:242–6.

130 Erkal H, Serin M, Cakmak A. Management of optic pathway and chiasmatic-hypothalamic gliomas in children: tumor volume response to radiation therapy. *Radiother Oncol* 1997; **45**:11–15.

131 Grabenbauer G, Schuchardt U, Buchfelder M, *et al.* Radiation therapy of optico-hypothalamic gliomas

(OHG) – radiographic response, vision and toxicity. *Radiother Oncol* 2000; **54**:239–45.

132 Harris J, Levene M. Visual complications following irradiation for pituitary adenomas and craniopharyngiomas. *Radiology* 1976; **120**:167–71.

133 Aristizabal S, Caldwell W, Avila J. The relationship of time-dose fractionation factors to complications in the treatment of pituitary tumors by irradiation. *Int J Radiat Oncol Biol Phys* 1977; **10**:667–73.

134 Atkinson A, Allen I, Gordon D, *et al.* Progressive visual failure in acromegaly following external pituitary irradiation. *Clin Endocrinol (Oxf)* 1979; **10**:469–79.

135 Kocks W, Kalff R, Reinhardt V, Grote W, Hilke J. Spinal metastasis of pilocytic astrocytoma of the chiasma opticum. *Childs Nerv Syst* 1989; **5**:118–20.

136 Obana W, Cogan P, Davis R, Edwards M. Metastatic juvenile pilocytic astrocytoma. *J Neurosurg* 1991; **75**:972–5.

137 Rutka J, George R, Davidson G, Hoffmann H. Low-grade astrocytoma of the tectal region as an unusual cause of knee pain: case report. *Neurosurgery* 1991; **29**:608–12.

138 McCowage G, Longee D, Fuchs H, Friedman H. Treatment of high-grade gliomas and metastatic pilocytic astrocytomas with high-dose cyclophosphamide. *Annual Meeting of the American Society of Clinical Oncologists* 1995; A290.

14

Astrocytic tumors, high-grade

JOHANNES E. A. WOLFF AND PASCAL CHASTAGNER

INTRODUCTION

High-grade gliomas (HGGs) are the most frequent malignant brain tumors in adults, but they are very rare in children. Patients become symptomatic with headaches, nausea, or vomiting, or present with focal neurological signs such as hemiplegia. The clinical situation deteriorates rapidly. A computed tomography (CT) or magnetic resonance imaging (MRI) scan will show the brain tumor, which is typically inhomogeneously contrast-enhancing. The final diagnosis is made by histology, which requires at least a biopsy as the surgical procedure. The treatment includes maximal possible surgery, irradiation, and chemotherapy. This standard approach can cure a few patients, but the general prognosis remains poor. Most tumors relapse within one or two years. HGG is therefore a major subject for medical research, including experimental treatments. This chapter will elucidate in more detail the classification, tumor biology, standard clinical management, and some of the experimental approaches.

CLASSIFICATION

HGGs comprise a group of tumors characterized by histological features of glial origin and of high malignancy, a grim prognosis, and lack of therapeutic improvement. The classification of HGG is based upon histological morphological criteria,[1] which have a high relevance for prognosis. In this definition, the term "high-grade glioma" summarizes a number of different entities. As classifications change, the number of diagnoses included in the group of HGG varies (Table 14.1).

The International Classification of Diseases – Oncology (ICD-O) classification is due to be modified soon, since, for instance, glioblastoma with sarcomatous component and gliosarcoma are no longer considered two different entities.

Table 14.1 *Histological diagnoses combined in the term "malignant glioma"*

Tumor	WHO grade	ICD-O	ICD-10
Glioblastoma multiforme	IV	M9440/3	C71.9
Giant-cell glioblastoma	IV	M9441/3	C71.9
Glioblastoma with sarcomatous component	IV	M9440/3	C71.9
Anaplastic astrocytoma	III	M9401/3	C71.9
Malignant glioma	not defined	M9380/3	C71.9
Anaplastic oligodendroglioma	III	M9451/3	C71.9
Malignant oligoastrocytoma	III	M9382/3	C71.9
Gliomatosis cerebri	III	M9381/3	C71.9
Gliosarcoma	IV	M9442/3	C71.9

ICD-10, International Classification of Diseases 10; ICD-O, International Classification of Diseases – Oncology; WHO, World Health Organization.

TUMOR BIOLOGY

Inherited defects in the regulation of cell proliferation and cell death, such as neurofibromatosis type 1 (NF-I) and Li–Fraumeni syndrome, can participate in glioma development. In addition, a number of external influences have been alleged to cause gliomas. Among these are viruses such as simian virus 40 and Jamestown Canyon (JC) virus,[2] chemicals, and irradiation. A few clinical cases, such as glioblastoma developing in a radiation field after therapeutic irradiation, confirm this method of glioma development. However, most gliomas in children appear to develop de novo without known external reason. Different from the primary or de novo glioblastomas that occur in older patients and exhibit epidermal growth factor receptor (EGFR) amplification or overexpression, HGGs occurring in children often belong to the family of secondary glioblastomas, which develop from pre-existing low-grade astrocytomas. These tumors have a more protracted clinical course, and frequently contain *p53* mutations and allelic loss of *17p*. Both types of tumor show deletions of chromosome 10 and possibly inactivating mutations of the *PTEN/MMAC1* gene as well as inactivation of the *p16* and *Rb* genes and overexpression of the *CDK4*, *EGFR*, and *VEGF* genes as an end-stage event.[3] The oligodendroglial phenotype has genetic abnormalities distinct from those of the astrocytic tumors: it is highly associated with loss of 1p ($P = 0.0002$), loss of 19q ($P < 0.0001$), and combined loss of 1p and 19q ($P < 0.0001$).[4] While the genetic alterations develop, the phenotype becomes more malignant. HGG cells produce cytokines that increase angiogenesis, such as vascular endothelial growth factor (VEGF) and scatter factor/ hepatocyte growth factor (SF/HGF),[5] modulate immune response,[6] and result in autocrine stimulation of glioma cell proliferation/invasion or inhibition of apoptotic cell death. The migration occurs predominantly along white-matter tracks. Heightened commitment to migrate and invade is accompanied by a glioma cell's reduced proliferative activity.[7] Once this commitment changes, the migrated cells can give rise to a second tumor far away from the primary lesion. Despite a high capacity to migrate, HGGs metastasize via the blood only very rarely. End-stage metastases may occur via the cerebrospinal fluid (CSF).

INCIDENCE AND LOCATION

HGGs are the most frequent brain tumors in adults, but they account for only 15 per cent of all central nervous system (CNS) tumors in children. The German population-based registry reports 0.13 cases per 100 000 people under the age of 15 years. This figure does not include brainstem glioma without biopsy, so the actual incidence might be significantly higher. HGG may occur at any age, including in newborn infants (some cases have been detected in utero by systematic ultrasound sonography during pregnancy). However, they are extremely rare in young children and the incidence increases with age until the sixth decade of life. In the pediatric population, the median age of HGG patients is nine years. The male/female ratio is about 1.2. In contrast to most other pediatric brain tumors, the tumor location of HGG is most frequently supratentorial. One-third to one-half are located in the cerebral hemispheres, the remainder being located in the deep midline structures of the diencephalon (thalamus, hypothalamus, third ventricle) and basal ganglia (half of those originating in the basal ganglia, the other half in the cerebral cortex or the superficial white matter). Infratentorial tumors are frequently located in the brainstem. Many are not biopsied and therefore are classified as brainstem glioma without histology. Cerebellar and spinal cord locations are rare.

SYMPTOMS AND SIGNS

First symptoms and signs of brain tumors depend more on the location and the age of the patient than on histology. Duration of symptoms before obtaining a diagnosis may vary from a few weeks to several years. Patients who harbor midline cerebellar tumors may have a shorter duration of symptoms. Infants and younger children also tend to have a brief history in comparison with older children. In one series, the mean time to diagnosis was as high as 43.4 weeks for supratentorial tumors, while it was 10.8 weeks for infratentorial locations.[8] Supratentorial HGGs frequently present with headaches, seizures, and hemiplegia. Seizures, which are observed in as many as one-third of these patients, are more frequent in patients harboring slowly evolving low-grade gliomas. Focal motor deficits and pyramidal tract findings may be observed in up to 40 per cent of patients with hemispheric and central tumors. Basal ganglia tumors may be diagnosed according to dysmetria and chorea. Posterior fossa tumors present with recurrent bouts of headache, nausea, or vomiting without focal deficits, except in the case of brainstem location. These symptoms suggest the presence of increased intracranial pressure related to the obstruction of the cerebral ventricles by the tumor, producing hydrocephalus.

The family history may exhibit one of the following: NF-1, neurofibromatosis type 2 (NF-2), Li–Fraumeni syndrome (breast carcinoma, sarcomas, brain tumors), Gorlin syndrome (multiple basal-cell carcinoma and other carcinoma), Turcot syndrome (inherited intestinal polyposis, brain tumors), Taybi–Rubinstein syndrome (short stature, mental retardation, dysmorphic features), Lindau syndrome (ocular angiomatosis), Bloom syndrome (short stature, teleangiectasia). However, if the diagnosis of a brain tumor in a child is suspected on

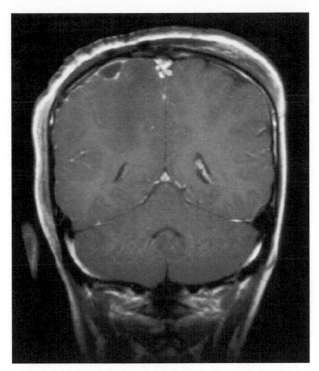

Figure 14.1 *A seven-year-old girl presented with headache, nausea, and focal seizures. The family history was significant, with a high incidence of malignant diseases in the family of the mother. Magnetic resonance imaging (MRI) showed a contrast-enhancing cortical lesion with significant perifocal edema. The lesion was completely resected and turned out to be a glioblastoma multiforme (World Health Organization grade IV). A p53 germ-line mutation was found in the family of the mother. Six months after diagnosis, the child is still being treated with intensive chemotherapy; there is no evidence of disease on repeated MRI scans.*

symptoms and signs or family history, then the definitive diagnosis is made by MRI (Figure 14.1).

DIAGNOSTIC IMAGING

Magnetic resonance tomography (MRT) is the most important diagnostic procedure for a child with a suspected brain tumor. It should not be delayed by other diagnostic procedures.

The MRI appearance of malignant glioma is an inhomogeneous space-occupying lesion localized in the cerebral cortex or in the basal ganglia with significant oedema and diffuse margins. Hemorrhagic and cystic areas are possible, but calcifications are rare. Contrast-enhancement is inhomogeneous but mostly high in at least some parts of the tumor. HGG may develop in a pre-existing diffuse low-grade glioma that is being watched with repetitive neuroimaging. Unfortunately, none of these characteristics is unique to HGG. The precise diagnosis of a pediatric HGG requires histological confirmation.

In addition to the primary diagnosis, MRI is required after each tumor surgery, since further treatment planning crucially depends on the neuroradiological evaluation of residual tumor. There is a small window of opportunity for this image. The first 24 hours after surgery seem to show more postoperative affects. The optimal window is 24–72 hours postsurgery.[9] If imaging is done later, then angiogenesis and gliosis can mimic residual tumor. Since these tissues shrink naturally, they can mimic tumor response to further treatment. This process may take up to six weeks after surgery. Images obtained during this period have to be interpreted cautiously. Even after this period, the assessment of tumor response to non-surgical treatment remains difficult in HGG. In clinical studies with adult patients, most frequently only the contrast-enhancing parts of the tumor are used for response criteria.[10] Since not all tumor parts of pediatric HGG are contrast-enhancing, this might not be useful for pediatric phase II studies. However, tumor edema might be reduced by glucocorticoids independently of tumor mass reduction caused by chemotherapy or irradiation, and has to be excluded from tumor response assessment. Most pediatric studies follow the Société Internationale d'Oncologie Pédiatrique (SIOP) criteria for describing tumor status and response.[11]

The investigation of neuraxis is often not done. However, up to ten per cent of spinal metastases have been reported at diagnosis.[12]

MRI spectroscopy and nuclear medicine methods such as thallium-single-photon-emission computed tomography (SPECT), Sestamibi (MIBI)-SPECT, and alpha-methyl-tyrosine-SPECT are of increasing academic importance. Metabolic information correlates with tumor grading and tumor proliferation. However, most of these methods require tumors larger than 2 cm, and they have not been validated in large populations.

SURGERY

According to tumor location, a temporary or permanent CSF diversion, usually by ventriculostomy, may be the first surgical step. This is appropriate for half of the deep tumors but less than ten per cent of hemispheric gliomas. Surgery is not only a therapeutic procedure but also necessary for diagnosis. The optimal extent of surgery differs for each patient. Recent data suggest significant differences between malignant glioma in adults and in pediatric patients with respect to the influence of gross total surgical resection. In adult patients, completeness of surgery is of minor importance for the prognosis. Far more important are age and Karnofsky index. Tumor resections are therefore done cautiously in an attempt to avoid further damage, which might jeopardize the remaining quality of life. While this is obviously an important aim in children as well, the completeness of resection plays a different role for the prognosis in this age group. In children, near-total resection (>90 per cent) is the most important prognostic factor. In the Children's Cancer Group CCG-945 trial, the multivariate analysis demonstrated that near-total tumor resection was the only therapeutic variable that significantly improved progression-free survival rates.[13] Long-term survivors have been described after gross total resection followed by intensive adjuvant treatment.[14] However, near-total tumor resection could be done in about only 40 per cent of cases. In the CCG-945 trial, it could be achieved in 49 per cent of the tumors in the superficial hemisphere and in 45 per cent of tumors in the posterior fossa, compared with only eight per cent of midline tumors.[13] In particular, in supratentorial cortical locations, a complete resection should be attempted in 40–80 per cent of cases. In diencephalic tumors, gross total resection is possible in less than 40 per cent of cases. However, with the availability of new adjuncts for operative planning, such as frameless stereotaxis and functional MRI, and modalities for mapping and monitoring brain function during surgery, many lesions that were once deemed unresectable are more frequently amenable to extensive resection rather than simple biopsy. For these, and for other selected deep-seated tumors for which the risks of open resection may be high, CT- or MRI-guided stereotactic biopsy is recommended. An attempt to resect might be advisable later during the treatment plan in multimodal approaches. The rare cerebellar HGG should be resected as far as possible. Some recommendations must be taken into account for improving the conditions of resection and surgical outcome. Corticosteroids could be administered before surgery to reduce peritumoral edema. Anticonvulsants could be initiated in case of supratentorial tumors to minimize the risk of perioperative seizures. Hormonal dysfunction must be investigated and treated by hormonal replacement for patients with tumors located in and around the hypothalamus. In this case, close monitoring of electrolytes and fluid infusions and volume status are usually required. The actual tumor resection is generally performed by ultrasonic aspiration, which facilitates internal debulking of the tumor.

PATHOLOGY

Objective grading of primary brain tumors in order to accurately reflect clinical behavior remains one of the most difficult problems facing the neuropathologist. It is crucial for treatment planning and academic evaluation in HGGs. Unfortunately, the fast-growing body of literature and various changing histopathological classification systems and schools of thinking make adequate and comparable histopathological diagnosis in childhood malignant glioma rather difficult. Conventional histopathology

with hematoxylin and eosin-stained slides supplemented with special stainings (Nissl for nuclear structure, and reticulin or collagen staining methods) are still the basis for further special methods. Similarly to low-grade glioma, tumor cells show some characteristics of differentiation in astrocytic or oligodendroglial direction. In addition to these, features of malignancy are seen in HGG, including cellular anaplasia, mitotic and apoptotic figures, high cellular density, angiogenesis, and necroses. However, the histological diagnosis does not depend solely on these single pieces of information, depending also on the pattern. The differential diagnosis of other primary brain tumors is supported by immunohistochemical stainings for glial fibrillary acid protein (GFAP), S100-protein, or neuronal and germ-cell markers. For assessment of malignancy, proliferation markers (MIB-1) are recommended. A major contribution to tumor diagnosis and understanding will occur as developments in molecular genetics are applied more directly to diagnostic tumor biopsies.

The need for a central review has been emphasized for gliomas. Of 250 gliomas described and treated as malignant gliomas according to the CCG-945 study, 46 (18.4 per cent) were deemed on central neuropathology review to be low-grade gliomas.[15] In a French pilot study, of 51 gliomas considered as malignant, 12 (24 per cent) were graded as low-grade gliomas after central review (personal communication). The intratumoral histologic heterogeneity of gliomas was described in a quantitative study investigating small and large biopsies punched from 50 unembedded supratentorial gliomas, with 48 per cent differently typed and 82 per cent differently graded samples among two observers who reviewed independently 1000 samples.[16] Therefore, most nations have developed pediatric neuropathology reference centers to support local pathologists or neuropathologists in these rare cases. For clinical studies, neuropathology review has become crucial.

PRINCIPLES OF POSTOPERATIVE TREATMENT

Since many more data regarding these tumors originate from adult patients, treatment principles developed in the adult patient population often influence the treatment of pediatric patients as well. The first finding in adult patients was that irradiation improves survival and quality of life.[17,18] When chemotherapy was added, the choice of drugs was guided by the permeability through the blood–brain barrier. Nitrosurea drugs such as carmustine (BCNU) and lomustine (CCNU) were tested and found to improve survival further.[17,19–22] The next series of controlled studies used irradiation and BCNU or CCNU as the standard arm.[23–26] In the following decade, nitrosoureas were combined with other drugs, and the combination of procarbazine, CCNU, and vincristine (PCV) was favored.[27–29] Most recently, there has been a trend towards the use of temozolomide,[30–36] which is based mainly upon its low toxicity in the recommended dose.[34,37,38] However, the evidence for superior efficacy is so far very limited.[39]

In pediatric patients, some differences have to be considered before using treatment concepts developed in adult patients. One difference is the treatment aim, which is more often curative in children, while a prolongation of remaining lifetime is often not considered a treatment success. The first step after the diagnosis of HGG in a child is therefore to make an informed decision about the main treatment aim. These tumors have a particularly poor prognosis, and most previous approaches have failed to produce a larger number of long-term survivors. Therefore, decisions for palliative care without tumor treatment may be quite reasonable, particularly in cases of non-resectable HGG located in the basal ganglia or the brainstem. Decisions for curative treatment goals as opposed to palliative care depend on individual ethical systems and culture; general recommendations cannot be given. However, if a decision for a curative treatment is made, then a general recommendation is possible: the patient should be enrolled in a modern multicenter treatment study. In those subgroups in which significant cure rates are absent, the treatment of HGGs is experimental in nature. Most curative treatment protocols have used maximal surgery, followed by radiation therapy and chemotherapy. Novel treatment elements may be a part of any of these treatment modalities.

Radiotherapy

It is generally accepted that radiation therapy increases median survival time by a few months for patients with malignant glioma, but the improvement of cure rates remains questionable. This assumption is based not on controlled randomized trials, as required for high-level evidence in modern medicine, but on the historical experience of increased survival times after introducing radiotherapy into the treatment plan, as well as on tumor responses reported frequently in individual cases and in numerous phase II studies. The amount of lower-level evidence supporting this assumption is so overwhelming that starting a phase III study to prove this would be considered unethical. Summarizing the available information, radiation therapy has to be recommended for patients with HGG and who are over three years of age. The standard radiotherapy follows conventional fractionation. This is five single fractions per week with 1.8 Gy (International Commission for Radiation Units (ICRU) 50 reference point) up to a total of 54 Gy (age three to six years) or 59.5 Gy (age seven years or older). The total dose is given over a period of six to seven weeks. The planning target volume typically includes the area of contrast enhancement with a 2-cm margin. The severe and constant adverse effects of ionizing radiation on the developing nervous system and, frequently, hormonal status have prompted physicians to tailor radiotherapy more accurately to the geometry of the tumor (conformal radiotherapy) and, for the youngest children, to defer irradiation by using chemotherapy.

Radiation side effects occurring during treatment are mild. They include headaches, nausea, vomiting, and lethargy. Depending on the treatment volume, brain edema might become a problem during and a few weeks after radiation. More concerning are late sequelae such as leukoencephalopathy and developmental delay without radiological correlate, which may occur months or years after irradiation. The likelihood of leukoencephalopathy depends on the dose, the treatment volume, and the age of the patient, being more prominent in younger children. This is why irradiation is not recommended for patients under three years of age. The second concerning late effect is secondary malignancy developing in the radiation field.[40–43] Experimental modifications of radiation treatments include different fractionation schemes, brachytherapy with I-125 implantation, proton therapy, boron-neutron capture therapy, pion irradiation, photodynamic therapy with porphyrins and visible light, and concurrent radiochemotherapy. Most of those methods have been evaluated in pilot studies for toxicity and should be confirmed in controlled studies to find out whether they are superior to conventional irradiation or other types of treatment. However, because of the small numbers of patients in most studies, this information will take a long time to accumulate. This problem is common to all experimental treatments for pediatric HGG. To some extent, it might be overcome by drawing conclusions from clinical studies with adult patients or for preclinical studies with pediatric tumor cell lines. However, there is still much information to be gained. This would be facilitated if all children with HGG could be enrolled in multicenter studies.

Chemotherapy

The contribution of chemotherapy to cure in HGG is less prominent than in other malignant CNS tumors such as medulloblastoma. However, as limited as it may be, the benefit from chemotherapy for some pediatric patients is well supported by controlled randomized trials (Tables 14.2 and 14.3). Despite these results, none of those protocols is generally recommended, because the benefit they create remains small while most of them cause some degree of harm to quality of life during the treatment.

The first randomized CCG study compared radiotherapy and adjuvant CCNU/vincristine/prednisone with radiotherapy alone. This trial showed the chemotherapy arm to be superior (46 per cent five-year event-free survival versus 18 per cent; $P = 0.026$).[73] These survival rates were not reproduced in the next randomized CCG phase III

Table 14.2 *Details of two armed (controlled) treatment studies in adult patients with newly diagnosed high-grade glioma*

Ref.	Standard arm	Experimental arm	Result
44	RT only	Mithramycin	No difference
17	No treatment	BCNU + RT	Treatment better than no treatment
19	RT only	RT + CCNU	CCNU better
19	RT only	RT + BCNU	No difference
45	RT only	RT + DHG	DHG better
20	RT only	RT + CCNU	CCNU marginally better (NS)
18	No treatment	RT only	RT better than no RT
18	RT only	RT + bleomycin	No difference
46	CCNU	CCNU + Prc	No difference
47	RT only	RT + DBD	RT + DBD marginally better
47	RT + DBD	RT + DBD + CCNU	With CCNU better
21	Mpred	BCNU	BCNU better
21	Mpred	Prc	Prc better
48	RT only	Miso + RT	Miso marginal better
49	Hyperfractionated RT	Hyperfractionated RT + Miso	No difference
50	BCNU	PCV	Tendency: PCV better (NS)
51	RT only	RT + ACNU	ACNU better
51	ACNU	ACNU + tegafur	No difference
52	RT only	RT + Miso	No difference
52	RT only	RT + CCNU	No difference
23	BCNU	BCNU + Miso	No difference
24	BCNU	Prc	No difference
24	BCNU	DTIC	No difference
53	ACNU	ACNU + picibanil	No difference
22	RT only	BCNU	In subgroups: BCNU better
54	RT only	RT + CCNU	No difference
25	CCNU	CCNU + Benzo	No difference
26	Convf RT + BCNU	Hyperfractionated RT + BCNU	No difference
26	BCNU	BCNU + Miso	No difference
55	BCNU	BCNU + Prc	No difference
55	BCNU	BCNU + HU + VM26	No difference
27	BCNU	PCV	PCV better
28	PCV + RT	PCV only	PCV + RT better
56	IA cisplatin subs RT	IA CDDP conc RT	No difference, not feasible
57	IV BCNU	IA BCNU	No difference, toxicity worse with IA BCNU
57	BCNU	BCNU + 5-FU	No difference
58	Convf RT	Hypof RT	Hypof in GBM better, convf in anaplastic astrocytoma better (NS)
59	BCNU	PCNU	No difference, different toxicity profile
60	Hyperfractionated RT + BCNU	Various RT doses	72 Gy best in hyperfractionated RT + BCNU
61	BCNU	AZQ	No difference, less toxicity with AZQ
62	IV PCNU	IA CDDP	IV PCNU marginally better
63	RT only	RT + Mit	No difference, toxicity worse with Mit
63	BCNU	BCNU + 6-MP	No difference
64	Placebo polymer	BCNU polymer	BCNU polymer better
65	BCNU	DBD	No survival difference, toxicity worse with BCNU
29	RT/PCV	RT + BudR/PCV	BudR worse
66	BCNU	PCV	No difference
67	Subs BCNU/CDDP	Conc BCNU/CDDP	No difference in survival, toxicity worse in conc
68	IV ACNU	IA ACNU	No difference
69	RT only	HSV/TK	No difference
70	PCV	PCV + DFMO	No difference
71	RT only	PCV	No difference
72	CCNU	CCNU + IFN-α	No difference, toxicity worse with IFN-α

ACNU, nimustine; AZQ, diaziquone; BCNU, carmustine; Benzo, benzonidazole; BudR, bromodeoxyuridine; CCNU, lomustine; conc, concurrent radiotherapy and chemotherapy; convf, conventionally fractionated; DBD, dibromodulcitol; DFMO, alpha-difluoromethyl ornithine; DHG, dianhydrogalactitol; DTIC, dacarbazine; 5-FU, 5-fluorouracil; GBM, glioblastoma multiforme; HSV/TK, herpes simplex virus/tyrosine kinase; HU, hydroxyurea; hypof, hypofractionated; IA, intra-arterial; IFN-α, interferon alpha; IV, intravenous; Miso, Misonidazole; Mit, mitomycin C; 6-MP, 6-mercaptopurine; Mpred, methylprednisolone; NS, not significant; PCV, procarbazine, CCNU (lomustine), and vincristine; RT, radiotherapy; Prc, procarbazine; subs, subsequential radiotherapy followed by chemotherapy; VM26, teniposide.

Table 14.3 *Details of two armed (controlled) treatment studies in children with high-grade glioma*

Ref.	Group	Standard treatment	Experimental arm	Result
73	CCG	RT only	RT + CCNU/VCR/Pred	Chemotherapy better
74	CCG	CCNU/VCR/Pred	8-in-1*	No difference
Unpublished	POG	BCNU/CDDP	Cyc/VP16	BCNU/CDDP better
75	GPOH	CDDP/CCNU/VCR	HIT-91S	HIT-91S better only after GTR

BCNU, carmustine; CCG, Children's Cancer Group; CCNU, lomustine; CDDP, cisplatin; Cyc, cyclophosphamide; HIT-91S, ifosfamide/VP16 + high-dose methotrexate + cysplatin/cytosine arabinoside; GPOH, Gesellschaft Pädiatrische Onkologie und Hämatologie; GTR, gross total resection; POG, Pediatric Oncology Group; RT, radiotherapy; VCR, vincristine; Pred, prednisone.
*8-in-1: vincristine, hydroxyurea, procarbazine, lomustine, cisplatin, cytosine arabinoside, high-dose methylprednisolone, and either cyclophosphamide or dacarbazine.

trial, which compared the CCNU/vincristine/prednisone regimen with the eight-drugs-in-one-day (8-in-1) regimen, associated with radiotherapy in both arms. The five-year progression-free survival was 26 per cent for the CCNU/vincristine/prednisone group versus 33 per cent ($P = NS$) for the 8-in-1 regimen.[74] A randomized comparison between BCNU/CDDP and cyclophosphamide/VP16 showed superiority of the BCNU/CDDP arm (Paediatric Oncology Group POG-9135: complete + partial response, 16/46 versus 8/48; two-year event-free survival, 29 per cent versus 11 per cent, $P = 0.03$; two-year overall survival 44 per cent versus 32 per cent, $P = 0.021$; personal communication 1999).

The German study group Gesellschaft Pädiatrische Onkologie und Hämatologie (GPOH) started a randomized trial comparing radiation treatment followed by CCNU/CDDP/vincristine with an intensive chemotherapy protocol before radiation therapy.[76] The results were not significant for the total group, but in the subgroup of patients who underwent a gross total resection, the sandwich chemotherapy appeared superior (median overall survival 5.2 years versus 1.3 years, $P = 0.015$).[75] Subsequently, a prospective cohort comparison study was initiated, including a series of one-armed treatment protocols.[77] In these data, a significant decrease of early progressive disease was observed for patients treated simultaneously with intensive chemotherapy and irradiation, as compared with patients treated with irradiation alone (228/58 versus 11/35, $P = 0.004$).[41] These data are still preliminary, and it remains questionable whether the response rates will translate into improved survival rates.

In the French experience, among 70 newly diagnosed patients enrolled in a pilot study evaluating the efficacy of two to six courses of the combination BCNU/CDDP/VP16 before radiotherapy, only 48 patients were considered to have a malignant glioma after central pathologic review. The response rate was 19 per cent, and the event-free survival rates were equivalent for responders and non-responders to the sandwich chemotherapy (median event-free survival, seven months). When combining published phase II data for children with HGGs, the overall response rate is 10–20 per cent.[78] Not all of these response rates translate into better survival times (Table 14.4).[79] Currently, there is no evidence that the responses observed could be translated into an increase in event-free survival.

Experimental chemotherapeutic protocols that showed some evidence of potential efficacy include alterations of the timeframe of chemotherapy with respect to the other treatment modalities (sandwich chemotherapy/phase-two windows studies or simultaneous radiochemotherapy);[80] new combinations of old drugs; old drugs in high doses with stem-cell support; novel drugs;[80] chemotherapy supported by molecular engineering/gene therapy; and interstitial chemotherapy with either polymers or direct installation of chemotherapy. Using high-dose chemotherapy can improve the delivery of drugs that do not cross the blood–brain barrier at conventional dosages and will achieve high concentrations within the tumor. The best role of autografting is most likely to be in consolidation therapy for children with chemoresponsive tumors and minimal residual disease. Indications for dose intensification have yet to be established. While the cumulative response rate of published series is 18 per cent,[80] it remains to be seen whether this method will improve event-free survival. Publications are scarce; in addition, they generally combine patients with measurable disease and patients who receive high-dose chemotherapy as a consolidation. International guidelines for conducting and reporting pediatric HGG studies that are in the process of development will help to overcome these problems.

Immunotherapy

Malignant brain tumors have long been considered model diseases for the development of immunotherapy concepts, since they develop in an immunoprivileged environment and it is far more likely to create an immune response to antigens that did not have prior contact with the immune system. The blood–brain barrier in HGG is leaky,[112] allowing effector cells and antibodies to penetrate tumor tissue.[113] However, by the time this penetration becomes possible, malignant gliomas have also developed immuno-suppressive mechanisms, such as transforming growth

Table 14.4 *Conventional-dose chemotherapy phase II trials/pilot studies for children with high-grade glioma*

Ref.	Relapsed (R) or newly diagnosed (N)	Drug and dose	Response
81	R	Carboplatin 175 mg/m^2	0/6
82	R	Carboplatin 560 mg/m^2	0/15
83	R	Carboplatin 560 mg/m^2	2/19
83	R	Iproplatin 270 mg/m^2	0/12
84	R	Cisplatin 120 mg/m^2	0/10
85	R	Cisplatin 120 mg/m^2	0/2
86	R	Cisplatin 120 mg/m^2	0/1
87	R	Cisplatin 120 mg/m^2	1/9
88	R	Cisplatin 120 mg/m^2	2/16
89	R	Ifosfamide 6000 mg/m^2	0/4
90	R	Ifosfamide 9000 mg/m^2	1/16
91	R, N	Cyclophosphamide 2–5000 mg/m^2	0/11
92	R	Cyclophosphamide 2–5000 mg/m^2	2/13
93	N	Cyclophosphamide 2000 mg/m^2 × 2	4/10
93	R	Cyclophosphamide 2000 mg/m^2 × 2	0/7
94	R	PCNU 70–125 mg/m^2	3/12
95	R	Thiotepa 65 mg/m^2	0/18
96	R	Procarbazine 2.1 g	0/1
97	R	Diazoquine 45 mg/m^2	1/13
98	R	Idarubicin 15 mg/m^2	3/19
99	R	Etoposide 375 mg/m^2	3/9
100	R	Etoposide 450 mg/m^2	0/14
101	R	VM26 155 mg/m^2	0/1
102	N, R	Topotecan 5.5–7.5 mg/m^2	0/9
103	R	Topotecan 3–3.75 mg/m^2	0/13
104	R	Methotrexate 18.45 mg/m^2/week	1/19
105	R	Methotrexate 5000 mg/m^2	0/1
106	N	Methotrexate 8000 mg/m^2	2/2
75	R	Trofosfamide + VP16	2/12
107	R	Ifosfamide + VP16	1/16
108	R	CCNU + VCR	0/5
109	R	MOPP	4/13
110	R, N	8-in-1*	5/15
111	R, N	8-in-1*	10/27
Total		All treatments	47/370 (11%)

CCNU, lomustine; MOPP, mechlorethamine, vincristine (Oncovin™), procarbazine, prednisone; VCR, vincristine; VM26, teniposide.
*8-in-1: vincristine, hydroxyurea, procarbazine, lomustine, cisplatin, cytosine arabinoside, high-dose methylprednisolone, and either cyclophosphamide or dacarbazine.

factor beta (TGF-β)[114–116] and interleukin 10 (IL-10).[117] If an immunological method could be developed that overcame those immunosuppressive mechanisms, then a major step forward could be made. Unfortunately, the first approaches using specific antibodies or non-specific immune stimulatory cytokines and killer cells have not yet been successful. At the time of writing, tumor vaccination with ex vivo purged autologous dendritic cells is being tested for clinical efficacy.[118]

Anti-angiogenesis and induction of differentiation

Malignant gliomas are highly vascularized and they may be an appropriate target for anti-angiogenic treatment.[119]

The approach is most likely to succeed in large, contrast-enhancing lesions that have their own vascular supply. Agents directly targeting endothelial cells or neutralizing angiogenic signals are in the clinical testing phase.[120–122] Another approach is to modify intracellular signaling of glioma cells, thus blocking the production of angiogenic signals.[123] Similarly, the malignant phenotype of the glioma cell can be altered, inducing a high degree of differentiation. Molecules such as valproic acid[124–126] and butyric acid[127] are in clinical testing.

Supportive care

Glucocorticoids can improve clinical symptoms and signs within a single day. The improvement appears most remarkable in tumors with large peritumoral edema, although it remains uncertain whether reducing edema is the predominant mechanism of action. Glucocorticoids do not increase survival time or cure rates. On the contrary, there is preclinical evidence that glucocorticoid treatments might diminish the efficacy of chemotherapy[128] or increase side effects.[129] Using glucocorticoids routinely, even in the absence of clinical signs, is therefore not advisable.

PROGNOSTIC CONSIDERATIONS

Age

Age does not seem to have an important impact on survival in childhood, except in children under three years of age.[12,74,130] In the series of Duffner and colleagues, which included 16 children under the age two of years and treated by chemotherapy until they reached three years of age, the response rate to chemotherapy was six per cent and the progression-free survival was 54 per cent.[131]

Histology

In contrast to adult studies in which the survival of patients with glioblastoma multiforme (GBM) is shorter than for patients with anaplastic astrocytoma, in series of children malignant gliomas, histology does not seem to have a major influence on survival.[12,74,130,132] While some reports demonstrate statistically significant differences of 30–50 per cent in favor of those with anaplastic astrocytoma,[73] older series and series in which no central pathology review was done must be viewed cautiously. In the CCG 945 study using World Health Organization (WHO) criteria, there is a significant difference in the five-year progression-free survival between grade III (28 per cent) and grade IV (16 per cent) gliomas. Interestingly, the five-year progression-free survival of "other" malignant gliomas is 64 per cent. The prognosis of oligoastrocytomas remains unclear, particularly in children. While the combined loss of 1p and 19q was identified as a univariate predictor of prolonged overall survival among patients with pure oligodendroglioma, this favorable association was not evident in patients with astrocytoma or mixed oligoastrocytoma.[4] The response rate – as high as 69 per cent in adult patients – and overall survival are not known in children. In the Société Francaise d'Oncologie Pédiatrique (SFOP) studies, the median progression-free survival of the 13 children reviewed as having a malignant oligodendroglioma was only seven months (P. Chastagner, personal communication).

Tumor location and extent of resection

Extent of resection is considered to be a dependent of tumor location. Most pediatric studies that suggest a strong correlation between extent of resection and outcome have not controlled for the possible confounding influence of tumor location. In the St Jude's and CCG 945 studies, extent of resection is an independently significant prognostic factor.[12,13]

CONCLUSIONS

Without treatment, the median progression-free survival of children with malignant glioma is six months. Radiation therapy doubles this time. Multimodal aggressive treatment, including radical resection irradiation and intensive chemotherapy, can result in cure, in particular in focal cortical tumors.[14,133]

HGGs remain a major therapeutic challenge. Prognosis remains very poor compared with the majority of tumors (CNS and non-CNS) arising in the pediatric population. HGGs are rare in children compared with adults. Therefore, although pediatric HGGs are not necessarily identical to adult HGGs in terms of biological behavior, it is important to take into account adult experience from the literature. In Europe, it will be essential to conduct international collaborative studies for children with HGG.

In the clinical setting, very difficult management decisions frequently have to be made. It is often necessary, particularly in the setting of the treatment of relapsed or progressive disease, to balance the likely morbidity of retrieval therapy versus the frequently poor outcome from this therapy.

One of the major priorities for collaborative groups is the identification of potentially useful new chemotherapeutic or novel biological agents. It is generally considered that the best opportunity for testing new agents and correctly identifying response is before radiotherapy in the form of an "up-front window study." However, at present, radiotherapy remains the main modality of therapy for extending the period of progression-free survival. It will be important to avoid continuing too long with ineffective systemic therapy and thus missing the opportunity to employ radiotherapy at a time when the child is at his or her optimum performance status.

In the multidisciplinary management of these children and their families, it is important to adopt a holistic approach, including supportive care and symptom control considerations.

REFERENCES

1   Kleihues PW, Cavenee K. *World Health Organization Classification of Tumors. Pathology and Genetics: Tumors of the Nervous System.* Lyon: IARC Press, 2000.
2   Caldarelli-Stefano R, Boldorini R, Monga G, *et al.* JC virus in human glial-derived tumours. *Hum Pathol* 2000; **31**:394.

3   Goussia AC, Agnantis NJ, Rao JS, Kyritsis AP. Cytogenetic and molecular abnormalities in astrocytic gliomas. *Oncol Rep* 2000; **7**:401–12.

4   Smith JS, Perry A, Borell TJ, *et al.* Alterations of chromosome arms 1p and 19q as predictors of survival in oligodendrogliomas, astrocytomas, and mixed oligoastrocytomas. *J Clin Oncol* 2000; **18**:636–45.

5   Lamszus K, Laterra J, Westphal M, Rosen EM. Scatter factor/ hepatocyte growth factor (SF/HGF) content and function in human gliomas. *Int J Dev Neurosci* 1999; **17**:517–30.

6   Hotfilder M, Knupfer H, Mohlenkamp G, *et al.* Interferon-gamma increases IL-6 production in human glioblastoma cell lines. *Anticancer Res* 2000; **20**:4445–50.

7   Berens ME, Giese A. ... those left behind. Biology and oncology of invasive glioma cells. *Neoplasia* 1999; **1**:208–19.

8   Flores LE, Williams DL, Bell BA, *et al.* Delay in the diagnosis of pediatric brain tumors. *Am J Dis Child* 1986; **140**:684–6.

9   Forsyth PA, Petrov E, Mahallati H, *et al.* Prospective study of postoperative magnetic resonance imaging in patients with malignant gliomas. *J Clin Oncol* 1997; **15**:2076–81.

10 Macdonald DR, Cascino TL, Schold SC, Jr, Cairncross JG. Response criteria for phase II studies of supratentorial malignant glioma. *J Clin Oncol* 1990; **8**:1277–80.

11 Gnekow AK. Recommendations of the Brain Tumour Subcommittee for the reporting of trials. SIOP Brain Tumour Subcommittee. International Society of Pediatric Oncology. *Med Pediatr Oncol* 1995; **24**:104–8.

12 Heideman RL, Kuttesch J, Gajjar AJ, *et al.* Supratentorial malignant gliomas in childhood. *Cancer* 1997; **80**:497–504.

13 Wisoff JH, Boyett JM, Berger MS, *et al.* Current neurosurgical management and the impact of the extent of resection in the treatment of malignant gliomas of childhood: a report of the Children's Cancer Group Trial CCG-945. *J Neurosurg* 1998; **89**:52–9.

14 Klein R, Molenkamp G, Sorensen N, Roggendorf W. Favorable outcome of giant cell glioblastoma in a child. Report of an 11-year survival period. *Childs Nerv Syst* 1998; **14**:288–91.

15 Norruddin L, Yates A, Becker L, *et al.* Outcome for children with centrally reviewed low-grade gliomas, treated with chemotherapy with or without irradiation: the malignant glioma study CCG-945. *J Pediatr Hematol Oncol* 1999; **21**:319.

16 Paulus W, Peiffer J. Intratumoral histologic heterogeneity of gliomas. A quantitative study. *Cancer* 1989; **64**:442–7.

17 Walker MD, Alexander E, Jr, Hunt WE, *et al.* Evaluation of BCNU and/or radiotherapy in the treatment of anaplastic gliomas. A cooperative clinical trial. *J Neurosurg* 1978; **49**:333–43.

18 Kristiansen K, Hagen S, Kollevold T, *et al.* Combined modality therapy of operated astrocytomas grade III and IV. Confirmation of the value of postoperative irradiation and lack of potentiation of bleomycin on survival time: a prospective multicenter trial of the Scandinavian Glioblastoma Study Group. *Cancer* 1981; **47**:649–52.

19 Solero CL, Monfardini S, Brambilla C, *et al.* Controlled study with BCNU vs. CCNU as adjuvant chemotherapy following surgery plus radiotherapy for glioblastoma multiforme. *Cancer Clin Trials* 1979; **2**:43–8.

20 Walker MD, Green SB, Byar DP, *et al.* Randomized comparisons of radiotherapy and nitrosoureas for the treatment of malignant glioma after surgery. *N Engl J Med* 1980; **303**:1323–9.

21 Green SB, Byar DP, Walker MD, *et al.* Comparisons of carmustine, procarbazine, and high-dose methylprednisolone as additions to surgery and radiotherapy for the treatment of malignant glioma. *Cancer Treat Rep* 1983; **67**:121–32.

22 Nelson DF, Diener-West M, Horton J, Chang CH, Schoenfeld D, Nelson JS. Combined modality approach to treatment of malignant gliomas – re-evaluation of RTOG 7401/ECOG 1374 with long-term follow-up: a joint study of the Radiation Therapy Oncology Group and the Eastern Cooperative Oncology Group. *NCI Monogr* 1988; **6**:279–84.

23 Nelson DF, Diener-West M, Weinstein AS, *et al.* A randomized comparison of misonidazole sensitized radiotherapy plus BCNU and radiotherapy plus BCNU for treatment of malignant glioma after surgery: final report of an RTOG study. *Int J Radiat Oncol Biol Phys* 1986; **12**:1793–800.

24 Eyre HJ, Eltringham JR, Gehan EA, *et al.* Randomized comparisons of radiotherapy and carmustine versus procarbazine versus dacarbazine for the treatment of malignant gliomas following surgery: a Southwest Oncology Group Study. *Cancer Treat Rep* 1986; **70**:1085–90.

25 Bleehen NM, Freedman LS, Stenning SP. A randomised study of CCNU with and without benznidazole in the treatment of recurrent grades 3 and 4 astrocytoma. Report to the Medical Research Council by the Brain Tumour Working Party. *Int J Radiat Oncol Biol Phys* 1989; **16**:1077–81.

26 Deutsch M, Green SB, Strike TA, *et al.* Results of a randomized trial comparing BCNU plus radiotherapy, streptozotocin plus radiotherapy, BCNU plus hyperfractionated radiotherapy, and BCNU following misonidazole plus radiotherapy in the postoperative treatment of malignant glioma. *Int J Radiat Oncol Biol Phys* 1989; **16**:1389–96.

27 Levin VA, Silver P, Hannigan J, *et al.* Superiority of post-radiotherapy adjuvant chemotherapy with CCNU, procarbazine, and vincristine (PCV) over BCNU for anaplastic gliomas: NCOG 6G61 final report. *Int J Radiat Oncol Biol Phys* 1990; **18**:321–4.

28 Sandberg-Wollheim M, Malmstrom P, Stromblad LG, *et al.* A randomized study of chemotherapy with procarbazine, vincristine, and lomustine with and without radiation therapy for astrocytoma grades 3 and/or 4. *Cancer* 1991; **68**:22–9.

29 Prados MD, Scott C, Sandler H, *et al.* A phase 3 randomized study of radiotherapy plus procarbazine, CCNU, and vincristine (PCV) with or without BUdR for the treatment of anaplastic astrocytoma: a preliminary report of RTOG 9404. *Int J Radiat Oncol Biol Phys* 1999; **45**:1109–15.

30 Bower M, Newlands ES, Bleehen NM, *et al.* Multicentre CRC phase II trial of temozolomide in recurrent or progressive high-grade glioma. *Cancer Chemother Pharmacol* 1997; **40**:484–8.

31 Yung WK, Albright RE, Olson J, *et al.* A phase II study of temozolomide vs. procarbazine in patients with glioblastoma multiforme at first relapse. *Br J Cancer* 2000; **83**:588–93.

32 Chinot OL, Honore S, Dufour H, *et al.* Safety and efficacy of temozolomide in patients with recurrent anaplastic oligodendrogliomas after standard radiotherapy and chemotherapy. *J Clin Oncol* 2001; **19**:2449–55.

33 Macdonald DR. Temozolomide for recurrent high-grade glioma. *Semin Oncol* 2001; **28** (4 suppl. 13):3–12.

34 Brada M, Hoang-Xuan K, Rampling R, et al. Multicenter phase II trial of temozolomide in patients with glioblastoma multiforme at first relapse. Ann Oncol 2001; 12:259–66.

35 Khan RB, Raizer JJ, Malkin MG, Bazylewicz KA, Abrey LE. A phase II study of extended low-dose temozolomide in recurrent malignant gliomas. Neuro-oncol 2002; 4:39–43.

36 Stupp R, Dietrich PY, Kraljevic SO, et al. Promising survival for patients with newly diagnosed glioblastoma multiforme treated with concomitant radiation plus temozolomide followed by adjuvant temozolomide. J Clin Oncol 2002; 20:1375–82.

37 Osoba D, Brada M, Yung WK, Prados M. Health-related quality of life in patients treated with temozolomide versus procarbazine for recurrent glioblastoma multiforme. J Clin Oncol 2000; 18:1481–91.

38 Paulsen F, Hoffmann W, Becker G, et al. Chemotherapy in the treatment of recurrent glioblastoma multiforme: ifosfamide versus temozolomide. J Cancer Res Clin Oncol 1999; 125:411–18.

39 Dinnes J, Cave C, Huang S, Milne R. A rapid and systematic review of the effectiveness of temozolomide for the treatment of recurrent malignant glioma. Br J Cancer 2002; 86:501–5.

40 Wolff JEA, Moelenkamp G, Westphal S, et al. Oral trofosfamide and VP16 in paediatric patients with glioblastoma multiforme. Cancer 2000; 89:2131–7.

41 Wolff JEA, Westphal S, Moelenkamp G, et al. Phase II study for children with high grade glioma and brain stem glioma. Med Pediatr Oncol 2000; 35:171.

42 Le Vu B, de Vathaire F, Shamsaldin A, et al. Radiation dose, chemotherapy and risk of osteosarcoma after solid tumours during childhood. Int J Cancer 1998; 77:370–7.

43 Pratt CB, Meyer WH, Luo X, et al. Second malignant neoplasms occurring in survivors of osteosarcoma. Cancer 1997; 80:960–5.

44 Walker MD, Alexander E, Jr, Hunt WE, et al. Evaluation of mithramycin in the treatment of anaplastic gliomas. J Neurosurg 1976; 44:655–67.

45 Eagan RT, Childs DS, Jr, Layton DD, Jr, et al. Dianhydrogalactitol and radiation therapy. Treatment of supratentorial glioma. J Am Med Assoc 1979; 241:2046–50.

46 Eyre HJ, Quagliana JM, Eltringham JR, et al. Randomized comparisons of radiotherapy and CCNU versus radiotherapy, CCNU plus procarbazine for the treatment of malignant gliomas following surgery. A Southwest Oncology Group Report. J Neuro-Oncol 1983; 1:171–7.

47 Afra D, Kocsis B, Dobay J, Eckhardt S. Combined radiotherapy and chemotherapy with dibromodulcitol and CCNU in the postoperative treatment of malignant gliomas. J Neurosurg 1983; 59:106–10.

48 Stadler B, Karcher KH, Kogelnik HD, Szepesi T. Misonidazole and irradiation in the treatment of high-grade astrocytomas: further report of the Vienna Study Group. Int J Radiat Oncol Biol Phys 1984; 10:1713–17.

49 Fulton DS, Urtasun RC, Shin KH, et al. Misonidazole combined with hyperfractionation in the management of malignant glioma. Int J Radiat Oncol Biol Phys 1984; 10:1709–12.

50 Levin VA, Wara WM, Davis RL, et al. Phase III comparison of BCNU and the combination of procarbazine, CCNU, and vincristine administered after radiotherapy with hydroxyurea for malignant gliomas. J Neurosurg 1985; 63:218–23.

51 Ushio Y, Abe H, Suzuki J, et al. [Evaluation of ACNU alone and combined with tegafur as additions to radiotherapy of the treatment of malignant gliomas – a cooperative clinical trial] No To Shinkei 1985; 37:999–1006.

52 Hatlevoll R, Lindegaard KF, Hagen S, et al. Combined modality treatment of operated astrocytomas grade 3 and 4. A prospective and randomized study of misonidazole and radiotherapy with two different radiation schedules and subsequent CCNU chemotherapy. Stage II of a prospective multicenter trial of the Scandinavian Glioblastoma Study Group. Cancer 1985; 56:41–7.

53 Shibata S, Mori K, Moriyama T, Tanaka K, Moroki J. Randomized controlled study of the effect of adjuvant immunotherapy with Picibanil on 51 malignant gliomas. Surg Neurol 1987; 27:259–63.

54 Trojanowski T, Peszynski J, Turowski K, et al. Postoperative radiotherapy and radiotherapy combined with CCNU chemotherapy for treatment of brain gliomas. J Neuro-Oncol 1988; 6:285–91.

55 Shapiro WR, Green SB, Burger PC, et al. Randomized trial of three chemotherapy regimens and two radiotherapy regimens in postoperative treatment of malignant glioma. Brain Tumor Cooperative Group Trial 8001. J Neurosurg 1989; 71:1–9.

56 Mortimer JE, Crowley J, Eyre H, Weiden P, Eltringham J, Stuckey WJ. A phase II randomized study comparing sequential and combined intra-arterial cisplatin and radiation therapy in primary brain tumors. A Southwest Oncology Group study. Cancer 1992; 69:1220–3.

57 Shapiro WR, Green SB, Burger PC, et al. A randomized comparison of intra-arterial versus intravenous BCNU, with or without intravenous 5-fluorouracil, for newly diagnosed patients with malignant glioma. J Neurosurg 1992; 76:772–81.

58 Glinski B. Postoperative hypofractionated radiotherapy versus conventionally fractionated radiotherapy in malignant gliomas. A preliminary report on a randomized trial. J Neuro-Oncol 1993; 16:167–72.

59 Dinapoli RP, Brown LD, Arusell RM, et al. Phase III comparative evaluation of PCNU and carmustine combined with radiation therapy for high-grade glioma. J Clin Oncol 1993; 11:1316–21.

60 Nelson DF, Curran WJ, Jr, Scott C, et al. Hyperfractionated radiation therapy and bis-chlorethyl nitrosourea in the treatment of malignant glioma – possible advantage observed at 72.0 Gy in 1.2 Gy B.I.D. fractions: report of the Radiation Therapy Oncology Group Protocol 8302. Int J Radiat Oncol Biol Phys 1993; 25:193–207.

61 Schold SC, Jr, Herndon JE, Burger PC, et al. Randomized comparison of diaziquone and carmustine in the treatment of adults with anaplastic glioma. J Clin Oncol 1993; 11:77–83.

62 Hiesiger EM, Green SB, Shapiro WR, et al. Results of a randomized trial comparing intra-arterial cisplatin and intravenous PCNU for the treatment of primary brain tumors in adults: Brain Tumor Cooperative Group trial 8420A. J Neuro-Oncol 1995; 25:143–54.

63 Halperin EC, Herndon J, Schold SC, et al. A phase III randomized prospective trial of external beam radiotherapy, mitomycin C, carmustine, and 6-mercaptopurine for the treatment of adults with anaplastic glioma of the brain.

CNS Cancer Consortium. *Int J Radiat Oncol Biol Phys* 1996; **34**:793–802.

64 Valtonen S, Timonen U, Toivanen P, *et al.* Interstitial chemotherapy with carmustine-loaded polymers for high-grade gliomas: a randomized double-blind study. *Neurosurgery* 1997; **41**:44–8, 48–9.

65 Elliott TE, Dinapoli RP, O'Fallon JR, *et al.* Randomized trial of radiation therapy (RT) plus dibromodulcitol (DBD) versus RT plus BCNU in high grade astrocytoma. *J Neuro-Oncol* 1997; **33**:239–50.

66 Prados MD, Scott C, Curran WJ, Jr, Nelson DF, Leibel S, Kramer S. Procarbazine, lomustine, and vincristine (PCV) chemotherapy for anaplastic astrocytoma: a retrospective review of radiation therapy oncology group protocols comparing survival with carmustine or PCV adjuvant chemotherapy. *J Clin Oncol* 1999; **17**:3389–95.

67 Kleinberg L, Grossman SA, Piantadosi S, Zeltzman M, Wharam M. The effects of sequential versus concurrent chemotherapy and radiotherapy on survival and toxicity in patients with newly diagnosed high-grade astrocytoma. *Int J Radiat Oncol Biol Phys* 1999; **44**:535–43.

68 Kochii M, Kitamura I, Goto T, *et al.* Randomized comparison of intra-arterial versus intravenous infusion of ACNU for newly diagnosed patients with glioblastoma. *J Neuro-Oncol* 2000; **49**:63–70.

69 Rainov NG. A phase III clinical evaluation of herpes simplex virus type 1 thymidine kinase and ganciclovir gene therapy as an adjuvant to surgical resection and radiation in adults with previously untreated glioblastoma multiforme. *Hum Gene Ther* 2000; **11**:2389–401.

70 Levin VA, Uhm JH, Jaeckle KA, *et al.* Phase III randomized study of postradiotherapy chemotherapy with alpha-difluoromethylornithine-procarbazine, N-(2-chloroethyl)-N'-cyclohexyl-N-nitrosurea, vincristine (DFMO-PCV) versus PCV for glioblastoma multiforme. *Clin Cancer Res* 2000; **6**:3878–84.

71 Medical Research Council. Randomized trial of procarbazine, lomustine, and vincristine in the adjuvant treatment of high-grade astrocytoma: a Medical Research Council trial. *J Clin Oncol* 2001; **19**:509–18.

72 Buckner JC, Schomberg PJ, McGinnis WL, *et al.* A phase III study of radiation therapy plus carmustine with or without recombinant interferon-alpha in the treatment of patients with newly diagnosed high-grade glioma. *Cancer* 2001; **92**:420–33.

73 Sposto R, Ertel IJ, Jenkin RD, *et al.* The effectiveness of chemotherapy for treatment of high grade astrocytoma in children: results of a randomized trial. A report from the Childrens Cancer Study Group. *J Neuro-Oncol* 1989; **7**: 165–77.

74 Finlay JL, Boyett JM, Yates AJ, *et al.* Randomized phase III trial in childhood high-grade astrocytoma comparing vincristine, lomustine, and prednisone with the eight-drugs-in-1-day regimen. Children's Cancer Group. *J Clin Oncol* 1995; **13**:112–23.

75 Wolff JE, Gnekow AK, Kortmann RD, *et al.* Preradiation chemotherapy for pediatric patients with high-grade glioma. *Cancer* 2002; **94**:264–71.

76 Kortmann RD, Kuhl J, Timmermann B, *et al.* Postoperative neoadjuvant chemotherapy before radiotherapy as compared to immediate radiotherapy followed by maintenance chemotherapy in the treatment of medulloblastoma in childhood: results of the German prospective randomized trial HIT '91. *Int J Radiat Oncol Biol Phys* 2000; **46**:269–79.

77 Wolff JE, Boos J, Kühl J. HIT-GBM: multicenter study of treatment of children with malignant glioma. *Klin Paediatr* 1996; **208**:193–6.

78 Chastagner P, Bouffet E, Grill J, Kalifa C. What have we learnt from previous phase II trials to help in the management of childhood brain tumours? *Eur J Cancer* 2001; **37**:1981–93.

79 Chastagner P, Kalifa C, Mechinaud-Lacroix F. Pilot study of combined BCNU, cisplatin and VP16 for the treatment of newly-diagnosed high grade glioma in children. *Med Pediatr Oncol* 1995; **25**:258.

80 Chastagner P, Kozin SV, Taghian A. Topotecan selectively enhances the radioresponse of human small-cell lung carcinoma and glioblastoma multiforme xenografts in nude mice. *Int J Radiat Oncol Biol Phys* 2001; **50**:777–82.

81 Allen JC, Walker R, Luks E, Jennings M, Barfoot S, Tan C. Carboplatin and recurrent childhood brain tumors. *J Clin Oncol* 1987; **5**:459–63.

82 Gaynon PS, Ettinger LJ, Baum ES, Siegel SE, Krailo MD, Hammond GD. Carboplatin in childhood brain tumors: a Children's Cancer Study Group phase II trial. *Cancer* 1990; **66**:2465–9.

83 Friedman HS, Krischer JP, Burger PC. Treatment of children with progressive of recurrent brain tumors with carboplatin or iproplatin: a Pediatric Oncology Group randomized phase II study. *J Clin Oncol* 1992; **10**:249–56.

84 Sexauer CL, Kahn A, Burger PC, *et al.* Cisplatin in recurrent pediatric brain tumors. *Cancer* 1985; **56**:1497–501.

85 Diez B, Monges J, Muriel FS. Evaluation of cisplatin in children with recurrent brain tumors. *Cancer Treat Rep* 1985; **69**:911–13.

86 Walker RW, Allen JC. Cisplatin in the treatment of recurrent childhood primary brain tumors. *J Clin Oncol* 1988; **6**:62–6.

87 Bertolone SJ, Baum ES, Krivit W, Hammond GD. A phase II study of cisplatin therapy in recurrent childhood brain tumors. A report from the Children's Cancer Study Group. *J Neuro-Oncol* 1989; **7**:5–11.

88 Khan AB, D'Souza BJ, Wharam MD, *et al.* Cisplatin therapy in recurrent childhood brain tumors. *Cancer Treat Rep* 1982; **12**:2013–20.

89 Chastagner P, Sommelet-Olive D, Kalifa C, *et al.* Phase II study of ifosfamide in childhood brain tumors: a report by the French Society Of Pediatric Oncology. *Med Pediatr Oncol* 1993; **21**:49–53.

90 Heideman RL, Douglass EC, Langston JA, *et al.* A phase II of every other day high-dose ifosfamide in pediatric brain tumors: a pediatric oncology group study. *J Neuro-Oncol* 1995; **25**:77–84.

91 Abrahamsen TG, Lange BJ, Packer RJ, *et al.* A phase I and II trial of dose-intensified cyclophosphamide and GM-CSF in paediatric malignant tumors. *J Pediatr Hematol Oncol* 1995; **17**:134–9.

92 Lachance DH, Oette D, Schold SC, *et al.* Dose escalation of cyclophosphamide with sargramostim in the treatment of central nervous system neoplasms. *Med Pediatr Oncol* 1995; **24**:241–7.

93 McCowage GB, Friedman HS, Moghrabi A, *et al.* Activity of high-dose cyclophosphamide in the treatment of childhood malignant gliomas. *Med Pediatr Oncol* 1998; **30**:75–80.

94 Allen JC, Hancock C, Walker R, Tan C. PCNU and recurrent childhood brain tumors. *J Neuro-Oncol* 1987; **5**:241–4.

95 Heideman RL, Packer RJ, Reaman GH, *et al.* A phase II evaluation of thiotepa in pediatric central nervous system malignancies. *Cancer* 1993; **72**:271–5.

96 Van Eys J, Cangir A, Pack R, Baram T. Phase I trial of procarbazine as a 5-day continuous infusion in children with central nervous system tumors. *Cancer Treat Rep* 1987; **71**:973–4.

97 Ettinger LJ, Ru N, Krailo M, Ruccione KS, Krivit W, Hammond GD. A phase II study of diaziquone in children with recurrent or progressive primary brain tumors: a report from the Children's Cancer Study group. *J Clin Oncol* 1990; **9**:69–76.

98 Arndt CAS, Krailo MD, Steinherz L, Scheithauer B, Liu-Mares W, Reaman GH. A phase II clinical trial of idarubicin administered to children with relapsed brain tumors. *Cancer* 1998; **83**:813–16.

99 Tirelli U, D'Incalci M, Canetta R, *et al.* Etoposide (VP-16-213) in malignant brain tumors: a phase II study. *J Clin Oncol* 1984; **2**:432–7.

100 Kung F, Hayes FA, Krischer J, *et al.* Clinical trial of etoposide (VP-16) in children with recurrent malignant solid tumors. A phase II study from the Pediatric Oncology Group. *Invest New Drugs* 1988; **6**:31–6.

101 Bleyer WA, Krivit W, Chard RL, Jr, Hammond D. Phase II study of VM-26 in acute leukemia, neuroblastoma, and other refractory childhood malignancies: a report from the Children's Cancer Study Group. *Cancer Treat Rep* 1979; **63**:977–81.

102 Blaney SM, Phillips PC, Packer RJ, *et al.* Phase II evaluation of topotecan for pediatric central nervous system tumors. *Cancer* 1996; **78**:527–31.

103 Kadota RP, Stewart CF, Horn M, *et al.* Topotecan for the treatment of recurrent or progressive central nervous system tumors – a pediatric oncology group phase II study. *J Neuro-Oncol* 1999; **43**:43–7.

104 Mulne AF, Ducore JM, Elterman RD, *et al.* Oral methotrexate for recurrent brain tumors in children: a Pediatric Oncology Group study. *J Pediatr Hematol Oncol* 2000; **22**:41–4.

105 Djerassi I, Kim JS, Reggev A. Response of astrocytoma to high-dose methotrexate with citrovorum factor rescue. *Cancer* 1985; **55**:2741–7.

106 Allen JC, Walker R, Rosen G. Preradiation high-dose intravenous methotrexate with leucovorin rescue for untreated primary childhood brain tumors. *J Clin Oncol* 1988; **6**:649–53.

107 Miser JS, Kinsella TJ, Triche TJ, *et al.* Ifosfamide with mesna uroprotection and etoposide: an effective regimen in the treatment of recurrent sarcomas and other tumors of children and young adults. *J Clin Oncol* 1987; **5**:1191–8.

108 Lefkowitz IB, Packer RJ, Sutton LN, Siegel KR, Bruce DA, Evans AE, Schut L. Results of the treatment of children with recurrent gliomas with lomustine and vincristine. *Cancer* 1988; **61**:896–902.

109 Van Eys J, Baram TZ, Cangir A, Bruner JM, Martinez-Prieto J. Salvage chemotherapy for recurrent primary brain tumors in children. *J Pediatr* 1988; **113**:601–6.

110 Chastagner P, Olive D, Philip T, *et al.* Efficacité du protocole "8 drogues en un jour" dans les tumeurs cérébrales de l'enfant. *Arch Fr Pediatr* 1988; **45**:249–54.

111 Pendergrass TW, Milstein JM, Geyer JR, *et al.* Eight drugs in one day chemotherapy for brain tumors: experience in 107 children and rationale for preradiation chemotherapy. *J Clin Oncol* 1987; **5**:121–31.

112 Seitz RJ, Wechsler W. Immunohistochemical demonstration of serum proteins in human cerebral gliomas. *Acta Neuropathol* 1987; **73**:145–52.

113 Gingras MC, Roussel E, Roth JA, Moser RP. Little expression of cytokine mRNA by fresh tumour-infiltrating mononuclear leukocytes from glioma and lung adenocarcinoma. *Cytokine* 1995; **7**:580–8.

114 Roszman TL, Brooks WH, Elliot LC. Inhibition of lymphocyte responsiveness by glial tumor cell-derived suppressive factor. *J Neurosurg* 1987; **67**:874–9.

115 Roszman T, Elliot L, Brooks W. Inability of mitogen activated lymphocytes obtained from patient's malignant primary intracranial tumors to express high affinity IL-2 receptors. *J Clin Invest* 1990; **86**:80–6.

116 Kuppner MC, van Meir E, Hamou MF, de Tribolet N. Cytokine regulation of intercellular adhesion molecule-1 (ICAM-1) expression on human glioblastoma cells. *Clin Exp Immunol* 1990; **81**:142–8.

117 Huettner C, Paulus W, Roggendorf W. Messenger RNA expression of the immunosuppressive cytokine IL-10 in human gliomas. *Am J Pathol* 1995; **146**:317–22.

118 Yu JS, Wheeler CJ, Zeltzer PM, *et al.* Vaccination of malignant glioma patients with peptide-pulsed dendritic cells elicits systemic cytotoxicity and intracranial T-cell infiltration. *Cancer Res* 2001; **61**:842–7.

119 Wolff JEA, Laterra J, Goldstein GW. Steroid inhibition of neural microvessel morphogenesis in vitro: receptor mediation and astroglial dependence. *J Neurochem* 1992; **58**:1023–32.

120 Oikawa T, Ito H, Ashino H, *et al.* Radicicol, a microbial cell differentiation modulator, inhibits in vivo angiogenesis. *Eur J Pharmacol* 1993; **241**:221–7.

121 Lee CG, Heijn M, di Tomaso E, *et al.* Anti-vascular endothelial growth factor treatment augments tumor radiation response under normoxic or hypoxic conditions. *Cancer Res* 2000; **60**:5565–70.

122 Fine HA, Figg WD, Jaeckle K, *et al.* Phase II trial of the antiangiogenic agent thalidomide in patients with recurrent high-grade gliomas. *J Clin Oncol* 2000; **18**:708–15.

123 Wolff JEA, Guerin C, Laterra J, *et al.* Dexamethasone reduces vascular density and plasminogen activator activity in 9L rat brain tumours. *Brain Res* 1993; **604**:79–85.

124 Knuepfer M, Hernaiz-Diever P, Poppenborg H, *et al.* Valproic acid inhibits growth and changes expression of CD44 and CD56 of malignant glioma cells in vitro. *Anticancer Res* 1998; **18**:3585–9.

125 Knuepfer MM, Poppenborg H, van Gool S, *et al.* Interferon-gamma inhibits proliferation and adhesion of T98G human malignant glioma cells in vitro. *Klin Paediatr* 1997; **209**:271–4.

126 Driever PH, Knuepfer M, Cintatl J, Wolff JEA. Valproic acid for the treatment of pediatric malignant glioma. *Klin Paediatr* 1999; **211**:323–8.

127 Thibault A, Samid D, Cooper MR, *et al.* Phase I study of phenylacetate administered twice daily to patients with cancer. *Cancer* 1995; **75**:2932–8.

128 Wolff JEA, Denecke J, Jürgens H. Dexamethasone induces partial resistance to cisplatinum in C6 glioma cells. *Anticancer Res* 1996; **16**:805–10.

129 Wolff JEA Hauch H, Kuehl J, Egeler RM, Juergens H. Dexamethasone increases hepatotoxicity of MTX in children with brain tumours. *Anticancer Res* 1998; **18**:2895–9.

130 Marchese MJ, Chang CH. Malignant astrocytic gliomas in children. *Cancer* 1990; **65**:2771–8.

131 Duffner PK, Krischer JP, Burger PC, *et al.* Treatment of infants with malignant gliomas: the Pediatric Oncology Group experience. *J Neuro-Oncol* 1996; **28**:245–56.

132 Al-Mefty O, Kersh JE, Routh A, Smith RR. The long-term side effects of radiation therapy for benign brain tumors in adults. *J Neurosurg* 1990; **73**:502–12.

133 Scott JN, Rewcastle NB, Brasher PM. Which glioblastoma multiforme patient will become a long-term survivor? A population-based study. *Ann Neurol* 1999; **46**:183–8.

15

Brainstem tumors

DAVID A. WALKER, JONATHAN A. G. PUNT AND MICHAEL SOKAL

INTRODUCTION

Tumors located in the brainstem are difficult to diagnose initially because of their fluctuating and frequently indistinct symptomatology. There are difficulties in correlating imaging characteristics with histological and biological features because of clinical controversies surrounding the risks and benefits of diagnostic biopsy within the brainstem. They are difficult to treat, as surgery has a role limited to the relief of raised intracranial pressure in some situations and tumor resection in a small and specific minority. Adjuvant therapy with radiation is curative in the minority and therefore is only palliative in the remainder. Apart from steroids, chemotherapy and other drug treatments are given only within clinical trials, which have yet to identify an effective agent or combination of agents in this major anatomical tumor subgroup (diffuse intrinsic pontine). Steroids can provide temporary relief of the signs and symptoms at presentation, but their sustained use leads inevitably to worsening disability and distressing side effects, including personality change. These facts, when put together for a child and family facing up to the diagnosis, provoke strong emotion, which can lead to disbelief and an overwhelming urge to seek alternative opinions and treatments. Skills in communication therefore are central to the management of a child with a tumor

in this region of the brain. Most of all, however, reliable selection of patients for whom there is effective treatment, coupled with the development of research strategies to investigate tumor biology and novel therapies for whom there are no current effective treatments, must be the goal shared by those who are referred these patients for specialist advice.

In this chapter, we aim to demonstrate how careful assessment of anatomical and, where appropriate, imaging and histological characteristics will guide the multidisciplinary neuro-oncology team to predict outcomes and select patients for curative, palliative, or experimental treatments. We will review evidence for the effectiveness of diagnostic and therapeutic approaches. We will use case scenarios to illustrate key points and conclude with recommendations for future avenues of research/clinical trials.

EPIDEMIOLOGY

Brainstem gliomas (BSGs) account for about 8–15 per cent of all brain and spinal tumors.[1] They occur most commonly in mid to late childhood, although they can occur in the first months of life. There is no sex predominance. From the UK Children's Cancer Study Group (UKCCSG) registry, data concerning the histology and survival of

Table 15.1 *UKCCSG brainstem tumors, 1977–1999*

Tumor type	Age at diagnosis (years)				
	0	1–4	5–9	10–14	Total
Gliomas					
Low-grade astrocytoma	0	34	32	19	85
High-grade astrocytoma	0	17	45	16	78
Unspecified astrocytoma	2	9	22	16	49
Other and unspecified glioma	5	80	179	46	310
Unspecified tumor	1	6	9	7	23
Total	8	146	287	104	545
Other tumors					
Ependymoma	0	6	5	3	14
PNET	2	4	1	0	7
Ganglioglioma	0	1	1	0	2
Rhabdomyosarcoma	0	1	0	0	1

PNET, primitive neuroectodermal tumor.

brainstem tumors are emerging. The registry cannot currently discriminate between tumors of different anatomical locations within the brainstem. However, it does show that the majority (56.9 per cent) of patients with brainstem tumors are not being biopsied and are presumed, therefore, to be typical pontine gliomas (Table 15.1). Of the biopsied cases, 90 per cent are astrocytic tumors, a third of which are labeled as high-grade; the remainder are labeled with other histologies, including ependymoma, primitive neuroectodermal tumor (PNET), ganglioglioma, and rhabdomyosarcoma. Astrocytic tumors in the brainstem account for 13 per cent of all central nervous system (CNS) astrocytic tumors, just over a third (36.2 per cent) of which are labeled as high-grade. Using these categories in the registry over a prolonged time period, five-year survival rates range from eight to 53 per cent (Figure 15.1). High-grade astrocytoma and unspecified tumors have the poorest prognosis (nine and eight per cent five-year survivals, respectively), while low-grade astrocytomas have a 53 per cent five-year survival. There may be an emerging trend for improving survival rates in the more recent time period. However, these figures do coincide with recent increases in registration rates for CNS tumors in the UK, generally, as well as the introduction of a national study of low-grade astrocytoma, which may, by expanding recruitment, be introducing a favorable bias to the register compared with previous time periods.

HISTOLOGICAL TYPES ENCOUNTERED

All variants of low-grade (fibrillary/pilocytic/protoplasmic) astrocytic tumors and high-grade (anaplastic/glioblastoma multiforme) astrocytic tumors occur in this location. The true incidence is not known, since diffuse intrinsic tumors have not been biopsied routinely and postmortem examination is a rare event. In our own limited series of biopsied ($n = 18$) diffuse intrinsic tumors, glioblastoma multiforme accounted for 44 per cent, anaplastic astrocytoma for 28 per cent, and low-grade astrocytoma for 28 per cent (Table 15.2).[2] The presence of 28 per cent low-grade tumors in this group raises the possibility that the diffuse intrinsic phenotype is not reliably predictive of high-grade tumors. This may account for the small number of long-term survivors reported in most series (e.g. see Tables 15.6 and 15.7). Secondly, the transient nature of post-biopsy complications in experienced hands justifies further consideration being given to the use of this technique in clinical trials of novel therapies in this disease. Other histologies in this part of the brain include PNET, ependymoma, and other rare glioma variants (ganglioglioma/oligodendroglioma). A more diverse range of histologies is observed in patients in the adult age range.[3] Tumors arising within the tectal plate are most commonly low-grade astrocytic tumors, as are those identified at the cervicomedullary junction.[4–15]

ANATOMY OF BRAINSTEM TUMORS

We define the brainstem as extending from the junction with the midbrain (tectal plate) to the medullary cervical junction (Figure 15.2). "Brainstem glioma," (BSG) therefore, is a term describing a collection of anatomically related tumors with characteristic appearances on computed tomography (CT) scanning and magnetic resonance imaging (MRI). This part of the brain, whilst being only one-fifth of the volume of total brain, contains all of the cranial nerve nuclei that are involved in appreciating taste, hearing, and cutaneous sensations of touch,

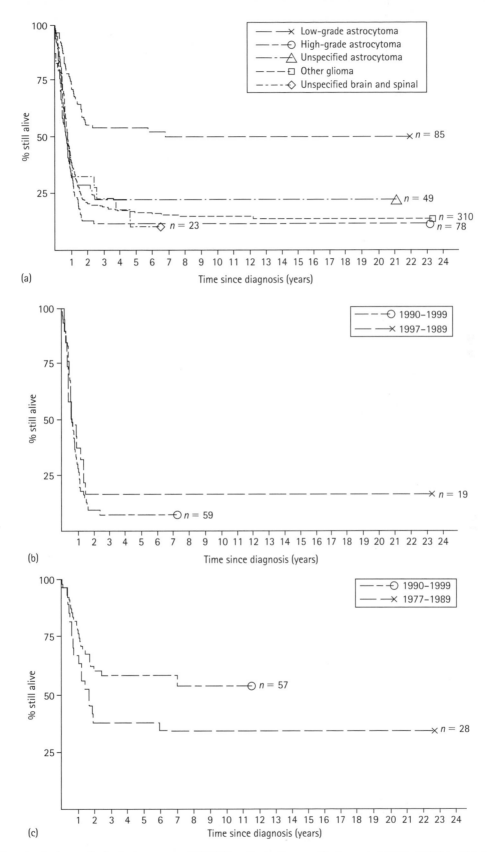

Figure 15.1a,b,c *Survival rates for brainstem tumors (UKCCSG patients diagnosed in the period 1977–1999) by histology and time period: (a) diagnosis group brainstem tumors; (b) diagnosis group high-grade brainstem astrocytoma; (c) diagnosis group low-grade brainstem astrocytoma.*

Table 15.2 *Histology, deficits, and survival following stereotactic biopsy of diffuse brainstem gliomas*[2]

Patient	Age (years)	Sex	Site	Symptom duration	Histology	No. of targets	No. of biopsies	Additional surgery	Added postoperative deficit	Duration of new deficit	Survival (months)
1	7	M	Pons/midbrain	2 months	GBM	3	3	–	Nil	–	2
2	9	F	Pons/midbrain	4 months	AA	1	1	–	Nil	–	48
3	0.5	M	Midbrain	6 months	GBM	3	4	Cyst aspiration	Nil	–	4
4	5	F	Pons	6 weeks	GBM	3	3	Cyst aspiration	Hemiparesis VII palsy	2 days	18
5	3	M	Pons	2 weeks	GBM	3	3	VP shunt	Nil	–	3
6	9	F	Pons	6 months	AA	3	3	VP shunt	Nil	–	16
7	5	F	Pons	2 months	GBM	3	3	VP shunt	Nil	–	5
8	4	F	Pons/midbrain	18 months	LGA	2	2	VP shunt	Eye movements	5 days	17
9	6	M	Pons	4 weeks	GBM	2	2	–	Nil	–	9
10	5	F	Pons	2 months	LGA	2	4	–	Nil	–	32
11	9	F	Pons	3 weeks	LGA	2	3	–	Nil	–	11
12	7	M	Pons	2 weeks	GBM	2	3	–	Nil	–	1
13	9	M	Midbrain	4 days	LGA	1	1	–	Eye movements	7 days	17
14	6	M	Pons	2 weeks	AA	1	1	–	Hemiparesis	3 days	4
15	9	F	Pons/midbrain	3 months	LGA	1	1	–	Nil	–	24
16	10	F	Midbrain	4 weeks	AA	2	2	VP shunt	Eye movements	5 days	19
17	4	F	Pons	4 months	GBM	3	4	–	Nil	–	7
18	6	F	Pons	5 weeks	AA	2	4	–	Nil	–	10

AA, anaplastic astrocytoma; GBM, glioblastoma multiforme; LGA, low-grade astrocytoma; VP, ventriculoperitoneal.

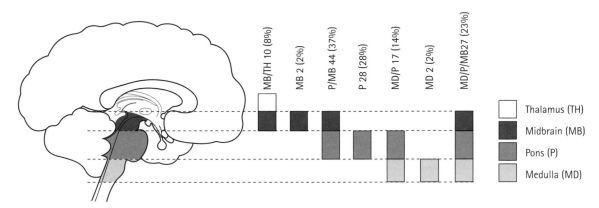

Figure 15.2 *Anatomical distribution and frequency of brainstem tumors in a childhood series.*[50]

pressure, and pain, particularly of the anterior scalp and face. The brainstem nerve fibers carry messages for balance and coordination of movement and speech as well as eye movements, facial expression, chewing, swallowing, protective mechanisms of the upper airway, and movement of the neck, upper and lower limbs, and trunk. The reticular system in the brainstem controls levels of consciousness and a variety of visceral functions, including heart rate, respiratory rate, and vomiting.

SYMPTOMATOLOGY AT PRESENTATION

Common presenting symptoms are those of cranial nerve dysfunction, producing any or all of the following: dysconjugate eye movements, diplopia, facial weakness, facial sensory loss, dysphagia, and dysarthria.[16] Other symptoms may include weakness and/or ataxia of one or more limbs, signifying involvement of the corticospinal pathways and cerebellar connections, respectively. Headache and vomiting can occur, although clinically significant raised intracranial pressure and papilledema are relatively unusual, except in later stages of disease progression. A fluctuating course is common and may include fluctuations in mood and behavior, which can give rise to confusion with inflammatory pathologies.[17] More prolonged histories (several weeks to several months) indicate slower-growing tumors. Faster-growing tumors can precipitate dramatic neurological deterioration over a few days or weeks. In younger children (under three years of age), failure to thrive, often associated with unexplained vomiting, may be mistaken for a gastrointestinal or nutritional problem. The motor symptoms can then be regarded incorrectly as developmental delay secondary to the poor state of nutrition, and a further delay in diagnosis follows. The exceptions to the above patterns of presentation are tumors of the tectal plate of the midbrain and dorsally exophytic growths of the medulla, both of which produce raised intracranial pressure due to hydrocephalus as the major symptom.

ESTABLISHING THE DIAGNOSIS

The ready availability of modern neuroimaging makes confirmation of the clinical diagnosis of a brainstem tumor in a child disarmingly simple, provided that the need for such imaging is identified by correct attention to the presenting clinical features. Diagnosis by CT and MRI gives clear definition of the site, extent, and direction of growth, as well as the nature of the tumor, e.g. focal, diffuse, solid, or cystic.[18–20] Symptoms at presentation are dictated by the level of the lesion in the brainstem (midbrain, pons, medulla) and by the rate and direction of growth of the tumor. Delays in diagnosis may be a problem if there is a lack of appreciation of the significance of symptoms and signs[21–24] and can lead to enhanced distress for the child and parents.

NEUROFIBROMATOSIS TYPE 1

Patients with neurofibromatosis type 1 (NF-1) have a predisposition to develop astrocytic tumors, which most commonly occur in the region of the hypothalamus/optic chiasm. They can also occur, less frequently, in the brainstem.[25–27] They may be confused with unidentified bright objects (UBOs) on MRI; furthermore, enlargement of the brainstem is a recognized feature of patients with NF-1. These abnormal appearances can enlarge and recede asymptomatically during childhood and adolescence. Magnetic resonance spectroscopy (MRS) has been shown to assist in differentiation between UBOs and tumor.[28] Brainstem tumors associated with NF-1 are more commonly medullary in location. Indications for treatment are based predominantly on the severity and rate of progression of symptoms. Selection of patients for surgery in order to relieve raised intracranial pressure and biopsy/debulk tumor is discussed below. Treatment with radiotherapy is associated with enhanced risk of serious neurotoxicity, characterized by clinical deterioration due to progressive neurological symptoms centered upon brainstem function and necrotic deterioration of the tumor. A cautious approach is recommended, reserving radiotherapy for patients with troublesome and progressive symptoms that are linked clearly to tumor progression.[26,27,29,30]

INITIAL ASSESSMENT

The first step to successful clinical management is to establish an effective clinical working relationship between the multidisciplinary team and the family. There must be a consensus on the anatomical and imaging classification of the tumor within the clinical team before meaningful parental counseling can be commenced. Where there is not consensus, the team must resolve this by seeking other opinions and agreeing a strategy. If the agreed diagnosis is diffuse intrinsic pontine glioma, then parental counseling is not easy, since with conventional treatment there is so little hope to offer. The scene for success or failure in this process is often set at the outset by the approach taken by the individual who breaks the initial bad news. The "Right from the Start Principles" should be followed (see Chapter 28).[31] Neurosurgical options are often an early subject of discussion. The use of phrases such as "inoperable tumor" is likely to bias the rest of the emotional management strongly towards frustration and failure. It is crucial that the neurosurgeon takes the time to explain the rationale behind the surgical decisions; in the case of diffuse intrinsic pontine glioma, it helps the family to understand that operation is not "impossible" but rather "unhelpful." Neurosurgeons dealing with these cases must accept the need for a child- and family-centered approach, otherwise they should pass the case to a neurosurgical colleague who understands that the pediatrics is as important as the neurosurgery. Families appreciate an early introduction to the concept of the pediatric neuro-oncology team and its links to national and international trials groups.[32,33] These organizations provide a network of pediatric specialists through whom alternative opinions can be sought in the knowledge that they are linked to recognized children's cancer centers.

In cases where intracranial pressure is controlled yet there is rapid progression of symptoms, emergency/urgent radiotherapy may be needed to preserve life and therefore initiate effective palliation.

SYMPTOM CARE

The nursing and rehabilitation teams face considerable difficulties in supporting an increasingly disabled child and severely shocked family. They have to provide advice and support for a child who develops severe progressive neurological disability, which can lead rapidly to death. Symptoms can fluctuate widely in severity, despite treatment, without clear reason. The full range of focal neurological symptoms can occur. Pain is not common, except where there is raised intracranial pressure or cervical/exophytic extension. Fluctuating levels of consciousness are common, and periodic breathing can persist for days or weeks as the tumor advances. Alterations in personality or behavior are also common, due to the effects of prolonged steroid use or changes of disciplinary boundaries in the family or as a result of frustration or boredom with reduced neurological performance. Cognitive abilities are generally preserved: the authors have witnessed remarkable children who, despite severe and progressive neurological disabilities, have insisted on attending school throughout their illness. Efforts to maintain involvement in normal activities are often the most effective way of relieving the distress. Effective liaison with schools can assist greatly in this area. Parents and family members frequently acquire and endure considerable personal disability linked to the inevitable emotional burden as well as the heavy nursing load that these children present. Access to social, psychological, and financial support is critical to maintain effective palliation. Back pain among parents is common from lifting and carrying the disabled child. Urgent provision of aids and home adaptations to support home care are high priorities, requiring assessments by occupational therapists and physiotherapists early in the child's illness (see Chapter 25).

Corticosteroids in symptom management

The use of corticosteroids (principally dexamethasone) is a widespread yet poorly defined clinical practice.[34,35] There is no doubt that prolonged use of dexamethasone leads inevitably to the development of Cushing's syndrome. Furthermore, in children with BSG, it also ultimately leads to worsening disability due to a combination of excessive weight gain, proximal myopathy, metabolic disturbance, cutaneous striae, and facial and body disfigurement. This set of symptoms is extremely distressing for the child and family. The change in personality can severely disrupt the child's relationship with parents and siblings. The excess weight gain in a disabled child reduces their capacity for independent mobility and can lead to parental musculoskeletal injuries from the physical burden of lifting and carrying a heavy and disabled child.

It is our practice to explain to all families that prolonged courses of steroids will be used only while arrangements are made to deliver specific treatments to relieve raised intracranial pressure, e.g. neuroendoscopic third ventriculostomy (NTV), shunt insertion, or radiotherapy. If, at other times, symptoms of raised intracranial pressure occur due to tumor progression, which is a rare event in the brainstem, then we use steroids in short courses of three to five days so that their benefits can be assessed by the child, family, and physician. If there is symptomatic improvement, then dexamethasone is stopped after five days with no tailing period and restarted only when the symptoms recur. Commonly, we see more than a week of symptom stability with this approach. We do not initiate steroids for progressive neurological symptoms as a routine, although if the symptoms are severe and progressive during or immediately after radiotherapy, then a three- to five-day (sometimes longer) trial of steroids is used to try to control these symptoms; the steroids are then stopped. We provide the family with a further supply of medication so that they can be started with minimal difficulty, at their own instigation, or after telephone consultation. This approach requires cooperation by all members of the clinical team. The prompt, transient neurological improvements that occur with the use of corticosteroids in the very difficult circumstances before radiotherapy/surgery are often, understandably but mistakenly, grasped by parents and doctors alike as a sign of a treatment effect. We routinely give an antacid with dexamethasone to limit dyspeptic symptoms (Table 15.3).

By adopting this policy, the family has the opportunity to assess the benefits of steroids and is given a supply of steroids that allows them to initiate further treatment if they feel it is indicated. We have found that families frequently choose to withhold steroids when neurological improvements are seen to be minimal. The severely steroidal, terminally ill child with a brainstem tumor is no longer a feature of our clinical practice.

THE ROLE OF SURGERY

General

As with all CNS tumors in childhood, the role of surgery is directed at the control of raised intracranial pressure, the provision of tissue for accurate histological diagnosis, and the physical reduction of tumor burden, with the intention of improving focal neurological dysfunction. The actual role of surgery relates to the site of the lesion and its gross morphological characteristics, as judged on MRI. Detailed gross morphological classification of brainstem

Table 15.3 *Steroid schedule for control of symptoms of raised intracranial pressure due to brainstem tumor*

Indications	Symptoms of raised intracranial pressure Preparation for neurosurgery Antiemetic Control of symptoms during delivery of radiotherapy
Drug	Dexamethasone
Route	Oral/intravenous
Starting dose	5–10 mg/m^2/day in divided doses, or 0.16–0.32 mg/kg/day in divided doses
Maximum dose	16 mg/day; keep doses as low as possible
Notes	For raised intracranial pressure, where no other strategy is to be employed, use short courses (3–5 days) and repeat, if effective, when symptoms return For prolonged courses, use concomitant antifungal and antacid preparations

tumors is now possible with both CT[18] and MRI.[19,20] Subgroups identified by site and imaging characteristics require specific management (Table 15.4). Whenever tumor debulking is being considered, the neurosurgeon needs to consider the risks and benefits as regards operative mortality and worsening neurological disability.

Midbrain tumors

TECTAL PLATE TUMORS

Focal tumors of the tectal plate are often small and produce hydrocephalus with or without midbrain eye signs. They are usually low-grade astrocytomas, and surgery is restricted to control of the hydrocephalus, preferably by NTV[36] rather than by insertion of a ventricular shunt, so as to avoid the morbidity associated with the latter.[37] Although typically indolent,[38] careful follow-up with annual MRI is required, as a number of tumors will progress,[39] at which time open operation to establish a firm diagnosis and to reduce tumor bulk is indicated. The occasional tumor will be large at presentation, spanning the pineal region and midbrain. Estimation of serum levels of alpha-fetoprotein (AFP), beta-human chorionic gonadotrophin (β-HCG), and placental alkaline phosphatase (PLAP) will detect the small numbers that are non-germinomatous germ-cell tumors. It is critical that these tumors are identified correctly, as their treatment is specific and often highly effective, delayed surgery after chemotherapy being associated with reduced morbidity.[40] Biopsy may be feasible at the time of NTV. For the remainder, which are usually low-grade astrocytomas or gangliogliomas, open operation is indicated.

Table 15.4 *Consensus for surgical management of brainstem tumors (UK Paediatric Neurosurgical Group)*

Anatomical site/imaging characteristics	Likely pathology	Surgical management
Midbrain		
Tectal plate	Low-grade astrocytoma; exclude non-germinomatous germ-cell tumors by measuring tumor markers	Observe/CSF diversion if necessary, consider debulking if tumor progresses
Other	As for pons	As for pons
Pons		
Diffuse	High-grade astrocytoma	No biopsy; proceed to radiotherapy
Focal solid/cystic	Low/high-grade astrocytoma	Drain cysts/debulk solid component, RT depending on severity of neurological signs
Exophytic	Low/high-grade astrocytoma	Debulk
Medulla	As for pons	Neurological; results of surgery poor
Cervicomedullary	Low-grade astrocytoma	Radical removal

CSF, cerebrospinal fluid; RT, radiotherapy. From Richard Hayward, personal communication.

Tectal plate tumors

A six-year-old boy presented with intermittent signs of raised intracranial pressure, with headache, vomiting, and intermittent sixth nerve palsy. This precipitated a CT scan, which showed a tumor in the midline around the tectal plate, obstructing the exit of the third ventricle, and associated with triventricular hydrocephalus (Figure 15.3). The patient was treated initially with intraventricular shunting, but he had problems with multiple shunt revisions due to infection and blockage. Subsequent NTV was performed successfully, decompressing the ventricular system. After a period of five years, there has been no progression of the tumor. Biopsy was not performed, but the tumor is assumed to be a low-grade glioma.

Tectal plate tumors present due to obstructive hydrocephalus and frequently do not progress. Therefore, specific therapy to remove or treat the tumor is not justified on the basis of benefits versus risks. Relief for the hydrocephalus is a primary course of action, as is close observation of the tumor to look for evidence of progression. Surveillance scans will identify the character of the lesion with respect to its capacity for progression.

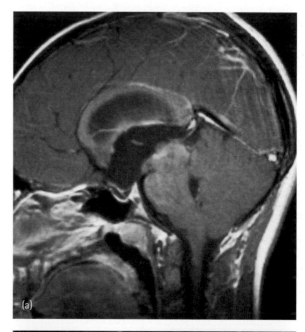

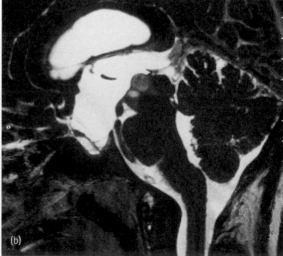

Figure 15.3a,b *Tectal plate tumor: (a) sagittal views T1 and (b) Ciss.*

TEGMENTUM TUMORS

Focal tumors of the tegmentum are usually low-grade astrocytomas or gangliogliomas and should be resected.[8] Diffuse tumors confined to the tegmentum are rare and should undergo image-guided stereotactic biopsy.

Pontine and medullary tumors

DIFFUSE TUMORS

These are by far the most common brainstem tumors. They are assumed to be high-grade, although our own series suggests that up to 25 per cent may be low-grade. Surgery of any sort, beyond that occasionally needed to relieve hydrocephalus, is not normally carried out, as the typical appearances on MRI are considered characteristic and reduction in tumor bulk serves only to add to the child's misery.[41] Although biopsy can be performed safely by image-guided stereotaxy (Table 15.2),[2] there are currently no indications for such a procedure in children with a short history and typical MRI appearances, as it will not alter management strategy.[42] This view may change if biological or imaging markers are identified that can predict more precisely the sensitivity of the tumor to therapy or other biological characteristics that are important for planning therapy, e.g. risk of metastasis.[43–45]

Diffuse intrinsic pontine tumors

A five-year-old boy was referred to a child neurologist with a short history (two weeks) of increasing leg weakness, to the point that he could walk for only a few meters and was incapable of going up the stairs in his home. His medical history was unremarkable, except for febrile seizures during the first four years of life, for which, at the age of 3.5 years, he had a head CT, which was negative. Talking with the parents, a subsequent history of voice change and drooling was elicited as well as some episodes of difficulties in starting urination.

On neurological examination, multiple cranial nerve deficits, involving the right VI and VII cranial nerves, loss of corneal and gag reflexes, and a bilateral lower extremities paresis, worse on the left, with brisk reflexes and a positive Babinsky sign on the left were noted. A head MRI was obtained, and a huge, totally intrinsic, hypointense, non-enhancing pontine mass was identified (Figure 15.4). No biopsy was requested, due to the unequivocal MRI findings and the fears of performing a biopsy of an intrinsic pontine lesion and of not obtaining sufficient material to be representative of the entire mass. Thus, based on the neuroradiological findings, the diagnosis of an intrinsic pontine glioma was formulated.

The child was put on steroids, and he rapidly improved neurologically. He was then treated with external beam irradiation according to the conventional 54 Gy daily fractionated regime. Concurrently, he was also treated with a cisplatin-based chemotherapy regimen, according to the local institutional protocol. He tolerated the entire treatment well, and at the end of radiotherapy he was off steroids, but on neuroradiological assessment the mass had not changed significantly in size.

Three months after stopping radiotherapy, the child's neurological condition deteriorated, with increased motor weakness and cranial nerve deficits. The parents, aware of the severe prognosis of their child, refused any further therapy, and the child died of his disease eight months after diagnosis.

This is a familiar story for a child with diffuse intrinsic pontine glioma. The histological grade of the tumor is unknown, but in Cartmill's series of 18 patients, eight were glioblastoma multiforme (GBM), five were anaplastic astrocytoma, and five were low-grade astrocytoma.[2] The short history in this case is compatible with a high-grade lesion (and the previously normal CT scan). Steroids produced an early symptomatic response, prolonged by radiotherapy, although post-radiation scanning failed to identify signs of tumor shrinkage and symptoms recurred within three months, leading to progressive neurological deterioration and death.

FOCAL TUMORS

These are either solid or partially cystic, have an aspect abutting on the fourth ventricle, and are not associated with alteration in speech or swallowing. This is especially so in tumors with a long clinical history, which are usually low-grade astrocytomas or gangliogliomas. Operation with a view to resection should be considered. Complete removal is not possible, but the residuum may not progress and an expectant policy is recommended following surgery. By contrast, if the history is short, there are bulbar symptoms, and the tumor is solid and placed low in the brainstem, then the morbidity of intervention is likely to be high and resection is best avoided.[10] The limiting factor will always be the concern regarding serious morbidity consequent upon loss of bulbar function. Recent and anticipated advances in intraoperative neurophysiological mapping may assist in reducing neural damage.[46] Once the surgical techniques have been optimized, there will be a requirement for a prospective randomized study to establish the approach that achieves

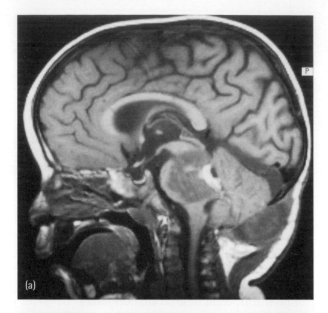

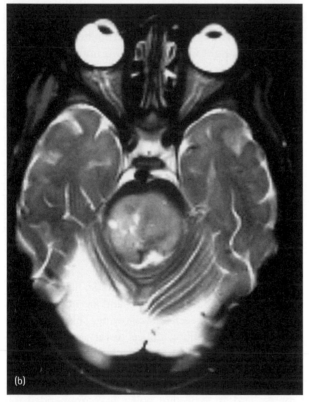

Figure 15.4a,b *Diffuse intrinsic pontine glioma: (a) saggital and (b) axial views.*

the best balance of toxicity, quality of life, and survival. This remains an area in which the surgeon has a very special responsibility to focus on the best interests of the child, which are paramount.

Children with a focal lower brainstem lesion and with a short, rapidly progressive history and very focal signs should undergo biopsy, as the lesion may be a PNET.[47]

DORSALLY EXOPHYTIC TUMORS

These are low-grade astrocytomas or gangliogliomas that have grown out of the brainstem into the fourth ventricle. The symptoms are slowly progressive and usually include features of raised intracranial pressure. Partial resection is indicated, and long-term remission without the need for adjuvant therapy is the rule.[8,30]

Exophytic medullary brainstem tumor: the importance of detailed counseling

A three-year-old girl presented with a year's history of intermittent head tilt, "funny" eye movement, fine tremor, and absence attacks. This constellation of neurological signs precipitated the performance of a CT scan and an MRI scan, which demonstrated an enhancing mass arising from the medulla, involving the cerebellar peduncle, and growing down to the foramen magnum (Figure 15.5a).

This was reviewed by the neuro-oncology multidisciplinary team. They could see no evidence of raised intracranial pressure requiring surgical treatment. They discussed, during counseling with the family, the pros and cons of considering biopsy. The family was reluctant to subject the child to an operation when neurological damage was a risk. The prognosis for this brainstem tumor was considered to be poor. The family elected to treat the child palliatively with analgesia, antiemetics, and sedatives in order to alleviate any symptoms. This clinical course of action was pursued for more than a year, during which time the child started to attend school. There were behavioral problems.

Re-imaging 14 months after diagnosis showed no change in the size of the exophytic medullary tumor. Further re-imaging 26 months after diagnosis, however (Figure 15.5b), showed spontaneous regression of the exophytic tumor. During the second year of follow-up, medications that had been in use to relieve pain and discomfort were discontinued. The girl continued at school and made good progress. She now has no residual neurological abnormality.

This remarkable case emphasizes the importance of being clear in the anatomical definition of brainstem tumor and the importance of histological diagnosis outside the diffuse pontine category for predicting outcome. We cannot be sure what the appearances on this scan represent in this child. It could be a low-grade glioma growing from the medulla and involving the cerebellar peduncles that has involuted spontaneously; these are described clearly in the literature. It could have been a localizing encephalomyelitis that has resolved

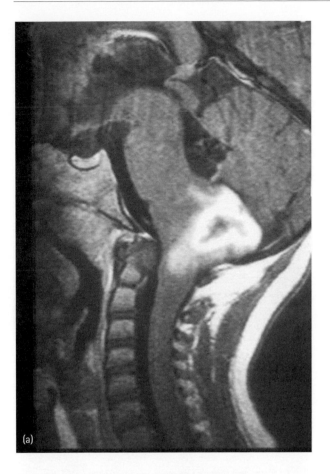

spontaneously with time. The absence of a tissue diagnosis in this case, coupled with a negative view taken by the parents, resulted in a prolonged period of "palliative therapy" using powerful analgesics, antiemetics, and other medications to control the symptoms for a young girl. Had a clear histological diagnosis been made, this may have been avoided, although if it had been diagnosed as a low-grade tumor, chemotherapy may have been offered to control tumor progression. In this case, this would have occurred anyway.

Successful management of these children requires careful, detailed parental counseling. The use of second opinions can often help families come to terms with and develop an understanding of the meaning of the information they have been given and, thereby, optimize the chances for a good outcome for their child with a minimum of toxicity.

CERVICOMEDULLARY TUMORS

These are essentially very rostral intrinsic spinal cord tumors and are amenable to radical resection[48] and subsequent adjuvant therapy according to histological grading and age of the patient.

Low-grade astrocytoma: medulla

A 12-year-old boy was admitted with a three-month history of headaches, nausea, and dizziness, culminating in a blackout. There were no seizures or localizing neurological signs. On examination, there were papilledema, horizontal nystagmus, and mild ataxia. A CT scan showed a large cystic posterior fossa lesion arising from the medulla and crushing the fourth ventricle (Figure 15.6). A decision to operate was made with the purpose of obtaining histological material and deflating the cyst. NTV was performed to relieve hydrocephalus. At the same operation, the posterior fossa cyst was partially removed and deflated. The fourth ventricle drained postoperatively, but the tumor appeared to arise from the top of the medulla oblongata and was not considered resectable without significant neurological risk. There were no neurological deficits postoperatively. His symptoms resolved.

Postoperative MRI showed complete drainage of the cyst but persistence of the mass in the medulla oblongata. The hydrocephalus was controlled well. Histology showed this to be a pilocytic astrocytoma. Because of the residual disease and the severe symptoms, which, if worsened, would significantly detract

Figure 15.5a,b *Exophytic medullary brainstem tumor (a) at diagnosis and (b) two years later.*

from quality of life, it was decided to initiate radio-therapy postoperatively to prevent further progression of this tumor, given the child's older age. He was treated with 51 Gy in 31 fractions over 6.5 weeks. He became unwell with headaches during the course of radiotherapy, and it became apparent that the third ventriculostomy had closed off. A ventriculo-peritoneal shunt was therefore inserted, which resolved the symptoms, and radiotherapy was completed.

Two and a half years after treatment, this patient remains well. He is attending school full-time. The only residual neurological signs are nystagmus, double vision on right gaze, a mild degree of ataxia, and occasional intermittent ptosis on the left side.

This case demonstrates the value of obtaining histological diagnosis in a tumor that could not be graded on imaging alone, the importance of managing the symptoms of raised intracranial pressure with third ventriculostomy or ventriculoperitoneal shunting, and the decision-making surrounding the need to select observation or treatment in tumors at the age of 12 years. Radiotherapy would be the conventional first-line adjuvant therapy for a low-grade astrocytoma. In this case, it was justified by the existence of severe and debilitating symptoms as a result of the large cystic component of the tumor, as well as the solid component within the medulla. Further progression of this solid component would have caused further severe symptoms and justified the use of radiotherapy at this time. We are hopeful that this treatment will lead to long-term control.

THE ROLE OF RADIOTHERAPY

Sadly, the majority of children with BSGs for which radiotherapy is indicated have a poor prognosis. Nevertheless, extreme care in the planning and delivery of the radiation therapy is essential, the more so if novel strategies are to be employed.

Traditionally, treatment has involved external beam irradiation using mega-voltage equipment, treating with 1.8-Gy daily fractions to a total of 54–55 Gy via a parallel pair of opposed fields. The clinical aims of such treatment range from palliation of neurological symptoms in diffuse intrinsic tumors to eradication of the tumor residuum after subtotal resection of focal tumors. In all patients, radiotherapy should start as soon as possible. For those with disabling symptoms, the urgency is even greater. The logistics of treating these children as regards their cooperation, the time taken to make their mask, identifying machine time, etc., makes the ideal of the current UKCCSG protocol for BSG to start radiotherapy

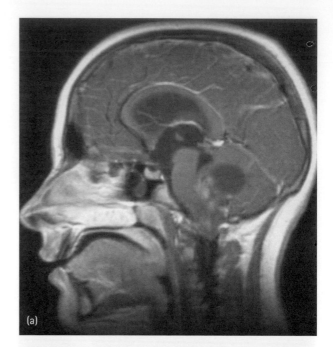

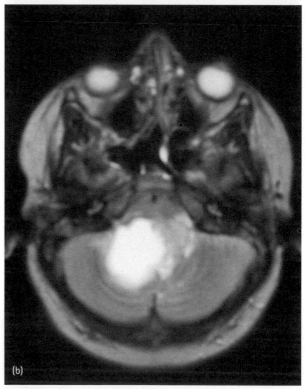

Figure 15.6a,b *Medullary cystic low-grade astrocytoma at diagnosis: (a) saggital and (b) axial views.*

within one week of diagnosis (Eric Bouffet, personal communication) hard to achieve. In practice in the UK, a recent audit identified that the time to start is usually three to four weeks (Elaine Sugden, personal communication, 2001). Steroids may be able to control life-threatening symptoms for a brief period, but longer-lasting benefits

Table 15.5 *Phase I studies in brainstem glioma*

Ref.	Drug	Dose/schedule	Evaluable patients (n)	Response method	Response: CR and PR/SD/PD	Duration of response/survival
74	Beta-interferon	Dose escalation 50–600 × 10^6 IU/m^2	8 rec	CT/MRI	2/3/3	2 PR: 8 and 16 weeks/ns 3 SD: 16, 20 and 32 weeks/ns
75	Temozolomide	500–1200 mg/m^2/5-day cycle every 28 days	10 rec	CT	1/2/7	1 PR: 54 weeks 2 SD: 27 and 20 weeks/ns

CR, complete response; CT, computerized tomography; MRI, magnetic resonance imaging; ns, not specified; PD, progressive disease; PR, partial response; rec, recurrent disease; SD, stable disease.

can be expected only once radiotherapy has been completed. Symptomatic improvement does not always occur during radiotherapy, since some patients, particularly those with NF-1, may experience considerable neurological deterioration. This is thought to be related to the radiation therapy and in some cases is associated with the development of necrotic cyst within the tumor.[29,30]

Delivery of radiotherapy

The preparation and immobilization of these children follow the principles laid out in Chapter 10. The indications for general anesthesia will depend on the age, cooperation, ability, and wishes of the child and their parents. A supine cast is required. As a general principle, the treatment volume of the radiation field should encompass all the site(s) of disease, with a defined margin to allow for non-imageable tumor spread into adjacent brain or upper cervical spine. The pediatric radiation oncologist is hampered particularly by often not having histological confirmation of the tumor type (low- or high-grade glioma). Thus, the margin between the planning target volume (PTV) and gross tumor volume (GTV), be it 1–2 cm for low-grade tumors or 2–3 cm for high-grade tumors, may have to be judged differently for each child. This is not such a problem when relatively large parallel opposed fields are used to cover the whole brainstem. However, if conformal techniques are used, even if aided by image fusion, then lack of knowledge of the degree of differentiation of the tumor may lead to under- or overdosage of the irradiated volume. This requires, particularly in trials of novel approaches, unambiguous, tightly written protocols with real-time review of proposed field placements by the trial coordinators. Similarly, the delivery of each fraction of irradiation must be accurate: machine quality assurance (QA), in vivo dosimetry, and portal imaging must adhere to the principles described in Chapter 10. The dose/fractionation schedule dictates the balance between tumoricidal efficacy and the risks of normal tissue damage.

The optimal target volume and dose/fractionation schedule has been studied extensively.[49] Unfortunately, conventional treatment (54–55 Gy in 30 fractions over six weeks) still yields poor results.[50] Theoretically, higher total doses may produce greater control rates, but in practice a higher cure rate has not been achieved for conventionally delivered doses of 66 Gy. Even biologically higher doses of radiation can be used. Thus, hyperfractionated radiotherapy (HFRT), in which multiple, smaller fractions are given, usually twice per day, has been the focus of much research over the past decade. The therapeutic ratio is likely to be very narrow. Total doses of up to 72 Gy using HFRT can be given safely,[51] but unacceptable toxicity ensues at doses of 75.6 Gy.[52]

These US results (shown in Table 15.8) have been confirmed in a similar study of twice-daily accelerated radiotherapy in the UK.[53] Occasionally, children with multifocal/metastatic BSGs require radiotherapy. Doses and techniques are as for PNET (see Chapter 10). This is a fast-moving area. At the time of writing, the traditional 54–55 Gy in 30 fractions remains the standard dose/fractionation regimen.

Results of treatment

Most BSGs respond transiently to radiotherapy, as judged by the alleviation of neurological symptoms; too low a dose (<50 Gy as opposed to >50 Gy) is definitely ineffective. There is evidence for improved duration of survival in patients given higher doses (>50 Gy as opposed to <50 Gy) of radiotherapy,[54,55] but some of these older studies did not use the McDonald criteria to assess response (see Chapter 8). For patients with diffuse pontine gliomas, the duration of response is brief, and progressive symptoms can be expected at a median of about nine months after diagnosis (Tables 15.5–15.7). Patients with localized and histologically benign disease may have a longer-lasting response, with a 50 per cent five-year survival rate (see Figure 15.1a).[56]

Tables 15.8 and 15.9 summarize published reports of studies of radiotherapy alone and in combination with a variety of chemotherapy regimens, many of which have included hyperfractionated accelerated radiotherapy

Table 15.6 *Single-agent phase II chemotherapy studies: brainstem glioma*

Ref.	Drug	Dose/schedule	Evaluable patients (*n*)	Response method	Response: CR and PR/SD/PD	Duration of response/survival
76	Aziridinyl-benzoquinone	9 mg/m² /day × 5 days every 3 weeks	12 rec	CT/MRI	0/1/11	ns
		18 mg/m² /week × 4 every 6 weeks	24 rec	CT	1/2/21	1 PR: 8 weeks/ns 2 SD: 20 weeks and >144 weeks/ns
77–80	Carboplatin	560 mg/m² every 4 weeks	18 rec	CT/MRI	1/4/13	1 PR: >132 weeks/ns 4 PD: 36, 64, >152 and >184 weeks/ns
		560 mg/m² every 28 days × 2 courses	23 rec	CT/MRI	1/ns/ns	PR: 20 weeks/ns
		175 mg/m² weekly × 4 every 3 weeks	8 rec	CT/MRI	1/1/6	SD: 16 weeks/ns
81–83	Cisplatin	120 mg/m² 6-h infusion	7 rec	Neurological examination	0/2/5	2 SD: 4 and 16 weeks/ns
84, 85	Etoposide (oral)	50 mg/m² /day × 21 days, every 28 days, × 2 courses	3 rec	CT/MRI	0/1/2	ns
86	Idarubicin	5 mg/m² /day × 3 IV every 21 days	13 rec	ns	0/ns	
87	Ifosfamide	3 g/m² /day × 3 IV, every 21 days, × 2 courses	10 rec	CT/MRI	0/2/8	2 SD: 10 and 16 weeks/ns
78	Iproplatin	270 mg/m² every 21 days, × 2 courses	14 rec	CT/MRI	0/ns/ns	ns
88	Methotrexate	8 g/m² IV (4 h) + folinic acid rescue q14 days, × 2–4 courses	5 nd	CT/MRI/neurological examination	0/4/1	4 SD: 28–164 weeks/32–>164 weeks 1 PD: 80 weeks/96 weeks
89	PCNU	100–125 mg/m² or 70–90 mg/m² IV every 6–7 weeks, × 2 courses	17 rec	CT	3/2/12	PR + SD: mean 22 weeks/ns
90	Thiotepa	65 mg/m² IV every 3 weeks, × 2 courses	14 rec	CT/MRI	0/4/ns	4 SD: 12–20 weeks/ns
91	Thiotepa	75 mg/m² IV every 21 days, × 2 courses.	1	CT/MRI	0/1/0	ns/ns
92	Topotecan	Dose escalation 5.5–7.5 mg/m² 24-h IV infusion, every 21 days, × 2 courses	14 nd	MRI or CT	0/3/0	3 SD: 12–28 weeks/ns

CR, complete response; CT, computed tomography; IV, intravenous; MRI, magnetic resonance imaging; nd, newly diagnosed; ns, not specified; PD, progressive disease; PR, partial response; rec, recurrent disease; SD, stable disease.

Table 15.7 *Multiagent phase II chemotherapy studies*

Ref.	Drug	Dose/schedule	Evaluable patients	Response method	Response: CR and PR/SD/PD	Duration of response/survival
93	8-in-1	Vincristine 1.5 mg/m², methylprednisolone 100 mg/m² × 3, hydroxyurea 1.5–3 g/m², procarbazine 75 mg/m², CCNU 75 mg/m², cisplatin 60/90 mg/m² (6 h), Ara-C 300 mg/m² (4 h), DTIC 150 mg/m² (30 min), cyclophosphamide 300 mg/m² every 14–21 days	13 nd	CT/MRI	3/ns	3 PR: 24, 24 and 28 weeks/ns
94	Mustine/vincristine/procarbazine/prednisolone					
95	PAE	Cisplatin 40 mg/m² (4 h) IV, Ara-C 400 mg/m² (30 min) IV, VP16 150 mg/m² (3 h)/day × 3, every 3–4 weeks × 2 courses	2 rec	CT/MRI	0/0/2	0/ns
96	Thiotepa + etoposide + ABMT	Thiotepa 300 mg/m²/day × 3 IV, etoposide 500 mg/m²/day × 3 and ABMT	2 nd 2 rec	CT/MRI	2/2/0	2 PR: 1 alive > 240 weeks, 1 dod 16 weeks 2 SD: ns/24 and 36 weeks
97	Thiotepa + etoposide alone or with BCNU/carboplatin + ABMT	Thiotepa 300 mg/m²/day × 3 IV, etoposide 250–500 mg/m²/day × 3, BCNU 100 mg/m²/dose bd days 1–3 or carboplatin 500 mg/m²/day days 1–3	10 rec 6 nd	MRI	ns	Rec patients: 4.7 weeks/0% nd patients: 11.4 weeks/0%
98	Thiotepa/etoposide + ABMR	Thiotepa 300 mg/m²/day × 3, etoposide 500 mg/m²/day × 3 + ABMR	6 rec	CT/MRI	1/3/2	1 MR: 68/94 weeks 3 SD: 8, 12 and 32 weeks/17, 22 and 46 weeks 2 PD: 0 and 4 weeks/6 and 11 weeks

ABMR, autologous bone marrow reinfusion; ABMT, autologous bone marrow transplant; Ara-C, cytosine Arabinoside; BCNU, carmustine; CCNU, lomustine; CR, complete response; CT, computerized tomography; dod, died of disease; DTIC, dacarbazine ([dimethyltriazeno] imidazole-carboxamide); IV, intravenous; MR, minor response; MRI, magnetic resonance imaging; nd, newly diagnosed; ns, not specified; PAE, cisplatin, Ara-C and etoposide; PD, progressive disease; rec, recurrent disease; SD, stable disease.

Table 15.8 *Collaborative group studies of hyperfractionation for brainstem glioma*

Study group	Study entry period	Ref.	No. of Patients	Dose/fraction (Gy)	Total dose (Gy)	Predicted equivalent dose (late effects)*	Predicted equivalent dose (anti-tumor)**	Median survival (months)	Median time to progression (months)	One-year survival (%)	Two-year survival (%)
POG	1984-1986	2	34	1.1 twice daily	66	53.84	62.08	11	6.5	47	6
POG	1986-1988	3	57	1.17 twice daily	70.2	58.56	66.45	10	6	40	23
POG	1989-1990	4	39	1.26 twice daily	75.6	64.86	72.14	10	7	39	7
CCG	1984-1986	5	15	1.2 twice daily	64.8	54.57	61.51	11	7	48	–
CCG	1988-1989	6	53	1.0 twice daily	72	56.84	67.12	9	5.5	38	14
CCG	1990-1991	7	66	1.0 twice daily	78	61.58	72.71	9.5	8	35	22
POG 9239***	1992-1996	8	66	1.8 daily	54	–	–	8.5	6	30.9	7.1
POG 9239***	1992-1996	8	64	1.17 twice daily	70.2	58.56	66.45	8	5	27	6.7

CCG, Children's Cancer Group; POG, Pediatric Oncology Group. *Equivalent dose at 1.8 Gy/fraction, predicted from linear quadratic formula assuming alpha/beta ratio of two for CNS late effects. **Equivalent dose at 1.8 Gy/fraction predicted from linear quadratic formula assuming alpha/beta ratio of ten for anti-tumor effect. ***Randomized study of hyperfractionated radiotherapy versus conventional radiotherapy; in both arms, patients received cisplatin 100 mg/m² on day 1 of weeks 3 and 5.

Table 15.9 *Combined-therapy studies in brainstem glioma*

Ref.	Treatment	Drug and RT regimen	No of patients	Response assessment	Radiological responses to chemotherapy: CR/PR/MR and SD/PD	Median overall survival/two-year overall survival
99	8-in-1 + RT	Vincristine 1.5 mg/m², methylprednisolone 100 mg/m² × 3, hydroxyurea 1.5–3 g/m², procarbazine 75 mg/m², CCNU 75 mg/m², cisplatin 60/90 mg/m² (6 h), Ara-C 300 mg/m² (4 h), DTIC 150 mg/m² (30 min), cyclophosphamide 300 mg/m² every 4–21 days; RT mean tumor dose 47.75 Gy	10 nd		ns	12 months/0%
100	RT followed by busulfan +thiotepa with ABMT	RT 50–55 Gy conventional fractionation, 60–65 Gy hyperfractionated Busulfan 150 mg/m²/day days 1–4 orally, thiotepa 300 mg/m²/day days 1–3 IV, ABMR 48 h after completion of chemotherapy	36 nd	MRI/neurological assessment	OR 1, otherwise ns	10 months/4%
101	Tamoxifen + RT	Tamoxifen 200 mg/m²/day for 52 weeks; RT mean tumor dose 54 Gy	29 nd recruited, 27 completed RT, 22 assessable for response	MRI 4–8 weeks after completion of RT	11/8/3	10.9 months/28%
102	Cisplatin + cyclophosphamide + HFRT	Cisplatin 100 mg/m², cyclophosphamide 3 g/m², HFRT 66 Gy	36 nd, 32 eligible	MRI/CT/neurological assessment	3/23/6	9/10 months/14%; 3 long-term survivors (>38, >44, 40 months)
103	Carboplatin concurrent with HFRT	Carboplatin IV dose escalation 20 mg/m² × 2/week for 7 weeks, dose increments 15 mg/m² to DLT	34 nd 29 evaluable	MRI/neurological assessment	15/8/6	12 months/15% >46 months overall survival
104	Dose-intensive, time-compressed PCV + PBSC + RT	CCNU 130 mg/m² IV day 1, procarbazine 150 mg/m² days 1–7, vincristine 1.5 mg/m² day 1 + PBSC reinfusion day 9; RT 5.4–5.94 Gy	6 nd	MRI	3/ns/ns	8 months/ns
105	Carboplatin/etoposide + HFRT	Etoposide 120 mg/m²/day days 1–3 IV, carboplatin IV dose escalation, AUC 2 mg/ml × minutes from 8–12 mg/ml × minutes × 2 courses before RT; RT 70.2 Gy over six days, 2×/day	9 nd	MRI/neurological assessment	ns	11 months/10%
106	Concurrent carboplatin + RT	Before RT: carboplatin 350 mg/m²/day × 3 every 21–28 days, × 2 courses; concurrent with RT: carboplatin 200 mg/m²/week, × 5 courses; RT 54 Gy	38 nd	MRI	ns	11 months/5%

ABMR, autologous bone marrow reinfusion; ABMT, autologous bone marrow transplant; Ara-C, cytosine Arabinoside; AUC; area under curve; BCNU, carmustine; CCNU, lomustine; CR, complete response; CT, computed tomography; DLT, dose-limiting toxicity; DTIC, dacarbazine ([dimethyltriazeno] imidazole-carboxamide); HFRT, hyperfractionated radiotherapy; IV, intravenous; MR, minor response; MRI, magnetic resonance imaging; nd, newly diagnosed; ns, not specified; PBSC, peripheral blood stem cell; PCV, procarbazine, PD, progressive disease; PR, partial response; rec, recurrent disease; RT, radiotherapy; SD, stable disease; VCR, vincristine.

(HART) and continuous hyperfractionated accelerated radiotherapy (CHART) regimens, but even these have not produced median survival times of more than one year. Most recently, concern has been expressed that cisplatin, when used as a radiosensitizing agent concomitantly with HFRT, may lead to worse outcomes when compared with HFRT alone. This highlights the importance of considering both risks and benefits of any new approaches to treatment in this disease.[57]

Editorial comment
Hyperfractionated radiotherapy for diffuse pontine glioma

Compared with conventionally fractionated radiotherapy, HFRT involves giving a smaller dose per fraction, usually with fractions administered twice daily. The total dose is increased and the total duration of treatment remains approximately the same. Small doses given more than once a day, usually six to eight hours apart, produce a redistribution of proliferating tumor cells, with some cells entering a radiosensitive stage. Other, non-proliferating issues, such as normal CNS, will potentially be spared this effect of redistribution. HFRT exploits the differences in repair capacity between tumor and late-responding normal tissues, such as the CNS. Thus, the aim of HFRT is to improve the therapeutic ratio by enhancing the antitumor effect, without an increase in late effects.

The optimal target volume and dose/fractionation schedule has been reviewed extensively.[49] Unfortunately, the outcome following conventional radiotherapy (54 Gy in 30 fractions) remains poor. Progression of diffuse pontine glioma is nearly always local rather than metastatic. This provides the rationale for aiming to improve the local control from radiotherapy. The use of HFRT has been investigated thoroughly in a series of North American single-center and collaborative group (Pediatric Oncology Group (POG), Children's Cancer Group (CCG)) studies (Table 15.8).[51,52,58–62] The radiation dose that can be delivered to the brain in conventionally fractionated radiotherapy is limited by tolerance of the CNS, particularly the brainstem. The aim of HFRT is to improve the therapeutic ratio of radiotherapy by increasing the biological effect on the tumor without an increase in normal tissue morbidity. In these series, escalating total radiation doses from 64.8 Gy to 78 Gy has been investigated. Early studies from the University of California, San Francisco, employing a dose of 1 Gy twice daily to a total of 72 Gy suggested an improved outcome compared with conventional fractionation.[63] In the intermediate dose range of 70.2 Gy given in fractions of 1.17 Gy twice daily (POG)[3] and for 72 Gy given in fractions of 1 Gy twice daily (CCG),[51] there

was evidence of a marginal benefit compared with conventional fractionation and lower doses of HFRT (66 Gy). However, this benefit was lost at the higher dose levels of 75.6 Gy (POG)[52] and 78 Gy (CCG).[61] In addition, unacceptable toxicity, including steroid dependency, white-matter changes, hearing loss, and epileptic disorders, were experienced in the few long-term survivors.[52,64]

Between 1992 and 1996, POG conducted a randomized study comparing HFRT 70.2 Gy given in fractions of 1.17 Gy twice daily with conventionally fractionated radiotherapy 54 Gy given in fractions of 1.8 Gy. Patients received cisplatin 100 mg/m^2 on day 1 of weeks 3 and 5 during radiotherapy in both arms of the study. There was no difference in outcome, which was poor in both arms (median survival eight months for HFRT and 8.5 months for conventional radiotherapy).

In the UK, the alternative approach of accelerated radiotherapy using a conventional fraction size (1.8 Gy) given twice daily to a dose of 50.4 Gy has been investigated.[53] In this study, the outcome was no better than would have been expected from conventional fractionation. Treatment was completed within three weeks as opposed to the usual six weeks. It has been suggested that this was an advantage for the patient and family. However, travelling for twice-daily radiotherapy is disruptive and time-consuming. In addition, for many families, completing radiotherapy within three weeks did not allow sufficient time with members of the multidisciplinary team to help them come to terms with the diagnosis.

Why has HFRT not been of value? The radiobiological parameters of tumor cells can be assessed from either in vitro studies or in vivo "iso-effect" studies comparing different dose/fractionation regimens. These data do not exist for diffuse pontine glioma, and therefore the HFRT series provided an empirical attempt to exploit a radiobiological mechanism. Presumably the radiobiological parameters of diffuse pontine glioma, possibly due to tumor heterogeneity, do not favor a lower dose per fraction. In addition, even though the equivalent dose in these studies was escalated to a significantly higher level than for conventional radiotherapy, there was no improvement in outcome, even at dose levels that resulted in excess late toxicity. However, the series of North American HFRT studies was a success in the sense that the potential for exploiting a radiobiological mechanism was evaluated thoroughly and radiotherapy quality assurance procedures continued to evolve and improve. Interest was generated in trying to improve outcome for a disease with a very poor prognosis, and outcome data provide a useful baseline for comparison with current and future studies.

Toxicity during and after treatment

For most children and their families, the logistics of radiotherapy should present few difficulties, as the treatment is painless and tolerated well. Very young children (under three to five years of age) may require daily anesthetics (see Chapter 10), but older children seldom require sedation, providing that the initial planning process is coordinated smoothly. Clear explanations through play therapy, training videos, and departmental visits before treatment ensure good cooperation in the majority (see Chapter 10). If parallel opposed fields are used, then hair loss in the radiation fields is inevitable. It usually regrows well, but there is an impression that hair recovery is less good if concomitant chemoradiotherapy is used. The other critical structures adjacent to the PTV are the midbrain, the occipital and parietal lobes, the middle and inner ears, and the hypothalamic/pituitary axis. Conformal radiotherapy obviously seeks to reduce the dose to these areas while retaining dose homogeneity within the PTV. Radiation brain necrosis is rare (two per cent) and usually untreatable, other than with steroids to reduce the surrounding edema. It can be difficult to distinguish from recurrence unless scanning directed at estimating tissue metabolism is employed, e.g. thallium or single-photon-emission computed tomography (SPECT) scanning.[65] Deafness may be exacerbated by concomitant or sequential cisplatin chemotherapy. Hypopituitarism should be assessed prospectively and hormone replacement given to the few long-term survivors who develop this complication.

THE ROLE OF CHEMOTHERAPY

Nowhere is the inherent optimism and the restless therapeutic enthusiasm of individuals working through institutional and cooperative groups in pediatric oncology demonstrated more clearly than in the investigation of novel drug treatments in brainstem glioma, the focus having been the typical diffuse pontine glioma. The past two decades have seen a massive scientific effort to study new treatment techniques in a wide range of study settings (see Tables 15.5–15.7 and 15.9), yet there has been no demonstrable evidence that outcomes using the new techniques being tested are superior in any way, regarding survival outcome compared with the use of conventional radiotherapy alone (Table 15.8).[66–68] Relatively few papers have reported the outcome for children without typical diffuse pontine tumors. The UK registry data (see Table 15.1 and Figure 15.1) highlight the importance for histological grading of brainstem tumors where those identified as low-grade histology have a 53 per cent five-year survival rate. Detailed review of the results of treatment on low-grade astrocytomas is provided in Chapter 13b.

Phase 3 study of chemotherapy in brainstem glioma

Only one randomized study of adjuvant chemotherapy has been carried out in this tumor group. Seventy of 74 eligible patients with pontine and medullary gliomas were randomized to receive or not receive prednisolone, lomustine, and vincristine after conventional dose radiotherapy (dose ranges given 42–59 Gy) or radiotherapy alone. Tissue specimens were obtained in 32 patients and were diagnostic in 23, of which 11 were low-grade astrocytoma, nine were glioblastoma multiforme, one was ganglioglioma, and two were mixed histologies. The chemotherapy was tolerated well. The five-year overall survival rate for the whole group was 20 per cent. The five-year overall survival rates for radiation only and radiation plus adjuvant therapy group, respectively, were 17 per cent and 23 per cent. The five-year relapse-free survival rates, respectively, were 17 per cent and 17 per cent. The median times to relapse, respectively, were eight months and seven months. The authors concluded that vincristine did not contribute to enhanced survival in BSG in contrast to the experience in high-grade astrocytomas of the cerebral hemispheres.[50]

Phase 2 studies of single-agent and combined-agent regimens

Phase 2 studies of single and multiple agents, in conventional doses and in high doses with stem cell/bone marrow rescue, have been conducted (Tables 15.6 and 15.7). The studies extend over a prolonged time period and include patients diagnosed in the CT era when the definitions of brainstem tumor were less clear-cut. Conventional imaging criteria of response in these tumors have been modified to accept stable disease as evidence of effectiveness for the purposes of this analysis of an extensive literature review. The limitations of this approach must be stated, as there is uncertainty of the natural history of the appearances of these tumors when they have been irradiated. Cystic change can lead to tumor enlargement and clinical deterioration because of direct effects on the surrounding brainstem. However, the cystic change can be linked to tumor necrosis, which may, in some cases, be a product of tumor response.[69] Time to progression is used as a second criterion for assessing response in this analysis. From this, a number of conclusions can be advanced. Response rates with multiple agents are generally higher than in those using single agents; however, the times to progression do not seem to differ. Secondly, there are a few patients who have very prolonged survival, for which there is no clear explanation. Whether this is due to bias in case selection or heterogeneity of biological sensitivity to treatment is not clear. Our own series of biopsied diffuse pontine tumors identified

28 per cent low-grade tumors with acceptable transient morbidity (Table 15.2).

Novel approaches to drug treatment

Other treatments have been tried in this resistant tumor, including beta-interferon and tamoxifen (Table 15.5). The latter has been studied in combination with radiotherapy. Neither has produced remarkable responses, suggesting that their non-cytotoxic pedigree offers little hope of an alternative effective treatment strategy.

COMBINED CHEMOTHERAPY AND RADIOTHERAPY

In this review, we have summarized the experience of trials of combined treatments in newly diagnosed patients (Table 15.9). Drug combinations varied but were generally intensive for the time period in which the study was conducted and were given before, in parallel with, or after radiotherapy. Response rates for chemotherapy regimens were not generally recorded, as radiotherapy was integral to the protocol and it was not possible to differentiate the effect on the tumor of one treatment from the other. Time to progression was the most widely reported outcome, although a number of studies reported overall survival rates. What is remarkable is that despite these intensive efforts with chemotherapy and radiotherapy, the reported median times to progression are remarkably constant (four to eight months, where reported) and the overall survival is similarly constant (8–12 months, where reported). These results are also remarkably similar to those of the randomized study conducted by the UKCCSG.[50]

FUNCTIONAL IMAGING OF RESPONSE

It is hoped that positron-emission tomography (PET), SPECT, and/or magnetic resonance spectroscopy (MRS) will, in the future, help to identify metabolic changes indicative of tumor response. Such techniques, when standardized and available widely, may provide a more precise way of determining qualitative changes indicative of tumor response to new treatments, which may help to select better treatment approaches.[43–45,65]

OUTCOMES FOR SURVIVORS

For the minority of patients who survive a typical diffuse pontine glioma, and for those children who have the more

indolent or low-grade tumors that are amenable to resection and/or adjuvant therapy, predicting the future quality of survival is a critical factor in weighing up the risks and benefits of either surgical or non-surgical therapies. Only a few studies have been published regarding long-term quality of survival in these patient groups. Where outcomes have been described, they have been reported mainly in institutional series after only operative intervention, and comments have been limited to neurological outcomes using crude classifications of mild, moderate, and severe.[10,12–15,70–72] In the study of Mulhern and colleagues, they attempted to correlate quality of life, measurements of IQ, neurological sequelae, academic achievement, and behavioral characteristics with the treatments used.[70] They studied a cohort of 11 children with dorsally exophytic tumors, treated by surgery alone ($n = 7$) and conventionally fractionated radiotherapy. They compared these with a second cohort of patients who had diffusely infiltrative pontine lesions ($n = 5$) and had been treated with HFRT after biopsy or limited resection ($n = 4/11$). Both cohorts were studied at a median of 2.5 years (range 1.5–5.6 years) after diagnosis. The group who had had surgical resection alone had the best quality-of-life outcomes, having higher IQs and fewer neurological defects than those who had been treated with conventional or hyperfractionated radiotherapy. Further analysis led the authors to conclude that the variance in health outcomes was linked primarily to the severity of neurological deficits rather than to the additional impact of radiation therapy. This would support the view that patient selection for surgical intervention is a critical factor in predicting long-term outcome in these groups. The work by Morota and colleagues in predicting patterns of cranial nerve nuclei displacement may help in this regard.[73] As trials groups develop studies of novel adjuvant therapies in these patients, optimizing both duration and quality of survival must be the endpoints for study as long-term survival with poor neurological function is to be avoided if at all possible.

CONCLUSION

Over the past two decades, CT and MRI techniques have allowed a much clearer correlation between anatomical imaging and clinical characteristics to be defined. This in turn has allowed a consensus to be established with regard to individualized management approaches and to identify those for whom tumor resection is most justified and those for whom it is not justified. In the case of tumors associated with NF-1, exercising caution when considering radiotherapy is strongly recommended, as the natural history of these tumors is more benign than comparable tumors in non-NF-1 patients. In the case of low-grade astrocytomas, the evidence of good long-term

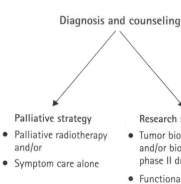

Diagnosis and counseling

Palliative strategy
- Palliative radiotherapy and/or
- Symptom care alone

Research strategy
- Tumor biopsy for histology grading and/or biological targets for phase II drug trials
  - Functional imaging study: natural history study, tumor response study
  - Palliative radiotherapy
  - Palliative use of steroids study
  - Postmortem tissue study/postmortem organ donation programme (cornea, heart valves)

Figure 15.7 *Diffuse intrinsic pontine glioma: a proposed clinical and research strategy from the UKCCSG Working Party (February 2003).*

outcome in survivors coupled with the increasing evidence from clinical trials that chemotherapy can control tumor progression provides hope that outcomes will continue to improve. The greatest challenge is to develop better understanding of the biological factors that give the typical diffuse pontine glioma its highly resistant phenotype. The appalling survival rates for this subgroup justify the use of research-based strategies for these patients. As conventional chemotherapy agents have not been shown to be effective, novel agents with different biological targets must be studied, justifying a strong commitment to obtaining tumor tissue at diagnosis or at postmortem for research purposes. Our experience of the distress of families being told the gloomy prognosis in these cases justifies such approaches, as one cannot predict at what point greater understanding of this disease will be achieved. It is as likely to be with the next child entered into a clinical trial, asking an important therapeutic or biological question, as in ten years' time, with the current track record and approaches to biopsy (Figure 15.7).

ACKNOWLEDGMENTS

The views expressed in this article have resulted from extensive discussions with colleagues from the Kids Neuro-Oncology WorkShop (KNOWS) at the University Hospital, Nottingham, UK, the UKCCSG Brain Tumour and Radiotherapy Committees, the UK Paediatric Neurosurgical Group of the Society of British Neurological Surgeons, and the Brain Tumour Committee of the Société Internationale d'Oncologie Pédiatrique (SIOP). We are grateful to our friends and colleagues for their commitment and wisdom in these discussions. We would like to acknowledge Dr Tim Jaspan for provision and selection of images for this chapter.

REFERENCES

1   Stiller CA, Nectoux J. International Incidence of Childhood Brain and Spinal Tumours. *Int J Epidemiol* 1994; **23**:458–64.

2   Cartmill M, Punt J. Brain stem gliomas, the role of biopsy. *Br J Neurosurg* 1997; **11**:177.

3   Steck J, Friedman W. Stereotactic biopsy of brainstem mass lesions. *Surg Neurol* 1995; **43**:563–7.

4   Sun B, Wang C, Wang J. MRI characteristics of midbrain tumours. *Neuroradiology* 1999; **41**:158–62.

5   Hamilton M, Lauryssen C, Hagen N. Focal midbrain glioma: long term survival in a cohort of 16 patients and the implications for management. *Can J Neurol Sci* 1996; **23**:204–7.

6   Squires L, Allen J, Abbott R, Epstein F. Focal tectal tumors: Management and prognosis. *Neurology* 1994; **44**:953–6.

7   Grant R, Naylor B, Junck L, Greenberg HS. Clinical outcome in aggressively treated meningeal gliomatosis. *Neurology* 1992; **42**:252–4.

8   Hoffman HJ. Dorsally exophytic brain stem tumors and midbrain tumors. *Pediatr Neurosurg* 1996; **24**:256–62.

9   Felice KJ, DiMario FJ. Cervicomedullary astrocytoma simulating a neuromuscular disorder. *Pediatr Neurol* 1999; **20**:78–80.

10 Abbott R, Shiminski-Maher T, Epstein F. Intrinsic tumors of the medulla: Predicting outcome after surgery. *Pediatr Neurosurg* 1996; **25**:41–4.

11 Teo J, Goh K, Rosenblum M, Muszynski C, Epstein F. Intraparenchymal clear cell meningioma of the brainstem in a 2-year-old child. Case report and literature review. *Pediatr Neurosurg* 1998; **28**:27–30.

12 Behnke J, Christen H, Mursch K, Markakis E. Intra-axial enophytic tumors in the pons and/or medulla oblongata II. Intraoperative findings, postoperative results, and 2-year follow up in 25 children. *Childs Nerv Syst* 1997; **13**:135–46.

13 Constantini S, Miller D, Allen J, Rorke L, Freed D, Epstein F. Radical excision of intramedullary spinal cord tumors: surgical morbidity and long-term follow-up evaluation in 164 children and young adults. *J Neurosurg* 2000; **92** (2 suppl.): 183–93.

14 Poussaint T, Yousuf N, Barnes P, *et al.* Cervicomedullary astrocytomas of childhood: clinical and imaging follow-up. *Pediatr Radiol* 1999; **29**:662–8.

15 Robertson PL, Allen JC, Abbott IR, Miller DC, Fidel J, Epstein FJ. Cervicomedullary tumors in children: a distinct subset of brainstem gliomas. *Neurology* 1994; **44**:1798–803.

16 Galbraith JG, Sahni P. Diagnosis of brainstem tumours. *Hosp Med* 1970; **6**:134–41.

17 Sarkari NBS, Bickerstaff ER. Relapses and remissions in brain stem tumours. *Br Med J* 1969; **2**:21–3.

18 Stroink AR, Hoffman HJ, Hendrick EB, Humphreys RP. Diagnosis and management of pediatric brain-stem gliomas. *J Neurosurg* 1986; **65**:745–50.

19 Barkovich AJ, Krischer J, Kun LE, et al. Brain stem gliomas: a classification system based on magnetic resonance imaging. Pediatr Neurosurg 1990; 16:73–83.

20 Fischbein NJ, Prados MD, Wara W, Russo C, Edwards MSB, Barkovich AJ. Radiologic classification of brain stem tumors: correlation of magnetic resonance imaging appearance and clinical outcome. Pediatr Neurosurg 1996; 24:9–23.

21 Edgeworth J, Bullock P, Bailey A, Gallagher A, Crouchman M. Why are brain tumours still being missed? Arch Dis Child 1996; 74:148–51.

22 Saha V, Love S, Eden T, Mitchell-Eynaud P, McKinlay G. Determinants of symptom interval childhood cancer. Arch Dis Child 1993; 68:771–4.

23 Pollock B, Krischer JP, Vietti TJ. Interval between symptom onset and diagnosis of pediatric solid tumors. J Pediatr 1991; 119:725–32.

24 Flores LE, Williams DL, Bell BA, O'Brien M, Ragab A. Delay in diagnosis of pediatric brain tumors. Am J Dis Child 1986; 140:684–6.

25 Hughes R. Neurological Complications of Neurofibromatosis 1. London: Chapman & Hall, 1994.

26 Molloy P, Bilaniuk L, Vaughan S, et al. Brainstem tumors in patients with neurofibromatosis type 1: A distinct clinical entity. Neurology 1995; 45:1897–902.

27 Raffel C, McComb JG, Bodner S, Gilles FE. Benign brain stem lesions in pediatric patients with neurofibromatosis: case reports. Neurosurgery 1989; 25:959.

28 Broniscer A, Gajjar A, Bhargava R, et al. Brain stem involvement in children with neurofibromatosis type 1: role of magnetic resonance imaging and spectroscopy in the distinction from diffuse pontine glioma. Neurosurgery 1997; 40:331–8.

29 Milstein JM, Geyer R, Berger MS, Bleyer W. Favourable prognosis for brainstem gliomas in neurofibromatosis. J Neuro-Oncol 1989; 7:367.

30 Pollack IF, Shultz B, Mulvihill JJ. The management of brainstem gliomas in patients with neurofibromatosis 1. Neurology 1996; 46:1652–60.

31 Lingam S. Right from the Start. The Way Parents are Told that Their Child has a Disability. London: British Paediatric Association [now Royal College of Paediatrics & Child Health], 1996.

32 Walker DA, Hockley A, Taylor R, et al. Guidance for Services for Children and Young People with Brain and Spinal Tumours. London: Royal College of Paediatrics and Child Health, 1997.

33 Duffner PK, Cohen ME, Flannery JT. Referral patterns of childhood brain tumors in the State of Connecticut. Cancer 1982; 50:1636–40.

34 Weissman DE. Glucocorticoid treatment for brain metastases and epidural spinal cord compression: a review. J Clin Oncol 1988; 6:543–51.

35 Glaser AW, Buxton N, Hewitt M, Punt J, Walker DA. The role of steroids in paediatric central nervous system malignancies. Br J Neurosurg 1996; 10:123–4.

36 MacArthur D. The role of neuroendoscopy in the management of brain tumours. Br J Neurosurg 2002; 16:465–70.

37 Punt J. Principles of CSF diversion and alternative treatments. In: Schurr P, Polkey C (eds). Hydrocephalus. Oxford: Oxford Medical Publications, 1993, pp. 139–60.

38 Chapman PH. Indolent gliomas of the mid-brain tectum. In: Marlin A (ed.). Concepts in Pediatric Neurosurgery. Basel: Karger, 1989, pp. 97–107.

39 Pollack IF, Pang D, Albright AL. The long-term outcome in children with late onset aqueduct stenosis resulting from benign intrinsic tectal tumors. J Neurosurg 1994; 80:681–8.

40 Calaminus G, Bamberg M, Baranzelli MC, et al. Intracranial germ cell tumors: a comprehensive update of the European data. Neuropediatrics 1994; 25:26.

41 Epstein F, Constantini S. Practical decisions in the treatment of pediatric brain stem tumors. Pediatr Neurosurg 1996; 24:24–34.

42 Albright AL, Wisoff JH, Zeltzer PM, et al. Effects of medulloblastoma resections on outcome in children: a report from the Children's Cancer Group. Neurosurgery 1996; 38:265–71.

43 Bruggers CS, Friedman HS, Fuller GN, et al. Comparison of serial PET and MRI scans in a pediatric patient with a brainstem glioma. Med Pediatr Oncol 1993; 21:301–306.

44 Nadvi SS, Ebrahim ES, Corr P. The value of 201 thallium-SPECT imaging in childhood brainstem gliomas. Pediatr Radiol 1998; 28:575–9.

45 Maria BL, Drane WB, Quisling RJ, Hoang KBN. Correlation between gadolinium-diethylene-triaminepentaacetic acid contrast enhancement and thallium-201 chloride uptake in pediatric brainstem glioma. J Child Neurol 1997; 12:341–8.

46 Morota N, Deletis V, Epstein F, et al. Brain stem mapping: neurophysiological localisation of motor nuclei on the floor of the fourth ventricle. Neurosurgery 1995; 37:922–30.

47 Molloy P, Yachnis A, Rorke L, et al. Central nervous system medulloepithelioma: a series of eight cases including two arising from the pons. J Neurosurg 1996; 84:430–6.

48 Epstein F. Intra-axial tumors of the cervico-medullary junction in children. Concept Pediatr Neurosurg 1987; 7:117.

49 Freeman C, Farmer J-P. Pediatric brain stem gliomas: a review. Int J Radiat Oncol Biol Phys 1998; 40:265–71.

50 Jenkin R, Boesel C, Ertel I, et al. Brain-stem tumors in childhood: a prospective randomized trial of irradiation with and without adjuvant CCNU, VCR, and prednisone. J Neurosurg 1987; 66:227–33.

51 Packer RJ, Boyett JM, Zimmerman RA, et al. Hyperfractionated radiation therapy (72 Gy) for children with brain stem gliomas. Cancer 1993; 72:1414–21.

52 Freeman C, Krischer J, Sanford R, et al. Final results of a study of escalating doses of hyperfractionated radiotherapy in brain stem tumors in children: a Pediatric Oncology Group study. Int J Radiat Oncol Biol Phys 1993; 27:197–206.

53 Lewis J, Lucraft H, Gholkar A. UKCCSG study of accelerated radiotherapy for pediatric brain stem glioma. Int J Radiat Oncol Biol Phys 1997; 38:925–9.

54 Lee F. Radiation of infratentorial and supratentorial brainstem tumors. J Neurosurg 1975; 43:65–8.

55 Halperin EC, Wehn SM, Scott JW, et al. Selection of a management strategy for pediatric brainstem tumors. Med Pediatr Oncol 1989; 17:116–25.

56 Albright AL, Guthkelch AN, Packer RJ, et al. Prognostic factors in pediatric brainstem gliomas. J Neurosurg 1986; 65:751–5.

57 Freeman C, Kepner J, Kun L, et al. A detrimental effect of a combined chemotherapy-radiotherapy approach in children

with diffuse intrinsic brain stem gliomas? *Int J Radiat Oncol Biol Phys* 2000; **47**:561–4.

58 Freeman C, Krischer J, Sanford R, Burger P, Cohen M, Norris DG. Hyperfractionated radiotherapy in brain stem tumors: results of a Pediatric Oncology Group study. *Int J Radiat Oncol Biol Phys* 1988; **15**:311–18.

59 Freeman C, Krischer J, Sanford R, *et al*. Hyperfractionated radiation therapy in brain stem tumors. *Cancer* 1991; **68**:474–81.

60 Packer RJ, Littman PA, Sposto RM, *et al*. Results of hyperfractionated radiation therapy for children with brainstem gliomas. *Int J Radiat Oncol Biol Phys* 1987; **13**:1647–51.

61 Packer R, Boyett JM, Zimmerman R, *et al*. Outcome of children with brain stem gliomas after treatment with 7800 cGy of hyperfractionated radiotherapy. A Children's Cancer Group phase I/II trial. *Cancer* 1994; **74**:1827–34.

62 Mandell L, Kadota R, Freeman C, *et al*. There is no role for hyperfractionated radiotherapy in the management of children with newly diagnosed diffuse intrinsic brainstem tumors: results of a pediatric oncology group phase III trial comparing conventional vs hyperfractionated radiotherapy. *Int J Radiat Oncol Biol Phys* 1999; **43**:959–64.

63 Edwards MSB, Wara WM, Urtasun RC, *et al*. Hyperfractionated radiation therapy for brain-stem glioma: a phase I-II trial. *J Neurosurg* 1989; **70**:691–700.

64 Freeman C, Bourgouin P, Sanford R, *et al*. Long term survivors of childhood brain stem gliomas treated with hyperfractionated radiotherapy. Clinical characteristics and treatment related toxicities. The Pediatric Oncology Group. *Cancer* 1996; **77**:555–62.

65 Sonoda Y, Kumabe T, Takahashi T, *et al*. Clinical usefulness of 11C-MET PET and 201Tl SPECT for differentiation of recurrent glioma from radiation necrosis. *Neurol Med Chir (Tokyo)* 1998; **38**:342–8.

66 Birch J, Marsden HB, Morris Jones PH, Pearson D, Blair V. Improvements in survival from childhood cancer: results of a population-based survey over 30 years. *Br Med J* 1988; **296**:1372–6.

67 Draper GJ, Birch JM, Bithell JF, *et al*. Childhood cancer in Britain – incidence, survival and mortality. In: *Studies on Medical and Population Subjects*, report no. 37. London: HMSO, 1982.

68 Stevens MC, Cameron AH, Muir KR, Parkes SE, Reid H, Whitwell H. Descriptive epidemiology of primary central nervous system tumours in children: a population-based study. *Clin Oncol* 1991; **3**:323–9.

69 Packer RJ, Zimmerman RA, Kaplan A, *et al*. Early cystic/necrotic changes after hyperfractionated radiation therapy in children with brain stem gliomas. *Cancer* 1993; **71**:2666–74.

70 Mulhern RK, Heideman RL, Khatib Z. Quality of survival among children treated for brain stem glioma. *Pediatr Neurosurg* 1994; **20**:226–32.

71 Mandigers CMPW, Lippens RJJ, Hoogenhout J, Meijer E, v Wieringen PMV, Theeuwes AGM. Astrocytoma in childhood: survival and performance. *Pediatr Hem Oncol* 1990; **7**:121–8.

72 Mundinger F, Braus DF, Krauss JK, Birg W. Long-term outcome of 89 low-grade brain-stem gliomas after interstitial radiation therapy. *J Neurosurg* 1991; **75**:740–6.

73 Morota N, Deletis V, Lee M, Epstein F. Functional anatomic relationship between brain-stem tumors and cranial motor nuclei. *Neurosurgery* 1996; **39**:787–93.

74 Allen J, Packer RJ, Bleyer A, Zeltzer P, Prados M, Nirenberg A. Recombinant interferon beta: a phase I-II trial in children with recurrent brain tumors. *J Clin Oncol* 1991; **9**:783–8.

75 Estlin E, Lashford LS, Ablett S, *et al*. Phase I study of temozolomide in paediatric patients with advanced cancer. *Br J Cancer* 1998; **78**:652–61.

76 Ettinger L, Ru N, Krailo M, Ruccione KS, Krivit W, Hammond GD. A phase II study of diaziquone in children with recurrent or progressive primary brain tumors: a report from the Children's Cancer Study Group. *J Neuro-Oncol* 1990; **9**:69–76.

77 Gaynon PS, Ettinger LJ, Baum ES, Siegel SE, Krailo MD, Hammond GD. Carboplatin in childhood brain tumors. A Children's Cancer Study Group phase II trial. *Cancer* 1990; **66**:2465–9.

78 Friedman H, Krischer JP, Burger P, *et al*. Treatment of children with progressive or recurrent brain tumors with carboplatin or iproplatin: a Paediatric Oncology Group randomized phase II study. *J Clin Oncol* 1992; **10**:249–56.

79 Allen JC, Walker R, Luks E, Jennings M, Barfoot S, Tan C. Carboplatin and recurrent childhood brain tumors. *J Clin Oncol* 1987; **5**:459–63.

80 Zeltzer PM, Epport K, Nelson MD, Jr, Huff K, Gaynon P. Prolonged response to carboplatin in an infant with brain stem glioma. *Cancer* 1991; **67**:43–7.

81 Walker RW, Allen JC. Cisplatin in the treatment of recurrent childhood primary brain tumors. *J Clin Oncol* 1988; **6**:62–6.

82 Sexauer CL, Khan A, Berger PC, *et al*. Cisplatin in recurrent pediatric brain tumors: a POG phase II study. *Cancer* 1985; **56**:1497–501.

83 Diez B, Monges J, Sackmann Muriel F. Evaluation of cisplatin in children with recurrent brain tumors. *Cancer Treat Rep* 1985; **69**:911–13.

84 Needle MN, Molloy PT, Geyer JR, *et al*. Phase II study of daily oral etoposide in children with recurrent brain tumors and other solid tumors. *Med Pediatr Oncol* 1997; **29**:28–32.

85 Chamberlain MC. Recurrent brainstem gliomas treated with oral VP-16. *J Neuro-Oncol* 1993; **15**:133–9.

86 Arndt CAS, Krailo MD, Steinherz L, Scheithauer B, Liu-Mares W, Reaman GH. A phase II clinical trial of idarubicin administered to children with relapsed brain tumors. *Cancer* 1998; **83**:813–16.

87 Heideman RL, Douglass EC, Langston JA, *et al*. A phase II study of every other day high dose ifosfamide in pediatric brain tumors: a Pediatric Oncology Group Study. *J Neuro-Oncol* 1995; **25**:77–84.

88 Allen JC, Walker R, Rosen G. Preradiation high-dose intravenous methotrexate with leucovorin rescue for untreated primary childhood brain tumors. *J Clin Oncol* 1988; **6**:649–53.

89 Allen JC, Hancock C, Walker R, Tan C. PCNU and recurrent childhood brain tumors. *J Neuro-Oncol* 1987; **5**:241–4.

90 Heideman RL, Packer RJ, Reaman GH, *et al*. A phase II evaluation of thiotepa in pediatric central nervous system malignancies. *Cancer* 1993; **72**:271–5.

91 Razzouk BI, Heideman RL, Friedman HS, *et al*. A phase II evaluation of thiotepa followed by other multi-agent regimens in infants and young children with malignant brain tumors. *Cancer* 1995; **75**:2762–7.

92 Blaney SM, Phillips PC, Packer RJ, *et al.* Phase II evaluation of topotecan for pediatric central nervous system tumors. *Cancer* 1996; **78**:527–31.

93 Chastagner P, Olive D, Philip T, *et al.* Efficacy of the "8 drugs in 1 day" regimen for the treatment of brain tumors in children. *Arch Fr Pediatr* 1988; **45**:249–54.

94 Van Eys J, Baram TZ, Cangir A, Bruner JM, Martinez-Prieto J. Salvage chemotherapy for recurrent primary brain tumors in children. *J Pediatr* 1988; **113**:601–6.

95 Corden BJ, Strauss LC, Killmond T, *et al.* Cisplatin, ara-C and etoposide (PAE) in the treatment of recurrent childhood brain tumors. *J Neuro-Oncol* 1991; **11**:57–63.

96 Bouffet E, Mottolese C, Jouvet A, *et al.* Etoposide and thiotepa followed by ABMT (autologous bone marrow transplantation) in children and young adults with high-grade gliomas. *Eur J Cancer* 1997; **33**:91–5.

97 Dunkel IJ, Garvin JH, Jr, Goldman S, *et al.* High dose chemotherapy with autologous bone marrow rescue for children with diffuse pontine brain stem tumors. *J Neuro-Oncol* 1998; **37**:67–73.

98 Finlay JL, Goldman S, Wong MC, *et al.* Pilot study of high-dose thiotepa and etoposide with autologous bone marrow rescue in children and young adults with recurrent CNS tumors. *J Clin Oncol* 1996; **14**:2495–503.

99 Ilveskoski I, Saarinen UM, Perkkio M, *et al.* Chemotherapy with the "8 in 1" protocol for malignant brain tumors in children: a population-based study in Finland. *Pediatr Hematol Oncol* 1996; **13**:69–80.

100 Bouffet E, Raquin M, Doz F, *et al.* Radiotherapy followed by high dose busulfan and thiotepa. *Cancer* 2000; **88**:685–92.

101 Broniscer A, da Costa Leite C, Lanchote VL, Machado TMS, Cristofani LM, Brainstem Glioma Co-operative Group. Radiation therapy and high-dose tamoxifen in the treatment of patients with diffuse brainstem gliomas: Results of a Brazilian co-operative study. *J Clin Oncol* 2000; **18**:1246–53.

102 Kretschmar CS, Tarbell NJ, Barnes PD, Krischer JP, Burger PC, Kun L. Pre-irradiation chemotherapy and hyperfractionated radiation therapy 66 Gy for children with brain stem tumors. *Cancer* 1993; **72**:1404–13.

103 Allen J, Siffert J, Donahue B, *et al.* A phase I/II study of carboplatin combined with hyperfractionated radiotherapy for brain stem gliomas. *Cancer* 1999; **86**:1064–9.

104 Jakacki R, Siffert J, Jamison C, Velasquez L, Allen J. Dose-intensive, time-compressed procarbazine, CCNU, vincristine (PCV) with peripheral blood stem cell support and concurrent radiation in patients with newly diagnosed high-grade gliomas. *J Neuro-Oncol* 1999; **44**:77–83.

105 Walter AW, Gajjar A, Ochs JS, *et al.* Carboplatin and etoposide with hyperfractionated radiotherapy in children with newly diagnosed diffuse pontine gliomas: a phase I/II study. *Med Pediatr Oncol* 1998; **30**:28–33.

106 Doz F, Neuenschwander S, Bouffet E, *et al.* Carboplatin before and during radiation therapy for the treatment of malignant brain stem tumors: a study by the Societe Francaise d'Oncologie Pediatrique. *Eur J Cancer* 2002; **38**:815–19.

16

Embryonic tumors

JOACHIN KÜHL, FRANÇOIS DOZ AND ROGER E. TAYLOR

INTRODUCTION

Embryonic tumors account for approximately 25 per cent of all childhood brain tumors.[1] They originate from pluripotent progenitor cells of the central nervous system (CNS) and share similar characteristic features of morphology and biology. They are classified by the World Health Organization (WHO) as highly malignant (grade IV) tumors.[2] Primitive neuroectodermal tumor (PNET) is the most frequent embryonic tumor. About 85 per cent of PNETs arise in the cerebellum, where they are referred to as medulloblastomas.

Rare tumors such as cerebral neuroblastoma, ependymoblastoma, and pineoblastoma can be classified together with the PNETs. The rhabdoid/atypical teratoid tumor (RT/ATT) and the medulloepithelioma have to be distinguished from PNETs because of different histogenesis.

MEDULLOBLASTOMA

Definition

Medulloblastoma is the most frequent malignant brain tumor of childhood, with an annual incidence of 0.5–0.7 cases per 100 000 children under the age of 15 years (peak five to seven years) and a slight male predominance of 1.1–1.7 to one.[3] The classical medulloblastoma usually arises from the cerebellar vermis. The desmoplastic type arises more often from the cerebellar hemispheres and occurs more frequently in adolescents and adults.[4]

Towards the end of the twentieth century, the population survival rate at ten years remained below 50 per cent for all children with medulloblastoma.[5–7] With modern techniques of neurosurgery and radiotherapy, between 50 and 60 per cent of these children are expected to be alive and free of progression five years following diagnosis.[8,9] The addition of a three-drug adjuvant chemotherapy regimen has resulted in five-year progression-free survival (PFS) rates of approximately 80 per cent or higher, in particular in children with localized disease.[10,11] Unfortunately, children who survive medulloblastoma are at high risk of developing serious neurocognitive, endocrine, and neuropsychological deficits. This is related to a variety of factors, including the direct and indirect effects of the tumor and the effects of surgery. However, one of the most significant factors is the brain irradiation received.[12–14] The long-term sequelae are more dramatic in young children who received high doses of whole-brain irradiation.[15–17]

Pattern of spread

By definition, medulloblastoma is a PNET arising in the cerebellum. The majority (80 per cent) arise in the vermis and the median part of the cerebellum; only 20 per cent arise in the cerebellar hemispheres. The hemispheric location is proportionally more frequent in adults, and the desmoplastic histological form is more frequent in this situation.

Locally, dissemination of medulloblastoma very often involves the fourth ventricle, sometimes reaching the supratentorial area through the aqueduct of Sylvius. It may involve the brainstem, the most frequent area of involvement being the floor of the fourth ventricle. Involvement deep within the brainstem is less frequent. Laterally, cerebellar peduncles, and rarely the cerebellopontine angles, may also be involved.

Meningeal and cerebrospinal fluid (CSF) dissemination is frequent in this disease. Local meningeal involvement may be observed within the posterior fossa, and CSF dissemination may also occur through the involvement of the fourth ventricle. The most frequent distant metastatic sites are in the subarachnoid space, either in the spinal canal and/or in the supratentorial area. Parenchymal metastases within the brain or the spinal cord are possible but less frequent. Metastases outside the CNS are possible in medulloblastoma but are observed very rarely at diagnosis. The less rare sites of hematogenous metastasis are bone and bone marrow. Dissemination within the peritoneal cavity following ventriculoperitoneal shunting has been described but is rare.

Clinical investigation/staging

Correct staging in medulloblastoma is very important in order to make appropriate therapeutic decisions. Postoperative imaging of the tumor bed is often difficult to interpret because of the frequent uncertainty regarding the significance of postsurgical abnormalities on imaging. The best early postoperative imaging is magnetic resonance imaging (MRI), but computed tomography (CT) scanning is often employed. It is important to have an early postoperative exam with and without contrast in order to attempt to differentiate non-pathological postoperative changes from residual tumor. Residual disease is best demonstrated by comparing the patient's preoperative MRI imaging with that obtained postoperatively. It is accepted that the postoperative scan is best performed between 24 and 72 hours after surgery, after which postoperative changes render interpretation of residual disease difficult.

With regard to local disease, several recent series have demonstrated the prognostic importance of achieving a gross total or near gross total surgical excision.[18] This was demonstrated clearly by the North American Children's Cancer Group CCG-921 study, which showed a survival advantage for patients having less than $1.5 \, cm^2$ residual disease on postoperative imaging compared with those patients with $1.5 \, cm^2$ or more of residual disease.[19] Thus, presently the Children's Oncology Group (COG) defines standard-risk patients in respect of local disease as those having $1.5 \, cm^2$ or less of residual disease after surgery. However, the definition of local residual disease has been

heterogeneous in the literature, which makes it still more difficult to know the prognostic value of this parameter. It is possible that prognosis may be affected adversely by residual tumor volume of more than $1.5 \, cm^2$,[19] more than $1.5 \, cm^3$,[20] more than 50 per cent of the preoperative tumor volume more,[11] or no identifiable or measurable residual tumor on early postoperative imaging without and with contrast enhancement.[21]

The Chang staging classification is the most widely used system for medulloblastoma:

Chang staging system for medulloblastoma

M1: positive CSF cytology.
M2: meningeal metastases within the posterior fossa or supratentorial area.
M3: spinal-canal metastases.
M4: metastases outside the CNS.

With regard to the extent of disease, the presence of metastatic disease at presentation as diagnosed by the presence of meningeal enhancement on MRI of the brain (Chang stage M2) or spine (Chang stage M3) clearly carries a poor prognosis.[22] In the MRI era, metastases are now looked for using the craniospinal MRI images. The use of preoperative spinal axis MRI scanning in the case of a posterior fossa tumor has been advocated in order to avoid postoperative artifacts in the cervical region. Good-quality imaging avoiding movement artifacts and incomplete staging (especially the missing of cervical or lower end of the thecal sac) is mandatory in order to determine the appropriate risk group.

The prognostic significance of Chang stage M1 disease, in which tumor cells are found within the CSF and without radiological evidence of metastasis, is less clear, although several studies have shown that patients with M1 disease do have a worse prognosis than those without evidence of such tumor spread.[19,23,24]

Other imaging examinations need not be used at diagnosis in the usual clinical presentation of medulloblastoma. Indeed, bone or bone marrow metastases at diagnosis are rare, thus isotopic bone scanning and bone marrow examination should not be systematically studied initially.

Summary of diagnostic procedures for children with medulloblastoma

- Pre- and postoperative brain MRI, without and with contrast.
- Full spinal axis MRI (if possible preoperatively).
- Postoperative CSF cytology, through lumbar puncture (usually about 15 days after surgery).

Risk grouping

Collaborative groups now generally classify patients according to the presence or absence of prognostic factors:

Medulloblastoma risk groups

- *Standard risk*: <1.5 cm^2 postsurgical residual disease on MRI scan 24–72 hours after surgery, no metastase, and negative CSF cytology (M0).
- *High risk*: >1.5 cm^2 postsurgical residual disease on MRI scan 24–72 hours after surgery, and/or metastases (M1–4).

Common signs and symptoms

Headaches, morning vomiting on an empty stomach resulting in transient improvement of the headaches, and lethargy are often the earliest clinical signs and are caused by increased intracranial pressure. Unfortunately, these symptoms are frequently not recognized early, and less than half of children with medulloblastoma are diagnosed within four weeks, compared with about 80 per cent of children with acute lymphoblastic leukemia (ALL) or nephroblastoma.[25] Some children present with only declining academic performance at school or personality changes.

Further typical signs and symptoms are ataxic gait, unsteadiness, and squint due to a sixth cranial nerve palsy. Symptoms due to local tumor invasion within the posterior fossa include dysarthria, dysphonia, dysphagia (deficits of cranial nerves), and gait disturbance (invasion of long tracts). In infants, developmental delay, irritability, increasing head circumference, and the "setting sun sign" are characteristic features.

Clinical assessment

Good clinical practice includes prospective evaluation of sensorineural and neurocognitive impacts of the disease. Ophthalmic assessment, including looking for papilledema and visual acuity, should be performed initially, at least in the postoperative period, and repeated later because of the frequency of raised intracranial pressure at diagnosis. Furthermore, because of treatment morbidity (radiation therapy as well as chemotherapy),[26] hearing should be studied initially and repeated.[27] Assessment of neurocognitive function initially and prospectively during follow-up appears necessary in medulloblastoma, although optimal timing is not yet determined. Because of the usual delay of cognitive function alteration, and because of the difficulty in assessing cognition in the preoperative or early postoperative period, it is often proposed that these evaluations should be performed at least a few weeks after surgery. However, a better understanding of these alterations in cognitive function necessitates a thorough prospective evaluation with long-term follow-up.[15,17] Health Utility Index (HUI) methodology has also been proposed to prospectively evaluate neurocognitive sequelae[28,29] and to screen for the most important late effects.[15] Finally, although prospective neuroendocrine assessment is part of the good clinical practice in children followed up after treatment for medulloblastoma, it does not appear necessary to have an early postoperative evaluation. Long-term endocrine follow-up starting at one or two years after surgery is usually sufficient to detect neuroendocrine damage, and a baseline evaluation soon after diagnosis does not seem to be justified.[30–32]

Therapy of medulloblastoma: introduction

Medulloblastoma is a highly malignant tumor that cannot be cured by neurosurgical resection.[33] Even a so-called total resection is not a radical resection in terms of general oncological standards. However, the disease is characterized by its radiosensitivity and chemosensitivity, and adjuvant non-surgical treatment is essential. Over the past three or four decades, it has become standard for children to receive craniospinal radiotherapy (CSRT). The omission of CSRT results in a dramatic increase of relapses and a poor outcome, because in almost all patients at least occult microscopic dissemination along the CSF pathway has to be assumed.[34,35]

Although medulloblastoma is radiosensitive, the potential for long-term sequelae associated with craniospinal irradiation is a limiting factor, particularly in young children.

Medulloblastoma is also a chemosensitive tumor.[36–38] However, the blood–brain barrier in the tumor area adjacent to the normal brain and the blood–CSF barrier remains a therapeutic problem, when craniospinal irradiation should be reduced, delayed, or even omitted.

The major targets of our efforts are not only to increase the cure rates of our patients but also to ensure that children cured of a medulloblastoma are healthy and will have a place within our society and not on its fringe. Supportive care and individual rehabilitation have to be part of the modern management of these children to compensate for the neurological, intellectual, endocrine, psychological, and social deficits of long-term survivors for a better quality of life.

Medulloblastoma: radiotherapeutic aspects of management

See also Chapter 10.

CSRT is one of the most complex techniques delivered in the majority of radiotherapy departments. The target volume for CSRT has an irregular shape that includes the whole of the CNS and the meninges. It is generally delivered using a technique in which the lower borders of lateral whole-brain fields are matched to the upper border of the spinal field.

Technical accuracy of planning and delivery of CSRT is essential for optimal results. Careful attention to coverage of the entire target volume is essential. In the most recent North American and French cooperative group studies, the frequency of major deviations from protocol is still approximately 30 per cent; such deviations have been shown to correlate with outcome. In a series of French medulloblastoma studies, the risk of recurrence has been demonstrated to relate to the accuracy of planning, particularly in the region of the cribriform fossa.[39,40]

Traditionally, shielding blocks have been used in the lateral fields to shield not only the nasal and oral structures and teeth but also the lens in order to minimize the risk of cataract. However, the cribriform plate lies between the eyes in young children. It may be preferable to risk the development of a cataract rather than underdose the cribriform fossa, with the increased risk of relapse.[41]

Another major issue in treatment planning for medulloblastoma is the choice of the volume and technique for the posterior fossa boost. Currently, it is standard to irradiate the entire posterior fossa. Using posterior oblique fields planned with CT scanning, it is possible to reduce the dose to the inner ear. This may be of benefit for patients also receiving cisplatin-containing adjuvant chemotherapy.[42]

From several studies, it has emerged that it is important to avoid unnecessary gaps in treatment due to machine servicing, public holidays, etc. The Société Internationale d'Oncologie Pédiatrique (SIOP) PNET-3 study has shown a significantly worse outcome when the duration of treatment exceeds 50 days as compared with the results for children treated as planned over 45–47 days.[43]

The "standard" dose of CSRT for medulloblastoma has been 35–36 Gy with a boost to the posterior fossa, giving a total dose to this area of 54–56 Gy.

Role of chemotherapy in medulloblastoma

INTRODUCTION

Since the 1950s, the standard treatment of medulloblastoma has been surgery followed by craniospinal radiotherapy. The introduction of chemotherapy in the treatment of medulloblastoma was justified to try to improve prognosis. The drugs chosen were those usually used for brain tumors in adults, especially the nitrosoureas.[5,7] The justification for using lipophilic drugs was their ability to cross the blood–brain barrier better. Although the blood–brain barrier is often disrupted by meningeal involvement by medulloblastoma, this is still a potential problem in normal brain, where it is necessary to treat occult distant locally invasive or metastatic tumor cells. The use of "sandwich chemotherapy" between surgery and radiotherapy has been advocated to allow better drug penetration in the tumor bed as well as better hematological tolerance and lower neurotoxicity and ototoxicity compared with giving following craniospinal irradiation.[44–46] Until recently, the benefit of such timing of chemotherapy was not demonstrated in prospective randomized trials.[19,47] However, the PNET-3 study has reported a significant advantage in event-free survival for the use of intensive pre-radiotherapy chemotherapy compared with radiotherapy alone.[43]

In recent years, the role of chemotherapy has become increasingly important for several reasons, including:

- the tumor response rates observed in phase II studies;
- the therapeutic benefit demonstrated in metastatic medulloblastoma;
- the aim to decrease late effects by decreasing the dose of radiation to the CNS in standard-risk medulloblastoma;
- attempts to postpone or avoid CNS radiotherapy in very young children.

PHASE II STUDIES

Medulloblastoma is clearly a chemosensitive tumor, as demonstrated in numerous phase II studies of relapsed patients[48–54] and in the initial treatment of metastatic disease.[9,44,46,55,56] Some of these phase II studies reported only small numbers of patients, and most of them have studied drug combinations rather than single-agent drug therapy (Table 16.1). Thus, there is a degree of unreliability of response rates and the demonstration of individual drugs. However, the chemosensitivity of this tumor is well recognized, and the main drugs that are currently in use are platinum compounds, alkylating agents, etoposide, vincristine, and lomustine. Using active drugs or drug combinations, a complete response rate of approximately 50 per cent can be achieved. The role of methotrexate (high-dose intravenous,[47] intrathecal, or intraventricular) is debated. Its value in the prevention of leptomeningeal relapse is advocated, but the risk of neurological toxicity is well recognized.[45] The outcomes of phase II chemotherapy studies are summarized in Table 16.1.

PHASE III STUDIES

Fundamental prospective randomized trials of the 1970s (adjuvant chemotherapy)

Three large randomized clinical trials involving patients with medulloblastoma explored the addition of adjuvant

Table 16.1 *Phase II chemotherapy studies in primitive neuroectodermal tumor (PNET)*

Ref.	Chemotherapy regimen	Response rate
44	Carboplatin 175 mg/m^2/week	6/14 (43%)
45	Oral etoposide 50 mg/m^2/day	PR 6/7
50	Carboplatin 560 mg/m^2 every 4 weeks	6/9
51	Carboplatin 160 mg/m^2 × 5 days, etoposide 100 mg/m^2 × 5 days	18/26 (72%): CR 8, PR 10
52	Vincristine 1.5 mg/m^2, CCNU 100 mg/m^2, cisplatin 90 mg/m^2	6 evaluable: CR 4, PR 2
53	Cyclophosphamide 1–2.5 g/m^2 × 2 days/sargramostim	PR 9/10 (90%)
55	Carboplatin 500 mg/m^2 × 2 days, etoposide 100 mg/m^2 × 2 days	5/6 (CR 2)
46	Cisplatin, etoposide	10/11: CR 2, PR 8

CR, complete response; PR, partial response.

chemotherapy regimens to CSRT in an attempt to improve survival. The SIOP and the Children's Cancer Study Group (CCSG) both conducted trials in which chemotherapy utilizing vincristine and lomustine given after radiotherapy was compared with the use of radiotherapy alone.[5, 7] Patients randomized to the chemotherapy arm also received vincristine given concurrently with CSRT. Early results of SIOP-I suggested that the group of children receiving chemotherapy achieved survival advantage. However, further follow-up has shown that this initial significant advantage has been lost.

The Pediatric Oncology Group (POG) tested adjuvant post-irradiation chemotherapy using the methochloroethamine, oncovin (vincristine), procarbazine, and prednisone (MOPP) regimen versus radiation therapy alone.[9] Patients treated with irradiation plus MOPP had a statistically significant increase in overall survival at five years (74 versus 56 per cent). The benefit appears to lessen after seven years post-treatment. Together, these trials demonstrated the feasibility of post-irradiation chemotherapy and a slight survival advantage for patients receiving chemotherapy (56 per cent versus 42 per cent five-year disease-free survival (SIOP-1); 59 per cent versus 50 per cent five-year event-free survival (CCG-942); 68 per cent versus 57 per cent five-year event-free survival (POG)).

Prospective randomized trials of the 1980s (neoadjuvant chemotherapy)

These trials were designed to explore the principle of the delivery of chemotherapy during the interval between neurosurgery and radiotherapy, i.e. "sandwich chemotherapy." There are theoretical advantages for giving chemotherapy before radiotherapy. The time between surgery and radiotherapy is when the tumor has its maximal blood supply and the blood–brain barrier is disrupted

maximally. The delivery of intensive chemotherapy may be more difficult after CSRT because of myelosuppression and due to the neurotoxicity and ototoxicity of drugs.

The second European study (SIOP II, 1984–1989) was constructed in order to discover in all patients whether the introduction of a pre-radiotherapy chemotherapy module improved disease-free survival. The sandwich chemotherapy consisted of procarbazine, vincristine, and methotrexate (2 g/m^2 six-hour infusion). There was no benefit observed from the addition of the sandwich chemotherapy. The five-year event-free survival rate for patients receiving sandwich chemotherapy was 57.9 per cent; for those not receiving sandwich chemotherapy, the five-year event-free survival was 59.8 per cent.[57] In the light of modern results of the pharmacokinetics of methotrexate, the sandwich therapy administered in the SIOP II study was almost certainly suboptimal, which may account for the lack of therapeutic efficacy observed.

Between 1992 and 2000, patients were entered into a further SIOP study (PNET-3). All children, with the exception of those with demonstrable metastatic disease, were assigned randomly to receive standard radiotherapy (35 Gy CSRT, 55 Gy to the posterior fossa) alone or to receive chemotherapy with carboplatin, cyclophosphamide, etoposide, and vincristine given before radiotherapy. Event-free survival was significantly better for patients treated by pre-radiotherapy chemotherapy compared with radiotherapy alone (78.7 versus 64.2 per cent at three years; 73.4 versus 60.0 per cent at five years; $P = 0.0419$). Although previous studies had not shown an advantage for sandwich chemotherapy, the regimen used in this study was of the maximum intensity that could be employed before CSRT and included a relatively high dose of carboplatin, a drug that had shown an apparent dose–response effect in phase II studies.[43]

The CCG conducted a trial (CCG-921, 1986–1992) that used neoadjuvant chemotherapy using an eight-drug combination with vincristine, methylprednisolone, lomustine, hydroxyurea, procarbazine, cisplatin, cyclophosphamide, and cytarabine ("8-in-1") and standard radiotherapy to treat patients with high-risk medulloblastoma.[19] The major question of this study was whether neoadjuvant 8-in-1 chemotherapy given two cycles before and eight cycles after radiotherapy was superior to adjuvant chemotherapy used in the CCG-942 trial. The five-year progression-free survival of 63 per cent versus 45 per cent of patients demonstrated the superiority of radiotherapy followed by adjuvant chemotherapy over neoadjuvant 8-in-1 chemotherapy plus radiotherapy for high-stage patients. The major criticism of the inferior 8-in-1 regimen concerned the suboptimal dose prescription of drugs, in particular vincristine and lomustine.

When the disadvantages of dose intensity of 8-in-1 became apparent, the German Society of Paediatric Oncology (GPOH) conducted a single-arm trial HIT '88/'89 to investigate the utility of a more intensive chemotherapy regimen given after neurosurgery but before standard irradiation.[37] The five-year progression-free survival of 57 per cent for high-risk patients who had a complete response encouraged the HIT group to investigate the HIT regimen in a phase III study. In the HIT '91 trial, patients were assigned randomly to receive either the HIT regimen or eight cycles of adjuvant chemotherapy according to the so-called Philadelphia protocol after standard radiotherapy.[47] There was no difference between the Philadelphia and the HIT arms, the three-year progression-free survival rates being 68 and 64 per cent, respectively. Focusing on patients without metastatic disease (M0–1), adjuvant chemotherapy was superior over neoadjuvant chemotherapy (three-year progression-free survival 78 versus 65 per cent).

The POG compared neoadjuvant versus adjuvant chemotherapy on the basis of sequential phase II trials with encouraging response rates.[46,54,58] Patients who were at high risk received three cycles of cisplatin and etoposide before or after radiotherapy and eight cycles of cyclophosphamide plus vincristine. Preliminary results of POG-9031 have demonstrated no significant differences in treatment outcomes between the two arms.[59]

In summary, no randomized trial has demonstrated a benefit for neoadjuvant (pre-radiotherapy) chemotherapy compared with adjuvant (post-radiotherapy) chemotherapy for patients with medulloblastoma. Delaying radiotherapy for patients with average-risk medulloblastoma may even have a negative impact on disease control. However, the PNET-3 study has shown a significant advantage in terms of event-free survival compared with radiotherapy alone, and it appears that if chemotherapy is sufficiently intensive, then the benefit from this is not offset by the short-term delay to radiotherapy. The outcomes of major phase III trials of chemotherapy for medulloblastoma are summarized in Table 16.2.

Prospective single-arm trials (intense adjuvant chemotherapy)

In order to increase the efficacy of CCNU and vincristine, this combination was supplemented with cisplatin, an agent that had demonstrated high efficacy in phase II studies. The combination of CCNU, vincristine, and cisplatin was used successfully in previously untreated patients with high-risk medulloblastoma at the Children's Hospital of Philadelphia.[60] This trial was expanded to include three institutions for the treatment of children aged between 1.5 and 21 years and who were at high risk for disease relapse. Six weeks after postoperative standard radiotherapy, the children received eight six-week cycles of adjuvant chemotherapy consisting of CCNU (75 mg/m^2 on day one), cisplatin (68 mg/m^2 on day one), and vincristine (1.5 mg/m^2, maximum 2 mg, on days one, eight, and 15). During radiotherapy, weekly vincristine (1.5 mg/m^2, maximum 2 mg) was given. The excellent five-year PFS of 85 per cent and event-free survival of 83 per cent demonstrated again the high efficacy of the adjuvant three-drug chemotherapy.[10] The chemotherapy has been tolerated relatively well. However, over half of the patients required modification to the dose of cisplatin, usually because of ototoxicity. The ototoxicity of cisplatin after radiotherapy could be reduced by employing dose-modification criteria to the chemotherapy protocol.

Role of chemotherapy in standard–risk patients

Data relating to the role of chemotherapy in the treatment of standard-risk medulloblastoma are conflicting. Until recently, no benefit of chemotherapy in addition to surgery and conventional radiotherapy had been demonstrated in a randomized fashion for the treatment of standard-risk medulloblastoma.[5,7,57] However, the preliminary results of the most recent SIOP study suggest the benefit of chemotherapy using the combination of etoposide and carboplatin alternating with etoposide and cyclophosphamide in patients that were then all treated by 35 Gy CSRT.

Chemotherapy added to surgery and reduced-dose CSRT with a classical dose on the posterior fossa seems to allow a high disease-free survival rate in standard-risk medulloblastoma. The best ever published disease-free survival in patients with standard-risk medulloblastoma treated with surgery and reduced-dose CSRT was reported by Packer and colleagues using vincristine during postoperative radiotherapy and the combination of vincristine, cisplatin, and lomustine after completion of radiotherapy.[11] This combination is currently accepted as a gold-standard regimen. However, data regarding the immediate toxicity and necessity for dose adjustment in more than 50 per cent of patients as well as concerns regarding late toxicity, especially auditory toxicity,[26] underline the necessity of developing alternative chemotherapy regimens.

Currently, the use of chemotherapy in standard-risk medulloblastoma is accepted by the large majority of pediatric neuro-oncology teams, with two main justifications:

- to allow a reduced craniospinal radiation radiotherapy dose;
- to decrease the risk of development of metastases outside the CNS.

Table 16.2 *Phase III chemotherapy studies for medulloblastoma*

Ref.	Study period	Radiotherapy dose	Standard arm	Experimental arm	Outcome
5	1975–1981	35–40 Gy CSRT, 50–55 Gy PF	RT alone	Post-RT VCR/CCNU/prednisolone 8 cycles 6-weekly	Experimental arm better (NS): 5-year EFS 59% v. 50%; significant advantage for patients with both T3/4 primary and M1-3 ($P = 0.006$)
7	1975–1979	30–35 Gy CSRT, 35–45 Gy brain, 50–55 Gy PF	RT alone	Post-RT CCNU/VCR 6-weekly for 1 year	Experimental arm better (NS) ($P = 0.07$): significant advantage for partial surgery ($P = 0.007$), brain stem involvement ($P = 0.001$), T3/4 primaries ($P = 0.007$)
57	1984–1989	35 Gy CSRT, 55 Gy PF, standard risk randomized to 25 Gy v. 35 Gy CSRT	RT (+ post-RT CCNU/VCR 6 cycles for high risk)	Pre-RT Proc/VCR/MTX (+ post-RT CCNU/VCR for high risk)	5-year EFS 57.9% standard arm, 59.8% experimental arm (NS); no statistically significant difference in outcome between standard-risk and high-risk patients. Standard-risk patients randomized to pre-RT chemotherapy, and low dose RT had worse outcome
19	1986–1992	36 Gy CSRT, 54 Gy PF	RT + post-RT VCR/CCNU/ prednisolone 8 cycles 6-weekly	2 cycles pre-RT and 8 cycles post-RT "8 in 1"	Standard arm better: 5-year PFS 63% v. 45% ($P = 0.006$). Prognostic factors identified: better prognosis for postsurgical residue <1.5cm², age >3, M stage M0 > M1 > M2-3
47	1991–1997	35.2 Gy CSRT, 55.2 Gy PF	Post-RT cisplatin/CCNU/VCR 8 cycles 6-weekly	Pre-RT 2 cycles ifosfamide/etoposide/ MTX/cisplatin/Cyt Post-RT cisplatin/ CCNU/VCR if not in CR after RT	Standard arm better: for M0–1 3-year PFS 78% v. 65% ($P < 0.03$). RFS at 3 years 72% for M0, 65% for M1, 30% for M2-3
59	1990–1996	CSRT M0–1 35.2 Gy, M2-3 40 Gy, 55.8 Gy PF	Post-RT cisplatin/etoposide/ cyclophosphamide/VCR, 1 year	Pre-RT cisplatin/etoposide + post-RT cyclophosphamide/VCR 3 cycles + post-RT chemotherapy, total duration 1 year	No statistically significant difference in 2-year EFS, 78% for pre-RT chemotherapy, 80% for pre- and post-RT chemotherapy. For M1–4 patients, 2-year EFS 61% for pre-RT chemotherapy and 74% for pre- and post-RT chemotherapy
43	1992–2000	35 Gy CSRT, 55 Gy PF	RT alone	Pre-RT carboplatin/etoposide/VCR/ cyclophosphamide 4 cycles 3-weekly	Experimental arm better: 3-year EFS 78.7% v. 64.2% ($P = 0.0419$). Duration of RT >50 days resulted in worse 3-year EFS ($P = 0.0184$)

CR, complete response; CSRT, craniospinal radiotherapy; Cyt, cytoxan (cyclophosphamide); EFS, event-free survival; MTX, methotrexate; NS, not significant; PFS, progression-free survival; PF, posterior fossa; Proc, procarbazine; RFS, relapse-free survival; RT, radiotherapy; VCR, vincristine.

CASE STUDY 1

A four-year-old boy presented with a five-day history of severe occipital headaches, nausea and vomiting, unsteadiness on his feet, a right convergent squint, and diplopia. CT scanning revealed a large tumor arising in the vermis of the cerebellum and filling the fourth ventricle. In addition, there was marked hydrocephalus. There was no evidence of supratentorial or spinal metastases on preoperative magnetic resonance scanning of the head and spine.

The primary tumor was resected using a cavitron ultrasonic aspirator (CUSA), leaving a very tiny area of tumor in the floor of the fourth ventricle. The boy was randomized in the UKCCSG/SIOP PNET-3 study and received four courses of chemotherapy with vincristine ($1.5 \, mg/m^2$) and etoposide ($100 \, mg/m^2 \times 3$ days) and alternating carboplatin ($500 \, mg/m^2 \times 2$ days) and cyclophosphamide ($1.5 \, g/m^2$). Following this, he received radiotherapy 35 Gy in 21 fractions to the craniospinal axis followed by 20 Gy in 12 fractions to the whole posterior fossa using lateral opposed fields. The total dose to the primary tumor was 55 Gy in 33 fractions of 1.67 Gy.

At follow-up five years following diagnosis, the boy remains well, with no evidence of recurrence. However, in school he has some difficulties with concentration. He requires growth hormone supplementation. Psychometric testing has confirmed that he has a full-scale IQ of 68 and a verbal IQ of 81.

This case illustrates the clinical problem of hydrocephalus developing in patients with medulloblastoma. The patient received chemotherapy and standard-dose CSRT at a relatively young age. Although he is free of recurrence, there are significant neuropsychological sequelae. Current aims of multicenter collaborative studies are to employ chemotherapy to allow a reduction in the CSRT dose, hopefully leading to a reduction in neuropsychological sequelae.

Role of chemotherapy in high-risk patients

The most important result of the three fundamental randomized trials of the 1970s in Europe and the USA was that children with high-risk disease had a significant benefit from adjuvant chemotherapy. A benefit for chemotherapy persisted in the SIOP1 trial even at ten years in subgroups characterized by brainstem involvement,

tumor stage T3/T4, and partial or subtotal resection (disease-free survival about 52 versus 33 per cent[7]). A small group of 30 patients with advanced disease (T3 or T4 and M1–M3) of the CCG-942 trial showed a striking effect of chemotherapy: the five-year event-free survival was 46 per cent versus zero ($P = 0.006$).[5] In the POG trial, each of the high-risk subgroups receiving irradiation plus MOPP had a better survival rate than those receiving irradiation alone.[9] The survival advantage was statistically significant among males and in patients aged five years or older (five-year overall survival 82 versus 50.1 per cent).

The results of the SIOP II trial confirmed the benefit from irradiation and adjuvant chemotherapy in patients assigned to the high-risk group defined by incomplete resection, brainstem involvement, or metastatic disease.[57] The five-year event-free survival of high-risk patients who received additionally adjuvant lomustine and vincristine was not inferior to that of low-risk patients. Patients with metastatic disease still did worst.

Less than total or near-total resection, and in particular residual disease after neurosurgery on early postoperative CT or MRI scanning, was an important predictor of worse outcome in children who were treated by postoperative radiotherapy only.[8,61] Efficacious adjuvant chemotherapy could overcome the negative impact on survival.[10,47] The progression-free survival of patients who received the three-drug adjuvant chemotherapy consisting of lomustine, cisplatin, and vincristine was not affected adversely by subtotal resection, brainstem involvement, or younger age.[10] In the HIT '91 trial, the progression-free survival of patients who had a residual tumor after neurosurgery but not metastatic disease of M2–4 stage was 68 per cent at three years, equivalent to the 72 per cent three-year progression-free survival for those patients who had no detectable residual tumor on early postoperative CT or MRI scanning.[47] Adjuvant three-drug chemotherapy had a significant positive impact on these results.

A subgroup that seemed not to benefit from the three-drug chemotherapy were those patients with disseminated disease. Five-year progression-free survival of patients with metastatic disease at the time of diagnosis was 67 per cent compared with 90 per cent for high-risk patients with localized disease. The results achieved with this particular regimen remained excellent in comparison with other experiences of multicenter trials reporting progression-free survival rates below 50 per cent.[19,47]

There has been considerable interest in trials of neoadjuvant or pre-irradiation chemotherapy, an ideal setting in which to test the efficacy of chemotherapy by determination of response in patients with measurable disease. Single-arm trials of pre-irradiation chemotherapy in high-risk medulloblastoma have shown reasonable tolerance and apparent efficacy.[37,38,51,62] Patients who showed a complete response seven weeks after the six-drug regimen of the pilot trial HIT '88/'89 achieved a five-year progression-free survival of 57 per cent, equivalent to the 61 per cent five-year progression-free survival for standard-risk patients.[37,38] These results supported the hypothesis of an increased curative potency of radiation therapy after a significant cell kill due to pre-radiation chemotherapy, but it was never confirmed by other multicenter trials.[63]

Investigators in Europe designed and conducted studies that used pre-irradiation chemotherapy. The French M7 protocol accrued 37 infants and older children with metastatic disease. Pre-irradiation chemotherapy consisted of two cycles of the 8-in-1 regimen and two courses of high-dose methotrexate ($12 \, g/m^2$) followed by conventional radiotherapy and four cycles of 8-in-1. The seven-year disease-free survival was 57 per cent for all high-risk patients and 45 per cent for patients with metastatic disease.[45]

The North American CCG-921 study included patients with higher-stage (M1–4, Chang T3B–4, $<1.5 \, cm^2$ residual tumor on CT/MRI) medulloblastoma and who were aged 1.5 years or older. In the setting of combined intense sandwich or adjuvant chemotherapy with conventional radiotherapy, metastatic disease of stage M2/M3 did worse (five-year progression-free survival 40 per cent). In patients who had no metastases at diagnosis (M0) but at least $1.5 \, cm^2$ of residual tumor, the five-year progression-free survival of 54 per cent was also dismal.[19] Neither 8-in-1 nor lomustine plus vincristine, with a five-year progression-free survival of 45 and 63 per cent, respectively, was able to reproduce the excellent results achieved in high-risk patients who received lomustine, cisplatin, and vincristine.[10]

In summary, pre-irradiation chemotherapy did not improve the progression-free survival of high-risk patients as expected, considering the high objective response rates that had been observed. Even with relatively high response rates, most trials also note a 20–30 per cent rate of disease progression during a three- to four-month pre-radiation chemotherapy regimen.[37,58,63]

The results of studies investigating pre-irradiation chemotherapy were not encouraging and raise the question of the appropriate duration of neoadjuvant chemotherapy before radiotherapy. It is difficult to conclude whether these disappointing experiences reflect a negative impact of delaying radiotherapy or the still suboptimal design of pre-irradiation chemotherapy. Nevertheless, high-risk medulloblastoma patients are the subject in particular of single-arm pilot trials to investigate the feasibility, efficacy, and toxicity of new cytotoxic drugs and drug combinations, especially in an up-front "therapeutic window" setting. Patients considered for treatment with neoadjuvant chemotherapy are young children, generally under three or four years of age. This is given with the aim of delaying or possibly even avoiding irradiation.

In addition, children with metastatic disease (stages M2 and M3) may benefit from high-dose chemotherapy.

Another approach in the high-risk medulloblastoma population whose survival rate was worse was an intensive multimodality protocol using hyperfractionated CSRT and adjuvant chemotherapy consisting of cyclophosphamide/vincristine, cisplatin/ etoposide, and carboplatin/vincristine.[64] The results were disappointing, particularly in patients with metastatic disease. A recent study (CCG-9931) employed multiagent neoadjuvant chemotherapy in a short window before hyperfractionated radiotherapy.

A more direct approach to improving the worse prognosis of children with metastatic disease is the intrathecal or even intraventricular administration of cytotoxic drugs such as methotrexate, etoposide, and topotecan.[65] Encouraging results were seen in patients with dissemination at relapse using the chemical substance mafosfamide, a metabolite of cyclophosphamide used for purging bone marrow before transplantation.[66]

Prevention of systemic dissemination

Improved control of CNS disease by newer techniques and better quality of radiotherapy was followed by an increase in clinically apparent systemic recurrence of disease in up to 20 per cent of patients with treatment failure.[67] In 50 patients treated with postoperative radiation therapy alone, 25 relapsed, six of whom had systemic metastases and died. In a consecutive series of 39 patients treated additionally with pre-radiation chemotherapy, there were nine recurrences, none of whom developed a recurrence outside the CNS.[68] The use of chemotherapy in this series decreased systemic relapses and consequently increased the relapse-free survival rate. In the SIOP II trial, 115 patients had a relapse.[57] Relapse outside the CNS occurred in five cases without a CNS relapse and in two cases with a CNS relapse. Six of these occurred in therapy groups that did not include chemotherapy.

No child has developed extraneural disease at the time of first relapse, when treated by adjuvant three-drug chemotherapy.[10,47] Hopefully in the future, when even more children will achieve a disease control in the CNS by effective local therapy, the prevention of extraneural relapse may become increasingly important.

Recent chemotherapy protocols

Increased understanding of the biology of medulloblastoma, more appropriate use and better knowledge concerning the acute toxicity and long-term-sequelae of the three treatment modalities neurosurgery, radiotherapy, and chemotherapy, and established prognostic factors useful for the stratification of patients have formed the base of more sophisticated treatment protocols. The major goal of not only almost all phase III trials but also pilot trials is to investigate the optimal risk adopted therapeutic concept for medulloblastoma patients providing high effectiveness but low short- and long-term toxicity, thus resulting in a good quality of life of children cured from medulloblastoma.

Patients at standard risk should benefit from reduced-dose craniospinal irradiation in combination with adjuvant chemotherapy. In North America, a recently closed, large, prospective study used reduced-dose craniospinal irradiation (23.4 Gy) for patients with average-risk disease and then assigned them randomly to either the very active lomustine-based or a cyclophosphamide-based three-drug chemotherapy regimen. The experimental regimen is thought to be less myelotoxic and less carcinogenic.

In Europe, a radiotherapeutic question that is recently a part of the German HIT 2000 trial will be asked in standard-risk patients. The SIOP trial PNET-4 will investigate whether hyperfractionated radiation therapy is able to further increase the event-free survival without increasing the acute toxicity and long-term sequelae in comparison with conventionally fractionated radiotherapy using a reduced dose to the craniospinal axis.

In high-risk patients, trials are under way to investigate more effective delivery of radiation therapy using hyperfractionated radiotherapy and of more intense chemotherapy using high-dose regimens and intrathecal administration of cytotoxic drugs.

Almost all clinical trials are accompanied by biological, long-term, and quality-of-life studies to prepare trials that will investigate, prospectively, individually guided therapy.

Randomized studies of craniospinal radiotherapy dose

For CSRT the conventional dose is in the region of 35–36 Gy given in fractions of approximately 1.8 Gy. Concern over the degree of long-term sequelae after CSRT has led to the attempt to reduce the dose of craniospinal irradiation in children with non-metastatic disease.

Two randomized studies of CSRT dose have demonstrated a worse outcome following a reduction of CSRT dose. In the North American POG 8631/CCG 923 study for standard-risk medulloblastoma, patients were randomized to a CSRT dose of either 36.0 Gy or 23.4 Gy.[20] The study was opened in 1986 and closed early in 1990. An excess of relapses was seen in the 23.4-Gy group. In the SIOP II study, standard-risk patients were randomized to two different radiotherapy dose regimens, namely 25 Gy and 35 Gy. There was an advantage for the higher-dose regimen, with a 67.6 per cent five-year event-free survival for 35 Gy compared with 55.3 per cent five-year event-free

survival for 25 Gy. Bailey and colleagues suggested that it was likely that part of this disadvantage for the reduced-dose radiotherapy may be explained by the relatively poor survival in the group receiving sandwich chemotherapy followed by reduced-dose CSRT, and that the poor outcome resulted from a delay to radiotherapy from "ineffective" chemotherapy.[57] In addition, there was variability in the application of strict staging, and it is likely that the "standard-risk" group included some high-risk patients.

In summary, two randomized studies of reduced-dose CSRT have demonstrated a worse outcome when no chemotherapy is given. It is now accepted in North America that the CSRT dose can be reduced safely, provided adjuvant chemotherapy is also given.

Reduced-dose CSRT has also been investigated in single-arm studies. The consecutive study (CCG-9892) was undertaken at 26 institutions to determine the feasibility of treating children between aged three and ten years and who have non-metastatic medulloblastoma with reduced-dose craniospinal irradiation (23.4 Gy), standard local tumor dose (55.2 Gy), and adjuvant three-drug chemotherapy. The five-year progression-free survival of 65 eligible patients was 79 per cent.[11] This confirmed that three-drug adjuvant chemotherapy was able to allow a dose reduction of CSRT in non-metastatic medulloblastoma.

A prospective comparison between patients treated with standard-dose irradiation alone and those treated with reduced-dose irradiation and adjuvant three-drug chemotherapy had the potential to confirm the hypotheses that CSRT can be reduced under the escort of chemotherapy. This study was commenced in North America but had to be closed because of poor accrual.

Medulloblastoma: trials of radiotherapy fractionation

Conventionally fractionated radiotherapy for medulloblastoma involves giving daily fractions usually of 1.67–1.8 Gy. Hyperfractionated radiotherapy (HFRT) involves giving a smaller dose per fraction, with fractions administered at least twice a day. The total radiotherapy dose is increased but the total duration of treatment remains about the same. The aim of HFRT is to improve the therapeutic ratio, either by enhancing the anti-tumor effect without an increase in late effects or by maintaining the same level of anti-tumor effect and reducing late morbidity. The radiation dose–response relationship for medulloblastoma is well known, and it seems that increasing the dose without increasing the late effects on CNS tissue might additionally improve local and metastatic tumor control. Several clinical pilot studies of HFRT for patients with PNET have been carried out.

In one series, following surgery, 23 patients with high stage PNET were treated between 1989 and 1995 with

HFRT 36 Gy in 1-Gy twice-daily fractions to the craniospinal axis, followed by a further 36 Gy in 1-Gy twice-daily fractions to the posterior fossa, giving a total dose to the posterior fossa of 72 Gy in 72 fractions.[64] This was followed by adjuvant chemotherapy for a total of nine months. Of 15 patients with non-metastatic medulloblastoma, 14 were in continuous complete response at a median follow-up of 78 months. The one patient who relapsed in this group had a solitary spinal relapse. Patients with metastases and with non-cerebellar primaries did less well.

In a series from the University of California, San Francisco, 25 patients with medulloblastoma, five with pineoblastoma, five with cerebral PNET, one with a spinal cord PNET, and three with malignant ependymoma received HFRT.[69] The CSRT dose was 30 Gy and the posterior fossa dose was 72 Gy. Patients with standard-risk disease received radiotherapy only, while those with high-risk disease also received post-radiotherapy adjuvant chemotherapy with cisplatin, vincristine, and lomustine. Three-year progression-free survival for 16 standard-risk patients with medulloblastoma was 63 per cent; for nine patients with high-risk disease, it was 56 per cent. For the 25 patients with medulloblastoma, there were only two relapses in the posterior fossa. The results of this study suggest that a CSRT dose of 30 Gy given in a 1-Gy twice-daily dose without chemotherapy is inadequate to control spinal disease.

In another small series, between 1986 and 1991, 13 high-risk patients, 11 with medulloblastoma and two with supratentorial PNET, were treated with a variety of HFRT and chemotherapy regimens.[70] This study suggested that HFRT to the craniospinal axis was feasible. A study of HFRT has been carried out by the Italian group (AIEOP SNC91 protocol). The CSRT dose was 30–36 Gy in 1-Gy twice-daily fractions, followed by a boost to the posterior fossa, up to a total dose of 66 Gy. All patients were given chemotherapy before and following HFRT. Preliminary data reported by Ricardi and colleagues on 23 patients showed clearly that 30 Gy given in 1-Gy twice-daily fractions does not adequately prevent leptomeningeal spinal relapses, even with chemotherapy.[71]

SUPRATENTORIAL PRIMITIVE NEUROECTODERMAL TUMORS

Supratentorial PNETs are rare, accounting for approximately two to three per cent of all childhood brain tumors. They arise predominantly in the cerebral hemispheres and also in the pineal region, where they are referred to as pineoblastoma. It is now acknowledged that the outcome for supratentorial PNETs is significantly worse than for medulloblastoma. A retrospective analysis of 36 children treated between 1970 and 1995 showed an overall survival rate of only 18 per cent at five years.[72] The six surviving patients all received craniospinal radiation therapy; four patients also received chemotherapy. At recurrence, disease remained local in 54 per cent of patients. Local failure only was observed in 71 per cent of 38 patients with progressive disease and who received either neoadjuvant HIT chemotherapy or adjuvant Philadelphia regimen.[73]

Supratentorial PNETs share similar biological and clinical features with medulloblastoma, but the locally invasive growth behavior seems to be more aggressive. This relates to the younger age of children with supratentorial PNET.[37,72,74]

In the CCG-921 trial, more than half of the patients with supratentorial PNETs were younger than five years, compared with only one-third of patients with medulloblastoma. Seven of 18 patients who had undergone complete staging procedures in the Toronto series had evidence of intracranial or spinal dissemination. Metastatic disease at diagnosis (27 per cent) was detected in ten (M1), seven (M3), and four (M2) patients in the HIT series. All patients in the CCG-921 trial and who had metastatic disease at diagnosis (18 per cent) failed treatment.[74]

Using pre-irradiation chemotherapy, the five-year survival rates of supratentorial PNET and medulloblastoma patients were 30 per cent and 57 per cent, respectively.[37] There was no difference regarding stage M2/M3 (ten versus 12 per cent), but supratentorial PNET patients were younger.

The survival rates and progression-free survival of 44 children aged 1.5 years or older and who received neoadjuvant 8-in-1 or adjuvant lomustine, vincristine, and prednisone were 57 and 45 per cent, respectively, at three years.[74]

The neuropathological concept of the WHO to distinguish pineoblastoma/pineal PNET from the other supratentorial PNETs because of a different histogenesis is supported by the clinical finding of a significantly better prognosis for patients with pineoblastoma using the same treatment. A pineal location for the primary was observed in 17.5–30 per cent of patients with supratentorial PNET.[73,74] Children with pineal PNETs (17 of 44 trial patients) did better, with survival and progression-free survival rates of 73 and 61 per cent, respectively, compared with non-pineal supratentorial PNETs.[74] On the contrary, all eight children with pineal tumors and who were less than 1.5 years of age had progressive disease.[75]

There is only a little evidence that the degree of surgical resection has an impact on outcome. While the role of chemotherapy is unclear, radiotherapy (CSRT with a boost to the primary tumor bed) might be the most important backbone of treatment. In a phase II setting using up-front multidrug chemotherapy in high-risk patients, the objective (complete response plus partial response) response rate was 57 per cent for supratentorial PNET and 67 per cent for medulloblastoma.[37] Similar findings in other trials have confirmed that supratentorial PNETs are chemosensitive tumors.[44,76] A significant impact of quality of radiation therapy was observed in the HIT trials. The overall survival rate of 63 children between the ages of three and 17 years with supratentorial PNETs was 48.4 per cent at three years. Reducing the CSRT or total tumor dose or omitting CSRT were associated with a frequently fatal outcome.[73] Because of the poor survival of children with supratentorial PNET, all children should receive postoperative craniospinal irradiation and chemotherapy. Even in infants, at least local irradiation has to be discussed for better tumor control.

Encouraging results were obtained using hyperfractionated craniospinal irradiation with escalating local tumor doses, and adjuvant chemotherapy.[77] Worse outcome in patients with metastatic disease indicates the need for a more aggressive treatment, such as high-dose chemotherapy, which has been used successfully in pineal tumors.[45]

CASE STUDY 2

A nine-year-old boy presented with a one-week history of right hemiparesis and symptoms related to increased intracranial pressure. A CT head scan demonstrated an area of calcification in the left superior temporal lobe and several intraventricular masses in the bodies of both lateral ventricles and the atrium of the left lateral ventricle. There was also an isodense mass anteriorly in the left temporal lobe, which showed minimal enhancement after contrast. The findings were confirmed by magnetic resonance scanning (Figure 16.1) and were consistent with multifocal tumor. The biopsy of the main mass was performed and revealed features consistent with PNET. In order to relieve the pressure, biooccipital shunting was performed. The patient underwent a left-sided burr hole and stereotactic biopsy and then formal decompression of the left temporal lesion with partial excision.

He was treated according to the SIOP/UKCCSG PNET-3 recommendations for supratentorial PNET. He received four cycles of chemotherapy with vincristine ($1.5 \, \text{mg/m}^2$), etoposide ($100 \, \text{mg/m}^2 \times 3$ days), and alternating cyclophosphamide ($1.5 \, \text{g/m}^2$) and carboplatin ($500 \, \text{mg/m}^2 \times 2$ days). Magnetic resonance scanning performed after chemotherapy and before radiotherapy showed an overall reduction in tumor volume. His medication was sodium valproate. Following this, he was planned to receive CSRT 35 Gy in 21 fractions followed by a boost of 20 Gy in 12 fractions to the primary. His

radiotherapy was complicated by thrombocytopenia, and he developed clinical evidence of progression of his primary tumor. He received 35 Gy to the whole brain, 25 Gy to the spine, and only one fraction of 1.67 Gy to the primary area. Owing to his hemiparesis, he required regular physiotherapy during his treatment and had a home tutor to maintain his education.

Unfortunately, progression continued and he died 11 months after diagnosis.

This case illustrates several features of supratentorial PNET, namely the extensive nature of the primary tumor and the poor response to therapy with progression and death despite intensive chemotherapy.

MANAGEMENT OF INFANTS WITH MEDULLOBLASTOMA

The management of infants with medulloblastoma and PNET is problematic. Historically, prognosis in this age group has been poor, but in addition there are serious risks of neuropsychological long-term effects associated particularly with the use of radiotherapy.[78] In an attempt to overcome this problem, all major collaborative groups have employed chemotherapy in an attempt to at least delay or possibly avoid radiotherapy. In the first POG study, children under two years of age were treated with two years of alternating cycles of vincristine/cyclophosphamide and cisplatin/etoposide; following this, they received radiotherapy. Children aged two to three years were treated with one year of chemotherapy followed by radiotherapy. A total of 62 patients with medulloblastoma were treated. The five-year progression-free survival was 31.5 per cent and overall survival was 39.7 per cent. Of the 62 per cent of patients who underwent a less than complete resection, 48 per cent achieved a complete or partial response to the first two cycles of chemotherapy with vincristine and cyclophosphamide. Overall survival was better (60 per cent) for the 20 patients who underwent complete resection (60 per cent). Thirteen patients had M0 disease and underwent complete resection and reduced-dose or no radiotherapy; these had a 69 per cent overall survival at five years.[79,80] In the CCG study that employed 8-in-1 chemotherapy, most patients did not receive radiotherapy; the three-year progression-free survival was only 22 per cent. In this study, patients who underwent complete resection and had M0 disease had a relapse-free survival of only 30 per cent at a median follow-up of six years.[81,82]

The second "Baby POG" study has tested the role of more intensive chemotherapy. Radiotherapy was used only for patients with persistent or progressive disease.

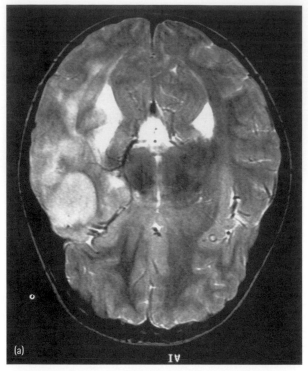

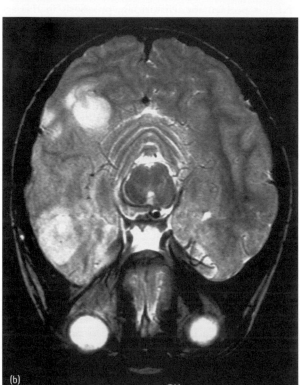

Figure 16.1a,b *Magnetic resonance scan, showing multifocal supratentorial primitive neuroectodermal tumor.*

progression-free survival was 77 per cent if no residual tumor was present (without the use of radiotherapy), 42 per cent for patients with residual tumor, and 27 per cent for patients with metastatic disease.[83] The excellent outcome for patients without residual tumor has to be balanced against the likely risk of leukoencephalopathy and possible neuropsychological sequelae as a result of the use of intraventricular methotrexate. In the German and North American studies, the presence of postoperative residual tumor has been an important prognostic variable for progression-free survival if radiotherapy has not been used.

With the exception of the German HIT SKK '92 study, investigations of the treatment of infants with medulloblastoma have demonstrated a high rate of relapse following chemotherapy alone. Priorities for collaborative groups will be to continue to use intensive chemotherapy with either low-dose CSRT (e.g. 18 Gy), or posterior fossa radiotherapy only. In the recently opened UKCCSG study, the intensive chemotherapy is supported by the use of peripheral blood stem cells, followed by posterior fossa radiotherapy.

FUTURE DIRECTIONS/EXPERIMENTAL APPROACHES OF MEDICAL TREATMENTS

New prognostic factors

Future therapeutic decisions will be based not only on staging but also on tumor parameters, including histological characteristics,[84] immunohistochemical characterization,[85] and biological criteria.[86–88] For example, the unfavorable large-cell type of medulloblastoma is often associated with the amplification of the oncogene *c-myc*. The demonstration or confirmation of some of these prognostic criteria is ongoing in multicenter prospective studies. The definition of biological risk factors will allow the classification of new categories, with less intensive treatment in low-risk patients while maintaining the intensity of treatment in high-risk patients. Currently, the definition of these prognostic risk factors is especially warranted in standard-risk patients, where radiation therapy doses as well as intensity of chemotherapy might be adapted.

Radiotherapy

A priority for collaborative groups in North America and Europe is to aim to reduce the morbidity from CSRT. Following the craniospinal dose reduction from 35 Gy to 23.4 Gy in standard-risk medulloblastoma, as well as the demonstration that full CNS radiotherapy may be

Results of this study are awaited. In the German HIT SKK '92 protocol, in which 45 patients were treated, an intensive chemotherapy regimen was used but with the addition of intraventricular methotrexate. The four-year avoided in young children under certain circumstances,[37,28,89] the next steps should be:

- to continue to decrease the neuraxis prophylactic dose, possibly from 23.4 Gy to 18 Gy;
- to extend the upper age limit for the definition of "young children" from three years to five years, and in the future probably older.

Other attempts, such as HFRT, in order to decrease late effects of radiation therapy without losing efficacy have been tested in limited series and are planned to be tested in a prospective randomized study within Europe.

Chemotherapy and other medical treatments

The recently completed COG trial compared two chemotherapy combinations after reduced-dose postoperative CSRT in standard-risk medulloblastoma. The standard arm was the lomustine, cisplatin, and vincristine combination;[11] the experimental arm comprised cyclophosphamide, cisplatin, and vincristine. The role of preoperative chemotherapy also needs to be explored, after histological documentation of the tumor, especially in metastatic medulloblastoma and in cases where complete surgery is difficult (involvement of the brainstem visible on preoperative MRI). The value of intrathecal or intraventricular chemotherapy is being evaluated in terms of efficacy[47] and toxicity.[37,38] Finally, the role of high-dose chemotherapy in metastatic medulloblastoma is also being evaluated; this approach should be introduced with caution since the survival rate for patients with metastatic medulloblastoma treated with chemotherapy and conventional CSRT is not negligible.[19,45,47,90] This technique is also under evaluation for the treatment of relapse after radiotherapy.[91]

New cytotoxic drugs, such as topoisomerase-1 inhibitors, might be useful in these patients; phase II studies of these drugs are ongoing. Furthermore, new drugs with new mechanisms of action, such as the tyrosine kinase inhibitors, might be helpful and more specific to achieve more frequent tumor control in these patients.

CONCLUSIONS

PNETs, of which cerebellar medulloblastomas are the most frequent, are important tumors characterized by their propensity for metastasis via the CSF. They are "radiocurable," and CSRT is an essential part of their management. This is a complex radiotherapy technique, the accuracy of which contributes to the survival and quality of survival of treated children. It is possible that optimizing fractionation may improve outcome further. In the past 25 years, European and North American collaborative studies have investigated the role of adjuvant chemotherapy. This is aimed at both improving outcome in terms of overall and recurrence-free survival, and also at reducing the dose of CSRT and hopefully long-term sequelae. In this respect, the management of infants with medulloblastoma remains a particular challenge.

REFERENCES

1 Kaatsch P, Spix C, Michaelis J. *20 years German Childhood Cancer Registry. Annual Report 1999.* Mainz: Institute for Medical Statistics and Documentation of the University, 2000, www.kinderkrebsregister.de.

2 Kleihues P, Cavenee WK. *World Health Organization Classification of Tumours of the Nervous System: Pathology and Genetics.* Lyon: IARC Press, 2000.

3 Parkin DM, Kramarova E, Draper GJ, *et al. International Incidence of Childhood Cancer,* vol. II. IARC scientific publication no. 144. Lyon: IARC Press, 1998.

4 Prados, MD, Warnick RE, Wara WM, Larson DA, Lamborn K, Wilson CB. Medulloblastoma in adults. *Int J Radiat Oncol Biol Phys* 1995; **32**:1145–52.

5 Evans AE, Jenkin RDT, Sposto R, *et al.* The treatment of medulloblastoma: results of a prospective randomized trial of radiation therapy with and without CCNU, vincristine and prednisone. *J Neurosurg* 1990; **72**:572–82.

6 Kaatsch P, Rickert CH, Kühl J, Schütz J, Michaelis J. Population-based epidemiologic data on brain tumors in German children. *Cancer* 2001; **92**:3155–64.

7 Tait DM, Thornton-Jones H, Bloom HJG, Lemerle J, Morris-Jones P. Adjuvant chemotherapy for medulloblastoma: the first multi-centre control trial of the International Society of Paediatric Oncology (SIOP I). *Eur J Cancer* 1990; **26**:464–9.

8 Jenkin DK, Goddard D, Armstrong L, *et al.* Posterior fossa medullo-blastoma in childhood: treatment results and a proposal for a new staging system. *Int J Radiat Oncol Biol Phys* 1990; **19**:265–74.

9 Krischer JP, Ragab AH, Kun L, *et al.* Nitrogen mustard, vincristine, procarbazine and prednisone as adjuvant chemo-therapy in the treatment of medulloblastoma. *J Neurosurg* 1991; **74**:905–9.

10 Packer RJ, Sutton LN, Elterman R, Lange B, Goldwein J, Nicholson HS. Outcome for children with medulloblastoma treated with radiation and cisplatin, CCNU and vincristine chemotherapy. *J Neurosurg* 1994; **81**:690–8.

11 Packer RJ, Goldwein J, Nicholson HS, *et al.* Treatment of children with medulloblastomas with reduced-dose craniospinal radiation therapy and adjuvant chemotherapy: a Children's Cancer Group study. *J Clin Oncol* 1999; **17**:2127–36.

12 Hoppe-Hirsch E, Brunet L, Laroussinie F, *et al.* Intellectual outcome in children with malignant tumors of the posterior fossa: influence of the field of irradiation and quality of surgery. *Childs Nerv Syst* 1995; **11**:340–6.

13 Roman DD, Sperduto PW. Neuropsychological effects of cranial radiation: current knowledge and future directions. *Int J Radiat Oncol Biol Phys* 1995; **31**:983–98.

14 Marx M, Beck JD, Müller H, Kühl J, Langer T, Dörr HG. Endocrine late-effects of brain tumour therapy in childhood

and adolescence: concept of a prospective endocrinological follow-up. *Klin Paediatr* 2000; **212**:224–8.

15 Mulhern RK, Kepner JL, Thomas PR, Armstrong FD, Friedman HS, Kun LE. Neuropsychologic functioning of survivors of childhood medulloblastoma randomized to receive conventional or reduced-dose craniospinal irradiation: a pediatric oncology group study. *J Clin Oncol* 1998; **16**:1723–8.

16 Radcliffe J, Bunin GR, Sutton LN, Goldwein JW, Phillips PC. Cognitive deficits in long-term survivors of childhood medulloblastoma and other noncortical tumors: age-dependent effects of whole brain radiation. *Int J Dev Neurosci* 1994; **12**:327–34.

17 Grill J, Kieffer-Renaux V, Bulteau C, *et al.* Long-term intellectual outcome in children with posterior fossa tumors according to radiation doses and volumes. *Int J Radiat Oncol Biol Phys* 1999; **45**:137–45.

18 Albright AL, Wisoff JH, Zeltzer PM, Boyett JM, Rorke LB, Stanley P. Effects of medulloblastoma resections on outcome in children: a report from the Children's Cancer Group. *Neurosurgery* 1996; **38**:265–71.

19 Zeltzer PM, Boyett JM, Finlay JL, *et al.* Metastasis stage, adjuvant treatment and residual treatment are prognostic factors for medulloblastomas in children: conclusions from the Children's Cancer Group 921 randomized phase III study. *J Clin Oncol* 1999; **17**:832–45.

20 Thomas PR, Deutsch M, Kepner JL, *et al.* Low-stage medulloblastoma: final analysis of trial comparing standard-dose with reduced-dose neuraxis irradiation. *J Clin Oncol* 2000; **18**:3004–11.

21 Gnekow A. Recommendations of the Brain Tumor Subcommittee for the reporting of trials. SIOP Brain Tumor Subcommittee. International Society of Pediatric Oncology *Med Pediatr Oncol* 1995; **24**:104–8.

22 Chang CH, Housepian EM, Herbert C, Jr. An operative staging system and a megavoltage radiotherapeutic technique for cerebellar medulloblastomas. *Radiology* 1969; **93**:1351–9.

23 Fouladi M, Heideman R, Langston JW, Kun LE, Thompson SJ, Gajjar A. Infectious meningitis mimicking recurrent medulloblastoma on magnetic resonance imaging. *J Neurosurg* 1999; **91**:499–502.

24 Miralbell R, Bieri S, Huguenin P, *et al.* Prognostic value of cerebrospinal fluid cytology in pediatric medulloblastoma. Swiss Pediatric Oncology Group. *Ann Oncol* 1999; **10**:239–41.

25 Flores LE, Williams DL, Bell AB, O'Brien M, Ragab AH. Delay in the diagnosis of pediatric brain tumors. *Am J Dis Child* 1986; **140**:684–6.

26 Schell MJ, McHaney VA, Green AA, *et al.* Hearing loss in children and young adults receiving cisplatin with or without prior cranial irradiation. *J Clin Oncol* 1989; **7**:754–60.

27 Brock PR, Bellman SC, Yeomans EC, Pinkerton CR, Pritchard J. Cisplatin ototoxicity in children: a practical grading system. *Med Pediatr Oncol* 1991; **19**:295–300.

28 Glaser AW, Furlong W, Walker DA, *et al.* Applicability of the Health Utilities Index to a population of childhood survivors of central nervous system tumours in the UK. *Eur J Cancer* 1999; **35**:256–61.

29 Le Gales C, Costet N, Gentet JC, *et al.* Cross-cultural adaptation of a health status classification system in children with cancer. First results of the French adaptation of the Health Utilities Index Marks 2 and 3. *Int J Cancer Suppl* 1999; **12**:112–18.

30 Spoudeas HA, Hindmarsh PC, Matthews DR, Brook CG. Evolution of growth hormone neurosecretory disturbance after cranial irradiation for childhood brain tumours: a prospective study. *J Endocrinol* 1996; **150**:329–42.

31 Lannering B, Marky I, Lundberg A, Olsson E. Long-term sequelae after pediatric brain tumors: their effect on disability and quality of life. *Med Pediatr Oncol* 1990; **18**:304–10.

32 Adan L, Sainte-Rose C, Souberbielle JC, Zucker JM, Kalifa C, Brauner R. Adult height after growth hormone (GH) treatment for GH deficiency due to cranial irradiation. *Med Pediatr Oncol* 2000; **34**:14–19.

33 Rutka JT, Hoffman HJ. Medulloblastoma: a historical perspective and overview. *J Neuro-Oncol* 1996; **29**:1–7.

34 Bouffet E, Bernard JL, Frappaz D, *et al.* M4 protocol for cerebellar medulloblastoma: Supratentorial radiotherapy may not be avoided. *Int J Radiat Oncol Biol Phys* 1992; **24**:79–85.

35 Landberg TG, Lindgren ML, Cavallin-Stahl EK, *et al.* Improvements in the radiotherapy of medulloblastoma. *Cancer* 1980; **45**:670–8.

36 Kramer ED, Packer RJ. Chemotherapy of malignant brain tumors in children. *Clin Pharmacol* 1992; **15**:163–85.

37 Kühl J, Müller HL, Berthold F, *et al.* Pre-radiation chemotherapy of children and young adults with malignant brain tumors: results of the German pilot trial HIT '88/'89. *Klin Paediatr* 1998; **210**:227–33.

38 Kühl J. Modern treatment strategies in medulloblastoma. *Childs Nerv Syst* 1998; **14**:2–5.

39 Carrie C, Alapetite C, Mere P, *et al.* Quality control of radiotherapeutic treatment of medulloblastoma in a multicentric study: the contribution of radiotherapy technique to tumour relapse. The French Medulloblastoma Group. *Radiother Oncol* 1992; **24**:77–81.

40 Carrie C, Hoffstetter S, Gomez F, *et al.* Impact of targeting deviations on outcome in medulloblastoma: study of the French Society of Pediatric Oncology (SFOP). *Int J Radiat Oncol Biol Phys* 1999; **45**:435–9.

41 Taylor RE. UKCCSG radiotherapy and brain tumour groups. Medulloblastoma/PNET and craniospinal radiotherapy (CSRT). Report of a workshop held in Leeds 30 June 99. *Clin Oncol* 2001; **13**:58–64.

42 Fukunaga-Johnson N, Sandler HM, Marsh R, Martel MK. The use of 3D conformal radiotherapy (3D CRT) to spare the cochlea in patients with medulloblastoma. *Int J Radiat Oncol Biol Phys* 1998; **41**:77–82.

43 Taylor RE, Bailey CC, Robinson K, *et al.* Results of a randomised study of pre-radiotherapy chemotherapy vs radiotherapy alone for non-metastatic (M0-1) medulloblastoma. The SIOP/UKCCSG PNET-3 study. *J Clin Oncol* 2003; **21**:1581–91.

44 Pendergrass TW, Milstein JM, Geyer JR, *et al.* Eight drugs in one day chemotherapy for brain tumors: experience in 107 children and rationale for preirradiation chemotherapy. *J Clin Oncol* 1987; **5**:1221–31.

45 Gentet JC, Bouffet E, Doz F, *et al.* Preirradiation chemotherapy including "eight drugs in 1 day" regimen and high dose methotrexate in childhood medulloblastoma: results of the M7 French cooperative study. *J Neurosurg* 1995; **82**:608–14.

46 Kovnar EH, Kellie SJ, Horowitz ME, *et al.* Preirradiation cisplatin and etoposide in the treatment of high-risk medulloblastoma and other malignant embryonal tumors of the central nervous system: a phase II study. *J Clin Oncol* 1990; **8**:330–6.

47 Kortmann RD, Kühl J, Timmermann B, *et al*. Postoperative neoadjuvant chemotherapy before radiotherapy as compared to immediate radiotherapy followed by maintenance chemotherapy in the treatment of medulloblastoma in childhood: results of the German prospective randomized trial HIT '91. *Int J Radiat Oncol Biol Phys* 2000; **46**:269–79.

48 Allen JC, Walker R, Luks E, Jennings M, Barfoot S, Tan C. Carboplatin and recurrent childhood brain tumors. *J Clin Oncol* 1987; **5**:459–63.

49 Ashley DM, Longee D, Tien R, *et al*. Treatment of patients with pineoblastoma with high dose cyclophosphamide. *Med Pediatr Oncol* 1996; **26**:387–92.

50 Gaynon PS, Ettinger LJ, Baum ES, Siegel SE, Krailo MD, Hammond GD. Carboplatin in childhood brain tumors. A Children's Cancer Study Group phase II trial. *Cancer* 1990; **66**:2465–9.

51 Gentet JC, Doz F, Bouffet E, *et al*. Carboplatin and VP 16 in medulloblastoma: a phase II study of the French Society of Pediatric Oncology (SFOP). *Med Pediatr Oncol* 1994; **23**:422–7.

52 Lefkowitz IB, Packer RJ, Siegel KR, Sutton LN, Schut L, Evans AE. Results of treatment of children with recurrent medulloblastoma/primitive neuroectodermal tumors with lomustine, cisplatin, and vincristine. *Cancer* 1990; **65**:412–17.

53 Moghrabi A, Fuchs H, Brown M, *et al*. Cyclophosphamide in combination with sargramostim for treatment of recurrent medulloblastoma. *Med Pediatr Oncol* 1995; **25**:190–6.

54 Friedman HS, Mahaley S, Schold SC, *et al*. Efficacy of vincristine and cyclophosphamide in the therapy of recurrent medulloblastoma. *Neurosurgery* 1986; **18**:335–40.

55 Castello MA, Clerico A, Deb G, Dominici C, Fidani P, Donfrancesco A. High-dose carboplatin in combination with etoposide (JET regimen) for childhood brain tumors. *Am J Pediatr Hematol Oncol* 1990; **12**:297–300.

56 Strauss LC, Killmond TM, Carson BS, Maria BL, Wharam MD, Leventhal BG. Efficacy of postoperative chemotherapy using cisplatin plus etoposide in young children with brain tumors. *Med Pediatr Oncol* 1991; **19**:16–21.

57 Bailey CC, Gnekow A, Wellek S, *et al*. Prospective randomised trial of chemotherapy given before radiotherapy in childhood medulloblastoma. International Society of Pediatric Oncology (SIOP) and the (German) Society of Pediatric Oncology (GPO): SIOP II. *Med Pediatr Oncol* 1995; **25**:166–78.

58 Heideman RL, Kovnar EH, Kellie SJ, *et al*. Preirradiation chemotherapy with carboplatin and etoposide in newly diagnosed embryonal pediatric CNS tumors. *J Clin Oncol* 1995; **13**:2247–54.

59 Tarbell NJ, Friedman H, Kepner J, *et al*. Outcome for children with high stage medulloblastoma: results of the Pediatric Oncology Group 9031. *Int J Radiat Oncol Biol Phys* 2000; **48** (suppl. 3):179.

60 Packer RJ, Sutton LN, Goldwein JW, *et al*. Improved survival with the use of adjuvant chemotherapy in the treatment of medulloblastoma. *J Neurosurg* 1991; **74**:433–40.

61 Bourne JP, Geyer R, Berger M, Griffin B, Milstein J. The prognostic significance of postoperative residual enhancement on CT scan in pediatric patients with medulloblastoma. *J Neuro-Oncol* 1992; **14**:263–70.

62 Mastrangelo R, Lasorella A, Riccardi R, *et al*. Carboplatin in childhood medulloblastoma/PNET: feasibility of an in vivo sensitivity test in an "up-front" study. *Med Pediatr Oncol* 1995; **24**:188–96.

63 Mosijczuk AD, Nigro MA, Thomas PRM, *et al*. Pre-radiation chemotherapy in advanced medulloblastoma. A Pediatric Oncology Group Pilot Study. *Cancer* 1993; **72**:2755–62.

64 Allen JC, Donahue B, Da Rosso R, Nierenberg A. Hyperfractionated craniospinal radiotherapy and adjuvant chemotherapy for children with newly diagnosed medulloblastoma and other primitive neuroectodermal tumors. *Int J Radiat Oncol Biol Phys* 1996; **30**:1155–61.

65 Blaney SM, Poplack DG. New cytotoxic drugs for intrathecal administration. *J Neuro-Oncol* 1998; **38**:219–23.

66 Slavc I, Schuller E, Czech T, Hainfellner JA, Seidl R, Dieckmann K. Intrathecal mafosfamide therapy for pediatric brain tumors with meningeal dissemination. *J Neuro-Oncol* 1998; **38**:213–18.

67 Tomita T, Das L, Radkowski M. Bone metastases of medulloblastoma in childhood. *J Neuro-Oncol* 1990; **8**:113–20.

68 Tarbell NJ, Loeffler JS, Silver B, *et al*. The change in patterns of relapse in medulloblastoma. *Cancer* 1991; **68**:1600–4.

69 Prados MD, Edwards MS, Chang SM, *et al*. Hyperfractionated craniospinal radiation therapy for primitive neuroectodermal tumors: results of a phase II study. *Int J Radiat Oncol Biol Phys* 1999; **43**:279–85.

70 Marymont MH, Geohas J, Tomita T. Strauss L, Brand WN, Bharat BM. Hyperfractionated craniospinal radiation in medulloblastoma. *Pediatr Neurosurg* 1996; **24**:178–84.

71 Ricardi U, Besenzon L, Cordero di Montezemolo L, *et al*. Low dose hyperfractionated craniospinal radiation therapy for childhood cerebellar medulloblastoma: early results of a phase I–II study. Presented at ECCO 9, Hamburg, Germany, 14–18 September 1997.

72 Dirks PB, Harris L, Hoffman HJ, Humphreys RP, Drake JM, Rutka JT. Supratentorial primitive neuroectodermal tumors in children. *J Neuro-Oncol* 1996; **29**:75–84.

73 Timmermann B, Kortmann RD, Kühl J, *et al*. The role of radiation therapy in the treatment of supratentorial PNET in childhood: results of the prospective German brain tumor trials HIT '88/'89 and '91. *J Clin Oncol* 2002; **20**:842–9.

74 Cohen BH, Zeltzer PM, Boyett JM, *et al*. Prognostic factors and treatment results for supratentorial primitive neuroectodermal tumors in children using radiation and chemotherapy. A Children's Cancer Group randomized trial. *J Clin Oncol* 1995; **13**:1687–96.

75 Jakacki RI, Zeltzer PM, Boyett JM, *et al*. Survival and prognostic factors following radiation and/or chemotherapy for primitive neuroectodermal tumors of the pineal region in infants and children: a report of the CCG. *J Clin Oncol* 1995; **13**:1377–83.

76 Cohen BH, Packer RJ. Chemotherapy for medulloblastomas and primitive neuroectodermal tumors. *J Neuro-Oncol* 1996; **29**:55–68.

77 Halperin EC, Friedman HS, Schold S, *et al*. Surgery, hyperfractionated craniospinal irradiation, and adjuvant chemotherapy in the management of supratentorial embryonal neuroepithelial neoplasms in children. *Surg Neurol* 1993; **40**:278–83.

78 Silber JH, Radcliffe J, Peckham V, *et al*. Whole-brain irradiation and decline in intelligence: the influence of dose and age on IQ score. *J Clin Oncol* 1992; **10**:1390–6.

79 Duffner PK, Horowitz ME, Krischer JP, *et al*. Postoperative chemotherapy and delayed radiation in children less than

three years of age with malignant brain tumors. *N Engl J Med* 1993; **328**:1725–31.

80 Duffner PK, Horowitz ME, Krischer JP, *et al.* The treatment of malignant brain tumors in infants and very young children: an update of the Pediatric Oncology Group experience. *J Neuro-Oncol* 1999; **1**:152–61.

81 Geyer JR, Zeltzer PM, Boyett, JM, *et al.* Survival of infants with primitive neuroectodermal tumors or malignant ependymomas of the CNS treated with eight drugs in 1 day: a report from the Children's Cancer Group. *J Clin Oncol* 1994; **12**:1607–15.

82 Tao ML, Turner JA, Geyer JR, *et al.* Radiation therapy for malignant brain tumors in infants less than 36 months old: compliance and survival. *Int J Radiat Oncol Biol Phys* 2000; **48**:180.

83 Kühl J, Bode F, Deinlein H, *et al.* Cure of infants with medulloblastoma (M0/M1-stage) by postoperative chemotherapy only. *Med Pediatr Oncol* 1999; **33**:169.

84 Leonard JR, Cai DX, Rivet DJ, *et al.* Large cell/anaplastic medulloblastomas and medullomyoblastomas: clinicopathological and genetic features. *J Neurosurg* 2001; **95**:82–8.

85 Gilbertson RJ, Perry RH, Kelly PJ, Pearson AD, Lunec J. Prognostic significance of HER2 and HER4 coexpression in childhood medulloblastoma. *Cancer Res* 1997; **57**:3272–80.

86 Herms JW, Behnke J, Bergmann M, *et al.* Potential prognostic value of C-erbB-2 expression in medulloblastomas in very young children. *J Pediatr Hematol Oncol* 1997; **19**:510–15.

87 Scheurlen WG, Schwabe GC, Joos S, Mollenhauer J, Sörensen N, Kühl J. Molecular analysis of childhood PNET defines markers associated with poor outcome. *J Clin Oncol* 1998; **16**:2478–85.

88 Grotzer MA, Janss AJ, Fung K, *et al.* TrkC expression predicts good clinical outcome in primitive neuroectodermal brain tumors. *J Clin Oncol* 2000; **18**:1027–35.

89 Dupuis-Girod S, Hartmann O, Benhamou E, *et al.* High-dose chemotherapy in relapse of medulloblastoma in young children. *Bull Cancer* 1997; **84**:264–72.

90 Bouffet E, Gentet JC, Doz F, *et al.* Metastatic medulloblastoma: the experience of the French Cooperative M7 Group. *Eur J Cancer* 1994; **30A**:1478–83.

91 Kalifa C, Valteau D, Pizer B, Vassal G, Grill J, Hartmann O. High-dose chemotherapy in childhood brain tumours. *Childs Nerv Syst* 1999; **15**:498–505.

17

Ependymal tumors

ABHAYA V. KULKARNI, ERIC BOUFFET AND JAMES M. DRAKE

INTRODUCTION

Ependymomas are tumors of the central nervous system (CNS) that derive from the ependymal cells lining the ventricles of the brain. This chapter focuses on intracranial ependymomas; therefore, ependymomas that arise in the spinal cord or cauda equina will not be dealt with.

EPIDEMIOLOGY

Incidence

Ependymomas are relatively uncommon tumors, with an annual incidence of approximately 2.2 per million children.[1,2] They arise more frequently in children than in adults. They are the third most common pediatric brain tumor, behind astrocytomas and primitive neuroectodermal tumors (PNETs), which have incidence rates of approximately 16.8 and five per million children per year, respectively. Ependymomas account for roughly six to ten per cent of all intracranial tumors of children[1–3] and approximately 1.7 per cent of all childhood cancers.[3]

Age

Ependymomas occur most commonly in younger children, with the median age at diagnosis ranging from three to eight years, depending on the series.[4–7] The incidence rate for ependymomas in children under five years of age is approximately 3.9 per one million children per year, compared with only 1.1 for older children.[1] Approximately 70–80 per cent of ependymomas are seen in children under eight years of age, and nearly 40 per cent are seen in children under four years of age.[4,8–10]

Recently, the very large Childhood Brain Tumor Consortium study reported a large increase in the relative proportion of older children (aged over 11 years) with ependymomas, especially supratentorial ependymomas, over a 50-year period of observation.[8] This trend was also seen for pilocytic and fibrillary astrocytomas. While there is no clear explanation for this finding, various hypotheses, including a relative decrease in the prenatal exposures that contribute to early childhood cancer and a relative increase in environmental exposures that contribute to later childhood and adolescent cancer, have been proffered.

Gender

Most large pediatric series do not show any consistent gender predilection for ependymomas, with the tumors arising relatively equally in boys and girls. Although some series have shown a predilection for ependymomas to occur in boys,[2,4,5] this has not held up consistently, and it appears that these tumors do not demonstrate a significant gender bias.[6,7,9,11]

Location

Ependymomas, being of ependymal origin, arise almost invariably in association with a ventricular surface. In children, the most common site for intracranial ependymomas is in the posterior fossa, associated with the surface of the fourth ventricle. This accounts for the location of roughly two-thirds of childhood ependymomas, with the remainder arising from the supratentorial ventricular system.[4–6,12–14] In very rare cases, ependymomas may develop in an ectopic fashion without any direct association with a ventricular surface.[15]

SIGNS AND SYMPTOMS

Given the predominant location of these tumors in the posterior fossa and their intimate association with the fourth ventricle, the most common presenting signs and symptoms are usually due to raised intracranial pressure from obstructive hydrocephalus. Patients may also display signs and symptoms attributable to direct cerebellar or cranial nerve dysfunction.

Common symptoms, in approximate order of decreasing incidence, include vomiting, headache (in older children), irritability and lethargy (especially in very young children), and gait disturbance.[4,9] Clinical signs include increased head circumference or bulging fontanel (in very young children), papilledema, meningism, ataxia, cranial nerve palsy, and nystagmus.[4,9] The duration of these symptoms before presentation varies greatly and can range from just a few days to several months.[9] Very rarely, ependymomas may present very acutely following an intratumoral hemorrhage.[16]

A complicating factor in diagnosing young children in particular is that some may present in a relatively nonspecific fashion with, for example, vomiting and irritability. A high degree of clinical suspicion is needed in such cases. It has been recognized that the diagnosis of brain tumors in children is frequently delayed compared with other childhood tumors.[17]

PATHOLOGY

The latest World Health Organization (WHO) grading of ependymomas defines four major tumor subtypes, divided into three grades: subependymoma and myxopapillary ependymoma (grade I), low-grade ependymoma (grade II), and anaplastic ependymoma (grade III) (Table 17.1).[18] Within the low-grade ependymomas, there are four described variants: cellular, papillary, clear-cell, and tanycytic.

Table 17.1 *World Health Organization classification (2000) of ependymal tumors**

Ependymoma
Cellular ependymoma
Papillary ependymoma
Clear-cell ependymoma
Tanycytic ependymoma
Anaplastic ependymoma
Myxopapillary ependymoma
Subependymoma

*From Wiestler *et al.* 2000[18]

Subependymomas are benign, usually asymptomatic, nodules on the walls of the lateral or fourth ventricle. They are found most commonly as an incidental autopsy finding. In very rare cases, they may become clinically evident secondary to obstruction of cerebrospinal fluid (CSF) flow.[19] Myxopapillary ependymomas are found almost exclusively in the region of the cauda equina, arising from the filum terminale or conus medullaris.[20] The occurrence of either of these tumors as symptomatic intracranial lesions is exceedingly rare, especially in children.[19,21–23] These will not be discussed in this chapter.

Ependymoblastoma was once considered an aggressive form of ependymoma. However, the WHO classification considers ependymoblastoma among the broader group of embryonal tumors.[24] This group includes medulloblastoma and other PNETs, medulloepithelioma, and neuroblastoma. Ependymoblastoma is an aggressive tumor with a propensity for leptomeningeal metastasis;[25,26] this tumor is discussed in Chapter 16.

Classic low-grade ependymomas, the most common type, have certain histological, ultrastructural, and immunohistochemical features that aid in their diagnosis.[20,27] On light microscopy, features include perivascular pseudorosettes, clear zones around the blood vessels that represent cytoplasmic processes of the tumor cells terminating on vessels and typical of ependymomas (Plate 16). These are to be distinguished from true ependymal rosettes, in which the lumen of the rosette is circumscribed by the surface of the tumor cells themselves (Plate 17). Ependymomas may also contain structures that resemble central canals or ventricular linings, harking back to their ependymal origin. Although infrequent, they can be diagnostic.

The nuclei of ependymoma cells are usually round to oval and contain dense chromatin material. The neoplastic cells may contain eosinophilic cytoplasmic granules. Some of the tumor cells may have the appearance of oligodendrocytes, but these can be distinguished by electron microscopy. The tumor may also contain cartilage, calcium deposits, or dysplastic bone.[19,20]

Electron microscopy typically reveals gland-like lumens with microvilli and cilia, basal bodies, intracytoplasmic intermediate filaments, and long, zipper-like junctional complexes.[19,27,28] In addition, it may reveal many more true rosettes than might be appreciated on light microscopy.[28]

Ependymomas also display varying degrees of immunopositivity to glial fibrillary acid protein (GFAP) and vimentin.[19] These are rather non-specific and rarely help in the diagnosis.

The diagnosis of anaplastic ependymoma can be difficult, and no clear consensus on the required criteria exists. It is not uncommon for low-grade ependymomas to have occasional mitotic figures, mild cellular pleomorphism, or small, scattered areas of necrosis without pseudopalisading. Anaplastic ependymomas, however, display frequent mitoses, marked cellular pleomorphism, high nuclear/cytoplasmic ratio, extensive necrosis, and microvascular proliferation.[20,27] There obviously exists a spectrum of pathological changes, and the distinction between low-grade and anaplastic is not always clear. In addition, foci of anaplastic areas may be found scattered in an otherwise bland-looking tumor, but the significance of this is not known. The difficulty in grading ependymomas becomes especially significant if one is considering different adjuvant treatment options based on tumor grade and also when trying to analyze tumor grade as a prognostic factor for survival.

The difficulty in diagnosing and grading ependymomas can be readily appreciated by noting the inconsistent proportion of allegedly malignant ependymomas in different series, ranging from seven per cent to as high as 89 per cent.[5,7,12,29–31] In a recent prospective, randomized trial by the Children's Cancer Group (CCG), the pathological diagnosis of the treating institution and the central review was discordant in 69 per cent of cases.[6] The difficulties in standardizing pathological diagnosis are not only troublesome in the treatment of the individual child; they also bring into serious question the validity of any of the published series of purported ependymomas.

More recent work has concentrated on the molecular genetic abnormalities associated with ependymomas. The most common abnormalities involve aneuploid karyotypes and abnormalities of chromosomes 6, 17, and 22.[32–35] No single molecular genetic change has yet been found consistently enough to be considered the responsible genetic lesion.

NEUROIMAGING

Computed tomography (CT) imaging usually reveals a mass located within the ventricular system itself or, less commonly, in a periventricular location. The tumor frequently contains cystic areas and calcification and is typically hyperdense. It is well demarcated, with contrast enhancement.[36,37] Obstructive hydrocephalus is a common accompanying feature that can be quite prominent.

More commonly today, magnetic resonance imaging (MRI) is used to diagnose intracranial mass lesions. On MRI, ependymomas typically display iso- to hypointensity on T1-weighted images and hyperintensity on T2-weighted images. In addition, they enhance with gadolinium injection and may contain areas of signal heterogeneity, representing hemorrhage, necrosis, or calcification.[38,39]

DIFFERENTIAL DIAGNOSIS

In the most common situation, the differential diagnosis of interest is that of a posterior fossa mass lesion. Aside from ependymoma, the most common tumors in this location in children include astrocytoma, medulloblastoma, and brainstem glioma. Less common tumors include choroid plexus papilloma, dermoid cyst, and meningioma.

Occasionally, an ependymoma will distinguish itself from these other tumors by way of certain imaging features. For example, their midline location and hyperdensity on CT is typically shared only by medulloblastomas. However, extrusion into the cerebellopontine angle or, especially, into the foramen magnum or upper cervical spine is much more characteristic of ependymoma than of medulloblastoma.

PROGNOSTIC FACTORS

Determination of the prognostic factors associated with ependymomas is an area of great interest. However, this process is a very difficult one. One of the major limitations in determining prognostic factors is the difficulty in comparing patient outcomes between, or even within, series. Part of this problem stems from the relatively uncommon nature of this tumor, such that most single-institution series report only a limited number of patients who have been accrued over decades. This presents a major limitation, as these patients span many different eras in the treatment of ependymomas. Some of the potentially important milestones include the exclusion of ependymoblastomas from the ependymoma group, the use and dose of radiotherapy, the use of chemotherapy, the use of CT and MRI for diagnosis and postoperative residual tumor assessment, and the improvements in surgical techniques. These all represent potential confounding factors that can occur when comparing results that transgress these milestones. In addition, there is much difficulty in standardizing the pathological diagnosis and grading of ependymomas, leading to great inconsistency in the literature. A further limitation is that the vast majority of data come from retrospective case series. This leads to inevitable biases in the retrieval and analysis of data, particularly with respect to prognostic factors. While the following summarizes the available literature, it should be noted that the quality of the current evidence from the medical literature is quite limited.

Age

There are numerous studies that suggest that age is a prognostic factor in children with ependymomas. Most studies show that older children (over the age of three or four years) have longer survival. In these studies, the five-year survival rate for the older children ranges from 55 to 83 per cent compared with 12–48 per cent for the younger group.[4,9,11,14,40,41] Even among children under three years old, a recent prospective study suggested that those aged over 24 months have a better prognosis (five-year survival 63 versus 26 per cent).[42] Although the verdict on age is not unanimous (some studies have not demonstrated any convincing difference in prognosis[6,43]), the overall weight of evidence does seem to indicate that older age is likely to have some prognostic significance. One possible reason for this, however, may be the current policy of avoiding or delaying radiotherapy in very young children. Although there is no clear evidence that the tumor behaves more aggressively in young patients, it has been reported that the size of the tumor at presentation appears to be related inversely to age.[38]

Location

Most pediatric ependymomas are located in the posterior fossa, but there is little evidence to suggest that this location is associated with a better survival prognosis. The five-year survival rates range from 12 to 68 per cent for infratentorial tumors compared with 22–100 per cent for supratentorial tumors (Table 17.2).[4,5,11,14,29,30,41,44–52] However, among posterior fossa tumors, it has been suggested that patients with lateral extension into the cerebellopontine angle do worse.[53] This is attributed to the much greater difficulty in completely removing these tumors due to the involvement of the lower cranial nerves and major vascular structures, e.g. the posterior inferior cerebellar artery.

Tumor grade

There is great controversy regarding the prognostic significance of tumor grade for ependymomas. Numerous retrospective studies have shown that anaplastic ependymomas, or at least tumors with certain anaplastic features, carry a worse prognosis.[5,7,9,11,13,43,52,54,55] Other studies have found tumor grade to be a factor for supratentorial tumors only.[23,44,56] The lack of uniformity in the grading system used across series makes it difficult to conclude which histological features are most prognostic.

While such an association would intuitively make sense (following the pattern that has been well established for different grades of astrocytomas), several studies

Table 17.2 *Survival by location of ependymoma*

| Ref. | Total | Patients (*n*) | | Supratentorial 5-year overall survival (%) | Infratentorial 5-year overall survival (%) | *P* |
		Supratentorial	Infratentorial			
5	26	9	17	22	35	NS
4	51	18	33	35	50	0.1
52	93	40	53	48	53	NS
49	46	20	26	32	57	NI
11	80	17	63	46	59	0.31
47	20	10	10	40	60	NI
30	29	5	24	49	68	NI
48	24	7	17	28	23	NI
45	28	11	17	36	12	NI
14	41	15	26	40	26	NS
29	37	NI	NI	51	19	0.08
44	25	9	16	64	34	0.17
51	92	60	32	66	47	0.46
46	31	11	20	76	34	0.04
41	37	12	25	83	46	0.3
50	19	8	11	100	54	0.036
Total	679	252*	390*			

NI, not indicated; NS, not significant.

*Total numbers are missing data from Carrie *et al.*[29]

have found no difference in prognosis based on tumor grade for ependymomas.[4,6,14,42,57] Among these series are two prospective studies: a randomized trial from the CCG[6] and a prospective cohort study from the Pediatric Oncology Group (POG).[42] The relatively higher methodological quality of these works needs to be appreciated and taken into account when weighing the overall evidence, especially since there are so few such works in the ependymoma literature. However, it should also be said that these studies were not very large and were somewhat limited in scope. In addition, the CCG study was potentially biased, since it was designed to include only the anaplastic subgroup of ependymomas. Of further note is that in the same CCG study, pathological specimens underwent a formal, independent review process.[6] This process was particularly enlightening, since it demonstrated a discordant pathological diagnosis in 69 per cent of the cases. As mentioned previously, this is a rather disturbing finding that significantly limits the conclusions one can infer from most studies that have examined the influence of tumor grade on prognosis.

Tumor resection

The extent of tumor resection is a particularly important factor, since it is one that the surgeon has at least some control over. The vast majority of studies do seem to suggest that extent of resection, particularly gross total resection (GTR), is associated with improved prognosis.[5,6,9,11,14,41,42,52] Reported five-year survivals range from 60 to 89 per cent after GTR compared with 21–46 per cent following partial resection. A small number of studies have failed to demonstrate any survival advantage following GTR.[4,7,43]

It is important to determine exactly how one ascertains the degree of surgical resection and, therefore, the amount of postoperative residual tumor. Healey and colleagues demonstrated in their small series that while postoperative residual tumor, as assessed by radiological imaging, was associated with progression-free survival, the assessment by the surgeon of the extent of resection was not prognostically significant.[30] In fact, the surgical assessment of resection was refuted by the postoperative imaging in 32 per cent of cases. It is important to keep in mind that postoperative imaging is mandatory and is the only acceptable means of assessing residual tumor. Even in patients for whom complete resection cannot be obtained, the randomized trial from the CCG suggests that improved survival may be seen in patients with less than 1.5 cm^2 of residual tumor.[6]

Miscellaneous factors

While age, tumor location, tumor grade, and extent of surgical resection are by far the most well established potentially significant prognostic factors, other factors have been suggested in the literature. These include gender, race, and duration of symptoms.[4,41,52] There is very little evidence to suggest that any of these factors is, in fact, significantly prognostic.[6,7,11]

An article by Bouffet and colleagues provides a thorough assessment of the current state of knowledge regarding ependymomas and makes a plea for future cooperation, particularly in the form of prospective randomized trials.[58] Given the small numbers of such cases that are seen at any single institution, a multicenter cooperative effort would be needed in order to prospectively recruit a critical number of patients in a reasonable period of time. Data from such studies would help answer, in a much more definitive way, the many questions that have been asked regarding ependymomas.

TREATMENT

Surgical therapy

Following diagnosis of a posterior fossa tumor, any immediate threats to the child's life need to be dealt with urgently. Most commonly, this is severe obstructive hydrocephalus, which may warrant rapid ventricular drainage. If the child is severely obtunded as a result of hydrocephalus, then urgent external drainage should be performed. However, in most cases, the child will improve, sometimes dramatically, with the urgent administration of steroids, e.g. dexamethasone. This can obviate the need for external ventricular drainage and should be tried first. This usually provides an adequate temporizing measure until the tumor is resected and normal CSF flow patterns are re-established.

Preoperatively, it can be difficult to confirm the exact type of tumor one is dealing with. However, virtually all types of pediatric posterior fossa tumors will benefit, at least in the short term, from surgical decompression. It was stated above that complete surgical resection appears to be an important prognostic factor. Therefore, every effort should be made to perform as complete a resection as is safely possible. Some authors have recommended that if early postoperative imaging reveals residual tumor, then a second-look surgery is warranted, with the goal being GTR.[59] Unfortunately, a complete resection is very frequently extremely difficult, if not impossible. Attempts at a radical resection may be associated with the risk of surgical complications, including the increasingly recognized cerebellar syndrome, which includes cerebellar mutism[60] and visual impairment.[61] In a randomized trial from the CCG, the authors followed a standard protocol for postoperative staging, and all patients were operated on using relatively recent microsurgical techniques.[6] However, over half the cases (53 per cent) demonstrated residual tumor on postoperative imaging.

An important preoperative investigation is full neuraxis staging with MRI. The results of this may have a significant impact on the goals of surgery. Specifically, if distant metastases are clearly observed, then this will certainly dampen one's enthusiasm for performing a GTR. This can be the deciding factor in determining how aggressively to proceed in resecting a difficult adherent tumor, for example.

Radiation therapy

The principles of radiotherapy in ependymoma are guided by their natural history. Although the benefit of radiotherapy has not been shown by randomized trials, large series have provided strong evidence that local control is better when postoperative radiotherapy with local doses greater than 45 Gy is given.[11,51,62–65] There has been a long debate as to whether local, whole-brain, or craniospinal radiation fields should be used. Some authors introduce histological criteria in their decision-making process and reserve large-field irradiation for patients with anaplastic features.[31,43,66] However, given that local tumor recurrence is the primary pattern of failure in ependymoma regardless of histology or completeness of resection, most authors have now abandoned craniospinal irradiation and advocate focal fields when postoperative radiotherapy is considered.[67] Isolated neuraxis failure is distinctly uncommon.

Because of persistent problems with local failure, intensification of radiation treatment to the primary site has been advocated and is currently under investigation. The POG has conducted a study of hyperfractionated irradiation in children with posterior fossa ependymoma. The dose to the primary site was delivered in 58 fractions of 1.2 Gy for a total dose of 69.6 Gy over six weeks. The four-year event-free survival in this study is 74 per cent in patients with GTR and 52 per cent for those with subtotal resection.[68] The preliminary results of this study suggest improved outcome with hyperfractionated irradiation in patients with residual tumor, but no benefit for patients with complete resection. Aggarwal and colleagues have reported a limited series of five children with incompletely resected ependymomas treated with stereotactic radiosurgery given as a boost in addition to standard fractionated irradiation.[69] Four of the five patients demonstrated response to this treatment, and all five patients were alive at the time of the report, without evidence of treatment related sequelae.

Advances in radiotherapy techniques, and particularly the possibility of delivering high doses of radiotherapy with high precision to well-defined volumes, are influencing the management of ependymoma in infants and young children. For decades, the policy has been to avoid radiotherapy for children under the age of three

years. The use of conformal or stereotactic irradiation allows the treatment of small volumes with minimal damage to the surrounding tissues. These techniques are currently under investigation, particularly in children over 18 months of age and with posterior fossa ependymomas.

Re-irradiation using "radiosurgery" has also been proposed for patients with recurrent ependymoma in order to prolong local control. Dramatic responses have been reported, but radionecrosis is frequent and may require steroids or reoperation.[70] Despite an interesting rate of local control, most patients eventually progress outside the radiosurgery field.[71] Patients with small posterior fossa recurrences seem to benefit the most from this treatment modality.

DEFERRAL OF RADIOTHERAPY

Reports on long progression-free survival following GTR suggest that a subgroup of patients may benefit from deferral strategies avoiding immediate postoperative radiotherapy. However, the characterization of this subgroup remains to be defined. Initial evidence came from retrospective institutional studies reporting on heterogeneous groups of patients treated over a long period of time. In the series of 35 children with posterior fossa ependymoma from the Hospital for Sick Children in Toronto, Canada, Nazar and colleagues reported three long-term survivors out of six patients who did not receive postoperative treatment.[9] Two of five patients in the series from Papadopoulos and colleagues,[5] and three of six patients from the series from Ernestus and colleauges,[56] did not show evidence of progression after radical surgery alone. In a retrospective review of 20 patients with supratentorial ependymoma, Palma and colleagues reported six long-term survivors who did not receive postoperative radiotherapy.[23] They concluded that surgery alone was a reasonable option for patients with completely resected, non-cystic, low-grade ependymoma. More recently, Awaad and colleagues reported the results of a prospective study aimed at deferring radiotherapy in children with histologically confirmed low-grade ependymoma following surgically reported gross resection.[72] Seven of the 12 eligible patients (one posterior fossa tumor, six supratentorial tumors) were included in the study, and five were alive and progression-free at the time of the report. The authors concluded that deferral of radiotherapy following GTR is a safe option, particularly in patients with supratentorial ependymoma. This report suffers several criticisms, particularly the lack of definition of the histological classification used, and a higher than expected proportion of patients with supratentorial lesions (19 of 38) and with anaplastic features (18 of 38), suggesting some selection biases.

Deferral strategies are also part of the strategy in use in infants and young children. While the POG used a policy of delayed irradiation in its first cooperative infant protocol conducted between 1986 and 1990,[73] the aim of the Société Française d'Oncologie Pédiatrique (SFOP) study for infants and young children with ependymoma was to avoid radiotherapy in first-line treatment.[74] The results from this group showed a 22 per cent four-year progression-free survival rate in the 73 children registered. In the multivariate analysis, supratentorial location and complete resection were associated with a favorable outcome. Despite this two-stage strategy, the four-year overall survival reported by this group compared favorably with survival data observed in older children treated with early postoperative irradiation (74 per cent for patients with complete resection, 35 per cent for patients with incomplete resection).

These data suggest that a small proportion of children with intracranial ependymoma may avoid radiotherapy. Complete resection, supratentorial location, and benign histology appear to be three important criteria to consider in this regard. Prospective cooperative studies aiming at avoiding radiotherapy in older children fulfilling these criteria are pending.

Chemotherapy

The benefit of chemotherapy has never been demonstrated for patients with ependymomas. The only randomized study assessing the role of chemotherapy failed to show a survival advantage of post-radiotherapy chemotherapy with vincristine, prednisone, and lomustine.[75] In retrospective studies, chemotherapy has never shown any evidence of benefit in terms of overall or event-free survival. Response rates with chemotherapy are disappointing, and a recent review of phase II studies reported an 11 per cent response rate for single agents and a 26 per cent response rate for combination chemotherapy in ependymomas.[76] Reports on high-dose chemotherapy studies do not suggest any benefit.[77,78] Only one series using intensive chemotherapy with vincristine, carboplatin, ifosfamide, and etoposide after radiation therapy suggested a survival benefit, with a five-year progression-free rate of 74 per cent, regardless of the extent of resection.[50] However, another recent report using a very similar ifosfamide, carboplatin, etoposide combination did not confirm these data.[79]

Despite these facts, chemotherapy is still a standard postoperative treatment for infants with ependymoma, when the aim of the physician is to delay or avoid radiotherapy. The first cooperative infant protocol conducted by the POG has reported an impressive 48 per cent response rate among evaluable infants, using a combination of vincristine and cyclophosphamide.[73] A parallel study was conducted at the same period by the Children's Cancer Study Group (CCSG) for infants with malignant brain tumors. The chemotherapy regimen "8 in 1" was given for one year; radiotherapy was given, at the discretion of the physician, either after two courses or at the end of the year of treatment. Most children were not irradiated,

and the three-year progression-free survival was 26 per cent for infants with ependymoma in this experience.[80] Other cooperative experiences have pointed out the high recurrence rate observed despite the use of chemotherapy in infants, even after complete macroscopic resection.[81] The POG-9233 study randomized a standard versus an intensified regimen for infants with malignant brain tumors. The relative dose intensity between standard and intensive chemotherapy was 1.8.[82] A total of 84 patients with ependymoma were eligible, including 47 with evidence of residual tumor after initial surgery. Seventeen of 25 infants with evaluable tumors and allocated to the standard chemotherapy arm responded to standard chemotherapy. All 22 infants with measurable disease responded to chemotherapy in the intensive arm. In this experience, event-free survival was improved with intensive chemotherapy, but overall survival was not. The three-year event-free survivals for children who had a complete or incomplete resection were 41 and 17 per cent, respectively. Although they may be of some benefit among individuals, these results provide little support for the systematic use of chemotherapy in patients with ependymoma. Appendix 1 summarizes all of the recent single-agent and combination therapy trials for ependymoma.

The current policy is to recommend chemotherapy (i) in all infants when the aim is to delay or avoid radiotherapy and (ii) in patients with residual tumor after initial surgery. The aim of chemotherapy in this context is to facilitate second-look surgery. The systematic analysis of tumor specimens obtained following chemotherapy may provide useful information for future development.

Drug resistance in ependymoma appears to be multifactorial. At least two mechanisms of resistance to chemotherapy have been suggested: (i) the expression of the multiple resistance gene $MDR-1$[83] and (ii) the overexpression of the DNA protein O^6-methyl-guanine-DNA methyltransferase.[84] So far, drugs known to reverse $MDR-1$ expression in vitro have failed to show any clinical benefit. Modulation of O^6-methyl-guanine-DNA methyltransferase activity is currently under investigation.

RECURRENCE AND PATTERNS OF FAILURE

Ependymomas have a propensity to spread via the CSF system, and between five and 22 per cent of children present with documented leptomeningeal metastases at diagnosis.[4,6,10,41,52] Given this fact, full and proper staging of the entire CNS is mandatory early on in the child's evaluation. This includes full-neuraxis MRI and examination of CSF cytology. It has been suggested that the proportion of ependymomas diagnosed with evidence of distant metastases has increased since the early 1970s.[10] Improvements in preoperative staging technology have likely played a large part in this change.

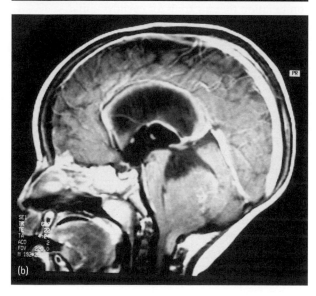

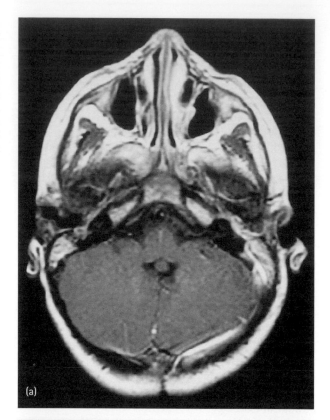

Figure 17.1a,b *Gadolinium-enhanced magnetic resonance axial (a) and sagittal (b) images, demonstrating a large posterior fossa ependymoma with minimal enhancement.*

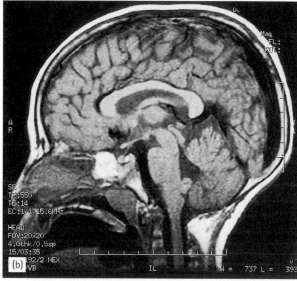

Figure 17.2a,b *Gadolinium-enhanced magnetic resonance axial (a) and sagittal (b) images, demonstrating a small nodular recurrence on the floor of the fourth ventricle.*

Although ependymomas do have the capacity for leptomeningeal spread, the vast majority of tumor recurrences occur as a result of local tumor relapse.[7,52,85–87] Tumor recurrence presenting as metastatic spread without any evidence of local recurrence is very rare, occurring in only seven to eight per cent of cases.[6,7]

Unfortunately, most childhood ependymomas do recur at some point. The five- and ten-year progression-free survivals are approximately 36–64 per cent and 47–48

per cent, respectively.[6,14,44,86] An unresolved issue is exactly what surveillance protocol is optimal for children with ependymomas, in order to maximize detection of recurrence without unduly wasting resources. The detection of asymptomatic recurrences through routine surveillance does appear to confer some benefit.[88] The CCG has recommended MRI of the brain (and spine, if there are documented metastases) every three months for the first year.[89] Others have suggested protocols, based on the pattern and timing of ependymoma recurrences, in which no imaging is performed in the first 18 months following resection. After this period, relatively frequent imaging (every four to six months) is performed for 3.5 years, with no further surveillance imaging thereafter.[90]

Treatment of recurrence

Once tumor recurrence has been identified, treatment options become relatively limited, both in scope and in efficacy. Initial consideration should be given to reoperation in cases of local recurrence. Since the local area, at least, has already been irradiated, further radiation therapy is usually no longer feasible, other than for isolated areas of remote metastases. However, some have recently suggested re-irradiation using radiosurgery.[70] Various chemotherapeutic regimens have been studied, with relatively poor results.[85,91–95] The only agent to show even mildly promising results has been cisplatin, but this is also associated with potentially significant renal and otological toxicity.[91,93,95] More recently, a very aggressive approach of high-dose, intensive chemotherapy with autologous bone-marrow transplant rescue has been investigated for recurrent ependymomas.[77,78] Unfortunately, the children in these small series experienced very little clinical response and there was a high incidence of fatal toxicity. The authors of both series concluded that this was not an effective means of treating recurrent ependymomas.

OUTCOME

Compared with many other childhood brain tumors, the outcome for ependymomas is relatively poor. The five-year survival rate ranges from 39 to 64 per cent.[4,6,7,9,12,30,52,53] The ten-year survival rate drops to approximately 45 per cent.[30,41,53] However, beyond the issue of just absolute survival, there is also the potential impairments that may occur in the quality of life of long-term survivors of childhood brain tumors.[96–98] These children frequently have relatively low intelligence quotients, along with poor general academic and psychosocial functioning. While current therapeutic modifications must be aimed at improving survival, the issue of quality of life must also be given strong consideration. Future therapeutic directions should be aimed at decreasing the long-term neurological morbidity that otherwise results from surgical-, chemotherapeutic-, and radiation-induced insults to the developing nervous system.

CASE STUDY

A 17-month old boy presented with a large posterior fossa tumor (Figure 17.1). A GTR was carried out without complication, and a diagnosis of ependymoma was made. Imaging did not reveal the presence of any metastases. The child received postoperative chemotherapy (Baby POG protocol). Although the child was doing well, surveillance imaging detected a small focal recurrence in the fourth ventricle four years after initial resection (Figure 17.2). This was treated with an operative exploration and another gross total resection of the small nodule of recurrence. Following surgery, the child, now five years old, received fractionated, local stereotactic radiotherapy. The child has continued to do well in follow-up.

REFERENCES

1 Gurney J, Severson R, Davis S, Robison L. Incidence of cancer in children in the United States. *Cancer* 1995; **75**:2186–95.
2 Kuratsu J, Ushio Y. Epidemiological study of primary intracranial tumors in childhood. *Pediatr Neurosurg* 1996; **25**:240–7.
3 Miller R, Young J, Novakovic B. Childhood cancer. *Cancer* 1995; **75**:395–405.
4 Goldwein J, Leahy J, Packer R, *et al.* Intracranial ependymomas in children. *Int J Radiat Oncol Biol Phys* 1990; **19**:1497–502.
5 Papadopoulos D, Giri S, Evans R. Prognostic factors and management of intracranial ependymomas. *Anticancer Res* 1990; **10**:689–92.
6 Robertson P, Zeltzer P, Boyett J, *et al.* Survival and prognostic factors following radiation therapy and chemotherapy for ependymomas in children: a report of the Children's Cancer Group. *J Neurosurg* 1998; **88**:695–703.
7 Shaw E, Evans R, Scheithauer B, Ilstrup D, Earle J. Postoperative radiotherapy of intracranial ependymoma in pediatric and adult patients. *Int J Radiat Oncol Biol Phys* 1987; **13**:1457–62.
8 Gilles F, Sobel E, Tavare C, Leviton A, Hedley-Whyte E. Age-related changes in diagnoses, histological features, and survival in children with brain tumors: 1930–1979. The Childhood Brain Tumor Consortium. *Neurosurgery* 1995; **37**:1056–68.
9 Nazar G, Hoffman H, Becker L, Jenkin D, Humphreys R, Hendrick E. Infratentorial ependymomas in childhood: prognostic factors and treatment. *J Neurosurg* 1990; **72**:408–17.
10 Polednak A, Flannery J. Brain, other central nervous system, and eye cancer. *Cancer* 1995; **75**:330–7.
11 Rousseau P, Habrand J, Sarrazin D, *et al.* Treatment of intracranial ependymomas of children: review of a 15-year experience. *Int J Radiat Oncol Biol Phys* 1994; **28**:381–6.
12 Pierre-Kahn A, Hirsch J, Roux F, Renier D, Sainte-Rose C. Intracranial ependymomas in childhood. Survival and functional results of 47 cases. *Childs Brain* 1983; **10**:145–56.

13 Schiffer D, Chio A, Cravioto H, *et al.* Ependymoma: internal correlations among pathological signs: the anaplastic variant. *Ncurosurgery* 1991; **29**:206–10.

14 Sutton L, Goldwein J, Perilongo G, *et al.* Prognostic factors in childhood ependymomas. *Pediatr Neurosurg* 1990; **16**:57–65.

15 Vernet O, Farmer J, Meagher-Villemure K, Montes J. Supratentorial ectopic ependymoma. *Can J Neurol Sci* 1995; **22**:316–19.

16 Ernestus R, Schroder R, Klug N. Spontaneous intracerebral hemorrhage from an unsuspected ependymoma in early infancy. *Childs Nerv Syst* 1992; **8**:357–60.

17 Flores L, Williams D, Bell B, Brien M, Ragab A. Delay in the diagnosis of pediatric brain tumors. *Am J Dis Child* 1986; **140**:684–6.

18 Wiestler O, Schiffer D, Coons S, Prayson R, Rosenblum M. Ependymoma. In: Kleihues P, Cavenee W (eds). *Pathology and Genetics of Tumours of the Nervous System.* Lyon: IARC Press, 2000, pp. 71–81.

19 Rosenblum MK. Ependymal tumors: a review of their diagnostic surgical pathology. *Pediatr Neurosurg* 1998; **28**:160–5.

20 Rorke L, Gilles F, Davis R, Becker L. Revision of the World Health Organization classification of brain tumors for childhood brain tumors. *Cancer* 1985; **56**:1869–86.

21 Artico M, Bardella L, Ciappetta P, Raco A. Surgical treatment of subependymomas of the central nervous system. Report of 8 cases and review of the literature. *Acta Neurochir* 1989; **98**:25–31.

22 Lombardi D, Scheithauer B, Meyer F, *et al.* Symptomatic subependymoma: a clinicopathological and flow cytometric study. *J Neurosurg* 1991; **75**:583–8.

23 Palma L, Celli P, Cantore G. Supratentorial ependymomas of the first two decades of life. Long-term follow-up of 20 cases (including two subependymomas). *Neurosurgery* 1993; **32**:169–75.

24 Kleihues P, Cavenee W. *Pathology and Genetics of Tumours of the Nervous System.* Lyon: IARC Press, 2000.

25 Mork S, Rubinstein L. Ependymoblastoma. A reappraisal of a rare embryonal tumor. *Cancer* 1985; **55**:1536–42.

26 Shyn P, Campbell G, Guinto F, Crofford M. Primary intracranial ependymoblastoma presenting as spinal cord compression due to metastasis. *Childs Nerv Syst* 1986; **2**:323–5.

27 Burger P, Scheithauer B, Vogel F. *Surgical Pathology of the Nervous System and its Coverings,* 3rd edn. New York: Churchill Livingstone, 1991.

28 Sara A, Bruner J, Mackay B. Ultrastructure of ependymoma. *Ultrastruct Pathol* 1994; **18**:33–42.

29 Carrie C, Mottolese C, Bouffet E, *et al.* Non-metastatic childhood ependymomas. *Radiother Oncol* 1995; **36**:101–6.

30 Healey E, Barnes P, Kupsky W, *et al.* The prognostic significance of postoperative residual tumor in ependymoma. *Neurosurgery* 1991; **28**:666–71.

31 Wallner K, Wara W, Sheline G, Davis R. Intracranial ependymomas: results of treatment with partial or whole brain irradiation without spinal irradiation. *Int J Radiat Oncol Biol Phys* 1986; **12**:1937–41.

32 Kotylo P, Robertson P, Fineberg N, Azzarelli B, Jakacki R. Flow cytometric DNA analysis of pediatric intracranial ependymomas. *Arch Pathol Lab Med* 1997; **121**:1255–8.

33 Kramer D, Parmiter A, Rorke L, Sutton L, Biegel J. Molecular cytogenetic studies of pediatric ependymomas. *J Neuro-Oncol* 1998; **37**:25–33.

34 Ransom D, Ritland S, Kimmel D, *et al.* Cytogenetic and loss of heterozygosity studies in ependymomas, pilocytic astrocytomas, and oligodendrogliomas. *Genes Chromosomes Cancer* 1992; **5**:348–56.

35 VonHaken M, White E, Daneshvar-Shyesther L, *et al.* Molecular genetic analysis of chromosome arm 17p and chromosome arm 22q DNA sequences in sporadic pediatric ependymomas. *Genes Chromosomes Cancer* 1996; **17**:37–44.

36 Centeno R, Lee A, Winter J, Barba D. Supratentorial ependymomas. Neuroimaging and clinicopathological correlation. *J Neurosurg* 1986; **64**:209–15.

37 VanTassel P, Lee Y, Bruner J. Supratentorial ependymomas: computed tomographic and pathologic correlations. *J Comput Tomography* 1986; **10**:157–65.

38 Comi A, Backstrom J, Burger P, Duffner P. Clinical and neuro-radiologic findings in infants with intracranial ependymomas. *Pediatr Neurol* 1998; **18**:23–9.

39 Spoto G, Press G, Hesselink J, Solomon M. Intracranial ependymoma and subependymoma: MR manifestations. *Am J Roentgenol* 1990; **154**:837–45.

40 Goldwein J, Corn B, Finlay J, Packer R, Rorke L, Schut L. Is craniospinal irradiation required to cure children with malignant (anaplastic) intracranial ependymomas? *Cancer* 1991; **67**:2766–771.

41 Pollack I, Gerszten P, Martinez A, *et al.* Intracranial ependymomas of childhood: long-term outcome and prognostic factors. *Neurosurgery* 1995; **37**:655–66.

42 Duffner P, Krischer J, Sanford R, *et al.* Prognostic factors in infants and very young children with intracranial ependymomas. *Pediatr Neurosurg* 1998; **28**:215–22.

43 Salazar O, Castro-Vita H, VanHoutte P, Rubin P, Aygun C. Improved survival in cases of intracranial ependymoma after radiation therapy. Late report and recommendations. *J Neurosurg* 1983; **59**:652–9.

44 Chiu J, Woo S, Ater J, *et al.* Intracranial ependymoma in children: analysis of prognostic factors. *J Neuro-Oncol* 1992; **13**:283–90.

45 Dohrmann G, Farwell J, Flannery J. Ependymomas and ependymoblastomas in children. *J Neurosurg* 1976; **45**:273–83.

46 Foreman NK, Love S, Thorne R. Intracranial ependymomas: analysis of prognostic factors in a population-based series. *Pediatr Neurosurg* 1996; **24**:119–25.

47 Imhof H, Hany M, Wiestler O, Glanzmann C. Long-term follow-up in 39 patients with an ependymoma after surgery and irradiation. *Strahlenther Onkol* 1992; **168**:513–19.

48 Jayawickreme D, Hayward R, Harkness W. Intracranial ependymomas in childhood: a report of 24 cases followed for 5 years. *Childs Nerv Syst* 1995; **11**:409–13.

49 Marks J, Adler S. A comparative study of ependymomas by site of origin. *Int J Radiat Oncol Biol Phys* 1982; **8**:37–43.

50 Needle M, Goldwein J, Grass J, *et al.* Adjuvant chemotherapy for the treatment of intracranial ependymoma of childhood. *Cancer* 1997; **80**:341–7.

51 Perilongo G, Massimino M, Sotti G, *et al.* Analyses of prognostic factors in a retrospective review of 92 children with ependymoma: Italian Pediatric Neuro-oncology Group. *Med Pediatr Oncol* 1997; **29**:79–85.

52 Vanuytsel L, Bessell E, Ashley S, Bloom H, Brada M. Intracranial ependymoma: long-term results of a policy of surgery and radiotherapy. *Int J Radiat Oncol Biol Phys* 1992; **23**:313–19.

53 Ikezaki K, Matsushima T, Inoue T, Yokoyama N, Kaneko Y, Fukui M. Correlation of microanatomical localization with postoperative survival in posterior fossa ependymomas. *Neurosurgery* 1993; **32**:38–44.

54 Figarella-Branger D, Gambarelli D, Dollo C, *et al.* Infratentorial ependymomas of childhood. Correlation between histological features, immunohistological phenotype, silver nucleolar organizer region staining values and post-operative survival in 16 cases. *Acta Neuropathol* 1991; **82**:208–16.

55 Rorke LB. Relationship of morphology of ependymoma in children to prognosis. *Progr Exp Tumor Res* 1987; **30**:170–4.

56 Ernestus R, Wilcke O, Schroder R. Supratentorial ependymomas in childhood: clinicopathological findings and prognosis. *Acta Neurochir (Wien)* 1991; **111**:96–102.

57 Ross G, Rubinstein L. Lack of histopathological correlation of malignant ependymomas with postoperative survival. *J Neurosurg* 1989; **70**:31–36.

58 Bouffet E, Perilongo G, Canete A, Massimino M. Intracranial ependymomas in children: a critical review of prognostic factors and a plea for cooperation. *Med Pediatr Oncol* 1998; **30**:319–29.

59 Foreman N, Love S, Gill S, Coakham H. Second-look surgery for incompletely resected fourth ventricle ependymomas: technical case report. *Neurosurgery* 1997; **40**:856–60.

60 Vancalenbergh F, Vandelaar A, Plets C, Goffin J, Casaer P. Transient cerebellar mutism after posterior fossa surgery in children. *Neurosurgery* 1995; **37**:894–8.

61 Liu G, Phillips P, Molloy P, *et al.* Visual impairment associated with mutism after posterior fossa surgery in children. *Neurosurgery* 1998; **42**:253–6.

62 Garrett P, Simpson W. Ependymomas: results of radiation therapy. *Int J Radiat Oncol Biol Phys* 1983; **9**:1121–4.

63 Kim Y, Fayos J. Intracranial ependymomas. *Radiology* 1977; **124**:805–8.

64 Phillips T, Sheline G, Boldrey E. Therapeutic consideration in tumors affecting the central nervous system: ependymomas. *Radiology* 1964; **83**:98–105.

65 Mork S, Loken A. Ependymoma. A follow-up study of 101 cases. *Cancer* 1977; **40**:907–15.

66 Scheurlen W, Kuhl J. Current diagnostic and therapeutic management of CNS metastasis in childhood primitive neuroectodermal tumors and ependymomas. *J Neuro-Oncol* 1998; **38**:181–5.

67 Goldwein J, Merchant, Vanuystel L, Brada M. The role of prophylactic spinal irradiation in localized intracranial ependymoma. *Int J Radiat Oncol Biol Phys* 1991; **21**:825–30.

68 Kovnar E. Hyperfractionated irradiation for childhood ependymoma: early results of a phase III Pediatric Oncology Group Study. Presented at the 8th International Symposium on Pediatric Neuro-Oncology, Rome, 6–9 May, 1998.

69 Aggarwal R, Yeung D, Kumar P, Muhlbauer M, Kun L. Efficacy and feasibility of stereotactic radiosurgery in the primary management of unfavorable pediatric ependymoma. *Radiother Oncol* 1997; **43**:269–73.

70 Stafford S, Pollock B, Foote R, Gorman D, Nelson D, Schomberg P. Sterotactic radiosurgery for recurrent ependymoma. *Cancer* 2000; **88**:870–5.

71 Jawahar A, Kondziolka D, Flickinger J, Lunsford L. Adjuvant stereotactic radiosurgery for anaplastic ependymoma. *Sterotact Funct Neurosurg* 1999; **73**:23–30.

72 Awaad YM, Allen JC, Miller DC, Schneider SJ, Wisoff J, Epstein FJ. Deferring adjuvant therapy for totally resected intracranial ependymoma. *Pediatr Neurol* 1996; **14**:216–19.

73 Duffner P, Horowitz M, Krischer J, *et al.* Postoperative chemotherapy and delayed radiation in children less than three years of age with malignant brain tumors. *N Engl J Med* 1993; **328**:1725–31.

74 Grill J, LeDeley M, Garambelli D, *et al.* Postoperative chemotherapy without irradiation for ependymoma in children under 5 years of age: a multicenter trial of the French Society of Pediatric Oncology. *J Clin Oncol* 2001; **19**:1288–96.

75 Evans A, Anderson J, Lefkowitz-Boudreaux I, Finlay J. Adjuvant chemotherapy of childhood posterior fossa ependymoma: cranio-spinal irradiation with or without adjuvant CCNU, vincristine, and prednisone: a Children's Cancer Group study. *Med Pediatr Oncol* 1996; **27**:8–14.

76 Bouffet E, Foreman N. Chemotherapy for intracranial ependymomas. *Childs Nerv Syst* 1999; **15**:563–70.

77 Grill J, Kalifa C, Doz F, *et al.* A high-dose busulfan-thiotepa combination followed by autologous bone marrow transplantation in childhood recurrent ependymoma. A phase-II study. *Pediatr Neurosurg* 1996; **25**:7–12.

78 Mason W, Goldman S, Yates A, Boyett J, Li H, Finlay J. Survival following intensive chemotherapy with bone marrow reconstitution for children with recurrent intracranial ependymoma – a report of the Children's Cancer Group. *J Neuro-Oncol* 1998; **37**:135–43.

79 Fouladi M, Baruchel S, Chan H, *et al.* Use of adjuvant ICE chemotherapy in the treatment of anaplastic ependymomas. *Childs Nerv Syst* 1998; **14**:590–5.

80 Geyer J, Zeltzer P, Boyett J, *et al.* Survival of infants with primitive neuroectodermal tumors or malignant ependymomas of the CNS treated with eight drugs in 1 day: a report from the Children's Cancer Group. *J Clin Oncol* 1994; **12**:1607–15.

81 Kellie S. Chemotherapy of central nervous system tumors in infants. *Childs Nerv Syst* 1999; **15**:592–612.

82 Strother D, Kepner J, Aronin P. Effects of degree of surgical resection and intensity of chemotherapy on event-free survival of children with ependymoma and medulloblastoma. Results from Pediatric Oncology Group Study 9233. Presented at the 9th International Symposium on Pediatric Neurooncology, San Francisco, 11–14 June, 2000.

83 Chou P, Barquin N, Gonzalez-Crussi F, Sanz C, Tomita T, Reyes-Mugica M. Ependymomas in children express the multidrug resistance gene: Immunohistochemical and molecular biologic study. *Pediatr Pathol Lab Med* 1996; **16**:551–61.

84 Hongeng S, Brent T, Sanford R, Li H, Kun L, Heideman R. O6-Methylguanine-DNA methyltransferase protein levels in pediatric brain tumors. *Clin Cancer Res* 1997; **3**:2459–63.

85 Goldweins J, Glauser T, Packer R, *et al.* Recurrent intracranial ependymomas in children. Survival, patterns of failure, and prognostic factors. *Cancer* 1990; **66**:557–63.

86 Kovalic J, Flaris N, Grigsby P, Pirkowski M, Simpson J, Roth K. Intracranial ependymoma long term outcome, patterns of failure. *J Neuro-Oncol* 1993; **15**:125–31.

87 Lyons M, Kelly P. Posterior fossa ependymomas: report of 30 cases and review of the literature. *Neurosurgery* 1991; **28**:659–64.

88 Good C, Wade A, Hayward R, *et al.* Surveillance neuroimaging in childhood intracranial ependymoma: how effective, how often, and for how long? *Neurosurgery* 2001; **94**:27–32.

89 Kramer E, Vezina L, Packer R, Fitz C, Zimmerman R, Cohen M. Staging and surveillance of children with central nervous system neoplasms: recommendations of the Neurology and Tumor Imaging Committees of the Children's Cancer Group. *Pediatr Neursurg* 1994; **20**:254–63.

90 Steinbok P, Hentschel S, Cochrane D, Kestle J. Value of post-operative surveillance imaging in the management of children with some common brain tumors. *J Neurosurg* 1996; **84**:726–32.

91 Bertolone S, Baum E, Krivit W, Hammond G. A phase II study of cisplatin therapy in recurrent childhood brain tumors. A report from the Children's Cancer Study Group. *J Neuro-Oncol* 1989; **7**:5–11.

92 Friedman H, Kirscher J, Burger P, *et al.* Treatment of children with progressive or recurrent brain tumors with carboplatin or iproplatin: a Pediatric Oncology Group randomized phase II study. *J Clin Oncol* 1992; **10**:249–56.

93 Khan A, D'Souza B, Wharam M, *et al.* Cisplatin therapy in recurrent childhood brain tumors. *Cancer Treat Rep* 1982; **66**:2013–20.

94 Ragab A, Burger P, Badnitsky S, Krischer J, VanEys J. PCNU in the treatment of recurrent medulloblastoma and ependymoma – a POG Study. *J Neuro-Oncol* 1986; **3**:341–2.

95 Sexauer C, Khan A, Burger P, *et al.* Cisplatin in recurrent pediatric brain tumors. A POG phase II study. *Cancer* 1985; **56**:1497–501.

96 Feeny D, Furlong W, Barr R, Torrance G, Rosenbaum P, Weitzman S. A comprehensive multiattribute system for classifying the health status of survivors of childhood cancer. *J Clin Oncol* 1992; **10**:923–8.

97 Hoppe-Hirsch E, Brunet L, Laroussinie F, *et al.* Intellectual outcome in children with malignant tumors of the posterior fossa: influence of the field of irradiation and quality of surgery. *Childs Nerv Syst* 1995; **11**:340–5.

98 Seaver E, Geyer R, Sulzbacher S, *et al.* Psychosocial adjustment in long-term survivors of childhood medulloblastoma and ependymoma treated with craniospinal irradiation. *Pediatr Neurosurg* 1994; **20**:248–53.

APPENDIX: CHEMOTHERAPY FOR EPENDYMOMA

Chemotherapy trials for ependymoma: single-agent therapy

Agent	Response/patients	CR	Ref.
AZQ	2/29	2	1–5
Carboplatin	4/31		6, 7
Cisplatin	11/33	6	8–11
Cyclophosphamide	1/2		12
Cytarabine	0/1		13
Dibromodulcitol	0/12		14
Etoposide	4/21	1	15–17
Idarubicin	0/13		18
Ifosfamide	1/20		19, 20
Interferon alpha	1/1		21
Interferon beta	0/2		22
Iproplatin	0/7		7
Irinotecan	1/5	0	23
Paclitaxel	0/14		24, 25
PCNU	1/11	1	26, 27
Procarbazine	0/3		13, 28, 29
Thiotepa	0/12		30, 31
Topotecan	0/4		32
Vincristine	0/1		13
Total	26/222 (11.7%)	10 (4.5%)	

AZQ, aziridinylbenzoquinone; CR, complete response; PCNU, [1-(2-chloroethyl)-3-(2,5-dioxo-3-piperidyl)-1-nitrosourea].

Chemotherapy trials for ependymoma: combination therapy

Combination	Response/patients	CR	Ref.
8-in-1	3/18	1	33–35
COPP	0/2		36
Cytarabine/ etoposide/cisplatin	0/2		37
Etoposide/carboplatin	1/11		38
Etoposide/ifosfamide	1/10		39
Etoposide/ifosfamide/ carboplatin	2/6	2	40
Etoposide/cisplatin	2/2	2	41
MOPP	3/3	3	42
Vincristine/ cyclophosphamide	12/25		43
Head Start	1/6		44
VETOPEC	6/7	NK	45
Baby SFOP (6-drug regimen)	0/27		46
Etoposide/thiotepa + carboplatin	0/7		47
Busulfan/thiotepa	0/15		48
Total	31/141 (22%)	8 (5.6%)	

COPP, cyclophosphamide, vincristine, procarbazine, and prednisone; CR, complete response; MOPP, mustine, vincristine, procarbazine, prednisone; NK, not known; SFOP, Société Francaise d'Oncologie Pédiatrique; VETOPEC, vincristine, etoposide, cyclophosphamide.

REFERENCES FOR APPENDIX

1   Schold SC, Jr, Friedman HS, Bjornsson TD, Falletta JM. Treatment of patients with recurrent primary brain tumors with AZQ. *Neurology* 1984; **34**:615–19.

2   Ettinger LJ, Ru N, Krailo M, Ruccione KS, Krivit W, Hammond GD. A phase II study of diaziquone in children with recurrent or progressive primary brain tumors: a report from the Children's Cancer Study Group. *J Neuro-Oncol* 1990; **9**:69–76.

3   Castleberry RP, Ragab AH, Steuber CP, *et al.* Aziridinyl-benzoquinone (AZQ) in the treatment of recurrent pediatric

brain and other malignant solid tumors. A Pediatric Oncology Group phase II study. *Invest New Drugs* 1990; **8**:401–6.

4 Chamberlain MC, Prados MD, Silver P, Levin VA. A phase I/II study of 24 hour intravenous AZQ in recurrent primary brain tumors. *J Neuro-Oncol* 1988; **6**:319–23.

5 Taylor SA, McCracken JD, Eyre HJ, O'Bryan RM, Neilan BA. Phase II study of aziridinylbenzoquinone (AZQ) in patients with central nervous system malignancies: a Southwest Oncology Group Study. *J Neuro-Oncol* 1985; **3**:131–5.

6 Gaynon PS, Ettinger LJ, Baum ES, Siegel SE, Krailo MD, Hammond GD. Carboplatin in childhood brain tumors. A Children's Cancer Study Group Phase II trial. *Cancer* 1990; **66**:2465–9.

7 Friedman HS, Krisher JP, Burger P, *et al*. Treatment of children with progressive or recurrent brain tumors with carboplatin or iproplatin: a Pediatric Oncology Group randomized phase II study. *J Clin Oncol* 1992; **10**:249–56.

8 Khan AB, D'Souza BJ, Wharam MD, *et al*. Cisplatin therapy in recurrent childhood brain tumors. *Cancer Treat Rep* 1982; **66**:2013–20.

9 Sexauer CL, Khan A, Burger PC, *et al*. Cisplatin in recurrent pediatric brain tumors. A Pediatric Oncology Group phase II study. *Cancer* 1985; **56**:1497–501.

10 Walker RW, Allen JC. Cisplatin in the treatment of recurrent primary brain tumors. *J Clin Oncol* 1988; **6**:62–6.

11 Bertolone SJ, Baum ES, Krivit W, Hammond GD. A phase II study of cisplatin therapy in recurrent childhood brain tumors. A report from the Children's Cancer Study Group. *J Neuro-Oncol* 1989; **7**:5–11.

12 Allen JC, Helson L. High-dose cyclophosphamide chemotherapy for recurrent CNS tumors in children. *J Neurosurg* 1981; **55**:749–56.

13 Goldwein JW, Glauser TA, Packer RJ, *et al*. Recurrent intracranial ependymomas in children. Survival, patterns of failure, and prognostic factors. *Cancer* 1990; **66**:557–63.

14 Levin VA, Edwards MS, Gutin PH, *et al*. Phase II evaluation of dibromodulcitol in the treatment of recurrent medulloblastoma, ependymoma, and malignant astrocytoma. *J Neurosurg* 1984; **61**:1063–8.

15 Needle MN, Molloy PT, Geyer JR, *et al*. Phase II study of daily oral etoposide in children with recurrent brain tumors and other solid tumors. *Med Pediatr Oncol* 1997; **29**:28–32.

16 Davidson A, Lewis I, Pearson AD, Stevens MC, Pinkerton CR. 21-day schedule oral etoposide in children – a feasibility study. *Eur J Cancer* 1993; **29A**:2223–5.

17 Chamberlain MC. Recurrent intracranial ependymoma in children: salvage therapy with oral etoposide. *Pediatr Neurol* 2001; **24**:117–21.

18 Arndt C, Krailo MD, Steinherz L, Scheitauer B, Liu-Mares W, Reaman GH. A phase II clinical trial of idarubicin administered to children with relapsed brain tumours. *Cancer* 1998; **83**:813–16.

19 Chastagner P, Sommelet Olive D, Kalifa C, *et al*. Phase II study of ifosfamide in childhood brain tumors: A report by the French Society of Pediatric Oncology (SFOP). *Med Pediatr Oncol* 1993; **21**:49–53.

20 Heideman RL, Douglass EC, Langston JA, *et al*. Phase II study of every other day high-dose ifosfamide in pediatric brain tumors: a Pediatric Oncology Group study. *J Neuro-Oncol* 1995; **25**:77–84.

21 Dorr RT, Salmon SE, Robertone A, Bonnem E. Phase I-II trial of interferon-alpha 2b by continuous subcutaneous infusion over 28 days. *J Interferon Res* 1988; **8**:717–25.

22 Allen J, Packer R, Bleyer A, Zeltzer P, Prados M, Nirenberg A. Recombinant interferon beta: a phase I-II trial in children with recurrent brain tumors. *J Clin Oncol* 1991; **9**:783–8.

23 Turner CD, Gururangan S, Eastwood J, *et al*. Phase II study of irinotecan (CPT-11) in children with high-risk malignant brain tumors: the Duke experience. *Neuro-oncol* 2002; **4**:102–8.

24 Hurwitz CA, Relling MV, Weitman SD, Ravindranath Y, Vietti TJ. Phase I trial of paclitaxel in children with refractory solid tumors: a Pediatric Oncology Group study. *J Clin Oncol* 1993; **11**:2324–9.

25 Hurwitz CA, Strauss LC, Kepner J, *et al*. Paclitaxel for the treatment of progressive or recurrent childhood brain tumors: a pediatric oncology phase II study. *J Pediatr Hematol Oncol* 2001; **23**:277–81.

26 Allen JC, Hancock C, Walker R, Tan C. PCNU and recurrent childhood brain tumors. *J Neuro-Oncol* 1987; **5**:241–4.

27 Ragab AH, Burger P, Badnitsky S, Krischer J, Van Eys J. PCNU in the treatment of recurrent medulloblastoma and ependymoma – a POG study. *J Neuro-Oncol* 1986; **3**:341–2.

28 Van Eys J, Cangir A, Pack R, Baram T. Phase I trial of procarbazine as a 5-day continuous infusion in children with central nervous system tumors. *Cancer Treat Rep* 1987; **71**:973–4.

29 Rodriguez LA, Prados M, Silver P, Levin VA. Reevaluation of procarbazine for the treatment of recurrent malignant central nervous system tumors. *Cancer* 1989; **64**:2420–3.

30 Heideman RL, Packer RJ, Allen JC. A phase II study of thiotepa in pediatric central nervous system tumors. *Pediatr Neurosci* 1989; **15**:146–7.

31 Razzouk BI, Heideman RL, Friedman HS, *et al*. A phase II evaluation of thiotepa followed by other multiagent chemotherapy regimens in infants and young children with malignant brain tumors. *Cancer* 1995; **75**:2762–7.

32 Blaney SM, Phillips PC, Packer RJ, Heideman RL, Berg SL, Adamson PC. Phase II evaluation of topotecan for pediatric central nervous system tumors. *Cancer* 1996; **78**:527–31.

33 Pendergrass TW, Milstein JM, Geyer JR, *et al*. Eight drugs in one day chemotherapy for brain tumors: experience in 107 children and rationale for preradiation chemotherapy. *J Clin Oncol* 1987; **5**:1221–31.

34 Chastagner P, Olive D, Philip T, *et al*. Efficacité du protocole "8 drogues en un jour" dans les tumeurs cérébrales de l'enfant. *Arch Fr Pediatr* 1988; **45**:249–54.

35 Geyer JR, Zeltzer PM, Boyett JM, *et al*. Survival of infants with primitive neuroectodermal tumors or malignant ependymomas of the CNS treated with eight drugs in 1 day: a report from the Children's Cancer Group. *J Clin Oncol* 1994; **12**:1607–15.

36 Ettinger LJ, Sinniah D, Siegel SE. Combination chemotherapy with cyclophosphamide, vincristine, procarbazine, and prednisone (COPP) in children with brain tumors. *J Neuro-Oncol* 1985; **3**:263–9.

37 Corden BJ, Strauss LC, Killmond T, et al. Cisplatin, ara-C and etoposide (PAE) in the treatment of recurrent childhood brain tumors. *J Neuro-Oncol* 1991; **11**:57–63.

38 Gentet JC, Bouffet E, Kalifa C, Doz F, Thyss A, Bernard JL. Phase II study of carboplatin and VP-16 in ependymoma: a report of the French Society of Pediatric Oncology. SIOP XXVI meeting. *Med Ped Oncol* 1994; **23**:215.

39 Miser J, Krailo M, Smithson W. Treatment of children with recurrent brain tumors with ifosfamide, etoposide and mesna. *Proc Am Soc Clin Oncol* 1989; **8**:84.

40 Fouladi M, Baruchel S, Chan H, *et al*. Use of adjuvant ICE chemotherapy in the treatment of anaplastic ependymomas. *Childs Nerv Syst* 1998; **14**:590–5.

41 Strauss LC, Killmond TM, Carson BS, Maria BL, Wharam MD, Leventhal BG. Efficacy of postoperative chemotherapy using cisplatin plus etoposide in young children with brain tumors. *Med Pediatr Oncol* 1991; **19**:16–21.

42 Van Eys J, Cangir A, Coody D, Smith B. MOPP regimen as primary chemotherapy for brain tumors in infants. *J Neuro-Oncol* 1985; **3**:237–43.

43 Duffner PK, Horowitz ME, Krischer JP. Postoperative chemotherapy and delayed radiation in children less than three years of age with malignant brain tumors. *N Engl J Med* 1993; **328**:1725–31.

44 Mason WP, Grovas A, Halpern S, *et al*. Intensive chemotherapy and bone marrow rescue for young children with newly diagnosed malignant brain tumors. *J Clin Oncol* 1998; **16**:210–21.

45 White L, Kellie S, Gray E, *et al*. Postoperative chemotherapy in children less than 4 years of age with malignant brain tumors: promising initial response to a VETOPEC-based regimen. A Study of the Australian and New Zealand Children's Cancer Study Group (ANZCCSG). *J Pediatr Hematol Oncol* 1998; **20**:125–30.

46 Grill J, Le Deley MC, Gambarelli D, *et al*. Postoperative chemotherapy without irradiation for ependymoma in children under 5 years of age: a multicenter trial of the French Society of Pediatric Oncology. *J Clin Oncol* 2001; **19**:1288–96.

47 Mason WP, Goldman S, Yates AJ, Boyett J, Li H, Finlay JL. Survival following intensive chemotherapy with bone marrow reconstitution for children with recurrent intracranial ependymoma – a report of the Children's Cancer Group. *J Neuro-Oncol* 1998; **37**:135–43.

48 Grill J, Kalifa C, Doz F, *et al*. A high-dose busulfan-thiotepa combination followed by autologous bone marrow transplantation in childhood recurrent ependymoma. A phase-II study. *Pediatr Neurosurg* 1996; **25**:7–12.

18a

Germ-cell tumors of the central nervous system

GABRIELE CALAMINUS AND MARIA LUISA GARRÉ

INTRODUCTION

The past two decades have been characterized by a dramatic improvement of the prognosis of malignant germ-cell tumors (GCTs) in all localizations, in both the adult and the pediatric populations. This can be attributed mainly to national and international cooperative therapeutic protocols that have utilized cisplatin-based combination chemotherapy integrated into a multimodal therapeutic approach. Although the first pediatric trials were designed in the light of the previous experience in malignant testicular GCTs in adults, these studies soon revealed the particular clinical and biological features of childhood GCT. Moreover, the early observations have allowed tailoring of therapy more specifically to the pediatric setting and the introduction of stratification of chemotherapy according to risk groups with respect to the parameters of age, histology, primary site, and stage.

Epidemiology

In the pediatric age group, malignant GCTs are rare tumors that contribute 2.9 per cent of all registered neoplasms in central children's cancer registries.[1] For example, in Germany the incidence of malignant GCT is 0.6/100 000 children aged 15 years or younger. Since teratomas contribute an additional 50 per cent, the overall incidence of GCT can be estimated as 0.9/100 000 children aged 15 years or younger. The distribution of GCTs with regard to tumor site and histology varies significantly with age. In neonates, mature and immature teratomas predominate (girls 0.9/100 000, boys 2.6/100 000). In the

first years of life, the overall incidence of GCT decreases (<0.1/100 000 for both sexes at five years of age), but among toddlers, the relative proportion of malignant tumors such as yolk-sac tumors (YSTs) increases. The incidence of gonadal tumors, mainly seminomas and dysgerminomas, increases with the onset of puberty. In patients under 15 years of age, there is a female predominance. In young men, GCTs represent the most common malignant tumor. Intracranial GCTs occur in children and adults and represent one per cent of all malignant neoplasms in children.

Natural history

According to the holistic concept of Teilum (Figure 18a.1),[2,3] GCTs arise from totipotent primordial germ cells

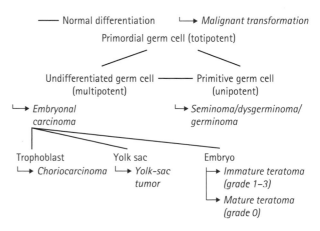

Figure 18a.1 *Holistic concept of germ-cell tumor histogenesis. (Modified according to Teilum[2] and Gonzalez-Crussi[3].)*

Table 18a.1 *Biological characteristics of germ-cell tumors*

Entity	Dignity	β–HCG	AFP	RT	CT
Germinoma	Malignant	(+)	–	+++	+++
Embryonal carcinoma	Malignant	–	–	+	+++
Yolk-sac tumor	Malignant	–	+++	+	+++
Choriocarcinoma	Malignant	+++	–	+	+++
Teratoma	Benign (potential malignant)	–	((+))	(+)	–

AFP, alpha-fetoprotein; β-HCG, beta-human chorionic gonadotrophin; CT, chemotherapy; RT, radiotherapy.

that are capable of embryonic and extraembryonic differentiation. YSTs and choriocarcinomas (CHCs) follow an extraembryonic differentiation pattern and are characterized by significant secretion of alpha-1-fetoprotein (AFP) and human choriogonadotrophin (HCG or β-HCG), respectively (Table 18a.1). Embryonal carcinomas represent tumors of immature totipotent cells. Teratomas display an embryonic differentiation and may mimic organ structures of all germ layers. In teratoma, the histologic grade of immaturity is defined by the extent of immature (predominantly neuroepithelial) elements.[4] Finally, germinomatous tumors (synonyms: seminoma (testis), dysgerminoma (ovary), germinoma (brain)) display morphological features of undifferentiated germ epithelium. In contrast to testicular GCTs of adult patients, pediatric GCTs do not develop from carcinoma in situ.[5]

Biology

Molecular studies of the imprinting status of GCTs have revealed that gonadal and non-gonadal GCTs share a common cellular origin, the primordial germ cell, although at different stages of their development.[6,7] These data substantiate the hypothesis that non-gonadal GCTs develop from germ cells that have become mislocated during their embryonic development. While no consistent correlation between cytogenetic aberration and primary site of the tumor has been observed, it is apparent that histology (teratoma versus malignant GCTs) and age (pre- versus postpubertal) both correlate significantly with distinct genetic profiles.[8]

Pediatric GCTs show a pattern of cytogenetic aberrations different from their adult counterparts. More than 80 per cent of adult malignant GCTs display a distinct and specific chromosomal aberration, the isochromosome 12p.[9] The remaining isochromosome 12p-negative tumors frequently show amplification of 12p (homogeneously staining regions or tandem repeats). These aberrations have been observed in gonadal and non-gonadal GCTs.

In children under ten years of age, an isochromosome 12p has been found in only a small minority of malignant GCTs.[8,9] On the other hand, aberrations at both the short and long arms of chromosome 1, at the long arm of chromosome 6, and in the sex chromosomes have been found frequently.[10] Finally, virtually all prepubertal teratomas are normal on conventional cytogenetic analysis and on comparative genomic hybridization.[11]

Diagnosis

Intracranial GCTs form a heterogeneous group of tumors that, although rare, present some peculiar features (sites of involvement and origin, hormonal activity, strict relationship of lesions with cerebrospinal fluid (CSF) and ventricular system, high chemo- and radiosensitivity) affecting the natural history, diagnostic approach, and treatment strategies. The accuracy of initial diagnosis and staging can influence significantly the treatment decisions and consequently the possibility of cure. Diagnosis of GCTs is based on clinical symptoms and signs, markers, neuroimaging, and cytological (CSF) and histological confirmation. All these aspects are important and are strongly recommended to be assessed fully by a multidisciplinary team (neurosurgeon, oncologist, neuroradiologist, pathologist) before treatment (including surgery) is initiated.[12–15]

The sequence of timing of decisions between diagnosis and the start of therapy is not always easy to adhere to, considering that the patient's clinical condition, especially in cases of pineal tumors, may not allow a long delay to start of therapy. However, it is very important to try to perform the correct staging and diagnosis before treatment is initiated, because this can positively influence the results of therapy and outcome.

Clinical aspects

The clinical symptoms and signs at presentation of GCTs, and their appearance, are strictly dependent on the particular site of involvement (suprasellar, pineal, or both) and with histological tumor types that can determine hormonal activity. Duration of symptoms before diagnosis is related to velocity of tumor growth and location,

Table 18a.2 *Intracranial germ-cell tumors in children: presenting clinical features*

Symptoms at diagnosis	Site (no. of cases)	
	Suprasellar (16)	Pineal (32)
Diabetes insipidus	11	5
Raised intracranial pressure	1	27
Visual changes	7	10 (Parinaud 8, loss of downward gaze 2)
Hypopituitarism	7	–
Changed level of consciousness	4	7
Seizures	–	1
Oculomotor palsies	1	–
Median duration before diagnosis (months)	21	4

Reprinted from H.J. Hoffman *et al.*[18] by permission of the *Journal of Neurosurgery.*

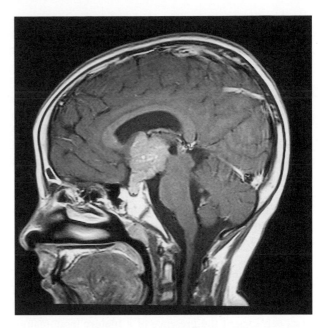

Figure 18a.2 *Example of a case with metastasis involving the ventricular system. The tumor is visible in the fourth ventricle of lateral ventricles.*

being longer in germinoma (especially of the suprasellar site) compared with malignant non-germinomatous germ-cell tumors (MNGGCTs). Median time from first symptom to diagnosis in suprasellar germinoma is reported to range from 20 to 30 months; this interval can be shorter, irrespective of histology, if the tumor is developing in a pineal site, where symptoms of increased intracranial pressure (caused by cerebral aqueduct obstruction) are more frequently apparent. Lesions in the pineal site may also cause compression and invasion of the tectal plate, producing the characteristic upward gaze and convergence paralysis known as Parinaud's syndrome. Other visual symptoms can be caused by invasion of the chiasm by suprasellar tumors, but visual signs and symptoms are usually less frequent.

Overall, the most frequent signs and symptoms at diagnosis are the endocrine abnormalities caused by several mechanisms: the disruption of the hypothalamo-hypophyseal structures (with consequent endocrine dysfunctions, e.g. diabetes insipidus, growth hormone deficiency) and direct production by the tumor of selected oncoproteins (β-HCG, HCG, a glycoprotein normally secreted by syncytiotrophoblasts) and a stimulant of testosterone secretion.[16,17]

The frequency and type of symptoms at diagnosis of intracranial GCTs have been reported by Hoffmann and colleagues (Table 18a.2)[18] and other authors.[19,20]

Of the endocrine symptoms, the most frequent at diagnosis for the tumors arising in the suprasellar location is diabetes insipidus, which is part of the classical triad: diabetes insipidus, symptoms and signs of hypothalamic-pituitary dysfunction, and visual disturbances. Diabetes insipidus is so common (between 93[18] and 100 per cent[21]) that a diagnosis of suprasellar germinoma should always be considered in the presence of so-called "idiopathic" diabetes insipidus. One study showed that of 79 cases of diabetes insipidus, 18 (20 per cent) were caused by a tumor (usually a germinoma) involving the hypophyseal peduncle.[22] The association of diabetes insipidus with other types of hypothalamic tumors that may be confused with germinoma, such as low-grade glioma, is extremely uncommon at diagnosis but is more common after surgery.[23,24] Diabetes insipidus is a result of the origin and development of the tumor in a specific area of the hypothalamus and the hypophyseal peduncle, from where the tumor can expand, as shown clearly by the case in Figure 18a.2.

Neuroimaging

Although not highly specific and not a substitute for histological diagnosis, which requires tumor tissue examination, the greater experience and the technical quality of modern imaging has contributed greatly to a more precise preoperative diagnosis of intracranial GCTs. Magnetic resonance imaging (MRI) is the most appropriate imaging modality, although computed tomography (CT) scanning can add information on the presence of calcification. Modern neuroradiology also contributes to insights into the natural history (site of origin, pattern of growth) of these diseases and is crucial for follow-up evaluation of response to treatment. MRI findings plus clinical signs and typical location (suprasellar, bifocal, pineal) can largely predict the presence of an intracranial GCT before biopsy. Correct interpretation of imaging should take into account the MRI appearance of the normal anatomy of the pineal and suprasellar regions at different ages and of that of other benign or malignant lesions typical in these sites (pineal cysts).[25–27] For a patient suspected of having a GCT, the appropriate radiological study is MRI, which should be performed as follows: pre-gadolinium axial study of the brain with T1, T2, and fluid attenuated inversion recovery (FLAIR) sequences; T1 axial, coronal, and sagittal sequences; and volumetric post-gadolinium T1 sequences. The study of the spine should be performed with both axial and sagittal post-gadolinium T1 sequences. At follow-up, the MRI study should be performed using the same procedure, making sure that the slices are comparable.

On MRI, GCTs usually appear as solid masses that are iso- or hyperintense relative to gray matter and show prominent enhancement following the administration of contrast media. Within the context of an otherwise bifocal GCT, the presence of fat and calcifications or intratumoral cysts can suggest the presence of a mature teratomatous component.[27–29]

The main neuroradiological features of pure germinomas are represented by their typical site of origin. Thirty per cent of cases are bifocal and less than ten per cent are metastatic with multifocal involvement, especially within the ventricular system. For patients with germinomas who present with endocrine symptoms, assessment with MRI is generally performed early, and thus diagnosis when the lesion is still small is becoming more frequent. In these cases, MRI can show the lack of the bright spot of the neurohypophysis on T1-weighted images and thickening of the hypothalamus and infundibular stalk. Larger masses usually demonstrate a homogeneous pattern. In contrast, secreting GCTs are isodense or hyperdense on CT. Evidence of calcifications may be present. They are hypoisointense on T1 MRI, and hyperintense or isointense on T2-weighted images.

In suprasellar sites, the differential diagnosis is from Langerhans cell histiocytosis and sarcoidosis for small lesions, and from low-grade gliomas for larger lesions. In the pineal location, differential diagnosis is from other, less frequent tumors in this site, such as primitive neuroectodermal tumors (PNETs), low-grade astrocytomas, and pineocytomas. For PNETs, the age of the patient can help in diagnosis, because they usually occur in younger children.[23]

The accuracy of MRI and CT scanning during follow-up is very important for the information that it can give regarding the response to treatment, and the presence, size, and location of residual tumor, which can influence subsequent treatment strategies.[30] Pure germinomas usually disappear completely after a relatively low dose of radiotherapy or a few cycles of chemotherapy. Germinomas with teratomatous components and MNGGCTs may have a more complex pattern of response, with slow

Table 18a.3 *Characteristics of beta-human chorionic gonadotrophin (β-HCG)*

Produced by placenta	Increases hormones to maintain pregnancy
Half-life	16 hours
Normal values	
Serum	<5 mUI/ml
Cerebrospinal fluid	Absent
Marker for	Placental tumors, fetal diseases (Down's syndrome)
	NG germ-cell tumors (choriocarcinoma, embryonal carcinoma, mixed)
	Pure germinomas (<5% of cases) with foci of trophoblastic tissue (levels <50)

NG, non-germinoma.

Table 18a.4 *Characteristics of alpha-fetoprotein (AFP)*

70 kDa-glycoprotein	
Binding protein in fetus (yolk sac, liver, intestine)	
Measurement technique	Immunoassay
Half-life	5 days
Normally elevated	• During gestation, in fetus and in mother
	• After birth; level decreases up to age 2 years
Marker for	• Liver tumors
	• NG germ-cell tumors (yolk sac, embryonal carcinoma, mixed)
Normal value	<15 mg/ml

regression of residual tumors despite markers of normalization or sometimes profound morphological regressive changes inside the lesions (increased necrosis and cystic component, increased volume of mature residual teratomatous component).

Markers

GCTs may secrete specific tumors markers such as β-HCG and alpha-fetoprotein (Tables 18a.3 and 18a.4).

Within the past five or ten years, due to the availability of more reliable laboratory tests to detect these oncoproteins in the serum and CSF and the greater experience achieved in the interpretation of tumor markers both in extracranial and intracranial GCTs, definite subgroups of patients with high or slight increases in serum and spinal fluid markers have been identified. High levels (>50 for β-HCG, >25 for alpha-fetoprotein) in so-called "secreting GCTs" are associated with a worse prognosis and the need for more aggressive treatment.[31–34] Pure germinomas and pure teratomas usually present with negative markers, although very low levels of β-HCG in pure germinomas, and of alpha-fetoprotein in pure teratomas, occur in a small percentage of cases (the real frequency of these cases is not completely clear, as the policy of determining markers systematically in both spinal fluid and serum in all cases at diagnosis was not recommended in the past). A relevant percentage of cases enrolled in the Société International d'Oncologie Pédiatrique (SIOP) GCTs study, which opened in Europe in 1996 and accounted for 259 cases at December 2000, had marker determination in spinal fluid and serum, but at the time of writing this information was not complete. Prognosis does not seem to be influenced negatively in patients presenting with a slight increase in β-HCG at diagnosis and having histologically proven germinoma. However, this is still controversial, and in the presence of slight elevation of levels of β-HCG, the presence of syncytiotrophoblastic foci in the tumor may be a worse prognostic factor.

Placental alkaline phosphatase (PLAP) is being used increasingly as a specific marker of seminomas in adults.[35] Its potential benefit in identifying specifically pure germinomas is under investigation. The main problem is that the techniques for detection of germinoma are not yet sensitive enough to guarantee the test for wider use.

In malignant non-germinomatous germ cell tumors (MNGGCTs), the presence of marker elevation at diagnosis is very frequent (80 per cent in serum, >60 per cent in CSF); this could even be underestimated, taking into account the high frequency of cases that are still staged incompletely. The presence of positive markers is then assumed to be an unequivocal sign of the presence of one or more malignant components needing a treatment different from that which is appropriate for germinoma, i.e. a need for chemotherapy without any histological confirmation if there is a typical clinical and neuroradiological picture of GCT. Modern treatment recommendations included in the international protocols designed for these tumors (SIOP CNS GCTs '96 study, International Germ Cell Tumor Study) recommend that if the history, endocrine signs, and imaging suggest a possible intracranial GCT, then markers should be performed before any treatment decision, including surgical removal, which can be postponed after chemotherapy in secreting tumors, probably with better results.

Marker determination is also very useful during treatment and follow-up in order to monitor response to chemotherapy or remission status. Marker levels decline after effective therapy and they are a sensitive diagnostic tool in detecting relapse.[36–38] β-HCG elevation unrelated to tumor regrowth was noted only in coincidence with hormonal replacement therapy.

Cerebrospinal fluid

The estimation assay of CSF for selected oncoproteins (β-HCG, alpha-fetoprotein) has become standard practice in the preoperative evaluation of patients suspected of harboring central nervous system (CNS) GCTs and for monitoring their response to treatment.[13,34] As shown by the SIOP preliminary data, a significant percentage of cases present with marker-positivity only in the CSF. CSF samples can be obtained during surgical procedures to treat hydrocephalus (positioning of ventriculoperitoneal shunt, third ventriculocisternotomy) or by lumbar puncture in cases without hydrocephalus or with small lesions and few symptoms. A cytological examination according to the techniques also used for detection of cancer cells in leukemia and medulloblastoma is strongly recommended, as cases with positive cytology are considered metastatic and eligible for more extended irradiation fields.

Histologic classification of intracranial germ-cell tumors

CNS GCTs are characterized by a profound heterogeneity in their histologic differentiation. They are classified according to the World Health Organization (WHO) grading for intracranial GCTs. As intra-tumor heterogeneity may be subtle, the initial diagnostic work-up should include the evaluation by an experienced pediatric pathologist. For instance, according to the guidelines of the German GCT protocols, a central reference histology is mandatory in order to achieve a standardized and reliable histopathological diagnosis and grading.

About 25 per cent of all pediatric CNS GCTs present as tumors with more than one histologic type. In this situation, therapy and prognosis depend on the component with the highest malignancy.

The final diagnosis of GCTs is made by histological examination of the tumor specimens obtained after surgical procedures. In the past, histological confirmation was made mainly after open biopsy or on tumor specimens obtained with tumor removal of the lesion. In the past ten years, several new techniques have become suitable for less invasive surgical procedures, such as stereotactic biopsy and biopsy during neuroendoscopy procedures.[39,40]

SURGICAL MANAGEMENT

Although there is a consensus that surgery is required in all patients with negative markers in serum and CSF or borderline secretion of markers for diagnosis, the value of extensive surgical resection, especially total or near-total resection, is unproven.[41]

If ventricular drainage is required, then one modern method of choice is neuroendoscopy by third ventriculostomy. In patients with involvement of the anterior third ventricle, thus making third ventriculostomy impossible, then ventriculoscopy at a procedure to establish external or internal ventricular drainage will still afford the opportunity to obtain biopsies and CSF sampling. Several papers have established the efficacy of neuroendoscopic biopsy in germ-cell and non-germ-cell tumors of the pineal[39] and of the third ventricle. Non-surgical treatment can be curative itself in most cases of germinomas, and patients with MNGGCTs can be treated by a policy involving a delayed surgical approach. A histological diagnosis by the least invasive technique is recommended whenever necessary (cases with markers negative, including patients with germinomas). The risks of surgery, including hemorrhage and oncological risks, such as tumor dissemination, should always be weighed against the benefits.

The use of stereotactic biopsy to obtain histological confirmation has become the standard diagnostic procedure.[41] However, it should be recognized that patients have to be treated as individuals in the acute situation, and particular circumstances may occasionally dictate the extent of surgery.

There are also situations in which the presence of a GCT is not considered high on the differential diagnosis, due to its location.

Surgery has a major role to play in the treatment of residual MNGGCT following chemotherapy and before consideration of radiotherapy. It also plays a dominant role in the treatment of intracranial mature teratoma.

Interesting histological aspects have been described increasingly since the wider use of delayed surgery for secreting GCTs. The tumor specimens after treatment are found to present significant histomorphological changes, such as disappearance of malignant components, maturation, and involutive changes, correlating to some MRI aspects, including increased necrosis and degenerative cystic changes.

NON–SURGICAL TREATMENT

General aspects

The treatment of malignant CNS GCTs in children and adolescents follows a multimodal concept that may include tumor resection irradiation, and chemotherapy. The response correlates with tumor histology. Germinomatous GCTs are exceptionally sensitive to both irradiation and platinum-based chemotherapy. Platinum-based chemotherapy is also highly effective in malignant non-germinomatous GCTs of children.[42,43]

Therapy for malignant intracranial GCTs is stratified according to the histologic differentiation (germinoma versus secreting GCT) and initial tumor stage (non-metastatic/metastatic).

The management scheme in the current European SIOP CNS GCT trial is summarized in Figure 18a.3.

Germinoma

Standard treatment for intracranial pure germinoma is craniospinal irradiation. The past decade of intracranial germinoma management has been characterized by a debate about the necessary dose and treatment volume of irradiation to achieve sufficient local tumor control and to treat subclinical disease in the whole ventricular and spinal CSF space. In the German MAKEI '89 protocol, a dose reduction from 36 to 30 Gy in the craniospinal axis was performed, and the five-year relapse-free survival rate was 88 per cent. It has been demonstrated that a five-year event-free survival of 91 per cent and a five-year overall survival of 94 per cent can be achieved by radiotherapy alone.[44]

With the combined chemo- and radiotherapy approach, a three-year relapse-free survival of 96 per cent and an overall three-year survival of 98 per cent have been reported. However, in this study, two of the four observed events occurred after the evaluated three-year observation period.[45] A recent analysis of recurrence in the Société Francaise d'Oncologie Pédiatrique (SFOP) studies and of the institutional experience of the Milan Cancer Institute revealed that most relapses after combined treatment and focal irradiation appeared in the ventricular area.[46,47] Finally, strategies that have utilized chemotherapy but that have excluded radiotherapy completely have resulted in insufficient local tumor control.[48]

The ongoing SIOP CNS GCT '96 protocol (Figure 18a.3) aims to evaluate two different therapeutic options in intracranial germinoma with regard to both their therapeutic impact and their specific acute and long-term toxicity. In pure intracranial germinomas, which account for 50 per cent of all intracranial GCTs, which may occur bifocally (30 per cent), and which do not secret significant amounts of β-HCG, histologic verification of the tumor is mandatory. According to the current SIOP CNS GCT '96 protocol, patients can be treated either

Non-metastatic

Germinoma → Craniospinal irradiation 24 Gy + 16 Gy tu
→ 2 × carboPEI → focal irradiation 40 Gy

Secreting GCT → 4 × PEI → focal irradiation 54 Gy

Metastatic

Germinoma → Craniospinal irradiation 24 Gy + 16 Gy tu
→ 2 × carboPEI → Craniospinal irradiation 24 Gy + 16 Gy tu

Secreting GCT → 4 × PEI → Craniospinal irradiation 30 Gy + 24 Gy tu

Figure 18a.3 *Société Internationale de Oncologie Pédiatrique (SIOP) 1996: central nervous system germ-cell tumor therapy. (carboPEI, carboplatin, etoposide, ifosfamide; PEI, cisplatin, etoposide, ifosfamide; tu, tumor.)*

with craniospinal irradiation with 24 Gy and a tumor boost of 16 Gy or with a multimodal treatment including two cycles of chemotherapy (carboplatin, etoposide, ifosfamide) followed by focal irradiation (40 Gy). The higher local dose at the primary tumor site also aims to control potential small foci of non-germinomatous histology, such as syncytiotrophoblastic cells that may have been missed by biopsy. As GCTs may arise adjacent to sensitive structures such as the optic chiasm, it is recommended that a reference radiation oncologist should be consulted for detailed recommendations on optimal treatment techniques. Preliminary data show a comparable event-free survival for both treatment arms.

Secreting germ–cell tumors

MNGGCTs (YSTs, CHC, embryonal carcinoma) show an inferior prognosis compared with germinoma.

The most effective chemotherapy and the optimal irradiation dose should provide the opportunity for cure in a majority of patients. A multimodal therapy combining chemotherapy and irradiation appears to be most promising. Observation of treatment with cisplatin, vinblastine, and bleomycin in combination with other drugs was reported in the late 1980s. A cumulative dosage of cisplatin of more than 300 mg/m^2 and irradiation with a tumor dose of approximately 50–54 Gy, together with craniospinal irradiation of approximately 40 Gy, seemed to be most effective.[49] Due to a synergistic effect of cisplatin and etoposide, this regimen was favored in the 1990s, with variable success.[41,50] These treatment strategies, investigated in several small series of patients, achieved survival rates between 30 and 60 per cent. The chemotherapy dosages and mode of administration, and the volumes and dose prescriptions of radiotherapy used, varied extensively. Strategies that excluded radiotherapy from first-line treatment yielded inferior results.[48]

In the SIOP CNS GCT '96 protocol for MNGGCTs, the effect of combined treatment with cisplatin, etoposide, and ifosfamide (PEI) and risk-adapted radiotherapy is being examined (non-metastatic/metastatic). In these patients, four cycles of cisplatin-based chemotherapy (PEI) are given, followed by delayed tumor resection and radiotherapy. The radiotherapy is stratified according to the initial staging. Non-metastatic tumors receive focal irradiation (54 Gy), while patients with intracranial or spinal metastases or tumor cells in the CSF receive craniospinal irradiation (30 Gy plus 24-Gy tumor boost).

The summary of several cooperative protocols and the preliminary data of the SIOP CNS GCT '96 protocol suggest that a long-term remission can be obtained in about two-thirds of patients.[49]

CASE STUDY 1

An 11-year-old boy presented with a short history of dizziness and diplopia. Clinical examination showed a right sixth nerve palsy. MRI revealed an infiltrative mass in the pineal area, with a non-communicating hydrocephalus (Figure 18a.4). The hydrocephalus was relieved with a right-sided ventriculoperitoneal shunt. CSF examination revealed no malignant cells. Blood and CSF for AFP and β-HCG were negative. A stereotactic biopsy of the lesion demonstrated germinoma. His symptoms resolved after the hydrocephalus was relieved.

The boy was treated according to the SIOP Germ Cell Tumor Study (GCT '96). He received craniospinal radiotherapy 24 Gy in 15 fractions of 1.6 Gy, followed by a boost to the primary of a further 16 Gy in ten fractions, giving a total dose to the primary area of 40 Gy. Four years after diagnosis he remains well. MRI confirms continued complete response (Figure 18a.5). He requires growth hormone supplementation. He is doing well at school, and he will soon be going to college to study a performing arts course. He has slight problems with short-term memory, but these do not affect his schoolwork. His height is 167.5 cm, just below the fiftieth centile.

This case illustrates the pathological behavior of intracranial germinoma with subependymal spread. This has to be taken into account when planning radiotherapy. The good prognosis following radiotherapy alone is illustrated. Long-term effects have been minimal, although so far the patient has required growth hormone supplementation.

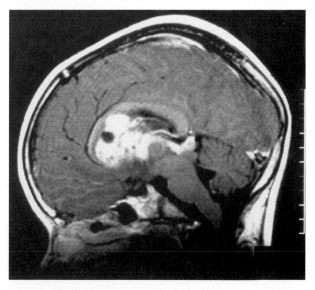

Figure 18a.4 *Magnetic resonance scan, showing extensive subependymal spread from pineal germinoma.*

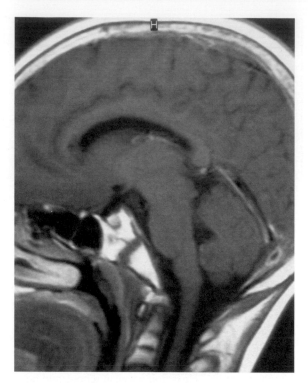

Figure 18a.5 *Resolution following craniospinal radiotherapy with a boost to the macroscopic tumor.*

Teratoma

Teratomas in the CNS are seen mainly in neonates and young infants, as is the case for sacrococcygeal teratoma. Complete resection is the most important therapeutic step. In immature teratomas, good results have been reported in some individuals treated with adjuvant chemotherapy.[21] The value of additional irradiation is described in a few case reports but has not been evaluated systematically. It is known that for treatment of teratomatous tumors from extracranial sites, a cumulative irradiation dose of over 50 Gy seems to show some effectiveness. Incompletely resected teratomas have a ten per cent (mature teratoma) or 20 per cent (immature teratoma) risk of relapse, irrespective of adjuvant chemotherapy.[51] Half of the recurrent tumors may display YST or embryonic carcinoma histology.

Side effects of chemotherapy

Pulmonary toxicity of bleomycin, which had also been reported as a problem in combination with reduced kidney function[52] and potentiated by anesthesia,[53] led to the use of regimens without this drug. The highly efficient combination of cisplatin, etoposide, and ifosfamide (PEI) is associated with a higher degree of myelosuppression and carries the risk of tubular nephropathy.[54] In the preliminary experience with this regimen, as used in the SIOP CNS GCT '96 protocol, we observed clinically apparent hearing impairment in approximately 10 per cent of patients. Although the auditory and renal toxicity of carboplatin regimen are less, carboplatin at effective doses ($600\,mg/m^2$/cycle) bears a substantial myelotoxicity.[55] Further attention should be drawn to the risk of therapy-related secondary leukemia, which depends on treatment intensity and modality, with an estimated cumulative risk of 1.0 per cent (three of 442 patients, Kaplan–Meier method at ten years' follow-up) for children treated with surgery and chemotherapy only and 4.2 per cent (three of 174 patients) for children treated with combined radio- and chemotherapy.[56] In children treated with cisplatin-containing polychemotherapy (especially with ifosfamide), the renal function has to be monitored carefully for tubular nephropathy. Prolonged phosphaturia may lead to renal rickets, with consecutive growth retardation, in children, while adolescents are at risk of renal osteomalacia.[54] These long-term sequelae can be avoided by supplementation of phosphate.

CASE STUDY 2

A nine-year old boy presented with a short history of headaches, vomiting, and impaired vision. Magnetic resonance scanning revealed a pineal area tumor and hydrocephalus. The tumor was biopsied via a third ventriculostomy. External ventricular drainage was also performed. Serum AFP was elevated, at 327 kU/l.

Biopsy confirmed a mixed GCT, with choriocarcinoma and yolk-sac differentiation. Immunohistochemistry showed positive staining for AFP and HCG and negative staining for PLAP, synaptophysin, and GFAP.

Staging investigations showed no evidence of supratentorial or spinal metastases.

The boy was treated according to the SIOP secreting GCT protocol (GCT '96). He received four courses of chemotherapy with cisplatin $20\,mg/m^2$ daily for five days, etoposide $100\,mg/m^2$ daily for three days, and ifosfamide $1500\,mg/m^2$ for five days. At diagnosis, he already had hypothyroidism and diabetes insipidus and was treated with desmopressin and thyroxine.

His serum AFP had returned to normal after two courses of chemotherapy. Following a total of four courses, he had underwent complete resection of residual tumor. Histology of the resected specimen revealed residual mature teratoma without any evidence of yolk-sac or choriocarcinomatous differentiation, which had been present in the initial histology.

Following this, he received radical radiotherapy with a planned margin of 1 cm to the surgical bed, giving a dose of 54 Gy in 30 fractions.

The boy continues on follow-up. One year and eight months after diagnosis, he remains well but has intermittent headaches. He remains on growth hormone replacement therapy, thyroxine, desmopressin, and hydrocortisone. The most recent MRI of his brain shows no evidence of recurrence of his pineal area tumor.

This case illustrates the importance of obtaining serum and CSF for AFP and β-HCG in patients with pineal area (and also for suprasellar and parasellar) tumors. Current protocols are based on intensive platinum-containing combination chemotherapy, resection of residual mass, and radical radiotherapy.

Side effects of radiotherapy

Alopecia as a long-term side effect of irradiation is reported infrequently. Cognitive impairment occurs as a lasting problem in some patients. Transient side effects that are reported relate mainly to moderate myelosuppression, such as symptoms of anemia. Headaches as a clinical symptom during radiotherapy are also reported. In a few cases, seizures are described; however, these are not necessarily related to irradiation, as they are seen mainly in patients with massive endocrine disturbances, such as diabetes insipidus.

Follow-up

A complete clinical remission is defined as normalization of the tumor markers within the age-related normal range and the absence of residual tumor on imaging, even in patients with normalized tumor markers, as residual masses on imaging may represent remaining mature teratoma. If any of these criteria is not fulfilled, then a diagnostic re-evaluation and, if necessary, a change or intensification of treatment is indicated urgently. Most relapses occur within the first two years after diagnosis. However, in some patients, late recurrences up to five years after diagnosis of intracranial germinoma have been observed. Therefore, the initial follow-up examinations after completion of chemotherapy must be performed at short intervals, including frequent (i.e. 4 weekly) estimations of tumor markers during early follow-up. In infants under two years of age, the interpretation of AFP may be difficult due to the physiologically elevated serum levels. In this context, it has been proven helpful to compare the AFP decline in neonates and infants.[57] A retarded decline or a secondary rise of the AFP levels strongly indicates the presence of incomplete tumor resection or a recurrence of YST.

In addition, the follow-up examinations must include repeated imaging of the primary tumor site. In the case of residual structures after chemotherapy, resection of these residues is indicated, since mature teratoma may have remained, with the risk of tumor progression.[58] Positron-emission tomography (PET) examinations have not been proven useful in this situation, as they cannot distinguish between mature teratoma and residual necrosis or scars.[59]

In intracranial tumors, repeated endocrinologic examinations at diagnosis and during follow-up are mandatory, since tumors of the suprasellar region can be associated with endocrinologic symptoms such as diabetes insipidus or panhypopituitarism.

Relapse treatment

In patients with recurrent or refractory tumors and who have been treated previously with a non-platinum or carboplatin therapy, cisplatin-based regimens (preferably PEI) have been applied successfully.[60,61] Therefore, cisplatin-containing regimens are preferred in patients with relapsed tumors, providing the organ toxicities related to the previous treatment allow further cisplatin therapy. Patients suffering from severe cisplatin-related toxicity may be treated with a combination of carboplatin and high-dose etoposide (400–600 mg/m^2 on three days). In our experience, high-dose chemotherapy with stem-cell support, as it has been applied in adult patients,[61] has resulted in long-term remissions only in patients in whom a clinical complete remission could be achieved before high-dose chemotherapy. Therefore, high-dose chemotherapy can be regarded as being indicated only for consolidation treatment.

In the experience of European trials of the past ten years, more than 90 per cent of relapses occur at the primary site of the tumor; 30 per cent of these relapses are combined with spinal relapses. Therefore, relapse chemotherapy should be accompanied by intensive local therapy, preferably complete resection of the recurrent tumor after tumor reduction by preoperative chemotherapy. The role of additional radiotherapy is not well defined, but experience in publications of relapse treatment in patients who received only chemotherapy has reflected a benefit of irradiation for survival after recurrence. Therefore, the possibility of additional irradiation in relapse patients should be considered.

Newly developed drugs, such as paclitaxel and gemcitabine, have not yet been studied in children with relapsing or refractory GCT.

As inadequate local tumor control at the primary site represents the main problem in most patients, further significant advances in relapsing GCT may be based on further improvement of local therapy.

LONG–TERM SEQUELAE OF TREATMENT

Before discussing the late sequelae of treatment, including surgery, it should be noted that tumor site and the related problems of resection also have an important influence on the appearance of short- and long-term sequelae.

Investigations in patients with GCTs have been reported by Kiltie and coworkers, who examined retrospectively 25 patients treated before the age of 16, nine of whom had non-germinomatous CNS GCTs.[62] All patients had received craniospinal irradiation. Of the long-term effects, endocrinologic impairment was most apparent, with a requirement for lifelong hormone replacement. Cranial nerve palsies and visual impairment were described in some patients. Learning disabilities were reported. Sutton and colleagues reported on quality of life in 22 patients with germinoma after craniospinal irradiation; the data showed a generally good quality-of-life rating.[63] In addition, patients were normally proportioned for height and weight. Patients showed educational achievements comparable to those of the normal population, which may reflect the fact that patients with germinoma are generally older than those with non-germinomatous malignant GCTs at the time of diagnosis. In our series, some patients had problems of obesity and growth, and there was a high incidence of endocrine impairment and frequent minor disabilities due to persistent central nerve palsies. One may conclude that because of older age at the time of diagnosis, patients with CNS GCTs do far better with respect to long-term rehabilitation, education, and employment prospects than patients with other malignant pediatric brain tumors.

Preliminary evaluation in patients treated within the SIOP CNS GCT protocol and who completed treatment at least one year previously show that patients with pineal tumors suffer mainly from visual impairment, central pareses, and motor impairment. Cognitive disturbances are more apparent compared to patients with suprasellar tumors.

In suprasellar tumors, endocrinologic problems such as diabetes insipidus are frequently seen in the long term due to the tumor location and tumor infiltration of the hypophyseal-hypothalamic area.

The impact of treatment such as chemotherapy and irradiation is difficult to access. Comparison of patients with germinoma treated either with craniospinal irradiation or with a combination of chemotherapy and irradiation in the SIOP study shows a slightly higher number of patients with endocrinologic problems in the combined treated group.

FUTURE AIMS

The future aims for treatment of pure germinoma will be to reduce treatment in good prognostic patients and to optimize local tumor control by increasing the irradiation volume to the ventricular area, which is the area of risk of developing locoregional relapse. These stratifications will also enable the omission of spinal irradiation in a high percentage of patients. Craniospinal irradiation will be the standard procedure for all patients with metastatic germinomas, since the available data have proven this to be able to achieve a greater than 90 per cent event-free survival, even in the presence of disseminated disease.

With MNGGCTs, locoregional tumor control remains the major problem, therefore complete staging and a more detailed response evaluation to chemotherapy will play a dominant role in the definition of risk groups. At an early stage, treatment intensification, such as surgery, high-dose chemotherapy, and more extensive radiotherapy, have to be discussed.

FINAL CONSIDERATIONS

Multidisciplinary treatment is the main challenge for patients with intracranial GCTs. Only such an approach will enable the responsible physicians to guarantee the best possible treatment, care, and support for the patient. Such a team requires an experienced pediatric oncologist, a neurosurgeon familiar with childhood brain tumors, a neuroradiologist, a radiation oncologist with experience in brain tumors, a pediatric neurologist, an endocrinologist, and a neuropathologist experienced in GCTs. Such a team is not always available, but it should be recommended because of the rareness of the disease. It is also appropriate to treat patients in larger centers with greater experience in the management of children with brain tumors. The SIOP Germ Cell Tumour Group has been established to develop common diagnostic and treatment guidelines and to establish national multidisciplinary groups, who are responsible in the different countries for promoting knowledge and cooperation in the management of this rare disease.

REFERENCES

1 Kaatsch P, Kaletsch U, Michaelis J. *Annual Report 2002: German Childhood Cancer Registry.* Mainz, Germany: Deutsches Kinderkrebsregister, 2003.

2 Teilum G. Classification of endodermal sinus tumour (mesoblastoma vitellinum) and so-called "embryonal carcinoma" of the ovary. *Acta Pathol Microbiol Scand* 1965; **64**:407–29.

3 Gonzalez-Crussi F. Extragonadal teratomas. In: *Atlas of Tumor Pathology*, second series, fascicle 18. Washington, DC: AFIP, 1970, pp. 129–38.

4 Gonzalez-Crussi F, Winkler RF, Mirkin DL. Sacrococcygeal teratomas in infants and children: relationship of histology and prognosis in 40 cases. *Arch Pathol Lab Med* 1978; **102**:420–5.

5 Hawkins E, Heifetz SA, Giller R, Cushing B. The prepubertal testis (prenatal and postnatal): its relationship to intratubular germ cell neoplasia: a combined Pediatric Oncology Group and Children's Cancer Study Group. *Hum Pathol* 1997; **28**:404–10.

6 Van Gurp RJ, Oosterhuis JW, Kalscheuer V, Mariman EC, Looijenga LH. Biallelic expression of the H19 and IGF2 genes in human testicular germ cell tumors. *J Natl Cancer Inst* 1994; **86**:1070–5.

7 Miura K, Obama M, Yun K, *et al.* Methylation imprinting of H19 and SNRPN genes in human benign ovarian teratomas. *Am J Hum Genet* 1999; **65**:1359–67.

8 Bussey KJ, Lawce HJ, Olson SB, *et al.* Chromosome abnormalities of eighty-one pediatric germ cell tumors: sex-, age-, site-, and histopathology-related differences – a Children's Cancer Group study. *Genes Chromosomes Cancer* 1999; **25**:134–46.

9 Chaganti RS, Houldsworth J. Genetics and biology of adult human male germ cell tumors. *Cancer Res* 2000; **60**:1475–82.

10 Perlman EJ, Hu J, Ho D, Cushing B, Lauer S, Castleberry RP. Genetic analysis of childhood endodermal sinus tumors by comparative genomic hybridization. *J Pediatr Hematol Oncol* 2000; **22**:100–5.

11 Schneider DT, Schuster AE, Fritsch MK, *et al.* Genetic analysis of mediastinal nonseminomatous germ cell tumors in children and adolescents. *Genes Chromosomes Cancer* 2002; **34**:115–25.

12 Diez B, Balmaceda C, Matsutani M, Weiner HL. Germ cell tumours of the CNS in children: recent advances in therapy. *Childs Nerv Syst* 1999; **15**:578–85.

13 Rosemblum MK, Matsutani M, Vanmeir EG. CNS germ cell tumours. In: Kleihues P, Cavenee WK (eds). *Pathology and Genetics of Tumours of the Nervous System*. Lyon: IARC Press, 2000, pp. 223–8.

14 Packer RJ, Cohen BH, Coney K. Intracranial germ cell tumors. *Oncologist* 2000; **5**:312–20.

15 Pomarede R, Czernichow P, Finidori J, *et al.* Endocrine aspects and tumoral markers in intracranial germinoma: an attempt to delineate the diagnostic procedure in 14 patients. *J Pediatr* 1982; **101**:374–8.

16 Aida T, Abe H, Fujieda K, Matsuura N. Endocrine functions in children with suprasellar germinoma. *Neurol Med Chir (Tokyo)* 1993; **33**:152–7.

17 Buchfelder M, Fahlbusch R, Walther M, Mann K. Endocrine disturbances in suprasellar germinomas. *Acta Endocrinol (Copenh)* 1989; **120**:337–42.

18 Hoffman HJ, Otsubo H, Hendrick EB, *et al.* Intracranial germ-cell tumours in children. *J Neurosurg* 1991; **74**:545–51.

19 Legido A, Packer RJ, Sutton LN, *et al.* Suprasellar germinomas in childhood. A reappraisal. *Cancer* 1989; **63**:340–4.

20 Packer RJ, Sutton LN, Rosenstock JG. Pineal region tumours of childhood. *Pediatrics* 1984; **74**:97–102.

21 Garre ML, El-Hossainy MO, Fondelli P, *et al.* Is chemotherapy effective therapy for intracranial immature teratoma? A case report. *Cancer* 1996; **77**:977–82.

22 Maghine M, Cosi GL, Genovese E, *et al.* Central diabetes insipidus in children and young adults. *N Engl J Med* 2000; **343**:998–1007.

23 Wilson JT. Primary diffuse chiasmatic germinomas: differentiation from optic chiasm gliomas. *Pediatr Neurosurg* 1995; **23**:1–5.

24 Cohen DN, Steinberg M, Buchwald R. Suprasellar germinomas: diagnostic confusion with optic gliomas. Case report. *J Neurosurg* 1974; **41**:490–3.

25 Zimmerman RA, Bilaniuk LT. Age-related incidence of pineal calcification detected by computed tomography. *Radiology* 1982; **142**:659–62.

26 Satoh H, Uozumi T, Kiya K, *et al.* MRI of pineal region tumours: relationship between tumours and adjacent structures. *Neuroradiology* 1995; **37**:624–30.

27 Fujimaki T, Matsutani M, Funada N, *et al.* CT and MRI features of intracranial germ cell tumors. *J Neuro-Oncol* 1994; **19**:217–26.

28 Tien RD, Barkovich AJ, Edwards MS. MR imaging of pineal tumors. *Am J Roentgenol* 1990; **155**:143–51.

29 Sumida M, Uozumi T, Kiya K, *et al.* MRI of intracranial germ cell tumours. *Neuroradiology* 1995; **37**:32–7.

30 Moon WK, Chang KH, Han MH, Kim IO. Intracranial germinomas: correlation of imaging findings with tumor response to radiation therapy. *Am J Roentgenol* 1999; **172**:713–16.

31 Saller B, Clara R, Spottl G, Siddle K, Mann K. Testicular cancer secrets intact human choriogonadotropin (hCG) and its free β-subunit: evidence that hCG (+hCG-β) assays are the most reliable in diagnosis and follow-up. *Clin Chem* 1990; **36**:234–9.

32 Mann K, Karl HJ. Molecular heterogeneity of human chorionic gonadotropin and its subunits in testicular cancer. *Cancer* 1983; **52**:654–60.

33 Oosterom R, Stoter G. Standardizing human chorionic gonadotropin measurements in serum of testicular cancer patients. *Clin Chem* 1992; **38**:601–2.

34 Allen JC, Nisselbaum J, Epstein F, Rosen G, Schwartz MK. Alphafetoprotein and human chorionic determination in cerebrospinal fluid: an aid to the diagnosis and management of intracranial germ-cell tumours. *Childs Nerv Syst* 1979; **51**:368–74.

35 Shinoda J, Yamada H, Sakai N, Ando T, Miwa Y. Placental alkaline phosphatase as a tumour marker for primary intracranial germinoma. *J Neurosurg* 1988; **68**:710–20.

36 Murphy BA, Motzer RJ, Mazundar M, *et al.* Serum tumour marker decline is an early predictor of treatment outcome in germ cell tumour patients treated with cisplatin and ifosfamide salvage chemotherapy. *Cancer* 1994; **73**:2520–6.

37 Trigo JM, Tabernero JM, Paz-Ares L, *et al.* Tumour markers at the time of recurrence in patients with germ cell tumours. *Cancer* 2000; **88**:162–8.

38 Gregory JJ, Finlay JL. α-Fetoprotein and β-human chorionic gonadotropin. Their clinical significance as tumour markers. *Drugs* 1999; **57**:463–7.

39 Pople IK, Athanasiou TC, Sandeman DR, Coakham HB. The role of endoscopic biopsy and third venrticulostomy in the management of pineal region tumors. *Br J Neurosurg* 2001; **15**:305–11.

40 Macarthur DC, Buxton N, Vioeberghs M, Punt J. The effectiveness of neuroendoscopic interventions in children with brain tumors. *Childs Nerv Syst* 2001; **17**:589–94.

41 Nam DH, Cho BK, Ahn HS. Treatment of intracranial non-germinomatous malignant germ cell tumors in children: the role of each treatment modality. *Childs Nerv Syst* 1999; **15**:185–91.

42 Einhorn LH, Donohue JP. Chemotherapy for disseminated testicular cancer. *Urol Clin North Am* 1977; **4**:407–26.

43 Herrmann HD, Westphal M, Winkler K, Laas RW, Schulte FJ. Treatment of non-germinomatous germ-cell tumors of the pineal region. *Neurosurgery* 1994; **34**:524–9.

44 Bamberg M, Kortmann RD, Calaminus G, *et al.* Radiation therapy for intracranial germinoma: results of the German cooperative prospective trials MAKEI 83/86/89. *J Clin Oncol* 1999; **17**:2585–92.

45 Bouffet E, Baranzelli MC, Patte C, *et al.* Combined treatment modality for intracranial germinomas: results of a multicentre SFOP experience. Société Francaise d'Oncologie Pédiatrique. *Br J Cancer* 1999; **79**:1199–204.

46 Cefalo G, Gianni MC, Lombardi F, Fossati-Bellani F. Intracranial germinoma: does a cisplatinum-based chemotherapeutic regimen permit to avoid whole CNS irradiation. *Med Ped Oncol* 1995; **25**:303.

47 Alapetite C, Carrie C, Brisse E, *et al.* Patterns of relapse following focal irradiation for intracranial germinoma. Critical review of TGM-TC90-SFOP protocol. *Med Pediatr Oncol* 2001; **37**:249.

48 Balmaceda C, Heller G, Rosenblum M, *et al.* Chemotherapy without irradiation – a novel approach for newly diagnosed CNS germ cell tumors: results of an international cooperative trial. The First International Central Nervous System Germ Cell Tumor Study. *J Clin Oncol* 1996; **14**:2908–15.

49 Calaminus G, Bamberg M, Baranzelli MC, *et al.* Intracranial germ cell tumors: a comprehensive update of the European data. *Neuropediatrics* 1994; **25**:26–32.

50 Yoshida J, Sugita K, Kobayashi T. Treatment of intracranial germ cell tumors: effectiveness of chemotherapy with cisplatin and etoposide (CDDP and VP16). *Acta Neurochir (Wien)* 1993; **120**:111–7.

51 Göbel U, Calaminus G, Engert J, *et al.* Teratoma in infancy and childhood. *Med Pediatr Oncol* 1998; **31**:8–15.

52 Dalgleish AG, Woods RL, Levi JA. Bleomycin pulmonary toxicity: its relationship to renal dysfunction. *Med Pediatr Oncol* 1984; **12**:313–7.

53 Goldinger PL, Schweizer O. The hazards of anesthesia and surgery in bleomycin-treated patients. *Semin Oncol* 1979; **6**:121–4.

54 Pratt CB, Meyer WH, Jenkins JJ, *et al.* Ifosfamide, Fanconi's syndrome, and rickets. *J Clin Oncol* 1991; **9**:1495–9.

55 Mann JR, Raafat F, Robinson K, *et al.* The United Kingdom Children's Cancer Study Group's second germ cell tumor study: carboplatin, etoposide, and bleomycin are effective treatment for children with malignant extracranial germ cell tumors, with acceptable toxicity. *J Clin Oncol* 2000; **18**:3809–18.

56 Schneider DT, Hilgenfeld E, Schwabe D, *et al.* Acute myelogenous leukemia after treatment for malignant germ cell tumors in children. *J Clin Oncol* 1999; **17**:3226–33.

57 Blohm ME, Vesterling-Hörner D, Calaminus G, Göbel U. Alpha 1-fetoprotein (AFP) reference values in infants up to 2 years of age. *Pediatr Hematol Oncol* 1998; **15**:135–42.

58 Stenning SP, Parkinson MC, Fisher C, *et al.* Postchemotherapy residual masses in germ cell tumor patients: content, clinical features, and prognosis. Medical Research Council Testicular Tumour Working Party. *Cancer* 1998; **83**:1409–19.

59 Stephens AW, Gonin R, Hutchins GD, Einhorn LH. Positron emission tomography evaluation of residual radiographic abnormalities in postchemotherapy germ cell tumor patients. *J Clin Oncol* 1996; **14**:1637–41.

60 Baranzelli MC, Bouffet E, Quintana E, Portas M, Thyss A, Patte C. Non-seminomatous ovarian germ cell tumours in children. *Eur J Cancer* 2000; **36**:376–83.

61 Bosl GJ. Germ cell tumor clinical trials in North America. *Semin Surg Oncol* 1997; **17**:257–62.

62 Kiltie AE, Gattamaneni HR. Survival and quality of life of pediatric intracranial germ cell tumor patients treated at the Christie Hospital, 1972–1993. *Med Pediatr Oncol* 1995; **25**:450–6.

63 Sutton LN, Radcliffe J, Goldwein JW, *et al*, Quality of life of germinomas treated with craniospinal irradiation. *Neurosurgery* 1996; **45**:1292–7, 1297–8.

Germ-cell tumors: a commentary

JONATHAN L. FINLAY

Chapter 18a summarizes the issues of clinical presentation; radiologic, tumor marker, and pathologic diagnosis; and the surgical, radiation therapeutic, and chemotherapeutic aspects of management. The purpose of this commentary is to highlight two issues that remain unresolved at this time.

DIAGNOSTIC AND PROGNOSTIC POWER OF SERUM VERSUS CEREBROSPINAL FLUID TUMOR MARKERS

Primary non-germinomatous germ cell tumors (GCTs) secrete into the serum and/or cerebrospinal fluid (CSF) alpha-fetoprotein (AFP) if they contain endodermal sinus tumor (EST) elements or beta-human chorionic gonadotrophin (β-HCG) if they contain choriocarcinomatous elements. So goes the dogma. However, there are several exceptions to these rules. First, embryonal carcinoma elements (fortunately rare in the central nervous system, CNS) may secrete – or not secrete – either or both of these tumor markers. Second, as the authors of Chapter 18a indicate, immature teratomatous elements may – or may not – secrete either or both of these tumor markers. This does *not* mean that within the immature teratomas are hiding elements of EST or choriocarcinoma. Adenocarcinoma or neuroectodermal cells within an immature teratoma may stain pathologically for AFP within these cellular elements.

The presence of "modest" elevations of β-HCG, as indicated in Chapter 18a, is recognized in a proportion of patients with otherwise pure CNS germinomas. These elevations are considered reflective of β-HCG-secreting syncytiotrophoblastic cells within the germinomas and are not an indicator of the presence of choriocarcinomatous elements. What is not resolved is whether the presence of such β-HCG-secreting cells and "modest" elevations of β-HCG in the serum and/or CSF of germinoma patients are adverse prognostic factors. A Japanese group has reported in the affirmative, but others have been unable to substantiate this. Part of the problem is the lack of determination of what constitute "modest" levels of β-HCG in the serum and/or CSF. How high a serum or CSF level of β-HCG is too high to be attributable to pure germinoma? Some studies accept a level below 50 iu/ml, but is this level true for both serum and CSF? I consider that significant elevations of CSF β-HCG may be observed in pure germinoma patients, even beyond 100 iu/ml, and that this invariably reflects leptomeningeal dissemination of tumor.

The lack of clarity in tumor marker elevation definition may impact significantly upon the interpretation of outcome in multicenter trials in which elevations of β-HCG are considered to confer poor prognosis status in the absence of pathological confirmation. This could likely produce a study population drift, in which the outcome for non-germinomatous GCT appears to be improved through "contamination" with pure β-HCG-secreting germinomas.

Although rare, adenocarcinomatous elements within primary CNS GCTs are well recognized. Their presence is associated with elevations of serum and/or CSF carcinoembryonic antigen (CEA) levels. Thus, it has become my practice to add this marker routinely in the diagnostic work-up of patients suspected of harboring primary CNS GCTs.

Some authors have suggested that the ratio of serum to CSF tumor markers is indicative of the presence or absence of leptomeningeal disease, i.e. the higher the CSF to serum ratio, the more likely the presence of leptomeningeal dissemination of tumor. In this situation, such patients might be at highest risk for leptomeningeal relapse, especially if treated with some current or proposed protocols attempting either to either avoid irradiation or to limit irradiation to local tumor sites. The prognostic importance of CSF versus serum tumor marker elevations and their ratios merit formal prospective evaluation in the multicenter trials currently under way.

Finally, what is the prognostic significance of the rate of decline of these tumor markers, if present at diagnosis in the serum and/or CSF, in response to treatment? Intuitively, one would anticipate that a relatively slow rate of disappearance would indicate a greater degree of relapse, based upon published experience with testicular GCTs. However, this again needs to be confirmed in the current multicenter trials, thereby providing a rational basis for therapy intensification in slow responders, be it higher-dose irradiation or myeloablative chemotherapy with stem-cell rescue, as used for slow-responding patients with testicular non-seminomatous tumors.

RADIATION THERAPY IN THE MANAGEMENT OF CENTRAL NERVOUS SYSTEM GERMINOMAS

Radiation therapy has been and continues to be the backbone of treatment for primary CNS germinomas. As the authors of Chapter 18a have indicated, the irradiation volumes required (craniospinal versus periventricular versus focal), as well as the doses required, remain the subject of debate among radiation therapists. What is crucial to recognize is that such questions are not simply an intellectual exercise. The median age of patients with primary CNS GCTs is approximately 13 years at diagnosis, thus the critical issue is the adverse impact of full-dose irradiation upon intellectual functioning and quality of life. As my own multicenter trials have demonstrated,[1] children who receive irradiation for primary CNS GCTs before the age of 13 years experience poorer quality of life and neuropsychometric function than those who either avoided irradiation or received irradiation in the teenage years or beyond. Current studies combining irradiation with chemotherapy seek to sustain the high cure rates achieved with full-dose irradiation while at the same time minimizing the late effects of irradiation by both dose and volume reductions. It is essential that late effects of irradiation are not replaced by irreversible chemotherapy-associated toxicities. Furthermore, the problem of secondary, treatment-related malignancies must not be overlooked. Radiation-induced malignant gliomas are well recognized in children, especially in the first decade of life, receiving brain irradiation for CNS GCT, other primary brain tumors, or acute leukemia. However, secondary leukemias due to chemotherapy (etoposide- or alkylator-related) have also been reported in children undergoing prolonged chemotherapy for CNS GCTs.

One major concern of current protocols designed to limit irradiation volumes to focal fields in conjunction with chemotherapy is that such patients would be at increased risk for failure within the ventricular system. Therefore, successful retrieval with radiation therapy would be hampered significantly by the prior focally administered irradiation. In our studies employing initial chemotherapy only, despite a high rate of relapse (almost 60 per cent), most of those patients could be cured successfully with irradiation alone or irradiation with short-course chemotherapy because of the absence of prior focal field irradiation to hamper the delivered dose and volume. Thus, the eight-year overall survival for patients in our first international study is not significantly different for germinoma patients from that achieved with irradiation – and with 40 per cent of patients avoiding irradiation. Nevertheless, our inability to document a significant adverse impact of irradiation upon those children in our studies who ultimately required irradiation beyond the age of 13 years old no longer supports the use of chemotherapy-only strategies in these older children with CNS germinomas. I anticipate that the outcome (in terms of both survival and neuropsychological functioning) of current and proposed studies employing reduced-dose irradiation with relatively less intensive chemotherapy – specifically that developed by the North American Children's Oncology Group (COG) – will ultimately negate the role for further chemotherapy-only trials, even in younger children with CNS germinomas.

REFERENCE

1 Sands SA, Kellie SJ, Davidow AL, *et al.* Long-term quality of life and neuropsychologic functioning for patients with CNS germ-cell tumors: from the First International CNS Germ Cell Tumor Study. *Neuro-Oncol* 2001; **3**:174–83.

19

Infant brain tumors

ANTONY MICHALSKI AND MARIA LUISA GARRÉ

INTRODUCTION

It is unusual to have a chapter categorized by age at diagnosis rather than histology, stage, or biology. However, in pediatric neuro-oncology, young children have been given special consideration for the past three decades.[1,2] This chapter will focus on the epidemiology of brain tumors in young children, the specific disease patterns that are seen most frequently, and the therapeutic considerations of balancing chances of cure against late effects of therapy.

EPIDEMIOLOGY

Based on epidemiological data from the available registries, such as the Surveillance, Epidemiological, and End Results (SEER) group in the USA, and population-based data from the UK, approximately one-third of all central nervous system (CNS) tumors occurring in children (age under 15 years) are diagnosed in children under three years of age (Figure 19.1).[3–5] This age has been chosen in order to distinguish a subgroup of patients that has peculiar features in terms of disease behavior, prognosis, and the risk of developing severe damage after irradiation due to incomplete brain development. The age of three years is not accepted universally as an appropriate cut-off, and many reports have used different age limits (under one year, under two years, under five years) for various purposes

(epidemiological studies, analysis of treatments results, protocols planning).[2,6,7]

Congenital tumors in infants (and perhaps those presenting within the first six months of age) possibly include a greater frequency of cases associated with genetic abnormalities related to cancer development or predisposition. Recent research has contributed information on the molecular genetic defects underlying inherited cancer syndromes.[8,9] Some syndromes specifically increase the risk of developing certain brain tumors, such as desmoplastic medulloblastoma in Gorlin syndrome and medulloblastoma (primitive neuroectodermal tumor,

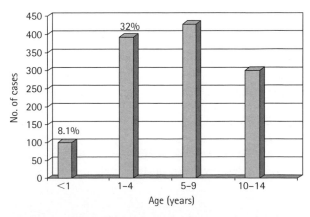

Figure 19.1 *Distribution of central nervous system tumors by age (all cases; US Surveillance, Epidemiological, and End Results (SEER) data 1983–1992).*

PNET) or glioblastoma in Turcot syndrome.[10–13] In other syndromes, such as Li–Fraumeni, which is due to constitutional inactivation of one copy of the *p53* gene, patients are predisposed to a wide variety of tumors, including choroid plexus tumors in the very young.[14,15]

HISTOLOGICAL SUBTYPES OF TUMOR IN YOUNG CHILDREN

The most common tumors encountered in this age group are gliomas (mainly midline, low-grade gliomas), PNETs, and ependymomas. Thirty per cent of cases of PNET and ependymoma occur in children under three years of age. A variant of PNET previously known as "cerebellar neuroblastoma" has been recently renamed "medulloblastoma with extensive nodularity", and described further as a new clinicopathological entity showing peculiar "grape-like" magnetic resonance imaging (MRI) features (Figure 19.2) and associated with young age and better prognosis compared with undifferentiated medulloblastoma.[8,16]

Several tumor types that are otherwise extremely rare are reported as occurring most commonly in the youngest patients. These include atypical rhabdoid/teratoid tumor (AT/RT), ependymoblastoma, desmoplastic infantile ganglioglioma, choroid plexus tumors, and both mature and immature pure teratomas. Conversely, common tumors of adult life, such as glioblastoma and meningioma, are rare in young children.

Regarding biological behavior, it is not always obvious whether, within the same histological type, youngest children comprise a subgroup of cases carrying tumors different in terms of response to treatment and histological features. Molecular genetic studies should be encouraged further in order to define age cut-off in a more objective and substantial way. The relative frequencies of CNS tumors in childhood are shown in Figure 19.3 and Table 19.1. These include data from the SEER registry (Figure 19.3) and from a series of 94 cases enrolled prospectively in the Italian cooperative study for children

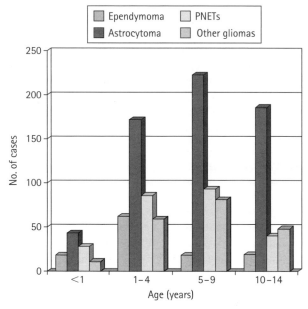

Figure 19.3 *Distribution of tumor types by age (1222 cases; US Surveillance, Epidemiological, and End Results (SEER) data 1983–1992).*

Table 19.1 *Italian cooperative study of malignant central nervous system tumors in children under three years of age (recruitment 1995–1999)*

Tumor*	Cases (*n*)	%
Medulloblastoma	36	38
PNET	11	12
AT/RT	15	17
Choroid plexus carcinoma	6	6
Ependymoma	20	21
Other (GBL, Uncl, AA)	6	6
Total	94	100

AA, anaplastic astrocytoma; AT/RT, atypical teratoid/rhabdoid tumor; GBL, glioblastoma; PNET, primitive neuroectodermal tumor; Uncl, unclear. *Histology reviewed in >80 per cent of cases by at least two neuropathologists.

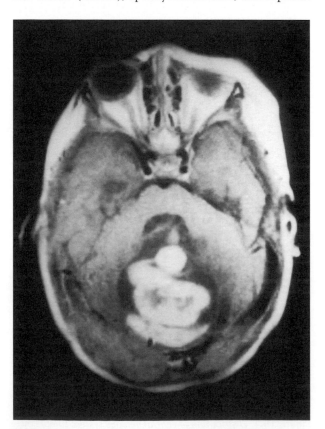

Figure 19.2 *Brain magnetic resonance image of a two-year-old girl with medulloblastoma with extensive nodularity.*

aged under three years and affected by malignant CNS tumors diagnosed in the period 1995–2000 (Table 19.1).

MAIN FEATURES AND TREATMENT OF RARE TUMORS SEEN PREDOMINANTLY IN INFANTS

Infantile desmoplastic ganglioglioma

This tumor is histologically grade 1 in the World Health Organization (WHO) classification. It typically occurs in the age range of 1–24 months, with a male/female ratio of 1.7 to one. Infantile desmoplastic gangliogliomas almost invariably involve the supratentorial region, with extension to more than one lobe (frontal and parietal most frequently). The appearance at MRI is quite typical, with the presence of a large, often multicentric cyst and a mural nodule attached to the dura.[17,18] The neuronal component inside the tumor can show aspects of immature neuroepithelial cell aggregates suggestive of desmoplastic neuroblastoma. Although worrying histologically, these clinicopathological characteristics do not change the favorable prognosis of this tumor, which rarely relapses after complete removal.[19] Surgical approach is then the treatment of choice, although the subsequent functional prognosis can be affected by surgical complications as well as the original extension of the lesion and cortical atrophy caused by tumor growth in fetal life or early childhood. In a series published by Vandenberg, none of the 14 cases died due to the disease, but the frequency of psychomotor delay and permanent neurological deficits was high.[20]

Mature and immature pure teratomas

Pure teratomas (not containing any malignant component) may occur in either the supratentorial or the infratentorial compartment. They represent up to four per cent of all brain tumors in infancy. The natural history and prognostic factors of intracranial pure teratomas are less well defined in the current literature than for extracranial tumors.[21,22] The extent of surgery remains the main prognostic factor, even for teratomas with partial or complete immature components, although complete excision is clearly more challenging in the CNS than in extracranial sites.[23,24] Careful follow-up after complete surgical removal is the recommended therapeutic strategy. Patients with residual immature teratoma after surgery and those who have residual disease following a relapse have been treated with chemotherapy according to protocols used for malignant germ-cell tumors. The efficacy is uncertain, but some authors have reported good responses.[24] Pure mature or immature teratomas are very often congenital tumors, presenting with giant intracranial masses causing irreversible brain damage and impairing quality of life in surviving patients even when radiotherapy or chemotherapy is not used. Thus, despite the fact that prognosis is good, with an overall survival of 80–90 per cent, long-term results in terms of quality of life may be disappointing.

Choroid plexus tumors

Tumors of choroid plexus epithelium are rare, accounting for 0.5 per cent of all tumors in adults and children. However, a reliable estimate of the real frequency of such tumors is not known, with a range of incidences being reported, from 0.5 to six per cent.[25–28] The true incidence of these tumors is likely to be higher than that quoted, since these rare entities tend to be underdiagnosed.[29] Almost 50 per cent of all cases occur in children under one year of age. The lateral ventricles are the most commonly involved sites. Neuropathologically, the WHO classification distinguishes choroid plexus papilloma (CPP, a grade I benign tumor) from choroid plexus carcinoma (CPC, a grade III malignant tumor), but in practice, grading tumors from small biopsies can be difficult.[8]

CPPs are composed of a simple or pseudostratified layer of cuboid to columnar cells resting on a basement membrane overlying papillary, vascularized, connective tissue cords. Cytological atypia, occasional mitoses, and rare foci of necrosis may be present. In CPC, there is clear evidence of anaplasia, increased mitotic activity, and brain invasion. Characteristically, these tumors may cause secreting hydrocephalus. A transitional form from CPP to CPC is increasingly recognized, known as atypical CPP, to describe a tumor with an increased mitotic activity and uncertain biological behavior compared with CPP. Few cases of atypical CPP have been reported in the past in older children; more recently, some authors have stressed these intermediate forms and the possibility of evolution from benign to malignant forms.[30] In the experience of the Italian cooperative group, the presence of atypical CPP in very young children with a clinicopathological pattern otherwise consistent with CPP is not associated with a worse prognosis.

For CPP and atypical CPP, the treatment of choice is surgical removal. Careful surveillance should follow in the atypical form. Neurosurgical problems during and following surgery are not uncommon due to the hydrodynamic imbalance, increased risk of bleeding due to hypervascularization of these lesions, and risk of subdural effusions.[27,28,31]

The natural history of CPC is not understood clearly, as the small number of published series each include only a few patients and have variable inclusion criteria. True CPC is associated with an unfavorable prognosis (ten-year overall survival rate of 25 per cent, from SEER data). The pattern of invasiveness (local versus metastatic) is controversial, as is the sensitivity of this tumor to chemotherapy and radiotherapy. However, there does seem to be evolving evidence that the use of preoperative chemotherapy may reduce the vascularity of the tumors, thereby decreasing the risks associated with attempted surgical removal.[32] Although the role of chemotherapy and radiotherapy in increasing the cure rate of CPC is not yet clarified sufficiently, long-term survivors are reported in all series after chemotherapy alone and after combined chemotherapy and radiotherapy. The most important prognostic factor appears to be whether the patient has had a total or a subtotal resection. An international cooperative study aiming to register a larger number of cases and test the chemosensitivity of the tumor has been approved recently by the Société International d'Oncologie Pédiatrique (SIOP).

Low-grade astrocytomas in infants

Low-grade gliomas, including pilocytic astrocytoma, represent a high proportion of brain tumors occurring in young children and are the second most frequently identified histological group (21 per cent of cases in the SEER series). Midline structures of the supratentorial compartment are involved most frequently. A substantial proportion (26 per cent in the SIOP Low Grade Study) of hypothalamic and chiasmatic low-grade astrocytomas are associated with neurofibromatosis type 1 (NF-1). Patients without NF-1 tend to have a worse prognosis and present with more extensive disease at diagnosis. In contrast to older children, only ten per cent of astrocytomas in infants arise in the cerebellum and only two per cent arise in the brainstem.

Histological features of low-grade gliomas that are useful prognostic tools may be different in infants compared with older children. For example, the percentage of cells staining with MIB-1 (a guide to tumor activity) is reported by neuropathologists to be higher in this age group.[8]

The myxoid variant of pilocytic astrocytoma has been described. This is characterized by a mucinous background and general cellular elongation; it may also show an increased number of mitoses and a lack of typical biphasic architecture. The tumors occur predominantly in the chiasmatic area in very young children and have been associated with more aggressive behavior, with a greater risk of a metastatic pattern at diagnosis, although some patients have survived for years after diagnosis.[33,34]

Optimal treatment for infants with low-grade glioma consists of "gentle" chemotherapy to delay or avoid irradiation (see Chapters 13a and 13b). It is uncertain whether more aggressive treatment can change the natural history in disseminated cases. Registration and prospective follow-up on an international basis, as proposed by the Low Grade SIOP study, could help in better defining these rare entities.

Ependymoblastoma

Ependymoblastoma is a rare embryonal brain tumor characterized histologically by distinctive multilayered rosettes. It manifests mainly in neonates and young children.[35,36] A real estimate of its incidence is lacking due to the fact that this tumor was previously diagnosed as anaplastic ependymoma or PNET. The preferred site of involvement is the lateral ventricles, but other sites, such as the posterior fossa, may be involved. Ependymoblastoma may arise from the neuroepithelial cells of the periventricular areas. The lesions grow very rapidly, with leptomeningeal dissemination and fatal outcome within six months to one year.[37,38] Because of the poor prognosis irrespective of staging (there is a bad outcome even in cases with complete removal and absence of metastasis), these cases should be treated aggressively up front, possibly with high-dose chemotherapy.[39] The rarity of this tumor and its poor outcome make it a candidate for cooperative international studies aiming to gain insight into the biology of the tumor and to define more effective treatment.

Atypical teratoid/rhabdoid tumor

Rhabdoid tumor was first described in the kidney as a sarcomatous variant of Wilms' tumor, but characterized by more aggressive behavior and poorer survival. In its initial description, this tumor showed areas of large round to polygonal cells, with eccentric nuclei and abundant eosinophilic cytoplasm, which resembled rhabdomyoblasts. Currently, rhabdoid tumors have been observed in almost every extrarenal site, including soft tissue, liver, pancreas, urinary bladder, uterus, gastrointestinal tract, retroperitoneum, mediastinum, orbit, skin, and the CNS.[40–44]

In about 10–15 per cent of young infants, renal rhabdoid tumor has been reported in association with malignant brain tumors. When the morphologic and immunohistochemical features of the two tumors are similar, the brain tumor is generally thought to represent a metastasis from the renal rhabdoid tumor, although synchronous or multifocal tumors cannot be excluded. In other cases, the association between systemic rhabdoid tumors and CNS malignancies with different histologic, immunohistochemical, and cytogenetic patterns, such as PNETs or gliomas of various types, has been noted.

The most frequent location outside of the kidney is the CNS, including the parenchyma and the meninges. In this site, rhabdoid tumors may be composed purely of rhabdoid cells or may display a combination of characteristic rhabdoid cells and a population of neuroepithelial, mesenchymal, and epithelial cells similar to but not typical of teratomas, as described by Rorke and colleagues,[42] who first termed this entity "atypical teratoid/rhabdoid tumor" (AT/RT).

The AT/RT of the CNS has been well characterized as a distinct clinicopathologic entity with an unusually poor prognosis and with the highest incidence in the first two years of life. It often arises in the posterior fossa (63–65 per cent). It has been misdiagnosed frequently as medulloblastoma, but its distinctive histological, immunohistochemical, and cytogenetic features permit an accurate diagnosis in most cases.[44,45]

The origin of this tumor is still open to speculation, and a variety of theories relative to the nature of the rhabdoid cell have been expressed. Different authors have postulated that it is of mesenchymal, neuroectodermal, histiocytic, neuroectomesenchymal, and meningeal lineage.[8] Combined cytogenetic, fluorescence *in situ* hybridization, and molecular genetic studies have demonstrated the presence of cytogenetic abnormalities, such as monosomy and deletion of chromosome 22, in some cases of CNS AT/RT as well as in renal and extrarenal rhabdoid tumors.[46] More recently, a gene within chromosome band 22q11, the *hSNF5/INI1* gene, has been identified as a candidate tumor-suppressor gene in the development of rhabdoid tumors of the kidney and soft tissue as well as of the CNS.[47,48] AT/RTs tend to have an intra-axial and extra-axial pattern of growth, confirming the possible mesodermal histogenesis.[49] The tumors tend to be multifocal, especially in congenital cases. A typical neuroimaging is shown in Figure 19.4.

AT/RT of the CNS is usually a fatal disease. Compared with medulloblastoma/PNET, it responds poorly to chemotherapy and radiotherapy. Rapid progression and frequent CNS dissemination have been reported. More recently, combined therapeutic regimens, including high-dose chemotherapy, have been used. It is uncertain whether these regimens are capable of prolonging survival and changing the natural history and aggressive behavior of this tumor.[50–52] Clearly, it is important to differentiate this entity from PNET, as different therapies need to be investigated. An international registry of cases has been proposed in order to pool experience of this rare and aggressive disease; pertinent data from this and other registries are presented in Table 19.2.

Malignant gliomas in infants

High-grade astrocytomas, i.e. anaplastic astrocytomas and glioblastomas, represent 11 per cent of tumors in the SEER series in young children and 12 per cent of the tumors in the Infant Study of the Pediatric Oncology Group (POG). The first Baby POG study treated 18 cases,

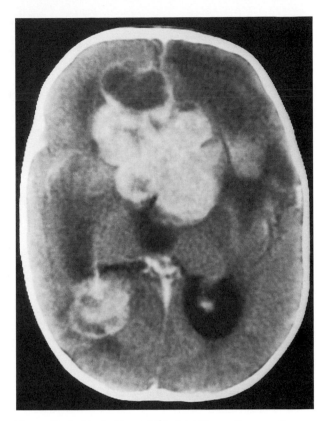

Figure 19.4 *Atypical teratoid/rhabdoid tumor four months after diagnosis, with multiple sites of involvement.*

while the Children's Cancer Study Group (CCSG) included 39 cases in their protocol for children aged under two years and treated with the "8-in-1" schema. In both studies, irradiation was delayed.[53,54] Both studies showed a better progression-free survival in anaplastic astrocytoma versus glioblastoma and a favorable impact of the extent of surgical resection. The results and response to chemotherapy of those patients that remained under follow-up are reported in Table 19.3.

Overall, despite the fact that these tumors tend to behave unfavorably, especially in children under one year of age, long-term survival and response to chemotherapy are reported more often than in older children. A mechanism of differentiation and maturation of the tumor induced by chemotherapy is reported to be possible. A genetic difference between younger and older children has been hypothesized, younger children having less frequent chromosomal aberrations and *TP53* mutations.[55–57] In several cases of supratentorial tumors of very young children (under one year old) for whom a diagnosis of malignant glioma can be considered in the differential diagnosis, the histopathological diagnosis is not always easy. In a few cases it is not possible to fit the tumor in any known histopathological entity; in this case, it may be defined as "malignant primitive neuroepithelial tumor not otherwise classifiable."[58]

Table 19.2 *Clinical features and survival of 160 reported cases with primary central nervous system atypical teratoid/rhabdoid tumor*

Parameter	Burger *et al.*[44] (%)	Rorke *et al.*[43] (%)	Other reports[41,42,45,51] (%)	Italian cooperative study[52] (%)	All reported cases (%)
Patients (*n*)	55	52	38	15	160
Age					
Range	2–60 months	NB–14.9 years	NB–18 years	6 days–28 months	NB–18 years
Median	17 months	16.5 months	24 months	10 months	18 months
Distribution ≤3 years	50 (91)	40 (77)	24 (63)	15 (100)	129 (81)
Distribution >3 years	5 (9)	12 (23)	14 (37)		
Sex					
Male	34 (62)	ND	21 (55)	7 (47)	62/108 (57)
Female	21 (38)	ND	17 (45)	8 (53)	46/108 (43)
Sex ratio	1.6:1	3:2	1.2:1	0.9:1	1.3:1
Site					
Posterior fossa	36 (65)	33 (63)	15 (39)	9 (60)	93 (58)
Cerebellum	ND	29 (56)	11 (29)	3 (20)	43/105 (41)
Cerebellopontine angle	ND	4 (7)	3 (8)	6 (40)	13/105 (12)
Brainstem	ND	1 (3)	1/105 (1)		
Hemisphere	8 (15)	10 (19)	19 (50)	4 (27)	40 (25)
Suprasellar/III/V	4 (7)	1 (2)	1 (3)	1 (7)	7 (4)
Pineal	3 (5)	3 (6)	2 (5)	1 (7)	9 (6)
Spinal	1 (2)	1 (1)			
Multifocal	2 (4)	4 (8)	3 (20)		10 (6)
Unknown	2 (4)	1 (3)	2 (1)		
Treatment					
Surgery	ND	52	38	14**	104/105
Total/subtotal resection	ND	16 (31)	21 (55)	4 (29)	41 (39)
Biopsy/partial resection	ND	36 (69)	15 (39)	10 (71)	61 (59)
ND	2 (5)	2 (2)			
Chemotherapy	ND	39 (75)	25 (66)	11/15 (73)	75 (71)
Radiotherapy	ND	10 (19)	28 (74)	0	38 (36)
Chemo/radiotherapy*	ND	6 (11)	20 (53)	2/15 (13)	28 (27)
Only surgery	ND	9 (17)	5 (13)	4/14 (29)	18 (17)
DOD	41 (75)	43 (83)	31 (82)	12 (80)	127 (79)
Survival (range)	ND	ND	1 week–26 months	2–58 months	1 week–58 months
Survival (mean or median)	11 ± 13 months	6 months	6 months	8 months	7 months

DOD, died of disease; NB, newborn; ND, not done.
*Radiation therapy following or preceding chemotherapy. **One patient with multifocal disease did not undergo surgery on primary SNC mass.

Table 19.3 *Outcome for studies of chemotherapy for infants with high-grade gliomas*

Study	Ref.	Cases (*n*)	% response to chemotherapy	Type of treatment	Progression-free survival (3 years)	% overall survival (5 years)
POG1	2, 54	18	59	CTX/VCR CDDP/VP16	43	50**
CCG	53	39	24	"8 in 1"	44*	

CCG, Children's Cancer Group; CDDP, cisplatin; CTX, cytoxan (cyclophosphamide); POG, Pediatric Oncology Group; VCR, vincristine; VP16, etoposide.
*In anaplastic astrocytomas, glioblastoma progression-free survival = 0. **Four cases without radiotherapy due to parental refusal.

HISTORICALLY POOR OUTCOME FOR INFANTS WITH CENTRAL NERVOUS SYSTEM TUMORS

Younger children with tumors of the CNS do not fare as well as older children. Data from the SEER studies (Figures 19.5 and 19.6) show that children under four years of age at diagnosis in the 1980s had a poorer survival than children in the age range above four years. In the first SIOP trial for medulloblastoma, the progression-free survival for children under two years of age was 38 per cent, compared with 58 per cent for older children.[59] There are

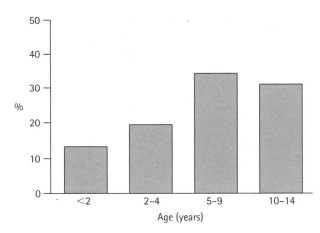

Figure 19.5 *Percentage distribution, by age, of all types of central nervous system tumors.*

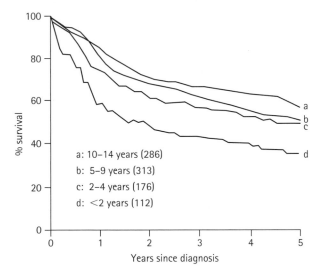

Figure 19.6 *Survival after central nervous system tumors, according to age at diagnosis.*

Table 19.4 *Change in awareness of late effects of treating central nervous system tumors*

Ref.	
82	70–75% live an active, useful life
83	45% educationally subnormal; most have some problems
62	50% IQ < 90, but educable; infants affected more severely

Table 19.5 *Effects of radiation on IQ in infants under three years of age*

Ref.	Patients (*n*)	IQ < 90	IQ < 70
62	9	7	7
63	7	7	4
64	5	3	3
61	18	14	7
Total	39	31 (79%)	21 (54%)

aggressive neurosurgery to be performed. However, as the late effects associated with radiotherapy in young children became recognized, parents and medical staff were no longer prepared to offer radiotherapy, and this was either omitted or given at a reduced dose or to reduced fields.

LATE EFFECTS OF RADIOTHERAPY

The late sequelae of craniospinal radiotherapy in young children are profound (see Chapter 24). Endocrinopathies and reduction of linear growth due to direct effect of spinal irradiation can affect adult height, but by far the most significant late effects are the neuropsychological problems that result from early radiotherapy. Jannoun and Bloom reported the results of IQ tests in children who received radiotherapy before the age of three years: of the 18 patients, 14 had an IQ of less than 90 and seven had an IQ of less than 70.[61] Similar results have been reported by other authors (Tables 19.4 and 19.5).[62–64] It appears that there is a dose relationship, with higher doses leading to more severe neuropsychological dysfunction.[65] Worse still is the fact that IQ appears to deteriorate with time, as shown in a cohort of patients treated with craniospinal irradiation for relapsed medulloblastoma: the patients' IQ scores continued to deteriorate at around four IQ points per year, and no plateau was reached at a median of almost five years of follow-up.[66]

IQ is probably a poor predictor of intellectual outcome. Indeed, Radcliffe and colleagues reported that 50 per cent of children who had no change in measured IQ post-craniospinal radiotherapy required extra school help.[67] Kiltie and colleagues described the late sequelae of 35 children who received craniospinal radiotherapy

three potential reasons why the outcome for young children may be different: the diseases could be different, the same histological disease may behave differently in the young, and therapy may be different. To some extent, all three reasons apply. Earlier in this chapter, we showed that high-risk tumors such as AT/RT and choroid plexus tumors occur at a higher frequency in this age group.

There is evidence from studies of medulloblastoma/PNET that younger children present with a higher incidence of metastatic disease.[60] Although this could be related to delayed diagnosis in preverbal children who cannot inform their parents about their symptoms, there is evidence that the diseases are more aggressive in the young; certainly, the median time to recurrence in young children with PNET is shorter than that in older children.

Historically, the surgical and anesthetic challenges of operating on very small children resulted in fewer children undergoing complete surgical resections of their tumors. Advances in technology and techniques now allow more

(CSRT) at a median age of 24 months: of 16 patients for whom there were adequate data, 15 required extra school help; only two of nine eligible for employment obtained work, and only one maintained this.[68]

Clearly, CSRT in young children is toxic, and many doctors and parents are not prepared to offer this potentially curative modality of therapy to children under three years of age.

BABY BRAIN STUDIES

Recognition of the severe adverse effects of radiotherapy prompted strategies that sought to delay the age at which radiotherapy was administered to allow further maturation of the brain before irradiation. The first of these studies was reported by Baram and colleagues, in which nine infants with medulloblastoma were treated with surgery and chemotherapy consisting of methylchlorethamine, vincristine, procarbazine, and prednisone (MOPP).[69] The original report showed that seven of the nine infants were alive, four of whom were more than a year off therapy. These results have never been bettered for a group of incompletely staged patients.

This report spawned a group of larger studies, all characterized by similar approaches and aims.[2,70–79] In most of these studies, all children with malignant tumors of the CNS were eligible and were treated with a regimen of multiagent chemotherapy. The chemotherapy combinations differed from study to study, and there were little or no phase II data for efficacy for each component of the regimens, let alone for the combination. The regimens were not particularly dose-intensive and were designed to be given over a period of at least one year. The aim of these studies was to delay radiotherapy until the end of the chemotherapy regimen, although some studies[76] aimed to withhold radiotherapy from patients who remained in complete remission at the end of the chemotherapy.

The biggest of these studies was reported by Duffner and colleagues on behalf of the POG.[2] This involved 132 children under 24 months of age at diagnosis and 66 children aged 24–36 months at diagnosis. The children were treated with two 28-day cycles of cyclophosphamide and vincristine followed by one 28-day cycle of cisplatin and etoposide. The sequence of three cycles was repeated for two years in patients under 24 months of age and for one year in children aged between 24 and 36 months, or until the disease progressed. The results were interesting in that the progression-free survival was 41 per cent at one year for children aged 24–36 months at diagnosis and 39 per cent at two years for those under 24 months of age at diagnosis. Not surprisingly, different histologies had different outcomes, with embryonal tumors doing badly. Complete resection conferred a survival benefit for the group as a whole. Preliminary analysis of neurocognitive

outcome in survivors showed no change from pre-chemotherapy levels. Further follow-up showed that the survival curves were not stable, and in many histologies later relapses continued to occur.[54]

It appeared that different chemotherapy regimens led to different results. For example, a regimen using eight drugs in one day reported by the Children's Cancer Group (CCG) had poorer results for embryonal tumors than the POG study noted above.[72] The survival for infants with PNETs in the study reported by Lashford and colleagues was particularly poor, with the majority of the recurrences occurring within a year of diagnosis when the children were still very young and susceptible to the worst effects of neuraxis radiotherapy.[76] Early results from the German study of infants with medulloblastoma show that for young children with no evidence of residual disease or metastases, survival rates in excess of 70 per cent can be achieved using a regimen of intravenous chemotherapy that did not differ substantially from that used in the study reported by Lashford and colleagues[76] but with the addition of intrathecal methotrexate.[75]

Of the children who had recurrences, some were offered CSRT, which resulted in cure for a variable percentage but at considerable cost in terms of neuropsychological sequelae.[66] Others were offered combinations of further chemotherapy, surgery, local radiotherapy, and high-dose chemotherapy.[72] The high-dose chemotherapy approaches showed some success in medulloblastoma/PNET but were disappointing in ependymoma and brain-stem glioma.[80]

CURRENT APPROACHES

Doctors and parents remain unwilling to treat very young children with neuraxis radiotherapy, even if the omission of irradiation compromises the chance of cure. The age at which radiotherapy is considered "acceptable" varies, with some groups using the age of five or six years[39,72,81] but others use the age of three years. It is clear that the use of a single protocol of therapy is not optimal for all histologies of tumor, and specific strategies are being developed for individual tumor types. Further risk stratification within a given histological subtype (e.g. presence or absence of metastases or residual disease) has led to a large number of patient groups, each with tiny numbers of patients eligible for the therapy under study. Even national or international studies will not be able to accrue sufficient numbers of patients in these restricted groups to end up with statistically valid comparisons of therapies, and so a number of single-arm studies are under way at national or institutional level. The use of high-dose chemotherapy is continuing to be explored in some studies,[80] but its role in cure seems to be limited to consolidating patients who have obtained complete remission by other means. The majority of these small studies have not, as yet, been reported, and it is hoped that successful strategies for individual disease groups will emerge, which can then be tested in the context of international studies.

SUMMARY

Young children with brain tumors present a particular challenge. The spectrum of diseases they suffer from differs from that seen in older children, and it may be that diseases that occur in older children have a more aggressive course in the very young. The sensitivity of the developing brain to insults, particularly to radiotherapy, results in profound neuropsychological consequences. Strategies that attempt to delay or avoid radiotherapy have been only partially successful and leave parents and their advisors facing difficult balances between chances of survival and quality of life. The plethora of different tumor subtypes makes large trials of therapy with homogeneous patient populations impossible to run, and progress is dependent on smaller, single-arm studies.

Editorial comment

The separation of long-term neuropsychological effects of therapy from those due to the direct or indirect effects of tumor remains problematic. The aim of delaying or possibly avoiding radiotherapy in the late 1980s and early 1990s led to a lumping together of infants with varying diagnosis into generic infant studies using the same chemotherapeutic approach. In some cases this approach was relatively successful (e.g. ependymoma), but in other cases it was detrimental (e.g. medulloblastoma/PNET). It has now become clear that infants should be treated with strategies related to their individual tumor type, but with relevant modifications according to their age. The use in certain circumstances of highly conformal radiotherapy (e.g. posterior fossa ependymoma) may, in some cases, obviate the need for wholesale avoidance or delay of radiotherapy. Collaborative groups are also discussing whether there is a "safe" dose of CSRT that can achieve reasonable disease control with acceptable, if not absent, sequelae. The scenario whereby survival is compromised in order to try to avoid radiotherapy may lead to ethical dilemmas that are impossible to resolve because of a lack of data on the relative impact of treatment and tumor-related parameters on long-term neuropsychological outcome. It is important to ensure that all future infant studies incorporate assessment of long-term functional outcome.

REFERENCES

1 Duffner PK. Brain tumours in infants and very young children. In: Cohen ME, Duffner PK (eds). *Brain Tumours in Children: Principles of Diagnosis and Treatment*, 2nd edn. New York: Raven Press, 1994.

2 Duffner PK, Horowitz ME, Krischer JP, *et al.* Postoperative chemotherapy and delayed radiation in children less than three years of age with malignant brain tumors. *N Engl J Med* 1993; **328**:1725–31.

3 Malcon AS, Lynn A, Gloecker R. Childhood cancer: incidence, survival and mortality. In: Pizzo PA, Popack DG (eds). *Principles and Practice of Pediatric Oncology*, 4th edn. Philadelphia: Lippincott William and Wilkins, 2002.

4 Ries L, Smith M, Gurney JG, *et al. Cancer Incidence and Survival Among Children and Adolescents: United States SEER Program 1975–1995*. NHI publication no. 99-4649. Bethesda, MD: National Cancer Institute, SEER program, 1999.

5 Parkin DM, Kramarova E, Draper GJ, *et al. International Incidence of Childhood Cancer*, vol. II. Lyon: IARC Scientific Publications, 1998.

6 Haddad SF, Menezes AH, Bell WE, Godersky JC, Afifi AK, Bale JF. Brain tumours occurring before 1 year of age: a retrospective review of 22 cases in a 11-year period (1977–1987). *Neurosurgery* 1991; **29**:8–13.

7 Choen BH, Packer RJ, Siegel KR, *et al.* Brain tumours in children under 2 years: treatment, survival and long term prognosis. *Pediatr Neurosurg* 1993; **19**:171–9.

8 Kleihues P, Cavenee WK. *World Health Organization Classification of Tumours: Pathology and Genetics of Tumours of the Nervous System*. Lyon: IARC Press, 2000.

9 Plon SE, Malkin D. Childhood cancer and heredity. In: Pizzo PA, Popack DG (eds). *Principles and Practice of Pediatric Oncology*, 4th edn. Philadelphia: Lippincott William and Wilkins, 2002.

10 Miyaki M, Nishio J, Konishi M, *et al.* Drastic genetic instability of tumours and normal tissues in Turcot syndrome. *Oncogene* 1997; **15**:2877–81

11 Pietsch T, Waha A, Koch A, *et al.* Medulloblastoma of the desmoplastic variant carry mutations of the human homologue of Drosophila patched. *Cancer Res* 1997; **57**:2085–8.

12 Zurawell RH, Allen C, Chiappa S, *et al.* Analysis of PTCH/SMO/SHH pathway genes in medulloblastoma genes. *Genes Chromosomes Cancer* 2000; **27**:44–51.

13 Huang H, Betania M, Mahler-Araujo M, *et al.* APC mutations in sporadic medulloblastoma. *Am J Pathol* 2000; **156**:433–7.

14 Yuasa H, Tokito S, Tokunaga M. Primary carcinoma of the choroid plexus in Li–Fraumeni syndrome: case report. *Neurosurgery* 1993; **32**:131–3.

15 Malkin D, Chilton-MacNeil S, Meister LA, Sexsmith E, Diller L, Garcea RL. Tissue specific expression of SV40 in tumours associated with the Li–Fraumeni syndrome. *Oncogene* 2001; **20**:4441–9.

16 Giangaspero F, Perilongo G, Fondelli MP, *et al.* Medulloblastoma with extensive nodularity: a variant with favourable prognosis. *J Neurosurgery* 1999; **91**:971–7.

17 Tenreiro-Picon OR, Kamath SV, Knorr JR, Ragland RL, Smith TW, Lau KY. Desmoplastic infantile ganglioglioma: CT and MRI features. *Pediatr Radiol* 1995; **25**:540–3.

18 Vanderberg SR, May EE, Rubistein LJ, *et al.* Desmoplastic supratentorial neuroepithelial tumours of infancy with divergent differentiation potential (desmoplastic infantile gangliogliomas). Report of 11 cases of a distinctive embryonal tumour with favourable prognosis. *J Neurosurgery* 1987; **66**:58–71.

19 Vanderberg SR. Desmoplastic infantile ganglioglioma: a clinicopathological review of sixteen cases. *Brain Tumour Pathol* 1991; **8**:25–31.

20 Vandenberg SR. Desmoplastic infantile ganglioglioma and desmoplastic cerebral astrocytoma of infancy. *Brain Pathol* 1993; **3**:275–81.

21 Gobel U, Haas RJ, Calaminus G, *et al.* Treatment of germ cell tumours in children: results of European Trials for testicular and non-testicular primary sites. *Crit Rev Oncol Hematol* 1990; **10**:89–98.

22 Flamant F. Baranzelli MC, Kalifa C, Lemerle J. Treatment of malignant germ cell tumours in children: experience of the Institute Gustave Roussy and the French Society of Pediatric Oncology. *Crit Rev Oncol Hematol* 1990; **10**:99–110.

23 Ferreira J, Eviatar L, Schneider S, Grossman R. Prenatal diagnosis of intracranial teratoma. Prolonged survival after resection of a malignant teratoma diagnosed prenatally by ultrasound: a case report and review of literature. *Pediatr Neurosurg* 1993; **19**:84–8.

24 Garrè ML, El-Hossainy MO, Fondelli P, *et al.* Is chemotherapy effective therapy for intracranial immature teratoma. *Cancer* 1996; **77**:977–82.

25 Berger C, Thiesse P, Lellouch-Tubiana A, Kalifa C, Pierre-Kahn A, Bouffet E. Choroid plexus ca in childhood: clinical features and prognostic factors. *Neurosurgery* 1998; **42**:470–5.

26 Duffner PK, Kun LE, Burger PC, *et al.* Postoperative chemotherapy and delayed radiation in infants and very young children with choroid plexus carcinomas. The Paediatric Oncology Group. *Pediatr Neurosurg* 1995; **22**:189–96.

27 Pencalet P, Sainte-Rose C, Lellouch-Tubiana A, *et al.* Papillomas and carcinomas of the choroid plexus in children. *J Neurosurg* 1998; **88**:521–8.

28 Mc Evoy AW, Harding BN, Phipps KP, *et al.* Management of choroid plexus tumours in children: 20 years experience at a single neurosurgical center. *Pediatr Neurosurg* 2000; **32**:192–9.

29 Chow E, Reardon DA, Shah AB, *et al.* Pediatric choroid plexus neoplasm. *Int J Radiat Oncol Biol Phys* 1999; **44**:249–54.

30 Diengdoh JV, Show M. Oncocytic variant of choroid plexus papilloma. Evolution from benign to malignant oncocytoma. *Cancer* 1993; **71**:855–8.

31 Garrè ML, Brisigotti M, Capra V, *et al.* Frequency and biological behaviour of choroid plexus (CP) tumours in children. *Neuro-Oncol* 2000; **2** (suppl. 1).

32 Sanford RA, Horowitz ME, Kun LE, Jenkins JJ, Simmons JCH, Kovnar EH. Preoperative chemotherapy to facilitate the total resection of paediatric brain tumours. In: Marlin AE (ed.). *Concepts in Pediatric Neurosurgery*, vol. 9. Basel: Karger, 1989, pp. 139–52.

33 Tihan T, Burger PC. A variant of pylocitic astrocytoma: a possible distinct clinicopathological entity with a less favourable outcome. *J Neuropathol Exp Neurol* 1998; **57**:495–500.

34 Cottingham SL, Bosel CP, Yates AJ. Pylocitic astrocytoma in infants: a distinctive histological pattern. *J Neuropathol Exp Neurol* 1996; **55**:654.

35 Becker LE, Cruz-Sanchez FF. Ependymoblastoma. In: Kleihues P, Cavenee WK. *Pathology and Genetics of Tumours of the Nervous System.* Lyon: IARC Press, 2000.

36 Mork SJ, Rubinstein LJ. Ependymoblastoma. A reappraisal of a rare embryonal tumour. *Cancer* 1985; **55**:1536–42.

37 Dorsay TA, Rovira MJ, Ho VB, Kelley J. Ependymoblastoma: MR presentation. A case report and review of literature. *Pediatr Radiol* 1995; **25**:433–5.

38 Wada C, Kurata A, Hirose R, *et al.* Primary leptomeningeal ependymoblastoma. Case report. *J Neurosurg* 1986; **64**:968–73.

39 Marec-Berard P, Jouvet A, Thiesse P, Kalifa C, Doz F, Frappaz D. Supratentorial embryonal tumours in children under 5 years an SFOP study of treatment with postoperative chemotherapy alone. *Med Pediatr Oncol* 2002; **38**:83–90.

40 Bonnin JM, Rubistein LJ, Palmer NF. The association of embryonal tumours originating in the kidney and in the brain. A report of seven cases. *Cancer* 1984; **54**:2137–46.

41 Parham DM, Weeks DA, Becwith JB. The clinico-pathological spectrum of putative extrarenal rhabdoid tumours. An analysis of 42 cases studied with immunohistochemistry or electron microscopy. *Am J Surg Pathol* 1994; **18**:1010–20.

42 Rorke LB, Packer RJ, Biegel JA. Central nervous system atypical teratoid/rhabdoid tumours of infancy and childhood. *J Neuro-Oncol* 1995; **24**:21–8.

43 Rorke LB, Packer RJ, Biegel JA. Central nervous system atypical teratoid/rhabdoid tumours of infancy and childhood definition of an entity. *J Neurosurg* 1996; **85**:56–65.

44 Burger PC, Yu IT, Friedman HS, *et al.* Atypical teratoid/rhabdoid tumour of the central nervous system. A highly malignant tumour of infancy and childhood frequently mistaken for medulloblastoma. A Paediatric Oncology Group Study. *Am J Surg Pathol* 1998; **22**:1083–92.

45 Giannini C, Garrè ML, Oka H. Atypical teratoid/rhabdoid tumour of the central nervous system: an aggressive pediatric brain tumour. *Path Case Rev* 1998; **3**:301–8.

46 Biegel JA. Cytogenetics and molecular genetics of childhood brain tumours. *Neurooncol* 1999; **1**:139–51.

47 Biegel JA, Zhou JY, Rorke L, Stenstrom C, Wainright, Fogelgren B. Germ-line and acquired mutations of INI1 in atypical teratoid and rhabdoid tumors. *Cancer Res* 1999; **59**:74–9.

48 Taylor MD, Gokgoz N, Andrulis IL, Mainprize TG, Drake JM, Rutka JT. Familial posterior fossa brain tumours of infancy secondary to germline mutation of the hSNF5 gene. *Am J Hum Genet* 2000; **66**:1403–6.

49 Tortori-Donati P, Fondelli MP, *et al.* Atypical teratoid/ rhabdoid tumours of the central nervous system in infancy – neuroradiological findings. *Int J Neuroradiol* 1997; **3**:327–38.

50 Olson TA, Bayar E, Kosnik E, *et al.* Successful treatment of disseminated central nervous system malignant rhabdoid tumour. *J Pediatr Hematol Oncol* 1995; **17**:71–5.

51 Hildel JM, Watterson J, Longee DC, *et al.* Central nervous system atypical teratoid tumour/rhabdoid tumour: response to

intensive therapy and review of literature. *J Neuro-Oncol* 1998; **40**:265–75.

52 Garrè ML, Giannini C, Brisigotti M, *et al*. Central nervous system (CNS) atypical teratoid/rhabdoid tumour (AT/RT): survival and prognostic factors in 15 cases included in the Italian Cooperative Study for children <3 yrs of age. *Neuro-Oncol* 2000; **2** (suppl. 1).

53 Geyer JR, Finlay JL, Boyett JM, *et al*. Survival of infants with malignant astrocytomas. A report from the Children's Cancer Group. *Cancer* 1995; **75**:1045–50.

54 Duffner PK, Horowitz ME, Krischer JP, *et al*. The treatment of malignant brain tumours in infants and very young children: an update of the Pediatric Oncology Group experience. *Neuro-Oncol* 1999; **1**:152–61.

55 Kunwar S, Mohapatra G, Bollen A, Lamborn KR, Prados M, Feuerstein BG. Genetic subgroups of anaplastic astrocytomas correlate with patient age and survival. *Cancer Res* 2001; **61**:7683–8.

56 Pollack IF, Finkelstein SD, Woods J, *et al*. Expression of *p53* and prognosis in children with malignant gliomas. *N Engl J Med* 2002; **7**; **346**:420–7.

57 Pollack IF, Finkelstein SD, Burnham J, *et al*. Age and TP53 mutation frequency in childhood malignant gliomas: results in a multi-institutional cohort. *Cancer Res* 2001; **61**:7404–7.

58 Cruz-Sanchez FF, Rossi ML, Hughes JT, Moss TH. Differentiation in embryonal neuroepithelial tumours of the central nervous system. *Cancer* 1991; **67**:965–76.

59 Tait DM, Thornton-Jones H, Bloom HJG, Lemerle H, Morris-Jones P. Adjuvant chemotherapy for medulloblastoma: the first multi-center control trial of the International Society of Pediatric Oncology (SIOPI). *Eur J Cancer* 1990; **26**:464–9.

60 Geyer R, Levy M, Berger MS, Milstein J, Griffin B, Bleyer WA. Infants with medulloblastoma: a single institution review of survival. *Neurosurgery* 1991; **29**:707–11.

61 Jannoun L, Bloom HJG. Long term psychological effects in children treated for intracranial tumours. *Int J Radiat Oncol Biol Phys* 1989; **18**:747–53.

62 Spunberg JJ, Chang CH, Goldman M, Auricchio E, Bell JJ. Quality of long-term survival following irradiation for intracranial tumors in children under the age of two. *Int J Radiat Oncol Biol Phys* 1981; **7**:727–36.

63 Duffner PK, Cohen ME, Thomas P. Late effects of treatment on the intelligence of children with posterior fossa tumors. *Cancer* 1983; **51**:233–7.

64 Danoff BF, Cowchock FS, Marquette C, Mulgrew L, Kramer S. Assessment of the long-term effects of primary radiation therapy for brain tumors in children. *Cancer* 1982; **49**:1580–6.

65 Grill J, Renaux VK, Bulteau C, *et al*. Long-term intellectual outcome in children with posterior fossa tumors according to radiation doses and volumes. *Int J Radiat Oncol Biol Phys* 1999; **45**:137–45.

66 Walter AW, Mulhern RK, Gajjar A, *et al*. Survival and neurodevelopmental outcome of young children with medulloblastoma at St Jude Children's Research Hospital. *J Clin Oncol* 1999; **17**:3720–8.

67 Radcliffe J, Bunin GR, Sutton LN, Goldwein JW, Phillips PC. Cognitive deficits in long-term survivors of childhood medulloblastoma and other noncortical tumors: age-dependent effects of whole brain radiation. *Int J Dev Neurosci* 1994; **12**:327–34.

68 Kiltie AE, Lashford LS, Gattamaneni HR. Survival and late effects in medulloblastoma patients treated with craniospinal irradiation under three years old. *Med Pediatr Oncol* 1997; **28**:348–54.

69 Baram TZ, Van Eys J, Dowell RE, Cangir A, Pack B, Bruner J. Survival and neurologic outcome of infants with medulloblastoma treated with surgery and MOPP chemotherapy – a preliminary report. *Cancer* 1987; **60**:173–7.

70 Agerlin N, Gjerris F, Brincker H, *et al*. Childhood medulloblastoma in Denmark 1960–1984. A population-based retrospective study. *Childs Nerv Syst* 1999; **15**:29–36.

71 Ater JL, van Eys J, Woo SY, Moore B, Copeland DR, Bruner J. MOPP chemotherapy without irradiation as primary postsurgical therapy for brain tumors in infants and young children. *J Neuro-Oncol* 1997; **32**:243–52.

72 Dupuis-Girod S, Hartmann O, Benhamou E, *et al*. Will high dose chemotherapy followed by autologous bone marrow transplantation supplant cranio-spinal irradiation in young children treated for medulloblastoma? *J Neuro-Oncol* 1996; **27**:87–98.

73 Geyer JR, Zeltzer PM, Boyett JM, *et al*. Survival of infants with primitive neuroectodermal tumors and malignant ependymomas of the CNS treated with eight drugs in 1 day: a report from the Children's Cancer Group. *J Clin Oncol* 1994; **12**:1607–16.

74 Kellie SJ. Chemotherapy of central nervous system tumours in infants. *Childs Nerv Syst* 1999; **15**:592–612.

75 Kuhl J. Modern treatment strategies in medulloblastoma. *Childs Nerv Syst* 1998; **14**:2–5.

76 Lashford LS, Campbell RH, Gattamaneni HR, Robinson K, Walker D, Bailey C. An intensive multiagent chemotherapy regimen for brain tumours occurring in very young children. *Arch Dis Child* 1996; **74**:219–23.

77 Massimino M, Gandola L, Cefalo G, *et al*. Management of medulloblastoma and ependymoma in infants: a single-institution long-term retrospective report. *Childs Nerv Syst* 2000; **16**:15–20.

78 Perilongo G, Massimino M, Sotti G, *et al*. Analyses of prognostic factors in a retrospective review of 92 children with ependymoma: Italian Pediatric Neuro-oncology Group. *Med Pediat Oncol* 1997; **29**:79–85.

79 White L, Kellie S, Gray E, *et al*. Postoperative chemotherapy in children less than 4 years of age with malignant brain tumors: promising initial response to a VETOPEC-based regimen. A study of the Australian and New Zealand Children's Cancer Study Group (ANZCCSG). *J Pediatr Hematol Oncol* 1998; **2**:125–30.

80 Kalifa C, Valteau D, Pizer B, Vassal G, Grill J, Hartmann O. High dose chemotherapy in childhood brain tumors. *Childs Nerv Syst* 1999; **15**:498–505.

81 Dunkel IJ, Finlay JL. High dose chemotherapy with autologous stem cell rescue for patients with medulloblastoma. *J Neuro-Oncol* 1996; **29**:69–74.

82 Bloom HJC, Wallace ENJ, Herk JM. The treatment and prognosis of medulloblastoma in children: a study of 82 verified cases. *Am J Roentgenol* 1969; **105**:43–62.

83 Bamford FN, Jones PM, Pearson O, *et al*. Residual disabilities in children treated for intracranial space-occupying lesions. *Cancer* 1976; **37**:1149–51.

20

Craniopharyngioma

RICHARD D HAYWARD, CATHERINE DEVILE AND MICHAEL BRADA

INTRODUCTION

Craniopharyngiomas are rare epithelial tumors of maldevelopmental origin. They account for approximately 6–13 per cent of all intracranial tumors in childhood, but they represent the commonest tumors to involve the hypothalamo-pituitary region. Although benign by histological criteria, they often follow a more malignant course in terms of both local disease progression and their associated morbidity.

The "modern" surgical management of craniopharyngioma is usually dated to Matson's observation that it was possible at surgery to identify a gliotic "capsule" that capped the tumor and, therefore, to remove the tumor completely without endangering the hypothalamus.[1] Early enthusiasm for attempts at curative surgery was tempered, however, by the difficulties often encountered in achieving this aim and by the resultant patient morbidity, particularly in relation to severe hypothalamic injury. Recognition of this morbidity by some but not all neurosurgeons prompted other treatment modalities to be explored – in particular, adjuvant radiotherapy following partial tumor resection. Advocates of primary aggressive surgical management have continued to argue that radiotherapy is difficult to justify as treatment for a histologically benign tumor with its unpredictable side effects, delayed toxicity, and doubtful efficacy. Consequently, one of the longest-standing controversies has arisen as to the place of radiotherapy in the treatment of craniopharyngioma and the optimal management approach in childhood.

The two extremes of management (radical surgery versus conservative surgery, e.g. cyst aspiration alone followed by radiotherapy) are best exemplified by the series presented by Yasargil and colleagues, who describe the results of treating 70 children by radical surgery,[2] and by Brada and colleagues, who describe their experience of treating 77 children aged between three and 16 years and referred for radiotherapy following only limited surgery.[3] Results from these studies are summarized later in this chapter.

More recently, the trend – particularly among neurosurgeons (to whom patients are usually referred initially) – has shifted again towards more radical surgery, using approaches that reflect advances in surgical technology, with the advent not only of the operating microscope but also of instrumentation designed to allow the removal of tumor bulk with as little interference to the surrounding (normal) tissues as possible. Thus, many neurosurgeons continue to advocate complete tumor excision as the gold standard and primary goal of treatment in every case, regardless of the age of the patient, tumor size, consistency (solid or cystic), and location. Whilst some surgeons have reported successful total surgical resection of tumors in 77–90 per cent of their patients, with apparent minimal mortality and diminished morbidity, others have continued to experience great difficulties, with complete tumor excision achieved in only 32–58 per cent of patients in studies including surgeons whose aim of surgery was attempted total tumor removal in all cases.[4]

It was against the background of a poor surgical outcome in four children who had presented to one particular unit as acute emergencies with large craniopharyngiomas that a series of in-depth studies were initiated in order to determine whether it was possible to predict the outcome following radical – usually attempted curative – surgery. The first findings to emerge from this study (which included the four children mentioned) made it possible to quantify the connection between hypothalamic damage (as demonstrated on magnetic resonance scanning) and clinical evidence of hypothalamic dysfunction, in this case obesity as measured by the body mass index (BMI). The analysis of three-dimensional, volume-acquisition magnetic resonance scans reconstructed in the sagittal plane confirmed that the greater the degree of hypothalamic damage, the greater the child's BMI – more than five times as great in those children with the most damage.[5]

The second part of the study looked at prognosis with regard to both morbidity and tumor recurrence.[6] For the former, a morbidity score, which incorporated a variety of neurological, psychological, ophthalmological, and endocrinological measures, was devised. These were set against details of the child's presentation and surgery (including any peroperative complications) and the results of imaging.

Of a total of 75 children studied, 29 of whom were under five years of age at diagnosis, there were no perioperative deaths, but nine patients subsequently died from their tumor or related sequelae at a median of 5.9 years (range 0.3–15.4 years) after initial surgery. Follow-up clinical and neuroimaging assessments were undertaken in the 66 survivors at a mean of seven years from initial surgery.

Predictors of poorer outcome (high morbidity) at study assessment included the grade of hydrocephalus, the occurrence of any peroperative complications and young age (≤5 years) at presentation. The presence of symptoms and signs of hypothalamic dysfunction at the time of diagnosis had a significant effect on the immediate postoperative morbidity score as well as being a predictive factor for longer-term hypothalamic injury, along with greater height of the tumor in the midline and attempts to remove adherent tumor from the region of the hypothalamus at operation.

From these data, we can conclude that younger children presenting as emergencies (usually with hydrocephalus and thus with larger tumors) are likely to have a poorer outcome following an attempt at a complete removal (which was the initial treatment policy in 58 of the patients – operated on transcranially – described above).

The study also demonstrated the relative risks of tumor recurrence and showed that they could be correlated with young age (≤5 years) at presentation and tumor size (as measured by the number of intracranial compartments involved by the tumor) whereas complete tumor excision (as determined by postoperative neuroimaging) and

external fractionated radiotherapy given electively after subtotal excision were significantly less likely to be associated with recurrent disease.[6,7]

From this experience, we can be reasonably sure of three things: (i) radical surgery, while being capable of providing long-term tumor control, can in certain (and predictable) cases be responsible for an unacceptable degree of hypothalamic damage; (ii) external beam fractionated radiotherapy may also provide long-term tumor control and largely predictable risk of late toxicity, particularly in children aged <4 years; and (iii) younger children fare worse than older children.

INCIDENCE

Overall, craniopharyngiomas constitute between 1.2 and four per cent of all brain tumors (adults and children). Peak age incidence is five to ten years, with a relatively constant percentage occurring throughout each decade of life, although there may be a second peak in the fifth to sixth decades.[8] A recent study from the USA suggested an incidence (for adults and children) of 0.13 per 100 000 patient years, an incidence which does not vary by gender or race.[9] The same authors calculated that 96 childhood cases (aged 15 years or under) might be expected out of the total number of 338 craniopharyngiomas predicted for the USA each year. Published articles on the subject are unusual if they contain more than 70 cases, and these are likely to have been accumulated over many years. Of the 75–80 pediatric intracranial tumors referred to Great Ormond Street Hospital for Children, London, each year for primary treatment (as opposed to recurrent tumors and referrals for second opinions), only three to five are likely to be craniopharyngiomas.

NEUROPATHOLOGY

Craniopharyngiomas are benign tumors (malignant transformation is extremely rare) that probably arise from remnants of Rathke's pouch, although an alternative origin from the adenohypophysis has been suggested.[10] They consist of squamous epithelium lining cystic cavities, and solid components that contain calcium and the keratin products of squamous cell activity. Although entirely cystic or entirely solid types are seen, most tumors have a mixture of the two components. From a histological point of view, craniopharyngiomas are sometimes subclassified as being of an adamantinomatous (more prone to calcium formation and the most common childhood form) or squamous papillary (less prone to calcium production) type. For a discussion of the possible effects of these variations on the surgical prognosis (and opposing views), see the articles by Adamson and colleagues[11] and Weiner and colleagues.[12]

The tumor's point of origin can be either the pituitary stalk or the tuber cinereum (the floor of the third ventricle). Each point of origin allows the tumor to expand in a different way and thus influences the morbidity (in terms of hypothalamic damage) associated with radical attempts at removal. Tumors that arise from the pituitary stalk typically extend downwards into the pituitary fossa itself (or else expand upwards from it), that part of the tumor immediately above the fossa possessing as a pseudo-capsule the attenuated dura of the sellar diaphragm. Tumors arising from the tuber cinereum are more likely to extend upwards through the hypothalamus and into the third ventricle, where they may cause hydrocephalus. Despite their midline origin, craniopharyngiomas can expand not only upwards but also laterally into one or both middle fossae, subfrontally, and even backwards and downwards into the posterior fossa. Occasional tumors invade the skull base. Figures 20.1–20.4 illustrate some of these variations.

Their relationship to the chiasm has always been of particular concern to neurosurgeons because of the influence this has on the operative approach used. A pre-fixed chiasm

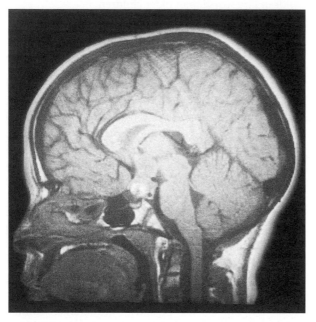

Figure 20.1 *Small craniopharyngioma arising just above the pituitary fossa.*

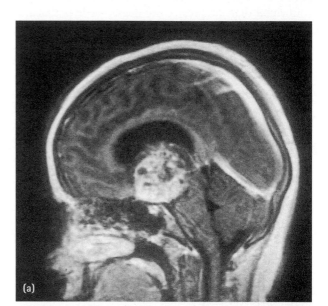

(a)

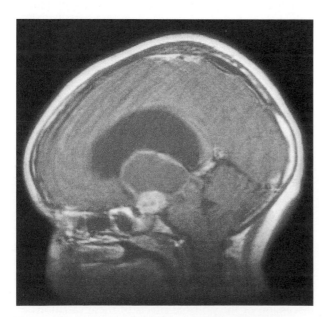

Figure 20.2 *Large, partly solid but predominantly cystic craniopharyngioma, associated with hydrocephalus.*

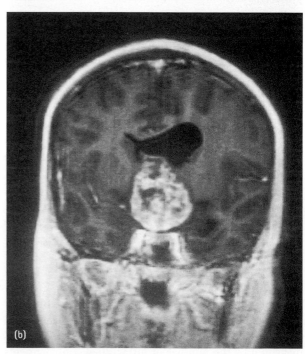

(b)

Figure 20.3a,b *Sagittal (a) and coronal (b) magnetic resonance scans of a large, solid craniopharyngioma.*

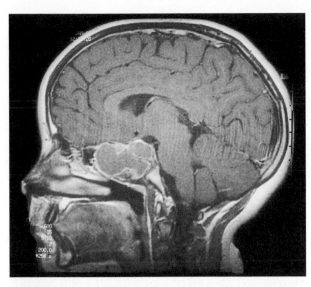

Figure 20.4 *Large, predominantly cystic craniopharyngioma involving the skull base.*

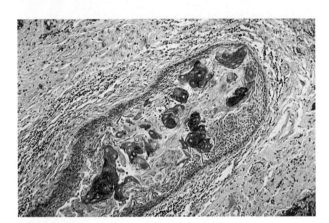

Figure 20.5 *Finger-like projection of craniopharyngioma tissue has invaded the adjacent hypothalamus (hematoxylin and eosin).*

Table 20.1 *Presenting features attributable to neurological, ophthalmic, and hypothalamo-pituitary dysfunction in 75 children treated for craniopharyngioma at Great Ormond Street Hospital for Children, London, from 1973 to 1994*

Presenting features	Patients (*n*, %)
Neurological	
Headaches	49 (65)
Vomiting	37 (49)
Somnolence	15 (20)
Developmental regression/delay	14 (19)
Unsteadiness	13 (17)
Decreased consciousness	12 (16)
Seizures	10 (13)
Hemiparesis	6 (8)
Total number with symptoms	62 (83)
Ophthalmic	
Gradual reduction in visual acuity	24 (32)
Acute reduction in visual acuity	11 (15)
Squint	13 (17)
Cranial nerve palsies	11 (15)
Documented field defects	33 (44)
Blindness	10 (13)
Optic atrophy	30 (40)
Papilloedema	24 (32)
Total number with symptoms	42 (56)
Hypothalamo-pituitary	
Growth failure/short stature	25 (33)
Anorexia/poor weight gain	23 (31)
Increased thirst/polyuria	21 (28)
Weight gain	11 (15)
Temperature intolerance	4 (5)
Frequent infections with lethargy	4 (5)
Delayed puberty	4 (5)
Precocious puberty	0 (0)
Total number with symptoms	53 (71)

leaves little space for surgical manipulation between it and the tuberculum sellae that lies immediately in front. A post-fixed chiasm has a convenient gap between the two structures through which a surgeon, using a traditional subfrontal approach, can remove some or all of the tumor.

Of equal importance is the degree of involvement of the hypothalamus. Although these tumors are, by histological criteria, benign, they may still project finger-like processes into the adjacent hypothalamus (Figure 20.5). At one time, it was believed that this invaded tissue adjacent to the tumor was reactive in nature and formed no part of the functioning hypothalamus. However, as the studies referred to above have demonstrated, radical surgery for tumors involving the hypothalamus is associated with an unacceptable morbidity and such "invasion" should be taken as an indication that a tumor is not amenable to a surgical cure regardless of the histological nature of the tissue involved.

DIAGNOSIS

Presenting symptoms and signs

Craniopharyngiomas are usually slow-growing, extra-axial tumors that produce symptoms by compression of adjacent neural structures, including visual pathways, hypothalamus, pituitary gland and stalk, cerebral cortex, major blood vessels, and rostral brainstem. In children, multiple symptomatology is often present by the time of diagnosis, although the commonest presenting complaints are those relating to raised intracranial pressure secondary to third ventricular compression and obstructive hydrocephalus (Table 20.1).

Neurosurgical studies show that while symptoms of visual disturbance are common at presentation, the reported incidence of reduced visual acuity and visual field loss in children, both preoperatively and at long-term follow-up, is very variable.[13,14] Thus, findings of impaired acuity range from 37–81 per cent of cases at presentation to 30–84 per cent at long-term follow-up, and visual field defects range from 22–68 per cent of cases at presentation to 33–68 per cent at long-term follow-up.[4]

Both the duration and degree of preoperative visual deficits have been shown to be significant factors influencing long-term visual outcome.[15] More recently, visual deterioration, papilledema, and hemianopia as presenting symptoms and signs have been shown to be significant factors associated with a poor overall outcome.[16] Prompt diagnosis is therefore essential but often difficult in children, as they are frequently inattentive to visual loss, as highlighted by the ten children in our series who were essentially blind at the time of referral, half of whom were aged six years or over at presentation. Symptoms of visual disturbance were present in 56 per cent of children at diagnosis, and 87 per cent of patients had ocular signs on preoperative ophthalmological examination (Table 20.1).

Ocular signs and symptoms may be misleading in children. Eight of 13 patients presenting with squints in our study had received treatment previously for an "idiopathic" concomitant strabismus, poor visual acuity being attributed to amblyopia. All had significant optic pathway involvement by tumor at diagnosis, with associated acuity and fundal abnormalities. Furthermore, the presence of significant optic atrophy – reflecting chronic compression of visual pathways – in all these cases at follow-up suggested that none of the squints was idiopathic. The marked biological heterogeneity of childhood craniopharyngiomas, with some tumors demonstrating long quiescent periods before renewed growth, supports this mode of presentation further.

Although symptoms related to hypothalamo-pituitary dysfunction are uncommon as the *presenting* complaint in children (21 of 75 patients followed up at Great Ormond Street Hospital), the majority (71 per cent) had symptoms to suggest an endocrinopathy at diagnosis (Table 20.1). A third of children presented with growth failure preceding the diagnosis by a mean of 2.9 years (range 0.5–5.0 years). The available data for preoperative endocrine status in children suggest that hypothalamo-pituitary dysfunction is present in 80–90 per cent of subjects, while growth hormone insufficiency occurs in approximately 75 per cent of patients tested. The prevalence of other pituitary hormone deficits before surgery has been summarized from the literature as 40 per cent for gonadotrophin insufficiency, 25 per cent for thyroid-stimulating hormone (TSH) and adrenocorticotropic hormone (ACTH) insufficiency, 9–17 per cent for antidiuretic hormone (ADH) insufficiency, and 20 per cent for a raised serum prolactin, although numbers reported are small. Higher figures for ADH insufficiency (34 per cent) have been reported, inclusive of those patients with concomitant ACTH insufficiency and in whom symptoms of diabetes insipidus were

masked completely or incompletely until the start of glucocorticoid replacement.

Hypothalamic symptoms at presentation are reported variably in the literature. In the Great Ormond Street Hospital series, 23 per cent of patients had evidence of hypothalamic dysfunction, with a history of weight gain for up to 3.5 years before diagnosis, extreme weight loss, or disturbances of behavior or memory as the predominant hypothalamic symptoms. In all of these patients, tumor was shown to extend into the hypothalamus on preoperative neuroimaging.

PREOPERATIVE ASSESSMENT

This is best divided into neuroimaging (discussed in the previous section) and endocrinological, ophthalmological, and cognitive assessment.

Endocrinological assessment

Due to the high prevalence of preoperative endocrinopathies, as discussed above, children should be covered perioperatively for the possibility of cortisol deficiency. In addition, they should be assessed for diabetes insipidus, hypothyroidism, and hyperprolactinemia on early-morning basal biochemistry, as outlined below. Most patients receive glucocorticoid cover as high-dose perioperative oral or intravenous dexamethasone (which may cause hyperglycemia in patients with a positive family history of type 2 diabetes); as the dose is reduced, hydrocortisone should be substituted and maintained in replacement doses until a full endocrine assessment has been performed approximately six to eight weeks after surgery and/or radiotherapy.

Preoperative endocrine investigations

- *Auxology:* height, weight, pubertal staging, calculation of surface area.
- *Biochemistry:* 0800 hours – paired plasma and urine electrolytes, glucose and osmolalities, serum cortisol, prolactin, free tri-iodothyronine (FT3), free tetra-iodothyronine (FT4), TSH, calcium, albumen. Luteinizing hormone (LH), follicle-stimulating hormone (FSH), testosterone/estradiol if aged nine years or older.
- *X-ray:* left hand/wrist for bone age.

Ophthalmological assessment

In view of the high incidence of ophthalmological symptoms at presentation, and the risk to vision posed by surgery (and radiotherapy), it is essential that all patients have a full assessment of their vision recorded before initiation of all but the most urgent treatment. This should include:

- visual acuity;
- visual field assessment;
- fundoscopy;
- visual electrophysiology, if available.

Psychological assessment

Because cognitive and behavioral problems can occur both before and after treatment, all children should, if time permits, have a psychometric assessment carried out before intervention.

DIFFERENTIAL DIAGNOSIS

There are three tumor types arising in the suprasellar region in children that need to be differentiated from a craniopharyngioma: pilocytic astrocytoma of the optic chiasm/hypothalamus, suprasellar germinoma, and Rathke's pouch cyst.

Pilocytic astrocytomas of the optic chiasm/hypothalamus occur more commonly than craniopharyngiomas. About a third are associated with neurofibromatosis type 1 (NF-1) (see Chapters 13a and 13b). Although they may contain cystic elements, these are not usually so prominent as in craniopharyngiomas. They tend to extend posteriorly along the optic tracts, a reflection of their origin intrinsic to the central nervous system (CNS). It is very unusual for these tumors to present with endocrine abnormalities. From a radiological point of view, it is their lack of any calcification that finally differentiates them from craniopharyngioma.

Suprasellar germinomas are more rare than craniopharyngiomas. They often present, like craniopharyngiomas, with diabetes insipidus (see Chapter 18a). However, like astrocytomas in this region, they do not contain calcium.

Rathke's pouch cysts – embryological cousins of craniopharyngiomas – are seen only rarely in childhood. They usually consist of both cystic and solid elements, they contain calcium, and they may present with many of the clinical features of craniopharyngioma. Differentiating the two preoperatively may, therefore, be difficult, but as the initial surgical management is likely to be the same for both, this does not pose a major clinical problem.

MANAGEMENT STRATEGY

General observations

The involvement of the hypothalamus is the reason why, before discussing management in terms of the therapeutic modalities employed (surgery and radiotherapy) it is appropriate to describe the clinical state of a child who has suffered hypothalamic damage (usually in addition to being rendered panhypopituitary as a result of treatment of a craniopharyngioma).[7] At the mildest end of the spectrum is so-called hypothalamic obesity, a condition observed so frequently after radical surgery that the parents of a child for whom such an operation is proposed should be warned specifically of its possibility. Obesity can occur with little or no evidence of other cognitive or behavioral problems; however, with increasing hypothalamic damage, there are worsening learning difficulties associated with defective short-term memory and limited concentration span. The child's behavior can also be affected severely. Hand in hand with the obesity is a desire to "feed," which may have the child stealing and fighting for food until everything edible in the home has to be locked away. Stealing of anything else that will supply an instant feeling of gratification can also occur. There is also a reversal of the normal circadian sleep patterns, which can leave the child awake for most of the night (and on the rampage for food) while during the day he or she can barely be roused.[17] Also, hypothalamic damage can destroy the child's sense of thirst, an essential sensation if the treatment of diabetes insipidus (which, if not present preoperatively, is almost inevitable following radical surgery) with desmopressin (nasal or oral) is to be successful. The combination of diabetes insipidus and lack of any sensation of thirst leaves the child with no idea of when they need to drink, and they therefore swing violently between states of over- and underhydration.

The net result of these disabilities can be a child, perhaps with seriously defective vision, whose personality has been changed completely by the combined effects of their tumor and its surgery, who is incapable of normal schooling, whose behavioral problems can have a severe effect upon the family unit, and whose life expectancy is shortened because of their vulnerability to hypothalamically-mediated metabolic crises.

The ultimate goals of treatment are therefore to decompress the visual apparatus and prevent further tumor growth while at the same time preserving not only hypothalamic function but also, if possible, pituitary function, i.e. to leave the child as normal as possible, physically, ophthalmologically, hormonally, and behaviorally.

Surgery

SURVIVAL AND TUMOR CONTROL

Summarizing the data from the literature:[4]

- A review of survival data corrected for number of patients at the beginning of each of the studies showed 81 per cent five-year and 69 per cent ten-year actuarial survival rates for all age groups following complete tumor excision.

- Similarly corrected five-year and ten-year survival data following incomplete surgical excision alone were 53 and 37 per cent, respectively.
- Corrected data for treatment with incomplete surgical excision plus radiotherapy showed 89 per cent five-year and 77 per cent ten-year actuarial survival rates, respectively.
- Reported incidences of tumor recurrence after apparent total tumor removal vary from zero to 50 per cent, with an overall tumor recurrence rate of 21 per cent. These data are derived from 16 studies that incorporate some of the more recent neurosurgical series. With improved neuroimaging techniques and by defining complete tumor excision by imaging criteria, this recurrence risk may be reduced to 5–11 per cent.
- Subtotal/partial tumor excision will be effective in the relief of immediate symptoms but is inadequate as curative management, as reported recurrence rates vary from 50 to 100 per cent, with an overall tumor recurrence rate of 67 per cent at a follow-up of 1–30 years. In the majority of cases, tumor progression will occur within five years from initial surgery.
- In the Great Ormond Street Hospital series, the five- and ten-year recurrence-free survival rates for patients with complete tumor excision, as defined on postoperative neuroimaging, were 89 and 78 per cent, respectively, compared with 32 and 28 per cent for patients with incomplete tumor excision.

NEUROSURGICAL CONSIDERATIONS

The aims of any operation can be to make the diagnosis (provide tissue for histopathological examination), to relieve symptoms, to provide a cure, and to aid other (not primarily surgical) treatments by reducing tumor load.

Surgery is not usually necessary solely to make the diagnosis of craniopharyngioma, which is usually obvious from the neuroimaging investigations. Relief of chiasmatic compression and raised intracranial pressure due to hydrocephalus may, however, be required urgently. Operative intervention is highly unlikely to reverse any endocrine problems present when the patient is first seen. Curative surgery is certainly possible in selected cases but, as has already been stated, at a not insignificant cost in terms of long-term morbidity due to hypothalamic damage in some children.

In this brief review of surgical management, it is not possible to do more than make some general observations to illustrate the complexity of the decision-making process. For the sake of simplicity, the operations that may need

to be considered can be divided into those aimed at relieving hydrocephalus and those aimed at the tumor itself. The latter can in turn be divided into those aimed at cyst drainage and instillations and those designed to remove tumor bulk (solid tumor and/or cyst wall).

Hydrocephalus

The conventional treatment for hydrocephalus is the insertion of a ventriculoperitoneal shunt (or, in an emergency, an external ventricular drain). However, as the third ventricular obstruction responsible for hydrocephalus in children with craniopharyngioma is often due to the upward expansion of a cystic component of the tumor (see Figure 20.2), it is sometimes possible to both decompress the cyst (and with it the chiasm) and relieve the hydrocephalus by aspirating the contents of the cyst, either stereotactically or endoscopically. This can save the patient the long-term problems associated with dependency upon a cerebrospinal fluid (CSF) shunt system (blockage, overdrainage, etc).

Direct tumor surgery

It is difficult to think of a particular operative approach that might not be required at some time for the most appropriate surgical management of a craniopharyngioma. A subfrontal/pterional approach is probably the most often used, although this author's (RDH) preference is for the bifrontal interhemispheric approach that recognizes the midline origin of the tumor regardless of whatever cranial compartments it may have expanded into.

Other approaches that are sometimes required and that should be mentioned are the trans-sphenoidal approach (particularly useful in the older child with a pneumatized sphenoid sinus and capable of allowing a complete removal of smaller tumors), a variety of skull-base procedures (aimed at optimizing the surgeon's angle of attack to the tumor), the transcallosal approach, and even – rarely – an approach through the posterior fossa.

For the attempted transcranial removal of a large tumor, it can sometimes be helpful to employ more than one approach, either at the same operation or at electively staged procedures. Staged surgical procedures, none of which is intended to achieve complete tumor removal, may also make it possible to buy time either until a child is old enough to be treated with external fractionated radiotherapy or (and this is conjecture), if radiotherapy has already been given, until a radical operation that aims for a complete removal may have a less destructive effect upon the hypothalamus.

Even a solid tumor that extends from the sella to the third ventricle can be dealt with in stages; if the lower part of the tumor is removed first, then subsequent magnetic resonance imaging (MRI) may reveal descent of the upper portion of the tumor into a more accessible position.

Surgery for cyst drainage and/or instillation

In addition to its use in an emergency situation (see above), cyst drainage may be used as the only surgical procedure for a patient in whom the decision has been made to relieve, say, optic chiasm compression and then treat the residual tumor (solid and cystic components) with radiotherapy. However, even in this situation it is advisable to leave a catheter (connected to a subcutaneous reservoir) within the cyst so that further aspirations can be carried out as necessary and also to allow direct instillations (see below under radiotherapy) to be made into the cyst in order to prevent further fluid accumulation. A variety of image-guidance techniques are now available to aid the optimal placement of the catheter within the cyst.[18]

It should be pointed out, however, that these instillation forms of treatment (which may spare both hypothalamic and pituitary function) will result in a cure only if the tumor is entirely cystic, a type that is not only comparatively rare but also is most likely to be cured (with an acceptably low hypothalamic morbidity) by radical surgery. Any solid component (being beyond the range of yttrium, ^{32}P, or bleomycin) will not be treated and will therefore still need to be dealt with by either surgery or external radiotherapy, assuming that radiotherapy has not already been given, if the patient is not to be deemed incurable.

Radiotherapy

OVERVIEW

Historically, it was the often poor outcome, particularly in children, following attempts at total surgical excision that prompted other treatment modalities to be explored. Carpenter and colleagues, in 1937, reported the long-term survival of four patients following the use of radiotherapy with less extensive surgery (tumor cyst aspiration).[19] In 1961, Kramer and colleagues, using more refined irradiation techniques following minimal surgery, reported that nine of their ten patients, including six children, were alive and well at follow-up more than six years after completion of treatment.[20] Thereafter, many reports appeared discussing the efficacy of radiotherapy for craniopharyngioma, including direct evidence that radiotherapy destroyed tumor cells with reports of complete necrosis of residual tumor within the irradiation field at postmortem.

SURVIVAL, TUMOR CONTROL, AND MORBIDITY

Summarizing the data from the literature:[4]

- Comparison of patients undergoing a putative total resection with those receiving radiotherapy after subtotal resection has shown similar outcomes in terms of survival. Older studies suggest marginally worse survival following complete resection compared to conservative surgery and radiotherapy.[21] However, most surgical studies report the outcome in patients where complete excision was achieved. The more appropriate comparative information should include all patients where radical excision was attempted, i.e., analyzing the results by treatment intent.

- Protracted follow-up data of 19 children treated 16–36 years previously (median follow-up 21 years) with combined surgery and external beam irradiation have shown an overall 20-year survival of 62 per cent.[22] When adjusted for disease status at the time of radiotherapy, the 20-year survival for those treated for primary disease was 78 per cent versus 25 per cent for those treated for recurrence.

- The largest series of 173 patients (77 children) treated with limited surgery and radiotherapy at the Royal Marsden Hospital reported ten- and 20-year progression-free survivals of 83 and 79 per cent, respectively, both overall and for children. Furthermore, these patients underwent a spectrum of surgical procedures, ranging from no surgery directed at tumor eradication to attempted radical tumor excision[23].

- The lack of demonstrable difference in progression-free survival according to extent of initial surgery suggested that radiotherapy was effective in controlling the progression of microscopic as well as macroscopic residual disease.

- In the Great Ormond Street Hospital series, actuarial ten-year recurrence-free survival after radiotherapy, including treatment given for recurrent disease, was 72 per cent at a median follow-up of 7.6 years (Figure 20.6). Nine patients developed tumor recurrences despite undergoing

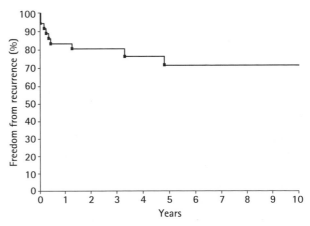

Figure 20.6 *Actuarial recurrence-free survival curve for 36 patients after conventional (external fractionated) radiotherapy, including treatment given for recurrent disease.*

radiation therapy; however, the "recurrences" (defined as evidence of tumor growth on neuroimaging with or without clinical symptoms) appeared either during treatment or within six months of irradiation in six cases, after which the tumor "stabilized" in five cases. This phenomenon has been reported by Brada and colleagues[24] as being due to tumor cyst enlargement, not representative of true tumor progression but an acute complication of radiotherapy, although the exact mechanism is unclear.

- Potential sequelae to radiation include optic neuropathy, hypothalamo-pituitary endocrine failure and radiation necrosis of surrounding brain causing neurological deficit. Hypothalamic damage from standard external beam irradiation alone has not been reported in the context of craniopharyngiomas. Following external beam radiotherapy with modern localized techniques to doses <50 Gy at <2 Gy per fraction, the incidence of radiation optic neuropathy is 1–2 per cent and the risk of necrosis less than 1 per cent. The incidence of radiation-induced hypothalamic-pituitary axis deficiency is poorly documented as the majority of children are hypopituitary prior to irradiation.[25] The estimate of new deficiency developing following irradiation is 20–30 per cent risk at ten years. High dose radiation to large volumes of normal brain in children less than four years of age is associated with cognitive impairment. The magnitude of long-term cognitive deficit following small volume irradiation to the sellar and suprasellar region has not been documented, and the additional impact of radiation to the effects of the tumor and surgery is not known.[26]

- Long-term sequelae of irradiation of benign sellar and parasellar tumors include the development of second brain tumors. By analogy with pituitary adenoma data the actuarial risk of second brain tumor is 2 per cent at 20 years; these consist of malignant gliomas and meningiomas.[27] Meningiomas may occur decades after radiotherapy. Potential impact of radiation on the risk of late cerebrovascular accident is not fully defined.[28,29]

- An overview by Brada and Thomas (1993) suggested that of 100 hypothetical patients treated with more conservative surgery and radiotherapy, 1–2 patients might die in the perioperative period; 17 cases would have subsequent tumor recurrence requiring salvage therapy (with present radiotherapy techniques and optimal dose regimens, recurrence risk may be reduced to 16 per cent). Overall, up to 7 per cent of patients might suffer long-term morbidity of surgery and radiotherapy, inclusive of second brain tumor, which would develop in one patient in 10 years.

- Fractionated irradiation can be given with higher precision using modern image guidance and stereotactic localization with improved fixation using relocatable devices and conformal treatment delivery. The resultant technique of fractionated stereotactic conformal radiotherapy (SCRT) leads to smaller volumes of normal brain receiving significant radiation doses. It is hoped that SCRT will further reduce the incidence of late sequelae, but proof is currently not available.

OTHER TREATMENT MODALITIES

Stereotactic techniques in the management of craniopharyngioma have been utilized increasingly in an attempt to achieve the dual goals of tumor control and enhanced quality of survival. These have included stereotactic radiosurgery for small solid tumors, stereotactic conformal radiotherapy, and intracavitary administration of radiocolloid or bleomycin through stereotactic positioning of an intracystic catheter.

Intracavitary irradiation

Intracavitary irradiation using either ^{90}Yttrium or ^{32}Phosphate has been advocated as a definitive procedure for solitary cystic craniopharyngiomas, initially by Backlund at the Karolinska Hospital in Stockholm. The ^{32}P colloidal suspension coats the inside of the cyst wall and the short-range of β-irradiation from ^{90}Yttrium and Phosphate suggest only localized irradiation. From a surgical point of view, this does not induce adhesions or scarring in the vicinity of the cyst and therefore, does not preclude later attempts at microsurgical dissection, should this become necessary.

The Pittsburgh group reported cyst regression in 28 of 32 patients (88 per cent) following intracystic chromic phosphate (^{32}P). However, 10 patients subsequently showed tumor progression and three died. While improvement in vision was reported in 19 of 30 patients (63 per cent), 11 (37 per cent) had deterioration.[30] Similar results were reported in 31 patients treated with Yttrium where over half had deterioration in vision.[31] In a UK report of 6 patients treated with Yttrium two patients died following therapy.[32]

Voges et al. reported 62 patients treated with intracystic colloidal chromic phosphate.[33] Three patients (5 per cent) had complete loss of vision and the survival rates were poor with 55 per cent 5 year and 45 per cent 10 year survival. While cyst response rate was reported as 80 per cent this was clearly an inappropriate surrogate endpoint of tumor control. On present evidence, intracystic instillation of radioisotope is not the appropriate primary therapy and should be reserved for patients with persistent symptomatic lesions following surgery and radiotherapy which keep re-accumulating despite repeat aspiration.

Stereotactic radiosurgery

Stereotactic radiosurgery is a highly accurate and precise technique which utilizes stereotactically directed convergent beams of ionizing radiation to treat small spherical volumes of tissue with a single dose. This technique is only applicable for small lesions (preferably less than 2 cm in greatest diameter) 0.5 cm or more away from the optic chiasm and other critical structures (brainstem, retina, motor cortex, cranial nerves), as ablation of normal and abnormal tissue will occur within the treatment volume with potentially devastating consequences. The tolerance of the optic nerve appears to be between 8 and 10 Gy in previously untreated patients and lower in those patients who have undergone prior fractionated external beam radiotherapy. Therefore, although precise in the administration of large single fractions, complications associated with larger volumes and certain locations limit the use of radiosurgery in the primary management of patients with craniopharyngioma.

Stereotactic radiotherapy

Stereotactic radiotherapy (SCRT as above) combines stereotactic localization and precise stereotactic head frame and support system for accurate relocation and conformal 3D planning and treatment delivery with fractionation, thereby providing focal and precise dose delivery to larger lesions with significantly reduced dose to adjacent non-target volume structures.

OUTCOME

Overview

The question of quality of survival following aggressive surgical treatment is very difficult to ascertain from the literature, particularly in relation to hypothalamic, neuropsychological, and psychosocial functioning. The occurrence of surgical morbidity is correlated strongly with extent of surgery. An overview of published surgical reports from 1966 to 1992 has indicated an average 12 per cent (range 2–43 per cent) risk of operative mortality and 30 per cent (range 12–61 per cent) incidence of severe morbidity. This includes 40 per cent (range 30–57 per cent) incidence of disabling hypothalamic damage and 19 per cent (range 10–35 per cent) risk of postoperative visual impairment. The largest single-center experience of 144 patients (70 children) using microsurgical techniques reported 17 per cent overall operative mortality, related to initial tumor size and whether primary or secondary microsurgery was being performed, 16 per cent significant morbidity, and 67 per cent "good" results.[2] However, 62 per cent of patients (62 per cent of children) had impairment of visual acuity at follow-up and 79 per cent (88 per cent of children) required permanent

hormone substitution therapy, with a further comment that intractable obesity (see below) continued to afflict some of the patients despite appropriate endocrine replacement therapy. Additionally, surgical mortality (at operation) included hypothalamic hemorrhage. Ten early and 11 late postoperative deaths included endocrinological causes, again suggesting significant hypothalamic injury.

Endocrine and hypothalamic morbidity

The majority of patients with craniopharyngiomas have multiple endocrine deficits regardless of the type of treatment employed, and reversal of previously abnormal endocrine function has not been observed with any treatment modality, with the rare exception of selected patients with cystic craniopharyngiomas treated with intracavitary radioisotope therapy alone. Much more contentious an issue is the irreversible hypothalamic morbidity that is associated closely with aggressive attempts at surgical excision of craniopharyngioma, as described earlier in this chapter.

ANTERIOR PITUITARY FUNCTION

Hypothalamo-pituitary dysfunction has been shown to be frequent at presentation and before any treatment. Following aggressive surgical resection of craniopharyngiomas, combined anterior and posterior pituitary dysfunction are almost universal, and as many as three-quarters of patients will have developed deficiencies of four or more hormones postoperatively. Apart from the rare finding of precocious puberty after craniopharyngioma surgery, the occurrence of spontaneous onset and progression through normal puberty is extremely uncommon in patients presenting prepubertally; therefore, appropriate and timely institution of growth hormone and exogenous sex steroids is particularly important in order to mimic normal pubertal development and to optimize final height prognosis.

Hypoadrenal crises in association with intercurrent illness are potential contributors to morbidity and mortality following craniopharyngioma surgery. The importance of repeated instruction to increase steroid replacement doses at times of illness, and warning adolescents about the potent hypoglycemic effects of alcohol, should be emphasized.

Posterior pituitary function

The incidence of permanent diabetes insipidus has shown a consistently closer correlation with extent of surgical resection; Sanford and colleagues reported a six per cent incidence of diabetes insipidus following limited surgery (<25 per cent tumor resection) and irradiation as compared with an incidence of 70–93 per cent in series pursuing a more radical surgical policy[34].

The combination of anterior (cortisol) and posterior (diabetes insipidus) pituitary deficiencies is potentially dangerous in both the acute situation and the longer term. Insufficient hydrocortisone cover in an emergency may aggravate dilutional hyponatremia caused by continuing desmopressin and an inability to excrete water.

The metabolic consequences of concomitant ADH insufficiency and absent thirst associated with severe, irreversible hypothalamic injury as a complication exclusive to radical surgery contribute significantly to the disabling hypothalamic damage found in up to 57 per cent of cases in various reported series and thus to overall morbidity and mortality. Despite appropriate management of patients with a fixed daily fluid intake and small, regular (two or three times daily) doses of desmopressin, maintenance of fluid and osmotic balance often remains precarious, as reflected by protracted hospital stays after surgery and high subsequent mortality.

HYPOTHALAMIC OBESITY

Excessive weight gain is one of the most distressing manifestations of hypothalamic injury and has been reported in up to 60 per cent of children following radical surgery for craniopharyngioma. In a minority of cases, extreme hyperphagia and obesity characterized by a total preoccupation with food and uncontrollable food-seeking behavior dominate the clinical course. Attempts at therapeutic intervention or behavior modification are usually unsuccessful, and the long-term outcome for control of weight is poor. Both hypothalamic infiltration by tumor and attempted surgical resection of craniopharyngioma from the basal diencephalon result in varying degrees of damage, which can be quantified using MRI. Severe postoperative obesity, as measured by BMI, occurs predominantly in patients who have significant, bilateral disruption of the normal hypothalamic anatomy, with either complete deficiency or extensive destruction of the floor of the third ventricle (Figure 20.7). Therefore, determination of the extent of hypothalamic injury on imaging may prove a useful discriminator of those children at greatest risk of problems with postoperative obesity. At a biochemical level, a rapid increase in serum leptin levels with respect to BMI has been observed in some patients following craniopharyngioma surgery, suggesting disruption of the feedback mechanism from hypothalamic leptin receptors to adipose tissue and a failure in the downregulation of appetite. Therefore, early postoperative serum leptin levels may additionally help to identify patients at risk of excessive weight gain following hypothalamic injury.

Visual outcome

Visual impairment remains one of the most significant sequelae preventing normal social reintegration of many

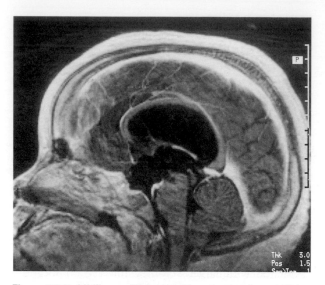

Figure 20.7 *Midline sagittal magnetic resonance image of the brain following radical surgical excision of craniopharyngioma (preoperative image shown in Figure 20.2), showing extensive destruction of the hypothalamo-pituitary region, which has been replaced by an expansive cerebrospinal fluid-filled void.*

children after craniopharyngioma surgery. In the series of 75 children followed up at Great Ormond Street Hospital for Children, 15 per cent of all patients were blind, 69 per cent had reduced visual acuity, and 68 per cent had visual field deficits (liable to considerable fluctuation over time) at a mean of seven years from initial surgery. Those patients with normal vision preoperatively rarely showed a deterioration in acuity at follow-up; 73 per cent of patients retained a visual acuity after treatment within two lines of their Snellen acuity (or equivalent) at presentation. Despite apparent damage to the anterior visual pathways in 81 per cent of cases on MRI, visual acuity was preserved (6/6 bilaterally) in 31 per cent of patients at follow-up. However, only 19 per cent of patients had both normal visual acuity and visual fields at follow-up assessment.

Our data showed that permanent damage to optic pathways by tumor was greater than that inflicted by treatment, although there was a propensity to cause further injury at surgery when the nerves and chiasm were already compromised. In a proportion of these cases, further visual compromise was accounted for by tumor recurrence. Comparison of results in other series becomes very difficult, as there are few definitions of what constitutes a progressive visual deficit and even fewer studies reporting on the visual sequelae after tumor recurrence.

In summary, visual status at presentation predominantly influences long-term visual outcome. Early detection of visual loss and prompt referral are therefore of paramount importance for prognosis. Despite almost all craniopharyngiomas impinging upon anterior visual pathways by the time of presentation, and the majority of patients showing evidence of structural injury to the optic nerves and chiasm on neuroimaging at follow-up, visual acuity may be well preserved, although most patients will have some degree of permanent visual dysfunction.

Neurological outcome

In terms of neurological sequelae, very few studies have detailed clinical and neuroimaging findings following treatment for childhood craniopharyngioma. In the Great Ormond Street Hospital series, almost 60 per cent of all patients (excluding patients with possible compressive injury by residual tumor or assessment of hypothalamic damage) had evidence of cerebral damage distant from the hypothalamo-pituitary region on cranial imaging at follow-up; in 23 per cent of cases, this was bilateral.[4] Right frontal lobe damage was present in 41 per cent of cases (Figure 20.8a); in 11 patients, damage to both frontal lobes had occurred as a consequence of surgery with or without radiotherapy. Radical tumor surgery by subfrontal exposure has been shown previously to be associated with significant frontal lobe dysfunction at follow-up.[35] However, the anatomical basis for this was not considered to be due entirely to operative trauma to the frontal lobe but also to concomitant hypothalamic injury. Our findings, therefore, suggest that direct cerebral hemisphere damage may be more significant than hypothesized previously.

Clinical examination of our patients confirmed abnormalities of motor function in 61 per cent of surviving patients (pyramidal signs predominating) and severe bilateral limb motor deficits occurred in 15 per cent. Seizures occurred in over half the patients at some time during the course of illness and remained an ongoing problem in a quarter at follow-up. Nine per cent of patients had seizures secondary to hypoglycemia in association with intercurrent infection, and nine per cent of patients had late-onset epilepsy (onset more than five years from surgery) of frontal lobe origin.

Neurological deficit before surgery contributed to postoperative morbidity in many of our patients, as did vessel injury incurred during attempts at tumor removal (Figure 20.8b). Dense adhesion of the tumor wall to adjacent neural and vascular structures is a major determinant of intraoperative complications,[21] and even the most fervent advocates of radical surgery agree that dissection should be curtailed if tumor is attached firmly to the internal carotid or posterior communicating arteries. Duff and colleagues have reaffirmed that tumor adhesiveness to surrounding neurovascular structures, as defined by observation of the operating surgeon, was a risk factor both for poor outcome and for tumor recurrence.[16]

In summary, both neurological impairment at diagnosis and the occurrence of intraoperative complications increase the likelihood of neurological sequelae in the postoperative period. Morbidity may also be increased by

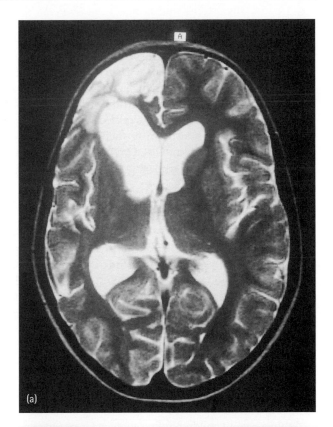

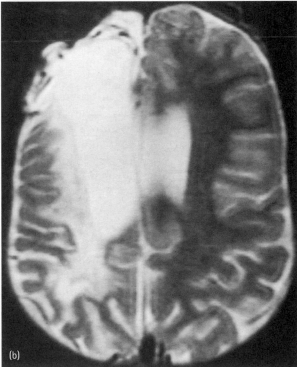

Figure 20.8a,b *Axial (T2-weighted) magnetic resonance images, showing (a) right frontal lobe damage with secondary dilatation of the anterior horn of the right lateral ventricle following surgical resection of a craniopharyngioma and (b) more extensive right hemispheric infarction in a central carotid distribution following intraoperative arterial hemorrhage.*

tumor recurrence, further surgery, adrenal crises with secondary hypoglycemia, and irradiation. Seizures are uncommon at presentation but are a frequent occurrence at some time during treatment and may persist in up to a quarter of patients at follow-up. Late-onset epilepsy, usually secondary to frontal lobe damage, may contribute further to long-term morbidity. Although transcranial operation usually involves a unilateral approach on the side of the non-dominant hemisphere, a significant proportion of children have bilateral neurological damage at long-term follow-up.

Neuropsychological outcome

Previous studies have recognized the increased risk of cognitive deficits and psychosocial dysfunction among survivors of childhood craniopharyngioma,[36–38] but few have addressed systematically the neuropsychological sequelae of this tumor and its treatment. The potential causes for neuropsychological morbidity are multifactorial; they include frontal lobe dysfunction, hypothalamic injury, multiple pituitary hormone deficiencies, epilepsy, and cranial irradiation, as well as the inevitable changes that occur in parental and peer relationships when a child is identified as having a serious, perhaps life-threatening disease.

In the series of children followed up at Great Ormond Street Hospital, assessment of intelligence and memory (excluding 18 per cent of survivors unable to attempt or complete psychometric testing because of the degree of intellectual and/or behavioral dysfunction) demonstrated a significant reduction of verbal, performance, and full-scale IQ, as well as global impairment of immediate and delayed verbal and non-verbal memory relative to the normal population. Subtest scores identified particular problems with attention, concentration, perceptual organization, and new verbal learning ability.[39] Patients with severe hypothalamic damage on brain MRI had significantly lower mean index scores for freedom from distractibility and perceptual organization than patients with no visible hypothalamic damage on neuroimaging.[39] As this group comprised those shown to have morbid obesity and usually associated hyperphagia, one could speculate that intrusive feelings of hunger and thoughts of food could be playing a significant part in their distractibility.

Risk factors for poor cognitive outcome included complications at the time of operation (inclusive of arterial or venous hemorrhage, arterial spasm, vessel damage, frontal lobe bruising, intraoperative cardiorespiratory problems) and multiple surgical procedures (inclusive of ventricular drainage procedures for hydrocephalus and operations for tumor recurrence). Figure 20.9 illustrates the number of surgical procedures some children had, both on the tumor itself and when including shunt-related operations. Treatment with radiotherapy (median follow-up 7.6 years), when added to the statistical model, did not

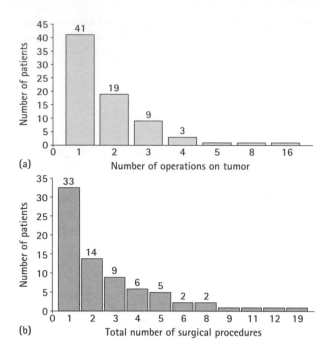

Figure 20.9a,b *Total number of surgical procedures performed on (a) tumor alone and (b) inclusive of ventricular drainage procedures in 75 children treated for craniopharyngioma at Great Ormond Street Hospital for Children, London, from 1973 to 1994.*

significantly influence cognitive outcome.[4] However, those children receiving irradiation following tumor recurrence, the majority of whom also had further surgery, had significantly lower mean performance and full-scale IQs at follow-up; although the mean verbal IQ was also lower, this did not achieve statistical significance.

Overall, educational difficulties occurred in 75 per cent of patients, a significant proportion of which had gone unrecognized until formal psychometric testing. Almost a third of children required special schooling for cognitive/behavioral impairment after treatment for their craniopharyngioma. Of those within mainstream education, almost half had significant schooling problems, including a combination of concentration and attention-span deficits, short-term memory problems, learning difficulties sufficient to warrant statementing, behavioral difficulties, and problems with being bullied over size, weight, and school attendance.

In summary, our data confirm the often profound adverse effects of this tumor and its subsequent management on psychosocial and intellectual functioning. Both complications at the time of surgery and the total number of operative procedures performed have the greatest influence on cognitive outcome, and these factors prevail over the known potential effects of cranial irradiation. It is therefore paramount for physician and surgeon to ensure optimal hormone replacement therapy, regular neuropsychological assessment, and close liaison between community pediatricians, parents, teachers, and educational psychologists so that the spectrum of possible cognitive, behavioral, and psychological deficits are identified early and acted upon promptly.

FOLLOW-UP

The follow-up care required for these children mirrors the investigations recommended before treatment was started: neuroimaging (aimed at the early detection of further or recurrent tumor growth), and endocrinological, ophthalmological, neurological, and psychological assessment. Although each aspect of morbidity has been considered separately, it is clear that many children may be multiply impaired, and the spectrum of possible visual, endocrine, neurological, cognitive, and behavioral pathology associated with the tumor and its management necessitates close liaison with a multidisciplinary, multiagency team.

Neuroimaging

The combination of a tumor that occurs infrequently and neuroimaging that is continuing to increase in sophistication means that it is still impossible to say with confidence exactly how long a child whose craniopharyngioma has received treatment intended to be curative (whether surgery, radiotherapy, or chemotherapy) should be followed up for. Our own policy is to continue with MRI six-monthly at first, and perhaps later at longer intervals until five years have elapsed since the last "definitive" treatment. These intervals may, of course, need to be modified to take into account the need to monitor the effects of particular treatments.

MANAGEMENT OF THE RECURRENT TUMOR

Recurrent tumors may present with the advent of new clinical symptoms and signs, or they may be detected before this stage if the patient has received appropriate surveillance imaging. Those presenting clinically are, by definition, larger than those presenting radiologically. Hopefully, the concentration of childhood craniopharyngiomas in centers where all the specialized care (including post-treatment imaging) required is available will mean that symptomatic recurrences will become a thing of the past and evidence of further tumor growth will be detected while it is small enough to be treated, with both a reduced risk of producing further ophthalmological and neurological damage and the possibility of effecting a cure.

For example, an intrasellar recurrence in a child who has previously undergone an apparently complete surgical excision may be suitable for radiosurgery, while a recurrent tumor after partial excision and radiotherapy

may have moved into a position that now makes it amenable to further surgery, preferably using a different operative approach. Patients receiving radiotherapy following surgical failure have tumor control and survival results in the same range as patients receiving radiotherapy after primary surgery.[40,41] This should not, however, be taken as justification to delay radiotherapy as survival in patients treated by incomplete excision not offered radiotherapy is significantly worse and policy of delayed radiotherapy frequently exposes the child to the morbidity of a second or subsequent surgical procedure.[21]

In this context, it should be pointed out that the continuing expansion of a cystic component for up to nine months following external fractionated radiotherapy is well described, does not necessarily mean that treatment has failed, and requires treatment (e.g. cyst aspiration) only if it becomes symptomatic.

There remain, however, some tumors (usually large when first diagnosed) whose hypothalamic component grows again some years after radiotherapy. If there is a prominent cyst, then it can be treated with some form of instillation therapy, but this will not touch any solid portion of the tumor. Direct surgery on the hypothalamus can be predicted to produce all the problems that a policy of selective treatments has, until now, been successful in avoiding and should be undertaken only after a frank discussion with the patient's family and the patient if they are sufficiently competent to be included. For these patients, unfortunately, the outlook remains gloomy, although there is anecdotal evidence from the fact that adult craniopharyngioma patients do not have the same incidence of devastating hypothalamic problems following attempted radical removals of large tumors that the adult hypothalamus may be more resilient than its childhood counterpart.

CONCLUSIONS

Despite considerable refinement in the management of craniopharyngioma, a significant proportion of children suffer the sequelae of disease and treatment. Management remains complex and controversial and should be undertaken in a multidisciplinary setting with highly experienced neurosurgeons and precision-localized radiotherapy given in a fractionated manner according to safe practice and aiming to provide long-term tumor control with the lowest morbidity.

Despite the reluctance on the part of some neurosurgeons to acknowledge the role of radiotherapy in the management of these tumors, it has been shown that modern fractionated external beam radiotherapy is effective both as adjuvant therapy after subtotal tumor excision and as a treatment modality for tumor recurrence. Risk factors for cognitive outcome further support the findings that radiotherapy should be considered early following subtotal tumor excision, rather than waiting for tumor recurrence, when additional surgical intervention is also likely to be required. However, the risks of multiple surgical procedures on cognitive outcome need to be balanced against the risks of irradiation to the young brain in children less than five years of age. Newer techniques of dose optimization, namely stereotactic radiotherapy, may help to further refine the management of these difficult tumors in the foreseeable future.

From what has been described, it can be seen that successful treatment in terms of preserving quality of life without sacrificing the best opportunity for tumor cure is dependent on recognizing the implications of many variables. For this reason we have formulated an algorithm (Figure 20.10) that has proved helpful. This should not be taken as definitive therapeutic advice for what is one of the most difficult tumors in pediatric neurosurgery to treat satisfactorily. Rather, it is an example of how knowledge of the factors that determine the outcome both with regard to

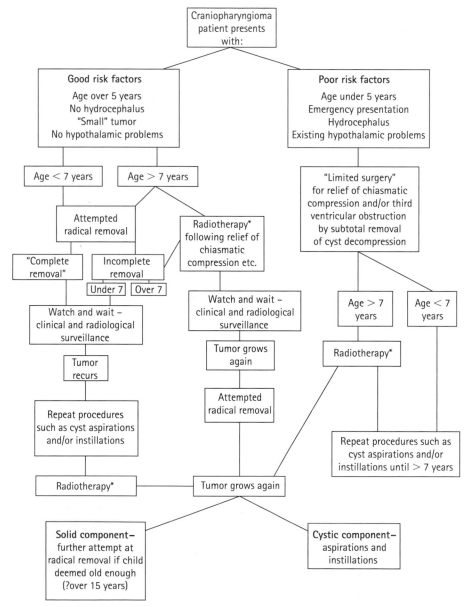

Figure 20.10 *Suggested algorithm for the management of childhood craniopharyngioma that takes into account the presence or absence of certain risk factors at the time of presentation and the child's age when radiotherapy is being considered. An age limit of seven years has been illustrated here, but in general the policy should be to postpone radiotherapy for the child's brain for as long as is practically possible. (*Radiotherapy in this context usually refers to external fractionated treatment (preferably conformal, stereotactically focused), but some tumors may be suitable for "radiosurgery" if sufficiently delineated from the optic apparatus, hypothalamus, and brainstem.)*

tumor recurrence and the functional condition of the child can be used to place treatment on a more rational basis.

The rarity of childhood craniopharyngiomas makes it difficult not only for a single neurosurgical unit to accumulate experience but also for the pediatric endocrinologists, ophthalmologists, and radiation (and medical) oncologists whose input is essential for their care to do the same, and then for all these specialties to share their experience in a useful way. This is not a problem that can be overcome merely by pooling data from multiple centers. The differences between patients and their tumors as well as in the various treatments deployed are too great to allow for any meaningful conclusions to be drawn. Only the concentration of cases into a small number of pediatric centers in which the complete team of experts can be deployed offers any opportunity for improving their outlook.

REFERENCES

1 Matson DD. *Neurosurgery of Infancy and Childhood.* Springfield, IL: Thomas, 1969.

2 Yasargil MG, Curcic M, Kis M, *et al.* Total removal of craniopharyngiomas: approaches and long-term results in 144 patients. *J Neurosurg* 1990; **73**:3–11.

3 Rajan B, Ashley S, Gorman C, *et al.* Craniopharyngioma – long-term results following limited surgery and radiotherapy. *Radiother Oncol* 1993; **26**:1–10.

4 DeVile CJ. A follow-up study of the outcome of children's post-craniopharyngioma surgery. MD thesis. London: University of London, 1998.

5 DeVile CJ, Grant DB, Hayward RD, *et al.* Obesity in childhood craniopharyngioma: relation to postoperative hypothalamic damage shown by magnetic resonance imaging. *J Clin Endocrinol Metab* 1996; **81**:2734–7.

6 DeVile CJ, Grant DB, Kendall BE, Hayward RD. The management of childhood craniopharyngioma: can the morbidity of radical surgery be predicted? *J Neurosurg* 1996; **85**:73–81.

7 DeVile CJ, Grant DB, Hayward RD, *et al.* Growth and endocrine sequelae of craniopharyngioma. *Arch Dis Child* 1996; **75**:108–14.

8 Sanford RA, Muhlbauer MS. Craniopharyngioma in children. *Neurol Clin* 1991; **9**:453–65.

9 Bunin G, Surawicz T, Witman P, *et al.* The descriptive epidemiology of craniopharyngioma. Presented at the 8th International Symposium on Pediatric Neuro-oncology, Rome, 1998.

10 Tachibana O, Yamashima T, Yamashita J, *et al.* Immunohistochemical expression of human chorionic gonadotrophin and P glycoprotein in human pituitary glands and craniopharyngiomas. *J Neurosurg* 1994; **80**:79–84.

11 Adamson TE, Wiestler OD, Kleihues P, *et al.* Correlation of clinical and pathological features in surgically treated craniopharyngiomas. *J Neurosurg* 1990; **73**:12–17.

12 Weiner HL, Wisoff JH, Rosenberg ME, *et al.* Craniopharyngiomas: a clinicopathological analysis of factors predictive of recurrence and functional outcome. *Neurosurgery* 1994; **35**:1001–11.

13 Choux M, Lena G, Genitori I. Craniopharyngioma in children. *Neurochirurgie* 1991; **37**:4–11;166–74.

14 Hoffman HJ, De Silva M, Humphreys RP, *et al.* Aggressive surgical management of craniopharyngiomas in children. *J Neurosurg* 1992; **76**:47–52.

15 Cabezudo Artero JM, Vaquero Crespo J, Zabalgoitia GB. Status of vision following surgical treatment of craniopharyngiomas. *Acta Neurochir* 1984; **73**:165–77.

16 Duff JM, Meyer FB, Ilstrup DM, *et al.* Long-term outcomes for surgically resected craniopharyngiomas. *Neurosurgery* 2000; **46**:291–302, 302–5.

17 Palm L, Nordin V, Elmqvist D, *et al.* Sleep and wakefulness after treatment for craniopharyngioma; influence on the quality and maturation of sleep. *Neuropaediatrics* 1992; **23**:39–45.

18 Vitaz TW, Hushek S, Shields C, *et al.* Changes in cyst volume following intraoperative MRI-guided Ommaya reservoir placement for cystic craniopharyngioma. *Pediatr Neurosurg* 2001; **35**:230–4.

19 Carpenter RC, Chamberlin GW, Frazier CH. The treatment of hypophyseal stalk tumors by evacuation and irradiation. *Am J Roentgenol* 1937; **38**:162–77.

20 Kramer S, McKissock W, Concannon JP. Craniopharyngiomas: treatment by combined surgery and radiation therapy. *J Neurosurg* 1961; **18**:217–26.

21 Brada M, Thomas DG. Craniopharyngioma revisited. *Int J Radiat Oncol Biol Phys* 1993; **27**:471–5.

22 Regine WF, Kramer S. Pediatric craniopharyngiomas: long term results of combined treatment with surgery and radiation. *Int J Radiat Oncol Biol Phys* 1992; **24**:611–17.

23 Rajan B, Ashley S, Gorman C, *et al.* Craniopharyngioma – long-term results following limited surgery and radiotherapy. *Radiotherapy and Oncology* 1993; **26**:1–10.

24 Rajan B, Ashley S, Thomas D, *et al.* Craniopharyngioma: improving outcome by early recognition and treatment of acute complications. *Int J Radiat Onc Biol Phys* 1997; **37**:517–21.

25 Honegger J, Buchfelder M, Fahlbusch R. Surgical treatment of craniopharyngiomas: endocrinological results. *J Neurosurg* 1999; **90**:251–7.

26 Carpentieri SC, Waber DP, Scott RM, *et al.* Memory deficits among children with craniopharyngiomas. *Neurosurgery* 2001; **49**:1053–7; discussion 1057–8.

27 Brada M, Ford D, Ashley S, Bliss JM, Crowley S, Mason M, Rajan B, Traish D. Risk of second brain tumour after conservative surgery and radiotherapy for pituitary adenoma. *Br Med J* 1992; **304**:1343–6.

28 Brada M, Burchell L, Ashley S, Traish D. The incidence of cerebrovascular accidents in patients with pituitary adenoma. *Int J Radiat Oncol Biol Phys* 1999; **45**:693–8.

29 Brada M, Dorward N, Thomas DGT. *Tumours of the Central Nervous System; tumours of the brain and spinal cord in adults.* 2001;

30 Pollock BE, Lunsford LD, Kondziolka D, Levine G, Flickinger JC. Phosphorus 32 intracavitary irradiation of cystic craniopharyngiomas: current technique and long term results. *Int J Radiat Oncol Biol Phys* 1995; **33**:437–46.

31 Van den Berge JH, Blaauw G, Breeman WA, Rahmy A, Wijngaarde R. Intracavitary brachytherapy of cystic craniopharyngiomas [see comments]. *J Neurosurg* 1992; **77**:545–50.

32 Blackburn TP, Doughty D, Plowman PN. Stereotactic intracavitary therapy of recurrent cystic craniopharyngioma by instillation of 90yttrium. *Br J Neurosurg* 1999; **13**:359–65.

33 Voges J, Sturm V, Lehrke R, Treuer H, Gauss C, Berthold F. Cystic craniopharyngioma: long-term results after intracavitary irradiation with stereotactically applied colloidal beta-emitting radioactive sources. Neurosurgery 1997; **40**:263–9.

34 Sanford RA. Craniopharyngioma: results of survey of the American Society of Pediatric Neurosurgery. *Ped Neurosurg* 1994; **21**(s):39–43.

35 Cavazzuti V, Fischer EG, Welch K, Belli JA, Winston K R. Neurological and psychophysiological sequelae following different treatments of craniopharyngioma in children. *J Neurosurg* 1983; **59**:409–17.

36 Clopper RR, Meyer WJ, III, Udvarhelyi GB, *et al.* Postsurgical IQ and behavioral data on twenty patients with a history of childhood craniopharyngioma. *Psychoneuroendocrinology* 1977; **2**:365–72.

37 Fischer EG, Welch K, Shillito J, *et al.* Craniopharyngiomas in children – long-term effects of conservative surgical procedures combined with radiation therapy. *J Neurosurg* 1990; **73**:534–40.

38 Galatzer A, Nofar E, Beit-Halachmi N, *et al.* Intellectual and psychosocial functions of children, adolescents and young adults before and after operation for craniopharyngioma. *Child Care Health Dev* 1981; **7**:307–16.

39 Wechsler D. *Manual for the Wechsler Intelligence Scale for Children*, 3rd edition. Sidcup, UK: Psychological Corporation, 1992.

40 Jose CC, Rajan B, Ashley S, Marsh H, Brada M. Radiotherapy for the treatment of recurrent craniopharyngioma. *Clin Oncol R Coll Radiol* 1992; **4**:287–9.

41 Kalapurakal JA. Goldman S, Hsieh YC, Tomita T, Marymont MH. Clinical outcome in children with recurrent craniopharyngioma after primary surgery. *Cancer J* 2000; **6**:388–93.

21

Intradural spinal tumors

HAROLD L. REKATE AND TRIMURTI D. NADKARNI, with contributions from ASTRID K. GNEKOW, ROGER J. PACKER AND ROLF D. KORTMANN

GENERAL CONSIDERATIONS

Spectrum of disease

See Table 21.1.[1]

Tumors of the spinal cord, exiting nerve roots, and enveloping meninges are very rare in childhood. Because of the high likelihood that these tumors are benign in nature and that their treatment should result in long survival times with the possibility of significant neurological morbidity, finding the optimal management is very important. The primary tumor pathologies that exist within the spinal cord proper include astrocytomas and ependymomas, but other types of tumors, including gangliogliomas, lipomas, and metastatic tumors, may also be found in this location. Complicated congenital defects related to occult spinal dysraphism may lead to teratomas and dermoids within the spinal cord.

Tumors that arise outside the spinal cord but within the dural sac are extremely rare in children, except in the context of neurofibromatosis. These tumors include meningiomas and nerve sheath tumors (NSTs). The latter may be either neurofibromas or schwannomas, which are also called neurilemmomas. Neurosurgeons do not expect to see these tumors as isolated findings before the fifth decade of life. However, in the context of both neurofibromatosis type 1 (NF-1) and neurofibromatosis type 2 (NF-2), it is common to see these intradural extramedullary tumors early in the second decade of life, and they have been reported in even younger children. In the context of NF-2, these tumors are usually multiple, making the management of each individual tumor more difficult. As many as five per cent of intramedullary spinal cord gliomas may occur in children with NF-1.[2]

Table 21.1 *Tumor types and location in 635 pediatric spinal tumors*

Location	Tumor type	*n*	Total (%)
Intramedullary			189 (29.7)
	Astrocytoma	114	
	Ependymoma	50	
	Lipoma	25	
Intradural extramedullary			156 (24.6)
	Dermoid	39	
	Neurofibroma	28	
	Schwannoma	20	
	Meningioma	17	
	Epidermoid	14	
	PNET	30	
	Hemangioepithelioma	8	
Extradural			219 (34.5)
	Sarcoma	67	
	Neuroblastoma	64	
	Teratoma	35	
	Metastasis	29	
	Ganglioneuroma	19	
	Lymphoma	5	
Others			71 (11.2)

From Yamamoto Y, Raffel C.[1] Intraspinal extramedullary neoplasms. In: Albright A, Pollack I, Adelson P (eds) *Operative Techniques in Pediatric Neurosurgery*. New York: Thieme, 2001, pp. 189–92. Reprinted by permission.

Incidence and location

Spinal cord tumors comprise two to five per cent of primary central nervous system (CNS) tumors in childhood.[2,3] The ratio of intracranial to intraspinal tumors has been reported to be between 20 and five to one. It is likely that the proportion of intramedullary spinal cord tumors to intrinsic brain tumors follows the ratio of the volume of tissue in the two compartments. Low-grade astrocytic tumors occur sporadically throughout childhood, with a median age around six to ten years. Sex distribution is even.[2,4,5]

In adults, 20 per cent of spinal tumors are intramedullary; these tumors account for at least 35 per cent of intraspinal tumors in children. The most common location for intramedullary spinal cord tumors in general is the cervicomedullary junction, followed by the thoracic spinal cord. Low-grade astrocytomas are distributed evenly along the spinal cord,[2] although in some series there appears to be a predilection for the cervical and thoracic segments.[4,6–8] Up to five or even ten per cent of cases in some series of intramedullary spinal cord tumors in children have extended from the upper cervical spinal cord to the conus medullaris and are regarded as holocord tumors.[4,9]

Apart from holocord tumors, it is sometimes stated that low-grade gliomas of the spinal cord rarely involve the conus medullaris or cauda equina. Sacral intradural metastases from primary low-grade astrocytoma of the chiasmatic-hypothalamic region have been reported.[10]

In children benign astrocytomas (grades I and II) account for the majority of intramedullary spinal cord tumors, but in adults ependymomas predominate. Except in the context of neurofibromatosis, intradural extramedullary tumors are very rare in children. Meningiomas account for only five per cent of spinal tumors in children. Neurofibromas (seen only in the context of neurofibromatosis) and schwannomas are usually linked together as NSTs because they tend to behave similarly and are indistinguishable on imaging.

The commonest extradural spinal tumor in childhood is paraspinal neuroblastoma (NBL) extending in an hourglass fashion into the spinal canal. As a cause of neoplastic spinal compression in childhood, NBL is second only to astrocytoma in frequency. Other extradural spinal tumors include various sarcomas, "blue-cell tumors," and lymphoma.

Clinical presentation

See Chapter 6.

Imaging

See Chapter 7 (in particular, Figures 7.37–7.42).

THERAPEUTIC OPTIONS

Extradural spinal tumors

The role of surgery is simply to provide decompression and tissue for histological diagnosis. Many cases of malignant extradural spinal tumor in childhood can be treated by chemotherapy without the need for neurosurgical intervention. The treatment of these tumors needs to be viewed in the context of the overall management strategy of the disease and will not be considered further here.

Intradural extramedullary spinal tumors

Although the histological distribution of intraspinal tumors in children differs from that in adults, the operative indications are similar. Most intradural extramedullary tumors are benign lesions that are best treated by complete surgical excision. The surgical decisions in the context of NF-2 are very complicated, but asymptomatic tumors almost regardless of size should be observed for signs of neurological involvement. If the symptomatic tumor involves a nerve root with important neurological function, then it is probably better to debulk the tumor surgically to decompress the spinal cord while leaving the nerve functional. In the case of schwannomas (about 52 per cent of the total) and meningiomas (35 per cent), it may be possible to gain a complete removal while leaving the parent nerve intact; however, in the case of neurofibromas (13 per cent), this is never the case. It is also rarely if ever possible to distinguish between these three tumor types before obtaining tissue at operation for pathological analysis.[11]

Intradural intramedullary spinal tumors

The management of intramedullary spinal cord tumors is quite controversial and will be dealt with below in the context of evidentiary review. While most tumors that are asymptomatic in the context of NF-2 should simply be observed, this may not be the case with intramedullary spinal cord tumors. The outcome of surgical resection in terms of postoperative neurological function depends greatly on the function of the patient before surgical intervention. This observation led Epstein and colleagues to question the value of operating on non-ambulatory patients. Because of the insidious nature of the slow-growing intramedullary tumor, it seems reasonable to remove these tumors prophylactically before the development of incapacitating symptoms. In the context of ependymomas, the most frequent intramedullary spinal cord tumor in NF-2, a gross total removal should be possible. Whatever management protocol is adopted for individual patients, the application of a standardized functional grading system, such as that proposed by McCormick and colleagues,[12] has considerable merits (Table 21.2).

Surgical technique

See Chapter 9.

The evidence base for management of intradural spinal tumors in children

The methodology used is that described in detail previously[13] and summarized in Tables 21.2–21.4. Of 445 articles concerning intramedullary spinal tumors in childhood, 74 were valuable for the purposes of this review. There were no class I studies.

INTRAMEDULLARY TUMORS

Feasibility of resection and its effect on outcome
Blind radiation of intramedullary tumors without a tissue diagnosis cannot be supported by the literature, and all children with intramedullary spinal cord tumors showing symptomatic or radiological progression should undergo surgical exploration. A significant percentage of low-grade intramedullary astrocytomas are amenable to extensive or gross total resection, with acceptable morbidity.[14–22] There is, however, a wide range of experience in this regard, with gross total, or subtotal, resection ranging from 49 per cent of cases in one European series[4] to 77 per cent in a North American series.[2] Other authors have advocated more conservative surgical approaches followed by radiation therapy, with good results in a large proportion of patients.[23–31]

Analysis of the literature leads to the conclusion that low-grade intramedullary astrocytomas should be explored and that if gross total removal is feasible, then no further adjunct treatment is necessary. This approach

should be viewed as a guideline for the management of this tumor.[13]

Because of the benignity and long periods of time to progression, direct comparisons of patients treated with radical surgery as compared with limited surgery with adjunctive radiation therapy are not available. Based on the literature reviewed, it is not possible to determine the best long-term outcome as a function of extent of resection. Enthusiasm for attempting gross total removal of these

Table 21.2 *Functional neurologic scale*

Grade	Functional status
I	Neurologically normal, mild focal deficit not significantly affecting function of involved limb; mild spasticity or reflex abnormality, normal gait
II	Presence of sensorimotor deficit affecting function of involved limb, mild to moderate gait difficulty, severe pain or dysesthetic syndrome impairing patient's quality of life, still functions and ambulates independently
III	More severe neurological deficit, requires cane/brace for ambulation or significant bilateral upper extremity impairment, may or may not function independently
IV	Severe deficit, requires wheelchair or cane/brace with bilateral upper extremity impairment, usually not independent

Reprinted from McCormick *et al.*[12] by permission of the *Journal of Neurosurgery.*

Table 21.3 *Classification of quality of data in clinical studies*

Class	Type of data
I	Randomized prospective studies
II	Comparison of results of two forms of treatment as they impact on a specified outcome
III	Everything else, including retrospective reviews of personal series, expert opinion, and case reports

From Nadkarni N, Rekate H.[13] Paediatric intramedullary spinal cord tumors: critical review of the literature. *Childs Nerv Syst* 1999; **15**: 17–28. Reprinted by permission.

Table 21.4 *Categories of management options*

Standards	Guidelines	Options
Accepted principles of patient management that reflect a high degree of clinical certainty	Reflect a moderate degree of clinical certainty	Outcomes are uncertain
Based on class I evidence or multiple strong class II studies	Based on class II data or a large number of concordant good class III studies	Based on class III evidence
Clinicians must act in conformity	Optimal choice is uncertain	Clinician may employ at own discretion
	Clinician should follow the guideline or inform the patient of the rationale underlying a different choice	

tumors has, until recently, been limited to a very few centers with large experiences.[14,15,17,18,32–35] A major question, such as whether a child with a residual spinal cord astrocytoma should receive adjunctive radiation or be observed for tumor growth, cannot be addressed objectively by a review of the literature.

Radical surgery has been performed in the case of malignant astrocytomas of the spinal cord.[31] However, there is little evidence that the outcome for these unfortunate patients can be improved in terms of survival or neurological morbidity. These tumors tend to be more vascular and hemorrhagic and lack a distinguishable plane between the tumor and the spinal cord.

Even the most aggressive group in terms of surgical removal now recommends a rather conservative approach to the resection of these tumors, to be followed by radiation therapy and chemotherapy as indicated.[17] As little information exists relative to the management of these tumors, and all that does exist should be considered as class III data, the above recommendation should be considered an option.

In the case of intramedullary ependymomas, however, the situation is significantly clearer. There is a clearly defined plane between the tumor and the surrounding spinal cord. An attempt should be made to radically excise these tumors. Several authors have reported excellent results with total excision of spinal cord ependymomas, with minimal morbidity in ambulatory patients.[12,19,28,36,37] Presumably with a higher level of confidence and experience, most if not all spinal cord ependymomas can be resected in their entirety. Late-outcome data exist and support the concept that in patients in whom gross total removal of an intramedullary ependymoma can be achieved, immediate postoperative radiation therapy is not warranted.[12,18,21,22,24,26,33,36,38–40]

Gross total removal of intramedullary ependymomas should be attempted in all patients who are ambulatory at the time of presentation and, if achieved, should be followed by long-term surveillance of the patient rather than radiation therapy. This recommendation should be considered as a standard.

What should be done if the surgeon believes that they have performed a gross total removal of the tumor and the postoperative magnetic resonance imaging (MRI) reveals that tumor remains? In the case of ependymoma, the patient should be re-explored early in an attempt to obtain a gross total removal unless there were elements of the surgical procedure that would put the patient at high risk of morbidity. If the tumor cannot be removed because there was no surgical plane or because of intraoperative deterioration of the evoked potentials, then it is unlikely that repeat surgery will result in further resection, and the patient could either be observed over time or be submitted to radiation therapy as options for care.

In the case of low-grade astrocytoma, total resection of the tumor is not an expected outcome of the procedure, even in the case of the inability to see residual tumor on postoperative MRI. For this reason, small amounts of residual tumor in the case of the intramedullary astrocytoma should simply be observed over time with sequential imaging. This is in line with an observational policy for incompletely excised low-grade astrocytoma elsewhere in the CNS.

Until recently, the extent of resection has been taken to be that described by the operating surgeon at the time of the resection. The availability of MRI has added a significant degree of objectivity to that assessment, particularly with respect to tumors that take up contrast material. Two studies have compared the surgeon's assessment of the degree of surgical removal of the tumor with the postoperative MRI. The conclusion of these studies is that the surgeon has an excellent chance of predicting extent of resection in the case of intramedullary ependymoma but is significantly less likely to be correct when dealing with astrocytomas.[8,41] Follow-up MRI is important not only to document residual tumor but also to detect asymptomatic recurrence. Minute residues of astrocytomas may be beyond the limits of resolution of MRI, and in this case residual tumor should be assumed despite a negative postoperative scan.[22]

Adjuncts to surgery

Very few techniques or surgical adjuncts have been subjected to scientific scrutiny to determine their efficacy and safety. Removal of spinal cord tumors, whether intramedullary or extramedullary, carries with it significant risk to the patient. Any surgical adjuncts that will lead to safer and more effective surgery should be utilized if possible. We have attempted to analyze the literature regarding the management of intramedullary spinal cord tumor to determine which are useful in improving the outcome of the patient. What follows is an attempt to determine objectively the value of various surgical adjuncts that have been advocated for the management of these tumors.

Ultrasonic aspirator Ultrasonic aspiration emulsifies tissue right at its tip, with little of the energy transmitted to surrounding structures. It is useful for removing tumors rapidly while leaving the sensitive neural structures in the vicinity at minimal risk of damage or distortion. Laboratory studies have shown that blood flow to tissues as little as 1 mm away from the point of the instrument is maintained without measurable distortion.[42] The power setting of the instrument can be adjusted, giving the surgeon some tactile input regarding the tissue being resected. The tumor is debulked internally until the normal white matter is seen; the dissection stops at this tumor–spinal cord interface.[18,31,43]

The device is reported to be excellent for the removal of intramedullary spinal cord tumors, but it is entirely possible to achieve the same results without its use. There are no outcome studies comparing the results with the device with those in which it was not used. Its use should therefore be considered an option.

Surgical laser The surgical laser is a precise tool that vaporizes tissue over a small, precisely controlled volume with little effect on surrounding tissues. It does not create any distortion of surrounding tissues. Most authors who recommend it use it to perform the initial myelotomy and then use it at the end of the procedure to remove small pieces of tumor at the interface of the normal cord. The major disadvantage of the surgical laser relates to its precision. It is a very slow instrument for this application. It is time-consuming to vaporize large volumes of tumor, and the char that remains may make it difficult to discern the interface between the spinal cord and the tumor that remains. In general, enthusiasm for the use of the surgical laser in neurosurgery has waned over the past decade, and its use should be considered an option.

Intraoperative ultrasound The intraoperative utilization of ultrasonography has proved useful for determining the location and extent of tumors as well as the identification of intratumoral cysts and syringes. Its use is advocated strongly by a number of authors.[21,26,31–33,36,41–45] Ultrasonography in experienced hands is also useful in determining the extent of resection intraoperatively. The use of intraoperative ultrasound should be viewed as a guideline.

Evoked potential monitoring Two types of evoked potential monitoring have been utilized in the intraoperative resection of intramedullary spinal cord tumors. Somatosensory-evoked potentials (SSEPs) rely on the integrity of the dorsal columns of the spinal cord and are the most widely available monitoring tool available worldwide. The theoretical objection to the use of SSEPs is that because of the reliance on the dorsal columns of the spinal cord, significant damage to the corticospinal tracts could lead to major deterioration without change in the evoked potential. False-negative results have been recorded in the case of scoliosis surgery, but as far as we have been able to determine, there is not a published confirmed case of a patient who suffered neurological deterioration during the resection of an intramedullary spinal cord tumor without seeing significant changes in the SSEPs. The major difficulty with SSEPs is the frequency of false-positive changes in the recordings.

The placement of the pial sutures, irrigation with cold irrigant, the use of the bipolar coagulator or laser, and changes in level of anesthesia or blood pressure may give false readings of general diminution or loss of SSEPs. In such cases, the irrigant is warmed and other manipulation ceased for a short time until the potentials resume; the procedure then continues.[43] The fact that SSEP monitoring is very likely to notify the surgeon that the patient may be being harmed before the development of permanent morbidity results in the use of SSEP monitoring during the removal of intramedullary spinal cord tumors being recommended as a guideline.

The monitoring of motor-evoked potentials (MEPs) is becoming more widespread and available in an increasing number of neurosurgical centers. This technique involves measuring the electrical activity of the corticospinal tracts, the structures that the surgeon wishes to protect. The use of MEP monitoring requires the availability of sophisticated neurophysiological support, but it has proved very helpful in the management of intramedullary spinal cord tumors.[18,46] The recommendation is that if the MEPs deteriorate below 50 per cent of the baseline, then surgery is discontinued to allow the potentials to recover; if they do not recover, then surgery is discontinued.[35,46] The limited clinical availability of this modality, and the limited number of controlled studies on the use of MEPs, make its use an option.

Adjuvant therapy

Until the relatively recent enthusiasm for radical resection of intramedullary spinal cord tumors, the majority of these lesions were managed by decompression, limited resection or biopsy, and radiation therapy. There have been no class I trials comparing radical surgery with limited surgery and radiation therapy, and it is very unlikely that such a study will ever be done. The rarity of the tumors, the passions of the individual investigators, and the long times to progression of these tumors make it almost impossible to perform a proper study to answer this question in terms of tumor control. Such a study might, however, address neurological and skeletal morbidity, especially that consequent upon therapies.

Radiation therapy The role of radiation therapy in the management of intramedullary spinal cord tumors in general, and especially low-grade astrocytomas, is certainly the most controversial aspect of this condition. Radiation therapy has been shown to be effective in a large number of patients harboring intramedullary astrocytomas with substantial tumor burdens in controlling the growth of tumors leading to many years of asymptomatic, progression-free survival.

The threshold for radiation injury of tumor containing spinal cord is encountered at 45–50 Gy using conventional fractionation,[47,48] and the risk of radiation-induced myelopathy limits the dose that can be delivered to a maximum of 50 Gy in 1.8–2.0-Gy fractions, which carries a very low incidence of myelopathy.[49,50] There is a presumed shallow dose–response curve: it appears that total doses in excess of 45 Gy are sufficient for tumor control, whereas total doses of less than 40 Gy may be associated with an increased failure rate; beyond 50 Gy, there is no additional therapeutic benefit.[4,7,8,47] The optimal length of the spinal cord field has not been determined (Table 21.5).[51]

Table 21.5 *Effect of radiotherapy for low-grade spinal tumors in children*

Ref.	Patient characteristics	Radiation dose (Gy)	Fractionation (Gy/fraction)	10-year survival (irradiated *v.* non-irradiated)
4	21 irradiated of 49 low-grade glioma	30–50	Not given	83% v. 70%, NS
9	9 irradiated of 18, 4/11 with low-grade glioma	43–50	Not given	3/4 alive v. 7/7 alive at 3–18 years
7	14 children <20 years/79 patients all ages	49.8 median (range 13.1–66.6)	1.8 (range 1.44–2.5)	80–85% v. 55–60% (pilocytic astrocytoma all ages, n = 43), NS
8	12 low-grade glioma/31 children	30–56	Not given	83% (all irradiated)

NS, not significant.

Radiation therapy should be withheld from patients following total removal of ependymomas as a standard. It should also be withheld from patients with low-grade astrocytomas undergoing radical removals, even though the removal falls short of a gross total removal as a guideline. Radiation therapy should be used after any degree of resection of a malignant (grade III or IV) astrocytic tumor as a guideline. Radiation therapy may be used at the time of progression of intramedullary spinal cord astrocytomas, either with or without prior repeat surgical exploration, as a guideline.

Chemotherapy The use of chemotherapy to treat intramedullary ependymomas and benign astrocytomas has not been studied in a prospective randomized trial and remains poorly defined. Chemotherapy has been utilized especially for infants with progressive low-grade tumors. There are only case reports, or very small series, suggesting that various chemotherapy regimes produce responses in either incompletely resected or unresectable tumors, with marked functional improvement.[4,52–56] As in other sites, chemotherapy may delay the need for radiotherapy or even obviate its use.[52,54,55] Close monitoring is required.[57]

Several authors have recommended the use of chemotherapy for malignant intramedullary tumors, but there seems to be no evidence that any of these regimens has altered the outcome of these devastating tumors.[25,58] The use of chemotherapy for any aspect of the treatment of intramedullary spinal cord tumors should be considered an option.

Laminectomy versus laminotomy As stated above, we use laminotomy in children because it is faster, results in a reconstruction of the spinal canal, and is safe.[59] This technique was originally recommended as a way of preventing spinal deformity;[60,61] there was some scepticism at the time.[62] Spinal deformities are a common problem in patients with both intra- and extramedullary tumors and occur with or without surgical intervention. Kyphosis as a result of multilevel laminectomy is the most common problem related to spinal stability faced by these patients.[14,15,31,43] The extent of spinal deformity relates to many factors, including the age of the patient at the time of the surgical intervention, the number of laminae that are removed, and whether the laminae are in the cervical, thoracic, or lumbar levels. The lack of purchase of the paraspinal musculature in the absence of spinous processes and laminae combines with the weakness of these muscles due to the effects of the tumor, to lead to the destabilization of the spine at the laminectomized level.

Radiation therapy has multiple effects leading to loss of the vertebral endplates and failure of the vertebral bodies to grow if they are in the radiation field.[18,31,63–66] The use of osteoplastic laminotomy returns the posterior elements to the spine, which may serve to stabilize the spine itself and serve as a site to be used later for subsequent spinal fusion, should it be needed.[59,60] Very long-term studies comparing spinal deformity in children following laminectomy or laminotomy have not been carried out, and some children do develop deformity of the spine despite the use of laminotomy.[18] Therefore, the efficacy of laminotomy to prevent spinal deformity has not been established, and its use should be considered an option at this point. Spinal deformity can occur many years following the treatment of children for spinal cord tumors. It can lead to pain, deformity, and neurological deterioration by compression of the spinal cord without signaling recurrence or progression of the tumor. Patients who have undergone laminectomy or laminotomy for spinal cord tumors should be followed until adulthood for the development of such deformity. This recommendation should be taken as a guideline.

Summary

In summary, only three recommendations can be made that carry the strength of certainty to be considered as standards. First, an attempt should be made to resect intramedullary ependymomas in their entirety. Second, if residual ependymoma is seen on the postoperative MRI, and the reason for the remaining tumor was that the surgeon did not identify it at operation, then the patient should be re-explored for removal of the remaining tumor. Finally, if gross total removal of intramedullary ependymomas and low-grade astrocytomas can be demonstrated, then radiation therapy should be withheld and the patient followed clinically and with surveillance MRI for the development of recurrent tumor.

INTRADURAL EXTRAMEDULLARY TUMORS

Of 48 articles regarding intradural extramedullary tumors in children, 18 were of value in this review. There were no class I or class II data. Intradural extramedullary tumors are extremely rare tumors in children, except in the context of neurofibromatosis. A thorough review of the previous literature on intraspinal tumors in children identified ten articles, with a total of 635 patients with spinal tumors, including intramedullary, intradural extramedullary, and extradural tumors (Table 21.1).[1,67] Overall, intradural extramedullary tumors represent about 25 per cent of tumors affecting the spine in children. If those mass lesions that are essentially congenital defects, such as dermoids and epidermoids are excluded, then a total of 65 patients with primary tumors are identified, representing approximately ten per cent of intraspinal tumors in childhood. Most of the tumors in this discussion occurred in the context of neurofibromatosis.

While spinal meningiomas and NSTs must occur as isolated events in children, these occurrences are so rare that they do not lend themselves to review using evidence-based medicine.

Meningiomas

Isolated meningiomas of the spine in children as an isolated event, as distinct from those found in the context of NF-1 or NF-2, tend to be more aggressive and probably represent meningeal sarcomas.[68,69] Meningiomas in the context of NF-2 are usually found when there are a large number of other intraspinal and intracranial tumors. The decision to operate on a meningioma of the spine should be based on the symptoms that the patient is experiencing and the relationship of the meningioma to the spinal cord. Complete resection is usually possible and should be curative of that meningioma. Due to the complex nature of the overall management of NF-2 spinal meningiomas that are found on routine imaging studies without overt spinal cord compression and without associated symptoms, an observational strategy should be viewed as a guideline.

Nerve sheath tumors

There are two types of tumors arising from the nerve sheath of the exiting spinal nerve roots, schwannomas (also called neurilemmomas) and neurofibromas. Schwannomas are made up exclusively of Schwann cells and grow from the sheath surrounding the nerve. It is often possible to remove the tumor whilst leaving the nerve functional.

In the case of neurofibromas, however, there is a mixture of Schwann cells and fibroblasts and an abundance of collagen. These tumors circumferentially expand the nerve itself, and total resection of necessity involves the parent nerve. The same principles of management as discussed above in relation to meningiomas in the context of neurofibromatosis applies equally well as a guideline to the management of schwannomas and neurofibromas in the context of NF-1 and NF-2.[70] If the nerve from which the tumor is formed is functionally important, such as the nerves forming the brachial and lumbosacral plexi, then debulking rather than complete excision should probably be performed; this should be seen as an option.

Prognosis

Overall survival rates for all types and grades of childhood intramedullary spinal cord tumors are between 39 and 90 per cent at five years, with event-free survival rates between 14 and 77 per cent. Overall survival rates for low-grade tumors regardless of treatment are reported at 76 per cent at ten years, and 83 per cent at ten years for regimes including radiation therapy.[4] For patients undergoing aggressive resection alone, five-year progression-free survival of 79 per cent has been reported.[71] Approximately 50 per cent of the tumors that have been deemed unresectable progress following chemotherapy.[53–55,57]

Factors influencing outcome have been the duration of presenting symptoms before diagnosis (specifically, the development of spinal deformity), the preoperative neurological condition, and the histology.[4,6] The extent of disease at diagnosis, as judged by the number of vertebral segments involved, has not been a significant factor.[7] Similar five-year progression-free survival has been observed in low-grade tumors that have been subtotally (80–95 per cent) resected compared with those that have been totally resected.[2] Although most relapses and progressions occur within five years of diagnosis, late recurrence beyond ten years is observed.

The principal prognostic determinant of postoperative functional status is the degree of preoperative neurological deficit. Patients with no or only mild deficits before surgery rarely deteriorate. Of 164 patients aged 21 years or younger, of whom 131 had low-grade tumors, and who underwent aggressive surgery with intention to achieve total resection if possible, clinical symptoms were unchanged in 60 per cent, improved in 16 per cent, and aggravated in 24 per cent.[2,71]

The risk of spinal deformity relates to age, anatomical level, and the number of spinal levels operated upon. For patients under 15 years of age and undergoing multilevel procedures, the risk is approximately eight times that for patients aged over 15 years. The risk is very high in the cervical region, less in the thoracic region, and negligible in the lumbar region.[66] Radiation therapy without surgery also carries a risk of spinal deformity, with incidences of up to 71 per cent.[72,73] This is also age-related, young age being a risk factor. Corrective orthopedic spinal surgery may be required.[6,51]

An incidence of second malignancy of 13 per cent at ten and 20 years has been reported.[8]

SUMMARY

Intradural tumors of childhood, whether intramedullary or extramedullary, are rare tumors whose management is primarily surgical. None have been treated using a randomized trial or even according to a standardized strategy-based protocol. Many of the larger series comprise patients encountered at single institutions and treated over a considerable period of time, during which the philosophy of management, as well as equipment and techniques, have changed. Furthermore, as with many institutional series, these series cannot include data from more than a highly selected proportion of the population at risk. It is sometimes difficult to know exactly why particular patients gravitated towards particular hospitals. Most of the management issues remain subject to debate. A small number of conclusions can be gained from a thorough review of the literature as it relates to intramedullary tumors. Thus, if a gross total removal of the tumor can be achieved, then postoperative adjuvant treatment using radiation or chemotherapy should await the diagnosis of recurrence. While this standard is limited to intramedullary tumors, it can almost certainly be extrapolated to meningiomas and NSTs seen in children.

REFERENCES

1 Yamamoto Y, Raffel C. Intraspinal extramedullary neoplasms. In: Albright A, Pollack I, Adelson P (eds) *Operative Techniques in Pediatric Neurosurgery*. New York: Thieme, 2001, pp. 183–92.

2 Constantini S, Miller DC, Allen JC, Rorke LB, Freed D, Epstein FJ. Radical excision of intramedullary spinal cord tumors: surgical morbidity and long-term follow-up evaluation in 164 children and young adults. *J Neurosurg* 2000; **93**:183–93.

3 Stiller CA, Nectoux J. International incidence of childhood brain and spinal tumours. *Int J Epidemiol* 1994; **23**:458–64.

4 Bouffet E, Pierre-Kahn A, Marchal JC, *et al.* Prognostic factors in pediatric spinal cord astrocytoma. *Cancer* 1998; **83**:2391–9.

5 Merchant TE, Kiehna EN, Thompson SJ, Heidman RL, Sanford RA, Kun LE. Pediatric low-grade and ependymal spinal cord tumors. *Pediatr Neurosurg* 2000; **32**:30–6.

6 Epstein F, Constantini S. Spinal cord tumors of childhood. In: Pang D (ed.) *Disorders of the Pediatric Spine*. New York: Raven Press, 1995, pp. 55–76.

7 Minehan K, Shaw EJ, Scheithauer BW, Davis DL, Onofrio BM. Spinal cord astrocytoma: pathological and treatment considerations. *J Neurosurg* 1995; **83**:590–5.

8 O'Sullivan C, Jenkin R, Doherty M, Hoffman H. Greenberg M. Spinal cord tumors in children: long-term results of combined surgical and radiation treatment. *J Neurosurg* 1994; **81**:507–12.

9 Przbylski GJ, Albright AL, Martinez AJ. Spinal cord astrocytomas: long term results comparing treatments in children. *Childs Nerv Syst* 1997; **13**:375–82.

10 Akar Z, Tanriover N, Kafadar AM, Gazioglu N, Oza B, Kuday C. Chiasmatic low-grade glioma presenting with sacral intradural spinal metastases. *Childs Nerv Syst* 2000; **16**:309–11.

11 Mautner VF, Tatagiba M, Lindenau M, *et al.* Spinal tumors in patients with neurofibromatosis type 2: MR imaging study of frequency, multiplicity, and variety. *Am J Roentgenol* 1995; **165**:951–5.

12 McCormick PC, Torres R, Post KD. Stein BM. Intramedullary ependymoma of the spinal cord. *J Neurosurg* 1990; **72**:523–32.

13 Nadkarni N, Rekate H. Pediatric intramedullary spinal cord tumors: critical review of the literature. *Childs Nerv Syst* 1999; **15**:17–28.

14 Epstein F, Epstein N. Surgical management of holocord intramedullary spinal cord astrocytomas in children. *J Neurosurg* 1981; **54**:829–32.

15 Epstein FJ, Epstein N. Surgical treatment of spinal cord astrocytomas of childhood. A series of 19 patients. *J Neurosurg* 1981; **57**:685–9.

16 Epstein FJ. Surgical treatment of intramedullary spinal cord tumors of childhood. In: Pascual-Castroviejo I (ed.) *Spinal Tumors in Children and Adolescents.* New York: Raven Press, 1990.

17 Epstein FJ, Farmer JP, Freed D. Adult intramedullary astrocytomas of the spinal cord. *J Neurosurg* 1992; **77**:355–9.

18 Goh KY, Velasquez L, Epstein FJ. Pediatric intramedullary spinal cord tumors: is surgery alone enough? *Pediatr Neurosurg* 1997; **27**:34–9.

19 Garrido E, Stein BM. Microsurgical removal of intramedullary spinal cord tumors. *Surg Neurol* 1977; **7**:215–19.

20 Brotchi J, Noterman J, Baleriaux D. Surgery of intramedullary spinal cord tumours. *Acta Neurochir (Wien)* 1992; **116**:176–8.

21 Cooper PR. Outcome after operative treatment of intramedullary spinal cord tumors in adults: intermediate and long-term results in 51 patients. *Neurosurgery* 1989; **25**:855–9.

22 Cristante L, Herrmann HD. Surgical management of intramedullary spinal cord tumors: functional outcome and sources of morbidity. *Neurosurgery* 1994; **35**:69–74.

23 Ahyai A, Woerner U, Markakis E. Surgical treatment of intramedullary tumors (spinal cord and medulla oblongata). Analysis of 16 cases. *Neurosurg Rev* 1990; **13**:45–52.

24 Guidetti B, Mercuri S, Vagnozzi R. Long-term results of the surgical treatment of 129 intramedullary spinal gliomas. *J Neurosurg* 1981; **54**:323–30.

25 Hardison HH, Packer RJ, Rorke LB, Schut L, Sutton LN, Bruce DA. Outcome of children with primary intramedullary spinal cord tumors. *Childs Nerv Syst* 1987; **3**:89–92.

26 Innocenzi G, Raco A, Cantore G, Raimondi AJ. Intramedullary astrocytomas and ependymomas in the pediatric age group: a retrospective study. *Childs Nerv Syst* 1996; **12**:776–80.

27 Innocenzi G, Salvati M, Cervoni L, Delfini R, Cantore G. Prognostic factors in intramedullary astrocytomas. *Clin Neurol Neurosurg* 1997; **99**:1–5.

28 Malis LI. Intramedullary spinal cord tumors. *Clin Neurosurg* 1978; **25**:512–39.

29 Lunardi P, Licastro G, Missori P, Ferrante L, Fortuna A. Management of intramedullary tumours in children. *Acta Neurochir (Wien)* 1993; **120**:59–65.

30 Rauhut F, Reinhardt V, Budach V, Wiedemayer H. Nau HE. Intramedullary pilocytic astrocytomas – a clinical and morphological study after combined surgical and photon or neutron therapy. *Neurosurg Rev* 1989; **12**:309–13.

31 Steinbok P, Cochrane DD, Poskitt K. Intramedullary spinal cord tumors in children. *Neurosurg Clin North Am* 1992; **3**:931–45.

32 Constantini S, Houten J, Miller DC, *et al.* Intramedullary spinal cord tumors in children under the age of 3 years. *J Neurosurg* 1996; **85**:1036–43.

33 Cooper PR, Epstein F. Radical resection of intramedullary spinal cord tumors in adults. Recent experience in 29 patients. *J Neurosurg* 1985; **63**:492–9.

34 Goy AM, Pinto RS, Raghavendra BN, Epstein FJ, Kricheff II. Intramedullary spinal cord tumors: MR imaging, with emphasis on associated cysts. *Radiology* 1986; **161**:381–6.

35 Kothbauer K, Deletis V, Epstein FJ. Intraoperative spinal cord monitoring for intramedullary surgery: an essential adjunct. *Pediatr Neurosurg* 1997; **26**:247–54.

36 Epstein FJ, Farmer JP, Freed D. Adult intramedullary spinal cord ependymomas: the result of surgery in 38 patients. *J Neurosurg* 1993; **79**:204–9.

37 Fischer G, Mansuy L. Total removal of intramedullary ependymomas: follow-up study of 16 cases. *Surg Neurol* 1980; **14**:243–9.

38 Lee M, Rezai AR, Freed D, Epstein FJ. Intramedullary spinal cord tumors in neurofibromatosis. *Neurosurgery* 1996; **38**:32–7.

39 Samii M, Klekamp J. Surgical results of 100 intramedullary tumors in relation to accompanying syringomyelia. *Neurosurgery* 1994; **35**:865–73.

40 Stein BM. Surgery of intramedullary spinal cord tumors. *Clin Neurosurg* 1979; **26**:529–42.

41 Xu QW, Bao WM, Mao RL, Yang GY. Aggressive surgery for intramedullary tumor of cervical spinal cord. *Surg Neurol* 1996; **46**:322–8.

42 Constantini S, Epstein F. Ultrasonic aspiration in neurosurgery. In: Wilkins R, Rengechary S (eds) *Neurosurgery.* New York: McGraw-Hill, 1996, pp. 607–8.

43 Constantini S, Epstein F. Intraspinal tumors in infants and children. In: Youmans J (ed.) *Neurological Surgery.* Philadelphia: Saunders, 1996, pp. 3123–33.

44 Epstein FJ, Farmer JP, Schneider SJ. Intraoperative ultrasonography: an important surgical adjunct for intramedullary tumors. *J Neurosurg* 1991; **74**:729–33.

45 Kawakami N, Mimatsu K, Kato F. Intraoperative sonography of intramedullary spinal cord tumours. *Neuroradiology* 436 9.

46 Morota N, Deletis V, Constantini S, Kofler M, Cohen H, Epstein FJ. The role of motor evoked potentials during surgery for intramedullary spinal cord tumors. *Neurosurgery* 1997; **41**:1327–36.

47 Linstadt DE, Wara WM, Leibel SA, Gutin PH, Wilson CB, Sheline GE. Postoperative radiotherapy of primary spinal cord tumors. *Int J Radiat Oncol Biol Phys* 1989; **16**:1397–403.

48 Mccunniff AJ, Liang MG. Radiation tolerance of the cervical spinal cord. *Int J Radiat Oncol Biol Phys* 1989; **16**:675–8.

49 Kopelson G, Linggood RM. Intramedullary spinal cord astrocytoma versus glioblastoma. The prognostic importance of histologic grade. *Cancer* 1982; **50**:732–5.

50 Kopelson G, Linggood RM, Kleinman GM, Doucette J, Wang CC. Management of intramedullary spinal cord tumors. *Radiology* 1980; **135**:473–9.

51 Marcus RB, Jr, Million RR. The incidence of myelitis after irradiation of the cervical spinal cord. *Int J Radiat Oncol Biol Phys* 1990; **19**:3–8.

52 Bouffet E, Amat D, Devaux Y, Desuzinges C. Chemotherapy for spinal cord astrocytoma. *Med Pediatr Oncol* 1997; **29**:560–2.

53 Fort DW, Packer RJ, Kirkpatrick GB, Kuttesch JF, Jr, Ater JL. Carboplatin and vincristine for pediatric primary spinal cord astrocytomas. *Childs Nerv Syst* 1998; **14**:484.

54 Doireau, V, Grill J, Chastagner P, *et al.* Chemotherapy for intramedullary glial tumors. *Childs Nerv Syst* 1998; **14**:484–5.

55 Doireau V, Grill J, Zerah M, *et al.* Chemotherapy for unresectable and recurrent intramedullary glial tumours in children. Brain Tumour Subcommittee of the French Society of Pediatric Oncology (SFOP). *Br J Cancer* 1999; **81**:835–40.

56 Lowis SP, Pizer BL, Coakham H, Nelson RJ, Bouffet E. Chemotherapy for spinal cord astrocytoma: can natural history be modified? *Childs Nerv Syst* 1998; **14**:317–21.

57 Foreman NK, Hay TC, Handler M. Chemotherapy for spinal cord astrocytoma. *Med Pediatr Oncol* 1998; **30**:311–2.

58 Cohen A, Wisoff J, Allen J, Epstein F. Malignant astrocytomas of the spinal cord. *J Neurosurg* 1989; **70**:50–4.

59 Abbott RF, Eldstein N, Wisoff J, Epstein F. Osteoplastic laminotomy in children. *Pediatr Neurosurg* 1992; **18**:153–5.

60 Raimondi A, Gutierrez F, Di Rocco C. Laminotomy and total reconstruction of the posterior spinal arch for spinal canal surgery in childhood. *J Neurosurg* 1976; **45**:555–60.

61 Gutierrez FA, Oi S, McClone DG. Intraspinal tumors in children: clinical review, surgical results and follow-up in 51 cases. *Concepts Pediatr Neurosurg* 1983; **4**:291–305.

62 Humphreys RP. Editor's comment. *Concepts Pediatr Neurosurg* 1983; **4**:304–5.

63 Cattell H, Clark G. Cervical kyphosis and instability following multiple laminectomies in children. *J Bone Joint Surg (Am)* 1967; **49**:713–20.

64 Lonstein J. Post-laminectomy kyphosis. *Clin Orthop* 1977; **128**:93–103.

65 Yasuoka S, Peterson H, Laws E, Maccarty C. Pathogenesis and prophylaxis of post-laminectomy deformity of the spine after multiple level laminectomy: difference between children and adults. *Neurosurgery* 1981; **9**:145–52.

66 Yasuoka S, Peterson H, Maccarty C. Incidence of spinal column deformity after multilevel laminectomy in children and adults. *J Neurosurg* 1982; **57**:441–5.

67 Yamamoto Y, Raffel C. Spinal extradural neoplasms and intradural extramedullary neoplasms. In: Albright A, Pollack I, Adelson P. *Principles and Practice of Pediatric Neurosurgery.* New York: Thieme, 1999, pp. 685–96.

68 Liu H, Armond S, Edwards M. An unusual spinal meningioma in a child: case report. *Neurosurgery* 1985; **17**:313–16.

69 Zwartverwer F, Kaplan A, Hart M. Meningeal sarcoma of the spinal cord in a newborn. *Arch Neurol* 1978; **35**:844–6.

70 Schut L, Duhaime A, Sutton L. Phakomatoses: surgical considerations. In: Cheek W (ed.) *Pediatric Neurosurgery: Surgery of the Developing Nervous System*, 3rd edn. Philadelphia: W. B. Saunders, 1994, pp. 473–84.

71 Constantini S, Miller DC, Allen JC, Rorke LB, Freed D, Epstein F. Radical excision of intramedullary spinal cord tumors: surgical morbidity and long-term follow-up evaluation in 164 children and young adults. *J Neurosurg* 2000; **93** (suppl. 2):183–93.

72 Katzman H, Waugh T, Berdon W. Skeletal changes following irradiation of childhood tumors. *J Bone Joint Surg Am* 1969; **51**:825–42.

73 Mayfield JK, Riseborough EJ, Jaffe N, Nehme Ame. Spinal deformity in children treated for neuroblastoma. *J Bone Joint Surg Am* 1981; **63**:183–93.

22

Rare tumors

RICHARD GRUNDY AND CONOR MALLUCCI

INTRODUCTION

A chapter on rare pediatric brain tumors is arguably one of the more essential components of any textbook of brain and spinal cord tumors of childhood. In writing this chapter, our aim was to provide a comprehensive and practical overview to help the practicing clinician deal with uncommon situations. In doing so, we have extensively reviewed the literature and attempted to draw some sensible conclusions, highlighting what is, and is not, known. Clearly, there is much to learn about these tumor types; given their rarity, this will best be achieved by international cooperation.

MIXED NEURONAL-GLIAL TUMORS

Gangliogliomas

Gangliogliomas and ganglioneuromas comprise 0.4 per cent of brain tumors in all ages, but in some large series they represent up to four per cent of all childhood brain tumors.[1,2] Most tumors occur before the age of 30 years, with presentations as young as six months and as old as 80 years.[3,4]

HISTOLOGY

The term "ganglioglioma" was first used to describe tumors consisting of ganglion (neuronal) and glial elements.[5] As differentiation is complete, these tumors are usually considered to be benign. However, the histological appearance is often highly variable, with the proportion of glial and ganglionic cells varying widely. The glial component usually shows increased cellularity and nuclear hyperchromasia, but mitoses are uncommon. The neuronal component often shows abnormal cell clustering and binucleate cells. Lymphocytic infiltration is often seen.

No clear relationship exists between the histological features, the clinical course, or the outcome.[4] However, differences in the histopathological features between midline and hemispheric tumors have led one group to suggest that these tumors should be divided into two entities.[6] Rarely, anaplastic gangliogliomas are reported, often with a long history of malignant evolution and poor outcome.[3,7,8]

CLINICAL FEATURES

Gangliogliomas are slow-growing lesions that typically develop from structures that normally contain nerve cells, such as the cerebral cortex. They occur most commonly in the temporal regions, but they may also develop in the cerebellum, basal ganglia, brainstem, and spinal cord.[2,3,6,9,10] Optic nerve gangliogliomas have also been reported.[11] The median age at presentation is ten years and there is a male predominance. The clinical presentation reflects the tumor location. Supratentorial tumors usually present with increasingly severe and poorly controlled epilepsy, often over significant time periods.[2,6] The electroencephalogram (EEG) is usually focally abnormal. Learning disability and behavioral problems are reported in about a third of cases.[2,6] Slowly evolving neurological signs may be present in up to half of the cases; most commonly with midline tumors.[2,6] Seizure control is usually improved following complete resection, indicating that seizure activity is related to the tumor.[2,6]

IMAGING

Computed tomography (CT) imaging studies reveal hypodense, well-circumscribed lesions that are frequently predominantly cystic. Calcification is present in up to 25 per cent of cases.[2,12] Magnetic resonance imaging (MRI) confers advantages in determining the extent and nature of these tumors, which are hyperintense on T2-weighted images. MRI also reveals a solid component.[9] Involvement of the leptomeninges is common,[2] but leptomeningeal spread is uncommon.[12]

TREATMENT

The management of ganglion cell tumors is surgical, aiming for complete resection.[2,6] Indeed, the extent of resection is the major prognostic factor, complete resection equating to a good prognosis. Second-look surgery may therefore play a role in the management of gangliogliomas. In most series, midline brainstem and spinal cord tumors have a worse prognosis, reflecting difficulties in achieving a complete resection.[4,13] Radiotherapy should be reserved for recurrent or progressive disease.[1,2,4,6,12] No reports of response to chemotherapy have been reported.

Dysembryoplastic neuroepithelial tumors

Dysembryoplastic neuroepithelial tumors (DNTs) were first described in 1988. They represent a rare form of mixed neuronal-glial tumor, which should probably be considered as a subcategory of ganglioglioma, described above. DNTs are essentially slow-growing hemispheric tumors, usually presenting with epilepsy.

HISTOLOGY

The DNT is differentiated from the ganglioglioma by demonstrating a multinodular architecture, including elements of cortical dysplasia in addition to the glioneuronal elements seen in ganglioglioma. The criteria for a diagnosis of DNT rest on the following features: (i) intracortical location of nodules, and (ii) loose, myxoid, hypocellular fields of mucopolysaccharide material, within which are small cells resembling oligodendroglial cells and in which neurons appear to float.

IMAGING

DNTs appear as hypodense lesions on T1 MRI and CT. They often do not enhance, and have very little mass effect. They are usually hemispheric, and frequently temporal in location.

CLINICAL FEATURES

DNTs were first described by Daumas-Duport and colleagues,[14] who separated them from other histologically benign tumors found in resection specimens from patients who had intractable epilepsy. DNTs therefore commonly manifest as a seizure disorder. They can present in the whole pediatric age range, but the mean age of presentation is nine years. There is a male preponderance. Occasionally, DNTs are present with headache and sometimes coincidental findings on scans performed for other reasons.

TREATMENT

DNTs are often well-circumscribed and amenable to complete surgical resection. The prognosis is generally excellent. Surgical resection is usually the mainstay of treatment. However, even after incomplete resection, long-term progression-free survival is common, and adjuvant therapy is commonly deferred. As these tumors often present with seizure disorders, postoperative seizure control sometimes plays a role in long-term functional outcome.

As with any of these hemispheric tumors, in which complete surgical resection is the goal, preoperative and intraoperative measures, such as image-guided systems and intraoperative imaging, can play an important role in achieving complete surgical resection with minimal deficit.[14–18]

Desmoplastic infantile ganglioglioma and desmoplastic astrocytoma of infancy

Desmoplastic infantile ganglioglioma (DIG) and desmoplastic infant astrocytoma (DIA) are very rare, unusual mixed astroglial tumors reported mainly on children under the age of one year. They are classically very large superficial tumors, often with aggressive histological findings that do not correspond to the generally good outcome.

HISTOLOGY

These tumors are almost identical histologically, except for the presence of neuronal cell differentiation in DIGs, which may be evident only on immunohistochemical staining. The exact nosology of desmoplastic tumors has been the subject of much discussion over the past two decades.[22–34] The reports of Taratuto and colleagues in 1984, describing "superficial cerebral astrocytoma," in infants followed by the description of a similar tumor with the added feature of ganglion cells in 1987, describing the desmoplastic infantile ganglioglioma, both led the way in identifying massive superficial tumors in children with dural attachment and characterized by the presence of a combination of both astrocytes and mesenchymal tissue such as fibrocollagen, which, despite showing malignant-looking areas, demonstrated a surprisingly benign clinical course.[27,32,34]

Both these tumors characteristically demonstrate intense desmoplasia, are glial fibrillary acid protein (GFAP)-positive, and demonstrate either cellular or nuclear pleomorphism, or both.[27] Focal areas with poorly differentiated cells and mitoses and primitive blast cells surrounded by areas of well-differentiated, benign-looking tissue is common. Some tumors demonstrate brain or dural infiltration. Some demonstrate a remarkable variety of cellular differentiation in different cell lines, with one, for example, demonstrating not only the astrocytoma and mesenchymal elements but also neuronal cells, Schwann cells, oligodendrocytes, and melanocytes. Large specimens are therefore important, as small biopsy specimens may be misleading.[18,22,26,27,31–46]

CLINICAL FEATURES

These tumors classically present as very large, hemispheric, superficial tumors in infants. The symptoms and signs of any large space-occupying supratentorial lesions in infants can be expected to include, most commonly, enlarging head circumference, bulging fontanelle, and hemiparesis. In children over one year of age, the duration of symptoms may vary, but symptoms of raised intracranial pressure may dominate.

Often remarkable is the sheer size of these tumors on the radiological imaging and the relative lack of obtundation in a child with such large masses, suggesting very slow growth of the tumor and a probable congenital origin.

On reviewing the literature, of the 18 or so DIA that have been reported to date, they had a median age of 6.4 months (range 1.5–18 months). DIGs are slightly more common, with 45 or more cases found in the reported literature; the median age is five months (range 2–48 months).[22,26–28,31–46]

IMAGING

In addition to large size, the superficial hemispheric location, and dural proximity, cystic and heterogeneous appearance and intense contrast enhancement should alert one to the diagnosis. MRI is the preferred investigation. In addition, one should look for flow voids on MRI, suggesting large vessels and caution at surgery. Angiography, or magnetic resonance angiography (MRA), and venography may be indicated in surgical planning. The radiological characteristics have been described well in previous reports.[27,47–50]

The differential diagnosis of these tumors on presentation is often difficult. Most commonly, they resemble meningiomas. The important differentiating factor is that meningiomas in childhood are more common in the second decade of life and are more frequently intraventricular in location, while fewer are cystic in nature. Other possibilities are pure astrocytomas, gangliogliomas, which are more commonly calcified, choroid plexus papillomas, primitive neuroectodermal tumors (PNETs), and DNTs.

TREATMENT

The mainstay of treatment for these tumors is surgical resection. These tumors represent a formidable surgical challenge due to their size, intense vascularity, and dural attachments. However, the prognosis is excellent if full surgical excision can be achieved, despite the often high-grade nature of the histological specimens. Adjuvant chemo- or radiotherapy should not be necessary. It is important that these tumors are managed with a similar surgical strategy, and that one is aware of their histological nature, as they behave in a biologically similar manner.

The typical surgical characteristics of these tumors are of a firm tumor coming to the surface of the hemisphere, which is either stuck to or infiltrating the dura, and often involving venous sinuses. They are frequently highly vascular, but a good plane of cleavage usually exists. Sometimes, second-look surgery may have to be planned if the threat of blood loss is too much for a small infant.

On reviewing the literature with regards to adjuvant treatment, only a few reports have commented on its use, with too few cases to draw definitive conclusions. Duffner and colleagues report on four cases of DIG, all of which received adjuvant chemotherapy.[22] One patient had a complete resection, and the remaining three patients had debulking procedures only. In those with measurable residual disease, one had a complete response, one had a partial response, and one remained stable, with a follow-up of 32–60 months. The authors concluded that following complete resection, adjuvant treatment might not be necessary. In a review paper, VandenBerg comments on an 8.7-year median follow-up on 14 cases of DIG from different institutions.[33] In these cases, in which the treatment modality was known in 90 per cent, 31 per cent had near-total resection and no further treatment, 38 per cent had surgery and radiotherapy, 23 per cent had surgery and chemotherapy, and eight per cent had surgery and both chemo- and radiotherapy. There were no deaths from either residual or recurrent tumor in this group. There was, however, one recurrence, which went on to have a repeat complete surgical resection and adjuvant radiotherapy, after which there was no sign of recurrence after eight years of follow-up.

Pleomorphic xanthoastrocytomas

Pleomorphic xanthoastrocytomas (PXAs) (first reported in 1979 by Kepes and colleagues[24]) are rare tumors of mixed neuronal-glial differentiation. They classically present in the second decade of life as large supratentorial hemispheric masses.

HISTOLOGY

Histologically, these tumors have been classified previously as astrocytic tumors, because most of their cells are GFAP-positive. More recently, however, it has been recognized that they commonly express features of neuronal differentiation and desmoplasia and have much in common with the DIAs and DIGs described above. In fact, the common term of "desmoplastic neuroepithelial tumor" has been proposed for PXA, DIA, and DIG. De Chadarevian and coworkers proposed that pleomorphic xanthoastrocytomas might represent a lipidized form of desmoplastic cerebral astrocytomas seen in older children and young adults.[51] The heterogeneous nature of these tumors is similar to that of DIA and DIG, with large areas of GFAP-positive astrocytic cells and with more focal areas of aggressive growth. The cytoplasm of these cells is often vacuolated, representing spaces occupied by fat globules. The prominent mesenchymal or desmoplastic feature is usually present.[24,51–56]

MOLECULAR BIOLOGY

A limited genetic screen of eight tumors for *TP53* mutations revealed missense mutations in two cases occurring outside of the conserved domain. Neither of these cases progressed. Loss of heterozygosity analysis for 10q and 19q revealed no evidence of allelic imbalance. The unusual constellation of *TP53* mutations and lack of allelic loss suggests that the genetic events resulting in PXA formation are different from those involved in diffuse astrocytoma formation.[57]

CLINICAL FEATURES

This tumor presents most commonly in the second and third decades of life. It is typically located, like DIAs and DIGs, in the superficial region in association with the leptomeninges. The temporoparietal region is the most common location. Cysts are not uncommon. Macroscopically the tumors may have a yellow tinge because of their high intracellular fat content. They tend to present as any large hemispheric tumor in an older child, with symptoms combining raised intracranial pressure, focal neurological deficits, and sometimes fits.

IMAGING

The imaging features are essentially similar to those for DIA and DIG, although not generally meeting the same massive size as in younger children. These are hemispheric, heterogeneous, intensely enhancing cystic masses on MRI and CT. Angiography or MRI/MRA may be indicated for surgical planning.[12,27,47,48,58–62]

TREATMENT

The mainstay of treatment is complete surgical resection. The same rules apply as for DIG and DIA. Second-look surgery may be appropriate in the case of initial incomplete resection. Preoperative chemotherapy has been used, with good effect, to facilitate surgical resection, and it should be considered in patients in whom primary surgery is difficult.[63]

Information regarding the clinical behavior of PXAs suggests that they usually have a benign clinical course, with survival times of up to 25 years being documented by Kepes and colleagues,[64] and actuarial survival at five years reported at 90 per cent. There are, however, some reports of aggressive recurrences of these tumors, and therefore caution and careful follow-up are necessary, especially if only subtotal resection has been achieved. There have also been reports of frankly malignant variants and even of metastases. Adjuvant treatment in these tumors, therefore, although not usually indicated, may have to be considered when aggressive histology is found and the surgeon feels that a complete resection is not possible. In this case, a low-grade glioma strategy should be adopted.[24,25,47,62–75]

Oligodendrogliomas

Oligodendrogliomas in childhood differ from their adult counterparts. They are less common, accounting for just under one per cent of all pediatric intracranial neoplasms, and they are more frequently of a higher histological grade.[76–80] Recent literature indicates that these tumors may be the second most common adult glioma.[81]

Oligodendrogliomas are usually well-differentiated, diffusely infiltrating tumors. They occur preferentially in the cerebral cortex, although occurrences in the posterior fossa, brainstem, and spinal cord have been reported.[76–80] Seizures are the most common presenting sign, followed by raised intracranial pressure (headaches, nausea, vomiting, papilledema). Duration of symptoms varies, but it may be prolonged.[76–80] Some reports have suggested a gender bias towards males,[80] but others have found equal incidence.[78,79]

PATHOLOGY

The tumor cells are arranged as sheets of cells with small, round homogenous nuclei, surrounded by a clear zone, giving a "fried egg" appearance. Microcalcification is often seen. Histologically, these tumors range from well-differentiated, World Health Organization (WHO) grade II to anaplastic WHO grade III, the distinction being made on the basis of mitotic activity, prominent microvascular proliferation, and necrosis. The recent description of OLIG2 as a specific marker of oligodendroglial tumor cells should provide a useful marker for the diagnosis of these tumors.[82]

MOLECULAR BIOLOGY

Tumor-specific allelic loss has been thought to represent the second hit resulting in the inactivation of a tumor suppressor gene and can be detected by loss of heterozygosity (LOH) analysis.[83,84] Molecular studies have found LOH for polymorphic markers on chromosomes 19q and 1p in up to 80 per cent of both low-grade and anaplastic tumors.[85,86] Additional, but less frequent, losses are seen on chromosomes 9q (involving the *P16/CDKN2A* locus) and 10q, where *PTEN* is one of the target genes.[87,88] Recent evidence suggests that there are two distinct molecular pathways, the first involving loss of 1p and 19q and the second involving the *P16/CDKN2A* locus, 10q loss, and *EGFR* amplification.[89] This also correlates with response to treatment, as discussed below.

IMAGING

CT appearances are usually of low-density lesions with as many as 50 per cent showing calcification. MRI reveals mixed isointense and hypointense T1-weighted images and hyperintense T2-weighted images.[77,78]

TREATMENT AND OUTCOME

Complete resection provides the best chance of long-term progression-free survival. In pediatric series, histological grade is a strong predictor of survival, as are tumor location and clinical features, with posterior fossa tumors having a particularly poor prognosis.[77,78] A close correlation between clinical presentation with raised intracranial hypertension, anaplasia, and poor outcome has also been reported.[79]

Oligodendrogliomas in adults are characterized by their sensitivity to chemotherapy with procarbazine, lomustine, and vincristine. However, up to a third of tumors do not respond to this regime. Interestingly, the molecular profile of the tumors is more predictive of response than either histopathology or clinical features. LOH for 1p and 19q is a statistically significant predictor of chemosensitivity and a longer relapse-free survival. Conversely, tumors with deletions involving the *P16/CDKN2A* locus fare badly.[90] The importance of these specific molecular signatures in pediatric tumors has not yet been established.

Radiotherapy has been used variably. In one pediatric series, all intermediate-grade tumors were irradiated,[78] while in others radiotherapy was reserved for recurrence.[79,80] In posterior fossa tumors, craniospinal radiotherapy is indicated due to the risk of leptomeningeal dissemination.[77]

Table 22.1 *Anatomical localization of gliomatosis cerebri*[91]

Location	%
Cerebral hemispheres	76
Mesencephalon	52
Pons	52
Thalamus	43
Basal ganglia	34
Cerebellum	29
Leptomeningeal involvement	17
Hypothalamus/optic pathway/spinal cord	9

GLIOMATOSIS CEREBRI

Gliomatosis cerebri is characterized by a diffuse neoplastic proliferation of glial cells distributed through neural structures, whose anatomical configuration remain intact. The disease process is usually extensive, often involving both cerebral hemispheres and infratentorial structures (Table 22.1). Gliomatosis cerebri has been divided into two forms: type I, the classic, diffusely infiltrative glioma, with no obvious tumor mass, and type II, where diffuse infiltrative disease coexists with a tumor mass.[91] The term "secondary gliomatosis cerebri" has also been used to describe the remote, contiguous infiltration of tumor cells from a previously diagnosed glioma.[92,93]

Although gliomatosis cerebri had been described previously by other authors, it was Samuel Nevin who first coined the term to describe a group of cases with similar pathological and clinical signs.[94] Gliomatosis cerebri is now considered a distinct and separate clinicopathological entity rather than a non-specific pattern of glial infiltration.

Clinical features

The clinical diagnosis of gliomatosis cerebri is very difficult because of the variability of the symptoms (which include mental changes, ataxia, headaches, seizures, and nausea) and the lack of focal neurological signs in the early course of the disease.[91,93–99] The pre-diagnostic symptomatic interval ranges from days to 23 years, although the majority of patients are symptomatic for less than 12 months (Table 22.2).[91] In the pre-modern imaging era, gliomatosis cerebri was usually diagnosed at postmortem.

The peak age incidence is 40–50 years, but gliomatosis cerebri has been reported in the neonatal period.[91] Gliomatosis cerebri has been reported in association with neurofibromatosis type 1 (NF-1), and in one review almost ten per cent of patients were reported to have this

Table 22.2 *Presenting symptoms of gliomatosis cerebri[91]*

Clinical sign	% (*n* = 110)
Cortical spinal tract deficits	58
Dementia/mental changes	44
Headache	39
Seizures	38
Raised intracranial pressure	37
Cranioneuropathies	33
Spinocerebellar deficit	33
Mental status changes/behavioral changes/psychoses	20
Sensory changes	18
Visual alterations	17
Pain	3

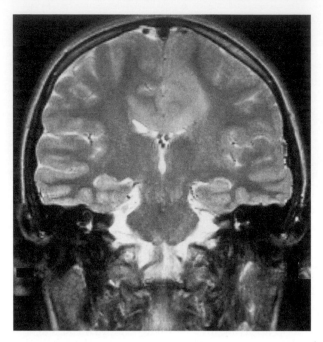

Figure 22.1 *Gliomatosis cerebri.*

condition.[96,100] An association with epidermal nevus syndrome has also been reported.

Overall, the prognosis is poor. Given the difficulties in making this diagnosis of exclusion, survival is best determined from the onset of symptoms. In the largest series analyzed, 52 per cent of patients were dead within 12 months, with only 15 per cent surviving more than 36 months.[91]

Imaging

MRI is superior to CT scanning in detecting gliomatosis cerebri.[98] MRI findings include poorly defined and diffuse high signal intensity on T2-weighted images. A mass effect is often apparent. Gadolinium enhancement is suggestive of malignant transformation.[101,102,103] It is the extensive infiltrative appearances that suggest the diagnosis of gliomatosis cerebri (Figure 22.1).

Positron-emission tomography (PET) scanning in gliomatosis cerebri has shown that the cortical gray matter is hypometabolic compared with normal gray matter.[101] Hypometabolic regions corresponding to the most obvious MRI abnormality have also been reported in two cases of childhood gliomatosis cerebri, with a third case showing a hypermetabolic signal.[91] These findings suggest that the cerebral cortex becomes functionally disconnected owing to the infiltrative nature of gliomatosis cerebri, which in turn may account for the high incidence of dementia noted in the course of this disease.

Histology

Gliomatosis cerebri is characterized by the widespread infiltration of neoplastic glial cells, with minimal destruction of pre-existing structures. Perineuronal, perivascular, or subpial tumor collections may be seen. The infiltrating cells may vary from small cells with little cytoplasm to cells with moderate cytoplasm. The nuclei vary from elongated, to oval, to round. A wide variation in cellularity and cytological composition is often seen. The histological features generally associated with localized anaplastic astrocytoma and glioblastoma multiforme, such as vascular proliferation in necrosis, are not usually seen in gliomatosis cerebri.[99] Mitotic activity is variable. GFAP is reported to be positive in the majority of cases.[96] Electron microscopic study reveals a neoplastic process of small, undifferentiated elements, transitional forms of astroglial to oligodendroglial, and anaplastic cells of astrocytic origin in all stages of development.[104]

The KI-67 labeling index has been shown to have a prognostic value in one study. An increased staining pattern was associated significantly with poor prognosis.[98] This factor therefore deserves further evaluation.

Nevin hypothesized that gliomatosis cerebri comprised mainly blastomatous malformations arising from a congenital defect, but he recognized the difficulty in determining where malformation ended and true tumor formation began.[94] Whether gliomatosis cerebri arises as a diffuse infiltrating lesion from a single focus,[105] as a multicentric origin with centrifugal infiltration,[94,106] or as a process of diffuse malignant transformation[93] is unclear.

The cell of origin is unknown, although most cases show similar phenotypic features to astrocytomas. There are occasional cases in which the predominant cell type is oligodendroglial.[93,96,107–111] Gliomatosis cerebri is therefore still included in the group of neuroepithelial tumors of unknown origin.[112] Classic and molecular cytogenetic analysis of one case of gliomatosis cerebri from a 12-year-old boy revealed 44.XY, del(6)(q25), del(14) (q21), del(15,21)(q10;q10), add18(q22), del(19)(p12), add(20) (p13),-21. A smaller proportion of cells had 88 chromosomes, with a doubling of the abnormal karyotype, consistent with a clonal neoplasm arising from a single cell.[111] However, in one other case investigated at the molecular level, opposite patterns of chromosome X inactivation in tissue sampled from different regions of an apparently contiguous lesion suggest at least a dual origin of this condition instability.[112] Gliomatosis cerebri may therefore result from "collision gliomas." Microsatellite instability was also noted in the latter case, a finding common to other malignant gliomas.[113] Interestingly, in the one case analyzed at the cytogenetic level, the chromosomal changes are distinct from those normally seen in malignant gliomas.[111] More research is needed to determine whether gliomatosis cerebri belongs to a separate category of brain tumors. Why the transformed glial cells lose anchorage dependence to become migratory as well as proliferative is unclear.

Treatment and management

Gliomatosis cerebri is a diagnosis of exclusion and therefore requires biopsy confirmation, which should ideally be performed stereotactically. However, there is often a poor correlation between biopsy and autopsy findings.[94,96,114,115] Diagnosis from cerebrospinal fluid (CSF) has been reported, but lumbar puncture may be hazardous in this condition.[116] The management of raised intracranial pressure is important and may provide relief of symptoms, either by inserting a shunt or resecting areas of edematous brain tissue to relieve the mass effect. However, because of the diffuse infiltrative nature of this disease, surgery is rarely more than palliative.

The role of radiation therapy remains unclear. Three papers suggest that radiotherapy may at least provide a survival advantage.[97,98,117] Twelve of a group of 16 adult patients with imaging- and biopsy-proven gliomatosis cerebri and receiving more than 50 Gy of whole-brain radiotherapy were surviving, with a median follow-up of 80 months.[98] Whole-brain radiotherapy using 50 Gy would therefore appear to have some merit and is recommended therapy, but it requires further evaluation.

Whether gliomatosis is indeed a distinct entity or just one end of the spectrum of glioblastoma multiforme is unclear. Further research may help to unravel this conundrum.

HYPOTHALAMIC HAMARTOMAS

Hypothalamic hamartomas are congenital malformations consisting of ectopic neurons of variable maturity and glial cells arranged irregularly in a fibrillary matrix.

They arise from cells forming the hypothalamic sulcus, which divide the diencephalon into a dorsal (thalamus) and a ventral (hypothalamic) region. These tumors typically form below the tuber cinerium, posterior to the pituitary stalk. The tumors may be pedunculated or sessile.[118] Hypothalamic hamartomas have been categorized, on the basis of the MRI appearance, into panhypothalamic and intrahypothalamic.[119]

Hypothalamic hamartomas are frequently seen in the context of congenital syndromes associated with craniofacial and skeletal anomalies.[120] Screening for hypothalamic hamartomas by MRI scanning is recommended in the Pallister–Hall syndrome (an autosomal dominant condition characterized by oral-facial, cardiac, lung, renal, genital, anal, and limb malformation). Other predisposition syndromes include the oral-facial-digital syndrome type 5 (Varadi syndrome) and several cases of holoprosencephaly.[121,122]

Hypothalamic hamartomas can be asymptomatic, but they are frequently associated with precocious puberty and/or gelastic seizures. High-quality neuroimaging is therefore mandatory in any child with either symptom. Behavioral problems such as aggression and impairment of memory are also reported. Panhypothalamic tumors tend to be associated with precocious puberty, while intrahypothalamic tumors are more frequently associated with epilepsy and developmental delay/behavioral disorders.[119]

Hypothalamic hamartomas appear as well-defined, non-enhancing lesions that are isointense on T1 but may be hyperintense on T2 MRI (Figure 22.2).[123] These lesions usually remain the same size for considerable periods of time.[124]

Both precocious puberty and gelastic epilepsy can be controlled medically. Gonadotrophin-releasing hormone (GnRH) agonist analogs effectively and safely control precocious puberty with few long-term side effects.[125–127] The management of gelastic seizures may be more difficult, especially with increasing time,[126] and there has been an

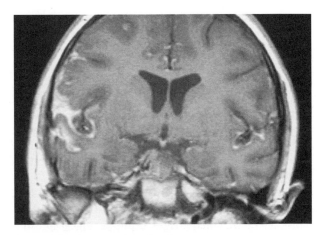

Figure 22.2 *Leptomeningeal melanoma.*

increasing trend for symptomatic lesions to be removed surgically.[128–130] Although complete resection can reverse precocious puberty and cure the gelastic seizures, a number of reports have found that surgery was only partially effective in controlling seizures.[123,130] The procedure is not without surgical risk, although the use of surgical navigational devices may have favored better surgical results.[130,131]

The successful use of focal radiotherapy (radio surgery) has also been reported in a few cases, but the late effects of this form of treatment are unclear and warrant careful consideration before recommending this approach.[132]

PINEAL PARENCHYMAL TUMORS

Pineal parenchymal tumors account for between two and eight per cent of pediatric brain tumors. Approximately half of these are germ-cell tumors, a third are pineal parenchymal tumors, and most of the others are astrocytomas. The management of germ-cell tumors is discussed in Chapter 18a and that of astrocytomas in Chapters 13a, 13b, and 14.

Pineal parenchymal tumors arise from pineocytes. These are cells with neuroendocrine and photosensory functions. The WHO classification includes pineocytoma (WHO grade II), pineoblastoma (WHO grade IV), and pineal parenchymal tumors of intermediate differentiation.

Pineoblastomas

Pineoblastomas are malignant primitive embryonal tumors that are now considered to be within the group of PNETs. They are managed along the same lines as other PNETs (see Chapter 16).

Pineocytomas

Pineocytomas account for approximately 45 per cent of pediatric pineal parenchymal tumors. They are typically slow-growing and composed of small, uniform, mature cells resembling pineocytes, with occasional large pineocytomatous rosettes. They generally occur in older children, particularly in the teenage years. Patients often present with symptoms and signs of raised intracranial pressure. As with other pineal area tumors, patients often present with Parinaud's syndrome, which consists of paralysis of upward gaze, nystagmus, eyelid retraction, and pupils that react more to light than to accommodation. On MRI, pineocytomas are generally well-circumscribed, contrast-enhancing, and hypodense on T1- and hyperdense on T2-weighted images. Leptomeningeal spread is rare[133] but has been described.[134]

Treatment should be with surgical resection where feasible. If complete or subtotal resection is achieved, then the outcome is generally good; it is uncertain whether adjuvant treatment is appropriate in these circumstances.[135] Following partial resection or biopsy, postoperative radiotherapy is generally employed using focal fields to a dose of 50–55 Gy. Following this approach, five-year survival of 86 per cent has been achieved.[136]

Pineal parenchymal tumors of intermediate differentiation

Pineal parenchymal tumors of intermediate differentiation are rare. They account for approximately ten per cent of pineal parenchymal tumors. Management has varied from surgery alone[135] to craniospinal radiotherapy.[136] It is unclear as to how these rare tumors are best managed.

INTRACRANIAL MELANOMAS AND OTHER MELANOTIC TUMORS

Primary melanoma arising in the central nervous system (CNS) may present as a focal mass in the brain or spinal cord or as diffuse leptomeningeal disease.[137–139] Approximately 20 per cent of children with primary cutaneous melanoma develop brain metastases.[140]

Primary leptomeningeal melanomas

Primary leptomeningeal melanomas arise from malignant transformation of melanocytes that are normally found distributed sparsely throughout the leptomeninges.[137–139] Approximately 25 per cent of cases occur in association with neurocutaneous melanosis (NCM), which is characterized by numerous and/or large congenital nevi in association with pigmentation of the leptomeninges. NCM commonly occurs before the age of ten years, with most patients presenting below the age of two years.[137,139,141,142] The majority of patients are asymptomatic until the time of presentation, which is usually with an acute intracerebral event. In view of the rarity of the condition, the association between cutaneous and cerebral melanosis is not always appreciated immediately. Patients with nevi in a posterior axial location on the neck, head, back, and/or buttocks are at a greater risk of developing malignant CNS manifestations of NCM.[143,144]

Diffuse involvement of the basal leptomeninges from meningeal melanosis, whether or not it is associated with cutaneous signs, may be associated with a communicating hydrocephalus. NCM is associated with the Dandy–Walker syndrome. The clinical presentation in infancy tends to be more acute, while children presenting later in life may have more chronic symptoms. Neuropsychiatric presentations including depression and psychosis have also been reported.[145,146] The development of symptoms related to raised intracranial pressure can predate the appearance of malignant change of the leptomeningeal lesions. Progression of neurological symptoms is usually rapid, even in the absence of malignant transformation, and the overall prognosis is poor.[147]

Primary leptomeningeal melanoma is a highly malignant tumor characterized by marked cellular pleomorphism, mitoses, necrosis, and hemorrhage. Metastases may be propagated by a ventricular peritoneal shunt.[148]

CSF examination can help to make the diagnosis, as large pigment-bearing cells can be identified microscopically. Immunohistochemical analysis and electron microscopy may also help to confirm the diagnosis.

IMAGING

MRI is the investigation of choice, most cases exhibiting a high signal on T1-weighted images (Figure 22.2). Gadolinium enhancement can be suggestive of malignant transformation.[103] Intracranial melanomas are prone to bleeding, and the signals seen on MRI can therefore vary considerably.

Diagnostic criteria for neurocutaneous melanosis[141]

- Large (diameter 20 cm) or multiple (more than 3) congenital nevi with meningeal melanosis or melanoma.
- No evidence of cutaneous melanoma, except in patients with benign meningeal lesions.
- No evidence of meningeal melanoma, except in patients with benign skin lesions.

TREATMENT

The surgical management is limited to achieving a histological diagnosis, as the widespread involvement of the CNS usually precludes total excision. However, melanomas forming a discrete mass tend to have a better prognosis, particularly if complete surgical resection is possible.[138,149,150]

Chemotherapy is therefore the main mode of tumor control. Numerous chemotherapy agents and regimes have been employed in treating CNS melanoma. Temozolamide, dacarbazine (DTIC), tamoxifen, cisplatin, fotemustine, and interferon alfa-2b have all been used.[151] Nearly all patients with NCM and with CNS melanomas will have multifocal or widespread involvement. Long-term survival from this disease is rare.[139] Malignant melanoma is widely considered to be a radio-resistant tumor.[152] However, dexamethasone and radiotherapy may offer a useful form of palliation.[153]

Benign melanocytic tumors in infancy

These primary melanotic tumors of the meninges usually present as extra-axial, intradural masses that may compress the adjacent brain. The lesions occur most frequently in the posterior fossa and upper cervical spine. They show a local aggressive behavior, but distant metastasis is extremely unusual. Intracranial lesions are more likely to recur than spinal cord tumors.[154]

Melanotic neuroectodermal tumors of infancy

Melanotic neuroectodermal tumors of infancy (MNTIs) are predominantly benign, pigmented neoplasms occurring in the first year of life. They are derived from the neural crest.[155–161] Table 22.3 shows the distribution of cases of MNTIs according to the site of origin of disease. Although considered benign, MNTIs may demonstrate locally invasive behavior, and a number of case reports have documented overt malignant potential.[155,160,162,163] However, it is possible that these cases may now be diagnosed as neuroblastomas or PNETs. CNS involvement of MNTIs is controversial. The local recurrence rate is reported to be 10–15 per cent.[164]

The majority of intracranial lesions occur within the cerebellum, and many authors believe them to be a variant of medulloblastoma. In addition, the age distribution and malignant behavior of these tumors are different from MNTIs at other sites.[158]

PATHOLOGY

MNTIs usually present as firm, lobulated, well-circumscribed masses, compressing but not infiltrating local structures. Microscopically, these tumors are arranged in irregular alveolar, pseudoglandular, and tubular structures separated by dense collagenous stroma.[158] Electron microscopy may aid diagnosis.[160]

Table 22.3 *Distribution of cases of melanotic neuroectodermal tumors of infancy (MNTIs) by site of origin of disease[155–159]*

Site of disease	Cases (*n*)
Maxilla	125
Skull	26
Epididymis	19
Mandible	12
Brain	12
Mediastinum	2
Other (single case reports)	10
Total	206

The immunohistochemical profile adds weight to the argument that MNTIs are of neural crest origin. MNTIs stain positively for neuron-specific enolase (NSE) and S-100 protein. HMB-45 positivity in the epithelial cells of MNTIs demonstrates them to be melanocytes actively producing melanin.[158] There are no distinguishing gross or histological characteristics that are useful in predicting which tumors have aggressive or malignant potential.

It is essential that MNTIs are distinguished from melanomas and from other neural-crest-derived tumors, such as neuroblastoma. Molecular cytogenetic studies are therefore mandatory.

CLINICAL PRESENTATION AND TREATMENT

Although the mainstay of treatment for MNTI is surgery, the extent of surgical resection is controversial. Numerous reports have advocated allowing residual portions of tumor to remain if radical excision would be mutilating.[165,166] Other authors have recommended more aggressive treatment with wide excision of the primary tumor, including a layer of normal bone around the margins.[167] As conservative surgery is so successful, an aggressive approach has to be questioned, particularly as the majority of cases are eventually cured with repeated surgery even when recurrences arise.

Cytotoxic chemotherapy has been used, with limited success, in the treatment of MNTI. Active agents include cisplatin, doxorubicin, vincristine, etoposide, and cyclophosphamide.[168] Radiotherapy has no proven role in the treatment of MNTI.

PEDIATRIC MENINGEAL TUMORS

Primary tumors of the meninges are uncommon in childhood and adolescence, and their characteristics in comparison with their adult counterparts are controversial. The incidence of adult meningiomas in most series of intracranial tumors varies between 13 and 27 per cent. However, in children, the reported incidence of meningeal tumors in primary CNS tumors is much lower, varying between 0.5 and 4.2 per cent, with up to 38 per cent of these being reported as meningeal sarcomas.[169–193]

The broadly grouped meningioma patients presenting after ten years of age behave like adults, although there are differences in their location and sex distribution. The malignant meningeal group, on the other hand, usually presents in the first few years of life, and has a significantly worse survival.

Histology

The histology of many pediatric meningiomas is indistinguishable from their adult counterparts, falling into the usual subtypes of meningioma, which have been well described, including meningothelial, papillary, fibroblastic, transitional, syncytial, angioblastic, and psammomatous. The relevance of subtype to prognosis is less well established.

Some reports suggest a higher incidence of malignant behavior, although in one review of the combined series, incidences of four per cent for malignant meningiomas and 11 per cent for sarcomas were reported.[182] It is interesting that in a large series of 936 adult meningiomas, Jaaskelainen and colleagues reported an incidence of 94.3 per cent benign, 4.7 per cent atypical, and one per cent anaplastic tumors.[194] Part of the confusion is because many, although not all, pediatric series have included meningeal sarcomas or other malignant meningeal neoplasms in their series, lending weight as a whole to the argument that meningeal tumors are more commonly malignant in children. These pediatric meningeal sarcomas are reported to varying degrees, but they would appear to be relatively more common, with reports ranging from four to 16 per cent. [171–193]

The definition of malignant meningiomas is not clear. Neither the classification of meningiomas by Russell and Rubinstein[8] nor that by the WHO includes sarcomas. Jaaskelainen and colleagues propose a cytological grading and classification for meningiomas, including sarcomas (1, benign; 2, atypical; 3, anaplastic; 4, sarcomatous).[194] Another histological subtype reportedly more common in children is the papillary meningioma. This is characterized by perivascular pseudorosettes, separated from vessels by a fine reticulin border. These are usually associated with cytological features suggestive of malignancy and carry a worse prognosis.[194–206]

CLINICAL FEATURES

The meningiomas present with a median age of 11–13 years, and the malignant group presents with a median age of two to three years. Sixty to 80 per cent of patients with meningiomas in adults are female, a predominance that is lacking in pediatric series. In fact, a slight male preponderance has been observed in several series, as summarized by Drake and colleagues, in which 53 per cent of 278 pediatric meningiomas reviewed collectively since 1972 were male.[182] This difference may be due to the presence of circulating estrogens in adult females affecting the development of meningiomas later in life.

The commonest presenting symptoms are those of raised intracranial pressure (headache, vomiting, drowsiness) and focal neurological deficit affecting the limbs or cranial nerves. Epilepsy is also a presenting symptom in up to 25 per cent of meningiomas and 40 per cent of malignant meningeal tumors. Other symptoms include gross frontal bossing, proptosis with optic nerve sheath meningioma, visual disturbance, deafness, and ataxia.

The median duration of symptoms is around four to eight months for meningiomas and four to nine weeks for the malignant tumors. It is clear that the malignant group has a more rapid onset of symptoms, and all present with focal neurological deficit and symptoms of raised intracranial pressure, suggesting advanced disease at presentation.

With regard to location, 90 per cent of the tumors in this age group are supratentorial, and a high proportion (11–31 per cent) of the meningiomas are intraventricular. Adult series of meningiomas have reported an incidence of between two and five per cent for an intraventricular location.

NF-1 and neurofibromatosis type 2 (NF-2) are relatively common in meningiomas. Large series of pediatric meningiomas report an incidence of 23–24 per cent for neurofibromatosis, with spinal and optic nerve sheath meningiomas being more common.[172,174,182,183,187,195,207]

Imaging

Radiological features of childhood meningiomas do not differ significantly in adults. They are typically hemispheric and superficial, with dural attachment. Around 50 per cent show calcification, cystic transformation being more common in children. The solid portion of a meningioma typically shows strong and uniform enhancement on both CT and MRI. One must be aware of more unusual locations in children, e.g. intraventricular, and occasionally with no dural attachment.[48,192,198,199,202,208–210]

Treatment and results

The treatment of choice for these tumors is complete surgical resection, even if this is done in two stages. The operative mortality in early series of pediatric meningiomas was high, probably because of the lack of modern medical support. Thankfully, this has dropped significantly, but one must be mindful of blood loss and attachment to vessels and neurological structures, such as cranial nerves, at surgery. Preoperative angiography and/or embolization may have a role in large tumors. Complete resection is effected in only 54–58 per cent of reported cases due to these difficulties.

In the case of complete resection of meningiomas, no further adjuvant treatment is indicated.

The role of radiotherapy is difficult to evaluate in pediatric meningiomas in subtotal resections due to the small numbers. Second-look surgery should always be considered if possible. In the more histologically aggressive tumors, adjuvant therapy is usually indicated, either as conventionally delivered or as stereotactic radiotherapy to small residuals.

Jaaskelainen and colleagues found that four of five adult anaplastic meningiomas recurred despite complete

excision and radiotherapy.[194] Wilson has reported improved survival for malignant meningiomas in adults when adjuvant radiotherapy has been given.[211] Wilson also reports improved progression-free survival of adults with subtotally removed meningiomas and receiving radiotherapy in the post-1980 era.[211] Similar results have been observed by Goldsmith and colleagues.[212] One of the problems with the pediatric group, however, is that patients with poorly differentiated tumors are often under three years of age, and therefore radiotherapy is generally contraindicated. Hence, there are few data on the role of radiotherapy in pediatric series of meningiomas.

In their review of the literature, Drake and colleagues reported that calculated survival rates of 76 per cent at five years and 55 per cent at 15 years were obtained. These rates increased to 84 and 63 per cent, respectively, when meningeal sarcomas were excluded. The presence of recurrence lowers the survival rates to 64 and 35 per cent for five and 15 years, respectively, in meningiomas. The other factor in outcome is the completeness of tumor removal.[182]

The survival rates for sarcomatous meningiomas are much lower: five- and 15-year survival rates are at best 44 and 27 per cent, respectively.[172,177,181,182,184,195,201,213]

In conclusion, although pediatric meningeal tumors include a relatively high proportion of malignant, poorly differentiated neoplasms that are associated with poor prognosis, meningiomas themselves are associated with good long-term survival following complete resection.

SKULL AND SKULL-BASE TUMORS

Chordoma

As the name would suggest, chordomas develop from vestigial remnants of the primitive notochord.[214] However, their aggressive clinical behavior belies the suffix "–oma." Chordomas present as slow-growing, locally invasive masses, often with extensive bony destruction. Less than five per cent of all chordomas are diagnosed within the pediatric population.[215] Chordomas are more common in boys than girls, and familial clusters have been described. The gene for familial chordoma has been linked to 7q33 by linkage analysis.[216]

Chordomas can arise anywhere within the axial skeleton, but they occur most frequently at either end of the spinal cord, i.e. at the base of the skull (predominantly in the spheno-occipital region) and in the sacrococcygeal region.[217–219] They can also occur in vertebral and extra-axial sites, such as the facial bones, sinuses, and mediastinum.[217–219] Most chordomas are extradural in origin.

There is a greater tendency for chordomas of childhood to metastasize, particularly those presenting in children under five years of age.[217–219] Metastasis is predominantly to lung and then bones.[217–219] A report has identified loss of heterozygosity for the retinoblastoma gene in highly aggressive chordomas.[220]

HISTOLOGY

Histologically, chordomas can be divided into classic and atypical variants. The classic form consists of cords, strands, and clusters of small polygonal cells, with eosinophilic cytoplasm and small hyperchromatic or larger vesicular nuclei in a myxoid matrix. The atypical form, which is more common in childhood, has a sarcomatoid appearance, with round epitheloid or spindle cells arranged in sheets, clusters, or solid nodular masses. Areas of necrosis may be seen. Immunohistochemical profile reveals reactivity, with antibodies to vimentin, cytokeratin, epithelial membrane antigen, and S100.[218,219,221] Electron microscopy is a useful diagnostic adjunct.

Clinical presentation is often late, with a prolonged history of symptoms related to tumor invasion or pressure on local structures. Intracranial hypertension and sixth cranial nerve palsies are the most common presenting features. There may be quadriparesis, dysphagia, dysarthria, and torticollis, reflecting anterior or posterior extension of a clival primary tumor.[217,218] Lower cranial nerve palsies are also reported.[217,218]

Investigation with X-rays and CT/MRI will define the extent of the tumor and is essential for radiotherapy planning.[222]

Surgery has a definitive role in the management of chordomas. Radical local excision is associated with a better outcome.[223,224] In predominantly adult series, a radical total or near-total excision is achieved in 40 per cent of cases; although different surgical approaches have been reported, the overall success and morbidity are similar.[223–225] The restrictions on wide surgical excision, imposed by the tumor site, lead to a high incidence of local recurrence and a poor prognosis.[223]

Most series show a survival advantage to adjuvant radiotherapy, but the optimal conventionally delivered dose is unclear.[222] Charged-particle radiation therapy (proton-beam radiotherapy) appears to give the best local control.[222,226] How this is best delivered is still debatable.[225,226] Salvage treatment following radiotherapy is rarely successful.

Chemotherapy using regimes that incorporate ifosfamide and doxorubicin has been reported as active. Treatment on a sarcoma protocol that includes ifosfamide and an anthracycline, such as the six-drug arm of the malignant mesenchymal tumor (MMT) '95 trial, is therefore appropriate.[227] This raises the possibility that preoperative chemotherapy may lead to tumor shrinkage, thereby improving the surgical resection rate and permitting less extensive radiation fields. Given the risks of extensive surgery and radiation, we feel that a trial of preoperative chemotherapy is justified in patients in whom there is no immediate risk of neurological deterioration.

Proton radiotherapy for skull-base tumors

This physical dose distribution from proton radiotherapy with its sharp cut-off beyond the target volume (Bragg peak) has been used in adults to treat chordomas of the base of skull. These tumors are generally difficult to irradiate because of their close proximity to the brainstem. However, the dose distribution from protons allows an escalation of radiation dose adjacent to radiosensitive structures. The role of proton radiotherapy in skull-base chordoma has been established in a number of series from the Massachusetts General Hospital. In one report, actuarial local control rates for 115 adult patients with base-of-skull chordomas and treated between 1978 and 1993 were 59 per cent at five years and 44 per cent at ten years.[228] Treatment of children with base-of-skull and cervical-spine chordomas has also been shown to be effective. Eighteen children aged between four and 18 years were treated at the Massachusetts General Hospital and Harvard Medical School with a mixed photon/proton regimen.[229] With a median follow-up of 72 months, the five-year actuarial overall and disease-free survival rates were 68 and 63 per cent, respectively. Long-term effects were acceptable. Two children developed growth hormone deficiency, three developed impaired hearing, and one required surgical excision of an area of temporal necrosis, which had resulted in epilepsy. A later series of children aged between one and 19 years and treated with proton radiotherapy for a variety of skull-base tumors has been reported from the same institution.[230] The malignant diagnoses in this group included chordoma (ten), chondrosarcoma (three), rhabdomyosarcoma (four), and other sarcomas (three). The benign diagnoses included giant-cell tumors (six), angiofibroma (two), and chondroblastoma (one). Radiotherapy doses ranged between 50.4 and 78.6 cobalt gray equivalent (CGE). With a median follow-up of 40 months (range 13–92 months), local tumor was controlled in six (60 per cent) patients with chordoma, three (100 per cent) with chondrosarcoma, four (100 per cent) with rhabdomyosarcoma, and two (66 per cent) with other sarcomas. One patient with a giant-cell tumor has experienced a local failure, and the other patients with benign diagnoses have maintained local tumor control. Proton radiotherapy is available in very few institutions, and further clinical research seems justified.

Chondrosarcomas

Chondrosarcomas are less common than chordomas. Apart from the mesenchymal variant,[231,232] these tumors have an indolent behavior warranting their consideration separate from chordomas.[233,234] These tumors are thought to originate from either primitive mesenchymal cells or cartilaginous rests that have failed to ossify.[235] Most arise along the base of the skull, where the chondrocranium is formed. There is a male predominance in most case series.[233,234] An association with Ollier's and Maffucci syndromes has been reported.[236,237]

Radical surgical resection is the treatment of choice, with the caveat of minimizing potential side effects in this indolent tumor. The role of radiotherapy in chondrosarcoma is unclear. Although radiotherapy is often delivered, there is no clear indication for its use.[225,238]

Mesenchymal chondrosarcomas

It is important to distinguish mesenchymal chondrosarcomas from the more benign chondrosarcomas. Although predominantly a bone tumor, a significant number of cases arise from the meninges.[231,239,240] Almost half of the reported cases have occurred in childhood.

The clinical signs are predominantly of headache and focal neurology dictated by the tumor location. Histologically, two predominant components are apparent: undifferentiated mesenchymal cells and bland cartilage.

Radical surgical resection is indicated. Due to the propensity to local recurrence, radiotherapy is indicated, particularly in incomplete resections.[231] Distant metastasis have been reported. Although chemotherapy has been advocated, its efficacy is unclear.[240]

Schwannomas and acoustic neuromas

Neuromas or schwannomas are benign neoplasms presumed to arise from the normal Schwann cells that surround peripheral nerve axons. They are very rare in children, and they are most commonly, but not always, associated with NF-2.[241] Acoustic neuromas usually arise from the sensory component of the eighth (vestibular part) cranial nerve.[242–4]

HISTOLOGY

Typically, these tumors grow in the epineurium of the nerve, leaving the normal nerve tissue separate from the truly encapsulated tumor. This results in gradual attenuation of the nervous tissue. Infiltration is rare but has been reported, especially associated with NF-2. Typical schwannomas have biphasic growth patterns, with solid tissue (Antoni A) composed of spindle cells in fascicles and loose tissue (Antoni B) composed of stellate cells with smaller, rounder nuclei. Sometimes, these tumors demonstrate the classic palisading of nuclei Verocay bodies, which are pathognomic and present in Antoni A areas.

The schwannoma cells are invariably immunopositive for S100 protein, low-affinity nerve growth factor receptor, and Leu-7 antibodies. Occasionally, they display some cells positive for GFAP and other unusual histological features, such as melanin formation (melanotic schwannomas have been described). NF-2 is known to result from mutations in the 22 chromosomes, the normal gene product of which is called merlin. The majority of sporadic schwannomas, and indeed meningiomas, also have a somatic mutation in this gene.

CLINICAL FEATURES

The classic schwannoma seen in the CNS is the acoustic neuroma. This classically presents in the cerebellopontine angle of the posterior fossa. The most usual age of presentation in children is the second decade of life. The most common presenting features are tinnitus and slow, gradual sensineural hearing loss. These tumors are commonly seen in NF-2 as bilateral tumors. However, they have been reported in isolation as sporadic unilateral disease, albeit extremely rarely, with only 39 reports in the literature in children under 16 years of age.

The next most common site for CNS neuromas is on the fifth cranial nerve. Schwannomas have also been described arising in the parenchyma of the CNS. Thus, there are case reports of schwannomas in the cerebral hemispheres, brainstem, ventricles, and spinal cord. These unusual locations can be rationalized by the presence of peripheral nerve fibers (usually autonomic) in vascular walls and leptomeninges.

Among adults with acoustic neuromas, 90 per cent present with unilateral hearing loss and tinnitus. In children, this often goes unnoticed for months and years, until they develop cerebellar signs, facial and other cranial nerve palsies, or symptoms of raised intracranial pressure from obstructive hydrocephalus.

In cases associated with NF-2, the children may have other manifestations of the disease, including neurofibromas, meningiomas, gliomas, posterior subcapsular lens opacity, and cerebral calcification. NF-2 has an autosomal dominant pattern of inheritance with high penetrance. Fifty per cent of new cases of NF-2, however, present as new mutations. The presence of bilateral acoustic neuromas in a child is diagnostic of NF-2. In the presence of unilateral disease, other features of NF-2 should be looked for. The screening process should include whole-CNS MRI with contrast, skin examination for café-au-lait spots, eye examination for posterior capsular cataracts and Lisch nodules, and genetic studies for germ-line mutations. This screening should be offered to first-degree relatives of the affected child.[179,241–258]

TREATMENT

Although these tumors are usually benign, treatment can be associated with a high morbidity. As they are very slow-growing, the timing of treatment in terms of preservation of function is very important, especially in bilateral acoustics.

Surgical management is very much a multidisciplinary approach. The participation of the neurophysiologist is extremely important. Preoperative assessment of seventh and eight nerve functions is very important. Intraoperative monitoring of both facial and acoustic nerve functions is also important. Because pediatric neurosurgeons will come across these tumors very rarely, it is recommended that adult neurosurgical and otological surgeons are consulted and involved in the surgery. These skull-base teams will have a much greater experience with removing these tumors safely and with minimum morbidity.

Acoustic neuromas can be approached by a variety of surgical routes, the lateral suboccipital and translabyrinthine approach being the most common. The aim should be complete resection with facial nerve preservation. The preservation of hearing is now also commonly reported in non-NF-2 patients, at least with smaller tumors. Unfortunately, the results for NF-2 patients are not so good, which impacts further on the fact that these patients have bilateral disease. In these patients, an initial conservative approach to management is often recommended initially, with six-monthly MRI over a few years to establish rate of growth. Surgery can be deferred until (i) rapid tumor growth is established (>1 cm/year), (ii) there are signs of brainstem compression, (iii) the presence of hydrocephalus is detected, and (iv) the presence of hearing discrimination in the affected ear is detected.

The other main treatment that is being evaluated is stereotactic radiotherapy. This has been established, at least in adults, as a useful alternative in the management of these tumors. Most series report tumor control rates with this technique of 90 per cent. There is variation in the reported risk to facial nerve and acoustic nerve damage, based on different tumor sizes and techniques. However, preservation of hearing, so important to NF-2 patients, is still poor.[241–243,247,248,251,252,255,257]

REFERENCES

1 Garrido E, Becker LF, et al. Gangliogliomas in children. A clinicopathological study. Childs Brain 1978; 4:339–46.
2 Sutton LN, Packer RJ, et al. Cerebral gangliogliomas during childhood. Neurosurgery 1983; 13:124–8.
3 Hall WA, Yunis EJ, et al. Anaplastic ganglioglioma in an infant: case report and review of the literature. Neurosurgery 1986; 19:1016–20.
4 Johannsson JH, Rekate HL, et al. Gangliogliomas: pathological and clinical correlations. J Neurosurg 1981; 54:58–63.
5 Courville GB. Ganglioglioma. Tumour of the central nervous system: review of the literature and report of two cases. Arch Neurol Psychiatry 1930; 24:439–91.
6 Haddad SF, Moore SA, et al. Ganglioglioma: 13 years of experience. Neurosurgery 1992; 31:171–8.
7 Sasaki A, Hirato J, et al. Recurrent anaplastic ganglioglioma: pathological characterisation of tumour cells. J Neurosurg 1996; 84:1055–9.
8 Russell DS, Rubenstein LJ. Ganglioglioma: a case with a long history and malignant evolution. J Neuropathol Exp Neurol 1962; 21:185–93.
9 Demierre B, Stichnoth FA, et al. Intracerbral ganglioglioma. J Neurosurg 1986; 65:177–82.
10 Garcia CA, McGarry PA, et al. Ganglioglioma of the brain stem. J Neurosurg 1984; 60:431–4.
11 Chilton J, Caughron MR, et al. Ganglioglioma of the optic chiasm: case report and review of the literature. Neurosurgery 1990; 26:1042–5.
12 Tien R, Tuori L, et al. Ganglioglioma with leptomeningeal and subarachnoid spread: results of CT, MR and PET imaging. Am J Radiol 1992; 159:391–3.
13 Lang FF, Epstein FJ, et al. Central nervous system gangliogliomas. Part 2: Clinical outcome. J Neurosurg 1993; 79:867–73.
14 Daumas-Duport C, Varlet P, et al. Dysembryoplastic neuroepithelial tumors: nonspecific histological forms – a study of 40 cases. J Neuro-Oncol 1999; 41:267–80.
15 Aronica E, Leenstra S, et al. Glioneuronal tumors and medically intractable epilepsy: a clinical study with long-term follow-up of seizure outcome after surgery. Epilepsy Res 2001; 43:179–91.
16 Blumcke I, Wiestler OD. Gangliogliomas: an intriguing tumor entity associated with focal epilepsies. J Neuropathol Exp Neurol 2002; 61:575–84.
17 Celli P, Scarpinati M, et al. Gangliogliomas of the cerebral hemispheres. Report of 14 cases with long-term follow-up and review of the literature. Acta Neurochir (Wien) 1993; 125:52–7.
18 Kim SK, Wang KC, et al. Intractable epilepsy associated with brain tumors in children: surgical modality and outcome. Childs Nerv Syst 2001; 17:445–52.
19 Komori T, Scheithauer BW, et al. Papillary glioneuronal tumor: a new variant of mixed neuronal-glial neoplasm. Am J Surg Pathol 1998; 22:1171–83.
20 Pollack IF, Claassen D, et al. Low-grade gliomas of the cerebral hemispheres in children – an analysis of 71 cases. J Neurosurg 1995; 82:536–47.
21 Taratuto AL, Pomata H, et al. Dysembryoplastic neuroepithelial tumor: morphological, immunocytochemical, and deoxyribonucleic acid analyses in a pediatric series. Neurosurgery 1995; 36:474–81.
22 Duffner PK, Burger PC, et al. Desmoplastic infantile gangliogliomas: an approach to therapy. Neurosurgery 1994; 34:583–9.
23 Giannini C, Scheithauer BW. Classification and grading of low-grade astrocytic tumors in children. Brain Pathol 1997; 7:785–98.
24 Kepes JJ, Rubinstein LJ, et al. Pleomorphic xanthoastrocytoma: a distinctive meningocerebral glioma of young subjects with

relatively favorable prognosis. A study of 12 cases. *Cancer* 1979; **44**:1839–52.

25 Kepes JJ. Astrocytomas: old and newly recognized variants, their spectrum of morphology and antigen expression. *Can J Neurol Sci* 1987; **14**:109–21.

26 Louis DN, von Deimling A, *et al.* Desmoplastic cerebral astrocytomas of infancy: a histopathologic, immunohistochemical, ultrastructural, and molecular genetic study. *Hum Pathol* 1992; **23**:1402–9.

27 Mallucci C, Lellouch-Tubiana A, *et al.* The management of desmoplastic neuroepithelial tumours in childhood. *Childs Nerv Syst* 2000; **16**:8–14.

28 Paulus W, Schlote W, *et al.* Desmoplastic supratentorial neuroepithelial tumours of infancy. *Histopathology* 1992; **21**:43–9.

29 Powell SZ, Yachnis AT, *et al.* Divergent differentiation in pleomorphic xanthoastrocytoma. Evidence for a neuronal element and possible relationship to ganglion cell tumors. *Am J Surg Pathol* 1996; **20**:80–5.

30 Prayson RA. Composite ganglioglioma and dysembryoplastic neuroepithelial tumor. *Arch Pathol Lab Med* 1999; **123**:247–50.

31 Rushing EJ, Rorke LB, *et al.* Problems in the nosology of desmoplastic tumors of childhood. *Pediatr Neurosurg* 1993; **19**:57–62.

32 VandenBerg SR, May EE, *et al.* Desmoplastic supratentorial neuroepithelial tumors of infancy with divergent differentiation potential (desmoplastic infantile gangliogliomas). Report on 11 cases of a distinctive embryonal tumor with favorable prognosis. *J Neurosurg* 1987; **66**:58–71.

33 VandenBerg SR. Desmoplastic infantile ganglioglioma and desmoplastic cerebral astrocytoma of infancy. *Brain Pathol* 1993; **3**:275–81.

34 Taratuto AL, Monges J, *et al.* Superficial cerebral astrocytoma attached to dura. Report of six cases in infants. *Cancer* 1984; **54**:2505–12.

35 Chintagumpala MM, Armstrong D, *et al.* Mixed neuronal–glial tumors (gangliogliomas) in children. *Pediatr Neurosurg* 1996; **24**:306–13.

36 Craver RD, Nadell J, *et al.* Desmoplastic infantile ganglioglioma. *Pediatr Dev Pathol* 1999; **2**:582–7.

37 De Munnynck K, Van Gool S, *et al.* Desmoplastic infantile ganglioglioma: a potentially malignant tumor? *Am J Surg Pathol* 2002; **26**:1515–22.

38 Miller DC, Lang FF, *et al.* Central nervous system gangliogliomas. Part 1: pathology. *J Neurosurg* 1993; **79**:859–66.

39 Kordek R, Liberski PP. Infantile desmoplastic ganglioglioma and desmoplastic cerebral astrocytoma of infancy. *Pol J Pathol* 2001; **52** (4 suppl.):95–8.

40 Mizuno M. Desmoplastic infantile ganglioglioma (DIG). *Ryoikibetsu Shokogun Shirizu* 2000; **28**:75–6.

41 Olas E, Kordek R, *et al.* Desmoplastic cerebral astrocytoma of infancy: a case report. *Folia Neuropathol* 1998; **36**:45–51.

42 Rothman S, Sharon N, *et al.* Desmoplastic infantile ganglioglioma. *Acta Oncol* 1997; **36**:655–7.

43 Rout P, Santosh V, *et al.* Desmoplastic infantile ganglioglioma – clinicopathological and immunohistochemical study of four cases. *Childs Nerv Syst* 2002; **18**:463–7.

44 Setty SN, Miller DC, *et al.* Desmoplastic infantile astrocytoma with metastases at presentation. *Mod Pathol* 1997; **10**:945–51.

45 Taguchi Y, Sakurai T, *et al.* Desmoplastic infantile ganglioglioma with extraparenchymatous cyst – case report. *Neurol Med Chir (Tokyo)* 1993; **33**:177–80.

46 Torres LF, Reis Filho JS, *et al.* Infantile desmoplastic ganglioglioma: a clinical, histopathological and epidemiological study of five cases. *Arq Neuropsiquiatr* 1998; **56**:443–8.

47 Bucciero A, De Caro M, *et al.* Pleomorphic xanthoastrocytoma: clinical, imaging and pathological features of four cases. *Clin Neurol Neurosurg* 1997; **99**:40–5.

48 Finizio FS. CT and MRI aspects of supratentorial hemispheric tumors of childhood and adolescence. *Childs Nerv Syst* 1995; **11**:559–67.

49 Martin DS, Levy B, *et al.* Desmoplastic infantile ganglioglioma: CT and MR features. *Am J Neuroradiol* 1991; **12**:1195–7.

50 Tenreiro-Picon OR, Kamath SV, *et al.* Desmoplastic infantile ganglioglioma: CT and MRI features. *Pediatr Radiol* 1995; **25**:540–3.

51 De Chadarevian JP, Pattisapu J, *et al.* Desmoplastic astrocytoma of infancy. Light microscopy, immunohistochemistry, and ultrastructure. *Cancer* 1990; **66**:173–9.

52 Grant JW, Gallagher PJ. Pleomorphic xanthoastrocytoma. Immunohistochemical methods for differentiation from fibrous histiocytomas with similar morphology. *Am J Surg Pathol* 1986; **10**:336–41.

53 Giannini C, Scheithauer BW, *et al.* Pleomorphic xanthoastrocytoma: what do we really know about it? *Cancer* 1999; **85**:2033–45.

54 Chou SM. Pleomorphic xanthoastrocytoma versus glioblastoma multiforme. *Zhonghua Bing Li Xue Za Zhi* 1986; **15**:277–8.

55 Brown JH, Chew FS. Pleomorphic xanthoastrocytoma. *Am J Roentgenol* 1993; **160**:1272.

56 Bayindir C, Balak N, *et al.* Anaplastic pleomorphic xanthoastrocytoma. *Childs Nerv Syst* 1997; **13**:50–6.

57 Paulus W, Lisle DK, *et al.* Molecular genetic alterations in pleomorphic xanthoastrocytoma. *Acta Neuropathol* 1996; **91**:293–7.

58 Cervoni L, Salvati M, *et al.* Pleomorphic xanthoastrocytoma: some observations. *Neurosurg Rev* 1996; **19**:13–16.

59 Davies KG, Maxwell RE, *et al.* Pleomorphic xanthoastrocytoma – report of four cases, with MRI scan appearances and literature review. *Br J Neurosurg* 1994; **8**:681–9.

60 Lipper MH, Eberhard DA, *et al.* Pleomorphic xanthoastrocytoma, a distinctive astroglial tumor: neuro-radiologic and pathologic features. *Am J Neuroradiol* 1993; **14**:1397–404.

61 Sundaram C, Naidu MR, *et al.* Pleomorphic xanthoastrocytoma – a clinicopathological study. *Indian J Pathol Microbiol* 2000; **43**:357–61.

62 Tonn JC, Paulus W, *et al.* Pleomorphic xanthoastrocytoma: report of six cases with special consideration of diagnostic and therapeutic pitfalls. *Surg Neurol* 1997; **47**:162–9.

63 Cartmill M, Hewitt M, *et al.* The use of chemotherapy to facilitate surgical resection in pleomorphic

xanthoastrocytoma: experience in a single case. *Childs Nerv Syst* 2001; **17**:563–6.

64 Kepes JJ, Rubinstein LJ, *et al.* Histopathological features of recurrent pleomorphic xanthoastrocytomas: further corroboration of the glial nature of this neoplasm. A study of 3 cases. *Acta Neuropathol (Berl)* 1989; **78**:585–93.

65 Bucciero A, De Caro MI, *et al.* Atypical pleomorphic xanthoastrocytoma. *J Neurosurg Sci* 1998; **42**:153–7.

66 Prayson RA, Morris HH, 3rd. Anaplastic pleomorphic xanthoastrocytoma. *Arch Pathol Lab Med* 1998; **122**:1082–6.

67 Pai MR, Kini H, *et al.* Pleomorphic xanthoastrocytoma. *Indian J Pathol Microbiol* 1996; **39**:329–31.

68 Ohta S, Ryu H, *et al.* Eighteen-year survival of a patient with malignant pleomorphic xanthoastrocytoma associated with von Recklinghausen neurofibromatosis. *Br J Neurosurg* 1999; **13**:420–2.

69 Kordek R, Biernat W, *et al.* Pleomorphic xanthoastrocytoma and desmoplastic infantile ganglioglioma – have these neoplasms a common origin? *Folia Neuropathol* 1994; **32**:237–9.

70 Maleki M, Robitaille Y, *et al.* Atypical xanthoastrocytoma presenting as a meningioma. *Surg Neurol* 1983; **20**:235–8.

71 Loiseau H, Rivel J, *et al.* Pleomorphic xanthoastrocytoma. Apropos of 3 new cases. Review of the literature. *Neurochirurgie* 1991; **37**:338–47.

72 Kros JM, Vecht CJ, *et al.* The pleomorphic xanthoastrocytoma and its differential diagnosis: a study of five cases. *Hum Pathol* 1991; **22**:1128–35.

73 Jones MC, Drut R, *et al.* Pleomorphic xanthoastrocytoma: a report of two cases. *Pediatr Pathol* 1983; **1**:459–67.

74 Heyerdahl Strom E, Skullerud K. Pleomorphic xanthoastrocytoma: report of 5 cases. *Clin Neuropathol* 1983; **2**:188–91.

75 Fouladi M, Jenkins J, *et al.* Pleomorphic xanthoastrocytoma: favorable outcome after complete surgical resection. *Neurooncol* 2001; **3**:184–92.

76 Nam D-H, Cho B-K, *et al.* Intramedullary anaplastic oligodendroglioma in a child. *Childs Nerv Syst* 1998; **14**:127–30.

77 Packer RJ, Sutton LN, *et al.* Oligodendrogliomas of the posterior fossa in children. *Cancer* 1985; **56**:195–9.

78 Razak N, Baumgartner J, *et al.* Pediatric oligodenrogliomas. *Pediatr Neurosurg* 1998; **28**:121–9.

79 Rizk T, Mottolese C, *et al.* Cerebral oligodendrogliomas in children: an analysis of 15 cases. *Childs Nerv Syst* 1996; **12**:527–9.

80 Dohrmann GJ, Farwell JR, *et al.* Oligodendrogliomas in children. *Surg Neurol* 1978; **10**:21–5.

81 Coons SW, Johnson PC, Scheithauer BW, Yates AJ, Pearl DK. Improving the diagnostic accuracy and interobserver concordance in the classification and grading of primary gliomas. *Cancer* 1997; **79**:1381–93.

82 Marie Y, Sanson M, *et al.* OLIG2 as a specific marker of oligodendroglial tumour cells. *Lancet* 2001; **358**:298–300.

83 Knudson AG. Mutation and cancer: statistical study of retinoblastoma. *Proc Natl Acad Sci USA* 1971; **68**:820–3.

84 Cavenee WK, Dryja TP, *et al.* Expression of recessive alleles by chromosomal mechanisms in retinoblastoma. *Nature* 1983; **305**:779–84.

85 Deimling AV, Louis DN, *et al.* Evidence for a tumour suppressor gene on chromosome 19q associated with human astrocytomas, oligodendrogliomas and mixed gliomas. *Cancer Res* 1992; **52**:4277–9.

86 Kraus JA, Koopman J, *et al.* Shared allelic losses on chromosomes 1p and 19q suggest a common origin of oligodendroglioma and oligoastrocytoma. *J Neuropathol Exp Neurol* 1995; **54**:91–5.

87 Reifenberger J, Reifenberger G, *et al.* Molecular genetic analysis of oligodendroglial tumours shows preferential alleleic deletions on19q and 1p. *Am J Pathol* 1994; **145**:1175–90.

88 Sasaki H, Zlatescu MC, *et al.* PTEN is the target of chromosome 10q loss in anaplastic oligodendrogliomas and PTEN alterations are associated with poor prognosis. *Am J Pathol* 2001; **159**:359–67.

89 Huong-Xuan K, He J, *et al.* Molecular heterogeneity of oligodendrogliomas suggests alternative pathways in tumour progression. *Neurology* 2001; **57**:1278–81.

90 Cairncross JG, Ueki K, *et al.* Specific genetic predictors of chemotherapeutic response and survival in patients with anaplastic oligodendrogliomas. *J Natl Cancer Inst* 1998; **90**:1473–9.

91 Jennings MT, Frenchman M, *et al.* Gliomatosis cerebri presenting as intractable epilepsy during early childhood. *J Child Neurol* 1995; **10**:37–45.

92 Burger PC, Dubois PJ, *et al.* Computerised tomographic and pathologic studies of untreated quiescent and recurrent glioblastoma multiforme. *J Neurosurg* 1983; **58**:159–69.

93 Ross IB, Robitaille Y, *et al.* Diagnosis and management of gliomatosis cerebri – recent trends. *Surg Neurol* 1991; **36**:431–40.

94 Nevin S. Gliomatosis cerebri of the brain. *Brain* 1938; **61**:170–91.

95 Couch JR, Weiss SA. Gliomatosis cerebri: reports of four cases and review of the literature. *Neurology* 1974; **24**:504–11.

96 Artigas J, Cervosnavarro J, *et al.* Gliomatosis cerebri – clinical and histological-findings. *Clin Neuropathol* 1985; **4**:135–48.

97 Hejazi N, Witzmann A, *et al.* Gliomatosis cerebri: intra vitam stereotactic determination in two cases and review of the literature. *Br J Neurosurg* 2001; **15**:396–401.

98 Kim DG, Yang HJ, *et al.* Gliomatosis cerebri: clinical features, treatment and prognosis. *Acta Neurochir* 1998; **140**:755–62.

99 Kandler RH, Smith CM, *et al.* Gliomatosis cerebri a clinical, radiological and pathologial report for cases. *Br J Neurosurg* 1991; **5**:187–93.

100 Scharenberg E, Jones E. Diffuse glioma of the brain in von Recklinghausen's disease. A study with silver carbonate. *Neurology* 1956; **6**:269–74.

101 Plowman PN, Saunders CAB, *et al.* Gliomatosis cerebri: disconnection of the cortical grey matter, demonstrated on PET scan. *Br J Neurosurg* 1998; **12**:240–4.

102 Barkovich AJ, Frieden IJ, *et al.* MR of neurocutaneous melanosis. *Am J Neuroradiol* 1994; **15**:859–67.

103 Byrd SE, Darling CF, *et al.* MR imaging of symptomatic neurocutaneous melanosis in children. *Pediatr Radiol* 1997; **27**:39–44.

104 Cervos-Navarro J, Artigas J, et al. The fine structure of gliomatosis cerebri. *Virchows Arch A Pathol Anat Histopathol* 1987; **411**:93–8.

105 Russell, DS, Rubenstein LJ. *Pathology of Tumours of the Nervous System*. Baltimore: Williams and Wilkins, 1989.

106 Malamud N, Wise BL, et al. Gliomatosis cerebri. *J Neurosurg* 1952; **9**:409–17.

107 Balko MG, Blisard KS, et al. Oligodendroglial gliomatosis cerebri. *Hum Pathol* 1992; **23**:706–7.

108 Tancredi A, Mangiola A, et al. Oligodendrocytic gliomatosis cerebri. *Acta Neurochir* 2000; **142**:469–72.

109 Roberts P, Lockwood LR, et al. Cytogenetic abnormalities in mesoblastic nephroma: a link to Wilms tumour? *Med Pediatr Oncol* 1993; **21**:416–20.

110 Ortin TS, Shostak CA, et al. Gonadal status and reproductive function following treatment for Hodgkin's disease in childhood: the Stanford experience. *Int J Radiat Oncol Biol Phys* 1990; **19**:873–80.

111 Hecht BK, Turc-Carel C, et al. Chromosomes in gliomatosis cerebri. *Genes Chromosomes Cancer* 1995; **14**:149–53.

112 Kattar MM, Kupsky WJ, et al. Clonal analysis of gliomas. *Hum Pathol* 1997; **28**:1166–78.

113 Dams E, Van de Kelft EJ, et al. Instability of microsatellites in human gliomas. *Cancer Res* 1995; **55**:1547–9.

114 Schober R, Mai JK, et al. Gliomatosis cerebri: bioptical approach and neuropathological verification. *Acta Neurochir* 1991; **113**:131–7.

115 Wilson NW, Symon L, et al. Gliomatosis cerebri – report of a case presenting as a focal cerebral mass. *J Neurol* 1987; **234**:445–7.

116 Miller R, Lin F, et al. Cytologic diagnosis of gliomatosis cerebri. *Acta Cytol* 1981; **5**:37–9.

117 Cozad SC, Townsend P, et al. Gliomatosis cerebri: results with radiation therapy. *Cancer* 1996; **78**:1789–93.

118 Valdueza JM, Cristante L, et al. Hypothalamic hamartomas – with special reference to gelastic epilepsy and surgery. *Neurosurgery* 1994; **34**:949–58.

119 Arita K, Ikawa F, et al. The relationship between magnetic resonance imaging findings and clinical manifestations of hypothalamic hamartoma. *J Neurosurg* 1999; **91**:212–20.

120 Tsugu H, Fukushima T, et al. Hypothalamic hamartoma associated with multiple congenital abnormalities. Two patients and a review of reported cases. *Pediatr Neurosurg* 1998; **29**:290–6.

121 Stephan MJ, Brookes KL, et al. Hypothalamic hamartoma in oral facial digital syndrome type 6 (Varadi syndrome). *Am J Med Genet* 1994; **51**:131–5.

122 Strickler HD, Rosenberg PS, et al. Contamination of poliovirus vaccines with simian virus 40 (1955–1963) and subsequent cancer rates. *J Am Med Assoc* 1998; **279**:292–5.

123 Berkovic SF, Andermann F, et al. Hypothalamic hamartomas and ictal laughter: evolution of a characteristic epileptic syndrome and diagnostic value of magnetic resonance imaging. *Ann Neurol* 1988; **23**:429–39.

124 Mahachoklertwattana P, Kaplan SL, et al. The luteinizing-hormone-releasing hormone-secreting hypothalamic hamartoma is a congenital malformation – natural history. *J Clin Endocrinol Metab* 1993; **77**:118–24.

125 Feuillan PP, Jones JV, et al. Boys with precocious puberty due to hypothalamic hamartoma: reproductive axis after

126 Kramer U, Spector S, et al. Surgical treatment of hypothalamic hamartoma and refractory seizures. A case report and review of the literature. *Pediatr Neurosurg* 2001; **34**:40–2.

127 Ishii T, Sato S, et al. Treatment with a gonadotropin-releasing-hormone analog and attainment of full height potential in a male monozygotic twin with gonadotropin-releasing hormone-dependent precocious puberty. *Eur J Pediatr* 1999; **158**:933–5.

128 Albright AL, Lee PA. Neurosurgical treatment of hypothalamic hamartomas causing precocious puberty. *J Neurosurg* 1993; **78**:77–82.

129 Delalande O, Rodriguez D, et al. Successful surgical relief of seizures associated with hamartomas of the floor of the fourth ventricle in children: report of two cases. *Neurosurgery* 2001; **49**:726–31.

130 Rosenfeld JV, Harvey AS, et al. Transcallosal resection of hypothalamic hamartomas, with control of seizures, in children with gelastic epilepsy. *Neurosurgery* 2001; **48**:108–18.

131 Mottolese C, Stan H, et al. Hypothalamic hamartoma: the role of surgery in a series of eight patients. *Childs Nerv Syst* 2001; **17**:229–36.

132 Unger F, Schrottner O, et al. Gamma knife radiosurgery for hypothalamic hamartomas in patients with medically intractable epilepsy and precocious puberty. Report of two cases. *J Neurosurg* 2000; **92**:726–31.

133 Schild SE, Scheithauer BW, et al. Pineal parenchymal tumors. Clinical, pathologic, and therapeutic aspects. *Cancer* 1993; **72**:870–80.

134 D'Andrea AD, Packer RJ, et al. Pineocytomas of childhood. A reappraisal of natural history and response to therapy. *Cancer* 1987; **59**:1353–7.

135 Jouvet A, Fevre M, et al. Structural and ultrastructural characteristics of human pineal gland, and pineal parenchymal tumors. *Acta Neuropathol (Berl)* 1994; **88**:334–48.

136 Schild SE, Scheithauer BW, et al. Histologically confirmed pineal tumors and other germ cell tumors of the brain. *Cancer* 1996; **78**:2564–71.

137 Allcutt D, Michowiz S, et al. Primary leptomeningeal melanoma – an unusually aggressive tumor in childhood. *Neurosurgery* 1993; **32**:721–9.

138 Baena RRY, Gaetani P, et al. Primary solitary intracranial melanoma - case-report and review of the literature. *Surg Neurol* 1992; **38**:26–37.

139 Makin GW, Eden OB, et al. Leptomeningeal melanoma in childhood. *Cancer* 1999; **86**:878–86.

140 Rodriguez-Gallindo C, Pappo AS, et al. Brain metastases in children with melanoma. *Cancer* 1997; **79**:2440–45.

141 Kadonaga IN, Frieden IJ. Neurocutaneous melanosis: definition and review of the literature. *J Am Acad Dermatol* 1991; **24**:747–55.

142 Lopez-Castilla JD, Diaz-Fernandez F, et al. Primary leptomeningeal melanoma in a child. *Pediatr Neurol* 2001; **24**:390–2.

143 DeDavid M, Orlow SJ, et al. Neurocutaneous melanosis: clinical features of large congenital melanocytic nevi in

discontinuation of gonadotropin-releasing hormone analog therapy. *J Clin Endocrinol Metab* 2000; **85**:4036–8.

patients with manifest central nervous system melanosis. *J Am Acad Dermatol* 1996; **35**:529–38.

144 Kinsler VA, Aylett SE, *et al.* Central nervous system imaging and congenital melanocytic naevi. *Arch Dis Child* 2001; **84**:152–5.

145 Thomas CS, Toone BK, *et al.* Neurocutaneous melanosis and psychosis. *Am J Psychiatry* 1988; **145**:649–50.

146 Nicolaides P, Newton RW, *et al.* Primary malignant melanoma of meninges: a typical presentation of sub acute meningitis. *Paediatr Neurol* 1995; **12**:172–4.

147 Salisbury JR, Rose PE. Primary central nervous malignant melanoma in the basal trunk and naevus syndrome. *Post Grad Med J* 1989; **65**:387–9.

148 Hoffman HJ, Freeman A. Primary malignant leptomeningeal melanoma in association with giant hairy naevi. *J Neurosurg* 1967; **26**:62–71.

149 Helsketh A, Helsketh E, *et al.* Primary meningeal melanoma. *Acta Oncol* 1989; **28**:103–4.

150 Nagakawa H, Hawakawa T, *et al.* Long term survival after removal of primary intracranial malignant melanoma. *Acta Neurochir* 1989; **101**:84–8.

151 Hillner BE, Agarwala S, *et al.* Post hoc economic analysis of temozolomide versus dacarbazine in the treatment of advanced metastatic melanoma. *J Clin Oncol* 2000; **18**:474–80.

152 Gupta G, Robertson AG, *et al.* Cerebral metastases of cutaneous melanoma. *Br J Cancer* 1997; **76**:256–9.

153 Beresford H. Melanoma of the nervous system. Treatment with corticosteroids and radiation. *Neurology* 1969; **19**:59–65.

154 Oruckaptan HH, Soylemezoglu F, *et al.* Benign melanocytic tumor in infancy: discussion on a rare case and review of the literature. *Paediatr Neurosurg* 2000; **32**:240–7.

155 Johnson R, Scheithauer B, *et al.* Melanotic neuroectodermal tumour of infancy. A review of seven cases. *Cancer* 1983; **52**:661–6.

156 Ricketts R, Majmudarr B. Epididymal melanotic neuroectodermal tumour of infancy. *Hum Pathol* 1985; **16**:416–20.

157 Parizek J, Nemecek S, *et al.* Melanotic neuroectodermal tumour of infancy of extra-intra subdural right temporal location: CT examination, surgical treatment, literature review. *Neuropediatrics* 1986; **17**:115–23.

158 Carpenter B, Jiminez J, *et al.* Melanotic neuroectodermal tumour of infancy. *Pediatr Pathol* 1985; **3**:227–44.

159 Pettinato G, Manivel J, *et al.* Melanotic neuroectodermal tumour of infancy. A reexamination of a histogenetic problem based on immunohistochemical, flow cytometric, and ultrastructural study of 10 cases. *Am J Surg Pathol* 1991; **15**:233–45.

160 Navas-Palacios J. Malignant melanotic neuroectodermal tumour. Light and electron microscopic study. *Cancer* 1980; **46**:529–36.

161 Pierre-Kahn A, Cinalli G, *et al.* Melanotic neuroectodermal tumor of the skull and meninges in infancy. *Pediatr Neurosurg* 1992; **18**:6–15.

162 Shokry A, Briner J, *et al.* Malignant melanotic neuroectodermal tumour of infancy: a case report. *Pediatr Pathol* 1986; **5**:217–23.

163 Block JC, Waite DE, *et al.* Pigmented neuroectodermal tumour of infancy: an example of rarely expressed malignant behavior. *Oral Surg Oral Med Oral Pathol* 1980; **49**:279–85.

164 Stowens D, Lin TH. Melanotic progonoma of the brain. *Hum Pathol* 1974; **5**:105–12.

165 Hupp J, Topazian D, *et al.* The melanotic neuroectodermal tumour of infancy. Report of two cases and review of the literature. *Int J Oral Surg* 1981; **10**:432–46.

166 Crocket D, McGill T, *et al.* Melanotic neuroectodermal tumor of infancy. *Otolaryngol Head Neck Surg* 1987; **96**:194–7.

167 Nagase M, Ueda K, *et al.* Recurrent melanotic neuroectodermal tumour of infancy. Case report and survey of 16 cases. *J Maxillofac Surg* 1983; **11**:131–6.

168 Jenkinson HC, Raafat F, *et al.* Melanotic neuroectodermal tumour of infancy. Is there a role for chemotherapy? *Med Pediatr Oncol* 1997; **29**:466–9.

169 Chan RC, Thompson GB. Intracranial meningiomas in childhood. *Surg Neurol* 1984; **21**:319–22.

170 Ferrante L, Acqui M, *et al.* Paediatric intracranial meningiomas. *Br J Neurosurg* 1989; **3**:189–96.

171 Kolluri VR, Reddy DR, *et al.* Meningiomas in childhood. *Childs Nerv Syst* 1987; **3**:271–3.

172 Mallucci CL, Parkes SE, *et al.* Paediatric meningeal tumours. *Childs Nerv Syst* 1996; **12**:582–8, 589.

173 Merli GA, Benedetti A, *et al.* Supratentorial meningiomas in childhood. *Sist Nerv* 1966; **18**:124–41.

174 Crouse SK, Berg BO. Intracranial meningiomas in childhood and adolescence. *Neurology* 1972; **22**:135–41.

175 Merten DF, Gooding CA, *et al.* Meningiomas of childhood and adolescence. *J Pediatr* 1974; **84**:696–700.

176 Hooper R. Intracranial tumours in childhood. *Childs Brain* 1975; **1**:136–40.

177 Leibel SA, Wara WM, *et al.* The treatment of meningiomas in childhood. *Cancer* 1976; **37**:2709–12.

178 Numaguchi Y, Hoffman JC, *et al.* Meningiomas in childhood and adolescence. *Neurol Med Chir (Tokyo)* 1978; **18**:119–27.

179 Fortuna A, Nolletti A, *et al.* Spinal neurinomas and meningiomas in children. *Acta Neurochir (Wien)* 1981; **55**:329–41.

180 Sano K, Wakai S, *et al.* Characteristics of intracranial meningiomas in childhood. *Childs Brain* 1981; **8**:98–106.

181 Nakamura Y, Becker LE. Meningeal tumors of infancy and childhood. *Pediatr Pathol* 1985; **3**:341–58.

182 Drake JM, Hendrick EB, *et al.* Intracranial meningiomas in children. *Pediatr Neurosci* 1985; **12**:134–9.

183 Doty JR, Schut L, *et al.* Intracranial meningiomas of childhood and adolescence. *Prog Exp Tumor Res* 1987; **30**:247–54.

184 Davidson GS, Hope JK. Meningeal tumors of childhood. *Cancer* 1989; **63**:1205–10.

185 Hung PC, Wang HS, *et al.* Intracranial meningiomas in childhood. *Zhonghua Min Guo Xiao Er Ke Yi Xue Hui Za Zhi* 1994; **35**:495–501.

186 Erdincler P, Lena G, *et al.* Intracranial meningiomas in children: review of 29 cases. *Surg Neurol* 1998; **49**:136–40, 140–1.

187 Di Rocco C, Di Rienzo A. Meningiomas in childhood. *Crit Rev Neurosurg* 1999; **9**:180–8.

188 Demirtas E, Ersahin Y, *et al.* Intracranial meningeal tumours in childhood: a clinicopathologic study including MIB-1 immunohistochemistry. *Pathol Res Pract* 2000; **196**:151–8.

189 Turgut M, Ozcan OE, *et al.* Meningiomas in childhood and adolescence: a report of 13 cases and review of the literature. *Br J Neurosurg* 1997; **11**:501–7.

190 Rickert CH, Paulus W. Epidemiology of central nervous system tumors in childhood and adolescence based on the new WHO classification. *Childs Nerv Syst* 2001; **17**:503–11.

191 Bondy M, Ligon BL. Epidemiology and etiology of intracranial meningiomas: a review. *J Neuro-Oncol* 1996; **29**:197–205.

192 Herz DA, Shapiro K, *et al.* Intracranial meningiomas of infancy, childhood and adolescence. Review of the literature and addition of 9 case reports. *Childs Brain* 1980; **7**:43–56.

193 Sheikh BY, Siqueira E, *et al.* Meningioma in children: a report of nine cases and a review of the literature. *Surg Neurol* 1996; **45**:328–35.

194 Jaaskelainen J, Haltia M, *et al.* Atypical and anaplastic meningiomas: radiology, surgery, radiotherapy, and outcome. *Surg Neurol* 1986; **25**:233–42.

195 Martinez-Avalos A, Rivera-Luna R, *et al.* Meningeal sarcoma in childhood. Experiences with 17 cases. *Bol Med Hosp Infant Mex* 1989; **46**:47–50.

196 Perry A, Scheithauer BW, *et al.* Malignancy in meningiomas: a clinicopathologic study of 116 patients, with grading implications. *Cancer* 1999; **85**:2046–56.

197 Kaba SE, DeMonte F, *et al.* The treatment of recurrent unresectable and malignant meningiomas with interferon alpha-2B. *Neurosurgery* 1997; **40**:271–5.

198 Iseda T, Goya T, *et al.* Magnetic resonance imaging and angiographic appearance of meningioma of the fourth ventricle – two case reports. *Neurol Med Chir (Tokyo)* 1997; **37**:36–40.

199 Ginsberg LE. Radiology of meningiomas. *J Neuro-Oncol* 1996; **29**:229–38.

200 Milosevic MF, Frost PJ, *et al.* Radiotherapy for atypical or malignant intracranial meningioma. *Int J Radiat Oncol Biol Phys* 1996; **34**:817–22.

201 Verheggen R, Finkenstaedt M, *et al.* Atypical and malignant meningiomas: evaluation of different radiological criteria based on CT and MRI. *Acta Neurochir Suppl (Wien)* 1996; **65**:66–9.

202 Sgouros S, Walsh AR, *et al.* Intraventricular malignant meningioma in a 6-year-old child. *Surg Neurol* 1994; **42**:41–5.

203 McLean CA, Jolley D, *et al.* Atypical and malignant meningiomas: importance of micronecrosis as a prognostic indicator. *Histopathology* 1993; **23**:349–53.

204 Alvarez F, Roda JM, *et al.* Malignant and atypical meningiomas: a reappraisal of clinical, histological, and computed tomographic features. *Neurosurgery* 1987; **20**:688–94.

205 Jaaskelainen J, Haltia M, *et al.* The growth rate of intracranial meningiomas and its relation to histology. An analysis of 43 patients. *Surg Neurol* 1985; **24**:165–72.

206 Jellinger K, Slowik F. Histological subtypes and prognostic problems in meningiomas. *J Neurol* 1975; **208**:279–98.

207 Inoue Y, Nemoto Y, *et al.* Neurofibromatosis type 1 and type 2: review of the central nervous system and related structures. *Brain Dev* 1997; **19**:1–12.

208 Ersahin Y, Ozdamar N, *et al.* Meningioma of the cavernous sinus in a child. *Childs Nerv Syst* 1999; **15**:8–10.

209 Higer HP, Gutjahr P, *et al.* NMR studies of the central nervous system in pediatrics. *ROFO Fortschr Geb Rontgenstr Nuklearmed* 1985; **143**:137–45.

210 Hope JK, Armstrong DA, *et al.* Primary meningeal tumors in children: correlation of clinical and CT findings with histologic type and prognosis. *Am J Neuroradiol* 1992; **13**:1353–64.

211 Wilson C. Meningiomas: genetics, malignancy and the role of radiation in the induction and treatment. *J Neurosurg* 1994; **81**:666–75.

212 Goldsmith BJ, Wara WM, *et al.* Postoperative irradiation of subtotally irradiated meningiomas. A retrospective analysis of 140 patients treated from 1967–1990. *J Neurosurg* 1994; **80**:195–201.

213 Symons P, Tobias V, *et al.* Brain-invasive meningioma in a 16-month-old boy. *Pathology* 2001; **33**:252–6.

214 Salisbury JR, Deverell MH, *et al.* Three-dimensional reconstruction of human embryonic notocords: clue to the pathogenesis of chordoma. *J Pathol* 1993; **171**:59–62.

215 Matsumoto J, Towbin RB, *et al.* Cranial chordomas in infancy and childhood. A report of two cases and review of the literature. *Pediatr Radiol* 1989; **20**:28–32.

216 Kelley MJ, Korczak JF, Sheridan E, Yang XH, Goldstein AM, Parry DM. Familial chordoma, a tumor of notochordal remnants, is linked to chromosome 7q33. *Am J Hum Genet* 2001; **69**:454–60.

217 Borba LAB, Al-Mefty O, *et al.* Cranial chordomas in children and adolescents. *J Neurosurg* 1996; **84**:584–91.

218 Wold LE, Laws ER. Cranial chordomas in children and young adults. *J Neurosurg* 1983; **59**:1043–7.

219 Coffin CM, Swanson PE, *et al.* Chordoma in childhood and adolescence. *Arch Path Lab Med* 1993; **117**:927–33.

220 Eisenberg MB, Woloschak M, *et al.* Loss of heterozygosity in the retinoblastoma tumor suppressor gene in skull base chordomas and chondrosarcomas. *Surg Neurol* 1997; **47**:156–61.

221 Bonneville F, Sarrazin JL, Marsot-Dupuch K, *et al.* Unusual lesions of the cerebellopontine angle: a segmental approach. *Radiographics* 2001; **21**:419–38.

222 Tai PTH, Craighead P, *et al.* Management issues in chordoma: a case series. *Clin Oncol* 2000; **12**:80–6.

223 Gay E, Sekhar LN, *et al.* Chordomas and chondrosarcomas of the cranial base: results and follow up of 60 patients. *Neurosurgery* 1995; **36**:887–97.

224 Al-Mefty O, Borba LAB. Skull base chordomas a management challenge. *J Neurosurg* 1997; **86**:182–9.

225 Crockard HA, Steel T, *et al.* A multidisciplinary team approach to skull base chordomas. *J Neurosurg* 2001; **95**:175–83.

226 Hug EB, Loredo LN, *et al.* Proton radiation therapy for chordomas and chondrosarcomas of the skull base. *J Neurosurg* 1999; **91**:432–9.

227 Sciemeca PG, James-Herry, AG *et al.* Chemotherapeutic treatment of malignant chordoma in children. *J Pediatr Hematol Oncol* 1996; **18**:237–40.

228 Terahara A, Niermierko A, *et al.* Analysis of the relationship between tumor dose inhomogeneity and local control in patients with skull base chordoma. *Int J Radiat Oncol Biol Phys* 1999; **45**:351–8.

229 Benk V, Liebsch N, *et al.* Base of skull and cervical spine chordomas in children treated by high-dose irradiation. *Int J Radiat Oncol Biol Phys* 1995; **31**:577–81.

230 Hug EB, Sweeney R, *et al.* Proton radiotherapy in mangement of pediatric base of skull tumors. *Int J Radiat Oncol Biol Phys* 2002; **52**:1017–24.

231 Cho B-K, Chi JG, *et al.* Intracranial mesenchymal chondrosarcoma: a case report and literature review. *Childs Nerv Syst* 1993; **9**:295–9.

232 Kubota T, Hayashi M, *et al.* Primary intracranial mesenchymal chondrosarcoma: case report and review of the literature. *Neurosurgery* 1982; **10**:105–10.

233 Gerszten PC, Pollack IF, *et al.* Primary parafalcine chondrosarcoma in a child. *Acta Neuropathol* 1998; **95**:111–14.

234 Bosma JJD, Kirollos RW, *et al.* Primary intradural classic chondrosarcoma: case report and literature review. *Neurosurgery* 2001; **48**:420–3.

235 Heffelfinger MJ, Dahlin DC, *et al.* Chordomas and cartilaginous tumours at the skull base. *Cancer* 1973; **32**:410–20.

236 Lewis RJ, Ketcham AS. Maffucci syndrome: functional and neoplastic significance. Case report and review of the literature. *J Bone Joint Surg* 1973; **55**:1465–79.

237 Clifton AG, Kendall BE, *et al.* Intracranial chondrosarcoma in a patient with Ollier's disease. *Br J Neurosurg* 1991; **64**:633–6.

238 Watkins L, Khudados ES, *et al.* Skull base chordomas: a review of 38 patients. *Br J Neurosurg* 1993; **7**:241–8.

239 Nakashima Y, Unni KK, *et al.* Mesenchymal chondrosarcoma of bone and soft tissue: a review of 111 cases. *Cancer* 1986; **57**:2444–53.

240 Rollo JL, Green WR, *et al.* Primary meningeal mesenchymal chondrosarcoma. *Arch Pathol Lab Med* 1979; **103**:239–43.

241 Allcutt DA, Hoffman HJ, *et al.* Acoustic schwannomas in children. *Neurosurgery* 1991; **29**:14–18.

242 Charabi S, Thomsen J, *et al.* Acoustic neuroma/vestibular schwannoma growth: past, present and future. *Acta Otolaryngol* 1998; **118**:327–32.

243 Charabi S, Tos M, *et al.* Vestibular schwannoma growth – long-term results. *Acta Otolaryngol Suppl* 2000; **543**:7–10.

244 Evans DG, Birch JM, *et al.* Paediatric presentation of type 2 neurofibromatosis. *Arch Dis Child* 1999; **81**:496–9.

245 Fitz CR. Neuroradiology of posterior fossa tumors in children. *Clin Neurosurg* 1983; **30**:189–202.

246 Harada K, Nishizaki T, *et al.* Pediatric acoustic schwannoma showing rapid regrowth with high proliferative activity. *Childs Nerv Syst* 2000; **16**:134–7.

247 Jackson CG, Pappas DG, Jr, *et al.* Pediatric neurotologic skull base surgery. *Laryngoscope* 1996; **106**:1205–9.

248 Mattucci KF, Glass WM, *et al.* Childhood acoustic neuroma. *N Y State J Med* 1987; **87**:665–6.

249 Mautner VF, Tatagiba M, *et al.* Neurofibromatosis 2 in the pediatric age group. *Neurosurgery* 1993; **33**:92–6.

250 Mautner VF, Baser ME, *et al.* Vestibular schwannoma growth in patients with neurofibromatosis type 2: a longitudinal study. *J Neurosurg* 2002; **96**:223–8.

251 Pastores GM, Michels VV, *et al.* Early childhood diagnosis of acoustic neuromas in presymptomatic individuals at risk for neurofibromatosis 2. *Am J Med Genet* 1991; **41**:325–9.

252 Pothula VB, Lesser T, *et al.* Vestibular schwannomas in children. *Otol Neurotol* 2001; **22**:903–7.

253 Shaida AM, O DD, *et al.* Schwannomatosis in a child – or early neurofibromatosis type 2. *J Laryngol Otol* 2002; **116**:551–5.

254 Sznajder L, Abrahams C, *et al.* Multiple schwannomas and meningiomas associated with irradiation in childhood. *Arch Intern Med* 1996; **156**:1873–8.

255 Truy E, Furminieux V, *et al.* Acoustic neuroma in children. Report of 5 cases. *Ann Otolaryngol Chir Cervicofac* 1999; **116**:92–7.

256 Valeviciene N. Paediatric neurofibromatosis. *Acta Radiol* 2002; **43**:623–4.

257 Vassilouthis J, Richardson AE. Acoustic neurinoma in a child. *Surg Neurol* 1979; **12**:37–9.

258 Wiet RJ, Mamikoglu B, *et al.* Long-term results of the first 500 cases of acoustic neuroma surgery. *Otolaryngol Head Neck Surg* 2001; **124**:645–51.

23

Exploiting biology for therapeutic gain

RICHARD GILBERTSON AND DONALD M. O'ROURKE

THE THERAPEUTIC CHALLENGE OF PEDIATRIC BRAIN TUMORS

In recent decades, the formation of cooperative groups, including the Children's Oncology Group (COG) in North America and the Société International d'Oncologie Pédiatrique (SIOP), has brought together medical, scientific, and nursing professionals to provide coordinated care for children with malignancies. Their integrated efforts have given rise to a greater understanding of the biology of childhood cancers and enabled the development of effective multimodality treatments. As a result, the overall probability of cure for childhood malignancy has more than tripled in the past 30 years.[1] However, this success has not occurred equally in all pediatric cancers. Most notably, and with few exceptions, the outlook for children with brain tumors has remained largely unchanged.

There are many reasons why tumors derived from cells of the central nervous system (CNS) continue to resist conventional treatment strategies. Their intimate relation to critical structures within the CNS, and their capacity to infiltrate locally and distally within the neuraxis, significantly curtails the extent to which local treatments, including surgery and radiotherapy, may be used to achieve effective cure. The physicochemical and functional efflux pump mechanisms that characterize endothelial cells of the blood–brain barrier provide an additional obstacle to the use of systemic chemotherapy.[2] However, arguably the greatest hurdle to improving the outlook of children with brain tumors has been the lack of knowledge regarding the molecular mechanisms that govern the initiation and progression of these diseases. Understanding these biological processes would revolutionize our approach to the management of brain tumors, by improving disease risk assessment, increasing the efficiency with which conventional therapies are employed, and providing targets for the development of novel treatment strategies. In the light of this, the early decades of the twenty-first century are likely to be an exciting time for the field of pediatric neuro-oncology. Progress is now being made in our understanding of the biology of pediatric brain tumors. Coupled with advances in the fields of developmental neurobiology and cancer biology, these insights hold great promise for real improvements to be made in the future management of children with brain tumors. However, these new approaches bring their own unique challenges. These include determining the in vivo biological activity of these agents, predicting which patients will benefit most from these treatments, and discovering how these therapies can be best employed in the context of existing conventional chemo- and radio-therapy. The continued coordinated efforts of medical, scientific, and nursing professionals will therefore be crucial if we are to realize fully the promise of biology-based treatments.

TARGETING TUMORIGENESIS: THE FUTURE OF PEDIATRIC BRAIN TUMOR TREATMENT

Central to the accurate development, evaluation, and employment of novel therapeutics is an understanding of the biological processes to be targeted. Brain tumor cells proliferate and invade both locally and distally within the CNS. This aberrant behavior requires the malignant cell to bypass the mechanisms that govern normal cell proliferation, apoptosis, integrity of tissue boundaries, migration, and recruitment of vascular architecture. Many of the genes that direct these processes have been identified. They include oncogenes and tumor suppressor genes that encode the principal components of signal transduction cascades, cell cycle and apoptosis control machinery, and factors involved in angiogenesis and cell migration.

Signal transduction pathways as therapeutic targets

GROWTH FACTOR RECEPTOR SIGNALING NETWORKS

In recent years, evidence has accumulated implicating the deregulation of numerous growth factor receptor pathways in the development of CNS malignancies. Components of these signal cascades therefore represent attractive targets for novel therapeutic approaches. Among the growth factor receptor signaling pathways implicated

in the pathogenesis of brain tumors, the epidermal growth factor receptor (EGFR, also known as ERBB)[3,4] and platelet-derived growth factor-receptor (PDGF-R)[5] families appear to play particularly prominent roles.

Extracellular growth factors activate signaling pathways by binding to specific cell-surface receptors. These interactions induce changes in receptor conformation, leading to oligomerization and intrinsic kinase activity.[6,7] Resultant autophosphorylation of tyrosine residues within receptor cytoplasmic c-terminal regions allows the recruitment of adapter molecules to the inner membrane surface. These adapters, e.g. GRB2 and SOS, provide a molecular bridge between the active ligand–receptor complex and cytoplasmic signal pathways, allowing further propagation of the message through the cell. SOS, a guanine nucleotide exchange factor, activates membrane-bound RAS by switching it from the guanosine diphosphate (GDP)-bound to the guanosine triphosphate (GTP)-bound state.[8] RAS then triggers a sequential series of enzymatic phosphorylation reactions among members of the mitogen-activated protein kinase (MAPK) pathways, which ultimately transfer the message to the cell nucleus (Figure 23.1). The three known MAPK signaling

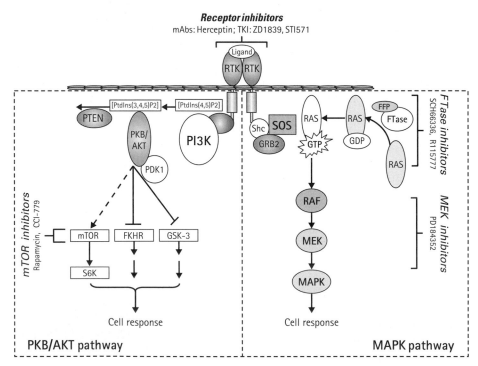

Figure 23.1 *Growth factor receptor signaling networks as a therapeutic target. Extracellular growth factors activate signaling pathways by binding to specific cell surface receptors (see text). These pathways include the protein kinase B (PKB)/AKT and RAS/ mitogen-activated protein kinase (MAPK) pathways shown on the left- and right-hand sides of the figure, respectively. Strategies that target the receptors themselves include small-molecule inhibitors of tyrosine kinase (TKI) activity and monoclonal antibodies (mAbs). Farnesyl transferase (FTase) plays a crucial role in the recruitment of RAS to the cell membrane. Agents that inhibit this enzyme are in clinical development. Drugs targeting the more distal components of the MAPK and PKB/AKT signal cascades are also shown. (GDP, guanosine diphosphate; GSK-3, glycogen synthase kinase-3; GTP, guanosine triphosphate; mTOR, mammalian target of rapamycin; PI3K, phosphatidylinositol-3-kinase; PTEN, phosphate tensin.)*

systems – the ERK, JNK, and p38 pathways – share this similar operating structure.[9] A great variety of cellular responses are elicited by these pathways, including proliferation, apoptosis, migration, and differentiation. The final readout depends largely on the activating receptor(s), the cell background, and the tissue environment.

In addition to MAPK cascades, growth factor receptors signal through a variety of other systems, including the protein kinase B (PKB/AKT)[10,11] and the signal transduction and activation of transcription (STAT) pathways.[7] The PKB/AKT pathway is activated following the recruitment of phosphatidylinositol 3-kinase (PI3K) to phosphorylated c-terminal receptor domains (Figure 23.1). Activated PI3K then generates 3'-phosphoinositides, which recruit PKB/AKT to the membrane. At least one additional kinase, PDK1, is required for PI3K-dependent activation of the PKB/AKT kinase. PKB/AKT then phosphorylates a number of protein substrates, including glycogen synthase kinase-3 (GSK-3) and the Forkhead family of transcription factors, thereby controlling a diverse array of cellular responses, including protein synthesis, cell growth, angiogenesis, and cell survival.[10,11]

The ability of cells to negatively regulate potent growth factor signaling pathways is crucial to normal control of cell proliferation and death. In this regard, the phosphatase tensin (*PTEN*) homolog tumor suppressor plays a critical role in PKB/AKT pathway control by limiting the availability of 3'-phosphoinositides and thus the activation of PKB/AKT. The importance of this gene for normal growth control is underscored by its frequent mutation in human tumors, including gliomas.[12,13]

ERBB RECEPTOR SIGNALING AS A THERAPEUTIC TARGET

The four members of the ERBB receptor family – ERBB1 (EGFR), ERBB2 (HER2/neu), ERBB3, and ERBB4 – interact to form homo- and heterodimers following ligand binding.[7] Receptor dimers then activate a variety of signal pathways, including the MAPK, STAT, and PKB/AKT networks. This normal signal system is deregulated in brain tumor cells by a variety of mechanisms.

ERBB1 is the most frequently amplified oncogene in adult glioma. Inhibition of ERBB1 kinase activity impairs glioma cell survival, angiogenesis, motility, and transformation.[14-17] About one-half of high-grade gliomas containing *ERBB1* amplification also possess an in-frame deletion of exons 2–7 of *ERBB1*, resulting in the expression of a constitutively active truncated receptor (EGFRvIII).[3,4,17] Elevated expression of the EGFRvIII and wild-type receptors at the cell surface appears to mediate transformation, at least in part, by constitutively activating the MAPK and PI3K pathways.[18,19] *ERBB1* amplification appears to be a rare event in pediatric glioma, but the incidence of *ERBB1* gene rearrangement

is not known. However, overexpression of the receptor has been reported to affect 80 per cent of high-grade gliomas in children,[20] including brainstem glioma.[21]

Other members of the ERBB kinase family play an important role in the pathogenesis of childhood CNS tumors. High-level tumor cell expression of ERBB2 and ERBB4 receptors has been shown to be an independent predictor of poor clinical outcome in medulloblastoma.[22-26] The ERBB2 receptor may play a particularly important role in the biology of medulloblastoma. While this receptor can be detected in up to 80 per cent of primary tumors,[22] it is undetectable in normal developing and mature human cerebellum.[24] Furthermore, its expression in primary tumors appears to identify patients with especially poor prognosis, even among cases with clinical standard-risk disease.[26] Efforts are under way to delineate the mechanism(s) by which *ERBB2* overexpression mediates poor prognosis in medulloblastoma. Recent evidence indicates that *ERBB2* overexpression increases the metastatic potential of medulloblastoma cells by upregulating a series of prometastatic genes.[27] Work in adult breast cancer, in which the *ERBB2* gene is amplified and/or overexpressed in around 25 per cent of cases, has also shown high expression of this receptor to mediate cell proliferation, resistance to chemotherapy and apoptosis, and enhanced metastatic potential.[7,28,29] High coexpression of ERBB2 and ERBB4 receptor mRNA and protein is also a feature of high-risk childhood ependymoma,[30] and signaling via *ERBB2* appears to promote the proliferation of ependymoma cells in vitro.

Because of their prominent role in adult malignancies, intense efforts have been made by pharmaceutical companies and academic institutions to identify effective inhibitors of ERBB receptor signaling. Consequently, these compounds represent some of the most numerous and advanced novel agents in clinical development. Two principal groups of compounds have been investigated: small-molecule inhibitors and monoclonal antibodies. These agents have demonstrated a diverse array of anti-tumor properties in preclinical studies, including growth inhibition, antibody-dependent cell-mediated cytotoxicity, and sensitization of tumor cells to chemo- and radiotherapy.[7,31] The anti-*ERBB2* monoclonal antibody Trastuzumab™ (Genentech inc.) has proved particularly useful in the management of some women with *ERBB2*-overexpressing breast cancer.[31,32] The limited penetration of systemically administered monoclonal antibodies (mAbs) into the cerebrospinal fluid (CSF) is likely to curtail the use of this approach to treat brain tumors. Efforts are therefore under way to evaluate small mimetics of full-length ERBB antibodies in brain tumor models. ERBB peptide mimetics have been developed that retain binding specificity and may penetrate solid tumors and body cavities (e.g. the blood–brain barrier) more readily than mAbs.[33]

ZD1839™ (AstraZeneca) is the most extensively studied ERBB kinase small-molecule inhibitor.[34,35] Originally developed as an ERBB1-specific agent, recent reports indicate that it also potently inhibits ERBB2 kinase.[35,36] This activity against both ERBB1 and ERBB2 may be particularly advantageous, since basic science and clinical studies indicate that ERBB heterodimers have greater transforming potency than homodimers.[7,22] In preclinical studies, ZD1839 demonstrated marked anti-tumor effects against *ERBB1*-expressing xenografts, although these responses were only maintained in the presence of continued drug administration. Therefore, these agents will likely require chronic dosage schedules or will have to be used in conjunction with conventional chemo- and radiotherapy.[34,35] Phase I studies indicate that ZD1839 has only moderate gastrointestinal and dermatological toxicity, and that doses as low as 400 mg/day (well below the maximum tolerated dose of 700 mg/day) generate trough plasma concentrations greater than that required to inhibit the growth of *ERBB1*-expressing tumor cells in culture by 90 per cent.[34,35] It is envisaged that phase I studies of small-molecule inhibitors such as ZD1839 will soon be conducted in children with *ERBB1*-expressing brain tumors. Critical questions to be answered in these studies will include not only issues of toxicity and pharmacokinetics, but also the most appropriate way to monitor biological response to these agents, which molecular factors accurately predict in vivo tumor sensitivity to these agents, and how to integrate their use with more conventional treatment approaches.

PLATELET–DERIVED GROWTH FACTOR RECEPTOR ALPHA SIGNALING AS A THERAPEUTIC TARGET

The platelet-derived growth factor receptor alpha (PDGFRA) system signals via the MAPK and PI3K pathways in a manner analogous to that of the ERBB receptor family. Evidence from a variety of different sources has implicated the PDGFR signaling system in the development of brain tumors, particularly glioma.[17] Gliomas that present in younger patients, especially tumors initially presenting as lower-grade neoplasms before progression to a higher-grade tumor, often display alterations of PDGF ligand and/or receptor(s).[17] PDGF signaling appears to play a significant role in glial cell differentiation[37] and angiogenesis. Somatic-cell gene transfer of *Pdgfb* in vivo results in the development of highly invasive murine gliomas.[38] Microarray analysis of pediatric medulloblastoma identified an apparent increase in the expression of *PDGFRA* and members of the MAPK cascade in primary tumors from patients with metastases at diagnosis.[39] However, these data have been challenged, and it appears that PDGFRB rather than PDGFRA might be more important in medulloblastoma invasion.[40]

These data suggest that PDGFRA or PDGFRB may represent useful therapeutic targets for pediatric brain tumors. STI571™ (Novartis) is a small-molecule tyrosine kinase inhibitor of the p210[BCR-ABL] and p190[BCR-ABL] fusion proteins associated with chronic myeloid leukemia and Philadelphia chromosome-positive acute lymphoblastic leukemia.[41] This agent also inhibits the PDGFR, and clinical evaluation of its activity in glioma and medulloblastoma has been proposed.[39,42]

MAPK AND PI3K PATHWAYS AS THERAPEUTIC TARGETS

The fact that a variety of cell-surface receptors, each with potential roles in the biology of brain tumors, utilize common second-messenger pathways to transmit their aberrant signals has led to investigation of these intracellular pathways as targets for novel therapies.[8,43] Furthermore, components of these pathways, most notably RAS, are frequent targets of oncogenic mutations in human cancer.[8] Therefore, a number of approaches that directly target downstream elements of receptor signaling pathways are in development. The most extensively investigated are those that target RAS.

RAS, like many cytosolic signal proteins, must locate to the cell membrane to participate in signal transduction (Figure 23.1). This is achieved through the process of prenylation, in which a farnesyl group is transferred from farnesyl pyrophosphate (FPP) to the cysteine residue of a CAAX motif on the c-terminus of RAS, a reaction that is catalyzed by farnesyl transferase (FTase).[8,44] The understanding that this process was critical for RAS-dependent signaling led to the development of FTase inhibitors (FTIs). FTIs may be divided into three groups: (i) CAAX competitive inhibitors e.g. SCH66336 and R115777, which compete with this motif on RAS for FTase; (ii) FPP competitive inhibitors, e.g. PD169451; and (iii) bisubstrate inhibitors, e.g. BMS-186511. Although FTIs inhibit RAS farnesylation, it is not clear whether this accounts for all their anti-tumor activity, and additional targets including RhoB and AKT2 have also been proposed.[8]

Evidence that FTIs may prove useful in the treatment of brain tumors has been provided by drug activity studies in preclinical models of human glioma.[45] Early clinical trials of R115777 and SCH66336 have also been conducted in adults with hematological and solid malignancies.[46,47] The principal dose-limiting toxicity associated with prolonged administration of these compounds appears to be myelosuppression. Complete and partial disease responses were observed in these studies, and their evaluation in phase I studies of pediatric brain tumors is planned.

Agents that target more distal components of the MAPK and PKB/AKT signal cascades are also in development. Rapamycin and its ester CCI-779 target mTOR (mammalian target of rapamycin), a protein downstream of PKB/AKT signaling (Figure 23.1). Rapamycin and CCI-779 were first proposed as potential treatments for pediatric brain tumors following reports of their activity against medulloblastoma xenografts.[48] Interestingly, cells transformed by GLI, a transcription factor that lies downstream of the *PTCH1* pathway, appear to be especially sensitive to rapamycin. Therefore, these agents may be of particular value in the treatment of medulloblastomas harboring *PTCH1* deletions.[49]

Aberrant cell–cycle and apoptosis control as a therapeutic target

Disease progression in adult astrocytomas is associated with a series of well-characterized genetic abnormalities, including critical components of the cell-cycle and apoptosis control machinery.[50] In contrast, remarkably little is known regarding which elements of these systems are disrupted in pediatric brain tumors. Nonetheless, overwhelming evidence indicates loss of cell-cycle control to be a key feature of most human malignancies,[51,52] and it is likely that further study of childhood brain tumors will identify abnormalities in this control system. Indeed, a number of groups have reported amplification and/or overexpression of *MYCC* in primary medulloblastoma, with some reporting an apparent relationship between high-level expression of this oncogene and poor clinical outcome.[53–55] Exploitation of the tumor necrosis factor (TNF)-related apoptosis-inducing ligand (TRAIL) pathway for therapeutic gain in primitive neuroectodermal tumors (PNETs) has also been proposed;[56] however, there are concerns regarding the toxicity of this approach.[57]

Angiogenesis as a therapeutic target

ANGIOGENESIS

Angiogenesis, the formation of new blood vessels from pre-existing vessels, plays a critical role in the early phases of tumor development.[58–60] This process, recognized histologically as microvascular proliferation, is a hallmark of anaplastic brain tumors.[17] These diseases have therefore been investigated increasingly as strong candidates for anti-angiogenic therapy.

Angiogenesis is activated by a number of cell-surface receptors and ligands.[61,62] Evidence suggests that vascular endothelial growth factor (VEGF) and its two receptors, VEGFR-1 and VEGFR-2, play particularly prominent roles in glioma-induced vascular regulation.[63,64] VEGF secreted by glioma cells stimulates receptor-expressing endothelial cells, activating a variety of signal pathways that promote cell proliferation, survival, vasopermeability, and migration, all of which contribute to angiogenesis (Figure 23.2).

INHIBITION OF ANGIOGENESIS

Anti-angiogenic agents may be divided into two broad groups: drugs that inhibit the signal pathways that stimulate angiogenesis and drugs that induce the death of existing endothelial cells. The first group of compounds includes SU5416 (Sugen), a selective inhibitor of VEGFR-1, and SU6668 (Sugen), a broader-acting agent that inhibits the kinase activity of the fibroblast growth factor (FGF) and PDGF receptors as well as VEGFR-1. Both agents inhibit the in vitro proliferation of endothelial cells and demonstrate in vivo anti-tumor activity against a range of human tumor xenografts, including gliomas.[65–67] Toxicity in phase I studies of SU5416 in adults included vomiting and headache.[68] Objective responses were also observed, and further clinical evaluations both as a single agent and in combination with chemotherapy, are ongoing.

A large number of agents with anti-endothelial cell activity have been identified. These include inhibitors of endothelial-specific integrin/survival signals, e.g. EMD 121974 and endostatin, a 20-kDa protein fragment of collagen XVIII, whose precise mechanism of action is still unclear. Novel delivery mechanisms for anti-angiogenic therapeutics in gliomas are also in development, including intratumoral delivery of endostatin-producing cells.[69]

The destruction of tumor vasculature is likely to account for a large component of the anti-tumor activity associated with anti-angiogenic agents. However, there is increasing evidence that these drugs also enhance tumor sensitivity to radio- and chemotherapy. This would seem contradictory, given that conventional treatments rely on an adequate blood supply to transport oxygen and drug to tumor cells. The concept of "normalization" of tumor vasculature has been proposed as a potential explanation for this observation.[60] This hypothesis suggests that while tumor vessels do provide a blood supply to malignant cells, their abnormal tortuous nature and compression by expanding tumor restrict this to a level below that required for optimal delivery of drugs and oxygen. However, anti-angiogenic agents appear to "normalize" the vasculature, eliminating excess endothelial cells and initially increasing the delivery of nutrients and therapeutics to tumor cells. If proved correct, this process may have a profound impact on the way anti-angiogenic drugs are used, particularly in combination with more conventional radio- and chemotherapy. Clinical trials of anti-angiogenic compounds in children with brain tumors are currently at the planning stage. However, the potential for these compounds to induce growth-related toxicity in the developing child will require particular attention as these agents enter clinical pediatric practice.

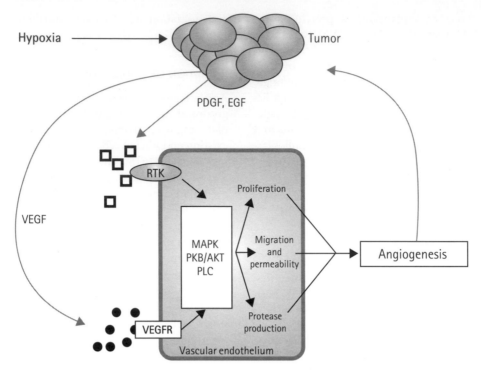

Figure 23.2 *Regulation of tumor angiogenesis. In response to a variety of stimuli, including hypoxia, tumor cells secrete growth factors, including platelet-derived growth factor (PDGF), epidermal growth factor (EGF), and vascular endothelial growth factor (VEGF). These ligands bind to their cognate receptors expressed on host vascular endothelial cells. VEGF binding to vascular endothelial growth factor receptors 1 or 2 (VEGFR-1, VEGFR-2) activates a receptor-signaling cascade, promoting the release of proteases, and inducing proliferation and migration toward the tumor, resulting in angiogenesis. A variety of anti-angiogenic agents have been developed that target various aspects of this pathway. Inhibitors of growth factor signaling, including the platelet-derived growth factor receptor (PDGFR) and ERBB systems, may also prove useful as anti-angiogenic agents. (MAPK, mitogen-activated protein kinase; PKB, protein kinase B.)*

Aberrant cell migration and invasion as a therapeutic target

BRAIN TUMOR CELL INVASION

High-grade gliomas disseminate widely in the brain along anatomical structures, including white-matter tracts and blood vessels. Other tumors, e.g. medulloblastoma and, more rarely, ependymoma, actively metastasize through the neuraxis. The balance between controlling malignant behavior, while preserving normal neuronal tissue, presents an enormous therapeutic challenge.

The process by which malignant cells spread beyond their site of origin involves a complex series of interactions between tumor cells and their tissue environment. Astrocytomas may migrate over stromal cells that elaborate extracellular matrix (ECM) proteins, including lamin, collagen-type IV, fibronectin, and vitronectin. There is also evidence to suggest that glioma cells themselves secrete an ECM-like substance that assists in their migration.[17] Other secreted proteins believed to promote the proliferation and migration of glioma cells include PDGF-AA, PDGF-BB, and ERBB and FGF ligands. The matrix metalloproteinases (MMPs) are a further group of proteins that contribute to the invasive potential of tumor cells. The production of these enzymes is induced by host tissue, under the regulation of growth factors and cytokines, in response to tumor cell invasion. MMPs contribute to a number of critical steps in tumor development, including local migration, basement-membrane degradation, and invasion and angiogenesis.[70]

TARGETING CELL MIGRATION AND INVASION

A variety of matrix metalloproteinases inhibitors (MMPIs) have entered clinical trial. Marimastat is one of the most extensively studied to date.[71,72] An inhibitor of MMPs 1–3, 7, 9, and 12, this agent demonstrated marked musculoskeletal side effects in phase I trials and failed to demonstrate objective responses in phase II studies.[71,73] Completed phase III trials for gastric cancer have also shown no survival advantage.[72] It remains to be determined whether this agent will prove useful in combination studies or whether the other MMPIs currently under investigation demonstrate more promising activity.

A novel mechanism by which glioma cells invade normal brain tissue has been proposed.[74] Termed "exocitotoxicity," this hypothesis suggests that the high levels of glutamate produced by glioma cells induce a cytotoxic/apoptotic cascade in surrounding neurons, thereby clearing

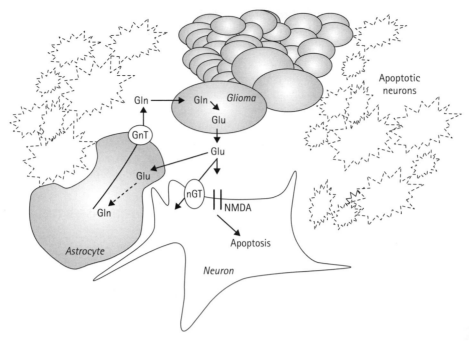

Figure 23.3 *Exocitotoxicity: a putative novel mechanism for glioma cell invasion of normal brain. Glutamate induces a cytotoxic response in normal neurons. Glioma cells generate glutamate (Glu) from glutamine (Gln). Signaling by Glu via its N-methyl-D-aspartate (NMDA) receptor expressed on nearby neurons results in a pro-apoptotic response. Thus, a path is cleared by the glioma, allowing further invasion of normal brain. Astrocytes may participate in this process through Glu reprocessing. A variety of components of this system may prove to be useful therapeutic targets. These include inhibitors of NMDA receptors or the GnT transporter. Alternatively, the neuronal Glu transporter (nGT, or its astrocytic counterpart gGT) may be stimulated, thus reducing the availability of Glu for signaling.*

a path for extension into the brain (Figure 23.3). As supporting evidence, Takano and colleagues demonstrated that the in vivo growth of brain tumors in their study model was related directly to the level of glutamate generated by tumors.[74] Furthermore, blockade of the N-methyl-D-aspartate (NMDA) glutamate receptor significantly abrogated the growth of tumors in a rat model. This observation opens up the possibility of a completely new avenue for brain tumor treatment, with potential sites of therapeutic action at all levels of glutamate signaling. Indeed, a number of glutamate receptor antagonists that proved ineffective in clinical trials of other neurological diseases, including stroke, are available for evaluation in CNS malignancies and may subsequently prove useful in the treatment of brain tumors.

Miscellaneous small–molecule inhibitors

INHIBITORS OF DNA METHYLATION AND HISTONE DEACETYLATION

A number of elements involved in the normal biology of DNA structure and function have been investigated as potential therapeutic targets in human disease, including cancer. In this regard, particular attention has been focused on DNA methylation and histone deacetylation. These two reactions appear to cooperate to silence the expression of certain genes, including tumor suppressors.[75,76] Briefly, the methylation of cysteine residues with CpG-rich gene promoter regions enables the recruitment of histone deacetylase complexes (HDAC), which modify the surrounding chromatin structure, resulting in repression of gene expression. A number of important growth and apoptosis control genes have been shown to be aberrantly methylated in human cancer cells, including $P16^{INK4A}$, $P14^{ARF}$, and *CASPASE 8*.[77–79] Importantly, silencing of *CASPASE-8* has been shown to affect medulloblastoma cells, resulting in increased resistance to apoptosis in vitro.[56]

A variety of DNA methylation and HDAC inhibitors are currently in clinical trials in adults and have demonstrated ability to alter gene expression in vivo.[80,81] While the assessment of each of these agents will be important, the apparent synergy between DNA methylation and HDAC in the silencing of genes suggests that the combination of methylation and HDAC inhibitors may prove especially exciting. Indeed, evidence already exists that such an approach is likely to prove more effective than single-agent therapy.[82]

HEAT SHOCK PROTEIN CHAPERONE SYSTEM AS A THERAPEUTIC TARGET

Heat shock protein-90 (HSP90) functions as a molecular chaperone for a number of protein kinases important in cell signaling, including the ERBB2 receptor and components of its downstream signaling pathway.[83] Novel therapeutics that target HSP90 therefore represent an attractive new approach for the management of human malignancies in which aberrant signaling plays an important pathological role. The benzoquinoid ansamycin 17-allylamino-17-demethoxygeldanamycin (17-AAG) represents the first HSP90 antagonist to enter clinical trials.

17-AAG is a novel structural analog of geldanamycin, a naturally occurring benzoquinoid ansamycin antibiotic. These drugs were first reported to possess potent anti-tumor activity following reports that geldanamycin and related compounds were active against solid-tumor xenografts in mice and could reverse the transformed phenotype in Rous sarcoma virus-transformed cells.[84] In vitro studies subsequently identified HSP90 and its endoplasmic reticulum homolog glucose-regulated protein-94 (GRP94) as the sole cellular targets for both geldanamycin[85,86] and 17-AAG.[87] HSP90 is a highly conserved and ubiquitously expressed stress protein that accounts for one to two per cent of the total cytosolic protein in mammalian cells. In eukaryotes, it has an important chaperone function, ensuring the conformational maturation of client cellular proteins.[83] X-ray crystallography has shown geldanamycin to compete with adenosine triphosphate (ATP) for the nucleotide binding site of HSP90, thereby inhibit the chaperoning of these clients.[88,89] Consequently, client molecules are targeted for polyubiquitination and proteolysis by the cytosolic ATP-dependent, 26S proteosome complex.

Both geldanamycin and 17-AAG[88] readily inhibit the growth and expression of cell signaling molecules by human tumor cell lines.[90] Initial studies of pediatric tumors suggest that the growth of pediatric PNET cells may be inhibited by benzoquinoid ansamycin treatment.[91] Subsequent studies have demonstrated that overexpression of the ERBB2 receptor sensitizes medulloblastoma cells to 17-AAG by upregulating MAPK signaling.[92] Further experiments are under way to determine in vivo growth-inhibitory and client protein degradation activity of 17-AAG against medulloblastoma xenografts. It is envisaged that data obtained from these experiments will assist in the planning of pediatric phase I studies once the ongoing early trials in adult cancer are complete.

Gene transfer approaches in the treatment of pediatric brain tumors

THE UNIQUE CHALLENGE OF DEVELOPING GENE-BASED TREATMENTS

The transfer of tumor suppressor genes, or genes encoding cytotoxic or immunomodulating products into tumor cells, has been the subject of a great deal of research and regulatory scrutiny over recent years.[93] Although this approach holds enormous therapeutic potential, it is the most controversial of novel biologic strategies. This relates in part to the considerable technical difficulties associated with the design, production, and effective employment of gene constructs and vectors. However, the safety of this approach has also raised concerns among the scientific community and general public. Careful future development of these treatments, within guidelines of accepted practice, will be vital to ensure that any benefits of this approach are obtained with the continued support of the wider community.

TARGETS OF GENE TRANSFER THERAPIES

Gene transfer therapy describes the delivery of DNA vectors that encode biological therapeutics, with a broad range of actions, to diseased tissues (Figure 23.4).[93–95] Therapeutic genes can serve to activate prodrugs, thus targeting drug action to disease sites,[96] or encode toxins fused to disease-relevant ligands, allowing local, disease-specific targeting of cytotoxic proteins.[95] Gene transfer can also be designed to work with conventional treatments. Such approaches may involve the use of expression vectors that either sensitize tissues to, or whose promoters and thus expression are activated by, radiotherapy.[97] Vectors may also be employed that express immunomodulators, including cytokines, thus boosting the host anti-tumor immune response. Finally, the vectors themselves can act as cytotoxic agents.[98]

Therapeutic genes that encode prodrug-metabolizing enzymes allow the potential to selectively concentrate cytotoxic metabolites within tumor cells (Figure 23.4). Within the context of brain tumor therapy, this approach employs non-toxic prodrugs that penetrate the brain parenchyma. One of the most widely used strategies has involved the combination of herpes simplex type 1 thymidine kinase (HSVTK) and ganciclovir. HSVTK phosphorylates inactive ganciclovir, enabling it to be incorporated into DNA and resulting in cell death.[99,100] Cytotoxic therapy can also be delivered to tumor cells by transferring genes that encode toxins fused to proteins, e.g. ligands, that bind selectively to tumor cells.[101] The delivery of tumor suppressor genes whose function has been lost in brain tumor cells, e.g. TP53,[102,103] or genes that encode proteins with dominant negative activity against oncoproteins, have also received much attention. In this regard, the elements of the angiogenic pathway including VEGF and VEGFR-1 have been investigated as potential targets.[104]

An intriguing use of replication-incompetent viruses involves the use of conditionally replicative vectors. ONYX-015 is an adenovirus in which the E1B gene is deleted and replicates only in certain cancer cells.[105] This appears to show a degree of selectivity for cells that are TP53-mutant, although preclinical data have been

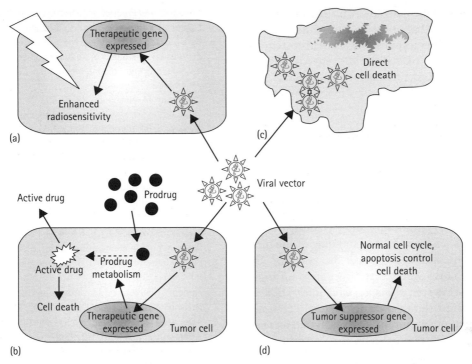

Figure 23.4a,b,c,d *Gene transfer therapies in brain tumors. A number of potential uses of gene transfer have been proposed for the treatment of brain tumors. (a) Viral vectors may contain therapeutic genes encoding radiosensitizing products, or they may include promoter regions that are activated by radiation. (b) "Suicide" gene therapy is one of the most widely studied approaches. Viral vectors encode enzymes, e.g. HSV-TK, that metabolize inactive prodrugs. The active drug is thus targeted only to transduced cells, reducing systemic side effects. The active drug may also diffuse locally to non-transduced cells, thereby increasing the anti-tumor effect. (c) Viruses may be directly cytopathic, e.g. ONYX-015 (see text). (d) Therapeutic genes may also include wild-type tumor suppressor genes, whose function has been lost in targeted tumor cells. The resulting restoration of cell-cycle/apoptotic control may lead to anti-tumor effects.*

somewhat controversial.[106] Nevertheless, combination studies of ONYX-015, cisplatin, and 5-fluorouracil have demonstrated promising results in patients with head/neck cancers,[107] and studies in adults with glioblastoma are under way.

VECTOR SYSTEMS

Vectors, the vehicle by which genes are transferred to their targets, fall into two broad groups: viral and non-viral. The latter essentially include naked DNA and DNA enclosed within lipid vesicles, or liposomes. Non-viral transfer systems are relatively inefficient, rendering them less attractive than viral systems. Viral vectors may be divided further into those that integrate DNA into host cell chromosomes and non-integrating vectors whose vector DNA remains as non-chromosomal episomes.

Retroviral vectors were among the first integrating vectors to be developed and have played an important role in the early development of gene therapy. Although their use in some disease states has been limited by their inability to infect non-dividing cells, their potential to avoid normal quiescent cells in the brain while infecting rapidly

proliferating tumor and neovascular endothelium has made them an attractive agent for brain tumors. Other viral vectors under investigation include the lentiviruses, the adenoviruses, and their dependent adeno-associated viruses. One additional application likely to be investigated in pediatric oncology is the use of gene therapy to protect normal tissues from high-dose chemotherapy. In particular, strategies to protect hemopoietic stem cells from cytotoxic agents are under investigation.

FUTURE CHALLENGES FOR GENE TRANSFER THERAPY

As the field of gene therapy has developed, the principal challenges facing those seeking to progress this novel approach have also changed. Now that viral vectors can be manufactured at high levels in forms that can deliver genes to diseased tissue, future challenges include issues of safety and maintenance of expression. The selective targeting of vectors to diseased tissue, with minimal delivery to normal cells, is an important component of protecting patients from adverse effects. Advances have been made in this area, with techniques including the design of viruses whose coats include engineered proteins that recognize tumor-specific antigens. A further major hurdle to be overcome is that of the host immune response to vector systems. This response serves both to remove transduced cells and to reduce the effectiveness of repeated administration of therapeutic viral vectors.

CONCLUSIONS

The failure of conventional treatment strategies to achieve effective cure for many children with brain tumors presents all professionals involved in the management of these children with a tremendous challenge. Central to this is the identification of new, effective treatment approaches. Increasing understanding of the biology of these diseases has opened the way for the introduction of novel agents that target aberrant brain tumor biology. However, the successful integration of these strategies into clinical practice will be a complex process. Biologists must continue to identify and increase our understanding of the pathways that are critical for tumor cell survival. Structural biologists and pharmacologists will be required to identify agents that target components of these pathways and provide additional insights into the molecular processes involved in drug–target interactions. Virologists, immunologists, and many other scientific disciplines will be crucial to the development of safe, effective ways of delivering biologics. Finally, all members of the medical community in association with these scientific specialists will participate in the evaluation of the toxicity and biological efficacy of these new treatments. Although this is a difficult challenge, it is far outweighed by the potential rewards for all the children and their families who are afflicted by these terrible diseases.

ACKNOWLEDGMENTS

Dr Gilbertson is supported by NIH grants CA 21765 and CA P01-96832, by a translational grant from the V-Foundation for Cancer Research, by a Distinguished Scientist Award from the Sontag Foundation, and by the American Lebanese Syrian Associated Charities (ALSAC).

Dr O'Rourke is supported by grants from the National Institutes of Health (RO1 CA 09586), The Department of Veterans Affairs (Merit Review Program) and by the Brain Tumor Society.

REFERENCES

1 Smith MA, Gloeckler Ries LA. Childhood cancer: incidence, survival and mortality. In: Pizzo PA, Poplack DG (eds). *Principals and Practice of Pediatric Oncology*. Philadelphia: Lippincott Williams & Wilkins, 2002, pp. 1–12.

2 Bart J, Groen HJ, Hendrikse NH, van der Graaf WT, Vaalburg W, de Vries EG. The blood–brain barrier and oncology: new insights into function and modulation. *Cancer Treat Rev* 2000; **26**:449–62.

3 Libermann TA, Nusbaum, HR, Razonn N, *et al*. Amplification, enhanced expression and possible rearrangement of EGF receptor gene in primary human brain tumours of glial origin. *Nature* 1985; **313**:144–7.

4 Ekstrand AJ, Sugawa N, James CD, Colins VP. Amplified and rearranged epidermal growth factor receptor genes in human glioblastomas reveal deletions of sequences encoding portions of the N- and/or C-terminal tails. *Proc Natl Acad Sci USA* 1992; **89**:4309–13.

5 Westermark B, Heldin CH, Nister M. Platelet-derived growth factor in human glioma. *Glia* 1995; **15**:257–63.

6 Blume-Jensen P, Hunter T. Oncogenic kinase signalling. *Nature* 2001; **411**:355–65.

7 Yarden Y, Sliwkowski MX. Untangling the ErbB signalling network. *Nature Rev Mol Cell Biol* 2001; **2**:127–37.

8 Adjei AA. Blocking oncogenic Ras signaling for cancer therapy. *J Natl Cancer Inst* 2001; **93**:1062–74.

9 Widmann C, Gibson S, Jarpe MB, Johnson GL. Mitogen-activated protein kinase: conservation of a three-kinase module from yeast to human. *Physiol Rev* 1999; **79**:143–80.

10 Brazil DP, Hemmings BA. Ten years of protein kinase B signalling: a hard Akt to follow. *Trends Biochem Sci* 2001; **26**:657–64.

11 Khwaja A. Akt is more than just a Bad kinase. *Nature* 1999; **401**:33–4.

12 Di Cristofano A, Pandolfi PP. The multiple roles of PTEN in tumor suppression. *Cell* 2000; **100**:387–90.

13 Bonneau D, Longy M. Mutations of the human PTEN gene. *Hum Mutat* 2000; **16**:109–22.

14 Wu CJ, Chen Z, Ullrich A, Greene MI, O'Rourke DM. Inhibition of EGFR-mediated phosphoinositide-3-OH kinase (PI3-K) signaling and glioblastoma phenotype by signal-regulatory proteins (SIRPs). *Oncogene* 2000; **19**:3999–4010.

15 O'Rourke DM, Qian X, Zhang HT, *et al*. Trans receptor inhibition of human glioblastoma cells by erbB family ectodomains. *Proc Natl Acad Sci USA* 1997; **94**:3250–5.

16 O'Rourke DM, Kao GD, Singh N, *et al*. Conversion of a radioresistant phenotype to a more sensitive one by disabling erbB signaling in human cancer cells. *Proc Natl Acad Sci USA* 1998; **95**:10842–7.

17 Cavenee WK, Furnari FB, Nagane M, Huang H, Newcomb EW, Bigner DD. Diffusely infiltrating astrocytomas. In: Kliehues P, Cavenee WK (eds). *World Health Organization Classification of Tumours: Pathology and Genetics of Tumours of the Nervous System*. Lyon: IARC Press, 2000, pp. 10–21.

18 Prigent SA, Nagane M, Lin H, *et al*. Enhanced tumorigenic behavior of glioblastoma cells expressing a truncated epidermal growth factor receptor is mediated through the Ras-Shc-Grb2 pathway. *J Biol Chem* 1996; **271**:25639–45.

19 Moscatello DK, Holgado-Madruga M, Emlet DR, Montgomery RB, Wong AJ. Constitutive activation of phosphatidylinositol 3-kinase by a naturally occurring mutant epidermal growth factor receptor. *J Biol Chem* 1998; **273**:200–6.

20 Bredel M, Pollack IF, Hamilton RL, James CD. Epidermal growth factor receptor expression and gene amplification in high-grade non-brainstem gliomas of childhood. *Clin Cancer Res* 1999; **5**:1786–92.

21 Gilbertson RJ, Hill A, Hernan R, *et al.* ERBB1 is amplified and overexpressed in high-grade diffusely infiltrative pediatric brain stem glioma. *Clin Cancer Res* 2003; **9**:3620–4.

22 Gilbertson RJ, Perry RH, Kelly PJ, Pearson AD, Lunec J. Prognostic significance of HER2 and HER4 coexpression in childhood medulloblastoma. *Cancer Res* 1997; **57**:3272–80.

23 Herms JW, Behnke J, Bergmann M, *et al.* Potential prognostic value of c-erbB-2 expression in medulloblastoma in very young children. *J Pediatr Hematol Oncol* 1997; **19**:510–15.

24 Gilbertson RJ, Clifford SC, MacMeekin W, *et al.* Expression of the ErbB-neuregulin signaling network during human cerebellar development: implications for the biology of medulloblastoma. *Cancer Res* 1998; **58**:3932–41.

25 Gilbertson R, Hernan R, Pietsch T, *et al.* Novel ERBB4 juxtamembrane splice variants are frequently expressed in childhood medulloblastoma. *Genes Chromosomes Cancer* 2001; **31**:288–94.

26 Gajjar A, Hernan R, Kocak M, *et al.* Clinical, histopathological and molecular markers of prognosis: toward a new disease risk stratification system for medulloblastoma. *J Clin Oncol* 2003; in press.

27 Hernan R, Fasheh R, Calabrese C, *et al.* The S100A4 metastasis-inducing gene is upregulated by ERBB2 in medulloblastoma. *Cancer Res* 2003; **63**:140–8.

28 Zhou BP, Liao Y, Xia W, Spohn B, Lee MH, Hung MC. Cytoplasmic localization of p21Cip1/WAF1 by Akt-induced phosphorylation in HER-2/neu-overexpressing cells. *Nature Cell Biol* 2001; **3**:245–52.

29 Yu D, Hung MC. Role of erbB2 in breast cancer chemosensitivity. *Bioessays* 2000; **22**:673–80.

30 Gilbertson RJ, Bentley L, Hernan R, *et al.* ERBB receptor signaling promotes ependymoma cell proliferation and represents a novel therapeutic target for this disease. *Clin Cancer Res* 2002; **8**:3054–64.

31 Wang SC, Hung MC. HER2 overexpression and cancer targeting. *Semin Oncol* 2001; **28**:115–24.

32 Cobleigh MA, Vogel CL, Tripathy D, *et al.* Multinational study of the efficacy and safety of humanized anti-HER2 monoclonal antibody in women who have HER2 overexpressing metastatic breast cancer that has progressed after chemotherapy for metastatic disease. *J Clin Oncol* 1999; **17**:2639–48.

33 Park BW, Zhang HT, Wu C, *et al.* Rationally designed anti-HER2/neu peptide mimetic disables P185HER2/neu tyrosine kinases in vitro and in vivo. *Nat Biotechnol* 2000; **18**:194–8.

34 Arteaga CL, Johnson DH. Tyrosine kinase inhibitors-ZD1839 (Iressa). *Curr Opin Oncol* 2001; **13**:491–8.

35 Baselga J, Averbuch SD. ZD1839 ("Iressa") as an anticancer agent. *Drugs* 2000; **60**:33–40.

36 Moasser MM, Basso A, Averbuch SD, Rosen N. The tyrosine kinase inhibitor ZD1839 ("Iressa") inhibits HER2-driven signaling and suppresses the growth of HER2-overexpressing tumor cells. *Cancer Res* 2001; **61**:7184–8.

37 McKinnon RD, Matsui T, Dubois-Dalcq M, Aaronson SA. FGF modulates the PDGF-driven pathway of oligodendrocyte development. *Neuron* 1990; **5**:603–14.

38 Uhrbom L, Hesselager G, Nister M, Westermark B. Induction of brain tumors in mice using a recombinant platelet-derived growth factor B-chain retrovirus. *Cancer Res* 1998; **58**:5275–9.

39 MacDonald TJ, Brown KM, LaFleur B, *et al.* Expression profiling of medulloblastoma: PDGFRA and the RAS/MAPK pathway as therapeutic targets for metastatic disease. *Nat Genet* 2001; **29**:143–52.

40 Gilbertson RJ, Clifford SC. PDGFRB is overexpressed in metastatic medulloblastoma. *Nat Genet* 2003; **35**(3):197–8.

41 Drucker B. Perspectives on the development of a molecularly targeted agent. *Cancer Cell* 2002; **1**:31–6.

42 Buchdunger E, Cioffi CL, Law N, *et al.* Abl protein-tyrosine kinase inhibitor STI571 inhibits in vitro signal transduction mediated by c-kit and platelet-derived growth factor receptors. *J Pharmacol Exp Ther* 2000; **295**:139–45.

43 Sebolt-Leopold JS. Development of anticancer drugs targeting the MAP kinase pathway. *Oncogene* 2000; **19**:6594–9.

44 Kato K, Cox AD, Hisaka MM, Graham SM, Buss JE, Der CJ. Isoprenoid addition to Ras protein is the critical modification for its membrane association and transforming activity. *Proc Natl Acad Sci USA* 1992; **89**:6403–7.

45 Bredel M, Pollack IF, Freund JM, Hamilton AD, Sebti SM. Inhibition of Ras and related G-proteins as a therapeutic strategy for blocking malignant glioma growth. *Neurosurgery* 1998; **43**:124–31.

46 Zujewski J, Horak ID, Bol CJ, *et al.* Phase I and pharmacokinetic study of farnesyl protein transferase inhibitor R115777 in advanced cancer. *J Clin Oncol* 2000; **18**:927–41.

47 Eskens FA, Awada A, Cutler DL, *et al.* European Organization for Research and Treatment of Cancer Early Clinical Studies Group. Phase I and pharmacokinetic study of the oral farnesyl transferase inhibitor SCH 66336 given twice daily to patients with advanced solid tumors. *J Clin Oncol* 2001; **19**:1167–75.

48 Geoerger B, Kerr K, Tang CB, *et al.* Antitumor activity of the rapamycin analog CCI-779 in human primitive neuroectodermal tumor/medulloblastoma models as single agent and in combination chemotherapy. *Cancer Res* 2001; **61**:1527–32.

49 Louro ID, McKie-Bell P, Gosnell H, Brindley BC, Bucy RP, Ruppert JM. The zinc finger protein GLI induces cellular sensitivity to the mTOR inhibitor rapamycin. *Cell Growth Differ* 1999; **10**:503–16.

50 Collins VP. Progression as exemplified by human astrocytic tumors. *Semin Cancer Biol* 1999; **9**:267–76.

51 Sherr CJ. The Pezcoller lecture: cancer cell cycles revisited. *Cancer Res* 2000; **60**:3689–95.

52 Sherr CJ. The ink4a/arf network in tumour suppression. *Nature Rev Mol Cell Biol* 2001; **2**:731–7.

53 Scheurlen WG, Schwabe GC, Joos S, Mallenhauer J, Sorensen N, Kuhl J. Molecular analysis of childhood primitive neuroectodermal tumours defines markers associated with poor outcome. *J Clin Oncol* 1998; **16**:2478–85.

54 Grotzer MA, Hogarty MD, Janss AJ, *et al.* MYC messenger RNA expression predicts survival outcome in childhood primitive neuroectodermal tumor/medulloblastoma. *Clin Cancer Res* 2001; **7**:2425–33.

55 Herms J, Neidt I, Luscher B, *et al.* C-MYC expression in medulloblastoma and its prognostic value. *Int J Cancer* 2000; **89**:395–402.

56 Grotzer MA, Eggert A, Zuzak TJ, *et al*. Resistance to TRAIL-induced apoptosis in primitive neuroectodermal brain tumor cells correlates with a loss of caspase-8 expression. *Oncogene* 2000; **19**:4604–10.

57 Nagata S. Steering anti-cancer drugs away from the TRAIL. *Nat Med* 2000; **6**:502–3.

58 Ferrara N, Alitalo K. Clinical applications of angiogenic growth factors and their inhibitors. *Nat Med* 1999; **5**:1359–64.

59 Carmeliet P, Jain RK. Angiogenesis in cancer and other diseases. *Nature* 2000; **407**:249–57.

60 Jain RK. Normalizing tumor vasculature with anti-angiogenic therapy: a new paradigm for combination therapy. *Nat Med* 2001; **7**:987–9.

61 Risau W. Mechanisms of angiogenesis. *Nature* 1997; **386**:671–4.

62 Korpelainen EI, Alitalo K. Signaling angiogenesis and lymphangiogenesis. *Curr Opin Cell Biol* 1998; **10**:159–64.

63 Plate KH, Breier G, Weich HA, Risau W. Vascular endothelial growth factor is a potential tumour angiogenesis factor in human gliomas in vivo. *Nature* 1992; **359**:845–8.

64 Millauer B, Shawver LK, Plate KH, Risau W, Ullrich A. Glioblastoma growth inhibited in vivo by a dominant-negative Flk-1 mutant. *Nature* 1994; **367**:576–9.

65 Kim KJ, Li B, Winer J, *et al*. Inhibition of vascular endothelial growth factor-induced angiogenesis suppresses tumour growth in vivo. *Nature* 1993; **362**:841–4.

66 Fong TA, Shawver LK, Sun L, *et al*. SU5416 is a potent and selective inhibitor of the vascular endothelial growth factor receptor (Flk-1/KDR) that inhibits tyrosine kinase catalysis, tumor vascularization, and growth of multiple tumor types. *Cancer Res* 1999; **59**:99–106.

67 Laird AD, Vajkoczy P, Shawver LK, *et al*. SU6668 is a potent antiangiogenic and antitumor agent that induces regression of established tumors. *Cancer Res* 2000; **60**:4152–60.

68 Stopeck A. Results of a phase I dose-escalating study of the anti-angiogenic agent, SU5416, in patients with advanced malignancies. *Proc Am Soc Clin Oncol* 2000; **19**:206a.

69 Read TA, Sorensen DR, Mahesparan R, *et al*. Local endostatin treatment of gliomas administered by microencapsulated producer cells. *Nat Biotechnol* 2001; **19**:29–34.

70 Chambers AF, Matrisian LM. Changing views of the role of matrix metalloproteinases in metastasis. *J Natl Cancer Inst* 1997; **89**:1260–70.

71 Steward WP. Marimastat (BB2516): current status of development. *Cancer Chemother Pharmacol* 1999; **43** (suppl.):S56–60.

72 Steward WP, Thomas AL. Marimastat: the clinical development of a matrix metalloproteinase inhibitor. *Expert Opin Investig Drugs* 2000; **9**:2913–22.

73 Rosemurgy A, Harris J, Langleben A, Casper E, Goode S, Rasmussen H. Marimastat in patients with advanced pancreatic cancer: a dose-finding study. *Am J Clin Oncol* 1999; **22**:247–52.

74 Takano T, Lin JH, Arcuino G, Gao Q, Yang J, Nedergaard M. Glutamate release promotes growth of malignant gliomas. *Nat Med* 2001; **7**:1010–15.

75 Nan X, Ng HH, Johnson CA, *et al*. Transcriptional repression by the methyl-CpG-binding protein MeCP2 involves a histone deacetylase complex. *Nature* 1998; **393**:386–9.

76 Jones PL, Veenstra GJ, Wade PA, *et al*. Methylated DNA and MeCP2 recruit histone deacetylase to repress transcription. *Nat Genet* 1998; **19**:187–91.

77 Robertson KD, Jones PA. The human ARF cell cycle regulatory gene promoter is a CpG island which can be silenced by DNA methylation and down-regulated by wild-type p53. *Mol Cell Biol* 1998; **18**:6457–73.

78 Esteller M, Corn PG, Baylin SB, Herman JG. A gene hypermethylation profile of human cancer. *Cancer Res* 2001; **61**:3225–9.

79 Teitz T, Wei T, Valentine MB, Vanin EF, *et al*. Caspase 8 is deleted or silenced preferentially in childhood neuroblastomas with amplification of MYCN. *Nat Med* 2000; **6**:529–35.

80 Yoshida M, Furumai R, Nishiyama M, Komatsu Y, Nishino N, Horinouchi S. Histone deacetylase as a new target for cancer chemotherapy. *Cancer Chemother Pharmacol* 2001; **48** (suppl 1):S20–6.

81 Szyf M. The DNA methylation machinery as a therapeutic target. *Curr Drug Targets* 2000; **1**:101–18.

82 Cameron EE, Bachman KE, Myohanen S, Herman JG, Baylin SB. Synergy of demethylation and histone deacetylase inhibition in the re-expression of genes silenced in cancer. *Nat Genet* 1999; **21**:103–7.

83 Pratt WB. The hsp90-based chaperone system: involvement in signal transduction from a variety of hormone and growth factor receptors. *Proc Soc Exp Biol Med* 1998; **217**:420–38.

84 Saski K, Ysuda H, Onodera, K. Growth inhibition of virus transformed cells in vitro and antitumour activity in vivo of geldanamycin and its derivatives. *J Antibiot* 1979; **32**:849–54.

85 Whitesell L, Mimnaugh EG, De Costa B. Inhibition of heat shock protein HSP90-pp60^{v-src} heteroprotein complex formation by benzoquinone ansamycins: essential role for stress proteins in oncogenic transformation. *Proc Natl Acad Sci USA* 1994; **91**:8324–8.

86 Chavany C, Mimnaugh EG, Miller P. p185(erbB2) binds to GRP94 in vivo-dissociation of the p185(erbB2)/GRP94 heterocomplex by benzoquinone ansamycins precedes depletion of p185(erbB2). *J Biol Chem* 1996; **271**:4974–7.

87 Schulte TW, Neckers L. The benzoquinone ansamycin 17-allylamino-17-demethoxygeldanamycin binds to HSP90 and shares important biologic activities with geldanamycin. *Cancer Chemother Pharmacol* 1998; **42**:273–9.

88 Prodromou C, Roe SM, O'Brien R. Identification and structural characterization of the ATP/ADP-binding site in the Hsp90 molecular chaperone. *Cell* 1997; **90**:65–75.

89 Scheibel T, Buchner J. The Hsp90 complex – a super-chaperone machine as a novel drug target. *Biochem Pharmacol* 1998; **56**:675–82.

90 Supko JG, Hickman RL, Grever MR, Malspeis L. Preclinical pharmacological evaluation of geldanamycin as an antitumour agent. *Cancer Chemotherapy Pharmacol* 1995; **36**:305–15.

91 Whitesell L, Shifrin SD, Schwab G, Neckers LM. Benzoquinoid ansamycins possess selective tumoricidal activity unrelated to *src* kinase inhibition. *Cancer Res* 1992; **52**:1721–8.

92 Calabrese C, Frank A, Maclean K, Gilbertson RJ. Medulloblastoma sensitivity to 17-allylamino 17-demethoxygeldanamycin requires MEK/ERK. *J Biol Chem* 2003; **278**:24951–9.

93 Somia N, Verma IM. Gene therapy: trials and tribulations. *Nat Rev Genet* 2000; **1**:91–9.

94 Alemany R, Gomez-Manzano C, Balague C, *et al*. Gene therapy for gliomas: molecular targets, adenoviral vectors, and oncolytic adenoviruses. *Exp Cell Res* 1999; **252**:1–12.

95 Lam PY, Breakefield XO. Potential of gene therapy for brain tumors. *Hum Mol Genet* 2001; **10**:777–87.

96 Aghi M, Hochberg F, Breakefield XO. Prodrug activation enzymes in cancer gene therapy. *J Gene Med* 2000; **2**:148–64.

97 Stackhouse MA, Buchsbaum DJ. Radiation to control gene expression. *Gene Ther* 2000; **7**:1085–6.

98 Wickman TJ. Targeting adenovirus. *Gene Ther* 2000; **7**:110–14.

99 Moolten FL, Wells JM. Curability of tumors bearing herpes thymidine kinase genes transferred by retroviral vectors. *J Natl Cancer Inst* 1990; **82**:297–300.

100 Culver KW, Ram Z, Wallbridge S, Ishii H, Oldfield EH, Blaese RM. In vivo gene transfer with retroviral vector-producer cells for treatment of experimental brain tumors. *Science* 1992; **256**:1550–2.

101 Puri RK. Development of a recombinant interleukin-4-*Pseudomonas* exotoxin for therapy of glioblastoma. *Toxicol Pathol* 1999; **27**:53–7.

102 Rosenfeld MR, Meneses P, Dalmau J, Drobnjak M, Cordon-Cardo C, Kaplitt MG. Gene transfer of wild-type p53 results in restoration of tumor-suppressor function in a medulloblastoma cell line. *Neurology* 1995; **45**:1533–9.

103 Estreicher A, Iggo R. Retrovirus-mediated p53 gene therapy. *Nat Med* 1996; **2**:1163.

104 Machein MR, Risau W, Plate KH. Antiangiogenic gene therapy in a rat glioma model using a dominant-negative vascular endothelial growth factor receptor 2. *Hum Gene Ther* 1999; **10**:1117–28.

105 Bischoff JR, Kirn DH, Williams A, *et al*. An adenovirus mutant that replicates selectively in p53-deficient human tumor cells. *Science* 1996; **274**:373–6.

106 Lane DP. Killing tumor cells with viruses – a question of specificity. *Nat Med* 1998; **4**:1012–13.

107 Khuri FR, Nemunaitis J, Ganly I, *et al*. A controlled trial of intratumoral ONYX-015, a selectively-replicating adenovirus, in combination with cisplatin and 5-fluorouracil in patients with recurrent head and neck cancer. *Nat Med* 2000; **6**:879–85.

PART VI

Late consequences and supportive care

24

Toxicity and late effects

HELEN SPOUDEAS AND FENELLA J. KIRKHAM

INTRODUCTION

One in 1000 young adults is a cancer survivor, 10–15 per cent of whom originally had a brain tumor. Thus, quality of life and any resulting long-term disabilities in these individuals have become important public health issues. Despite the recognition of endocrine, neurological, and cognitive deficits, there is little understanding of the underlying pathology or its evolution, whilst community awareness of potential secondary disease and/or remedial help is often limited. Early (and even preventive) psychological and rehabilitative intervention to improve not only physical and hormonal health but also social, educational, and independence skills may make the difference between an institutionalized, unhealthy, short life, and a fuller, independent adult life.

In terms of life-years lost by death from cancer, a suboptimal treatment in childhood has a high and much greater impact on society than in adults (average 68 years lost per case of childhood cancer, compared with ten years for adult cancers). For example, the incidence of medulloblastoma is 0.7 per 100 000 children under 14 years, per annum.[1] This equates to some 1000 cases per annum in Europe. With a current estimated survival of 70 per cent, and 50–90 per cent of survivors being affected by one or more disabilities, it can be predicted that 20 000 life-years will be lost and a burden of 30 000–50 000 life-years of disability gained by this group of children alone. The extent of acquired, lifelong neuropsychological, hormonal, physical, or other disability among survivors from current treatment regimens is thus a large potential economic, health, and social burden on families and society. This belies the flawed but frequently held perception that as childhood brain cancer is a low-risk disease, it has little significance in the health of nations. Any measures that together increase treatment efficacy and decrease long-term disability would carry huge advantages in human and economic terms.

In this chapter, endocrine and neurological consequences of brain tumors and their treatment will be identified, and the evidence for the current state of knowledge with respect to their diagnosis, etiology, long-term consequences and treatment will be reviewed. Within the context of treating children for these tumors, a model summarizing the factors that enhance risks of both neurological and endocrine consequences emphasizes the interplay between tumor, treatment, and host factors (Figure 24.1). This is a fast-changing field, and each year brings new data and new treatments that alter the balance with respect to the selection of anti-tumor treatments as well as the possibilities for preventing or treating the endocrine or neurological consequences.

ENDOCRINE CONSEQUENCES OF BRAIN AND SPINAL TUMORS AND THEIR TREATMENT

The control of the normal hormonal milieu is heavily dependent on central control of hormone release emanating from the hypothalamic-pituitary axis (HPA). Figure 24.2 and Table 24.1 summarize the current knowledge

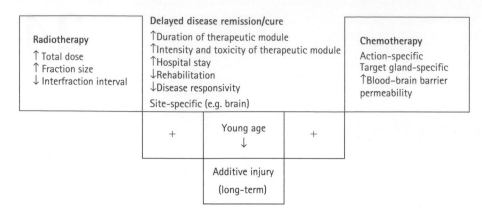

Figure 24.1 *Adverse factors contributing to long-term neurological and endocrine injury.*

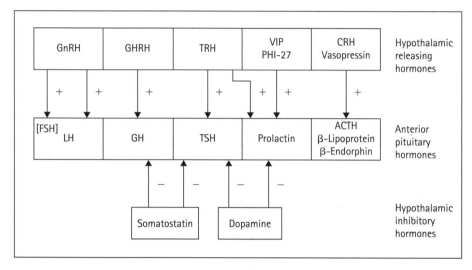

Figure 24.2 *Hormones in the anterior pituitary and the hypothalamus. This figure summarizes the current nomenclature and mechanisms regulating the release of hormones that are produced in the hypothalamus and anterior pituitary gland. (ACTH, adrenocorticotrophic hormone; CRH, corticotrophin-releasing hormone; FSH, follicle-stimulating hormone; GH, growth hormone; GHRH, growth hormone-releasing hormone; GnRH, gonadotrophin-releasing hormone; LH, luteinizing hormone; TRH, thyrotropin-releasing hormone; TSH, thyroid-stimulating hormone; VIP, vasoactive intestinal peptide.)*

Table 24.1 *Function of hypophysiotropic hormones*

Hormone	Function
GnRH	Releases LH and FSH
GHRH	Releases GH
TRH	Releases TSH and prolactin
VIP (PHI-27)	Releases prolactin
CRH	Releases ACTH, β-endorphin, and β-lipoprotein
Vasopressin	Antidiuretic action in kidney; releases ACTH through CRH
Dopamine	Inhibits pituitary TSH and prolactin release, with widespread distribution and effects
Somatostatin	Inhibits pituitary GH and TSH release, with widespread distribution and effects

ACTH, adrenocorticotrophic hormone; CRH, corticotrophin-releasing hormone; FSH, follicle-stimulating hormone; GH, growth hormone; GHRH, growth hormone-releasing hormone; GnRH, gonadotrophin-releasing hormone; LH, luteinizing hormone; TRH, thyrotropin-releasing hormone; TSH, thyroid-stimulating hormone; VIP, vasoactive intestinal peptide.

concerning the range of hormones released by these cerebral structures, the mechanisms controlling their release, and their normal actions. Detailed understanding of how these hormonal mechanisms become disrupted by brain tumors or their treatment, and the consequences for the growing child, have been the focus of clinical research over the past two decades. During this period, clinical practices with respect to decision-making and techniques employed in both neurosurgery and radiotherapy have changed and continue to be re-evaluated as the data concerning endocrine effects of treatment are collected and assimilated. This section will examine the evidence for etiology, pathophysiology, and clinical patterns of endocrine dysfunction in the immature child. The spectrum of endocrine disorders linked to brain tumors and their treatment includes damage to both the HPA and target glands, the consequences of which are lifelong and include gland failure, infertility, obesity, and impaired bone mineralization.

Pathophysiology of hypothalamo–pituitary dysfunction and growth hormone deficiency

Just as the adverse neuropsychological late effects have been attributed almost entirely to a dose-dependent effect of cranial irradiation,[2] so have the deficits in growth hormone (GH) secretion.[3] Hypopituitarism commonly occurs after surgery and radiation treatment for tumoral involvement of the pituitary (Figure 24.3a).[4] Nevertheless, late endocrine comparisons between adults and children irradiated for pituitary tumors and posterior fossa tumors suggest that the anatomical site of the tumor must make an important contribution to the number and hierarchical evolution of post-irradiation endocrinopathies. Despite similar estimated pituitary doses of 40 Gy, GH is often the only hormone affected in this group of children, with adrenocorticotropic hormone (ACTH) deficiency fortunately rare by comparison, although it may yet evolve (Figure 24.3b).[5]

Patterns of isolated growth hormone deficiency after cranial irradiation

Evaluation of GH physiology can be measured by 24-hour GH level monitoring, in which the pulsatile release pattern can be evaluated, or after stimulation of GH release in order to measure peak responses. Children exposed to cranial irradiation alone experience growth failure due to disturbances in both pulsatile GH secretion and/or attenuated stimulated peak GH responses. These effects are seen in 60–100 per cent of children within two to five years of fractionated (<2 Gy) cranial irradiation at total doses of more than 30 Gy.[6,7] The speed of onset is dose-dependent,[3]

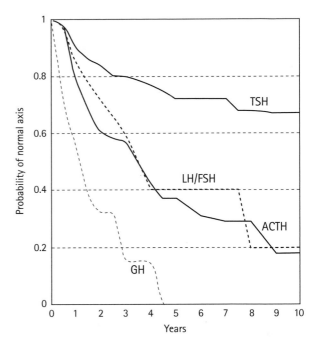

Figure 24.3a *Endocrinopathies after treatment for pituitary tumors (adults). Cumulative percentage of 37 adults experiencing endocrinopathies after radiotherapy (37.5–42.5 Gy) in 15 fractions over 20–22 days for pituitary tumors and who demonstrated postoperatively one or more intact pituitary hormones, from a total cohort of 165 surgically treated cases. The hierarchical loss demonstrates that growth hormone (GH) is the most sensitive, all adults being deficient within five years. Thyroid-stimulating hormone (TSH) is the least sensitive. Adrenocorticotrophic hormone (ACTH) and gonadotropin (luteinizing hormone (LH)/follicle-stimulating hormone (FSH)) deficiency are affected increasingly over time (80 per cent at ten years). (Redrawn from Littley et al.[4])*

but there is unlikely to be a lowest "safe" dose. The few studies of pulsatile 24-hour GH secretion before and after radiation (>30 Gy) for brain tumors distant from the hypothalamo-pituitary axis (HPA) suggest an evolving picture, with neurosecretory disturbances getting worse and more frequent with time and irradiation dose intensity. The changes in these circumstances become severe and permanent (Figure 24.3c).[6,8] In Figure 24.3c, note the wide variation in trough secretion across groups compared with controls, and the marked early discrepancy between spontaneous (preserved) and stimulated (attenuated) peaks, even in children treated with surgery only (Gp 1). This discrepancy becomes concordant with time and intensity of therapy, as spontaneous GH secretions fails.

At lower cranial irradiation doses, as seen in cranial irradiation for central nervous system (CNS) directed therapy in leukemia, discrepancies between growth velocity and the results of stimulated and 24-hour pulsatile GH-secretion measurements may occur.[9,10] Such discrepant findings may also be seen at early time periods after high

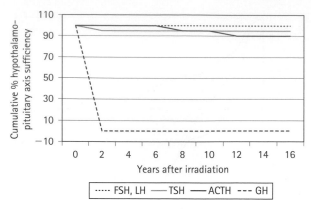

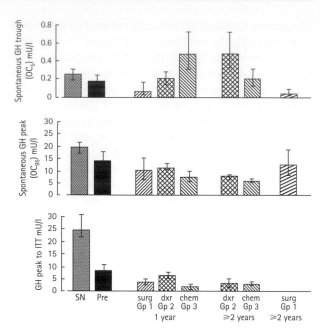

Figure 24.3b *Endocrinopathies after treatment for posterior fossa tumors. Cumulative percentage of 16 patients with posterior fossa tumors demonstrating normal anterior pituitary function during a median 11.0 (6.8–21.4)-year follow-up period. Despite the greater duration of follow-up than the study cited in (a) (more than eight years in 13 patients, more than 12 years in seven patients, 16 years in one patient) and similar biologically effective pituitary doses (at least 40 Gy in 1.8-Gy fractions), there were no cases of gonadotrophin deficiency and only two cases of (asymptomatic) borderline adrenal insufficiency. This suggests that ACTH deficiency is unusual where the primary tumor is well displaced from the pituitary area and is unlikely to be a radiation-induced endocrinopathy. (Redrawn from Spoudeas et al.[5])*

Figure 24.3c *Relationship of spontaneous GH troughs (OC_5) (upper panel), spontaneous GH peaks (OC_{95}) (middle panel), and stimulated peak GH responses to hypoglycemia insulin tolerance test (ITT) (lower panel) with increasing therapeutic intensity and time in short normal (SN) controls and in children with brain tumors before (pre) radiotherapy and at one and two to five years after neurosurgery alone (surg Gp1), or with additional >30 Gy cranial irradiation (dxr Gp 2), or >30 Gy cranial irradiation with adjuvant chemotherapy (chem Gp 3). (Redrawn from Spoudeas et al.[6])*

dose cranial irradiation for brain tumors but then disappear as the endocrine damage evolves with time and all measures become suppressed and thus concordant.[6] It is assumed that this is due to the higher radiation dose leading to a more rapid and complete GH deficiency. Subtle abnormalities in the pulsatile pattern of GH release can be particularly evident around the time of puberty.[11] Augmented GH secretion is necessary at this time to mount a normal (largely spinal) growth spurt. Failure of this pulsatile GH release probably accounts in part for the shorter adult spine that has remained unexplained in other studies.[12]

The lack of a gold standard for assessing GH secretory status after brain tumors makes it imperative that all slowly growing children have a full endocrinological assessment. Furthermore, adult survivors of brain tumors, with or without cranial irradiation, are at real risk of adult GH deficiency, with its attendant implications for bone mineralization, body composition, lipid profile, and quality of life (see box).

Diagnosing and treating growth hormone deficiency

- Discrepant growth rates and standard diagnostic tests of GH deficiency may confuse the diagnosis of GH deficiency in the cranially irradiated survivor, particularly if performed soon after cure.

- The imperative to treat early with recombinant hormone growth hormone (r-hGH) is greatest in the youngest and smallest children and those treated most intensively, because catch-up growth is incomplete and compounding over time.

- Children who receive spinal or total body irradiation, particularly with co-administered chemotherapy, deserve special attention because the spinal component of puberty is compromised, even with r-hGH.

- It is important to maximize the growth potential in the legs while this window of opportunity exists, i.e. prepubertally.

- With a proactive endocrine surveillance program, most childhood cancer survivors achieve adult heights within the normal centiles and an age-appropriate puberty.

- Treatment with r-hGH in replacement doses does not increase the disease relapse rate compared with untreated children.

Etiologies of tumor–related hypothalamic dysfunction

Research studies that reliably define the etiology of endocrine dysfunction after treatment for brain tumor are important, as the results will assist in the selection of new and hopefully less toxic strategies for therapy. Children with central optic, pineal, or pituitary/hypo-thalamic tumors are those most at risk of developing potentially life-threatening endocrinopathies. In such locations, the effects of the tumor itself, attempts at surgical removal or debulking, local and extended field irradiation, and chemotherapy can all add to the risk of endocrine damage. Nowhere is this demonstrated better than in the management of craniopharyngioma, where conservative surgery (e.g. cyst aspiration) followed by radiotherapy reduces the otherwise high incidence of pituitary failure seen after radical surgery (see Chapter 20). The evidence for independent and potentially addi-tive toxicities of multimodal therapy on the neuroen-docrine system comes from the few prospective and longitudinal studies of children with posterior fossa tumors. Subtle central deficits in the neuroregulatory secretion of GH exist after surgery alone, and are com-pounded by irradiation and increased further with the passage of time. Similarly, chemotherapy can potentiate this progressive disruption of the central hypothalamic GH release mechanisms, thereby further confounding the interpretation of dynamic GH provocation tests (Figure 24.3).[6]

The sustained augmentation and pulsatility of GH release, without downregulation, observed over a 24-hour continuous infusion of growth hormone-releasing hor-mone (GHRH), depends on the endogenous integrity of a second inhibitory hypothalamic hormone, somatostatin, important for both maintaining GH within a readily releasable pituitary pool and determining the timing of each pulse (on/off). The integrity of this GH-inhibitory hormone tone appears easily disturbed by cerebral insults in vivo,[6,13,14] which may explain both the disturbed rhythmicity of GH pulsatility and the reason why GHRH therapy is less effective than r-hGH in this situation (Figure 24.4). If the etiology and site of the damage were determined accurately, then pre-irradiation strategies for protecting the area might be attempted,[15] and/or more physiological, cost-effective, and user-friendly depot or oral peptide treatments may be developed.

Thus, hypothalamic disruption occurs first most probably then causing secondary pituitary atrophy; whether this is neural or vascular in origin is unclear from the few studies of hypothalamo-pituitary blood flow in this situation.[16] The importance of differentiating between hypothalamic and pituitary dysfunction is high-lighted, because therapeutic options, such as inducing fertility with hypothalamic releasing factors (e.g.

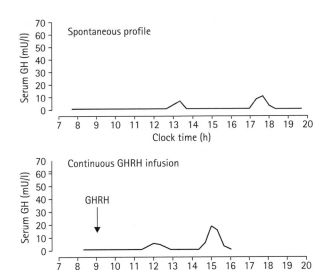

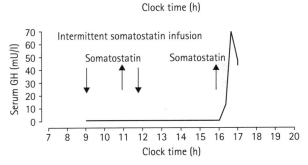

Figure 24.4 *One year after cranial radiotherapy for a cerebral tumor, a seven-year-old boy demonstrated very attenuated growth hormone (GH) pulsatility (upper panel). This can be manipulated and augmented by continuous growth hormone-releasing hormone (GHRH) therapy (middle panel) and somatostatin withdrawal, indicating that the pituitary remains responsive at this early stage. (Redrawn from Spoudeas.[13])*

The hypothalamic-pituitary-adrenal axis

- GH deficiency affects all cranially irradiated survivors eventually, but ACTH deficiency is rare if there has been no HPA disease.
- The hypothalamic and/or pituitary nature of the post-irradiation endocrinopathy is not understood fully.
- Cranial irradiation is not the only culprit: surgery and the presence of tumors are also significant factors.
- Systemic chemotherapy crosses the disrupted blood–brain barrier and causes additive central toxicity.
- The differentiation of hypothalamic from pituitary disease has important therapeutic and etiological implications.

gonadotrophin-releasing hormone (GnRH)),[17] would be limited severely by the existence of significant pituitary or gonadal disease.

PATTERNS OF ENDOCRINE DYSFUNCTION

Growth

Spinal irradiation (27–35 Gy in 22–27 days) independently impairs spinal growth.[18,19] The younger the child, the greater the deficit, which is estimated at 9 cm if irradiation is administered at one year, 7 cm if administered at five years, and 5.5 cm if administered at ten years.[19] Spinal growth is a major component of the pubertal growth spurt, so the disproportionate deficit, compounded by pubertal GH deficiency, may only then become apparent, at a time when growth promotion is limited.

Because irradiation damages both the epiphyses and the bony matrix, the skeleton may not demonstrate the growth response to GH treatment expected in children with idiopathic GH deficiency. Thus, it is important to maximize prepubertal growth potential in the legs while this is still possible by early GH replacement therapy. It is almost inevitable to anticipate some loss of spinal growth compromising final adult height, even with optimal replacement therapy (Figure 24.5).

Conventionally scheduled radiation is delivered in daily fractions five days per week. Typical fractions are less than 2 Gy. Giving radiation in smaller fractions more frequently (two or three times a day; see Chapter 10) may reduce the toxic effects of the radiation on normal tissues while preserving the anti-tumor effects; this is known as hyperfractionated radiotherapy. The effects of hyperfractionation of the radiation dose remain to be determined. Animal experiments support the view that such techniques may spare normal tissues.[20] Trials comparing conventional and hyperfractionated techniques in children have been launched, but their results with respect to late toxicities are awaited.

Additive injury at target gland (gonads, thyroid, skeleton)

The two adjuvant treatment modalities, chemotherapy and radiotherapy, are apparently additively toxic not only at the pituitary level[6] but also at both the glandular and the skeletal level.[21–23] With spinal irradiation techniques used during the early era of radiotherapy, subfertility and hypothyroidism affected approximately one-third of survivors. This figure was doubled by the added toxicity of chemotherapy.[21,22] While the evidence for the additive effect of chemotherapy is based on the observation of temporary

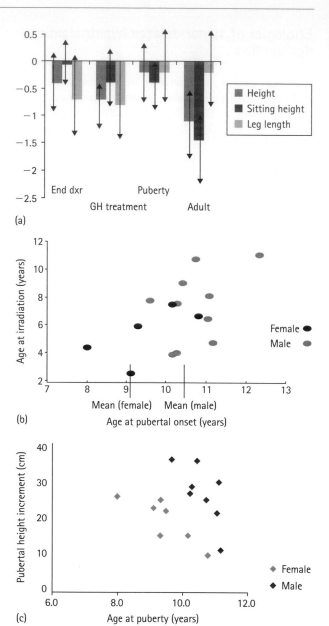

Figure 24.5a,b,c *(a) By the end of craniospinal irradiation (dxr), the cohort of prepubertal patients studied were already short. Despite the early (within two years from diagnosis) institution of growth hormone (GH) therapy, there was inadequate catch-up growth back to the original centile at adult height. The adult height deficit was incurred largely after onset of puberty, the pubertal spurt being early (b) and increasingly attenuated with age (c). It was due to incomplete spinal (not leg length) growth. The latter was normalized with prompt GH replacement therapy, allowing the majority of patients to achieve an adult height within the normal centiles. (Redrawn from Spoudeas)[19a]*

elevations in thyroid-stimulating hormone (TSH) after Hodgkin's disease chemotherapy, its independent role in the pathogenesis of sustained thyroid dysfunction is less evident. Hypothyroidism and gonadal dysfunction are much less common in young adult survivors of radiotherapy treated more recently,[5] with virtually no evidence so far of long-term adrenal dysfunction (Figure 24.3b).

Thyroid dysfunction

Radiation damage to the thyroid gland causes hypothyroidism, sometimes associated with autoimmunity usually compensated by increased TSH production, and thyroid tumors. Hypothyroidism is dose- and time-dependent. It has been well documented after fractionated doses to the neck in excess of 25 Gy.[24] It has also been documented in the longer term after scattered doses to the thyroid as low as 0.3 Gy for benign disease in childhood[25] and after natural radiation fall-out experiments, such as following the Chernobyl disaster.[26]

Elevations in TSH have been attributed to primary thyroid gland damage. Because of the carcinogenic potential of prolonged stimulation of the irradiated gland, annual thyroid function tests (with thyroxine replacement if TSH is persistently elevated), thyroid palpation (with ultrasound and needle biopsy of isolated nodules) are recommended. However, documented TSH normalization and thyroid recovery after craniospinal irradiation[22] raises the possibility that elevations in TSH may be evidence of higher hypothalamic irradiation damage, disturbing the normal day-to-night TSH variation by obliterating the nocturnal TSH surge (Figure 24.6).[13,27]

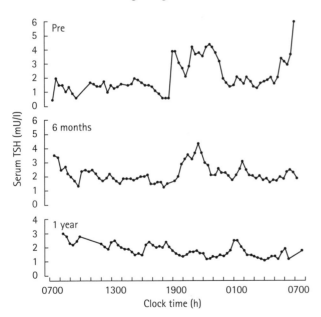

Figure 24.6 *The 24-hour 20-minute thyroid-stimulating hormone (TSH) profile of a five-year-old girl with medulloblastoma before (upper panel) and six (middle panel) and 12 (lower panel) months after craniospinal irradiation, indicating loss of the normal nocturnal TSH surge. Thyroxine and TSH levels remained well within the normal range. This pattern of disturbance has been thought to represent hypothalamic dysfunction. (Redrawn from Spoudeas.[13])*

Thyroid

- After craniospinal irradiation, with or without additional chemotherapy, primary thyroid and gonadal dysfunction may coexist with (and mask) thyrotropin-releasing hormone (TRH) or GnRH hypothalamo-pituitary disturbance.
- The loss of the nocturnal TSH surge and the possible "recovery" of compensated hypothyroidism after cranial irradiation may indicate higher hypothalamic disturbance.
- Compensated primary hypothyroidism after cranial or craniospinal irradiation deserves treatment to suppress TSH because of the risk of malignancy in the irradiated thyroid gland.
- Thyroid swellings should be assessed carefully with scans, needle biopsy, and a low threshold for thyroidectomy (according to forthcoming national BSPED/UKCCSG guidelines.)[28]

Precocious puberty

Precocious (early) puberty is a recognized presentation of optic, hypothalamic, and other "central" tumors, but it has also been detected after treatment for more laterally or inferiorly placed tumors.[7, 29] Possible coexistent gonadotoxicity induced by chemotherapy[30,31] or spinal irradiation[21] confounds the true prevalence. Gonadotrophin deficiency arresting pubertal development is also possible,[21] although this is more likely after high-dose irradiation of pituitary or closely located tumors.[4,32]

Early puberty, related directly to the age at irradiation,[29] occurs particularly but not exclusively in girls, whose hypothalamic gonadotrophin pulse generator is known to be more sensitive. It is more evident after lower cranial doses used in leukemia (24 or 18 Gy) than after the higher (>35 Gy) cranial irradiation doses used in brain tumors. This finding has become more evident since spinal irradiation, and thus scattered ovarian irradiation, was omitted from neuraxial prophylaxis. Early puberty also occurs after episodes of prolonged intracranial pressure due to obstructive hydrocephalus. Its importance in these situations is that it can severely limit growth potential. To the untrained eye, an early, albeit attenuated, growth spurt can mask GH deficiency (Figure 24.7) until it is too late for intervention with replacement therapy. A similar situation can exist with obesity.

Reproductive capacity

It is difficult to forecast the growth, pubertal progress, and ultimate reproductive potential of a prepubertal

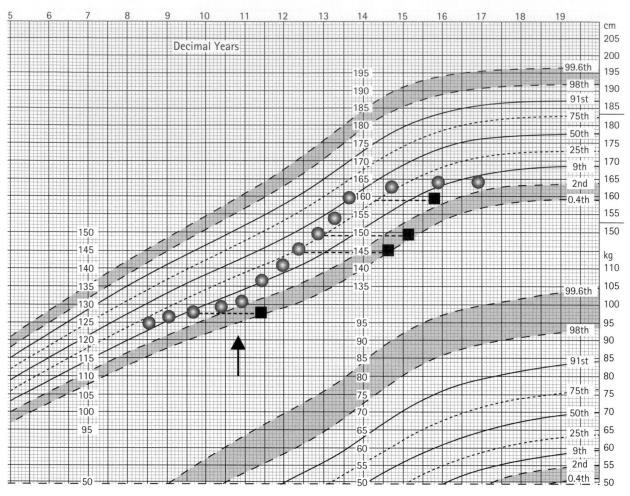

Figure 24.7 *This young boy's spinal irradiation, early puberty, and hence advanced skeletal maturation (indicated by solid squares) compromised the amount of "catch-up" growth he could achieve despite growth hormone replacement therapy (indicated by arrow).*

child receiving both cranial irradiation (with its potential effects on pituitary hormone secretion, both activating and depleting),and potentially gonadotoxic therapy, since many sites on the hypothalamo-pituitary target-gland axis may be affected simultaneously by multimodal therapies and/or disease. Subclinical target-gland toxicity (such as might occur after lower or scattered irradiation doses to the gonad[21]) may carry important implications for future reproductive capacity, which may not be detectable for many years. Indeed, the observation that early puberty is evident, despite gonadotoxic chemotherapy and scattered gonadal irradiation,[22] suggests that disrupted hypothalamic control predominates over peripheral target gland toxicity, at least at these low estimated scattered irradiation doses to the ovary (approximately 4 Gy)[31] or testis (<2 Gy).[30] For such reasons, it is important to ascertain, if possible, longitudinal growth, puberty, and hormonal data before treatment and at intervals thereafter until growth and puberty are complete. Such assessments are ideally performed together with questionnaire-derived

quality-of-life (QoL) outcomes (see Chapter 27). Despite the long follow-up required, final height data and long-term reproductive outcome are important outcome measures impacting on QoL, which are being addressed in the newest UK Children's Cancer Study Group (UKCCSG) and Société Internationale de Oncologie Pédiatrique (SIOP) protocols for primitive neuroectodermal tumor (PNET).

FACTORS INFLUENCING FERTILITY

All girls are born with a fixed ovarian pool of oocytes, which undergo progressive atresia from before birth until the menopause. Given the larger residual ovarian pool in younger (as opposed to older) girls, and the greater radiosensitivity of the testicular (sperm-producing) Sertoli cells as compared with the (hormone-secreting) Leydig cells,[33,34] it is likely that most children with brain tumors will experience a spontaneous puberty, often earlier than expected, despite scattered spinal irradiation and gonadotoxic chemotherapy.[7] However, this does not exclude the coexistent possibility of male subfertility or a premature menopause[35] at some time in the future, nor of bone demineralization due to subclinical sex steroid deficiency. In addition, there is evidence for dose-dependent recovery of sperm counts with time after graded irradiation doses to the testis[36] while after gonadotoxic chemotherapy the speed of recovery can be modulated hormonally,[37] provided the doses are not ablative.[38] Therefore, in the youngest patients, there may be a window for the application of assisted reproductive technology, which has revolutionized male infertility.[39] Early referral to an endocrine or reproductive center for both males and females is recommended for detailed counseling about future reproductive and sexual health. In selected cases, pre-treatment gamete cryopreservation is an effective insurance strategy being increasingly considered in adolescents.

Adult growth hormone deficiency

After treatment for brain tumor and cranial irradiation for leukemia, GH deficiency is common. Its prevalence increases with time and affects almost all cranially irradiated survivors within five years.[7,40] Its diagnosis is complicated by early puberty, obesity, and the confounding effects of spinal irradiation. Accurate diagnosis requires a high index of suspicion and careful growth and development surveillance. In a recent multicenter report, the prevalence of GH replacement therapy among 545 patients (age under 15 years at diagnosis) after treatment for medulloblastoma varied from five to 73 per cent and was commenced on average four years after diagnosis.[41] GH deficiency has also been blamed for osteopenia, obesity, atherogenic lipid profiles, decreased cardiac performance, and reduced QoL due to the adult GH deficiency syndrome.[42] Cardiac contractility may be reduced further by significant (30 per cent) irradiation scatter to the mediastinum from the spinal dose,[43] while the adjuvant toxicity of potentially cardiotoxic chemotherapeutic agents needs to be considered in this context and also in relation to the potential for lung fibrosis.[43]

Although GH replacement in physiological doses appears safe in these patients from the point of view of disease relapse,[41,44] there have been concerns that supraphysiological doses of GH may promote tissue overgrowth,[45] which could enhance the risk of tumor recurrence or second tumor development in adult life. However, there is as yet no evidence for this in childhood.

Obesity

Obesity may occur as a result of cranial irradiation and/or the brain tumor itself,[46] although it is harder to explain in those without hypothalamic lesions.[47] Untreated growth and thyroid hormonal deficiencies may contribute. Excessive weight gain is a recognized complication of suprasellar, but not intrasellar, tumors and their treatment. For some time, growth may be maintained in the face of GH deficiency by increased insulin-like growth factor (IGF)-bioavailability, modulated in turn by hyperinsulinemia, which further drives the obesity (Figure 24.8).[48] There is some evidence to suggest that obesity in these circumstances results from ventromedial hypothalamic lesions causing disinhibition of vagal tone at the level of the pancreatic beta cell. In extreme cases, truncal vagotomy has alleviated the obesity.[49]

The tendency to obesity observed in cranially irradiated youngsters without hypothalamic lesions is harder to explain and just as difficult to treat.[47] Whether the eventual insulin resistance is also primarily the result of increased vagal tone or secondary to hyperphagia involving central satiety centers is unknown. Corticosteroid use[50] and reduced exercise[51] may also be important contributory factors. Obesity and insulin resistance pose a real risk of premature death from diabetes and cardiovascular disease. GH deficiency aggravates obesity, while GH therapy decreases fat mass, increases lean mass through direct actions on adipocytes, and suppresses leptin in parallel.[52] Both insulin and leptin are suppressed by somatostatin, which paradoxically may improve short-term insulin resistance in this situation.[47] Leptin signaling modulates energy balance via effects on the hypothalamus and other tissues, maintaining adipose tissue mass within a finite physiological range. Any role that disturbances in this pathway might play in the evolution of obesity (or early puberty) after cranial irradiation still remains to be elucidated, but healthy lifestyle measures and possibly adult GH replacement therapy need to be considered in these circumstances, particularly if there are other significant endocrinopathies.

Impaired bone mineralization

Osteoporosis has been blamed on the adult GH deficiency syndrome, but skeletal changes observed in cancer survivors may also be attributable to other hormonal (sex steroid) deficiencies. Skeletal irradiation,[18] corticosteroids, and antineoplastic agents[53–55] may also impair mineralization directly or indirectly by inducing renal tubulopathies. Disease,[56] prolonged bedrest, and changes in vitamin D metabolism may also influence bone mineral density (BMD). Concern that a lower peak bone mass in adolescence will cause osteoporosis later in adult life is therefore valid. However, the interpretation of surrogate markers of BMD, such as dual energy x-ray absorptiometry (DEXA) measurements at the lumbar spine, needs to be undertaken with care. Sex- and age-standardized

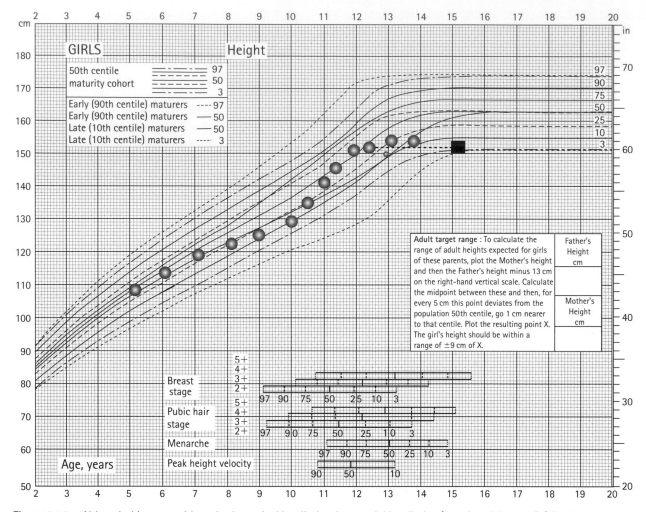

Figure 24.8a *Although this young girl received no spinal irradiation, her cranial irradiation (at reduced dose 24 Gy) for leukemia caused pubertal growth hormone deficiency, which was missed due to an early but suboptimal growth spurt and continued growth at the expense of excessive and inexorable weight gain. Her adult height potential was compromised significantly as a result.*

reference charts may be misleading in a population that is short because of GH deficiency and spinal irradiation, and with pubertal maturation delay.[57] In adults, other femoral and distal radial sites may be used, but corrections should still be made for size.[57] Volumetric densities, independent of bone size and measured with quantitative computed tomography (CT), are the current gold standard.[58] Future prospective studies are necessary to help delineate the multifactorial etiology of peak bone mass impairment and to encourage appropriate intervention strategies.

Osteoporosis

- Correction factors for size are needed when assessing BMD in the cancer survivor.

- Hormone and dietary replacement therapies should be optimized to aid peak bone mineral accretion, age-appropriate puberty, uterine enlargement, and hair regrowth, and to prevent obesity.
- Weight-bearing, aerobic exercise and a healthy calcium-containing diet should be encouraged to prevent osteopenia, obesity, and insulin resistance.
- GH replacement therapy should be considered in adult life for those with severe and multiple pituitary deficiencies.
- The benefit of GH replacement in the adult with isolated GH deficiency is not proven.

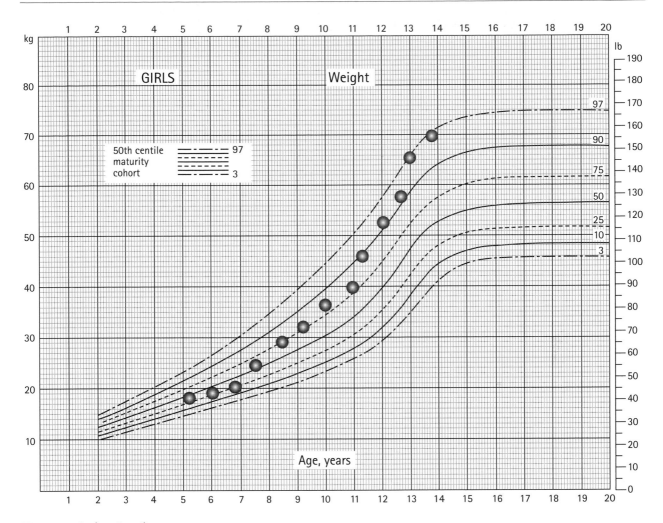

Figure 24.8b *(continued)*

SUMMARY

Figure 24.9 summarizes the endocrine consequences of CNS tumors and their treatments.

Effects in the immature individual

The endocrine system is highly vulnerable to damage from primary CNS tumors and their treatment. In planning any treatment aimed at the tumor, a number of consequences must be balanced against the predicted benefits of the planned treatment.

Sustained and uncontrolled raised intracranial pressure is common at the time of presentation, due to lag time between onset of symptoms and diagnosis. Sustained periods of raised pressure may contribute to the development of precocious puberty, particularly in girls, GH deficiency, and cognitive impairment.

Surgical attempts at tumor resection in the vicinity of hormone-secreting structures can cause severe damage, e.g. craniopharyngioma surgery, resection of hypothalamic, pineal, or pituitary tumors, and be additive to pre-existing endocrinopathies. Postoperatively, these children can have major life-threatening problems with hormone deficiencies of both anterior and posterior pituitary hormone production further complicated by adipsia and hyperphagia. Antidiuretic hormone (ADH)-deficiency presents particularly difficult short- and longer term management problems related to achieving fluid balance, in the cortisol-deficient, unconscious or hypodipsic child.

Craniospinal irradiation, used for treatment of malignant tumors with capacity for CSF dissemination, e.g. medulloblastoma, CNS involvement with acute lymphatic leukemia, or germ-cell tumors, has the capacity to profoundly affect both growth and pubertal development through hypothalamic pituitary damage, the inhibition of GHRH and somatostatin release, primary

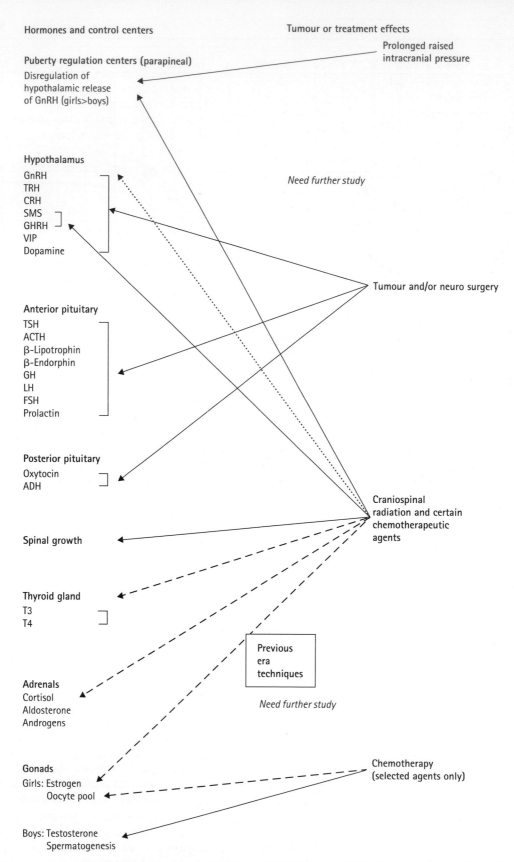

Figure 24.9 *Summary of the existing knowledge of tumor and treatment effects on endocrine and reproductive organs. Solid arrow indicates proven toxicity, dotted arrow indicates probable toxicity (ACTH, adrenocorticotrophic hormone; ADH, antidiuretic hormone; CRH, corticotrophin-releasing hormone; FSH, follicle-stimulating hormone; GH, growth hormone; GHRH, growth hormone-releasing hormone; GnRH, gonadotrophin-releasing hormone; LH, luteinizing hormone; SMS, somatostatin; T3, tri-iodothyronine; T4, thyroxine; TRH, thyrotropin-releasing hormone; TSH, thyroid-stimulating hormone; VIP, vasoactive intestinal peptide.)*

hypothyroidism from scattered thyroid irradiation, and the direct effect of spinal column irradiation, which compromises the adolescent spinal growth spurt. Taken together, the worst situation arises in the girls who are smallest and youngest; a poor prepubertal growth velocity, reduced sitting height, and early puberty can severely compromise the adult final height and put the individual at risk of exaggerated central obesity. Previously, radiotherapy techniques delivered scatter doses of radiation to the ovaries in some young girls, which could compromise both hormone and egg production.

Effects in the mature individual (late survivor)

The consequences of this endocrine damage in mature individuals must still be determined by long-term follow-up studies. Lifelong hormone deficiencies, including panhypopituitarism, primary hypothyroidism, and isolated GH deficiency, are well recognized after hypothalamic/pituitary surgery and/or craniospinal radiotherapy. They require lifelong hormone replacement therapy if symptoms attributable to the deficiency are identified or predicted. Disturbances of sexual function and/or fertility may be related to panhypopituitarism or may be due to direct gonadal damage by chemotherapy or radiotherapy. Obesity and osteoporosis, the possible end results of brain tumor therapy, cause long-term public health implications in relation to hypertension, diabetes, cardiovascular disease and osteoporosis.

Chemotherapy is not thought to cause profound effects on central endocrine control but the few early studies which do examine this aspect suggest a concern which requires further longitudinal assessment of children treated with chemotherapy alone in endocrine clinics. Selected chemotherapy agents, particularly in high cumulative doses, may cause a reduction in egg number in girls, which may lead to a predicted shortened fertile period and premature menopause. In boys, the damaging effects of selected chemotherapy agents, particularly in high cumulative doses, may cause oligospermia and azoospermia and therefore reduced natural fertility, although assisted fertility techniques are offering an increasing range of alternative approaches to this type of problem. The combined effects of pelvic irradiation (from spinal irradiation) and chemotherapy may be additionally and potentially more toxic to spinal growth and reproductive capacity.

Future goals

- National cross-specialty longitudinal studies of adequate duration to address QoL outcomes in specific tumor cohorts and treatments.
- Prospective clinical and biochemical growth, pubertal, bone mineralization, fertility, and QoL data collection in national studies.
- Comparison of endocrine outcomes between randomized groups conducted in parallel (rather than in series).
- More prospective physiological studies addressing causation and clinical consequences of HPA dysfunction, early puberty, obesity, and osteoporosis.
- More randomized therapeutic intervention studies to prevent obesity and osteoporosis.
- Randomized protective intervention strategies of the HPA or gonadal axes before/during cancer therapy.

Conclusion

- Cranial irradiation to the HPA usually results in endocrine dysfunction. Its incidence, time course, and severity are dependent not only on the dose, fractionation, and time elapsed since irradiation, but also on the sensitivity of each hormone and each site to the damaging mechanisms. In addition to radiation, tumor position, surgery, and chemotherapy also contribute to late toxicity at all levels of the hypothalamo-pituitary-target-gland axis and thus mandate endocrine follow-up for all patients with brain tumors, regardless of therapy.
- Lifelong endocrine follow-up, in an age-appropriate multidisciplinary setting, is certainly necessary after cranial irradiation, and possibly after any brain tumor therapy, to detect and differentiate evolving central from peripheral endocrinopathies.
- If tumors have not involved the "central" pituitary area, then the GH axis is the most sensitive and the adrenal axis the most resistant to the effects of direct irradiation.
- Interpreting growth rates of children with radiation-induced skeletal lesions in the face of disturbances of GH release and discrepancies between different provocation tests will help to define physiological abnormalities, target potential protective strategies, and the most appropriate replacement therapy.
- Instituting therapy early may be of especial benefit in promoting normal pubertal and social adjustment, growth, fertility, and bone mineralization. An increasing number of reports suggest an important role for GH therapy in aging hypopituitary adults to optimize atherogenic lipid profiles, body mass, and bone density, and therefore QoL. This is yet to be evaluated fully in younger populations.

- Resources directed at encouraging a healthy, active lifestyle and increased metabolic expenditure may delay the need for adult GH replacement in those with isolated GH deficiency.
- Oncologists and radiotherapists must plan the timing of treatment protocols with the intention of reducing neuroendocrine morbidity and prolonging survival.
- Reducing the neuroendocrine burden of morbidity, whether due to treatment or tumor damage, will lighten the load for the brain tumor survivor, who may also be struggling with the neurological or cognitive consequences of brain injury. These are discussed below.

NEUROLOGICAL FUNCTION

The wide variety of motor and sensory neurological deficits that children experience in relation to the anatomical site of the tumor and its treatment are beyond the scope of this chapter. However, some specific deficits of general relevance are considered below, with particular reference to strategies for prevention.

Specific patterns of neurological dysfunction

CEREBELLAR MUTISM

This is a well-recognized postoperative syndrome after cerebellar tumor surgery, with 29 per cent of children having clinical evidence in one prospective series.[1] Risk factors include the site (midline) and nature (medulloblastoma) of the tumor; patients with large medulloblastomas are particularly at risk.[1] The postoperative symptoms are usually dominated by lack of speech, but there may be other components of the posterior fossa syndrome, including ataxia, cranial nerve palsies, bulbar palsies, hemiparesis, cognitive impairment, and emotional lability. It develops a few days after surgery and may last for several months or longer, often to be followed by dysarthria. The most accepted cause for the condition is vascular spasm, with involvement of the dentate nucleus and the dentatorubrothalamic tracts to the brainstem and subsequently to the cortex. Diaschisis, reduction of blood flow in the contralateral hemisphere in relation to cerebellar pathology, may be involved in causing the loss of higher cerebral functions, although a recent single-photon-emission computed tomography (SPECT) study suggested that this was not the case.[59] It is also possible that complicating hydrocephalus plays a role, although there was little evidence for this in a large prospective series.[1]

HEARING LOSS

High-frequency hearing loss, progressing to involve the speech frequency range (500–3000 Hz), is a major dose-dependent toxicity of cisplatin. However, other factors such as the dose per course and drug scheduling may be important. This effect is compounded by young age, the tumor itself, preceding cranial irradiation, and dark eye color. Of the 65 patients treated in CCG 9892, 21 (32.3 per cent) developed grade 3 or 4 ototoxicity.[60] In these patients, hearing loss occurred from the third to seventh cycle of lomustine (CCNU), cisplatin, and vincristine chemotherapy. Ototoxicity was the principal reason for dose modification or curtailment of chemotherapy. By contrast, grade 3 or 4 ototoxicity occurred in only ten per cent of patients with medulloblastoma treated on the maintenance arm of the HIT 91 study, despite similar chemotherapy.[61]

VISUAL DISORDERS

In patients with anterior visual pathway optic gliomas, craniopharyngioma, or pituitary tumors, compromised vision often precipitates therapeutic intervention. Patients with optic glioma who do not have neurofibromatosis are particularly vulnerable (see Tables 13b.2 and 13b.3).[62] One study of optic gliomas demonstrated progressive deterioration in the worse eye over time and, despite treatment, no change in the better eye. This was independent, regardless of neurofibromatosis type 1 (NF-1) status, suggesting that the damage was earlier, tumor-induced damage evolving over with time.[63] Visual field or occipital cortex deficits can also compromise vision in a large number of cerebral and hypothalamic tumors. Paralytic squints and ophthalmoplegias may compromise functional visual ability and lower educational achievement.

CEREBROVASCULAR DISEASE AND STROKE

Perioperative stroke

Stroke may occur immediately after brain tumor surgery, either as a direct effect of surgical interference with the cerebral vessels or secondary to sinovenous thrombosis if the patient becomes relatively dehydrated.[64–68] Since thrombophilia and systemic venous thrombosis are both common in patients with brain tumor,[69,70] this complication may be more frequent than has been documented to date, as the symptoms and signs may be masked by those of the tumor. Reversible posterior leukencephalopathy in the context of fluctuations in blood pressure has been reported after surgery for a posterior fossa tumor[71] and again could be difficult to diagnose.

Non-perioperative stroke

Non-perioperative stroke has been well described and has an incidence of 4.03 per 1000 years of follow-up.[72]

Cerebrovascular disease and arterial stroke are well recognized associations with suprasellar tumors, including optic and hypothalamic glioma, germinoma, pituitary adenoma, and craniopharyngioma.[73–99] Occasionally, cerebrovascular disease has been described in tumors in other locations, such as brainstem glioma[100] and medulloblastoma/PNET.[101–103]

The basal cerebral vessels are usually stenosed or occluded, and there is often a network of collateral vessels similar to those seen in primary moyamoya. The pathology appears to be endothelial proliferation and thickening of the tunica intima and tunica muscularis of the internal carotid and basal cerebral arteries.[104,105] There may, however, be significant radiological and pathological differences from primary moyamoya.[95] The majority of patients present with transient ischemic attack (TIA) or infarctive stroke, but hemorrhagic stroke secondary to aneurysm has been described.[106]

Risk factors for cerebrovascular disease and stroke

Risk factors for cerebrovascular disease and stroke include the nature of the tumor, the extent of debulking surgery, and the radiotherapy dose (Table 24.2).[72,92] Vasculopathy appears to be commoner with optic glioma than with other tumors,[72] but some series have reported no cases.[62] In a large series from one center, radiotherapy was the strongest risk factor, with chemotherapy being of borderline significance.[72] In midline tumors, such as craniopharyngioma and hypothalamic or optic glioma, stroke may occur even in children who have not received radiotherapy.[72] Encasement of the cerebral vessels by tumor, which may necessitate additional surgery and handling

Table 24.2 *Investigation to identify possible risk*

Full blood count and differential white cell count
Iron, folate, red cell folate, vitamin B12
Erythrocyte sedimentation rate (ESR)
Hemoglobin electrophoresis if appropriate ethnic group
Thermolabile methylene tetrahydrofolate reductase (tMTHFR)
  gene
Total homocysteine
Fasting cholesterol and triglycerides, lipoprotein (a)
Infection screen, including *Mycoplasma*, *Chlamydia*,
  Helicobacter, and *Borrelia* titers
Serum and cerebrospinal fluid to look for intrathecal
production of antibodies to varicella zoster
Sleep study to look for obstructive sleep apnea or nocturnal
  hypoxemia
Protein S (total and free), protein C, anti-thrombin III, heparin
  co-factor II, plasminogen
Von Willibrand factor antigen, factor VIII, factor XII
Lupus anticoagulant
Anticardiolipin antibodies
Factor V Leiden and activated protein C resistance
Prothrombin 20210 gene

of the vessels, appears to increase the risk. It is possible that there are angiogenic growth factors related to the tumor.[107] Patients may have vascular risk factors,[99,108] and the process may be one of accelerated atherosclerosis.[108] There is evidence for abnormal flow-mediated dilation after radiotherapy, which suggests that the mechanism of vascular damage may involve nitric oxide bioavailability.[109] Genetic predisposition to vascular disease appears to be a risk factor, particularly NF-1,[85,86,110] which is associated with vasculopathy in the absence of tumor or radiation,[111] perhaps related to the gene for familial moyamoya disease close to the NF-1 gene on chromosome 17[112] or to the predisposition of patients with NF-1 to hypertension.[113] Other predisposing factors may include those for thrombosis, such as hyperfibrinogenemia and the factor V Leiden mutation,[114–117] and those for atherogenesis, such as hypertension,[118,119] diabetes,[108] hyperhomocysteinemia,[117,120] and hyperlipidemia;[99,117] however, there are very few data available at the present.[72] Cholesterol levels do appear to be higher in patients with brain tumors at the time of diagnosis than in the general population,[121–123] and hypertriglyceridemia has also been reported.[124,125] Although there may be no etiological link in terms of oncogenesis,[123] dyslipidemia may play a role in cerebrovascular disease. The secondary endocrine problems, such as hypopituitarism and Cushing's syndrome, and their treatment, e.g. with GH, may have as yet unidentified effects on endothelial function and the risk of small- or large-vessel disease.[125,126] It is also possible that relative immunodeficiency, exposure to infection, and the host reaction to infection play a role, as they appear to do in other etiologies for childhood stroke.[118] Other common childhood infections, such as varicella zoster,[118] also appear to be associated with vasculopathy and stroke in children and could exacerbate radiation-induced vascular disease. Anemia and hypoxia may be risk factors for cerebrovascular disease and stroke in children and are relatively common in those who are chronically sick.[127–130] The relative importance of various risk factors may vary with age, ethnicity, and underlying diagnosis, as is the case in childhood stroke in general,[118,131] but there is a good case for investigating for vascular risk factors not related to the tumor or its treatment, since recurrence and outcome are related to the number of risk factors[132] and many are modifiable.[131]

DIFFUSE BRAIN DAMAGE

Effects of radiotherapy

It is becoming increasingly clear that there is a significant cost in terms of neurological, behavioral, and cognitive sequelae for children who survive brain tumors (see Chapter 26). This appears to be due to widespread effects of radiotherapy on neuronal, glial, and endothelial cells, for which the pathological evidence is reviewed here before a discussion of strategies for neuroprotection that might be explored.

Pathology

The available evidence suggests that the oligodendrocytes and endothelial cells are involved in radiation damage.[133] Injury to the endothelium of the small vessels may result in a cascade of events, leading to increased vascular permeability and fibrinoid necrosis of the vessel wall.[134] In rabbits with hypercholesterolemia, 5 Gy of radiation caused small- and medium-sized-vessel disease, with deposition of lipophages and changes to the elastic structure.[135] Similar changes may occur in humans.[136,137] Large vessels may also be infiltrated by fat-laden macrophages.[138]

Imaging

Some, but not all, of the changes secondary to radiotherapy may be visualized on conventional magnetic resonance imaging (MRI).[139] Full-scale IQ, factual knowledge, and verbal and performance thinking (but not sustained attention or verbal memory) in patients with posterior fossa tumors is related to the volume of normal-appearing white matter (NAWM).[140] Compared with controls with low-grade cerebellar tumors, the volume of NAWM is lower in patients treated with chemotherapy as well as radiotherapy.[141] In one study the rate of loss of NAWM volume was 23 per cent lower in those receiving 24 Gy craniospinal radiotherapy (CSRT) than in those receiving 36 Gy.[142] Quantitative T1 mapping shows an effect on white matter at doses over 20 Gy and on grey matter at doses over 60 Gy.[143]

Imaging also provides some evidence for small-vessel vasculopathy. Lacunar infarcts were seen in 25 of 421 children who had radiotherapy or chemotherapy for brain tumor but in none of those treated with surgery alone.[144] However, IQ was not lower in those with lacunes than in age- and diagnosis-matched controls. Fourteen patients had craniospinal irradiation and 11 had local radiotherapy only. The strongest predictor of lacunar infarction was age under five years at the time of radiotherapy. Cerebral calcification shows high rather than low intensity on T1, suggesting a mineralizing microangiopathy.[145] Magnetic resonance spectroscopy (MRS) has also been performed in children who have undergone brain irradiation. In one study of children with leukemia, the N-acetyl aspartate/creatine ratio was not related to age at diagnosis but decreased progressively with time since diagnosis.[146] However, in another study, proton spectroscopy markers were not different from controls in 14 children irradiated for acute lymphatic leukemia (ALL) or tumor and only choline/water related to full-scale IQ.[147]

There is also evidence for reduced cerebral blood flow and metabolic rate in association with neurological and cognitive sequelae. For patients with leukemia and treated with radiotherapy and chemotherapy, there is evidence for reduced glucose metabolism in the white matter and thalami.[148] In adults, SPECT may show focal perfusion deficits that correlate with neuropsychological deficit in patients who have undergone radiotherapy.[149] Positron-emission tomography (PET) may help to distinguish between postsurgical or radiation damage and recrudescence of the tumor.[150,151] One case report suggests that diffusion-weighted MRI may also be useful in this context.[152]

Other risk factors for diffuse brain damage

Neurological and cognitive function may also be affected by associated hormonal deficiencies. Calcification of the basal ganglia was seen in five per cent of brain tumors in a Dutch center and was associated with a larger IQ loss and a higher incidence of hypothyroidism and GH deficiency, which might possibly have an etiological role.[153] As discussed above, hypopituitarism may be associated with dyslipidemias.[124,135] In adults, there is some evidence for an additional effect of anticonvulsants, especially carbamazepine,[154] and this possibility should be examined in children; it is certainly sensible to avoid polypharmacy for epilepsy.

Management of neurological complications

DIAGNOSIS AND ACUTE MANAGEMENT OF STROKE

MRI (including diffusion and perfusion), magnetic resonance arteriography (MRA), and magnetic resonance venography (MRV) are very useful in pediatric stroke, where there is a wide variety of possible pathologies.[155] Although it can be done with MRI, emergency CT may be needed to exclude hemorrhage. However, infarction is commonly not seen in the first few hours, and MRI is more likely to be able to define extent and territory, particularly if diffusion imaging is used to differentiate acute from chronic infarction or from tumor.[152,156] MRA may be used to define the vascular anatomy of the circle of Willis and neck vessels in the majority of cases, and avoids the complications associated with conventional angiography, although the latter may be needed to exclude small-vessel disease or if surgery is planned, e.g. for moyamoya. MRV may be required to exclude sagittal sinus thrombosis, which may occur after neurosurgery or chemotherapy. Perfusion imaging demonstrates areas of abnormal cerebral blood flow, blood volume, and mean transit time.[156,157]

In adults, the main focus of recent studies of treatment has been in looking at the possibility of minimizing the effect of the initial stroke, using either thrombolysis or neuroprotection. One controlled study of intravenous tissue plasminogen activator (t-PA), conducted in adults who could be randomized within three hours, showed significant benefit in terms of outcome at three months. However, thrombolysis in adults carries a ten per cent risk of hemorrhage, associated with considerable mortality. The results beyond a three-hour time window have been very disappointing, and only about five per cent of patients fulfil the criteria for treatment (no recent operative procedure, hemorrhage excluded on CT scan within three hours of onset of symptoms). Although children with a stroke often present to a doctor within three hours, because of the rarity of stroke, the low sensitivity of CT for acute infarction and the wide differential in this age group means that the diagnosis is rarely made with any degree of certainty at this stage. In addition, mortality is lower in children, and most children presenting with stroke can probably expect to lead independent lives as adults. It is therefore difficult to see a major role for t-PA in this age group at the present time, although it may occasionally be justified in children known to be at risk (e.g. because of brain tumor) and who develop stroke in hospital. Patients who have undergone a recent operative procedure are currently excluded. Infarct volume and outcome appear to be related to body temperature during the first few days of the stroke. A direct causative effect remains unproven, but maintaining body temperature just below 37°C is unlikely to do harm. Apart from preventing fever, there is currently no neuroprotective strategy available that can be recommended for use in children in the acute phase.

There are, nevertheless, a number of management strategies for individual patient groups that may make a difference, in addition to the need for clot removal in hemorrhage.[155] Seizures in the acute phase should be managed appropriately, although there is no evidence for a detrimental effect on outcome in adults. There is a case for surgical decompression[155] in children presenting in coma with large ischemic middle cerebral infarcts, which are almost always fatal if managed conservatively.

The acute management of the remaining patients remains controversial, and many physicians give no specific treatment. The question of anticoagulation remains a difficult one.[158] One large trial in adults suggested benefit, but others have demonstrated increased morbidity and mortality. Despite the risk of hemorrhage, there are some patient groups, e.g. those with vessel dissection, venous sinus thrombosis, and known prothrombotic abnormalities, who should probably be anticoagulated acutely to prevent early recurrence. Aspirin appeared to be associated with a modest improvement in outcome, probably because of a reduction in early recurrence and perhaps in addition via its antipyretic effect, in two very large controlled trials in adults, the results of which have now been combined.[159] The risk of hemorrhage appears to be lower with aspirin than with anticoagulants, and although there is no evidence of benefit in children, it is a reasonable option.

PREVENTION OF RECURRENT STROKE

Diet and lifestyle

Table 24.3 summarizes the dietary and lifestyle management of vascular risk factors.

B-complex vitamin supplementation is probably reasonable in those with hyperhomocysteinemia, although more research is required.[120] Children with hypercholesterolemia or high lipoprotein (a) should reduce cholesterol intake in childhood and might be candidates for prophylaxis with statins[160] if at particularly high risk of vascular pathology. A controlled trial has suggested that children with familial hypercholesterolemia, who are at high risk of cardiovascular and cerebrovascular disease, appear to have an improved lipid profile with few side effects,[160] but more long-term studies are needed. Blood pressure should be checked routinely, and consideration should be given to starting therapy for hypertension if blood pressure remains above the ninety-fifth centile for age as adolescence/adulthood is entered.[118] Advice should be given about the risks of smoking.

Table 24.3 *Management of vascular risk factors*

General advice about:
> improving diet, e.g. increasing intake of fruit and vegetables to five portions/day, decreasing consumption of fat in junk food
> taking more exercise, e.g. walking to school
> seeking immediate medical attention in hospital if further symptoms

Specific advice for patients with the following risk factors:
> *For moyamoya*:
>> Consider revascularization, particularly if transient ischemic attacks or cognitive decline
>> Exclude nocturnal hypoxaemia/obstructive apnoea
> *For those with blood pressure >90th centile for height and age*:
>> Low-salt diet
>> Consider antihypertensives
> *For homozygotes for the tMTHFR gene and patients with hyperhomocysteinemia (plasma level > 13.5 mM/l)*:
>> B-complex vitamin (especially folic acid) supplementation
> *For those with a persistent prothrombotic disorder, e.g. factor V Leiden*:
>> Consider warfarin with regular monitoring of INR (discuss with hematologist in individual case)
> *For those with hypercholesterolemia (> 5.5 mmol/l)*:
>> Low-cholesterol diet
>> Consider cholesterol-lowering agents, e.g. statins
> *For others with stroke in a vascular distribution and/or cerebrovascular disease*:
>> Low-dose aspirin (1 mg/kg)

Antiplatelet or anticoagulant prophylaxis

For ischemic stroke, long-term recurrence prevention is a controversial issue. The lifelong recurrence risk has not been defined for children, but as there is commonly cerebrovascular disease on follow-up MRA, a low-dose aspirin regime (approximately 1 mg/kg) is probably justified.[158] The relative risk of further stroke and life-threatening hemorrhage on long-term warfarin has not been assessed for patients with inherited thrombophilias such as factor V Leiden, but there is occasionally a case for cautious anticoagulation in some patients, particularly if there are ongoing symptoms.[158]

Revascularization surgery

Radiation-associated vasculopathy of the arteries of the circle of Willis is often associated with a network of collaterals not unlike those seen in primary moyamoya. A variety of direct and indirect extracranial/intracranial bypass procedures have been used in moyamoya (both primary and secondary to other conditions such as sickle cell disease), and such procedures have been used in patients with TIAs secondary to radiation-induced vasculopathy.[161] The transient ischemic events are often abolished or reduced by surgical procedures, but the effect on the risk of ischemic or hemorrhagic stroke or on cognitive function remains uncertain.

Experience of stroke after brain tumor at Great Ormond Street Hospital, London

Of 212 consecutive patients presenting to Great Ormond Street Hospital, London, between 1978 and 2000 with arterial stroke,[86] five (two per cent) had had a brain tumor (two craniopharyngioma, two optic glioma, one hypothalamic hamartoma). Four had had radiotherapy. The median age at stroke was ten years (range 15 months–17.5 years), and four were girls. The child who had not had radiotherapy had three strokes with infarcts along the border zone between the anterior and middle cerebral arteries, beginning a few days after complete excision of a craniopharyngioma (Figures 24.10–24.12). MRA and conventional angiography were normal, but the patient had familial hypercholesterolemia, was homozygous for the thermolabile variant of the methylene tetrahydrofolate reductase gene, which is associated with hyperhomocysteinemia, and had iron-deficiency anemia, leukocytosis, thrombocytosis, and a blood pressure above the ninety-fifth centile for height and weight. One other patient had a transient ischemic event after repeat surgery for a craniopharyngioma, which recurred despite partial resection and radiotherapy; she did not have vascular imaging, but she was heterozygous for the factor V Leiden mutation,[84] she was hypertensive, and she had a high fibrinogen. The other three children who had had radiotherapy had a bilateral vasculopathy (Figure 24.13) and were revascularized after the first stroke. One other patient was hypertensive and one other was anemic at the time of the stroke. Cholesterol and triglycerides were not measured in four children. All five children had recurrent ear and/or throat infections, three had a high white count at the time of the stroke, and three of the four asked had a clinical history suggestive of obstructive sleep apnea. A sixth child with a craniopharyngioma developed a left hemiparesis in the context of drowsiness and vomiting and was though to have had sinovenous thrombosis that resolved spontaneously.

TREATMENT OF RADIATION NECROSIS

Steroids

Steroids may improve the symptoms of radiation necrosis, probably by reducing local cerebral edema.[162] It has also been suggested that radiation-associated vasculopathy is in part an autoimmune phenomenon, which may be exacerbated by coexisting infection and may be treatable with steroids.[163] The presently available steroids would, however, produce unacceptable side effects if used long-term.

Hyperbaric oxygenation

There have been isolated reports of improvement in radiation necrosis with hyperbaric oxygenation performed soon after diagnosis,[164,165] but an animal study showed no benefit[166] and this therapy has not been pursued further.

REHABILITATION, COGNITIVE THERAPY, AND EDUCATION

The majority of children who have suffered a stroke have significant motor and or learning disabilities,[167] with implications for quality of life.[168] Appropriate rehabilitation with physiotherapy, occupational therapy, and reintegration into school is therefore essential. In children who have had a brain tumor, with or without an overt stroke, academic and social failure may reinforce cognitive and behavioral difficulties,[169] but, encouragingly, remediation may allow improvement, e.g. in literacy.[170,171] Adults receiving surgery and radiotherapy may experience a reduction in full-scale IQ, which may recover in those who return to work early. Late improvement may also be seen in children, perhaps secondary to targeted education for specific learning difficulties.[172]

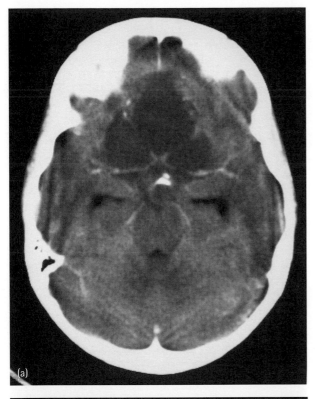

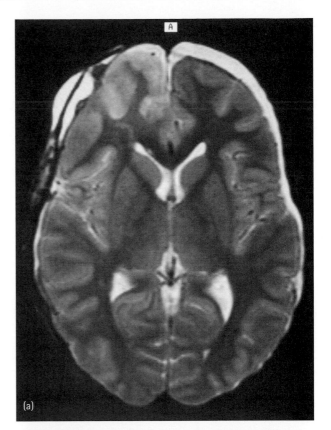

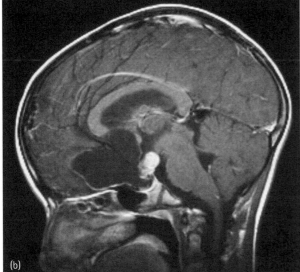

Figure 24.10a,b *(a) Axial unenhanced computerized tomography (CT) scan and (b) sagittal post-contrast T_1-weighted magnetic resonance imaging (MRI) scan, showing a large craniopharyngioma in a ten-year-old girl with a family history of hypercholesterolemia. Calcification in the cyst wall is seen on the axial CT scan. The tumor exerts pressure on and displaces the chiasm posterosuperiorly and inferiorly involves the pituitary fossa. The anterior cerebral arteries are elevated and splayed, and the middle cerebral arteries are attenuated by the cyst. The cyst was drained for immediate relief of pressure effects. Three weeks later, she underwent a right frontal craniotomy for removal of the cystic and enhancing solid component.*

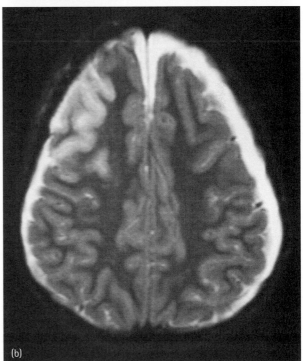

Figure 24.11a,b *(a) and (b) Ten days after surgery, the patient referred to in Figure 24.10 developed a left hemiparesis. A magnetic resonance image (MRI) obtained three days later showed bilateral shallow subdural collections over the frontal convexities, which are a common complication of craniotomy, and right frontal cortical edema.*

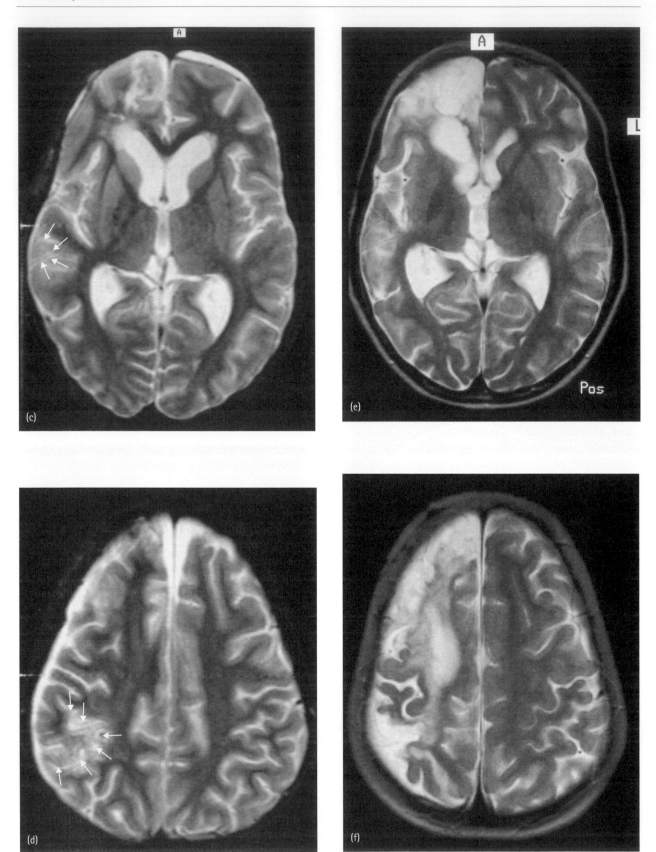

Figure 24.11c,d,e,f *(c) and (d) One month later, a repeat MRI showed a new right frontoparietal infarct in the middle cerebral artery territory (arrowheads). (e) and (f) Eighteen months later, she had a further episode of left hemiparesis and there was further extension of the infarction along the middle and posterior cerebral artery border zone.*

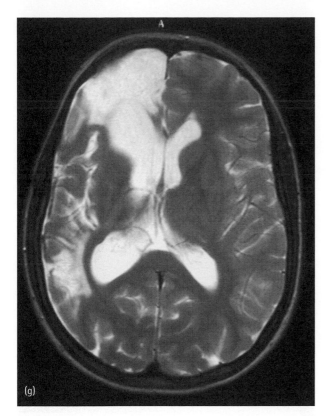
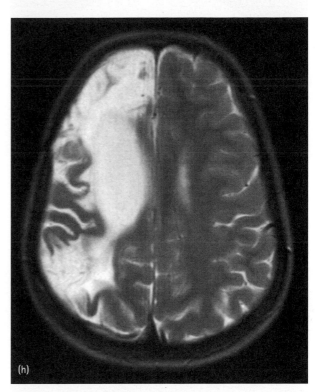

Figure 24.11g,h *(g) and (h) She continued to experience frequent headaches and seizures. The final scan, five years after the original presentation, shows maturation of the anterior and middle cerebral artery territory infarction.*

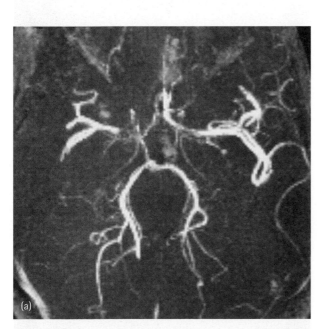
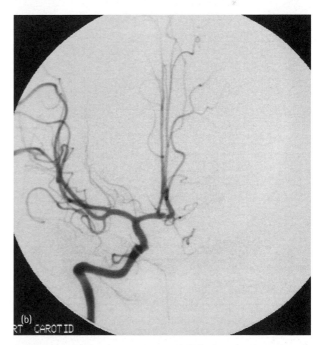

Figure 24.12a,b *The same girl referred to in Figures 24.10 and 24.11. (a) Magnetic resonance angiography (MRA) at the time of the first stroke showing complete loss of signal, indicating marked reduction in flow within the proximal right middle cerebral artery and reduced flow within the insular branches of the middle cerebral artery. Magnetic resonance venography (MRV) performed at the same time was normal (not shown). (b) Normal anteroposterior projection of the right carotid angiography performed 18 months later.*

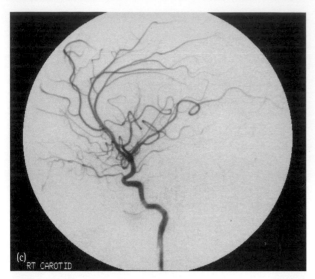

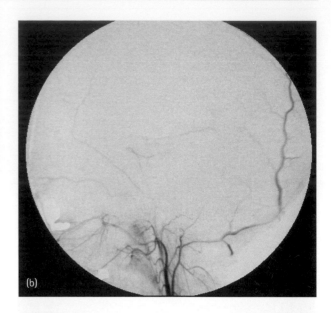

Figure 24.12c *Normal lateral projection of the right carotid angiography performed 18 months later.*

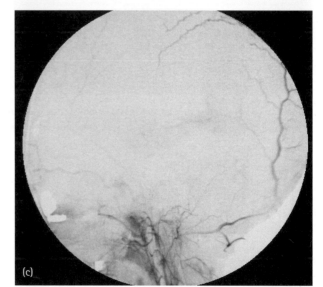

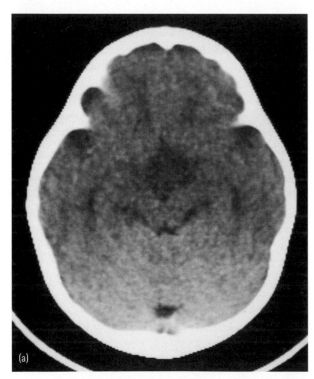

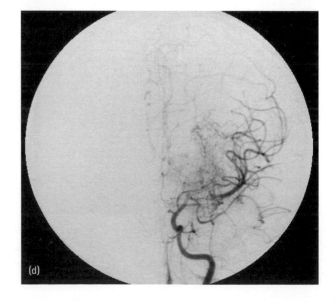

Figure 24.13a–d *(a) Computerized tomography (CT) scan showing a hypothalamic glioma in a boy aged 22 months. He was treated with radiotherapy and presented three years later with left- and right-sided transient hemiparesis and seizures. Magnetic resonance imaging (MRI) showed multiple areas of altered signal in the left frontal and temporal white matter. Formal angiography showed poor filling of the main vessels (b), with collateral formation (c,d,e).*

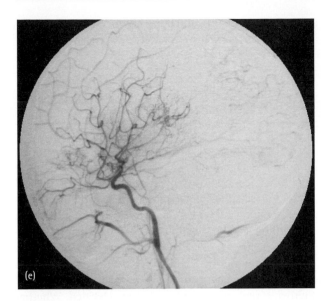

Figure 24.13e *(continued)*

Neuroprotection

Some studies have looked at the possibility of reducing the radiation dosage without increasing the mortality for the tumor. Substitution with chemotherapy has been investigated in the most vulnerable (under three years of age) patients and where five-year survival rates are already very high (e.g. leukemias). Increasing the poorer five-year survival rates (60 per cent) in children with brain tumors but without increasing intellectual morbidity is being attempted by substituting more aggressive chemotherapy and/or the reduction, hyperfractionation, or more focal (stereotactic) application of the cranial irradiation dose. However, these strategies carry their own risks of potentially compromising cure rates and causing later additive toxicity after salvage therapy. An alternative strategy is to attempt neuroprotection in those at highest risk, but at present these patients are difficult to identify, and there is no evidence-based therapy that reduces the brain injury associated with the treatment of brain tumors.

EARLY DIAGNOSIS AND OPTIMAL SURGICAL TECHNIQUE

There are still unacceptable delays in the diagnosis of brain tumors in some children,[173] and strategies to enable earlier diagnosis must be instituted as part of clinical governance. The surgical management of children with brain tumors is usually conducted by experienced neurosurgeons in centers with a large number of patients, but audit and research into the optimal strategy for each tumor type and presentation must continue.

REDUCTION OF THE RADIATION DOSE

The toxicity of radiotherapy may be reduced by lowering the dose or altering the fractionation.[174] As part of a controlled trial for low-grade medulloblastoma, Mulhern and colleagues provided evidence that a dose of 36 Gy was associated with greater neuropsychological decline than 23.4 Gy and that this effect was greater in younger children.[175] For children with posterior fossa tumors, Grill and colleagues found that the mean IQ was related most strongly to the dose of craniospinal irradiation, with full-scale IQs of 84.5, 76.9, and 63.7 for doses of 0, 25, and 35 Gy respectively, and significant loss of verbal comprehension for those receiving the higher dosage.[176] Kieffer-Renaux and colleagues, from the same group, found in a controlled trial of 25 versus 36 Gy of whole-brain irradiation that the higher dose of radiation was associated with more verbal and performance deficits in children with medulloblastoma.[177] Fuss and coworkers pooled data from 1938 children and found that, for whole-brain irradiation, IQ less than 85 was related to dose and age; thus, for children under three years old, the critical dose was 24 Gy and for those aged over six years it was 36 Gy.[178] Partial brain irradiation had a measurable effect only at doses over 50 Gy. Reduced-dose radiotherapy for medulloblastoma was associated with a decline in IQ in the whole group of about four points/year, i.e. still substantial but better than previous studies using a higher dose.[179] Certain subgroups may be more vulnerable, so that, for example, verbal IQ declined more in females, nonverbal IQ declined more in those treated at a younger age, and full-scale IQ declined most in those with a higher IQ at baseline. Another study using lower doses of radiation for medulloblastoma also shows a loss of 2.55 IQ points/year of follow-up.[180] The raw scores suggested that the ongoing problem is a failure to learn new information.[180]

The main concern currently is that any preservation of cognitive performance may be bought at the expense of a lower cure rate. For standard-risk medulloblastoma, five-year survival was lower with 24 Gy of CST than with 36 Gy,[181] but survival with adjuvant chemotherapy may be better.[182] However, tumor progression may be commoner in those in whom radiotherapy is delayed.[183]

The management of medulloblastoma in very young children and in those with disseminated disease is difficult, as the majority of children progress on chemotherapy and then require radiotherapy and there is a progressive reduction in IQ of −3.9 points/year, regardless of whether radiotherapy is required.[184]

PREVENTION OF THE VASCULOPATHY

There is evidence from animal studies and early pathological data in humans that small- and large-vessel disease occurs after irradiation for brain tumors, but the relative importance of this vasculopathy compared with direct damage to neurons and glial cells has received little attention. This is unfortunate, since there is considerable interest in reducing the impact of genetic and environmental risk factors for cerebrovascular disease in the context of stroke and of vascular dementia. Some of these strategies are low-risk for the patient, e.g. folate supplementation for hyperhomocysteinemia.[120] There is considerable evidence from adult studies that control of hypertension reduces the risk of stroke recurrence, and it is possible that raised blood pressure is important in the cognitive decline seen after radiotherapy for brain tumors.[185] One-half of children who have had a stroke have blood pressure higher than the ninetieth centile for height and age,[118] but this is rarely measured systematically or managed appropriately in children with brain tumors.

Since patients with brain tumors have higher cholesterol levels than the general population,[121–123] and since there is evidence from animal studies that the pathophysiology of radiation vasculopathy includes accumulation of lipids,[135] variation in lipid profiles might account for part of the risk of cerebrovascular disease and dementia. In elderly adults, there is a little evidence that prophylaxis with 3-hydroxy-3-methylglutaryl coenzyme A (HMG-CoA) reductase inhibitors (statins) reduces the risk of vascular dementia,[186] and there is a possibility that statin prophylaxis might reduce the cognitive consequences associated with radiotherapy. There are concerns over the risk of oncogenesis, cerebral hemorrhage, and the effect of widespread apoptosis with the use of statins.[185] There would then be an important question to be answered as to whether statins might have adverse effects by promoting tumor growth through angiogenesis,[187] or whether they might have a beneficial effect by reducing tumor bulk, because the rate-limiting step in the mevalonate pathway (hepatic HMG-CoA reductase) is inhibited, reducing the synthesis of cell-wall lipids and inducing apoptosis[188] but not arrest of the cellular proliferation.[189] Phase I/II trials have shown that statins may be tolerated in adults with very malignant brain tumors[190] and in children with hypercholesterolemia,[160,191] but a considerable amount of preclinical work would be needed before their use could be considered for children with malignant brain tumors.

It would be relatively easy to justify a study of the effect of cerebrovascular risk factors in those tumors with a higher risk of large vessel disease, e.g. craniopharyngiomas and optic and hypothalamic gliomas. Demonstration of the vasculopathy as a surrogate marker of disease is now possible non-invasively with transcranial Doppler ultrasound or magnetic resonance angiography. Advantages of the latter technique include the possibility of including it at the time of follow-up MRI and of performing perfusion imaging in addition, since in sickle cell disease, reduction in focal cerebral blood flow has been reported in the absence of cerebrovascular disease.[192] If part of the variation in cognitive function term outcome for pediatric brain tumors is related to the vasculopathy affecting the small vessels, then the rate of decline might be related to the number of vascular risk factors, e.g. hypertension, hypercholesterolemia, and hyperhomocysteinemia. Many of these risk factors are modifiable, and trials of prophylactic treatment might be worthwhile.

SECOND PRIMARY TUMORS

Early death may also occur from second primary tumors.[193] Brain tumor survivors may develop meningiomas at the edge of the radiation field or thyroid tumors after spinal irradiation. Because of the recognized carcinogenic potential of megavoltage irradiation and prolonged TSH stimulation, annual thyroid palpation (with further ultrasound and needle biopsy evaluation of any nodules) and thyroid function tests (fT4 and TSH) have always been advised, with institution of thyroxine replacement when TSH is elevated. Whether adjuvant chemotherapy will increase this risk, as documented for thyroid dysfunction, has not been tested to date.[22,194]

Summary

- Many children with brain tumors have significant CNS late effects that are difficult to predict or prevent at the present time.
- Modifications to the treatment regime to reduce the direct side effects can be justified only if the cure rate is equivalent.
- Strategies for prevention of CNS late effects might be targeted at vascular risk factors if these prove to be part of the pathophysiology.
- Early recognition of cerebrovascular disease, e.g. when a child presents with a TIA rather than stroke, and of the specific cognitive and behavioral problems, may allow targeted management of the individual patient.
- The long-term risks of cerebrovascular disease in survivors during adolescence and early adulthood are unknown.
- Due consideration will need to be given to clinical priorities for screening for risks, and to stratify preventive and therapeutic intervention for cerebrovascular disease in this patient group.

ACKNOWLEDGMENTS

Dr Kirkham was funded by the Wellcome Trust, Action Research, and the Stroke Association. She thanks Dr Dawn Saunders, consultant neuroradiologist, for assistance with the figures.

REFERENCES

1 Catsman-Berrevoets CE, Van Dongen HR, Mulder PG, Paz y Geuze D, Paquier PF, Lequin MH. Tumour type and size are high risk factors for the syndrome of "cerebellar" mutism and subsequent dysarthria. *J Neurol Neurosurg Psychiatry* 1999; **67**:755–7.

2 Silber J, Radcliffe J, Peckham Vea. Whole brain irradiation and decline in intelligence. The influence of dose and age on IQ scores. *J Clin Oncol* 1992; **10**:1390–96.

3 Clayton P, Shalet S. Dose dependency of time of onset of radiation induced growth hormone deficiency. *J Pediatr* 1991; **118**:226–8.

4 Littley M, Shalet S, CG B, Ahmed S, Applegate G, Sutton M. Hypopituitarism following external radiotherapy for pituitary tumours in adults. *Q J Med* 1989; **70**:145–60.

5 Spoudeas H, Charmandari E, Brook C. Hypothalamo-pituitary-adrenal axis integrity after cranial irradiation for posterior fossa tumours in childhood. *Med Pediatr Oncol* 2003; **40**:224–9.

6 Spoudeas H, Hindmarsh P, Matthews D, Brook C. Evolution of growth hormone (GH) neurosecretory disturbance after cranial irradiation for childhood brain tumours: a prospective study. *J Endocrinol* 1996; **150**:329–42.

7 Darendeliler F, Livesey E, Hindmarsh P, Brook C. Growth and growth hormone secretion in children following treatment of brain tumours with radiotherapy. *Acta Paediatr Scand* 1990; **79**:121–7.

8 Achermann J, Hindmarsh P, Brook C. The relationship between the growth hormone and insulin-like growth factor axis in long-term survivors of childhood brain tumours. *Clin Endocrinol* 1998; **49**:639–45.

9 Spiliotis B, August G, Hung W, Sonis W, Mendelson W, Bercu B. Growth hormone neurosecretory dysfunction: a treatable cause of short stature. *J Am Med Assoc* 1984; **251**:2223–30.

10 Ryalls M, Spoudeas H, Hindmarsh P, *et al.* Short term endocrine consequences of total body irradiation and bone marrow transplantation in children treated for leukaemia. *J Endocrinol* 1993; **136**:331–8.

11 Crowne E, Moore C, Wallace W, *et al.* A novel variant of growth hormone (GH) insufficiency following low dose cranial irradiation. *Clin Endocrinol* 1992; **36**:59–68.

12 Davies H, Didcock E, Didi M, Ogilvy-Stuart A, Wales J, Shalet S. Disproportionate short stature after cranial irradiation and combination chemotherapy for leukaemia. *Arch Dis Child* 1994; **70**:472–5.

13 Spoudeas H. The evolution of growth hormone neurosecretory disturbance during high dose cranial irradiation and chemotherapy for childhood brain tumours. MD thesis. London: University of London, 1995.

14 Achermann J. The pathophysiology of post-irradiation growth hormone insufficiency. MD thesis. London: University of London, 1997.

15 Chiarenza A, Lempereur L, Palmucci T, *et al.* Responsiveness of irradiated rat anterior pituitary cells to hypothalamic releasing hormones is restored by treatment with growth hormone. *Neuro-endocrinology* 2000; **72**:392–9.

16 Chieng P, Huang T, Chang Cea. Reduced hypothalamic blood flow after radiation treatment of nasopharyngeal cancer: SPECT studies in 34 patients. *Am J Nucl Radiol* 1991; **12**:661–5.

17 Hall J, Martin K, Whitney H, Landy H, Crowley WJ. Potential for fertility with replacement hypothalamic gonadotropin-releasing hormone in long term female survivors of cranial tumours. *J Clin Endocrinol Metab* 1994; **79**:1166–72.

18 Probert J, Parker B, Kaplan H. Growth retardation in children after megavoltage irradiation of the spine. *Cancer* 1973; **32**:634–9.

19 Shalet S, Gibson B, Swindell R, Pearson D. Effect of spinal irradiation on growth. *Arch Dis Child* 1987; **62**:461–4.

19a Spoudeas *et al.* Abstract. *Med Pediatric Oncol* 2002; **39**:306.

20 Hartsell W, Hanson W, Conterato D, Hendrickson F. Hyperfractionation decreases the deleterious effects of conventional radiation fractionation on vertebral growth in animals. *Cancer* 1989; **63**:2452–5.

21 Livesey E, Brook C. Gonadal dysfunction after treatment of intracranial tumours. *Arch Dis Child* 1988; **63**:495–500.

22 Ogilvy-Stuart A, Shalet S, Gattamaneni H. Thyroid function after treatment of brain tumors in children. *J Pediatr* 1991; **119**:733–7.

23 Olshan J, Gubernick J, Packer R, *et al.* The effects of adjuvant chemotherapy on growth in children with medulloblastoma. *Cancer* 1992; **70**:2013–17.

24 Samaan N, Vieto R, Schultz P, *et al.* Hypothalamic, pituitary and thyroid dysfunction after radiotherapy to the head and neck. *Int J Radiat Oncol Biol Phys* 1982; **8**:1857–67.

25 Ron E, Lubin J, Shore R, *et al.* Thyroid cancer after exposure to external irradiation: a pooled analysis of seven studies. *Radiat Res* 1995; **141**:259–77.

26 Rubino C, Cailleux A, De Vathaire F, Schlumberger M. Thyroid cancer after radiation exposure. *J Cancer* 2002; **35**:645–7.

27 Rose S, Lustig R, Pitukcheewanont P, *et al.* Diagnosis of central hidden hypothyroidism in survivors of childhood cancer. *J Clin Endocrinol Metab* 1999; **84**:4472–9.

28 *BSPED/UKCCSG consensus statement of the management of rare endocrine tumours in childhood*, in press.

29 Ogilvy-Stuart A, Clayton P, Shalet S. Cranial irradiation and early puberty. *J Clin Endocrinol Metab* 1994; **78**:1282–6.

30 Clayton P, Shalet S, Price D, Campbell R. Testicular damage after chemotherapy for childhood brain tumors. *J Pediatr* 1988; **112**:922–6.

31 Clayton P, Shalet S, Price D, Morris-Jones P. Ovarian function following chemotherapy for childhood brain tumours. *Med Pediatr Oncol* 1989; **17**:92–6.

32 Constine L, Woolf P, Cann D, *et al.* Hypothalamic pituitary dysfunction after radiation for brain tumors. *N Engl J Med* 1993; **328**:87–94.

33 Castillo L, Craft A, Kernhan J, Evans R, Aynsley Green A. Gonadal function after 12 Gy testicular irradiation in childhood acute lymphoblastic leukaemia. *Med Pediatr Oncol* 1990; **18**:185–9.

34 Shalet S, Tsatsoulis A, Whitehead E, Read G. Vulnerability of the human Leydig cell to radiation damage is dose-dependent. *J Endocrinol* 1989; **120**:161–5.

35 Wallace W, Shalet S, Hendry J, Morris-Jones P, Gattamaneni H. Ovarian failure following abdominal irradiation in childhood: the radiosensitivity of the human oocyte. *Br J Radiol* 1989; **62**:995–8.

36 Ash P. The influence of radiation on fertility in man. *Br J Radiol* 1980; **53**:271–8.

37 Masala A, Faedda R, Alagnas, *et al*. Use of testosterone to prevent cyclophosphamide-induced azoospermia. *Ann Intern Med* 1997; **126**:292–5.

38 Thompson A, Campbell A, Irvine D, Anderson R, Kelnar C, Wallace H.W. Semen quality and spermatozoal DNA integrity in survivors of childhood cancer: a case-control study. *Lancet* 2002; **360**:361–7.

39 Palermo G, Schlegel P, Scott Sills E, *et al*. Births after intracytoplasmic injection of sperm obtained by testicular extraction from men with non-mosaic Klinefelter's syndrome. *New Engl J Med* 1998; **338**:588–90.

40 Livesey E, Hindmarsh P, Brook C, *et al*. Endocrine disorders following treatment of childhood brain tumours. *Br J Cancer* 1990; **64**:622–5.

41 Packer R, Boyett J, Janns A, Stavrou T, Kun L, Wisoff Jea. Growth hormone replacement therapy in children with medulloblastoma: use and effect on tumour control. *J Clin Oncol* 2001; **19**:480–7.

42 Ter Maaten J. Should we start and continue growth hormone (GH) replacement therapy in adults with GH deficiency? *Ann Med* 2000; **32**:452–61.

43 Jakacki R, Goldwein J, Larsen R, Barber G, Silber J. Cardiac dysfunction following spinal irradiation during childhood. *J Clin Oncol* 1993; **11**:1033–8.

44 Swerdlow A, Reddinguis R, Higgins C, *et al*. Growth hormone treatment of children with brain tumours and risk of tumour recurrence. *J Clin Endocrinol Metab* 2000; **85**:4444–9.

45 Swerdlow A, Higgins C, Adlard P, Preece M. Risk of cancer in patients treated with human pituitary growth hormone in the UK, 1959–85: a cohort study. *Lancet* 2002; **360**:273–7.

46 DeVile C, Grant D, Hayward R, Kendall B, Neville B, Stanhope R. Obesity in childhood craniopharyngioma: relation to post-operative hypothalamic damage shown by magnetic resonance imaging. *J Clin Endocrinol Metab* 1996; **81**:2734–7.

47 Lustig R, Rose S, Burghen G, *et al*. Hypothalamic obesity caused by cranial insult in children: altered glucose and insulin dynamics and reversal by a somatostatin agonist. *J Pediatr* 1999; **135**:162–8.

48 Tiulpakov A, Mazerkina A, Brook C, Hindmarsh P, Peterkova V, Gorelyshev S. Growth in children with craniopharyngioma following surgery. *Clin Endocrinol* 1998; **49**:733–8.

49 Smith D, Sarfeh J, Howard L. Truncal vagotomy in hypothalamic obesity. *Lancet* 1983; **1**:1330–1.

50 Odame I, Reilly J, Gibson B, Donaldson M. Patterns of obesity in boys and girls after treatment of acute lymphoblastic leukaemia. *Arch Dis Child* 1994; **71**:147–9.

51 Reilly J, Ventham J, Ralston J, Donaldson M, Gibson B. Reduced energy expenditure in pre-obese children treated for acute lymphoblastic leukaemia. *Pediatr Res* 1998; **44**:557–62.

52 Randeva H, Murray R, Lewandowski K, *et al*. Effects of growth hormone on components of the leptin system. *J Endocrinol* 2000; **164** (suppl):135.

53 Crofton P, Ahmed S, Wade J, *et al*. Effects of intensive chemotherapy on bone and collagen turnover and the growth hormone axis in children with acute lymphoblastic leukaemia. *J Clin Endocrinol Metab* 1998; **83**:3121–9.

54 Robson H, Anderson E, Eden O, Isaksson O, Shalet S. Chemotherapeutic agents used in the treatment of childhood

malignancies have direct effects on growth plate chondrocyte proliferation. *J Endocrinol* 1998; **157**:225–35.

55 Robson H, Anderson E, Eden O, Isaksson O, Shalet S. Glucocorticoid pre-treatment reduces the cytotoxic effects of a variety of DNA-damaging agents on rat tibial growth-plate chondrocytes in vitro. *Cancer Chemother Pharmacol* 1998; **42**:171–6.

56 Arikowski P, Komulainen J, Riikonen P, Voutilainen R, Knip M, Kroger H. Alterations in bone turnover and impaired development of bone mineral density in newly diagnosed children with cancer: A one year prospective study. *J Clin Endocrinol Metab* 1999; **84**:3174–81.

57 Prentice A, Parsons T, Cole T. Uncritical use of bone mineral density in absorptiometry may lead to size-related artefacts in the identification of bone mineral determinants. *Am J Clin Nutr* 1994; **60**:837–42.

58 Gilsanz V, Carlson M, Roe T, Ortega J. Osteoporosis after cranial irradiation for acute lymphoblastic leukaemia. *J Pediatr* 1990; **117**:238–44.

59 Ersahin Y, Yararbas U, Duman Y, Mutluer S. Single photon emission tomography following posterior fossa surgery in patients with and without mutism. *Childs Nerv Syst* 2002; **18**:318–25.

60 Reddy AT, Witek K. Neurologic complications of chemotherapy for children with cancer. *Curr Neurol Neurosci Rep* 2003; **3**:137–42.

61 Kortmann RD, Kuhl J, Timmermann B *et al*. Postoperative neoadjuvant chemotherapy before radiotherapy as compared to immediate radiotherapy followed by maintenance chemotherapy in the treatment of medulloblastoma in childhood: results of the German prospective randomized trial HIT '91. *Int J Radiat Oncol Biol Phys* 2000; **46**:269–79.

62 Singhal S, Birch JM, Kerr B, Lashford L, Evans DG. Neurofibromatosis type 1 and sporadic optic gliomas. *Arch Dis Child* 2002; **87**:65–70.

63 Gayre GS, Scott IU, Feuer W, Saunders TG, Siatkowski RM. Long-term visual outcome in patients with anterior visual pathway gliomas. *J Neuroophthalmol* 2001; **21**:1–7.

64 Zimmerman RA, Bilaniuk LT, Hackney DB, Goldberg HI, Grossman RI. Magnetic resonance imaging of dural venous sinus invasion, occlusion and thrombosis. *Acta Radiol Suppl* 1986; **369**:110–12.

65 Nadel L, Braun IF, Muizelaar JP, Laine FJ. Tumoral thrombosis of cerebral venous sinuses: preoperative diagnosis using magnetic resonance phase imaging. *Surg Neurol* 1991; **35**:189–95.

66 Carvalho KS, Bodensteiner JB, Connolly PJ, Garg BP. Cerebral venous thrombosis in children. *J Child Neurol* 2000; **16**:574–80.

67 DeVeber G, Andrew M. Canadian Pediatric Ischemic Stroke Study Group. The epidemiology and outcome of sinovenous thrombosis in pediatric patients. *N Engl J Med* 2001; **345**:417–23.

68 Kiya K, Satoh H, Mizoue T, Kinoshita Y. Postoperative cortical venous infarction in tumours firmly adherent to the cortex. *J Clin Neurosci* 2001; **8** (suppl. 1):109–13.

69 Ruud E, Holmstrom H ,Natvig S, Wesenberg F. Prevalence of thrombophilia and central venous catheter-associated neck vein thrombosis in 41 children with cancer a prospective study. *Med Pediatr Oncol* 2002; **38**:405–10.

70 Goh KY-C, Tsoi WC, Feng C-S, Wickham N, Poon, WS. Haemostatic changes during surgery for primary brain tumours. *J Neurol Neurosurg Psychiatry* 1997; **63**:334–8.

71 Moriarity JL, Jr, Lim M, Storm PB, Beauchamp NJ, Jr, Olivi A. Reversible posterior leukoencephalopathy occurring during resection of a posterior fossa tumor: case report and review of the literature. *Neurosurgery* 2001; **49**:1237-9.

72 Bowers DC, Mulne AF, Reisch JS, *et al.* Nonperioperative strokes in children with central nervous system tumors. *Cancer* 2002; **94**:1094-101.

73 Painter MJ, Chutorian AM, Hilal SK. Cerebrovasculopathy following irradiation in childhood. *Neurology* 1975; **25**:189-94.

74 Wright TL, Bresnan MJ. Radiation-induced cerebrovascular disease in children. *Neurology* 1976; **26**:540-3.

75 Servo A, Puranen M. Moyamoya syndrome as a complication of radiation therapy. Case report. *J Neurosurg* 1978; **48**:1026-9.

76 Mori K, Takeuchi J, Ishikawa M, Handa H, Toyama M, Yamaki T. Occlusive arteriopathy and brain tumor. *J Neurosurg* 1978; **49**:2-35.

77 Rajakulasingam K, Cerullo LJ, Raimondi AJ. Childhood moyamoya syndrome. Postradiation pathogenesis. *Childs Brain* 1979; **5**:467-75.

78 Hirata Y, Matsukado Y, Mihara Y, Kochi M, Sonoda H, Fukumura A. Occlusion of the internal carotid artery after radiation therapy for the chiasmal lesion. *Acta Neurochir* 1985; **74**:141-7.

79 Ishibashi Y, Okada H, Mineura K, Kodama N. A case of radiation necrosis with vascular changes on main cerebral arteries. *No Shinkei Geka* 1982; **10**:337-41.

80 Naitoh H, Koizumi N, Nihei K, Taguchi N, Tanaka H. Cerebrovascular disorders after radiation therapy. *Shonika Rinsho* 1982; **35**:97-101.

81 Ono J, Mimaki T, Tagawa T, *et al.* Two case reports of cerebrovascular disorder after radiation therapy. *No To Hattatsu* 1985; **17**:64-70.

82 Kyoi K, Kirino Y, Sakaki T, *et al.* Therapeutic irradiation of brain tumor and cerebrovasculopathy. *No Shinkei Geka* 1989; **17**:163-70.

83 Benoit P, Destee A, Verier A, Giraldon JM, Warot P. Post-radiotherapy stenosis of the supraclinoid internal carotid artery: moyamoya network. *Rev Neurol (Paris)* 1985; **141**:666-8.

84 Montanera W, Chui M, Hudson A. Meningioma and occlusive vasculopathy: coexisting complications of past extracranial radiation. *Surg Neurol* 1985; **24**:35-9.

85 Okuno T, Prensky AL, Gado M. The moyamoya syndrome associated with irradiation of an optic glioma in children: report of two cases and review of the literature. *Pediatr Neurol* 1985; **1**:311-16.

86 Kestle JR, Hoffman HJ, Mock AR. Moyamoya phenomenon after radiation for optic glioma. *J Neurosurg* 1993; **79**:32-5.

87 Lau YL, Milligan DW. Atypical presentation of craniopharyngioma associated with moyamoya disease. *J R Soc Med* 1986; **79**:236-7.

88 Beyer RA, Paden P, Sobel DF, Flynn FG. Moyamoya pattern of vascular occlusion after radiotherapy for glioma of the optic chiasm. *Neurology* 1986; **36**:1173-8.

89 Nishizawa S, Ryu H, Yokoyama T, *et al.* Post-irradiation vasculopathy of intracranial major arteries in children: report of two cases. *Neurol Med Chir* 1991; **31**:336-41.

90 Mitchell WG, Fishman LS, Miller JH, *et al.* Stroke as a late sequela of cranial irradiation for childhood brain tumours. *J Child Neurol* 1991; **6**:128-33.

91 Sutton LN, Gusnard D, Bruce DA, Fried A, Packer RJ, Zimmerman RA. Fusiform dilatation of the carotid artery following radical surgery of childhood craniopharyngiomas. *J Neurosurg* 1991; **74**:695-700.

92 Bitzer M, Topka H. Progressive cerebral occlusive disease after radiation therapy. *Stroke* 1995; **26**:131-6.

93 Rudoltz MS, Regine WF, Langston JW, Sanford R, Kovnar EH, Kun LE. Multiple causes of cerebrovascular accidents in children with tumors of the suprasellar region. *J Neuro-Oncol* 1998; **37**:251-61.

94 Hasegawa S, Hamada J, Morioka M, Kai Y, Hashiguchi A, Ushio Y. Radiation-induced cerebrovasculopathy of the distal middle cerebral artery and distal posterior cerebral artery – case report. *Neurol Med Chir* 2000; **40**:220-3.

95 Aoki S, Hayashi N, Abe O, *et al.* Radiation-induced arteritis: thickened wall with prominent enhancement on cranial MR images – report of five cases and comparison with 18 cases of moyamoya disease. *Radiology* 2002; **223**:683-8

96 Al-Amro A, Schultz H. Moyamoya vasculopathy after cranial irradiation: a case report. *Acta Oncol* 1995; **34**:261-3.

97 Brada M, Burchell L, Ashley S, Traish D. The incidence of cerebrovascular accidents in patients with pituitary adenoma. *Int J Radiat Oncol Biol Phys* 1999; **45**:693-8.

98 Grattan-Smith PJ, Morris JG, Langlands AO. Delayed radiation necrosis of the central nervous system in patients irradiated for pituitary tumours. *J Neurol Neurosurg Psychiatry* 1992; **55**:949-55.

99 Katoh M, Kamiyama H, Abe H, Aida T, Takikawa S, Kuroda S. Complete occlusion of right middle cerebral artery by radiation therapy after removal of pituitary adenoma: case report. *No Shinkei Geka* 1990; **18**:855-9.

100 Kitano S, Sakamoto H, Fujitani K, Kobayashi Y. Moyamoya disease associated with a brain stem glioma. *Childs Nerv Syst* 2000; **16**:251-5.

101 Aihara N, Nagai H, Mase M, Kanai H, Wakabayashi S, Mabe H. Atypical moyamoya disease associated with brain tumor. *Surg Neurol* 1992; **37**:46-50.

102 Grenier Y, Tomita T, Marymont MH, Byrd S, Burrowes DM. Late postradiation occlusive vasculopathy in childhood medulloblastoma. *J Neurosurg* 1998; **89**:460-64.

103 Maher CO, Raffel C. Early vasculopathy following radiation in a child with medulloblastoma. *Pediatr Neurosurg* 2000; **32**:255-8.

104 Darmody WR, Thomas LM, Gurdjian ES. Postirradiation vascular insufficiency syndrome. *Neurology* 1967; **17**:1190-2.

105 Brant-Zawadzki M, Anderson M, DeArmond SJ, Conley FK, Jahnke W. Radiation-induced large intracranial vessel occlusive vasculopathy. *Am J Roentgenol* 1980; **134**:51-5.

106 Maruyama K, Mishima K, Saito N, Fujimaki T, Sasaki T, Kirino T. Radiation-induced aneurysm and moyamoya vessels presenting with subarachnoid haemorrhage. *Acta Neurochir* 2000; **142**:139-43.

107 Harris OA, Chang SD, Harris BT, Adler JR. Acquired cerebral arteriovenous malformation induced by an anaplastic astrocytoma: an interesting case. *Neurol Res* 2000; **22**:473-7.

108 Sinsawaiwong S, Phanthumchinda K. Progressive cerebral occlusive disease after hypothalamic astrocytoma radiation therapy. *J Med Assoc Thai* 1997; **80**:338-42.

109 Beckman JA, Thakore A, Kalinowski BH, Harris JR, Creager MA. Radiation therapy impairs endothelium-dependent vasodilation in humans. *J Am Coll Cardiol* 2001; **37**:761–5.

110 Grill J, Couanet D, Cappelli C, *et al*. Radiation-induced cerebral vasculopathy in children with neurofibromatosis and optic pathway glioma. *Ann Neurol* 1999; **45**:393–6.

111 Tomsick TA, Luskin RR, Chambers AA, Benton C. Neurofibromatosis and intracranial arterial occlusive disease. *Neuroradiology* 1976; **11**:229–34.

112 Yamauchi T, Tada M, Houkin K, *et al*. Linkage of familial moyamoya disease (spontaneous occlusion of the circle of Willis) to chromosome 17q25. *Stroke* 2000; **31**:930.

113 Virdis R, Balestrazzi P, Zampolli M, Donadio A, Street M, Lorenzetti E. Hypertension in children with neurofibromatosis. *J Hum Hypertens* 1994; **8**:395–7.

114 Ganesan V, Kelsey H, Cookson J, Osborn A, Kirkham FJ. Activated protein C resistance in childhood stroke. *Lancet* 1996; **347**:260.

115 Kenet G, Sadetzki S, Murad H, *et al*. Factor V Leiden and antiphospholipid antibodies are significant risk factors for ischemic stroke in children. *Stroke* 2000; **31**:1283.

116 Bonduel M, Hepner M, Sciuccati G, Torres AF, Tenembaum S, de Veber G. Prothrombotic disorders in children with moyamoya syndrome. *Stroke* 2001; **32**:1786–92.

117 Nowak-Gottl U, Strater R, Heinecke A, *et al*. Lipoprotein (a) and genetic polymorphisms of clotting factor V, prothrombin, and methylenetetrahydrofolate reductase are risk factors of spontaneous ischemic stroke in childhood. *Blood* 1999; **94**:3678–82.

118 Ganesan V, Prengler M, McShane MA, Wade A, Kirkham FJ. Investigation of risk factors in children with arterial ischemic stroke. *Ann Neurol* 2003; **53**:167–73.

119 Heikens J, Ubbink MC, van der Pal HP, *et al*. Long term survivors of childhood brain cancer have an increased risk for cardiovascular disease. *Cancer* 2000; **88**:2116–21.

120 Prengler M, Sturt N, Krywawych S, Surtees R, Kirkham F. The homozygous thermolabile variant of the methylenetetrahydrofolate reductase gene: a risk factor for recurrent stroke in childhood. *Dev Med Child Neurol* 2001; **43**:220–5.

121 Abramson ZH, Kark JD. Serum cholesterol and primary brain tumours: a case-control study. *Br J Cancer* 1985; **52**:93–8.

122 Smith GD, Neaton JD, Ben-Shlomo Y, Shipley M, Wentworth D. Serum cholesterol concentration and primary malignant brain tumors: a prospective study. *Am J Epidemiol* 1992; **135**:259–65.

123 Herrington LJ, Friedman DG. Serum cholesterol concentration and risk of brain cancer. *Br Med J* 1995; **310**:367–8.

124 Crook M, Robinson R, Swaminathan R. Hypertriglyceridaemia in a child with hypernatraemia due to a hypothalamic tumour. *Ann Clin Biochem* 1995; **32** (Pt 2):226–8.

125 Kearney T, Navas de Gallegos C, Chrisoulidou A, *et al*. Hypopituitarism is associated with triglyceride enrichment of very low-density lipoprotein. *J Clin Endocrinol Metab* 2001; **86**:3900–6.

126 Landin-Wilhelmsen K, Tengborn L, Wilhelmsen L, Bengtsson BA. Elevated fibrinogen levels decrease following treatment of acromegaly. *Clin Endocrinol* 1997; **46**:69–74.

127 Ohene-Frempong K, Weiner SJ, Sleeper LA, *et al*. Cerebrovascular accidents in sickle cell disease: rates and risk factors. *Blood* 1998; **91**:288–94.

128 Hartfield DS, Lowry NJ, Keene DL, Yager JY. Iron deficiency: a cause of stroke in infants and children. *Pediatr Neurol* 1997; **16**:50–3.

129 Tokunaga Y, Ohga S, Suita S, Matsushima T, Hara T. Moyamoya syndrome with spherocytosis: effect of splenectomy on stroke. *Pediatr Neurol* 2001; **25**:75–7.

130 Kirkham FJ, Hewes DKM, Hargrave D, *et al*. Nocturnal hypoxaemia predicts CNS events in sickle cell disease. *Lancet* 2001; **357**:1656–9.

131 Kirkham FJ, Prengler M, Hewes D, Ganesan V. Risk factors for ischemic stroke in childhood. *J Child Neurol* 2000; **15**:299–307.

132 Lanthier S, Carmant L, David M, Larbrisseau A, de Veber G. Stroke in children: the coexistence of multiple risk factors predicts poor outcome. *Neurology* 2000; **54**:371–8.

133 Schultheiss TE, Kun LE, Ang KK, Stephens LC. Radiation response of the central nervous system. *Int J Radiat Oncol Biol Phys* 1995; **31**:1093–12.

134 Glantz MJ, Burger PC, Friedman AH, Radtke RA, Massey EW, Schold SC, Jr. Treatment of radiation-induced nervous system injury with heparin and warfarin. *Neurology* 1994; **44**:2020–7.

135 Lamberts HD, de Boer WGRM. Contributions to the study of immediate and early X-ray reactions with regard to chemoprotection: VII. X-ray induced atheromatous lesions in the arterial wall of atheromatous rabbits. *Int J Radiat Biol* 1965; **6**:343–50.

136 Levinson SA, Close MB, Ehrenfeld WK, Stoney RJ. Carotid artery occlusive disease following external cervical irradiation. *Arch Surg* 1973; **107**:395–7.

137 Murros KE, Toole JF. The effect of radiation on carotid arteries. A review article. *Arch Neurol* 1989; **46**:449–55.

138 Glick B. Bilateral carotid occlusive disease following irradiation for carcinoma of the vocal cords. *Arch Pathol Lab Med* 1972; **93**:352–5.

139 Constine LS, Konski A, Ekholm S, McDonald S, Rubin P. Adverse effects of brain irradiation correlated with MR and CT imaging. *Int J Radiat Oncol Biol Phys* 1988; **15**:319–30.

140 Mulhern RK, Palmer SL, Reddick WE, *et al*. Risks of young age for selected neurocognitive deficits in medulloblastoma are associated with white matter loss. *J Clin Oncol* 2001; **19**:472–9.

141 Mulhern RK, Reddick WE, Palmer SL, *et al*. Neurocognitive deficits in medulloblastoma survivors and white matter loss. *Ann Neurol* 1999; **46**:834–41.

142 Reddickaij WE, Russell JM, Glass JO, *et al*. Subtle white matter volume differences in children treated for medulloblastoma with conventional or reduced dose craniospinal irradiation. *Magn Reson Imaging* 2000; **18**:787–93.

143 Steen RG, Koury BSM, Granja CI, *et al*. Effect of ionizing radiation on the human brain: white matter and grey matter T1 in pediatric brain tumor patients treated with conformal radiation therapy. *Int J Radiat Oncol Biol Phys* 2001; **49**:79–81.

144 Fouladi M, Langston J, Mulhern R, *et al*. Silent lacunar lesions detected by magnetic resonance imaging of children with brain tumors: a late sequela of therapy. *J Clin Oncol* 2000; **18**:824–31.

145 Suzuki S, Nishio S, Takata K, Morioka T, Fukui M. Radiation-induced brain calcification: paradoxical high signal intensity in T1-weighted MR images. *Acta Neurochir* 2000; **142**:801–4.

146 Chan YL, Roebuck DJ, Yuen MP, Yeung KW, Lau KY, Li CK, Chik KW. Long-term cerebral metabolite changes on proton magnetic resonance spectroscopy in patients cured of acute lymphoblastic leukemia with previous intrathecal methotrexate and cranial irradiation prophylaxis. *Int J Radiat Oncol Biol Phys* 2001; **50**:759–63.

147 Davidson A, Tait DM, Payne GS, *et al.* Magnetic resonance spectroscopy in the evaluation of neurotoxicity following cranial irradiation for childhood cancer. *Br J Radiol* 2000; **73**:421–4.

148 Phillips PC, Moeller JR, Sidtis JJ, *et al.* Abnormal cerebral glucose metabolism in long-term survivors of childhood acute lymphocytic leukemia. *Ann Neurol* 1991; **29**:263–71.

149 Dadparvar S, Hussain R, Koffler SP, Gillan MM, Bartolic EI, Miyamoto C. The role of Tc-99 m HMPAO functional brain imaging in detection of cerebral radionecrosis. *Cancer J* 2000; **6**:381–7.

150 Plowman PN, Saunders CA, Maisey M. On the usefulness of brain PET scanning to the paediatric neuro-oncologist. *Br J Neurosurg* 1997; **11**:525–32.

151 Langleben DD, Segall GM. PET in differentiation of recurrent brain tumor from radiation injury. *J Nucl Med* 2000; **41**:1861–7.

152 Biousse V, Newman NJ, Hunter SB, Hudgins PA. Diffusion weighted imaging in radiation necrosis. *J Neurol Neurosurg Psychiatry* 2003; **74**:382–4.

153 Lippens RJ, van Ooijen AG. Calcifications of the basal ganglia in children with brain tumours. *Eur J Paediatr Neurol* 1997; **1**:85–9.

154 Nieder C, Leicht A, Motaref B, Nestle U, Niewald M, Schnabel K. Late radiation toxicity after whole brain radiotherapy: the influence of antiepileptic drugs. *Am J Clin Oncol* 1999; **22**:573–9.

155 Kirkham FJ. Stroke in childhood. *Arch Dis Child* 1999; **81**:85–9.

156 Gadian DG, Calamante F, Kirkham FJ, *et al.* Diffusion and perfusion magnetic resonance imaging in childhood stroke. *J Child Neurol* 2000; **15**:279–83.

157 Calamante F, Ganesan V, Kirkham FJ, *et al.* MR perfusion imaging in moyamoya syndrome: Potential implications for clinical evaluation of occlusive cerebrovascular disease. *Stroke* 2001; **32**:2810–16.

158 Nowak-Gottl U, Straeter R, Sebire G, Kirkham F. Antithrombotic drug treatment of pediatric patients with ischemic stroke. *Paediatr Drugs* 2003; **5**:167–75.

159 Chen ZM, Sandercock P, Pan HC, *et al.* Indications for early aspirin use in acute ischemic stroke: a combined analysis of 40 000 randomized patients from the Chinese acute stroke trial and the international stroke trial. On behalf of the CAST and IST collaborative groups. *Stroke* 2000; **31**:1240–9.

160 De Jongh S, Ose L, Szamosi T, *et al.* Simvastatin in Children Study Group. Efficacy and safety of statin therapy in children with familial hypercholesterolemia: a randomized, double-blind, placebo-controlled trial with simvastatin. *Circulation* 2002; **106**:2231–7.

161 Ishikawa T, Houkin K, Yoshimoto T, Abe H. Vasoreconstructive surgery for radiation-induced vasculopathy in childhood. *Surg Neurol* 1997; **48**:620–6.

162 Martins AN, Johnston JS, Henry JM, Stoffel TJ, Di Chiro G. Delayed radiation necrosis of the brain. *J Neurosurg* 1977; **47**:336–45.

163 Groothuis DR, Mikhael MA. Focal cerebral vasculitis associated with circulating immune complexes and brain irradiation. *Ann Neurol* 1986; **19**:590–2.

164 Hart GB, Mainous EG. The treatment of radiation necrosis with hyperbaric oxygen (OHP). *Cancer* 1976; **37**:2580–5.

165 Guy J, Schatz NJ. Hyperbaric oxygen in the treatment of radiation-induced optic neuropathy. *Ophthalmology* 1986; **93**:1083–8.

166 Poulton TJ, Witcofski RL. Hyperbaric oxygen therapy for radiation myelitis. *Undersea Biomed Res* 1985; **12**:453–8.

167 Ganesan V, Hogan A, Shack N, Gordon A, Isaacs E, Kirkham FJ. Outcome after ischaemic stroke in childhood. *Dev Med Child Neurol* 2000; **42**:455–61.

168 Gordon AL, Ganesan V, Towell A, Kirkham FJ. Functional outcome following stroke in children. *J Child Neurol* 2002; **17**:429–34.

169 Riva D, Giorgi C. The neurodevelopmental price of survival in children with malignant brain tumours. *Childs Nerv Syst* 2000; **16**:751–4.

170 Anderson VA, Godber T, Smibert E, Weiskop S, Ekert H. Cognitive and academic outcome following cranial irradiation and chemotherapy in children: a longitudinal study. *Br J Cancer* 2000; **82**:255–62.

171 Zucchinelli V, Bouffet E. Academic future of children treated for brain tumors. Single-center study of 27 children. *Arch Pediatr* 2000; **7**:933–41.

172 Kun LE, Mulhern RK, Jr. Neuropsychologic function in children with brain tumors: II. Serial studies of intellect and time after treatment. *Am J Clin Oncol* 1983; **6**:651–6.

173 Edgeworth J, Bullock P, Bailey A, Gallagher A, Crouchman M. Why are brain tumours still being missed? *Arch Dis Child* 1996; **74**:148–51.

174 Habrand JL, De Crevoisier R. Radiation therapy in the management of childhood brain tumors. *Childs Nerv Syst* 2001; **17**:121–33.

175 Mulhern RK, Kepner JL, Thomas PR, Armstrong FD, Friedman HS, Kun LE. Neuropsychologic functioning of survivors of childhood medulloblastoma randomized to receive conventional or reduced-dose craniospinal irradiation: a Pediatric Oncology Group study. *J Clin Oncol* 1998; **16**:1723–8.

176 Grill J, Renaux VK, Bulteau C, *et al.* Long-term intellectual outcome in children with posterior fossa tumors according to radiation doses and volumes. *Int J Radiat Oncol Biol Phys* 1999; **45**:137–45.

177 Kieffer-Renaux V, Bulteau C, Grill J, Kalifa C, Viguier D, Jambaque I. Patterns of neuropsychological deficits in children with medulloblastoma according to craniospatial irradiation doses. *Dev Med Child Neurol* 2000; **42**:741–5.

178 Fuss M, Poljanc K, Hug EB. Full scale IQ (FSIQ) changes in children treated with whole brain and partial brain irradiation. A review and analysis. *Strahlenther Onkol* 2000; **176**:573–81.

179 Ris MD, Packer R, Goldwein J, Jones-Wallace D, Boyett JM. Intellectual outcome after reduced-dose radiation therapy plus adjuvant chemotherapy for medulloblastoma: a Children's Cancer Group study. *J Clin Oncol* 2001; **19**:3470–6.

180 Palmer SL, Goloubeva O, Reddick WE, *et al.* Patterns of intellectual development among survivors of pediatric medulloblastoma: a longitudinal analysis. *J Clin Oncol* 2001; **19**:2302–8.

181 Thomas PR, Deutsch M, Kepner JL, *et al*. Low-stage medulloblastoma: final analysis of trial comparing standard-dose with reduced-dose neuraxis irradiation. *J Clin Oncol* 2000; **18**:3004–11.

182 Packer RJ, Goldwein J, Nicholson HS, *et al*. Treatment of children with medulloblastomas with reduced-dose craniospinal radiation therapy and adjuvant chemotherapy: a Children's Cancer Group Study. *J Clin Oncol* 1999; **17**:2127–36.

183 Tornesello A, Mastrangelo S, Piciacchia D, *et al*. Progressive disease in children with medulloblastoma/PNET during preradiation chemotherapy. *J Neuro-Oncol* 1999; **45**:135–40.

184 Packer RJ, Cogen P, Vezina G, Rorke LB. Medulloblastoma: clinical and biologic aspects. *Neurooncol* 1999; **1**:232–50.

185 Cucchiara B, Kasner SE. Use of statins in CNS disorders. *J Neurol Sci* 2001; **187**:81–9.

186 Jick H, Zornberg GL, Jick SS, Seshadri S, Drachman DA. Statins and the risk of dementia. *Lancet* 2000; **356**:1627–31.

187 Ungvari Z, Pacher P, Csiszar A. Can simvastatin promote tumor growth by inducing angiogenesis similar to VEGF? *Med Hypotheses* 2002; **58**:85–6.

188 Macaulay RJ, Wang W, Dimitroulakos J, Becker LE, Yeger H. Lovastatin-induced apoptosis of human medulloblastoma cell lines in vitro. *J Neuro-Oncol* 1999; **42**:1–11.

189 Schmidt F, Groscurth P, Kermer M, Dichgans J, Weller M. Lovastatin and phenylacetate induce apoptosis, but not differentiation, in human malignant glioma cells. *Acta Neuropathol (Berl)* 2001; **101**:217–24.

190 Larner J, Jane J, Laws E, Packer R, Myers C, Shaffrey M. A phase I–II trial of lovastatin for anaplastic astrocytoma and glioblastoma multiforme. Am *J Clin Oncol* 1998; **21**:579–83.

191 Black DM. Statins in children: what do we know and what do we need to do? *Curr Atheroscler Rep* 2001; **3**:29–34.

192 Kirkham FJ, Calamante F, Bynevelt M, *et al*. Perfusion MR abnormalities in patients with sickle cell disease: relation to symptoms, infarction and cerebrovascular disease. *Ann Neurol* 2001; **49**:477–85.

193 Packer R, Goldwein J, Nicholson H, *et al*. Treatment of children with medulloblastomas with reduced-dose craniospinal radiation therapy and adjuvant chemotherapy: a Children's Cancer Group Study. *J Clin Oncol* 1999; **17**:2127–36.

194 Livesey E, Brook C. Thyroid dysfunction after radiotherapy and chemotherapy of brain tumours. *Arch Dis Child* 1989; **64**:593–5.

25

Physical care, rehabilitation, and complementary therapies

CARLOS DE SOUSA, LINDY MAY AND VIRGINIA MCGIVERN

INTRODUCTION

The modern management of the child with a brain or spinal tumor has as its goals:

- the return of the child to as normal function as is possible;
- the reintegration of the child into family life and into society.

Attention needs to be given from the earliest point to each and every aspect of the child's condition in order to succeed in these goals. Success also requires the expertise of a team of professionals. Some members of the team will be involved in the treatment of every child, while others will be involved only in selected cases. The multidisciplinary team should have an orchestrated approach, with the different professionals playing a greater or lesser role during different phases in the child's management. Good communication between professionals, and between professionals and the family, is essential. The benefits of early involvement by so many professionals must be offset against the risk of the child and family becoming overwhelmed and confused. Decisions will need to be made in individual cases about the priorities for that child's treatment. Ultimately, advances in treatment will improve the child's quality of life only if they are a part of holistic care provided by a well-performing multidisciplinary neuro-oncology team.

THE CHILD AND FAMILY DURING THE PROCESS OF ASSESSMENT, DIAGNOSIS, AND MANAGEMENT DECISIONS

The family's response to illness

For the family of a child with a newly diagnosed brain tumor, the shock of diagnosis, the grief and loss of a healthy child, and the uncertainty of outcome will rock the most stable of relationships. The family members may find themselves overwhelmed by information and explanations. Uncertainty occurs when there is not enough information to define or categorize an event adequately, and the diagnosis of a brain or spinal tumor produces a state of complete uncertainty, where nothing can be assumed and the future is an awesome and frightening unknown.[1] The family may have no sense of control or order. Despair and fear are common initial feelings, followed by anger and sadness, and allowances must be made by healthcare professionals for episodes of unpredictable or irrational behavior by the child's parents.

An experienced team will assist the family in reaching a stage of acceptance and active participation in their child's care, by providing support, honesty, explanation, and kindness. The family's response to illness and their ability to cope will depend partly on the existing sociocultural, political, economic, emotional, and physical framework within that family. Some families may be more positive in their outlook to serious illness and may have more supportive family networks or other resources available. Other families have a more pessimistic view, may be financially disadvantaged, or may have less supportive networks. Role changes, isolation, financial concerns, and family dynamics will all affect the family of a sick child. An appreciation of these responses and coping mechanisms will assist those involved with the child and family in providing improved care (see Chapter 28).

Staff caring for these children and their families will also be affected to some extent. Constant exposure to extreme experiences and emotions requires a supportive network for the team, and it is important to recognize that in any situation, our personal feelings will be present and must be addressed.[2] A caring work environment should be established, where staff feel supported and valued.

The professionals that will have a role in management

As an example, the Great Ormond Street Hospital, London, pediatric neuro-oncology team, which meets once a week to plan management and review progress of all patients, consists of the following professionals:

- *Nursing:*
  - pediatric neurosurgery ward nurse
  - pediatric oncology ward nurse
  - clinical nurse specialist
  - research nurse.
- *Medical:*
  - neurosurgeon
  - pediatric oncologist
  - radiotherapist
  - pediatric neurologist
  - pediatric endocrinologist
  - radiologist.
- *Professionals allied to medicine:*
  - clinical psychologist
  - physiotherapist.

These professional constitute the core pediatric neuro-oncology team. The following also have an important role in the extended team: anesthetist, pediatric intensivist, child psychiatrist, occupational therapist, speech therapist, dietician, social worker, and play specialist.

MANAGEMENT OF COMMON MEDICAL PROBLEMS

Hydrocephalus

In children with central nervous system (CNS) tumors, hydrocephalus may be caused by tumors of the posterior fossa, pineal region, choroid plexus, and structures adjacent to the lateral and third ventricles, as well as by spinal tumors.[3] If ventricular enlargement is shown on brain imaging, but the child has no symptoms or signs of hydrocephalus, then usually there is no need for an immediate cerebrospinal fluid (CSF) diversion procedure. However, there are different considerations to be made, according to the site and size of the tumor, its dissemination, and the age and size of the child. The majority of children with childhood posterior fossa tumors and associated hydrocephalus may be managed with perioperative extraventricular drainage and will not require a shunt or ventriculostomy, unless tumor resection has been only minimal.[4] Some surgeons favor the routine use of endoscopic third ventriculostomy before surgery in all children with hydrocephalus and posterior fossa brain tumors.[5] Children with thalamic tumors often present without hydrocephalus, so surgery may be required both to relieve intracranial pressure and to establish the histology of the tumor.[6]

Complications of ventricular shunts include shunt infection, shunt blockage, ascites,[7] and very rarely tumor dissemination.[8] The rate of shunt blockage in children with brain tumors may be less than in hydrocephalus due to other causes.[9] Complications of endoscopic third ventriculostomy include basilar artery perforation,[10] spontaneous closure, and tumor recurrence along an endoscope tract.[11] Although third ventriculostomy is as effective as a shunt in the treatment of hydrocephalus in children,[12] there are as yet insufficient quality-of-life and clinical outcome measures to establish its superiority.[13]

SEIZURES

Epilepsy is common in children with brain tumors (although less common than in adults), and it may be the sole manifestation of a tumor. In children under 14 years of age and with supratentorial tumors, seizures occur in around 22 per cent (increasing to 68 per cent in older teenagers). In those with posterior fossa tumors, seizures occur in around six per cent.[14] The occurrence of seizures is greatest in children with multiple neurological deficits as a result of their tumor (motor deficits, visual impairment, and altered conscious level). Patients with tumors located superficially in the cerebral hemispheres, especially those close to the motor strip and adjacent to the central sulcus, are the most likely to have seizures. Studies in adults have shown seizures to be associated more frequently with slowly growing and relatively benign tumors, such as low-grade glial tumors,[15] but there are no comparable data from children.

Tumor-associated epilepsy is due to multiple factors, including peritumoral amino acid disturbances, local metabolic imbalances, cerebral edema, pH abnormalities, morphological changes in the neuropil, changes in neuronal and glial enzyme and protein expression, altered immunological activity, cytokines (tumor necrosis factor (TNF) and nuclear factor-kappaB), and abnormal function of *N*-methyl-D-aspartate (NMDA) receptors.[16,17]

The electroencephalogram (EEG) shows focal abnormalities ipsilateral to the tumor in 62–73 per cent of children with brain tumors and epilepsy.[18,19] However, abnormalities, including focal epileptiform discharges, can also occur in children with brain tumors and no seizures, so that the diagnosis of epilepsy in this group must be a clinical one supported by the appropriate neurophysiological investigations.

Seizures may also occur for the first time in a child with a relapsed tumor, or tumor progression may be associated with an increase in the frequency of seizures that were occurring previously. In an infant or young child, the seizures due to a brain tumor may be difficult to recognize, especially subtle and non-convulsive partial seizures.[20]

Epilepsy contributes to behavioral disorders, confusion, stupor, and coma in children with brain tumors.[14,18] Status epilepticus carries with it a significant morbidity and mortality. The imperatives in a child with a brain tumor and seizures are to diagnose the seizures, to identify any reversible predisposing conditions (metabolic disturbance, hemorrhage, infection), to stop the seizures, and to prevent seizures from recurring.

The child with status epilepticus and a brain tumor will be treated using standardized guidelines for the management of the acutely ill child.[21] Children with raised intracranial pressure and seizures may be especially sensitive to the effects of respiratory-depressant drugs such as benzodiazepines, and therefore the treatment of a child with seizures and a tumor must be carried out with facilities available for assisted ventilation. Children with less severe seizures may be treated either with a loading dose of phenytoin followed by oral phenytoin or, if the seizures are less frequent, by commencing an oral antiepileptic drug such as sodium valproate or carbamazepine. Rectal diazepam, buccal or nasal midazolam, or rectal paraldehyde can be used to terminate seizures that occur despite prophylactic antiepileptic drug treatment. There is, however, no place for the routine use of antiepileptic drugs in children with brain tumors but who have not had seizures.

There is a potential for interaction between antiepileptic drugs and other treatments that the child is receiving, including analgesic, anti-inflammatory, and cytotoxic agents.[22,23] These agents may reduce the anticonvulsant effects of antiepileptic drugs.

Early postoperative seizures in a child with a brain tumor may be due to the tumor itself, metabolic disturbances, hemorrhage, cerebral infarction, or CNS infection. Later-onset seizures may be caused by radiation injury and chemotherapy-related encephalopathies.[24]

Following a subfrontal craniotomy, postoperative epilepsy occurs in less than 12 per cent of patients.[25] When seizures do occur in this setting, antiepileptic drugs can generally be decreased and then stopped one month postoperatively and should not be used for long-term prophylactic therapy.

Dysphagia

One of the effects of having a brain tumor, or of undergoing treatment for it, is an abnormality of the feeding process. This can include disturbances of appetite and satiety, behavioral disorders affecting feeding, and abnormalities of the oral and pharyngeal phases of swallowing, causing dysphagia and pulmonary aspiration. A lesion of the developing brain will affect not only fully developed functions but also those that are maturing and emerging. These disorders have been studied scarcely in adults with brain tumors and hardly at all in children.[26]

Brain tumors and their treatments can affect the feeding process in several different ways. Direct neurological effects of tumors and their treatments on the control of feeding and swallowing include the following:

- Cerebral tumors and those that impinge on corticobulbar neural pathways may cause impairment of control of mouth closure, chewing, and swallowing.
- Tumors of the diencephalon may cause disturbances in appetite and consequently weight gain. The diencephalic syndrome, which occurs most often as the result of low-grade gliomas of the hypothalamus and optic chiasm in infancy, is at one end of a spectrum of disorders caused by lesions in this region.[27]
- Tumors of the cerebellum may cause uncoordinated action of bulbar muscles, affecting chewing and swallowing.
- Brainstem tumors may impinge on cranial nerve nuclei, causing a bulbar palsy, with impairment of mouth closure, chewing, and swallowing.[28] Surgery for tumors, especially those close to the floor of the fourth ventricle, may have similar effects. Tumors of the brainstem may directly affect emetic centres, causing vomiting and gastroesophageal reflux.[29]

Brain tumors and their treatments may also have indirect neurological effects on the control of auxiliary functions necessary for feeding:

- Children with central motor deficits (due to lesions of the cerebral cortex, corticospinal pathways, basal ganglia, cerebellum, or brainstem), which cause ataxia, spasticity, or dystonia, and affect control of hand function, are less able to feed themselves. If they also have impaired control of trunk posture, they are less able to be positioned correctly for feeding.[30]

- Children with a visual impairment as a result of a brain tumor are likely to be delayed in the acquisition of normally coordinated self-feeding.[31]
- Hearing loss as a result of either the tumor or its treatment can contribute to communication difficulties, one of the causes of behavioral problems that can arise around feeding in childhood.

Brain tumors will also have developmental and psychosocial consequences that affect the feeding and swallowing process:

- Some children with brain tumors may have communication difficulties, making it difficult for them to express hunger or food preferences. This can also lead to frustration in the parent or carer, who may have difficulty in interpreting cues from the child.
- Brain tumors in infancy may disrupt a sensitive or critical learning period for the acquisition of feeding skills.[32] After such a critical period, a particular behavioral pattern can no longer be learned in the same way. To acquire such a pattern later will require a different learning process from that of normal infant development.
- The child with a brain tumor will go through many abnormal experiences following diagnosis. These may include diagnostic investigations, surgery, radiotherapy, and chemotherapy. Many of these will cause pain, fear, and upset. They will make it difficult to maintain or establish set routines, which are necessary for successful feeding, especially in young infants.[33]
- Many of the factors described here will affect the emotional interaction between the child and the parents. An additional factor is the emotional state of the parents, which will be affected by knowledge of their child's diagnosis and prognosis. These emotional factors may contribute to difficulties with successful feeding.[34] Some children may have a learned aversion to feeding as a result of these experiences and emotional interactions, which can persist after the removal of the unpleasant stimuli.

Some of the treatments for brain tumors have secondary effects, which are not related specifically to tumor location:

- Some agents used as part of a chemotherapy regime may cause anorexia, nausea, and vomiting. Children may feel lethargic during part of their treatment. If the child is treated with antiepileptic drugs, some of these may suppress appetite; others can worsen feeding and swallowing difficulties by promoting the production of saliva. Corticosteroids, which are often given to palliate the effects of a tumor soon after diagnosis, or while awaiting more definitive treatment, will cause abnormalities of appetite as well as having behavioral and metabolic effects.
- Radiotherapy will often cause a period of somnolence after treatment, which may contribute to difficulties with feeding and swallowing.
- Many children treated for brain tumors have endocrine late effects.[35] Some of these are due to the location of the tumor in the hypothalamus, while others are the result of surgery or radiotherapy that alter function of the hypothalamus and pituitary. Disturbances of growth hormone, sex hormones, thyroid hormone, and endogenous steroid production can affect appetite, mood, weight gain, and growth.
- Constipation may be a result of drugs (e.g. opiate analgesics, chemotherapy agents including vincristine) or alterations in diet, fluid intake, mobility, and normal routine. It will contribute to problems with lack of appetite.

Management of dysphagia in children with brain tumors first requires its recognition. This may be obvious if the child is an in-patient and the feeding disorder is severe. It may be less easy to diagnose in children who are at home, unless the right questions are asked or the parents volunteer information. Speech therapists and dieticians are key professionals working with the neuro-oncology team in the diagnosis and management of dysphagia. It is important to have a holistic approach to this problem, realizing that rarely is there a single cause, and that many factors, including emotional and behavioral ones, will need to be addressed.

Radiographic techniques, such as a barium cine-swallow, will assist with the clinical diagnosis of the reasons for swallowing difficulties. If gastroesophageal reflux is suspected, the child may require esophageal pH monitoring. Treatment of reflux with cimetidine and promotility agents such as domperidone can provide relief from the symptoms of reflux. In some cases, more intensive anti-reflux treatment, occasionally including surgery, will be required.

Artificial means of feeding are often necessary in young children undergoing combined modality treatment for brain tumors with surgery followed by radiotherapy and chemotherapy. It is best to identify problems at an early stage. Many children will be helped by the placement of a gastrostomy tube (which can be done endoscopically). This can remain in place for the duration of treatment or until the child is able to re-establish nutritionally adequate and safe oral feeding.

Gregory

At 11 years of age, Gregory was admitted to his local hospital with a six-week history of headache and vomiting. He was subsequently diagnosed as having a left frontoparietal primitive neuroectodermal tumor (PNET). This was treated by surgical resection, followed by chemotherapy and craniospinal radiotherapy. He made a good recovery from his surgery, with no apparent neurological deficits. He had an onset of somnolence during radiotherapy, which delayed his re-entry into school. There was initially some improvement in his symptoms, but a few months after finishing radiotherapy he had a flu-like illness, following which he developed fatigue and headache. These symptoms persisted, and he then also began to experience limb pain and episodes of absence and altered behavior. He commenced treatment with carbamazepine.

Gregory was readmitted to the child neurology unit for investigation of these symptoms. His magnetic resonance imaging (MRI) scan showed no evidence of tumor recurrence. EEG monitoring during episodes of absence showed that these were non-epileptic seizures and his carbamazepine was stopped. His endocrinological investigations showed that he had growth hormone deficiency and low plasma cortisol levels, and he was commenced on replacement treatment. Gregory and his parents refused to meet the clinical psychologist and child psychiatrist during this admission.

His symptoms improved, and he started to attend school on a part-time basis. Three months later, he had a further seizure, following which his symptoms of headache, limb pain, and fatigue returned with increased severity. He was also unable to hold a pen in his right hand. He was readmitted to hospital urgently, and he underwent further investigations, including an MRI brain scan. Again, there was no evidence of tumor recurrence. In hospital, he appeared unhappy and withdrawn. He was seen by a psychiatrist, and a plan was made to admit him to the regional child psychiatry unit for assessment and rehabilitation.

On the day of the proposed psychiatric admission, Gregory's father telephoned to say that he was too unwell to attend. Gregory remained at home. His father gave up work to help to look after him. Gregory was unable to return to school, and the local education authority arranged for a home tutor. Gregory attended for his follow-up appointments in the neuro-oncology clinic and saw the oncologists, neurologist, and endocrinologist. His surveillance brain imaging continued to show no evidence of tumor recurrence. His pain persisted and he commenced treatment with gabapentin.

Two and a half years after the original diagnosis, Gregory was still unable to return to school. His parents had divorced and his elder brother had left home. Gregory continued to be looked after by his father. In addition to his previous symptoms, Gregory now had a poor appetite and some weight loss. Gregory and his father finally agreed to his admission to a medical ward for a program of rehabilitation. This included physiotherapy, occupational therapy, attendance at the hospital school, clinical psychology, and child psychiatry. Two weeks into the admission, Gregory failed to return from weekend leave. A hospital social worker visited him at home and persuaded him to return. He was commenced on treatment with a selective serotonin reuptake inhibitor (SSRI). His mood improved, as did his appetite. He spent a total of six weeks in hospital. Meetings were held with his community pediatrician and a teacher from his school before his discharge from hospital.

Following his discharge from hospital, Gregory made a successful re-entry into full-time school, a year behind his age group. He required additional classroom help because of some specific learning difficulties. Over a six-month period, with support and encouragement from the community medical and nursing team, he successfully reintegrated into a full range of physical activities. All his drugs were eventually stopped, with the exception of growth hormone replacement treatment.

- Psychiatric and psychosomatic illness may complicate recovery after the successful treatment of a brain tumor.
- In order for functional improvement to occur, the patient and family need to accept the need for rehabilitation, including psychological and family therapy.
- Persistence in rehabilitation pays off.
- Long-term success depends upon effective working and cooperation between the specialist hospital team and those based locally (health, education, and social services).

POSTOPERATIVE MANAGEMENT

Where and how the child should be looked after following surgery

Following surgery for a brain tumor, children require high-dependency or intensive care from nurses and doctors with specialized skills. Depending on the type of procedure, the child's age, and the postoperative condition, this may necessitate the child's immediate care following surgery to be in the intensive care unit or in a high-dependency unit within the neurosurgical ward. During the postoperative period, the child progresses from a high level of dependency, to a greater emphasis on family-centered care provided alongside nursing support and advice.

The immediate requirements of the child following surgery include management of the airway and hemodynamic homeostasis. Regular neurological assessment is essential, and a recognized pediatric coma scoring system should be utilized, such as a pediatric adaptation of the Glasgow Coma Scale.[36,37] Early recognition and treatment of complications such as raised intracranial pressure are essential and require good communication and teamwork.

Hemodynamic and fluid management

In addition to neurological assessment, the visual assessment of the child and monitoring of physiological measures (blood pressure, pulse, temperature, central venous pressure, intracranial pressure) provide a continuous appraisal of the child's condition. Arterial and central venous pressure monitoring may be necessary, particularly in situations where major fluid imbalance is anticipated, such as following removal of a craniopharyngioma. Following removal of a cerebral tumor other than a craniopharyngioma, intravenous or oral fluid intake is initially restricted to 50–70 per cent of the normal maintenance requirements, in an attempt to reduce the effects of cerebral edema. A short course of dexamethasone following surgery is also given routinely in many centers.

Cardiovascular instability and cardiac arrhythmias may occur especially following surgery to the posterior fossa, probably because of direct effects on brainstem vasomotor centres. In such a situation, it is important to correct any plasma electrolyte abnormalities and fluid imbalances. These brainstem vasomotor disturbances usually correct spontaneously.

Postoperative respiratory depression is usually the result of anesthesia. However, prolonged or severe respiratory depression may result from surgical complications, including hemorrhage. If the lower cranial nerves (especially IX and X) are injured during surgery, then the child is at increased risk of aspiration of secretions, sometimes causing hypoxia, which has its onset some hours after emerging from anesthesia.

Raised intracranial pressure

A number of measures can be taken to treat elevated intracranial pressure. Hyperventilation has traditionally been the first measure, as hypocapnia leads to cerebral vasoconstriction. However, excessive hyperventilation may reduce cerebral blood flow to unacceptable levels, thus impairing cerebral metabolism and potentially compromising outcome. Other effective measures include the use of sedation or neuromuscular blockade, the effective

treatment of seizures, the minimization of stimulation, and the use of the osmotic diuretic mannitol.

Postoperative pain management

Postoperative pain should be anticipated and early treatment commenced. The use of rectal analgesia given before anesthesia is reversed (with parental consent) provides immediate relief from postoperative pain. The use of intravenous patient-controlled analgesia (PCA) or nurse-controlled analgesia (NCA) morphine pumps following craniotomy remains controversial. Herbert suggests that this is an outdated idea and that "titrated morphine has no inherent risk if the patient is well observed."[38] Once the child is conscious, a variety of "pain tools" can be utilized for measuring pain, e.g. the Children's Hospital of Eastern Ontario pain scale (CHEOPS),[39] the Faces Scale,[40] and the Eland Color Scale.[41] The tool used must give consistent results and be appropriate to the child's cognitive level.

Culture and gender may have an influence on perceptions of pain.[42] Adolescents may deny pain if they feel it is socially unacceptable to acknowledge it.[43] Good preoperative preparation and explanation help to counteract these feelings and to allay the fears and anxieties that contribute towards pain.[44]

Posterior fossa syndrome

This syndrome comprises a number of symptoms and signs that appear for the first time in a small proportion of children following posterior fossa surgery. It occurs most often following surgery involving the inferior cerebellar vermis and is seen very seldom in tumors confined to the cerebellar hemispheres. Any tumor type may be responsible, although medulloblastoma is the most frequent.[45] The symptoms usually have their onset between one and four days (rarely up to one week) after surgery. The foremost of these symptoms is mutism (hence the term "cerebellar mutism," which is sometimes used interchangeably for this syndrome). Many affected children display personality changes, emotional lability, and decreased initiation of voluntary movements.[46] Cranial nerve palsies, especially sixth and seventh nerve palsies, dysphagia, hemiparesis, and orofacial and limb dyskinesias (random, non-purposeful movements), occur in some children with this syndrome. Many of the symptoms resolve completely or improve considerably with time. This is especially true of the mutism and personality changes, which usually resolve within three months.[47] Ataxia, cranial nerve deficits, and dysarthria may be persisting problems in children with posterior fossa syndrome.

The first task in managing the syndrome is its differentiation from other postsurgical complications. The behavioral changes and abnormal movements result in some children being diagnosed incorrectly as having epilepsy, whereas seizures are in fact unusual postoperatively in children with posterior fossa tumors and who do not also have electrolyte disturbances. Both the child and the family will need great support and reassurance during this distressing time. A speech therapist can assess the child's communication ability and recommend aids such as a communication board. Speech therapy is an important part of the continuing rehabilitation of children with this syndrome. Because of the associated dysphagia, there must be meticulous attention to the child's feeding abilities and dietary intake during the time of recovery. Many children with this syndrome require a period of enteral feeding (nasogastric tube or gastrostomy).[48]

The precise cause of the posterior fossa syndrome is not known. The cerebellum has an important role in learning and language development, and these children have an apraxia (loss of learned activities) of the oral and pharyngeal musculature.[47] Although frequently associated with involvement of vermian and paravermian structures, there does not appear to be a single anatomical locus underlying the syndrome. It seems likely that the interruption of afferent and efferent connections to the cerebellum leads to this loss of learned speech and other complex motor activities as well as modifying behavior and the child's affective state.[46]

COMPLEMENTARY THERAPIES

Amy

Amy was diagnosed with an ependymoma at the age of 14 years. Vincristine was given as part of her treatment. The drug caused a peripheral neuropathy, which led to foot drop, constipation, and severe cramps in the legs and jaw. She was a strong and determined young lady, but some of the side effects of chemotherapy were making life trying for her and she wanted some relief. These symptoms were not relieved with any orthodox analgesia, and aromatherapy massage seemed to be the only therapy that could help her.

The nurse therapist saw Amy on a monthly basis to fit in with her medical treatments. The nurse therapist taught Amy's mother to massage Amy's legs in particular. This needed to be done on a regular basis to ease her discomfort. At the first consultation, Amy was excited about having a massage, as her mother had explained to her what the therapy involves. She was a very particular young lady and wished to know in great detail what was to happen. During the consultation and consent, Amy asked many questions. She chose her own oils – chamomile

---

Roman and lavender – because of their smell and properties. These oils were mixed with grapeseed oil.

During her full body massage, Amy relaxed very quickly and seemed very comfortable with the therapy. Her mother worked alongside the nurse therapist as she massaged Amy's legs. She picked it up well and appeared confident to continue at home.

By the time of the second consultation, Amy had had a difficult month due to nausea and vomiting following her previous course of chemotherapy. The nurse therapist discussed acupressure points on the wrist and the use of bracelets designed specifically to help people overcome nausea. Amy said she had thoroughly enjoyed her last massage and was looking forward to her next session. Amy also said her mother was doing very well with her daily leg massages and that her discomfort was considerably less. The nurse therapist massaged Amy's back, hands, arms, legs, and feet using the chosen oils. She had fallen asleep by the time the therapist reached her legs, and she stayed asleep until the hour's session ended.

At the third consultation, Amy said her previous visit had left her as if she was "floating on air, with muscles like jelly." She said every time she felt anxious or nauseous, she just closed her eyes and sniffed the tissue with a couple of drops of lavender oil on. This reminded her how relaxed she felt when she was having her massage. Amy had bought a relaxation tape, which she played at night to help her to sleep. Her sleeping had improved, also with the help of an electric aromatherapy lamp in her bedroom.

The acupressure bands had also been a success. Amy's mother was very pleased with the sessions and happy that she had learned a way to relieve her daughter's discomfort. The nurse therapist massaged Amy as before, with the same positive results.

By her fourth consultation, Amy was now taking more control in easing her own pain and nausea. She was very proud of this, but she said she would still like to come for monthly massages once her treatment had finished. The nurse therapist massaged her as before, but this time she talked all the way through about a forthcoming holiday.

Amy built up a special relationship with the therapist during their sessions, and this helped her and her family through what could have been a very frustrating and painful time. Amy had a total of 12 sessions before feeling that she did not require them as frequently. She benefited a great deal from these sessions on a physical and psychological level.

- Sometimes, conventional medication cannot relieve pain caused as a side effect of some chemotherapy drugs.

- Massage is an effective way of helping to relieve this pain while also allowing the child and family some control and satisfaction in helping to do so.

What are complementary therapies?

Complementary therapies are any therapies used in conjunction with orthodox medical and nursing treatments to enhance a patient's well-being and quality of life and to provide symptomatic relief. Interest about using complementary therapies is growing among nurses and healthcare professionals. The range of such therapies includes massage, aromatherapy, reflexology, hypnosis, visualization, reiki, music and color therapy, snoezelen, and relaxation techniques. Within pediatric multidisciplinary teams, more and more orthodox practitioners are keen to incorporate complementary therapies into their practice, thus enhancing their skills and training to the benefit of their patients. This section will describe a variety of techniques and discuss how these can be applied in a child- and family-centered multiprofessional team.

As interest grows, it is essential that the therapies are being carried out safely, following the policies and procedures set up by the employer and national professional organizations. A prerequisite is that the healthcare professional has a recognized qualification in the therapy they wish to practice.

The Royal College of Nursing of the United Kingdom Complementary Therapies in Nursing Special Interest Group: Statement of Beliefs

1 We believe that nurses using complementary therapies as part of their care should know and understand their responsibilities to the patient/client and the United Kingdom Central Council for Nursing, Midwifery and Health Visiting. Further we believe that the UKCC code sets the professional requirement to be met by all registered nurses using complementary therapies.

2 We believe that all patients and clients have the right to be offered and to receive complementary therapies either exclusively or as part of orthodox nursing practice.

3 We believe that all patients have the right to expect that their religious, cultural and spiritual beliefs will be observed by nurses practising complementary therapies.

4 We believe that all complementary therapies available to patients must have the support of the collaborative care team.

5 We believe that a registered nurse who is appropriately qualified to carry out a complementary therapy must agree and work to locally agreed protocols for practice and standards of care.

6 We believe that the patient/client, in partnership with the nurse complementary therapist, should determine the suitability of any proposed complementary therapy. Informed, documented consent will be obtained and detailed records kept with the patient/client's care record.

7 We believe that, where possible, research-based complementary therapy practices should be used. Where this is not possible then nurse complementary therapists, as accountable professionals, must be able to justify their actions.

8 We believe that nurse complementary therapists should, when appropriate, be prepared to instruct significant individuals in the patient's/client's life (including the patient/client) so that they can learn basic complementary therapy skills for self care.

9 We believe that nurse complementary therapists should seek to develop their self awareness and interpersonal skills and so enhance their role as reflective practitioners.

10 We believe that nurse complementary therapists have a responsibility to collect detailed information on all therapy sessions and to evaluate the outcomes of therapy on the patient/client.

11 We believe that the practice of complementary therapies by nurses should be the subject of at least an annual review by an appropriately constituted multidisciplinary committee. The review should take into account patients' measures of satisfaction and benefit.

Although there has been research into the use of complementary therapies for children, there is still a great deal to be done in this area. Some of the research involving children with cancer is negative, as the families decided to opt for alternative therapies rather than complementary therapies, shunning medical opinion. This can lead to a conflict of interest and can cause disharmony in the relationship between patient and physician. The intention in using complementary therapies is to support the child and family through their treatment, not to provide a cure.

Massage and aromatherapy

With massage and aromatherapy, the therapist is able to transform a clinical area into a calm, relaxing space with the aid of an aromatherapy lamp, fiber-optic lights, and soothing music (Figure 25.1). Young patients soon forget that they are in hospital and are able to lose some of the anxieties and stresses that may have built up during their stay. A ten-year-old girl with a spinal tumor commented: "The oils, the music, and the massage made me feel really relaxed; it made me feel like I was floating on air. The lights and the smells in the room were a great atmosphere. It made me feel special – to feel special makes me feel happy. I went to sleep and felt totally relaxed, it made me feel free."

Much research has gone into showing that touch is an essential part of a child's life. Babies, children, and adults all need touch.[49] It is a primary means of conveying caring.[50] Touch can promote the speed of recovery, self-esteem, self-worth, and personal integrity.[51]

Massage consists of a series of kneading, stroking, and percussive movements. "Massage is not only one of the most pleasant experiences that can happen to a person, it fulfils a necessary role – that of the need of human touch."[52] Massage makes touch more structured, offering boundaries to the child, giving them control to accept or reject any form of tactile care (Figures 25.2).

Benefits of massage for both child and carer

- Supports and builds a strong bond, improving emotional contact.
- Teaches both child and carer how to relax: it is quality sharing time.
- Reduces anxiety and stress.
- Improves sleep patterns.
- Provides pain relief (by the release of endorphins?).
- Shows the child that they are loved and valued and that the relationship is important.
- Can help to develop body awareness, coordination, suppleness, and alertness.
- Can provide relief from the discomforts of colic, constipation, and congestion.
- Helps the carer to learn to read and respond appropriately to their child's non-verbal communication.
- In a pediatric intensive care unit (PICU), parents are often wary of touching their child in case they disturb any of the equipment. By showing them a simple foot or hand massage, they feel they are continuing to give affection and reassurance.

We promote family-centered care within our children's services in Nottingham. We aim to involve parents and carers in all aspects of their care. If we teach them to

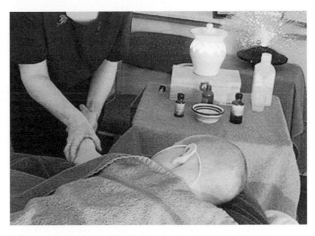

Figure 25.1 *Aromatherapy massage. (©Photography Department, Queen's Medical Centre, 2001.)*

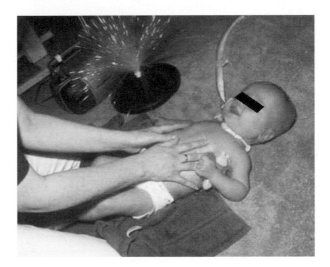

Figure 25.2 *Infant massage.*

flush central lines and give antibiotics, why not a simple foot massage? Massage is a medium in which parents can regain their parental role with a very ill child, promoting a more positive partnership and thereby empowering the carer. The transfer of parental anxiety to the child can be relieved effectively by giving a ten-minute Indian head, neck, and shoulder massage to the parent or carer. This shows the carer that they are being cared for, offering them something more than an analgesic and taking them away from a stressful situation. The fact that someone has recognized their stress and is offering them some care is very much appreciated and can break cycles of stress and anxiety during prolonged periods of hospitalization.

The points of practice that have been devised by the Royal College of Nursing Complementary Therapies in Nursing Forum advise that the therapist must ensure that the child's medical condition does not contraindicate touch/massage therapy and that the child/parent has received sufficient information and is able to provide the nurse with a clear indication of consent.

When implementing massage therapy, the nurse needs to:

- maintain dignity, privacy, care, individuality, comfort, safety, and confidentiality;
- monitor the child's response, recording and reporting responses during and after the session;
- evaluate the session with the child and parents, ensuring that the aim of relaxation is being met and leaving the child comfortable on completion;
- record the treatment on the child's care plan: documentation is very important!

Once in use, annual evaluations will be carried out to audit the service.

When planning any therapy, ensure that:

- you are confident that the child's medical condition does not contraindicate touch/massage therapy;
- the child and parents have received sufficient information and are able to provide the nurse with a clear indication of consent;
- a consultation card has been completed, ensuring a comprehensive medical history is documented. This includes any medication the child is taking, as it is important that you are aware of any adverse reactions that may occur;
- consideration has been given to the time, place, resources, and preparation of oneself and the child before starting any treatment.

Aromatherapy

Aromatherapy is a holistic therapy that uses oils of plants to heal and treat the body. The oils can be derived from shrubs, trees, and many parts of plants, including the fruit, leaves, wood, bark, and flowers. The essential oils can be used as inhalations and topically in baths, via skin massage treatments, and compresses. They can have an effect both physiologically and psychologically. Each oil is composed of many different organic molecules, which are responsible both for the unique aroma and the range of therapeutic values.[53] Aromatherapy is seen as being natural and is therefore assumed to be safe. This is not always the case, as some oils are contraindicated in all children or those with certain conditions.[54]

In pain management, aromatherapy can help in three ways – psychological, tactile, and analgesic support. For example *Lavendula angustifolia* works as an analgesic as well as a gentle sedative. *Chamomile roman* has a sedative effect that can promote relaxation and sleep and is also effective for neuralgic pain; like lavender oil, it has anti-inflammatory properties. Both of these oils are used

widely and safely in children. Aromatherapy can help to relieve much of the child's distress and anxiety. Children can be worn down by their pain, becoming miserable and anxious about their treatment. Aromatherapy can make them feel positive and more in control.[54]

Therapeutic touch

Although many people enjoy a massage or tactile reassurance, some find it uncomfortable: unwanted touch can be seen as threatening or an invasion of personal space. There may also be times when, because of discomfort and/or irritability, touch or massage may be painful. In these cases, therapeutic touch may be the complementary therapy of choice.

Therapeutic touch is concerned with the use of energy fields, balancing energy from a place of centeredness. A demonstration is the best way to explain therapeutic touch, as it is difficult to describe. Nurses and physiotherapists in the USA are taught therapeutic touch as part of their training. Research has shown it to be useful for relaxation and for relief of anxiety and reduction in pain and headaches.

Reflexology

Reflexology involves applying varying degrees of pressure to different parts of the body, usually the feet, in order to promote health and well-being. It is based on the belief that every part of the body is connected by reflex zones or pathways terminating in the soles of the feet, palms of the hands, ears, tongue, and head.[55] Reflexology has been in use for over 5000 years in India and China. Training is very involved, and a recognized qualification is essential. Reflexology has a variety of uses, from pain relief in acute and chronic stages, through control of anxiety, to relief of constipation.

Snoezelen

Snoezelen is a concept developed in Holland in 1975. It is now used widely internationally, particularly in children with special needs and learning difficulties. The idea stems from the basic human need of stimulation. It involves gentle sensory stimulation. The rooms are specially designed, with soothing lighting, music, and aromatherapy, creating an atmosphere that makes the best use of the senses and promotes rest and relaxation.

Indian head, neck, and shoulder massage

This is a simple, safe, and highly beneficial therapy that is popular throughout the Indian subcontinent (Figure 25.3). Massage of the scalp, face, neck, and shoulders soothes,

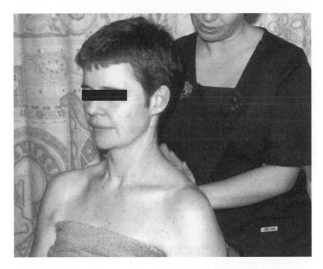

Figure 25.3 *Indian head, neck, and shoulder massage.*

comforts, and rebalances the energy flow to produce a feeling of peace, well-being, and tranquillity. (Healthcare professionals will be able to select the appropriate areas for massage from their knowledge of the medical condition and treatment.) This massage not only relieves stress but also stimulates the scalp, helping to eliminate muscular tension. It is very relaxing.

The massage can be done with the client fully clothed and in a sitting position. It is an excellent form of massage that can be useful if the client does not like aromatherapy oils or is perhaps unable to lie down. It can be a valuable introduction to massage for those who may feel inhibited with regards to undressing.

Discomfort due to the side effects of chemotherapy and postoperative pain can be relieved with massage therapy. By helping them to relax, the child and the family cope better with anxiety as a result of stressful situations, either at home or in hospital.

Application in oncology practice

Many children come to see their complementary therapy treatment for pain relief as something to look forward to during their treatment or stay in hospital. Following surgery, many children require intensive physiotherapy and occupational therapy. Liaison with other therapists and the child's carers enables some of the therapy exercises to be less painful, by teaching the child and carers to massage the areas with oils to warm up the muscles before commencing the exercises. Sometimes, for relaxation, the child will have a complementary treatment after the session with the physiotherapists; this can be seen as a treat.

People whose quality of life has been reduced by an illness or disease deserve tender loving care, with something to look forward to while they are experiencing what can be a very traumatic time. If they do not wish to have a massage, then the child and family can go to the snoezelen, where they can relax among the beanbags, and enjoy the soothing music and gentle ambiance.

With an ever-increasing workload, healthcare professionals may be feeling frustrated at not being able to give the quality time they would like to give their patients. By giving them an hour on their own, without interruption, this gap can be filled by performing what are basic human needs in the form of touch, massage, and attention. Healthcare professionals can thus make the treatment experience less traumatic and less frightening.

It can be very important to teach the rudiments of massage to the family so that they can continue the therapy at home or in hospital. The nursing profession is advancing its technical skills, but nurses are at risk of losing some of their fundamental nurturing qualities, which are the basic foundations of the profession.

Complementary therapies can be particularly beneficial for children and young adults receiving palliative care. They offer pain relief through gentle massage techniques, but they also show the child and family that healthcare professionals are still there for them, continuing to care for them in a supportive way.

"Giving people access to the skilful use of touch through massage can enhance the quality of the relationship between nurse and client. But touch is more than this; it has been identified as an essential component in achieving a state of physical and mental health."[50]

REHABILITATION OF CHILDREN WITH BRAIN AND SPINAL TUMORS

Principles of rehabilitation

Neurological rehabilitation begins at the time that a child is diagnosed as having a brain or spinal tumor. It continues while the child is undergoing treatments, some of which (in particular, surgery and radiotherapy) may temporarily worsen neurological abnormalities. In many cases, rehabilitation continues long after other treatments for a brain tumor are complete.

Patients with brain and spinal tumors will improve in their neurological function as a result of a rehabilitation program. This has been shown in studies of children with brain tumors[56] as well as in adults with brain and spinal tumors.[57] The results of rehabilitation following a brain tumor are as good as or better than those following brain injury[58] or stroke.[59]

As with other aspects of the child's treatment, the greatest benefits come from an approach that uses the expertise of a team of professionals, working in partnership with the family. The other key component is the development and maintenance of links with education, therapy, and medical services local to the child's home.

It is on these services that the child and family will need to rely for longer-term care and support, and it is vital that they are involved from the earliest point.

There are different models of rehabilitation, but they are not mutually exclusive. The choice between them depends on the nature and severity of the child's neurological disorder, the stage reached in treatment, the age of the child, parental and patient choice, and availability of and funding for services. The different models of rehabilitation include in-patient rehabilitation at a specialist or district hospital, specialist rehabilitation centers, and out-patient and community-based rehabilitation. In the earliest phases of treatment, and particularly when the child is undergoing frequent hospital-based treatments, rehabilitation takes place in a hospital setting. Older children with severe and continuing disability may require intensive and sometimes prolonged rehabilitation in a specialist center away from the acute hospital. Rehabilitation for children with neurological disorders can also be carried out successfully in a home and community setting.[60] Adolescents with acquired neurological disorders can successfully undergo programs of cognitive rehabilitation in a highschool setting.[61] All of these endeavors require dedicated teams, adequate resources, and partnerships with education and local services.

There are many factors involved in predicting a child's recovery and quality of life following treatment for brain tumor, and these will need to be considered when measuring the impact of an individualized package of support and rehabilitation on the long-term progress of a child with a brain tumor. Non-familial social support significantly predicts the adjustment of children newly diagnosed with cancer and may be enhanced through interpersonal social skills training.[62,63] School reintegration programs are highly rated by parents as being helpful both for parents and for the child.[64]

Major recovery of lost skills may not occur without specific neuropsychological or social training,[65] and there is a need for ongoing rehabilitation. Intensive and immediate physical rehabilitation has been demonstrated to be essential for laying down the foundations of cognitive rehabilitation.[56] Few studies have assessed the effects of providing an intensive support program on the long-term effects of brain tumors and their subsequent treatment on children.[66]

Occupational therapy

In the acute care phase, occupational therapy involvement is aimed primarily at maximizing functional abilities within the hospital and home environments. For children who have significant neurological deficits, rehabilitation will start while they are still undergoing medical intervention. This may include provision of positioning equipment to assist with postural stability in sitting, adaptive bathroom equipment to assist children and their caregivers in accessing the toilet or bath/shower, and modified car seats to promote safe transportation. The occupational therapist assists in providing suggestions and adaptations to allow the child to return to school. Sensorimotor intervention may be initiated to assist in compensating for sensory deficits, such as loss of vision, and motor deficits, such as hemiplegia and ataxia. The focus is on restoring or compensating for lost functions. Therapy is often provided on an outpatient basis or in the school setting to optimize generalization of skills within familiar and meaningful environments.

Motor deficits (including ataxia, hemiplegia, and paraplegia)

One of the effects of having a brain or spinal tumor, or of undergoing treatment for it, is a central motor deficit. This term is used here to describe abnormalities of control of posture and movement due to lesions of the brain and spinal cord. The term excludes motor deficits due to lesions of the peripheral nerves or muscle.

A central motor deficit can be defined by the predominant pattern of abnormality of posture and movement, by the part of the body most involved, and by its effects on motor function. Depending on the site of the brain or spinal lesion, the motor deficit will be characterized by predominant spasticity, or ataxia, or dystonia, or another abnormality of posture, tone, and movement; or there may be a mixed picture, with more than one of the above. The distribution of the abnormality will also differ, with mainly truncal or limb involvement, or both, and with greater involvement of one limb or the limbs of one side of the body. Central motor deficits may cause marked impairments of function, e.g. preventing walking or restricting the use of one limb. They may also cause less marked impairments, which, although more difficult to detect, may affect a range of daily living and educational activities, such as feeding, dressing, pencil skills, and keyboard skills.

Control of posture, tone, and movement is affected not only by lesions in the motor cortex, cerebellum, and pyramidal and extrapyramidal pathways: visual impairment, abnormalities of hand–eye coordination, vestibular dysfunction, and sensory and motor peripheral neuropathy, all of which may occur in children with brain and spinal tumors, will also contribute to the difficulties with motor control.

BRAIN PLASTICITY

A lesion of the developing brain affects not only fully developed functions but also those that are maturing and emerging. On the other hand, plasticity, the ability to recruit and use existing areas of brain to carry out functions lost as a result of lesions elsewhere, is more likely to occur in the developing than in the fully developed brain. This is one reason why the outcome from rehabilitation following neurological illness is often better in young children than in adults with comparable disorders.[67]

RELEARNING SKILLS

Practice and repetition are required to learn any motor skill, and this is equally true of the reacquisition of lost or deficient skills. Pediatric physiotherapists use a number of different treatment approaches. Among the most popular in the UK are those of Bobath,[68] which use a neurodevelopmental approach and whose techniques include the facilitation of normal patterns of movement through the handling of key points and the inhibition of abnormal reflexes and movements. The conductive learning approach, developed in Hungary by Peto,[69] aims to help the individual to function in society without the dependence on aids or devices. Through repetition and reinforcement, children are taught to master each of the component parts of functional activities. Many pediatric physiotherapists in the UK use an eclectic approach that combines elements of Bobath and conductive education with others, to reflect the needs of individual children with specific disorders.

Sandra

Sandra was 13 when she was diagnosed as having a multifocal cerebral glioma with spinal metastases, following a one-month history of headache, aphasia, and arm weakness. She underwent craniotomy and debulking of the cerebral tumor. Her postoperative course was complicated by hydrocephalus, which was treated by an intraventricular drain and did not require ventriculoperitoneal shunting.

Sandra had had moderate learning difficulties identified when she was ten years of age, although she had continued in mainstream education. Following surgery, she was treated with craniospinal irradiation. During this treatment, she had an onset of epileptic seizures, which were treated with phenytoin.

Two months after completing her radiotherapy, Sandra was readmitted to hospital because of ataxia and back and leg pain. Her phenytoin levels were above the therapeutic range, and her ataxia improved as soon as her dose was adjusted. Her brain and spinal MRI showed that the cerebral tumor was smaller. She was treated with a small booster course of radiotherapy to her lower spine and sacrum. Her pain improved.

Six months after her diagnosis, Sandra was admitted to hospital again. She was losing weight and experiencing limb pain, and she had decreased mobility. MRI scans showed a further decrease in the size of her cerebral and spinal tumors. She spent seven weeks in hospital, receiving an intensive assessment and treatment program of pain management, physiotherapy, speech therapy, occupational therapy, and psychology. Her pain improved following treatment with indomethacin and gabapentin. She was provided with a left ankle–foot orthosis and a knee brace. Her mobility improved. Her speech therapy assessment showed that she had a dysfluent expressive aphasia.

A planning meeting took place between hospital health professionals and community-based therapists. Recommendations were made to modify the family home in order to provide Sandra with a downstairs bedroom, toilet, and shower. It proved impossible for the local services to continue to provide the level of speech therapy and physiotherapy input recommended by the hospital team. An admission was planned to a brain injury rehabilitation unit. The health authority refused to fund this but made additional provision for speech and physiotherapy at home.

Six months after her discharge from hospital, Sandra was free of severe pain and walking better than before, with support. Funding for the modifications to the family home had been agreed, but the work had not yet started. Her parents had to carry her upstairs, and she came downstairs sitting on her bottom. Her physiotherapy was continuing, but speech therapy had stopped because of local staff shortages. Sandra was undergoing a local education authority assessment of special educational needs and had transferred to a school for children with physical and educational difficulties.

- Children with brain tumors can have pre-existing neurodevelopmental disorders.
- Effective management of symptoms often requires a combination of treatment modalities.
- Rehabilitation can be successful in children with incompletely cured tumors.
- The long-term success of rehabilitation depends on effective interagency working (including community health, education, and local government) and the availability of sufficient resources.

ATAXIA

Ataxia is common in children with tumors of the posterior fossa. In infants and younger children with posterior fossa tumors, hypotonia is often very marked, at least initially. Ataxia is characterized by abnormalities in executing voluntary movements at the required rate, to the required range, and of the required force. Voluntary movement is uncoordinated and there is dysmetria (error in estimating amplitude of movement, resulting in overshooting during the finger/nose test). In children with midline posterior fossa tumors, the ataxia is predominantly truncal. The child with ataxia may have an abnormality of gait. The feet are placed widely apart. As the child walks, he or she may stagger irregularly to both sides (or mainly to one side with unilateral cerebellar lesions). Minor degrees of ataxia are more evident when the child is asked to walk heel to toe or along a straight line. Often, there is also dysarthria. By providing stability to the trunk and proximal joints, the therapist improves the ability of the child with ataxia to stand and to walk. The child with severe and continuing ataxia may require supportive seating.

SPASTICITY

Spasticity is an abnormality of tone characterized by a velocity-dependent increase in the resistance to passive movement. It is caused by lesions of the pyramidal motor pathways. It results from tumors of the cerebral hemispheres (which will usually cause hemiplegia), brainstem, and spinal cord (causing spastic paraplegia). Spasticity limits function and leads to contractures. Spasticity can be reduced by the way in which the child is moved and handled by the physiotherapist and other carers. Seating and the child's lying position are very important. Soft-tissue length may be maintained by passive stretching, reducing the likelihood of contractures. Splinting may be necessary, particularly in unconscious, immobile patients with markedly increased tone. Drugs such as baclofen can be used to reduce spasticity, although their effects will not be restricted to the most severely affected muscles. Following treatment for a spinal cord tumor, severe spastic paraplegia can be improved in some cases by the use of intrathecal baclofen. Injection of botulinum toxin into target spastic muscles can significantly reduce tone for up to four months at a time.[70] The benefits in function, including improved ambulation, often persist.

DYSTONIA

Dystonia is a movement disorder arising as a result of lesions of the basal ganglia and characterized by sustained involuntary muscle contractions. A deeply placed cerebral tumor, often a glioma, can cause dystonia, which is usually unilateral.[71] The disorder may be very focal, affecting only the extremities of one limb, or it may be more generalized. Children with dystonia will be helped by a therapy program (from physiotherapists and occupational therapists) that encourages hand use and mobile weight-bearing and establishes realistic functional goals. Drugs such as benzhexol and levodopa help to reduce rigidity.

Cranial nerve palsies

Around a quarter of children with brain tumors have cranial nerve palsies at presentation.[72] Cranial neuropathy may be the result of a tumor arising from the nerves or the dissemination of an intracranial tumor, or may be due to raised intracranial pressure, or may be a result of treatments, including surgery, radiotherapy, and chemotherapy. With the exception of anterior visual pathway gliomas involving the optic nerves and chiasm,[73] primary tumors of the cranial nerves such as neurinomas and schwannomas are uncommon in children.[74,75] Multiple cranial abnormalities, especially involving the sixth, seventh, eight, ninth, and tenth cranial nerves, are common in children with diffuse intrinsic brainstem gliomas. Other posterior fossa tumors that involve the brainstem can also cause lower cranial nerve palsies. Surgery for brainstem tumors,[76,77] other posterior fossa tumors (including ependymoma) involving the brainstem,[78] or rarer skull-base tumors[79] can cause cranial nerve palsies. Radiotherapy can damage any of the cranial nerves, although this is a rare and usually late complication, with the exception of damage to the optic nerve. Some chemotherapeutic agents, including vincristine, can cause cranial neuropathies. The facial nerve is involved most frequently.

VISUAL LOSS

Tumors affecting the optic nerve usually cause progressive visual failure and may cause proptosis and pain. Facial palsy may put the child at risk of corneal damage; this will require early treatment with artificial tears and taping the eyelids closed. Permanent weakness of lid closure can be improved by surgical placement of a weight in the eyelid. Palsies of the third, fourth, and sixth nerves cause diplopia and sometimes compensatory head tilt in children. The child may require eye patching to minimize diplopia. Surgery can improve a persistent squint.

Neuropathies involving the ninth and tenth nerves cause dysphagia and hoarseness. The child will have difficulty swallowing secretions and may be at risk of pulmonary aspiration. In severe cases, a tracheostomy may be needed to manage this.

Sleep disorders

Sleep difficulties occur in many children with brain and spinal tumors, even when previous good sleeping habits had been established. The causes are multiple and include the effects of the tumor, its treatments, and changes in the child's and family's routine. It can be hard for parents to maintain any kind of regular pattern to the child's day during hospitalization. The strangeness of hospital and the absence of familiar bedtime rituals can easily disturb a child's sleep patterns. Young children who are undergoing treatment for brain tumors may also tire easily and may have a low tolerance for unusual or stressful situations.

As the child improves, parents often find it hard to be firm and consistent and re-establish usual bedtime routines. Establishing a sleep routine that is acceptable for the family and allows the child sufficient sleep for their needs is important for all members of the family, including the child.

With most sleep disturbances, particularly those involving night waking and bedtime settling problems, it is best to start making changes at bedtime rather than in the middle of the night. Night waking usually reduces once a settling routine has been established. For most parents, trying to change sleep patterns in the middle of the night is very stressful and usually not productive. A behavioral approach that reinforces good habits and is supported by a psychologist in regular contact with the family is often successful (Gumley D, personal communication, 2001). It helps to give parents some written reminders, such as these:

Good sleep habits checklist

- Establish a set bedtime routine
- Avoid extending the bedtime routine
- Do not include activities that could cause conflict or raise excitement
- Develop a regular bedtime and a regular time to awaken.
- Restrict activities in bed to those that induce sleep.
- Reduce noise in the bedroom.
- Avoid extreme temperature changes.
- It is very important to change only one thing at a time.

In some children, the use of melatonin alongside a behavioral approach can help to promote good sleeping habits.[80]

Illness behavior

Biological cure does not necessarily equate with physical and psychological well-being. Non-organic illness can be equally debilitating in its impact on the child and family. Children who re-present with new symptoms following treatment of a tumor may have a recurrence of the original tumor, or they may have complications of the original tumor or its treatment. They might have an unrelated disorder. In some cases, their new symptoms will be due to non-organic illness; this group presents a particular challenge to the clinician.

The new symptoms can include headaches, limb weakness, gait abnormalities, and non-organic seizures. As a result of these, the child may be unable to attend school or may function only abnormally in school. Families often find it very difficult to accept that their child does not have new organic disease. The symptoms provoke a similar response in these families on their reappearance as at the time of first diagnosis. Many families attempt to reorganize to help the child, e.g. separated parents may temporarily reunite or a parent may stop working to be at home with the child.

When evaluating new symptoms or the late effects of treatment, it is important to know about the premorbid state of the child. All patients should be investigated comprehensively for evidence of tumor recurrence or new disease. If no cause is found, then the new symptoms can be managed as psychosomatic symptoms, understandable in terms of the child's life situation.

A pragmatic approach to rehabilitation should be adopted, concentrating on:

- improvement in function;
- return to normal school;
- social reintegration.

This will require an in-patient and out-patient rehabilitation program with a multidisciplinary team, including the clinical nurse specialist, neurologist, oncologist, psychiatrist, and physiotherapist. Although non-organic disease following biological tumor cure has a major impact on quality of life, these symptoms can be improved successfully, and prognosis is good for this group.[81]

CONCLUSION

Advances in the treatment of children with brain and spinal tumors have led to improved outcomes, with the result that many more children survive to an older age. It is important that these children not only survive longer but also enjoy an improved quality of life. Approximately 80 per cent of children who have had brain tumors experience some subsequent morbidity, with more than one attribute affected in the great majority. Not only the tumor and its treatments but also family, social, and cultural factors affect outcome. It is essential that treatment is holistic from the beginning and that there is continuing surveillance for the late effects of the tumor and its treatments. It is also important that meaningful outcomes (those relating to independence, emotional well-being, social adjustment, schooling, and employment) are measured; the results of these outcomes help to determine new methods of treatment. The management of children with brain and spinal tumors must be based on the best available evidence about outcomes obtained from research, in order to strengthen the work of clinical and rehabilitation teams.

REFERENCES

1 Kibber S. Psychological support. In: Guerrero D (ed.). *Neuro-oncology for Nurses*. London: Whurr, 1998, p. 272.

2 Lewis C. Loss and change on the neonatal intensive care unit. *Paediatr Nurs* 1998; **10**:21–3.

3 Rifkinson-Mann S, Wisoff JH, Epstein F. The association of hydrocephalus with intramedullary spinal cord tumors: a series of 25 patients. *Neurosurgery* 1990; **27**:749–54.

4 Dias MS, Albright AL. Management of hydrocephalus complicating childhood posterior fossa tumors. *Pediatr Neurosci* 1989; **15**:283–9.

5 Sainte-Rose C, Cinalli G, Roux FE, *et al*. Management of hydrocephalus in pediatric patients with posterior fossa tumors: the role of endoscopic third ventriculostomy. *J Neurosurg* 2001; **95**:791–7.

6 Allen JC. Initial management of children with hypothalamic and thalamic tumors and the modifying role of neurofibromatosis-1. *Pediatr Neurosurg* 2000; **32**:154–62.

7 Gil Z, Beni-Adani L, Siomin V, Nagar H, Dvir R, Constantini S. Ascites following ventriculoperitoneal shunting in children with chiasmatic-hypothalamic glioma. *Childs Nerv Syst* 2001; **17**:395–8.

8 Rickert CH. Abdominal metastases of pediatric brain tumors via ventriculo-peritoneal shunts. *Childs Nerv Syst* 1998; **14**:10–14.

9 Jamjoom AB, Jamjoom ZA, Ur RN. Low rate of shunt revision in tumoural obstructive hydrocephalus. *Acta Neurochir (Wien)* 1998; **140**:595–7.

10 Brockmeyer D, Abtin K, Carey L, Walker ML. Endoscopic third ventriculostomy: an outcome analysis. *Pediatr Neurosurg* 1998; **28**:236–40.

11 Haw C, Steinbok P. Ventriculoscope tract recurrence after endoscopic biopsy of pineal germinoma. *Pediatr Neurosurg* 2001; **34**:215–17.

12 Macarthur DC, Buxton N, Vloeberghs M, Punt J. The effectiveness of neuroendoscopic interventions in children with brain tumours. *Childs Nerv Syst* 2001; **17**:589–94.

13 Tuli S, Alshail E, Drake J. Third ventriculostomy versus cerebrospinal fluid shunt as a first procedure in pediatric hydrocephalus. *Pediatr Neurosurg* 1999; **30**:11–15.

14 Gilles FH, Sobel E, Leviton A, *et al*. Epidemiology of seizures in children with brain tumors. The Childhood Brain Tumor Consortium. *J Neuro-Oncol* 1992; **12**:53–68.

15 Zentner J, Hufnagel A, Wolf HK, *et al*. Surgical treatment of neoplasms associated with medically intractable epilepsy. *Neurosurgery* 1997; **41**:378–86.

16 Beaumont A, Whittle IR. The pathogenesis of tumour-associated epilepsy. *Acta Neurochir (Wien)* 2000; **142**:1–15.

17 Albensi BC. Potential roles for tumor necrosis factor and nuclear factor-kappaB in seizure activity. *J Neurosci Res* 2001; **66**:151–4.

18 Williams BA, Abbott KJ, Manson JI. Cerebral tumors in children presenting with epilepsy. *J Child Neurol* 1992; **7**:291–4.

19 Patel H, Garg BP, Salanova V, Boaz JC, Luerssen TG, Kalsbeck JE. Tumor-related epilepsy in children. *J Child Neurol* 2001; **16**:141–5.

20 Acharya JN, Wyllie E, Luders HO, Kotagal P, Lancman M, Coelho M. Seizure symptomatology in infants with localization-related epilepsy. *Neurology* 1997; **48**:189–96.

21 Advanced Life Support Group. *Advanced Paediatric Life Support: The Practical Approach*, 3rd edn. London: BMJ Publications, 2001.

22 Gattis WA, May DB. Possible interaction involving phenytoin, dexamethasone, and antineoplastic agents: a case report and review. *Ann Pharmacother* 1996; **30**:520–6.

23 French JA, Gidal BE. Antiepileptic drug interactions. *Epilepsia* 2000; **41** (suppl. 8):S30–6.

24 Stein DA, Chamberlain MC. Evaluation and management of seizures in the patient with cancer. *Oncology (Huntingt)* 1991; **5**:33–9.

25 Wang EC, Geyer JR, Berger MS. Incidence of postoperative epilepsy in children following subfrontal craniotomy for tumor. *Pediatr Neurosurg* 1994; **21**:165–72.

26 Newton HB, Newton C, Pearl D, Davidson T. Swallowing assessment in primary brain tumor patients with dysphagia. *Neurology* 1994; **44**:1927–32.

27 Gropman AL, Packer RJ, Nicholson HS, *et al*. Treatment of diencephalic syndrome with chemotherapy: growth, tumor response, and long term control. *Cancer* 1998; **83**:166–72.

28 Straube A, Witt TN. Oculo-bulbar myasthenic symptoms as the sole sign of tumour involving or compressing the brain stem. *J Neurol* 1990; **237**:369–71.

29 Mahony MJ, Kennedy JD, Leaf A, Matthew DJ, Milla PJ. Brain stem glioma presenting as gastro-oesophageal reflux. *Arch Dis Child* 1987; **62**:731–3.

30 Trier E, Thomas AG. Feeding the disabled child. *Nutrition* 1998; **14**:801–5.

31 Kitzinger M. Planning management of feeding in the visually handicapped child. *Child Care Health Dev* 1980; **6**:291–9.

32 Ilingworth RS, Lister J. The critical or sensitive period, with reference to certain feeding and swallowing problems in infants and children. *J Pediatr* 1964; **65**:839–49.

33 Skuse D. Identification and management of problem eaters. *Arch Dis Child* 1993; **69**:604–8.

34 Reilly S, Skuse D. Characteristics and management of feeding problems of young children with cerebral palsy. *Dev Med Child Neurol* 1992; **34**:379–88.

35 Oberfield SE, Chin D, Uli N, David R, Sklar C. Endocrine late effects of childhood cancers. *J Pediatr* 1997; **131**:S37–41.

36 Ellis A, Cavanagh SJ. Aspects of neurosurgical assessment using the Glasgow Coma Scale. *Intensive Crit Care Nurs* 1992; **8**:94–9.

37 Warren A. Paediatric coma scoring researched and benchmarked. *Paediatr Nurs* 2000; **12**:14–18.

38 Herbert C. The use of morphine after intracranial surgery. *Prof Nurse* 2001; **16**:1029.

39 McGarth PJ, Johnson G, Goodman JT, Schillinger J, Dunn J, Chapman J. A behavioural scale for rating postoperative pain in children. In: Fields HL, Dubner R, Cervero F (eds) *Advances in Pain Research and Therapy*. New York: Raven Press, 1985, pp. 395–401.

40 Wong DL, Baker CM. Pain in children: comparison of assessment scales. *Pediatr Nurs* 1988; **14**:9–17.

41 Eland JM. Pain in children. *Nurs Clin North Am* 1990; **25**:871–84.

42 Parsons E. Cultural aspects of pain. *Surg Nurse* 1992; **5**:14–16.

43 Favaloro R. Adolescent development and implications for pain management. *Pediatr Nurs* 1988; **14**:27–9.

44 Henry C. Bone cancer in young people. In: Gibson F, Evans M (eds) *Paediatric Oncology: Acute Nursing Care.* London: Whurr, 1998, pp. 361–95.

45 Doxey D, Bruce D, Sklar F, Swift D, Shapiro K. Posterior fossa syndrome: identifiable risk factors and irreversible complications. *Pediatr Neurosurg* 1999; **31**:131–6.

46 Pollack IF. Posterior fossa syndrome. *Int Rev Neurobiol* 1997; **41**:411–32.

47 Dailey AT, McKhann GM, Berger MS. The pathophysiology of oral pharyngeal apraxia and mutism following posterior fossa tumor resection in children. *J Neurosurg* 1995; **83**:467–75.

48 Kirk EA, Howard VC, Scott CA. Description of posterior fossa syndrome in children after posterior fossa brain tumor surgery. *J Pediatr Oncol Nurs* 1995; **12**:181–7.

49 Adamson S. Teaching baby massage to new parents. *Complement Ther Nurs Midwifery* 1996; **2**:6.

50 Montague A. *Touching: The Human Significance of the Skin.* New York: Harper and Row, 1986.

51 Goodykoontz L. Touch: attitudes and practice. *Nurs Forum* 1975; **18**:4–17.

52 Tilton J. Massage in medicine. *J Comm Nurs* 1992, October.

53 Tisserand B, Balacs T. *Essential Oil Safety.* Edinburgh: Churchill Livingstone, 1995.

54 Price S, Price L. *Aromatherapy for Health Professionals.* Edinburgh: Churchill Livingstone, 1995.

55 Ashkenazi R. Multidimensional reflexology. *Int J Altern Complement Med* 1993; **8**:12.

56 Philip PA, Ayyangar R, Vanderbilt J, Gaebler-Spira DJ. Rehabilitation outcome in children after treatment of primary brain tumor. *Arch Phys Med Rehabil* 1994; **75**:36–9.

57 McKinley WO, Conti-Wyneken AR, Vokac CW, Cifu DX. Rehabilitative functional outcome of patients with neoplastic spinal cord compressions. *Arch Phys Med Rehabil* 1996; **77**:892–5.

58 Huang ME, Cifu DX, Keyser-Marcus L. Functional outcomes in patients with brain tumor after inpatient rehabilitation: comparison with traumatic brain injury. *Am J Phys Med Rehabil* 2000; **79**:327–35.

59 Huang ME, Cifu DX, Keyser-Marcus L. Functional outcome after brain tumor and acute stroke: a comparative analysis. *Arch Phys Med Rehabil* 1998; **79**:1386–90.

60 Pace GM, Schlund MW, Hazard-Haupt T, *et al.* Characteristics and outcomes of a home and community-based neurorehabilitation programme. *Brain Inj* 1999; **13**:535–46.

61 Brett AW, Laatsch L. Cognitive rehabilitation therapy of brain-injured students in a public high school setting. *Pediatr Rehabil* 1998; **2**:27–31.

62 Speechley KN, Noh S. Surviving childhood cancer, social support, and parents' psychological adjustment. *J Pediatr Psychol* 1992; **17**:15–31.

63 Katz ER, Varni JW. Social support and social cognitive problem-solving in children with newly diagnosed cancer. *Cancer* 1993; **71** (10 suppl.):3314–19.

64 Katz ER, Rubenstein CL, Hubert N, Blew A. School and social reintegration of children with cancer. *J Psychosoc Oncol* 1988; **6**:123–40.

65 Emanuelson I, von Wendt L, Beckung E, Hagberg I. Late outcome after severe traumatic brain injury in children and adolescents. *Pediatr Rehabil* 1998; **2**:65–70.

66 Riva D, Pantaleoni C, Milani N, Fossati BF. Impairment of neuropsychological functions in children with medulloblastomas and astrocytomas in the posterior fossa. *Childs Nerv Syst* 1989; **5**:107–10.

67 Kurihara M, Kumagai K, Watanabe M, Noda Y. [Prognosis of severe head injury in childhood: from the viewpoint of brain plasticity.] *No To Hattatsu* 1996; **28**:243–50.

68 Bobath B. The treatment of neuromuscular disorders by improving patterns of co-ordination. *Physiotherapy* 1969; **55**:18–22.

69 Cottam PJ, Sutton A. *Conductive Education: a System for Overcoming Motor Disorder.* London: Croom Helm, 1986.

70 Cosgrove AP, Corry IS, Graham HK. Botulinum toxin in the management of the lower limb in cerebral palsy. *Dev Med Child Neurol* 1994; **36**:386–96.

71 Vandertop WP, Kamphuis DJ, Witkamp TD. Hemidystonia as presenting symptom of an optic glioma. *Childs Nerv Syst* 1997; **13**:289–92.

72 Snyder H, Robinson K, Shah D, Brennan R, Handrigan M. Signs and symptoms of patients with brain tumors presenting to the emergency department. *J Emerg Med* 1993; **11**:253–8.

73 Shuper A, Horev G, Kornreich L, *et al.* Visual pathway glioma: an erratic tumour with therapeutic dilemmas. *Arch Dis Child* 1997; **76**:259–63.

74 Chinski A, Orfila D, Perata H, Lubochiner LJ, Bensur D, Romano Luna MF. Facial nerve neurinoma in a child. *Int J Pediatr Otorhinolaryngol* 1997; **40**:203–10.

75 Frim DM, Ogilvy CS, Vonsattal JP, Chapman PH. Is intracerebral schwannoma a developmental tumor of children and young adults? Case report and review. *Pediatr Neurosurg* 1992; **18**:190–4.

76 Cochrane DD, Gustavsson B, Poskitt KP, Steinbok P, Kestle JR. The surgical and natural morbidity of aggressive resection for posterior fossa tumors in childhood. *Pediatr Neurosurg* 1994; **20**:19–29.

77 Abbott R, Shiminski-Maher T, Wisoff JH, Epstein FJ. Intrinsic tumors of the medulla: surgical complications. *Pediatr Neurosurg* 1991; **17**:239–44.

78 Nagib MG, O'Fallon MT. Posterior fossa lateral ependymoma in childhood. *Pediatr Neurosurg* 1996; **24**:299–305.

79 Teo C, Dornhoffer J, Hanna E, Bower C. Application of skull base techniques to pediatric neurosurgery. *Childs Nerv Syst* 1999; **15**:103–9.

80 Jan JE, Tai J, Hahn G, Rothstein RR. Melatonin replacement therapy in a child with a pineal tumor. *J Child Neurol* 2001; **16**:139–40.

81 De Sousa C, Goldberg D, Prendergast M, Christie D, Michalski A. Remembering and moving on: non-organic symptoms after successful treatment of brain tumours. Presented at the 8th International Symposium on Pediatric Neuro-Oncology, Rome, 1998.

26

Cognitive development and educational rehabilitation

RONALD C. SAVAGE, BRADFORD J. ROSS, SUE WALKER AND BETH WICKS

INTRODUCTION

The impact of brain tumors on children's continuing neurological development and their ability to continue to learn can significantly affect their ability to function at home, in school, and in their communities. The sites of such tumors and the corresponding treatments may impact upon the overall functioning of children. This chapter discusses the neurobehavioral challenges that children experience, by examining cognitive and behavioral functioning, as well as the potential long-term impact of tumors on neurological development through the physical maturation of various brain stages. In addition, since schools are the long-term providers of services for children, the educational needs of children with brain tumors are presented, with guidelines for professionals to follow. Despite the medical therapies that exist for children, it is within their schools and families where their long-term functional needs are identified and met. This chapter addresses these needs and offers solutions to support these children and their families.

COGNITIVE/BEHAVIORAL EFFECTS OF BRAIN TUMORS AND TREATMENTS

Survival for children diagnosed with brain tumors has increased with the advent of improved imaging that provides earlier and more precise diagnosis and location of the tumor, new surgical techniques such as stereo tactic surgery, and new chemotherapy agents and radiation protocols. The fact that children are living longer after diagnosis of brain tumor also results in more children with acquired cognitive and behavioral deficits as the result of the tumor and/or treatment. Various research studies have examined the effects of brain tumors and treatment on children, but the results of these studies are often hampered by small sample sizes.[1] Several researchers have examined the direct damage caused by brain tumors in children. Castro-Sierra and colleagues found that for patients with inferior temporal cortex tumors, procedural learning was slower for sorting tasks.[2] Buono examined 123 children with brain tumors and found that 57 per cent had an academic deficit, with arithmetic difficulties 16 times more likely than reading difficulties.[3] These children with arithmetic deficits had characteristics similar to a non-verbal learning disability. Examination of treatment protocols, location, and pathology did not differentiate.

Type of surgical intervention has been examined. Anderson and coworkers reviewed 20 children with craniopharyngioma and who had subfrontal craniotomy and either partial or gross total resection.[4] Approximately three years post-surgery, only three of 20 children had good outcomes on neuropsychological testing, behavior, or school performance. Type of resection was not related to outcome.

The effects of chemotherapy on childhood cancers have shown various cognitive deficits. Chemotherapy effects have been studied most extensively in the treatment of leukemia. Central nervous system (CNS) prophylactic chemotherapy in children with leukemia has shown adverse effects in academic functioning. Brown and colleagues showed that children treated for three years had more adverse effects in the area of educational functioning in reading, spelling, and arithmetic compared with controls.[5] However, small sample size and poorer school attendance for those children treated were limitations in this study. Dowell and coworkers, with a small sample size, suggested that motor deficits resulting from chemotherapy in the treatment of acute lymphoblastic leukemia was dose-dependent, with a gain in functioning occurring after the end of treatment or adjustment in dosage.[6]

Several authors have studied the effects of irradiation. Late-delayed radiation effects can occur months or years after treatment, with necrosis of the white matter, vascular changes, and edema, although this appears in less than one per cent of children who develop necrosis.[7] Radcliffe and colleagues studied 19 children with brain tumors and who were treated with whole-brain radiotherapy, with 15 of the children also receiving chemotherapy.[8] For the group as a whole, there was a 12-point drop in IQ scores over a two-year period. Age was related inversely to change in IQ score, with children under seven years of age at diagnosis showing a 27-point loss and children over seven years not showing a significant decrease. Although they did not show a significant IQ score loss, 50 per cent of the children aged over seven years were receiving supplemental education services.

Mulhern and coworkers studied seven children treated for temporal lobe astrocytomas with surgery and irradiation.[1] Only two of the seven showed normal functioning on neuropsychological testing. The other children showed either cognitive deficits or psychopathology. Hemispheric location of the tumor did not appear to contribute to the type of deficit. Early age of onset, seizure control, tumor recurrence, and type and dose of radiation were suggestive of poorer outcome. The authors have recommended that a pooling of data from intergroup efforts is needed to control for the small sample size that is found in many research studies.

Bordeaux and colleagues, with a small sample size, found that children with brain tumors have deficits on tests of fine motor control, psychomotor, and timed language skills, but that these areas are not exacerbated further by surgery and radiotherapy.[9] However, follow-up in this study was limited to approximately one year. The authors suggest that these children may show more long-term decline on future follow-up, as has been shown in children treated for leukemia with chemotherapy and/or radiation.

Chapman and colleagues studied 15 long-term survivors of posterior fossa tumors who had been treated with irradiation and 14 children who were treated with surgery.[10] An early age of onset (under six years of age) was associated with more neurological and neuropsychological sequelae.

Anderson and coworkers studied the effects of cranial radiation and chemotherapy on 100 children and 50 survivors of cancers treated with chemotherapy only.[4] Cranial radiation and chemotherapy in combination were associated with reductions in intelligence, educational skill, immediate memory, processing speed, and executive function. Children treated with chemotherapy alone exhibited subtle information processing deficits. Younger age for receiving irradiation was predictive of deficits in nonverbal ability, educational skills, and executive functions. High-dose irradiation was associated with poorer information processing and lower arithmetic ability.

THE ROLE OF NEUROPSYCHOLOGICAL AND BEHAVIORAL ASSESSMENT

Damage to the brain from tumor and treatment can affect cognitive and behavioral functioning. Strengths and weaknesses in functioning need to be assessed in order to develop a treatment plan for remediation or compensation of acquired areas of weakness. The cognitive and behavioral effects of brain tumor and treatment can vary depending on the location of the tumor and specific brain areas affected by treatment.[11] The role of brain areas in the functioning of adults and children has been outlined by Gaddes and Edgell[12] and by Lezak.[13] A summary of brain functioning as related to cognitive and behavioral processes is presented in Table 26.1.

Professionals in neuropsychology and applied behavior analysis examine brain–behavior relationships. These examinations evaluate many areas of functioning, including basic sensation, perception, motor skills, verbal and visual problem-solving, attention, concentration, memory, organizational skills, and social and emotional functioning. Interpretation is based on the behavioral findings linked to information about a child's cerebral pathology.

A neuropsychological evaluation examines the way a child receives, processes, stores, and expresses information. A behavioral assessment includes the study of the "function" of unwanted behaviors (e.g., outbursts, aggression, impulsivity) and recommendations for their replacement with positive behaviors. Since cognition and behavior are so intertwined in a child's life, it is important to look at how the child functions at many levels. For example, a sensoriperceptual examination looks at the way sensory information is interpreted. Auditory, tactile, and visual senses are examined. Damage to the temporal

Table 26.1 *Functional, cognitive, and behavioral consequences of regional injury*

Brain structure	Function	Cognitive/behavioral symptoms that may occur
Cerebral cortex	Outermost layer of the cerebral hemispheres, and composed of gray matter. Cortices are asymmetrical. Both right and left hemispheres are able to analyze sensory data, perform memory functions, learn new information, monitor behavior and actions, form thoughts, and make decisions	Difficulty in: processing sensory information; storing/retrieving information; learning new information; inappropriate behaviors
Left hemisphere	Left cerebral cortex. Processes information sequentially through systematic analysis and logical interpretation of information. Interpretation and production of symbolic information (language, reading), mathematics, and abstract reasoning. Memory stored in a language format. Retention of appropriate behavior rules and consequences	Difficulty with: speech/language/communication; reading/writing/computation; sequencing/logical analysis; memory for semantic information (symbols, letters, numerals); monitoring social rules and appropriate actions
Right hemisphere	Right cerebral cortex. Processes information holistically through simultaneous multisensory input to provide visual spatial picture of one's environment. Memory is stored in auditory, visual, and spatial modalities. Behavior regulation via social engagement and emotions	Difficulty in: processing visuospatial and perceptual motor skills; orienting in space and drawing geometric shapes; recognizing peoples' faces and expressions and processing emotional data; discriminating non-verbal information
Frontal lobes	Higher-level cognition, behavior, and executive functioning. Prefrontal area: ability to concentrate, attend, and elaboration of thought; monitors judgment, inhibition, emotions, personality, and social actions. Motor cortex (Brodman's): voluntary motor activity. Premotor cortex: storage of motor patterns and voluntary activities. Language: motor speech	Difficulty with: recent memory (verbal and non-verbal), attention, concentration, monitoring personal and social behaviors; learning new information, comprehending music; controlling inhibitions (inappropriate social and/or sexual behaviors); emotional lability (flat affect); contralateral plegia, paresis; expressive/motor aphasia
Parietal Lobes	Processing of sensory input, sensory discrimination. Mediate tactile and kinesthetic perception. Body orientation. Primary/secondary somatic area.	Difficulty in: discriminating between sensory stimuli; recognizing objects by tactile sensitivity; locating and recognizing parts of the body (neglect), sometimes recognizing own self; orienting self in environmental space; skilled voluntary movements (sports, writing)

Temporal lobes	Perception, analysis, and evaluation of auditory stimuli. Reception and analysis of verbal and non-verbal memory. Expressed behavior and temperament	Difficulty with: verbal and non-verbal memory; processing auditory language, hearing; receptive/sensory aphasia; agitation, irritability, immature behavior
Occipital lobes	Visual functions, visual discrimination, analysis of language-related visual forms (words, numbers), and perception of non-verbal forms and colors	Difficulty with: integrating visual stimuli into a coherent whole or comprehending multiple aspects of a visual form; distinguishing color hues; reading/writing/arithmetic
Limbic system	Basic elemental emotions: fight, flight, sex, rage, fear. Integration of recent memory, biological rhythms, olfactory pathways. Amygdala: emotional memories and reactions. Hippocampus: memory functioning (short-/long-term). Hypothalamus: eating, drinking, sexual rhythms, endocrine levels, temperature regulation	Difficulty with: agitation, controlling emotions, anxiety, retaining new memories; basic life functions (endocrine, temperature regulation); how one perceives and feels about self; loss of sense of smell, problems eating
Basal ganglia	Subcortical gray matter nuclei. Processing link between thalamus and motor cortex. Initiation and direction of voluntary movement. Balance (inhibitory), equilibrium, postural reflexes. Part of extrapyramidal system: regulation of automatic movement	Difficulty with: movement – slowness, chorea, tremors at rest and with initiation of movement, abnormal increase in muscle tone, difficulty initiating movement; parkinsonian symptoms
Cerebellum	Controls movement and monitors impulses from the motor and sensory centers. Helps control direction, rate, force, and steadiness of movements	Difficulty with: eye–hand coordination, automatic motor routines; muscle tone, posture, and daily routines (getting dressed, riding a bike)
Brainstem	Reticular activating system (RAS) modulates arousal, alertness, concentration, and basic biological rhythms. Controls many basic metabolic responses (swallowing, vomiting, breathing, respiration, heart rate, blood pressure). Elementary forms of seeing and hearing	Difficulty with: attention, mental stamina, hyper- or hypoemotional responses; eating, drinking, sleeping, sexual functioning; hormonal/endocrine/neurochemical systems

lobes can affect perception of sounds. The left temporal lobe deals with verbal auditory information, while the right temporal lobe deals with non-verbal information such as intonation and pitch. Damage along the sensori-motor strip can result in imperceptions or lack of perception in the tactile modality. Damage of the optic nerve tract can result in visual problems, such as visual field deficits. Damage to the occipital lobe can result in other visual abnormalities. Damage to the posterior left hemisphere can result in difficulty with receiving verbal information correctly.

Other verbal skills can also be affected after a neurological event. Receptive language may be reduced, but some children may retain the same levels of comprehension as before their illness whilst having difficulties with expressive language. Verbal fluency or the rate of expression can be changed after a brain tumor. The child may know what they want to say but have difficulty in expressing it in a smooth, flowing manner. Intonation, rate of speaking, and slowness in producing words may result in a speech pattern that sounds unusual to the listener. Word finding or dyspraxic difficulties may be experienced. Some neurological conditions from tumors can result in loss of reading or spelling skills, even though speech appears normal.

Visual and perceptual skills can also be changed after a brain tumor. Visual field deficits can result in objects being difficult to see if they are placed in an area of the person's field of vision where information is not relayed to the brain for processing. Attention to visual details may be weak. The child may have difficulty in recognizing previously familiar objects. Visual construction, such as the ability to write, put together puzzles, or draw designs, may be altered. Motor planning may also be affected, and carrying out a sequence of coordinated movements may be difficult.

Attention and concentration are often affected after an acquired brain injury. Weaknesses in these areas result in difficulty in learning new information, even though previously learned information is intact. A neuropsychological evaluation assesses different types of attention. Sustained attention refers to the ability to attend and concentrate for longer periods of time. If a child cannot sustain attention, then only part of the information is processed. Alternating or dividing attention refers to the ability to follow more than one thing at a time. Some children after an acquired brain injury find it difficult to filter out extraneous noise in their environment. For example, a typical classroom full of children can make it difficult for the child with a brain injury to focus on his or her work.

Many people who have suffered a brain injury do not have significant difficulty in recalling previously learned information. However, the ability to recall newly learned information is often impaired. Neuropsychological and behavioral evaluations examine various kinds of verbal and visual memory and learning. Can the child repeat information immediately, such as telephone numbers or number/letter combinations? This type of information can be remembered briefly, but most people cannot hold on to the information for any significant length of time. The ability to remember more meaningful information, such as short sentences, is also examined, as is memory for longer amounts of verbal information, such as story recall. If the child has difficulty in recalling longer amounts of verbal information, then the examiner can determine whether the child benefits from cues, such as answering multiple-choice questions about the information. Charts can be posted, reminding children of the rules before errors are committed. If the child was successful in recalling information when given these cues, then this suggests that the child has learned the information but has difficulty retrieving it from memory. Verbal information learned over a series of attempts is also examined to assess whether the child can profit from repetition of material to be learned.

Visual information is assessed in various ways. Can the child scan a picture and remember various details? Are they able to reproduce a sequence of hand movements? Can the child draw or write information from memory? Functional visual memory, such as memory for faces, places, and directions, is also examined.

Executive skills refer to those higher order-processes that serve to adapt a child's affect, behavior, and thinking to the changing demands of complex environments. These processes include self-regulation, self-monitoring, problem-solving, goal formation, and learning from the consequences of one's behavior. Parents' and teachers' reports are helpful in determining whether the child has difficulty in regulating behavior. Is the child impulsive or showing a low tolerance for frustration? Does the child's mood change rapidly? Problem-solving is also an important part of executive skills. Does the child profit from feedback, including learning from mistakes? Can the child look at a problem from different viewpoints? How does the child deal with transitions and the changing environment?

Neuropsychological and behavioral examinations also attempt to look at the impact of social and emotional functioning on cognitive skills and interpersonal skills. Any change in brain status can result in social, emotional, and behavioral difficulties. Dependent on the severity of the brain insult, the adjustment period can be lifelong. Changes in physical appearance and loss of skills can result in a change in relationships with family and friends. A child who has survived a brain tumor differs from other children with learning difficulties in that they often remember that they were functioning in a relatively normal status before their injuries but now are presented with new cognitive weaknesses. A sense of loss of the old self and acceptance of the new self is a difficult process. Emotional lability, low tolerance for frustration, and poor self-regulation of behavior impacts on interactions in school and the community. Social isolation due to changes in friendships can lead to depression. These long-term effects can be seen in many children as they continue to develop and mature.

DEVELOPMENTAL ISSUES

It is important to understand the physical maturation stages of the brain through childhood in order to predict the long-term impact of tumors on continued development. Researchers in the past decade have been using the latest technology to understand how children's brains grow and mature. The concept of plasticity, for example, is much more complicated than many neuroscientists once thought.[14] Earlier beliefs that younger children recovered better than older children after treatment for a brain tumor or brain injury may only recognize the "medical recovery" of the brain. The long-term cognitive impact of tumors and tumor treatment is a concern for neuropsychologists and educators working with these children. Through developmental studies and techniques, such as neuropsychological testing, magnetic resonance imaging (MRI), and special uses of electroencephalography (EEG), critical discoveries are being made about how the brain grows and matures throughout childhood. New research utilizing advanced scanning technology and statistical analysis of EEGs has better identified how a child's brain matures from birth through adolescence. In particular, five peak maturation periods have been identified that have varying developmental increments depending on the region of the brain (Figure 26.1):

- *Age 1–6 years*: during this period of overall rapid brain growth, all regions of the brain – those governing frontal executive, visuospatial, somatic, and visuoauditory functions – show signs of synchronous development. Children are perfecting skills such as their ability to form images, use words, and place things in serial order. They also begin to develop tactics for solving problems.
- *Age 7–10 years*: at this point, only the sensory and motor systems continue to mature in tandem up to about age 7.5 years, when the frontal executive system begins accelerated development. Beginning at about age six years, the maturation of the sensory motor regions of the brain peaks just as children begin to perform simple operational functions, such as determining weight and logical mathematical reasoning.
- *Age 11–13 years*: this stage involves primarily the elaboration of the visuospatial functions, but it also includes maturation of the visuoauditory regions. By the age of ten years, while visual and auditory regions of the brain mature, children are able to perform formal operations, such as calculations, and perceive new meaning in familiar objects.
- *Age 14–17 years*: during these years, successive maturation of the visuoauditory, visuospatial, and somatic systems reach their maturational peak within one-year intervals of each other. In their early years, young people enter the stage of dialectic ability. They are able to review formal operations, find flaws with them, and create new ones. Meanwhile, the visuoauditory, visuospatial, and somatic systems of the brain are developing.
- *Age 18–21 years*: the final stage begins around age 17–18 years, when the region governing the frontal executive functions matures on its own. Young people begin to question information they are given, reconsider it, and form new hypotheses, incorporating ideas of their own. This development occurs in conjunction with rapid maturation of the frontal executive region of the brain.

It is important to recognize that this maturation occurs during childhood. Thus, depending on the age of the child when the tumor is treated, and the region of the brain that the tumor affects most, one may be able

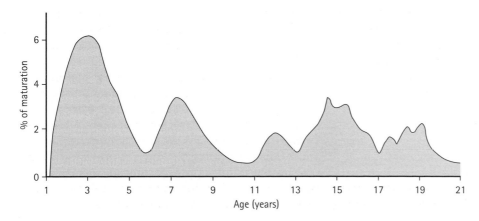

Figure 26.1 *Cerebral maturation stages.*

to predict the kinds of cognitive and learning challenges that the child may experience now and in the future. This knowledge will allow professionals working with the child to predict the resources they may need to better support the child, especially in the school system.

PLANNING SCHOOL REINTEGRATION

As mentioned previously, tumors and their treatments can significantly alter a child's level of functioning in many ways. Unsurprisingly, therefore, research also identifies considerable difficulties experienced by children when they return to school following treatment, with significant repercussions for their physical, educational, and social/emotional well-being.[15–19] It is important to consider the child's future educational needs well in advance of discharge from the hospital or rehabilitation setting.

Each child's recovery process is unique. The nature and extent of any difficulties will depend on a variety of factors, including the child's age and developmental stage, time away from school, pre-illness functioning, personality, the quality of family and other support systems, such as health and education services, the site of the tumor, and the effects of treatment. This, therefore, demands a highly individual approach to the planning for future school provision, based on each child's individual circumstances. However, there are some key features common to successful reintegration that should form the hospital discharge plan and be put into action at as early a stage as possible during the child's clinical treatment:[18]

- school personnel planning with family and hospital team;
- comprehensive assessment and identification of needs;
- appropriate identification of provision to meet needs;
- in-service training or provision of relevant information for school staff;
- helping child, family, and peers to prepare for and manage return to school;
- review and follow-up.

Planning for successful school return requires collaboration between all those involved in the child's health and educational welfare, including hospital and rehabilitation staff, family, and education personnel, each of whom brings a unique perspective and area of expertise.[17] The relationship between them all, and the quality of communication, will greatly influence the process. It is also important to remember that if the child has been diagnosed with a malignant tumor, then the word "cancer" may evoke highly emotive negative reactions in others, born mainly out of ignorance and fear. Exchanging and sharing information with the ill child, the rest of the

family, and other children at school, as well as between professionals, is crucial, and, to a large extent, will determine the ease with which the child reintegrates back to school. However, permission must be sought from the child's parents before sharing or disclosing any personal information.

Initial contact between school and hospital should be immediately after the child's admission. A plan for efficient and effective two-way flow of information needs to be established, and a key contact person from within both settings must be identified who is responsible for coordination and ensuring that information is conveyed. It is important to be aware that written reports alone may be the least efficient mode of communication, as they can be filed away without the advice and recommendations in them being brought to the notice of the members of staff for whom they are intended, i.e. those who work directly with the child.

Multidisciplinary assessment

Comprehensive multidisciplinary evaluation is an essential requirement for effective educational planning. This needs to include information from functional settings and from standardized assessment. Informal assessment techniques and the perceptions of those who know the child well are essential for obtaining a full picture of the child's abilities. Identifying a child's current strengths and needs will enable decisions about provision to be made before their return. Assessment of the learning environment is also important, as it is imperative that the school enables the child to experience success and feel positive from the first day of their return. Inevitably, adjustments may need to be made, but any attempt to delay an assessment of special educational needs with a wait-and-see approach is unacceptable. As the child's illness and treatment may have caused major side effects, including hair loss, weight alteration, scars, headaches, nausea, fatigue, and motor, behavioral, and cognitive changes, these can provoke dramatic and detrimental issues for a child. These include the effects of concomitant loss of skill, frailty, restricted autonomy, and loss of or change in familiar friendships resulting from prolonged absence from school. Experience of early failure on return to school may lead to loss of confidence and self-esteem. There is thus a risk of the child becoming demoralized and developing secondary behavioral difficulties.

Optimum timing of an assessment for informing the school of re-entry arrangements is an important consideration. It needs to be long enough to allow for arrangements to be put into place, but evaluation of cognitive, behavioral, and academic skills at an early period of a child's illness or recovery is unlikely to provide useful information in the longer term for identifying school-based support and an appropriate curriculum. Inconsistent performance is also commonly noted during the early stages of recovery, and changes in ability can occur rapidly. Continuing monitoring and evaluation are, therefore, essential.

Choosing the best educational environment

The usual expectation is for the child to return to the school that they were attending before their illness. For the great majority of children with special educational needs, this is highly desirable and there is never any reason to consider a different educational environment. Any additional provision required as a result of changing needs should ideally be made in the school that the child would otherwise have been attending. However, for some children, this may no longer be a viable option, e.g. particular facilities such as wheelchair access or specialist teaching provision may be required and only available elsewhere. However, there must always be assurance that decisions are based first and foremost on the child's individual needs and parental wishes, rather than on political, social, or financial policies. Consideration of the needs of the whole child is important, including the important issue of their age. Bax contends:[20] "... children with moderate or severe disabilities are more readily accepted by younger children. In the post pubescent years, children strongly identify with their own peer group and are often more reluctant to accept anyone who departs from their perceived norm."

Daniel

Following surgical intervention for a spinal tumor, which had affected his mobility, Daniel, aged 14 years, required the use of a wheelchair. He was very sensitive about his obvious physical differences and was exceedingly reluctant to return to his local mainstream school. Before his illness, he had been the subject of bullying, and he was scared about his additional vulnerability in that environment. His parents had also been unhappy about the way school staff had dealt with the issue, as well as the increasingly poor reputation and educational record of the school. Daniel and his parents were previously keen for him to enroll at another school, which had not been able to offer him a place. However, as it had a good reputation for pastoral care and also had two other wheelchair users at the school, Daniel's acquired special educational needs eventually enabled a fresh application to be viewed sympathetically. He was granted a place, but unfortunately not before Daniel and his parents had experienced much additional anxiety.

Information for school staff and parents

In effect, schools are the main providers of long-term rehabilitation for these children. The opportunities that schools offer for structured learning programs, close monitoring, regular support, and long-term planning make them well placed for providing ongoing services after discharge from the clinical setting. However, education personnel are often unaware of the effects that a brain or spinal tumor and its resulting treatment can have on a child's functioning, particularly in relation to cognitive skills and the impact on learning, behavior, and social communication. This often makes them unprepared to address the needs of such children re-entering school. There is also a commonly held assumption that children who make a relatively good physical recovery and demonstrate the surface features of language will make a smooth transition back to school. There is not a general understanding of the further sequelae that have a profound impact on cognitive ability.

There is little appreciation of the hidden or subtle deficits related to changes in memory, concentration, learning, and behavior that can create far more handicapping conditions than those that are immediately obvious. These facts are often least apparent to, and most easily misunderstood by, education personnel. Without appropriate information, it is all too easy to focus on the obvious or the easily observable effects without acknowledgment that a tumor and/or its treatment can alter academic ability. Regrettably, too few educators make the connection.

Before school return, therefore, provision of information for education staff and formal in-service training, if this is possible, needs to include basic details of the child's illness and treatment, and the effects that these have had and may continue to have on the child's functioning. Information needs to be presented in a way that is easily understood and that provides practical suggestions. Members of school staff also need to feel supported and to have an opportunity to deal with what may be strong emotional reactions to the prospect of working with a child who has a serious and possibly life-threatening disease. A teacher who has known the child well may be particularly distressed or upset by the child's condition. The child may have been displaying symptoms in school for some time before diagnosis, which were unrecognized by teachers and which may have invoked criticism and complaints relating to deterioration in standards of work. Teachers sometimes then feel guilt and can attempt to compensate for this. They may also be unsure about how actively involved they should be in coordinating with the child's family, some fearing that contact may put additional strain on the parents in an already difficult situation.[21] However, if the prognosis is poor, then school staff can do much to support parents during the process of anticipatory grieving as well as helping to improve the quality of life of children and families whose outlook is more promising. Blosser and DePompei emphasize the importance of flexibility, which can be encouraged through in-service training opportunities where teachers not only learn more about the medical issues but also "... how to talk to the student, how to observe and respond to his or her behaviors, how to re-evaluate and re-establish goals, and how to respond to their own frustrations as educators."[22]

It is important to encourage parental participation in planning educational provision and setting goals. Parents know their child best and care more about their well-being than anyone else. However, teachers need to be sensitive to the emotional and financial pressures that a parent may be under, and to respect their differing needs. Making plans and decisions about any special educational arrangements can be complicated and confusing for parents who may not have had any previous knowledge or experience in the arena of special education.[23] This process often needs to be undertaken at the very time that they are already overwhelmed and still struggling to acquire understanding about their child's illness and its uncertain progression, as well as juggling a host of other family and work commitments. Davis highlights the profound effect that children's illness has on parents, with as many as one-third of parents of children with cancer, even those in remission, having such severe depression and anxiety that they too require professional help.[24]

Key questions that professionals and family need to consider together can help to empower families to become active participants in the process of return to school:[16]

- What does the family know about the child's or adolescent's educational needs?
- What does the family know about policies, procedures, and provision for ensuring their child's needs are well met?
- What are the expectations of rehabilitation personnel for the school?
- What do families and peers expect about the social aspects of school return?

Information for the child and their peers

A critical component of the planning for school return is the child's involvement, which must be appropriate to their age and level of understanding. The extent to which an individual child is traumatized by their illness and treatment is difficult to quantify. Psychosocial (i.e. social, emotional, psychological, behavioral) sequelae significantly affect the quality of life for the child returning to school.[25] Children need help in communicating their needs and in understanding what has been happening to them. In addition to the essential support from trusted adults with whom there is a good relationship, books and interactive activities may be helpful tools for working with both young children[26,27] and adolescents.

Experience shows that many children initially respond, at least superficially, in a very stoical manner when they first receive diagnosis of a tumor. This may be related to a lack of awareness or knowledge in the case of a young child, to natural feelings of "invincibility" in the young, or to lack of acceptance or self-protective denial. There is also the fact that while the child is in hospital, particularly in an oncology ward, illness and treatments and the symptoms produced by these are the norm. These children are placed within a strange, abnormal situation in the midst of other children with bald heads, drips, and cannulas and talking about their current treatments. Newly admitted children take up the language and the rules of this otherwise frightening environment and begin to identify with other children there. After their initial hospital stay, they may return on a regular basis and meet with the same group of staff, patients, and parents. They need support to move away from this environment.

The most important points to remember when considering return to school are to allow the child to do so (even if, initially, this is on a part-time basis), to allow them to be as normal as possible, and to listen to what they are saying. It is also important to involve the child in setting some achievable goals that they want to accomplish after they go back to school. They will probably be unaware of the extent of their own changes, and thus they could quickly become demoralized when back in the real-world setting. Parents and children may need sensitive encouragement to re-evaluate their expectations.

Frequent or long absences from school can disrupt peer relationships. School personnel must take a lead role in keeping the relationships alive. While the child is away from school, contact by letter, card, fax, email, telephone, and video, as well as visits, can help sustain friendships and play an important part in maintaining the child's morale.

The involvement of other children also increases the likelihood of a successful return, but how this is dealt with must first be discussed and agreed with the child who is preparing to come back, or, in the case of a young child, with the parent(s). Some basic and simple information about the illness and treatment and the effect that it has had can help peers and the child's siblings to make adjustments and accommodate possible changes in relationships. It can be hard for them to understand how and why changes have occurred.

Consideration must be given to a phased return to school. The transition "... is often mistakenly thought of as a 1-day activity. In fact effective transition ... may take days, weeks, or even months."[28]

There must be awareness that, following discharge from hospital and carefully planned school reintegration, it will be very important to continue the multidisciplinary perspective and involvement in the review of the child's progress. Vigilant monitoring, good communication, and flexibility of response will help to ensure that the child's needs continue to be well met.

RETURN TO SCHOOL

Returning to school is perceived by many as the return to normality, but this represents another stage of rehabilitation that " ... is a long-term process that will continue throughout the child's development and has no defined end point."[28]

This can be a difficult time for the child. Once they are at home and back at school, even if they are returning to hospital, they have two worlds in which to integrate. Despite the often-seeming acceptance of the illness and treatment in the hospital situation, most of these children seek a continuation of "normality" as a mainstay to offset their insecurities. The most normal event in the world for children is to go to school. It is possible to see young people who may previously have been very reluctant to go to school or to engage in activities when they were there become very keen to return as soon as possible. Sometimes, parents and school staff have attempted to be helpful by suggesting that young people have additional time off school to rest and relax, but this is not necessarily what young people want or need. They are seeking something normal, non-threatening, and non-invasive, and, above all, a familiar environment that holds no surprises or uncertainties. Unknown clinical procedures can be very frightening for a child, even if explanations or other preparatory approaches have been used. In contrast, however much they used to think that they hated it, there are no surprises involved in working from their math book and they can predict how it will make them feel, even if all those feelings are negative.

Return to school "... mobilizes hope, encourages social contact, and reinforces the living child within them. Seriously ill and dying children often cope best with their condition by living as fully as they can until they die. During serious illness, school may represent one of the few areas where the child feels a sense of control and accomplishment."[21]

Luke

Luke, aged six years, was receiving treatment for an aggressive, high-grade tumor. Throughout his treatment, he maintained a wonderful, sunny disposition as long as he was able to interact with his peers and to engage in activities that he loved. As his illness progressed, the staff at his school became concerned that they may not be able to meet his needs and were frightened of encountering a medical emergency for which they thought that they would be ill equipped to cope. They suggested that he should no longer attend school, and he changed quickly to become a pale and withdrawn child, motivated to do very little at home. However, when the school staff was persuaded to allow him to return and to be involved in as much as he could, he returned to his original happy self. Despite the fact that the treatment was ultimately unsuccessful, the quality of the final months of his life was improved significantly.

Relationships in school

The young person's relationships with their friends are important. Initially, the child may be the center of attention of their peers, but this may be short-lived if the child is not as active or energetic as they had been previously and not able to join in with all the usual activities that enable acceptance within their particular peer group. The child with a tumor may also be missing from school on a regular basis for continued treatment and may find it difficult to keep up with the culture and current interests of the group. It is important that teachers are aware of this and, if possible, ensure that the child has appropriate ways to relate to their peers. Sometimes, the child will use their illness as a means to gain attention; the function and appropriateness of this should be considered carefully. For instance, some children have shaved heads with dramatic-looking scars from surgery, which they sometimes display as a "badge of honor" to attract the attention of other children. They sometimes recount stories relating to treatment and show "trophies" such as metal staples removed from surgical incisions. It may be appropriate for the child to share these accounts with their friends initially and to satisfy the natural curiosity of other children, but later it may be more appropriate for them to be positively redirected to continue to seek attention in alternative ways.

Practical considerations after return to school

Once classroom teachers have been given the vitally important accurate information regarding a child's current strengths and weaknesses, they must not be left to make assumptions on the basis of the child's previous ability or to draw conclusions about this child based on the levels of functioning of others. When a young person becomes aware of altered levels of ability, it can cause very significant additional frustration, confusion, and distress. When this is understood and addressed, further exacerbation of difficulties can often be avoided.

Angela

Angela, aged 15 years, returned to school after treatment with no physical difficulties and seemingly happy and enthusiastic. She was referred back to the treating hospital some time later with a range of physical symptoms. She had extreme mobility problems and was almost unable to walk unaided. Initially, no cause could be found for these symptoms, but it then became clear that, as a previously average student, she was experiencing difficulties in specific areas of school work. These were directly as a result of acquired cognitive difficulties. These were explained to Angela and to the school staff. She then understood why she was encountering these inexplicable problems, the staff understood how to help her, and an agreement was reached to focus more on her strengths within the curriculum and to work with her to develop appropriate strategies. As soon as this situation was addressed, her gait problems resolved spontaneously.

Although expectations are initially often reduced inappropriately, after this overprotection teachers can make assumptions that the young person has returned "to normal," leading to equally unrealistic expectations.

Adam

Adam, aged 14 years, was very determined to return to his academic course of study with no reduction in the content of the curriculum. He could have managed this, except that no one at the school had considered his physical access to this. He had mobility problems, severe back pain, and high levels of fatigue during his treatment. He had to walk around a large school, climb stairs frequently, and sit in uncomfortable plastic chairs. He was very upset and considered that he had "failed" when he had to give up full attendance at school as he was too exhausted and uncomfortable.

In terms of the further content and delivery of the school curriculum, it is vitally important that the full range of the young person's physical and cognitive strengths and weaknesses are taken into account and appropriate curricular or environmental adjustments made. These need to be monitored and re-evaluated on a regular and frequent basis. For instance, school personnel must show flexibility in allowing alterations to the environment or to the curricular content and enable young people to discover strengths within the limitations of their acquired difficulties.

Peter

Peter was 10 years old when he gradually lost most of his functional vision as a result of a brain tumor. He was very frustrated and demotivated by the fact that he could no longer complete independently work that he had previously enjoyed. However, he discovered that he was able to work with clay and produced many pottery items, including presents for friends and family with messages and personalized touches. He was allowed to spend additional time in art lessons, and his level of success and independence with that enabled him to cope with the frustration of receiving higher levels of support in other areas.

CONTINUED REVIEW AND MONITORING

School staff must be made aware that as tumors and their treatment can cause damage to the child's brain that is within a process of development, changes in the ability to learn may not be immediately obvious and are also likely to alter throughout subsequent years. Teachers must remain vigilant to detect and address any difficulties as they emerge. They must also be aware of the fact that altered levels of ability and acquired cognitive difficulties can affect the child's behavior. They should be informed of the implications of other related clinical factors that may affect a child's behavior at some time, such as hormonal imbalance.

BEST PRACTICE

The most important issues to optimize a successful future school placement are (Figure 26.2):

- To recognize the right of access to the known and the normal and the importance of this to recovery and rehabilitation.
- To consider social needs and peer relationships and to offer support in these.
- To consider the effects of the illness on the whole family and the ways in which these, in turn, may impact upon the child and their levels of functioning in school.
- To be aware of physical difficulties and symptoms and to make adaptations to address these.
- To be aware of the full spectrum of educational needs and not to focus purely on physical symptoms.
- To be aware that acquired cognitive difficulties will probably be specific and therefore affect only certain aspects of learning. Other skills may be intact. Help

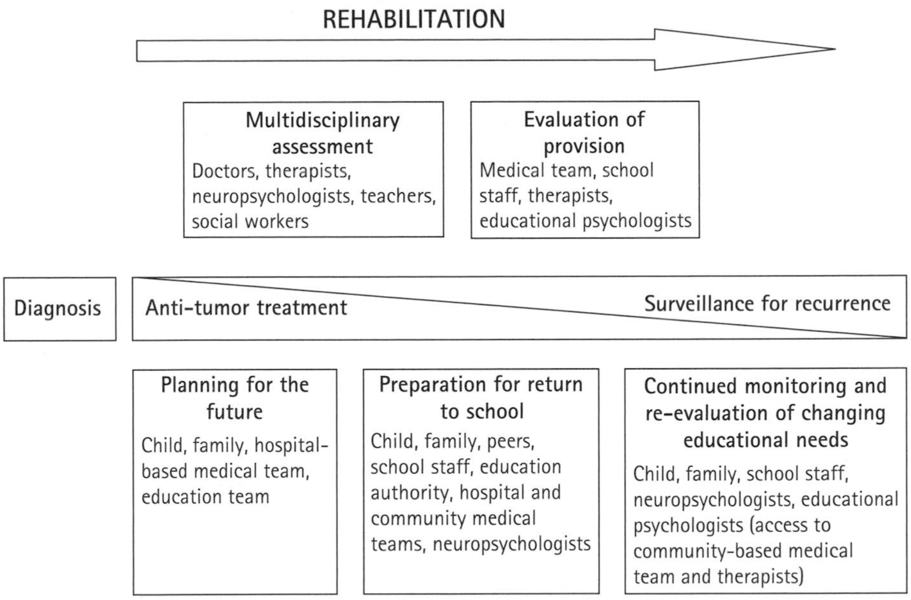

REHABILITATION

Multidisciplinary assessment	Evaluation of provision
Doctors, therapists, neuropsychologists, teachers, social workers	Medical team, school staff, therapists, educational psychologists

Diagnosis	Anti-tumor treatment	Surveillance for recurrence

Planning for the future	Preparation for return to school	Continued monitoring and re-evaluation of changing educational needs
Child, family, hospital-based medical team, education team	Child, family, peers, school staff, education authority, hospital and community medical teams, neuropsychologists	Child, family, school staff, neuropsychologists, educational psychologists (access to community-based medical team and therapists)

Figure 26.2 *Meeting the educational needs of children with brain tumors.*

may be needed in some areas despite good levels of ability in others.

- To be aware that environmental, cognitive, and organic factors may affect behavior.
- To accept the fact that adaptations may need to be made to:
  - the school environment;
  - the timetable and curriculum;
  - the teaching methods.
- To accept that future cognitive development may be affected by the illness or its treatment, and to ensure that performance continues to be monitored throughout the child's school career. Specific difficulties may only emerge in future years.
- To seek and expect appropriate and detailed information from the medical team responsible for the child's care, and to provide the team with pertinent information relating to functional and scholastic progress.

Adequate information is empowering, but school staff must remain flexible and adaptive in their approach. They must know that the needs of young people with acquired difficulties as a result of tumors are different from other special educational needs, and that the illness can impact in ways that are unfamiliar even to the experienced special needs teacher. The child faces the new and unknown, as does the teacher. Above all, educational staff must not make assumptions based on previous experience of different children with different special educational needs.

SUMMARY

The impact of brain tumors on the cognitive, developmental, and educational needs of students can be devastating unless professionals understand the long-term functional needs of these children and how to support them. By using neuropsychological and other evaluations to better understand how children are responding cognitively and behaviorally to the tumor and the treatment, we can identify ways to help children learn. Knowledge of brain maturation can enable professionals to predict the needs of children as they grow and develop. Using the resources that schools can provide will allow continued rehabilitation within a structured environment.

REFERENCES

1 Mulhern RK, Kovnar EH, Kun LE, Crisco JJ, Williams JM. Psychological and neurological function following treatment for childhood temporal lobe astrocytoma. *J Child Neurol* 1988; **3**:l47–52.
2 Castro-Sierra E, Paredes-Diaz E, Lazareff J. Short-term and procedural memory for colors and inferior temporal cortex activity. *Behav Neurol* 1997; **10**:83–92.
3 Buono L. Evidence for syndrome of nonverbal learning disabilities in children with brain tumors. *Child Neuropsychol*, 1998; **4**:144–57.
4 Anderson V, Godber T, Smibert E, Ekert H. Neurobehavioural sequelae following cranial irradiation and chemotherapy in children: an analysis of risk factors. *Pediatr Rehabil* 1997; **1**:63–76.
5 Brown RT, Sawyer MB, Antoniou G, *et al.* A 3-year follow-up of the intellectual and academic functioning of children receiving central nervous system prophylactic chemotherapy for leukemia. *Dev Behav Pediatr* 1996; **17**:392–8.
6 Dowell RE, Copeland DR, Judd BW. Neuropsychological effects of chemotherapeutic agents. *Dev Neuropsychol* 1989; **5**:17–24.
7 Warnick R, Edwards M. Pediatric brain tumors. *Curr Prob Pediatr* 1991; **21**:129–73.
8 Radcliffe JR, Packer RJ, Atkins TE, *et al.* Three and four year cognitive outcome in children with noncortical brain tumors

treated with whole-brain radiotherapy. *Ann Neurol* 1992;
32:551–4.

9   Bordeaux J, Dowell RE, Copeland DR, Fletcher JM, Francis DJ,
Van Eys J. A prospective study of neuropsychological sequelae
in children with brain tumors. *J Child Neurol* 1988; **3**:63–8.

10 Chapman CA, Bernstein JH, Pomeroy SL, La Vally B, Sallan SE,
Tarball N. Neurobehavioral and neurological outcome in long-
term survivors of posterior fossa brain tumors: role of age and
perioperative factors. *J Child Neurol* 1995; **10**:209–12.

11 Walsh K. *Neuropsychology: A Clinical Approach.* Edinburgh:
Churchill Livingstone, 1994.

12 Gaddes WH, Edgell D. *Learning Disabilities and Brain Function:
A Neuropsychological Approach.* New York: Springer-Verlag,
1994.

13 Lezak MD. *Neuropsychological Assessment.* Oxford: Oxford
University Press, 1995.

14 Alison M. The effects of neurologic injury on the maturing
brain. *Headlines* 1992; **3**:2–6, 9–10.

15 DePompei R, Blosser J, Savage R, Lash M. Back to school after
a moderate to severe brain injury. Wake Forest, NC: L&A
Publishing, 2001, pp. 1–5.

16 DePompei R, Blosser R. The family as collaborators for
effective school reintegration. In: Savage R, Wolcott G (eds).
Educational Dimensions of Acquired Brain Injury. Austin, TX:
Pro-Ed, 1994, pp. 489–506.

17 Ylvisaker M. *Traumatic Brain Injury Rehabilitation: Children
and Adolescents.* Boston, MA: Butterworth-Heinemann, 1998.

18 Savage R, Wolcott G. *An Educator's Manual.* Alexandria, VA:
Brain Injury Association, 1995.

19 Chang P. Psychosocial needs of long-term childhood cancer
survivors: a review of the literature. *Pediatrician* 1991; **18**:20–4.

20 Bax M. Joining the mainstream. *Dev Med Child Neurol*
1999; **41**:3.

21 Dyregrov A. *Grief in Children: A Handbook for Adults.* London:
Jessica Kingsley, 1991.

22 Blosser J, DePompei R. Creating an effective classroom
environment. In: Savage R, Wolcott G (eds). *Educational
Dimensions of Acquired Brain Injury.* Austin, TX: Pro-Ed, 1994,
pp. 413–52.

23 Lash M. *A Manual for Managing Special Education of Students
with Brain Injuries.* Wake Forest, NC: L&A Publishing, 1998.

24 Davis H. *Counselling Parents of Children with Chronic Illness
and Disability.* Leicester, UK: British Psychological Society, 1993.

25 Deaton A, Waaland P. Psychosocial effects of acquired brain
injury. In: Savage R, Wolcott G (eds). *Educational Dimensions
of Acquired Brain Injury.* Austin, TX: Pro-Ed, 1994, pp. 239–56.

26 Heegaard M. *When Someone Has A Very Serious Illness.*
Minneapolis: Woodland Press, 1991.

27 Mills J. *Little Tree. A Story for Children with Serious Medical
Problems.* Washington, DC: Magination Press, 1992.

28 Savage R, Mishkin LA. Neuroeducational model for teaching
students with acquired brain injuries. In: Savage R, Wolcott G
(eds). *Educational Dimensions of Acquired Brain Injury.* Austin,
TX: Pro-Ed, 1994, pp. 393–412.

27

Quality of survival

COLIN KENNEDY AND ADAM GLASER

INTRODUCTION

Quality of survival is an essential but often neglected variable when treating individuals for central nervous system (CNS) tumors. The direct effects of the tumor and therapies targeted at it may damage the young brain to the extent that in the past, only 30 per cent have lived independently without significant disability.[1] This damage is compounded further by the psychological distress consequent upon the diagnosis of a life-threatening illness and the inevitable family disturbances that occur, as well as disruption to the normal educational experience.[2] The high prevalence of additional central and/or peripheral hormonal dysfunction predisposes the child to growth and maturational disturbances,[3] further exaggerating peer differences and impacting on life experiences. In certain central tumors, these effects may be particularly severe and life-threatening (hypopituitarism),[4] whilst the tendency to obesity carries its own emotional and health-related concerns.[5]

Reintegration into society and maintenance of as normal a lifestyle as possible are two of the primary aims of children's cancer services.[6] As cancer survival rates have improved, so the concept of "cure at any cost" is increasingly being replaced by that of "cure at what cost?". Although survival figures for CNS tumors lag behind those for other groups of pediatric malignancies, the location of these tumors and the potential susceptibility of the developing brain oblige healthcare professionals to consider quality of life when looking after children during and after their treatment.

This chapter aims to explore the issues of quality of life, health-related quality of life, problems unique to children, specific late effects of therapy (neurological, endocrine), outcome assessments in the context of clinical trials, and finally a way forward to minimize the morbidity burden associated with survival from CNS tumors.

ASSESSMENT OF QUALITY OF LIFE

The concepts

Quality of life is an increasingly widely used outcome measure, although little consensus exists regarding its definition.[7] Many of the major sponsors of clinical trials, including the Medical Research Council in the UK and the National Cancer Institute in the USA, insist that new trials include built-in quality-of-life assessments if they are to be supported.[8,9] However, it is essential to define the term and included target domains.[10] The World Health Organization Quality of Life (WHOQOL) Group provides the following definition:

WHOQOL Group definition

Quality of life is defined as an individual's perception of their position in life in the context of the culture and value systems in which they live and in relation to their goals, expectations, standards,

---

and concerns. It is a broad-ranging concept affected in a complex way by the person's physical health, psychological state, level of independence, social relationships, and their relationships to salient features of their environment.[11]

A complex series of interactions between the intrinsic physical, emotional, social, and spiritual elements of an individual's life determine their overall quality of life at any given point in time. The American Cancer Society's workshop on quality of life in children's cancer acknowledged these issues in its definition:

> **American Cancer Society definition**
>
> Quality of life is multidimensional. It includes, but is not limited to, the social, physical, and emotional functioning of the child and adolescent, and when indicated his/her family, and it must be sensitive to the changes that occur through development.[12]

The goal of healthcare is to maximize the health-related component of an individual's quality of life. To simplify the measurement of quality of life as a medical outcome measure, health-related quality of life (HRQL) can be assessed (Figure 27.1). This has the advantage that factors not affected directly by health are excluded. Child

health can be defined as the ability to participate fully in developmentally appropriate activities and requires physical, psychological, and social energy.[13] Assessment of HRQL enables discrimination between individuals, evaluation, and prediction of outcome.[14]

Specific pediatric issues

Established measures of adult quality of life and HRQL may not be appropriate for use in children, due to the issues of growth and development, the dependence of children on carers and proxy respondents, and children's conceptualization of health.

Growth and development

Throughout childhood and adolescence, growth (an increase in size) and development (the acquisition of new skills) occur. Additionally, a rapid development of physical, mental, and social perspectives takes place.[15] These processes are susceptible to disruption when normality does not occur, be it secondary to illness or deprivation. They must be considered during the assessment of HRQL, which in turn must be developmentally appropriate for the individual.[16] A complicating factor is that for the majority of domains contributing to HRQL in childhood, there is not a predictable linear pattern of development.[17]

Cognition and conceptualization of health

The normal developmental process includes the evolution of cognitive skills. When applying questionnaires and outcome measures to children, the issues of comprehension of language and reading and writing skills need to be addressed. Position bias in children's responses, with a tendency to choose the first answer among response options, and confusion regarding questionnaire terminology (e.g. equating "diabetes" with "you are about to die") have been identified as major issues.[13]

Variations in cognitive capabilities can cause practical problems in evaluating responses to abstract ideas.[18] Both the understanding of health as a concept and the meaning of that concept change during childhood and adolescence. For instance, Natapoff found that approximately 20 per cent of six-year olds described feeling healthy as "not sick," whereas over 60 per cent of 12-year-olds responded in this way.[19] Progressively through the teenage years, the proportion of individuals who define health as "the absence of illness" decreases, and an increasing awareness of psychosocial and emotional implications of illness develops.[20,21] This indicates a change in appreciation of concepts and language of health and ill health as children mature.

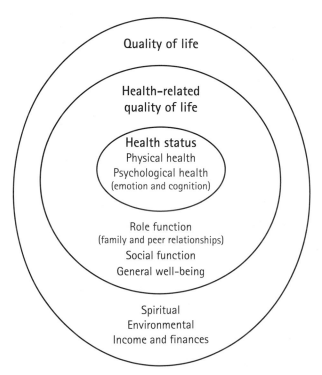

Figure 27.1 *Relationship between quality of life, health-related quality of life, and health status.*

Proxy respondents

The ideal person to judge an individual's quality of life is that person. However, the requirement for the assessment to be acceptable to, and appropriate for, children often precludes this. Few self-completed measures of childhood HRQL exist.[22] Accordingly, proxy respondents are needed for most generic instruments. Evidence exists that the more subjective domains of HRQL are measured less adequately by proxy respondents than the more objective domains, which include functional capacity.[23,24]

Adolescents in particular disagree with their parents' rating of anxieties and concerns.[25] Some studies have shown children to report more problems related to emotional distress, while their parents report more issues associated with observable behavioral reactions.[26] However, disagreement may be "healthy," and high levels of concordance between parents and offspring may in fact represent a poor quality of life, as childhood is normally associated with gaining autonomy and independence from parental views.[27]

Despite concerns relating to the use of proxy respondents, they can, nevertheless, provide informative details relating to children's HRQL.[28] Until such time as psychometrically valid, reliable, and reproducible measures for child self-completion become available, this should not be ignored.

Central nervous system and extracranial tumors

The exact cause of the neural toxicity that occurs after specific cancer therapies is still unclear, but its existence and certain characteristics are now well recognized. Awareness of this has led in some instances to reduction or omission of the neurotoxic components of the treatment strategies, e.g. using cranial radiotherapy fields or doses in young children. It is exceptional for these treatment modifications to be truly evidence-based in their justification. It is generally true in most countries that supportive community and educational strategies and services to support children with CNS toxicities to address the neural deficits in existing survivors are organized haphazardly.

CLINICAL TRIALS

Rationale

The requirement for scientific evidence (or reproducible experiment) as the rationale upon which most advances in medical treatments are based hardly seems to need stating, yet there are many exceptions to this rule. In particular, treatments that make a large and obvious improvement to outcome, such as antibiotics for meningitis, are rarely submitted to controlled scientific experiment; nor are treatments that may or may not make a reliably measurable clinical improvement but are felt to have sufficient face validity not to require it, such as provision of special educational support tailored to the needs of the child. Randomized, controlled clinical trials (RCTs) are generally considered to be the best way to determine which of two treatments that have a similar outcome is superior. Very few interventions, however, are all good, and decision-making involves a risk/benefit analysis that quantifies the degree of uncertainty[29] and, increasingly, needs to involve patients and carers.[30]

For a treatment to be adopted as a result of a clinical trial, the findings of the trial should be reliable and generalizable. These characteristics are harder to achieve in a single institution because of small numbers and selection of patients by local referral pattern. These difficulties lead logically to multicenter RCTs, which are necessary because of the rarity of the disorders and challenging because of the difficulty in obtaining agreement on the experimental question to be addressed. They are burdensome in their conduct between countries with barriers of language, ethics, and rules of research practice.

Selection of outcome measure

There are many variables that may affect the outcome and also many different outcomes to measure. Event-free survival at a time interval after diagnosis is clearly one important definable end point and is, historically, often the only kind of outcome that has been ascertained adequately in multicenter trials of treatment of children with brain tumors. However, long-term health status and associated quality of life, as detailed earlier in this chapter, are recognized by family, other carers, and health professionals to be critically important. This becomes increasingly the case as the overall long-term survival from brain tumors rises from its current rate of greater than 50 per cent overall.[31] Important variables at diagnosis that are predictive of quality of survival after diagnosis and treatment include the individual differences in intelligence, development, and disability between children before the presentation of their tumor, deficits caused by the tumor itself before treatment, morbidity associated with surgery, and the toxicities of chemotherapy and radiotherapy. These continue to cause deficits in neurological, behavioral, and endocrine functions, as well as other late-effect organ toxicities, e.g. in the kidneys, ears, heart, lungs, and skin.

Effect of individual therapies on quality of survival

Radiation therapy has been the easiest of these factors to study, both because it is the most standardized in its application and because its effects can be predicted by analogy with the use of whole-brain and craniospinal irradiation in the more common and more clinically stereotyped circumstances of acute lymphocytic leukemia without CNS involvement in the disease (see below).[32] Relatively little information has been collected systematically regarding the other therapies mentioned above, or their interactions with radiation effects, or tumor effects and other background variables in the social, psychological, and educational circumstances of the affected child, although the data that do exist suggest that these factors are important.[33–36]

The effects of cranial radiotherapy (18–24 Gy) have been studied in large numbers of survivors of acute childhood leukemia. Even with these lower doses, impaired school performance with a reduction of up to 20 points in IQ,[37] poor growth, disordered pubertal development,[38] and obesity[39] may all follow. These adverse effects are most severe in children under three years of age,[40] and there is some increased susceptibility to neuroendocrine toxicity in children under seven years of age,[41] not least because they have much of their growth, development, and education ahead of them.

Systemic and intrathecal chemotherapy may cause cerebral white-matter damage, with resultant morbidity.[42] Intrathecal chemotherapy may be responsible for compounding the cognitive consequences by cranial irradiation,[43] which manifests itself neuroradiologically.[44] Additive toxicity of the two modalities of treatment also affects the endocrine system (see Chapter 24).

In the case of primary CNS tumors, these mechanisms of injury are compounded further by the mass effects of the tumor itself, the consequences of raised intracranial pressure due to episodes of hydrocephalus, traumatic brain injury due to neurosurgery, a disrupted blood–brain barrier open to chemotherapeutic agents, and the use of focused high-dose (55 Gy) and whole-brain (35 Gy) radiation.[5,45,46] Although the damage is incurred at the time of diagnosis and treatment, its effects may appear to evolve over time.

To date, attempts to assess the impact of therapy on HRQL of survivors of childhood cancer have not revealed a clear-cut or simple picture. Survivors of CNS tumors are likely to experience a high overall morbidity burden and poor psychosocial outcome for multiple reasons.[47,48] They have often been excluded as a special case from studies of effects of a wide range of cancers on school behavior, performance, and health status,[48,49] perhaps reflecting low societal expectation of their achievements.

> It has been said that the gold standard is no radiotherapy.

Focusing on reducing irradiation toxicity alone to the exclusion of other therapeutic or tumor-induced harm may well not enhance eventual quality of survival and may compromise existing event-free survival rates. Since radiation is the most effective and proven treatment modality, it is imperative to examine longitudinally the effects of age, dose, tumor position, and time interval from treatment on specific aspects of quality of life and cognitive and endocrine outcomes. Only then can the exact etiology of neural toxicity be truly identified, and treatment and rehabilitation interventions (endocrine, psychotherapeutic, educational) be devised to increase autonomy, psychosocial function, and quality of life.

CONSTRAINTS ON TYPES OF MEASURE

Length of assessment

Conventional assessment of neuropsychological function by psychometric testing is time-consuming, costly, and therefore difficult to achieve across multiple institutions (see *Primitive neuroectodermal tumors*, below). It also fails to test a number of important domains of function. To be predictive of function in daily life, data on cognitive function must be considered within a standardized framework that also incorporates motor and sensory function, emotion, pain, hormonal and maturational status, behavior, educational provision and achievement, social integration, and the subjective experience of the growing child and their family. The need for this information has to be balanced against increasing risk of poor ascertainment of the data from families and medical staff with increasing length and complexity of assessment. In order to combine breadth with reliability and brevity, short questionnaires, preferably with a bias to information provided by the family and patient themselves, seem to be the logical solution.[50] Furthermore, there are data supporting the validity of this approach, in comparison with more in-depth testing. Thus, the Health Utilities Index (HUI), a 16-item questionnaire, was found to be at least as predictive of school performance as neuropsychological testing in one study of children with primitive neuroectodermal tumor (PNET).[51] Very good agreement has also been reported between in-depth neurodevelopmental testing and parent- or health-visitor-completed questionnaires in follow-up of premature infants in multicenter RCTs.[52,53]

Timing of assessments

Many assessments of morbidity in survivors of childhood brain tumors have been cross-sectional or retrospective, performed following completion of therapy.

Longitudinal studies have documented a high incidence of sensory motor disabilities at presentation or following surgery, so that survivors would be predicted to have a high incidence of developmental and endocrine problems, even if no further treatment were given.[46,54,55] It is therefore desirable to collect information not only about the postoperative and post-adjuvant therapy status but also about the presenting state, although the practicalities of the clinical situation mean that only postoperative assessment is achievable by direct observation as opposed to parental report.

At the time of any single assessment, the child's trajectory of developmental progress may be approaching or progressively deviating from the normal.[17] For this reason, data from a single set of assessments are difficult to interpret with respect to subsequent function, particularly when the short-term toxicities are significant or the long-term toxicities progressive over several years.[56] One published standardized framework for follow-up suggests assessments relating to time of diagnosis, following postoperative discharge, at one, three, and five years from diagnosis, and at the age of 25 years,[57] although more frequent measurements may be required for interpretation of endocrine data.

Infants and preschool children

Morbidity following brain tumors in preschool children is high, but reliable estimates of developmental status in very young children can be technically difficult to achieve, particularly during treatment.[54] Problems that can be defined at school age may be more predictive of the strengths and limitations of the future adult's functioning than earlier assessments. A picture of the early developmental trajectory of infants and preschool children can be obtained by the use of a standardized parental report measure, such as the Vineland Adaptive Behaviour Scale.[58]

ILLUSTRATIVE PROBLEMS IN TRIALS (EUROPEAN AND AMERICAN EXPERIENCE)

Primitive neuroectodermal tumors

PNET is the most common malignant brain tumor of childhood. The current standard of care includes surgery, radiotherapy, and chemotherapy, whose effects on long-term outcome are therefore all questions of immediate importance. For these reasons, it provides perhaps the most graphic illustration of the difficulties associated with assessing quality of survival in multicenter trials. Thousands of children have been enrolled in RCTs of treatment for PNET. In many cases, the two treatment arms

have been selected for comparison with an improvement in quality of survival as a primary or secondary aim of the trial, and yet the extent to which this was achieved is known incompletely and the findings are inconclusive. The efforts to obtain such information in two trials conducted in the USA are summarized below.

The Pediatric Oncology Group (POG) study 8631 for low-risk medulloblastoma (1986–1990) randomized patients to receive reduced-dose neuraxial radiotherapy (RRT) of 23.4 Gy in 13 fractions or standard-dose radiotherapy (SRT) of 36 Gy in 20 fractions. Patients in both arms received a 32.4-Gy boost to the posterior fossa. The protocol required serial psychological testing and measurement of achievement for 42 months, but "compliance with these studies was poor … therefore, the planned longitudinal analysis of intergroup data was abandoned."[47] Special funding to enable the testing psychologists to be reimbursed was obtained in 1996, and 22 of 35 (60 per cent) eligible surviving patients completed testing. Patients were divided into younger (Y) and older (O) groups according to their median age at diagnosis (8.85 years). Attention, reading, arithmetic, and verbal, performance, and full-scale IQ were assessed at a median time from diagnosis of 8.2 years. The group as a whole scored a low average level on these measures at their last assessment, but with a wide range (e.g. full-scale IQ median 85.8, range 55–105). Although younger age and higher radiation dose were expected to be associated with lower IQ, this was noted only as a progressive decline in both full-scale IQ and performance IQ across O/RRT, O/SST, Y/RRT, and Y/SST, but not in comparisons between any pair of these four groups. Longitudinal comparison of individual baseline scores with subsequent scores in the same patients did not confirm an age- or radiation-dose-dependent pattern. A (statistically non-significant) 15-point IQ point advantage was seen in the Y/RRT group ($n = 6$) compared with the Y/SRT group ($n = 4$). The authors commented that the poor ascertainment using their methods had been "unfortunate but instructive," and they recommended that "in future studies, alternative methodologies should be considered such as using well-validated parent or teacher questionnaires or abbreviated measures that can be administered by a variety of health care professionals."[47]

Another similar attempt to assess outcome of treatment for medulloblastoma was made in the Children's Cancer Study Group single-arm study 9892 (1989–1994), in which 43 of 61 (70 per cent) eligible patients underwent longitudinal intelligence testing (i.e. were tested at least twice).[56] They were all treated with RRT plus adjuvant therapy with vincristine, lomustine, and cisplatin. Using a statistical technique in which the predicted rate of change of IQ over time is defined by the average slope of all the individual subjects' curves, the authors reported a predicted fall of 17.4 points over four years from radiotherapy, from a baseline (measured after surgery) of 96.2. Similar results were reported for verbal and non-verbal subscores. Individuals with higher baseline scores had larger falls in IQ. Females ($n = 8$) and subjects aged less than seven years ($n = 27$) had larger falls in verbal IQ scores than males ($n = 32$) and those aged seven years or older ($n = 13$). The authors commented that the decline in IQ following reduced-dose radiotherapy in their patients did not appear to differ significantly from that reported in previous studies with standard-dose radiotherapy, but it corresponded to the rate of decline predicted from an earlier study of irradiation at the lower dose in leukemia.[32] They speculated that a follow-up period longer than four years was necessary, and that any subsequent further fall in IQ in their patients in the future might be less than that reported in some previous studies of SRT.[59] This might also be the case for growth and puberty outcomes.[38]

Despite the prospective and randomized design of these two trials in the commonest of brain tumors for which treatment choice exists, the logistical difficulties in obtaining the relevant information repeatedly has meant that comparisons had to be made between incomplete subgroups of, in some cases, fewer than ten children. The result is a lack of reliable evidence supporting the idea that reducing the dose of radiotherapy is beneficial, while the potentially detrimental effects of presenting status and surgery[60] remain untested.

It is regrettable that very little information on quality of survival is available on the large numbers of children enrolled in previous European trials of treatment for PNET. Attempts to rectify this omission for patients previously enrolled in two of these trials are currently in progress in a cross-sectional study, and health status, endocrine function, and health-related quality of life will be assessed longitudinally using standardized questionnaires in the International Society of Paediatric Oncology PNET 4 trial for children aged three years and over, which opened in 2002. Infants with PNET are at even greater risk of poor neurodevelopmental outcome,[61] and they may exhibit greater neurotoxicity and psychosocial consequences from chemotherapy followed by delayed irradiation.[62]

Intracranial germinoma

The difficulties described above in determining the quality of outcome in children with PNET are in contrast to the more complete ascertainment of outcome, albeit with less in-depth information, in the case of the much less common intracranial germinoma. This tumor can be treated effectively either with radiation therapy or with chemotherapy. A prevailing belief in the late 1980s that craniospinal irradiation must lead to poor quality of life prompted a move away from conventional radiation treatment towards a variety of chemotherapeutic regimens.

Some of the latter proved to have a lower event-free and overall survival than radiation therapy (UKCCSG review of patients registered from 1989 to 1994).

Two subsequent papers have obtained quality-of-life data on survivors treated over a 20-year period. Information was obtained on over 80 per cent of eligible patients by questionnaire. The findings suggested that their long-term health status and quality of life was, in fact, good, even in the large majority that had been treated with whole-brain or craniospinal irradiation ($n = 22, n = 20$, respectively, in the two studies).[63,64] Positive contributory factors are likely to include later age at presentation (usually adolescence) and relatively little tumor- or surgery-related disability. Thus, in this treatment context, the outcome of craniospinal irradiation is quite different from that reported in PNET, and the evidence seems to favor a different answer about irradiation toxicity than the prevailing belief in a high incidence of serious adverse effects. In this instance, changes for treatment have sometimes been driven more by belief or fashion than by evidence, even though useful data to inform treatment choice can be obtained, even in rare tumors, by brief questionnaire methods and simple endocrine surveillance.

Other tumor types

Similar controversies urgently require systematic data collection to inform treatment choices in many types of brain tumor, especially in the youngest children. These include low-grade glioma, including hypothalamic chiasmatic glioma (e.g. observation versus either chemotherapy or local radiation therapy), craniopharyngioma (e.g. radical surgery versus conservative surgery plus radiation therapy; see Chapter 20), and malignant tumors in infants (e.g. chemotherapy plus delayed local radiotherapy versus chemotherapy alone).

THE WAY FORWARD

Experiences such as that described above are now resulting in widening agreement on three issues:

- Information on quality of survival must be collected prospectively in trials of treatment for childhood brain tumors.
- Parent- and child-completed questionnaires are the most practicable method for achieving this.
- Functions such as hearing, vision, manipulative skills, mobility, cognition, growth, puberty and hormonal integrity, emotional well-being, behavior, and some measure of the parents' and child's perception of their health-related quality of life should be included in the assessment.

Detailed suggestions have been made (e.g. by Glaser and colleagues[57]) and continue to evolve, but firm recommendations must await the accumulation of more experience in using such methods. In general, it is likely that generic questionnaires will need to be supplemented by disease-specific questions, which will vary with the diagnosis and with the specific treatment-related toxicities expected.

The evidence base for rehabilitative interventions improving quality of outcome in these patient groups is, with the exception of hormone replacement, absent. Some would argue that multidisciplinary evaluation of, and provision for motor, sensory, cognitive, behavioral, and emotional difficulties are probably within the category of interventions with sufficient face validity not to require formal scientific evaluation, which would certainly be difficult to undertake. Similarly, communicating clear and comprehensible medical advice to schools and deployment of schooling support tailored to the needs of the individual, especially at important transitional phases (e.g. return to school, primary/secondary school transition, school/employment transition), seem clinically essential. However, these views remain a matter of commonsense rather than evidence. Ultimately, more specific information about the range and relative importance of different disabilities should not only inform anti-tumor treatment but also provide the basis for evaluation of specific rehabilitative strategies in several domains, perhaps including parenting, education, psychiatric intervention, and the acquisition of social skills.

REFERENCES

1 Jannoun L, Bloom H. Long-term psychological effects in children treated for intracranial tumors. *Int J Radiat Oncol Biol Phys* 1989; **18**:747.

2 Mulhern R, Wasserman A, Friedman A, Fairclough D. Social competence and behavioural adjustment of children who are long-term survivors of cancer. *Pediatrics* 1989; **83**:18–25.

3 Livesey E, Hindmarsh P, Brook C, *et al.* Endocrine disorders following treatment of childhood brain tumours. *Br J Cancer* 1990; **64**:622–5.

4 Littley M, Shalet S, CG B, Ahmed S, Applegate G, Sutton M. Hypopituitarism following external radiotherapy for pituitary tumours in adults. *Q J Med* 1989; **70**:145–60.

5 Lustig R, Rose S, Burghen G, *et al.* Hypothalamic obesity caused by cranial insult in children: altered glucose and insulin dynamics and reversal by a somatostatin agonist. *J Pediatr* 1999; **135**:162–8.

6 Société International de Oncologie Pédiatrique. Guidelines for School/education. *Med Pediatr Oncol* 1995; **24**:429–30.

7 Editorial. Quality of life. *Lancet* 1991; **338**:350–1.

8 Nayfield S, Ganz P, Moipour C, Cella D, Hailey B. Report from the National Cancer Institute (USA) workshop on quality of life assessment in cancer clinical trials. *Qual Life Res* 1992; **1**:203–10.

9 Medical Research Council. *The Assessment of MRC Trials 1996–97.* London: Medical Research Council, 1996.

10 Gill T, Feinstein A. A critical appraisal of the quality of life measurements. *J Am Med Assoc* 1994; **272**:619–26.

11 WHOQOL Group. *Measuring Quality of Life: The Development of the World Health Organization Quality of Life Instrument (WHOQOL).* Geneva: World Health Organization, 1993.

12 Bradlyn A, Ritchey A, Moore IEA. Quality of life research in pediatric oncology. *Cancer* 1996; **78**:1333–9.

13 Pantel R, Lewis C. Measuring the impact of medical care on children. *J Chronic Dis* 1987; **40** (suppl. 1):99–108S.

14 Guyatt G, Feeny D, Patrick D. Measuring health-related quality of life: basic sciences review. *Ann Intern Med* 1993; **118**:622–9.

15 Lindstrom B, Kohler L. Youth, disability and quality of life. *Pediatrician* 1991; **18**:121–8.

16 Jenney M, Campbell S. Measuring quality of life. *Arch Dis Child* 1997; **77**:347–54.

17 Jenney M, Kane R, Lurie N. Developing a measure of health outcomes in survivors of childhood cancer: a review of the issues. *Med Pediatr Oncol* 1995; **24**:145–53.

18 Rosenbaum P, Cadman D, Kirplani H. Pediatrics: assessing quality of life. In: Spiker B (ed.). *Quality of Life Assessments in Clinical Trials.* New York: Raven Press, 1990.

19 Natapoff J. Children's views of health: a developmental study. *Am J Publ Health* 1978; **68**:995–1000.

20 Perrin E, Gerrity P. There's a demon in your belly: children's understanding of illness. *Pediatrics* 1981; **67**:841–9.

21 Millstein S, Urwin C. Concepts of health and illness: different constructs or variations and a theme. *Health Psychol* 1987; **6**:515–24.

22 Eiser C, Morse R. Quality of life measures in chronic diseases of childhood. *Health Technol Assess* 2001; **5**:1–157.

23 Herjanic B, Reich W. Development of a structured psychiatric interview for children: agreement between child and parent on individual symptoms. *J Abnorm Psychol* 1982; **10**:307–24.

24 Glaser A, Davies K, Walker D, Brazier D. Influence of proxy respondents and setting on health status assessment following central nervous system tumours in childhood. *Qual Life Res* 1997; **6**:43–53.

25 Achenbach T, Edelbrock C. *Manual for the Child Behaviour Checklist and Revised Behaviour Profile.* Burlington, VT: University of Vermont, 1983.

26 Stone W, Lemanek K. Developmental issues in children's self-reports. In: La Greca A (ed.). *Through the Eyes of the Child: Obtaining Self-reports from Children and Adolescents.* Boston, MA: Allyn & Bacon, 1990, pp. 18–56.

27 Eiser C. Children's quality of life measures. *Arch Dis Child* 1997; **77**:347–54.

28 Glaser A, Furlong W, Walker D, *et al.* Applicability of the Health Utilities Index to a population of childhood survivors of central nervous system tumours in the UK. *Eur J Cancer* 1999; **35**:256–61.

29 Sackett D, Haynes R, Guyatt G, Tugwell P. *Clinical Epidemiology: A Basic Science for Clinical Medicine,* 2nd edn. Boston, MA: Little Brown, 1991.

30 Kee F. Patients' prerogatives and perceptions of benefit. *Br Med J* 1996; **312**:958–60.

31 Stiller C, Bunch K, Lewis I. Ethnic group and survival from childhood cancer: report from the UK Children's Cancer Study group. *Br J Cancer* 2000; **82**:1339–43.

32 Silber J, Radcliffe J, Peckham Vea. Whole brain irradiation and decline in intelligence. The influence of dose and age on IQ scores. *J Clin Oncol* 1992; **10**:1390–6.

33 Olshan J, Gubernick J, Packer R, *et al*. The effects of adjuvant chemotherapy on growth in children with medulloblastoma. *Cancer* 1992; **70**:2013–17.

34 Livesey E, Brook C. Gonadal dysfunction after treatment of intracranial tumours. *Arch Dis Child* 1988; **63**:495–500.

35 Ogilvy-Stuart A, Shalet S, Gattamaneni H. Thyroid function after treatment of brain tumors in children. *J Pediatr* 1991; **119**:733–7.

36 Kennedy C, Leyland K. Disability, emotional/behavioural disorders and health-related quality of life in survivors of childhood brain tumours. *Int J Cancer* 1999; **S12**:106–11.

37 Christie D, Leiper A, Chessells J, Vardga-Khadem F. Intellectual performance after presymptomatic cranial radiotherapy for leukaemia: effects of age and sex. *Arch Dis Child* 1995; **73**:136–40.

38 Uruena M, Stanhope R, Chessells J, Leiper A. Impaired pubertal growth in acute lymphoblastic leukaemia. *Arch Dis Child* 1991; **66**:1403–7.

39 Didi M, Didcock E, Davies H, Ogilvy-Stuart A, Wales J, Shalet S. High incidence of obesity in young adults after treatment of acute lymphoblastic leukemia in childhood. *J Pediatr* 1995; **127**:63–7.

40 Leiper A, Chessells J. Acute lymphoblastic leukaemia under two years. *Arch Dis Child* 1986; **61**:1007–12.

41 Anderson V, Smibert E, Ekert H, Godber T. Intellectual, educational and behavioral sequelae after cranial irradiation and chemotherapy. *Arch Dis Child* 1994; **70**:476–83.

42 Ball W, Prenger E, Ballard E. Neurotoxicity of radio/chemotherapy in children: pathologic and MR correlation. *Am J Neuroradiol* 1992; **13**:761–76.

43 Riva D, Giorgi C. The neurodevelopmental price of survival in children with malignant brain tumours. *Childs Nerv Syst* 2000; **16**:751–4.

44 Hertzberg H, Huk W, Uerball Mea. CNS late effects after ALL therapy in childhood. Part 1: neuroradiological findings in long-term survivors of childhood ALL – an evaluation of the interferences between morphology and neuropsychological performance. *Med Pediatr Oncol* 1997; **28**:387–400.

45 Darendeliler F, Livesey E, Hindmarsh P, Brook C. Growth and growth hormone secretion in children following treatment of brain tumours with radiotherapy. *Acta Paediatr Scand* 1990; **79**:121–7.

46 Spoudeas H, Hindmarsh P, Matthews D, Brook C. Evolution of growth hormone (GH) neurosecretory disturbance after cranial irradiation for childhood brain tumours: a prospective study. *J Endocrinol* 1996; **150**:329–42.

47 Mulhern R, Kepner J, Thomas P, Armstrong D, Friedman H, Kun L. Neuropsychological functioning of survivors of childhood medulloblastoma randomised to receive conventional or reduced dose craniospinal irradiation: a Pediatric Oncology Group study. *J Clin Oncol* 1998; **16**:1723–8.

48 Glauser T, Packer R. Cognitive deficits in long-term survivors of childhood brain tumours. *Childs Nerv Syst* 1991; **7**:2–12.

49 Gregory K, Parker L, Craft A. Returning to primary school after cancer. *Pediatr Hematol Oncol* 1994; **11**:105–9.

50 Johnson A. Follow-up studies: a case for a minimum data set. *Arch Dis Child* 1997; **76**:F61–3.

51 Mulhern R. Correlation of HUI2 cognition scale and neuropsychological functioning among survivors of childhood medulloblastoma. *Int J Cancer* 1999; **S12**:91–4.

52 Fooks J, Fritz S, Tin W, *et al*. A comparison of two methods of follow-up in a trial of prophylactic volume expansion in preterm babies. *Paediatr Perinat Epidemiol* 1998; **12**:199–216.

53 Fooks J, Mutch L, Yudkin P, Johnson A, Elbourne D. Comparing two methods of follow-up in a multi-centre randomised trial. *Arch Dis Child* 1997; **76**:369–76.

54 Mulhern R, Horowitz M, Kovnar E, Langston J, Sanford R, Kun L. Neurodevelopmental status of infants and young children treated for brain tumours with pre-irradiation chemotherapy. *J Clin Oncol* 1989; **7**:1660–6.

55 Mulhern R, Carpentieri S, Sherna S, Stone P, Fairclough D. Factors associated with social and behavioural problems among children recently diagnosed with brain tumour. *J Pediatr Psychol* 1993; **18**:339–50.

56 Ris M, Packer R, Goldwein J, Jones-Wallace D, Boyett J. Intellectual outcome after reduced-dose radiation therapy plus adjuvant chemotherapy for medulloblastoma: a Children's Cancer Group study. *J Clin Oncol* 2001; **19**:3470–6.

57 Glaser A, Kennedy C, Punt J, Walker D. A standardised strategy for qualitative assessment of brain tumour survivors treated within clinical trials in childhood. *Int J Cancer* 1999; **S12**:77–82.

58 Sparrow S, Balla D, Cicchetti D. *Adaptive Behavior Scales*. Minnesota: Circle Press, 1984.

59 Radcliffe J, Packer R, Atkins T, *et al*. Three and four year cognitive outcome in children with noncortical brain tumours treated with whole-brain radiotherapy. *Ann Neurol* 1992; **32**:551–4.

60 Kao G, Goldwein J, Schulz Dea. The impact of perioperative factors on subsequent intelligence quotient deficits in children treated for medulloblastoma/posterior fossa primitive neuroectodermal tumors. *Cancer* 1994; **74**:965–71.

61 Kiltie A, Lashford L, Gattamaneni H. Survival and late effects in medulloblastoma patients treated with craniospinal irradiation under three years old. *Med Pediatr Oncol* 1997; **28**:348–54.

62 Gajjar A, Mulhern R, Heidemann R, *et al*. Medulloblastoma in very young children: outcome of definitive craniospinal irradiation following incomplete response to chemotherapy. *J Clin Oncol* 1994; **12**:1212–16.

63 Kiltie A, Gattamaneni H. Survival and quality of life of paediatric intracranial germ cell tumour patients treated at the Christie Hospital 1972–1993. *Med Pediatr Oncol* 1995; **25**:450–6.

64 Sutton L, Radcliffe J, Goldwein Jea. Quality of life of adult survivors of germinomas treated with craniospinal irradiation. *Neurosurgery* 1999; **45**:1292–7.

28

Information needs for children and families

MARK L. GREENBERG, DARREN HARGRAVE AND JANE BOND

INTRODUCTION

There is no doubt that appropriate information to understand what is happening to them enables families to deal more effectively with the experience of childhood cancer, throughout treatment and follow-up. Families of children with brain tumors in New York identified medical information and education as one of the four key issues.[1] Other studies of family needs support this conclusion.[2,3]

The explanation of signs and symptoms of brain and spinal cord tumors, together with the rationale of treatment selection and prospects for follow-up, are overwhelming for parents and child. A systematic staged approach to the presentation of such a vast range of information carries the risk of adding to rather than alleviating the burden. The healthcare team has to understand the content and sources of information, the methods, process, and dynamics of information transfer, and the specific issues for each patient, parent, and family. The scope of information that is relevant, and the family's ability to understand, process and use it, evolve as the disease and its treatment unfold. Furthermore, new information derived from research emerges constantly and needs to be assimilated by the clinical team and the family. Acquisition and provision of information form a dynamic process that requires the active participation of both the healthcare team and the family. This chapter starts with a parent's view of information needs, describes a professional framework for meeting the information

needs of the child and family, and finally reviews current Internet techniques and sites relevant to the needs of the child with a brain tumor and their family.

A parent's view: closing the gaps

JANE BOND

It is three years since my daughter was diagnosed with a brain tumor at the age of nine. From the sunny uplands of remission, I can now look back on that time and see it demarcated into different stages, each with its attendant set of obstacles and emotions. This vantage point has been reached only after a benighted journey through a landscape so unfamiliar and so frightening that it was often possible to see only as far ahead as the next footstep.

My husband Chris and I were turned to rubble by the diagnosis. Work was out of the question; family life was instantly in tatters. There was a dislocating sense of unreality, as if we were floating in the corner of a room, watching a drama in which our bodily selves played foolish, bumbling characters that missed their cues and fluffed their lines. Everyone knew the plot except us.

Orienting ourselves in this alien landscape seemed impossible. The ground kept disappearing beneath our feet as we slid away, inexorably downwards, constantly overtaken by events, new complications, new disasters. First the bombshell news of the tumor, followed by surgery, then brain swelling and pneumonia, then further surgery, then back to intensive care with brainstem damage – cancer all the while sitting on the sidelines like the Grim Reaper sharpening his scythe.

The enormity of the diagnosis and rapidity of events swept away our ability to understand what was happening. Shock and grief establish their own priorities: only immediate information seemed relevant. Our underlying ignorance was too great to be addressed. Glasgow Coma Scale? We had never heard of it. It was nearly a week before I realized that Amy's pneumonia was not a "chill" with knobs on but a result of inhaling her own secretions during the operation. Either this had not been explained, or I had somehow missed the explanation.

Doctors and nurses imparted information in slow, simplistic, sound bites. While we were grateful for this, it also made us feel very stupid. It was the most catastrophic event in our daughter's life, yet instead of protecting and helping her we were reduced to the level of useless, passive cripples. Neither did it help to be asked if we had any questions. How can you ask a question when you have no vocabulary? Besides, the questions we could articulate – What is the reputation of this center? How qualified/experienced is the surgeon? – seemed too impolite to express. It takes a confident parent indeed to run the risk of alienating the medical professionals by questioning their very competence. It is astonishing how manners can get in the way of communications, even in extremis.

We needed to know who was who, what their status was, and where they fitted into the overall picture. A name and a job title were not enough. We wanted a diagram, a map of the whole maze. Without this overview, events seemed haphazard and arbitrary, and the comings and goings of doctors unfathomable. What to the professionals may have been a key meeting seemed to us like a snatched, accidental moment at the bottom of the bed. We had no access to the agenda, did not know what questions to ask. Everyone was busy with vitally important tasks, and there was no time at all for the basic, open-ended discussion we required.

If communications were hampered by lack of time, ignorance, and politeness, then they were stalled even more by the constant presence of my daughter, who for all but the first two days of the four months we were in hospital was unable to communicate. No one could guess what she might or might not want to hear, and our instinct was to protect her. Opportunities for discussion away from the bed were few and far between, and we frequently felt unable to hold the kind of frank discussion we wanted. It even felt sometimes as if the doctors knew this and used her presence as a way of inhibiting free and time-consuming debate. For me, if the price I had to pay for a direct exchange was that Amy, in her mute, paralyzed state, had to hear it too, then there was no option – I would have to do without.

What we needed at this time was access to independent, written material about the complications that can follow brain injury. We felt we were trying to piece together a picture when we had only a few bits of the jigsaw. We had the conflicting opinions implied by the behavior of the professionals, the undisguised dismay of the friends and relatives who came to visit Amy, as well as the unsought reactions of every Tom, Dick, and Harry who came into contact with us: the well-meaning parent who told me that six months after her son's brain injury in a road accident, she had finally accepted that miracles don't happen; the paramedic who assumed Amy had been "born that way;" the therapists keen to equip us with wheelchairs, feed machines, and stairlifts for the life ahead.

Without an overview to put things in perspective, small events took on a significance that they did not merit, and key information was obscured. My daughter's radiotherapy, for example, was carried out at a different hospital, and the practical arrangements for this were chaotic. Rationally, we knew that the quality of the actual treatment was not linked to these organizational difficulties. Emotionally, it undermined our confidence. In a vivid nightmare, a casual young radiographer shot indiscriminate bursts of radiation at all three of my children from a kind of machine gun, while I politely said nothing. Absurd, maybe, but it articulated my deepest fears that perhaps everything really was out of control and there was nothing I could do about it. Actions sometimes speak louder than words, and if the surface that the parents see is disorganized, confused, and contradictory, then this will drown out any verbal reassurances from doctors.

This tendency to fill the gaps with terrifying imaginings was a destructive and energy-sapping experience. Reading between the lines became a pastime, aggravated by the reticence of the professionals. The non-committal silence that descends on medical and nursing staff when the prognosis is uncertain creates a gulf so wide that you can feel the wind blow through it. The feeling of being excluded from some terrible professional secret is inescapable. It leaves parents stranded in a no-man's land of uninformed speculation. Chris and I would sit miserably having "What if ...?" conversations. What if her brain had been deprived of oxygen? What if the damage was irreparable? What if there was something we were not being told?

It was a land of inference and insinuation, full of "may," "might," "possibly," and "perhaps," where everything was implicit, nothing explicit. On the one hand we had nurses who treated our daughter as if she could hear, see, and understand everything; on the other we had those who clearly felt she had been reduced to the level of an infant. We had one doctor who referred obliquely to "miracles," another who repeatedly shook his head and said one word – "Terrible."

My first instinct on hitting any problem is to read around the subject. Trapped in hospital for weeks on end dealing with Amy's day-to-day care, we were cut off from other sources of information – books, friends, the Internet. We had no opportunity, time, or energy to research things for ourselves. Requests for written material from the hospital met with an apologetic shrug and a tiny leaflet on children's brain tumors that was pitched at a laughably low level. Any grown-up, whatever their educational status, would have required more information than this if they were taking out a mortgage or buying a new car, let alone dealing with a matter of life and death for their child. I had managed to get hold of an American booklet through the hospital patients' library. It was good, but it was short. Salvation came in the form of a book sent by my father. Written by Patricia M. Davies, it was called *Starting Again*, and it was about rehabilitation after brain injury. It was full of practical information, explanations, and graphic photos. One picture showed a boy of 12 with a twisted torso and useless arms. The frontispiece showed him as a young man ... windsurfing. The book was about brain damage, not brain tumors, but it was what I needed.

Further enlightenment came when a doctor gave us a book on neurosurgery, with a section marked for us to read. He was clearly worried that the pictures would upset us, that we would get confused or burden ourselves with irrelevant anxieties. We got the impression that giving us the book was a calculated risk. It came with a warning that we should not go reading the rest of it. It was a turning point. The marked section was about cerebellar mutism, the syndrome affecting Amy. All the worrying symptoms – the total inability to communicate, the obsessive, repetitive tics, the almost autistic withdrawal from the world – were described. We were not in uncharted waters after all. At last we had a map.

Of course, we scoured the rest of the book. Tell Pandora not to open the box and she will be delving away before you can say "sin." At an earlier stage, an officious doctor told me I could not see my daughter's notes or read a letter pertaining to her treatment. I would have to apply, I would have to pay, and in any case the notes might upset me.

Upset me? My daughter had cancer and brain damage. What possible piece of ink and paper could upset me more than this? What image could be more gruesome than the reality of my own child's flaccid, dribbling face? Or more confusing than the mixed messages that bombarded me every day on the ward? I was becoming increasingly irritated by the notion that other people seemed to think they knew what was best for me and that information was being rationed out, piecemeal, at what were deemed appropriate stages. Well-meaning though this approach was, helpful even in the first few days, it eventually made me feel that I was being kept in the dark.

There will never be an equal partnership between parents and doctors/nurses. Most parents would not wish for an equal partnership – we want a level of perfection and detachment from the professionals caring for our children that we do not possess ourselves – but there is one area where there can and should be a level playing field, and that is in the sharing of information. Current practices regarding the keeping of medical and nursing notes do nothing to nurture a culture of transparency and openness. The discovery that not only my daughter's condition but also my own state of mental distress had been recorded in the nursing notes left me feeling even more like a laboratory rat trapped in a maze. My emotional state had been recorded, but my opinions and concerns had not. It seemed that I was regarded as an honorary patient, not a partner.

The thing that would have made the single biggest difference to our experience in hospital is the thing most difficult to come by: more "parent-only" time with the doctors. Given that this is a tall order, there are two other simple steps that would have improved things: (i) a wide-ranging ward library of written background information, and (ii) access to and regular discussion of our child's notes.

Our hypocrisy knew no bounds when it came to sharing information with Amy. Everything we told her was edited carefully, with an upbeat, positive spin on it. If anyone said anything negative in front of her, I would whisper contradictions in her ear as soon as they had gone. The ghoulish radiotherapy doll and scary video I was supposed to show her stayed in the cupboard. I wasn't going to dump this load on a child who couldn't respond, and I hated everyone for suggesting that I should.

I think I would have felt and behaved differently if Amy had not been in such a passive state. Everything would have been easier if she had been able to react, ask questions, discuss things, cry. Maybe I would even have managed a bit of honesty. By the time she came back to us, things had moved on so far that there seemed little point in going back over old ground. When she was first able to communicate, which she did with the aid of a speaking machine, it became apparent that she had taken in quite a lot. She had acquired a medical vocabulary and could even spell most of the words. Yet to this day, she asks few questions about her illness and seems intent on getting on with her life. I think this is natural, healthy, and desirable. Burdening a child with adult notions of "honesty" and "truth" is pointless and seems to me to have more to do with preserving some abstract professional integrity than with providing what is constructive for the child and family.

Going home felt like escaping from prison. We wanted to pull up the drawbridge, batten down the hatches, and never speak to or see a doctor or nurse again. The horrible realization that we had become part of a "cancer network" that meant the unsought delivery of brown envelopes containing newsletters, magazines, and invitations to support groups made us feel like nailing up the letterbox too.

Radiotherapy over, all we could do was wait and see whether if had worked. We had had enough of cancer, and we didn't want to know any more. Practical help with rehabilitation was what we needed now. A meeting set up before we left hospital augured well for our return home. We were promised physiotherapy, speech therapy, occupational therapy, community nurses, a community pediatrician, a statement of special educational needs …

I have spent the past two and a half years trying to close the gap between this veneer of words and the crumbly, under-funded structure it covers. I have all the written information I need, enough words to sink a ship, when all I really want is a little bit of action.

It has taken every communication skill I possess to get my daughter what she needs to recover from her brain injury. I have negotiated by phone, by letter, and in person, I have begged, cried, used emotional blackmail, surfed the Internet, scoured the papers, got angry with people, and sought out complementary therapies. During the course of this process, I have grown a second head that babbles jargon and fluently rehearses the litany of my daughter's disabilities in order to secure her the help she needs.

I do not like this second head, but it is a necessary evil. If it has to do a lot of talking (for instance, if I am arguing the case for more educational support in school), I can end up getting depressed by my own punctilious enumeration of all Amy's difficulties, but the system will not deliver for children unless parents learn this role. Key people within the system have been invaluable in helping me learn to play this part. I just have to make sure I don't lose sight of my real feelings: my relief, joy, and gratitude that I still have Amy, whatever the problems.

Communications with hospital have improved since we escaped from its clutches. We were allowed to get off the knife-edge of constant scans as soon as we had a clear one. We have just enough appointments to reassure us that everything is well, and we know we will get an immediate response if we have any concerns. We have stopped putting *Contact* magazine (a UK parents' magazine concerned with childhood cancer) in the bin. We have even reached the stage where we feel pleased to see the hospital staff again. And I never thought I would say that!

Jane Bond's piece has described graphically the parents' experience as their child is diagnosed and treated and recovers. The first step is breaking the news that a brain tumor has been found.

SETTING THE CONTEXT FOR BREAKING THE NEWS

The context in which bad news is conveyed has significant impact on the reception and processing it receives.

Attempts have been made to define some of the components that facilitate the process and minimize the distress of the family. The Scope guidelines were developed by parents who had been told of their child's handicap/disability.[4] These guidelines identify conditions to be considered by the clinician when planning to break bad news. The SPIKES program defines a six-step protocol to be followed when breaking bad news to families.[5] SPIKES summarizes six successive steps in accomplishing complex communication: (i) creating appropriate interview *setting* and circumstances; (ii) determining the patient's *perception*, comprehension, and current state of mind regarding the medical situation to date; (iii) *inviting* patients/parents to identify how, when, and how much information they wish to receive; (iv) providing *knowledge* in small and understandable bites, with repeated inquiry as to patient/parent comprehension; (v) assessing and addressing the parents' and patient's *emotions* and reactions, with an emphasis on moving on to other issues only when the patients/parents are ready; and (vi) generating a *strategy* and *summary*, in which the patient is capable of discussing treatment options, the family's specific, disease-related goals are identified, and in which staff contend with their own difficult emotional reactions. Both approaches are well founded and provide a useful framework for the disclosure process, although they will need to be adapted for individual practitioners' styles of practice, having at the forefront of consideration the best interests of the child and family.

ESTABLISHING A COMMON LANGUAGE AND VOCABULARY

Central to the successful development of shared understanding is the establishment of a common language of healthcare. Most lay-directed guidebooks and self-help texts include glossaries to define words used in clinical practice and that have no meaning or anchor for the newly exposed families. Continued attention to these definitions will prevent misunderstanding of information obtained from outside sources and prove helpful to families at every stage.

THE MULTIDISCIPLINARY/MULTIPROFESSIONAL TEAM AND THEIR ROLES

The different roles of members of the multiprofessional team need early explanation, so that it is clear which specialists will make decisions regarding clinical strategies and treatments. The diversity of professional roles is confounding and requires careful explanation. It is important that families understand that any member of the team will reflect the consensus opinion of the team. Where advanced practice nurses are involved, the specific nature of their role must be clarified and differentiated from that of the bedside nurse. As different specialists become involved over the course of the illness, they should be introduced and their roles identified.

WHO PROVIDES THE INFORMATION AND EDUCATION?

There are at least two components to achieving understanding in parents and families. One is provision of information; the other is achieving their education. Providing information ensures that the family and the child are in possession of the facts that are relevant and appropriate to their circumstances. Achieving education implies that they have understood and are able to apply these facts in decision-making and understanding of their own situation.

Many people are involved in decision-making, and the use of consistent language is key to successful communication between specialists and with children and their families. Communication with the families is achieved best by designating a single individual who fulfils the role of the primary communicator. Where therapy involves multiple modalities of treatment, that individual will most often be the oncologist. Other team specialists will have roles explaining aspects of their own particular intervention, e.g. surgery or radiotherapy.

It is now naive to think that the primary source of information is the clinical professionals. While there is evidence to suggest that the primary physician is still the preferred source of information,[4] the Internet is a major secondary source. Awareness that information provided by the caregivers will be compared with that derived from the Internet or other sources requires health professionals to have knowledge of the content of key websites and other published literature.

The interpretation and assimilation of information can be facilitated by the advanced practice nurse or equivalent, with a view to enhancing understanding and modifying behaviors throughout the patient's journey.

WHO NEEDS WHAT INFORMATION AND IN WHAT FORMAT?

All members of the family need information appropriate for their needs at the time. Parents are the first targets, even when the patient is an adolescent. Material developed for children's understanding is often more effective in starting the adults along the right lines of comprehension. The level of complexity of information and the format in which it is most useful are determined by many factors. The level of education, the primary language of communication, and the cultural and social background are important determinants, as is familiarity with and access to the Internet. In general, providing access to a wide range of material allows people to choose that which is most useful.

It is helpful if parents have material, in whatever format, reflecting the content of the discussion to take away from interviews. This may be written material, drawings, diagrams, flow sheets, or video cassettes. This sort of information can provide a framework for subsequent discussions.

Siblings have a significant need for information.[5] Whether professionals or parents provide this will vary with the circumstances and preferences. Education of the extended family may help the parents cope; however, this is usually beyond the scope of the treatment team. This deficit can be addressed through educational symposia, public lectures, TV programs, and open forums addressing relevant topics in a general context. Inclusion of extended family members in contacts with the clinical team at certain stages of the treatment journey can be very helpful in achieving the goal of an educated family.

INFORMATION NEEDS OVER THE COURSE OF THE DISEASE

Before definitive diagnosis

THE PARENTS' NEEDS

Many, but not all, parents whose child develops neurological symptoms may consider a brain tumor as one of the likely diagnoses. The process of making or excluding this diagnosis should be the focus of the initial exchange of information. Explanations of reasons for symptoms and the likelihood of their permanence/capacity for recovery is critical, as are descriptions of forthcoming procedures and surgical procedures.

The results of the imaging studies must be communicated clearly. Description of these findings allows an explanation of the link between functional neuroanatomy and symptoms. Furthermore, it is central to planning surgery, which is most frequently the first intervention. The intent of the surgical procedure should be explained and may require the introduction of concepts such as biopsy, partial removal, and non-resectability. When surgical intervention is not planned, the reason for this requires explanation. The reasons for not resecting, for example, an optic pathway glioma differ from those for not resecting a brainstem glioma, but it is not uncommon for parents to draw incorrect conclusions.

The purpose and implications of shunt placement, if planned, requires explanation, as does any anticipated ancillary procedure, such as central-line placement. An outline of the most likely postoperative events, including how the child will look and behave when they wake up, whether the child will be on the intensive care unit, the need for postoperative investigations for staging, and again the anticipated delay while pathologic characterization occurs, is very important information for parents in limbo.

THE CHILD'S NEEDS

The principal need for most children at this stage is an answer to the question, "What is happening to me?" The underlying process is of less concern in the first instance than is the explanation of the immediate clinical events. A direct explanation of symptoms, and what will be done to relieve them, will achieve the most reassurance.

After the definitive diagnosis is established

THE PARENTS' NEEDS

There is a need to clarify and expand the common vocabulary in addition to providing specific information about this particular child and disease. Information groupings include:

- *The nature, biology, and behavior of brain tumors in general and the child's tumor in detail*: concepts of benign and malignant as they apply to brain tumors need clarification. Explanation of low-grade tumors that produce lethal effects by compression may be appropriate. A basic explanation of what cells are, and concepts of normal and disordered cell growth, will be understood by most parents and will allow a grasp of the biology that will determine therapy. The name and nature of the tumor must be specified clearly, in part to ensure that the search for information from the Internet targets the appropriate information. Differences between adult and pediatric tumors with the same name are important in this regard, most notably with regard to astrocytomas. When a specific diagnosis has been dependent on a particular molecular or immunophenotypic characteristic, then it is valuable to identify that characteristic. Where appropriate, the concepts of metastasis and cerebrospinal pathway axis spread need explanation, and the staging findings and their implications in this patient need to be made clear. Questions of causation merit particular attention. Most parents will ask about causation; while the question is in part a straightforward request for

information, there is also an implicit question – what did I do, or not do, to cause my child's cancer? It is important to address both components of the question. Where there are known associations, e.g. heritable conditions, careful explanation in a manner that avoids assumption of blame is appropriate. The other component addresses direct parental culpability, and articulating that neither anything done by the parents, nor anything not done by them, has any role in causation may answer the implicit question.

- *Neuroanatomy and its implications*: an understanding of the organization of brain structures is important. A grasp of structure–function relationships will allow better comprehension of the functional impact of the tumor and of the surgical and radiotherapy interventions. A basic explanation of where it was anatomically, and what the functional role of this part of the brain is, will allow an honest explanation of the nature of the resulting functional disability from the tumor or its treatment. The timing for this explanation will vary from family to family. A balance must be struck between giving honest predictions of disability and capacity for recovery, whilst maintaining a mood of optimism and hope. It is our experience that removal of hope is the single most devastating experience for families from which they sometimes never recover. The possible extent of the disability should not be understated, but reasonable optimism and hope should be both permitted and encouraged.

- *Therapeutic interventions*: treatment protocols that specify the overall aims of therapy, the program of investigation, and treatment events are often given to the parents. In general, their use by the team ensures shared understanding. However, in this discussion, a balance must be struck between casting the protocol as absolute, instilling the fear that any deviation is detrimental (a fear often triggered if therapy is delayed for complications) and framing it too casually as a general guide that can be changed arbitrarily.

- *Clinical trials*: clinical trials, as distinct from protocols, require careful explanation, since parents are encountering, probably for the first time, concepts of standard therapy, experimental arms, and randomization. Description of the process by which clinical trials are developed and monitored for safety may be reassuring. When approaching a newly diagnosed child and family for consent to participate in a clinical trial, the guidelines for obtaining informed consent laid out in the Helsinki Declaration must be followed. These include the obligation of the investigator/clinician to inform potential participants in a clinical research study of the aims, methods, sources of funding, possible conflicts of interest, institutional affiliations of the researcher, the anticipated benefits and potential risks of the study, and the discomfort it may entail. For legally incompetent minors, the legally authorized representative or guardian must consent; where the child is competent, assent should be obtained from the child in accordance with national guidelines. Where a trial is not currently open, then the standard therapy should be the best, currently available therapy based on established evidence. Surgical intervention will probably already have occurred by the time of definitive diagnosis. The limitations of surgery and the potential for future second-look procedures, where appropriate, merit explanation. Explanations of radiation and chemotherapies must be undertaken if they are to be applied. The depth with which each is approached may be modified according to the sequence within the protocol.

- *Radiation therapy*: radiation therapy is a complex and unfamiliar idea to most parents. The explanation needs to address a variety of technical and clinical issues in order to allay anxieties. It should include a description of the roles of staff involved in radiation delivery, the principles of high-energy directed beams, the machinery that produces them, and the systems used to ensure safety and accuracy (see Chapter 10). The processes of planning, simulation, and mould-creation should be described, and the number and frequency of individual fractions should be explained. The short- and long-term effects of radiotherapy on the tumor and the brain demand extensive discussion. Accurate description and methods of management of short-term toxicities will encourage parental participation in care. More difficult is an explanation of long-term neurotoxic, endocrine, and cosmetic consequences. This needs to be accurate but not overwhelming. Much skill and understanding is required to frame the cost–benefit ratio of its use; not all families will accept the justification, and discussions can be prolonged.
- *Chemotherapy*: principles underlying chemotherapy, mechanisms of action of various chemotherapeutic agents, the rationale for combination chemotherapy, and specific details of administration (including route and frequency) of the particular drugs involved must be described, including short-term and long-term toxicities. Other members of the multiprofessional team can assist, e.g. specialist nurses and clinical pharmacists support in-depth teaching of these principles in many centers, with evidence of effectiveness.[6] The initial description of the intended chemotherapy should come from the oncologist taking responsibility for the decision. The longer-term toxicities of some of the agents used may be of concern to parents, and a balanced discussion of major long-term effects, such as hearing loss, infertility, and second malignant neoplasms in the context of the contribution to survival, is necessary. Framing the balance between the risk of such adverse events offset against the proven benefits is key to parental perspective and understanding.

- *Family organization*: the diagnosis and therapy of a brain or spinal cord tumor predictably creates chaos in the lives of the parents involved. In addition to a functional understanding of the major components of therapy and of expectation of treatment outcomes, sharing information at the onset of the process should convey a sense of the major adaptations that will be necessary in the family's lifestyle. When communicated adequately, the information will allow families to plan the next period of their life and to draw on resources available to them.
- *Potential outcomes*: the prospect for survival is the foremost issue for parents initially. Probabilistic estimates are commonly used, but the uncertainty of prognosticating for any given patient should be emphasized. To endure the intensity of therapy that will ensue, most parents need to hear an estimate of survival probability and to incorporate that estimate within a belief that their particular child is likely to be in the group of survivors. Most parents need information about two other dimensions of outcome: the likelihood of disability and the long-term effects of therapy. Some parents need to have this information at the outset, but others prefer to deal with it later. One approach is to table these two outcomes at the beginning and then to follow the parents' lead as to the extent to which they wish to discuss long-term outcomes when survival is the principal issue. Where long-term outcomes of a particular treatment are so poor that they dictate the rejection of therapy, as was seen with craniospinal irradiation in young infants, this should be explained.

THE CHILD'S NEEDS

A simple, truthful, articulate, age-adjusted statement of the diagnosis begins the dialog effectively. The terms that will be encountered over the course of treatment should be explained.

There is value in diagrammatic, visual, and verbal descriptive explanations of tumors, cancer, chemotherapy, and the process of radiation therapy. The purpose is to provide information in an age-adjusted manner and to explain the frightening components of treatment that the child will have to endure. The acute side effects of treatment must be laid out in a manner that allows the child to understand and incorporate them into their life. It is possible to explain all of this without unduly scaring the child. Too much information may be overwhelming, and the child may do better with information that will allow him or her to deal effectively with the next step, rather than grappling with the multiple steps involved in the overall care.

The process of explaining both the disease and the treatment may be aided significantly when dealing with younger children by involving expertise in the use of therapeutic play (see Chapter 10). Child life specialists or equivalent experts are often able to convey non-verbally some of the information that might not be appreciated properly by a preverbal or young child when conveyed in words. Engagement in active play simulating some of the medical interventions that will occur often provides a safe context for transmitting information in this age group, which can translate into enhanced confidence and cooperation.

Preadolescent and adolescent children in particular may ask about prognosis. Most often, this is framed as a very direct question: am I going to die? For most children, the honest answer – without treatment you would die, but the treatment you will receive will hopefully stop that from happening – is reassuring. Honesty remains key, and although no absolute assurances should be given, a confident and assured reply to this question is usually enough to calm fears and stimulate trust and confidence.

During therapy

THE PARENTS' NEEDS

The duration of therapy is protracted in most central nervous system (CNS) tumors, and parental exhaustion and frustration are frequent. Periodic review of the child's status and course is helpful. The advanced practice nurse has a pre-eminent role to play in this process. Before each course of therapy, review of the drugs and the duration of treatment enables parents to review their planning and arrangements. Status reports and evaluation of response, clinical and radiologic, at strategic intervals provide the opportunity to identify concerns, to discuss information obtained from other sources, and to permit open discussion of complementary and alternative methods of treatment that may be in use (see Chapter 25).

The impact of delays in delivery treatment according to protocol therapy may concern parents, and it is important to discuss the inevitability of some delay, e.g. infections, and the fact that the next phase of treatment cannot start until the complications of the previous phase are settled. Furthermore, identifying the apparent lack of adverse impact on outcome is helpful.

At the outset of treatment on protocol, a commitment is made, and stated explicitly in informed consents, to updating parents on developments in the context of the response of the child's tumor and in the execution of the clinical trial. While new developments that are directly relevant may not occur, parents often read accounts of "breakthroughs" in the press; it is important for the treating team to be aware of these reports and to address them, either on request or, if important enough, pre-emptively.

THE CHILD'S NEEDS

For the majority of children, the focus during therapy is the therapy itself rather than the disease. All relevant information addressing each portion of therapy must be provided before the treatment. What will hurt or cause discomfort, and what will be done to alleviate that discomfort, should be laid out. Reminders of how effectively the symptom was controlled the last time it occurred are often reassuring. All anxiety cannot be forestalled, but a child informed of what they must deal with, and assisted to do so by such allied professionals as child life specialists, is more likely to tolerate interventions with less anxiety.

At the end of therapy

THE PARENTS' NEEDS

The end of therapy is both a time of elation and a very difficult time for families. Parents and children are facing the difficult task of balancing anxiety and hope. There is a transition from close and regular contact with the treating team to more irregular contact, and the withdrawal of therapy that has come to be perceived as crucial in maintaining remission. Families feel vulnerable, and the provision of factual information has the potential to ease this task substantially.

Formal review of factual information can be helpful. Summary of the treatment that has occurred, an explanation of the schedule for follow-up visits, imaging, and other monitoring studies, and reiteration of why continuing therapy offers no benefit can be helpful. Realistic appraisal of the likelihood of continued disease control is valuable and can be couched optimistically. Careful, sensitive instruction regarding the clinical signs and symptoms of recurrence, and reassurance that the normal complaints of childhood will occur and do not indicate recurrence, are important.

Questions about treatment options in the event of recurrence often arise at this juncture. The acknowledgment that options exist, if realistic, can be helpful, but in-depth discussion of those options and their likelihood of success is not.

THE CHILD'S NEEDS

For the younger child, the end of therapy is less stressful than for the parents. For preadolescents and adolescents, anxiety around discontinuation of therapy may be similar to that experienced by the parents. Similar reassurance about normal physical symptoms and their lack of sinister significance is especially important in this age group. The ongoing follow-up and monitoring schedule, and the plans for rehabilitation where appropriate, will maintain the sense of connection, and a realistic assessment of the child's potential and limitations, focusing on abilities rather than limitations, is important in orienting the child to a future. Connecting children to support groups may be of particular benefit at this time.

INFORMATION ADDRESSING THE LATE EFFECTS OF TREATMENT

As the active phase of treatment recedes, the anxiety around relapse may diminish and be replaced by concern about the late effects of treatment and the disease. While attempts will have been made to address some of these issues during the active phase of treatment, the focus during that time is directed most appropriately at treatment and survival. The late effects move into focus more dominantly when it appears that survival is likely. Many tertiary-care centers are developing late-effects or after-care clinics that monitor routinely for known late effects. Involvement of the parents and the child in monitoring for late effects and in addressing them requires that appropriate information about them be provided. Information might encompass growth failure as a result of irradiation, hypothyroidism, neurocognitive dysfunction, and chemotherapy consequences such as hearing loss, infertility, and second primary malignancy (see Chapter 24). Parental awareness of these late outcomes, in conjunction with organized programs to address them, may ameliorate their impact. Early intervention with regard to neurocognitive delay is imperative and is part of a continuum between active treatment and the after-care setting. If appropriate information is provided to parents and via them to educators, then the educational consequences may be mitigated. For patients in whom significant neurocognitive dysfunction becomes a reality, information about vocational opportunities, and the availability of vocational assessment and training programs, is likely to result in the most productive outcomes for the survivors of childhood brain tumors.

At relapse

THE PARENTS' NEEDS

Independent of the prospect of a second remission, relapse is described as more devastating than the original diagnosis. The optimism most parents find at initial diagnosis is replaced by the reality that despite all that has been endured, the tumor has recurred. The vocabulary and issues are no longer mysterious, parents are knowledgeable, and the communications by the treatment team must acknowledge this altered parental state.

The precise nature of the relapse must be defined for the parent. The implications of the relapse, whether it is local or distant, and the overall neurologic and general status of the child will be factors that will bear on the subsequent parental decision-making.

The recognition of relapse imposes a speed of decision-making that may pre-empt thoughtful consideration of the goals of subsequent therapy by parents and may therefore influence the choices they make. These goals must be clarified by provision of realistic information about potential outcomes and the implications of continuation of therapy after relapse that are likely to be non-curable.[7,8]

Available protocols for relapse are usually phase I or II studies (see Chapter 8). Where potential exists for cure or substantial prolongation of life, this should be defined clearly and realistically. Where the probability is for short-term prolongation of life, then that too should be defined clearly, as should the potential toxicity. Where a phase I study is the primary option, then the intent of phase I studies must be defined clearly. Parents may choose to enter their child into such a study out of the faint hope of cure or significant prolongation of life, or out of altruism, but they can do so knowledgeably only if the pertinent information has been presented unambiguously. The advent of agents that are targeted molecularly may alter the concept of phase I studies in a way that focuses on optimal dose to achieve biologic effect rather than on maximally tolerated dose, and may alter the decision-making process for parents.

Relapse is often a time when parents seek second opinions, which may be valuable to parents and treating physicians. It is preferable for the treating physician to request the second opinion and to provide all relevant information. Where parents choose to seek their own second opinion, the treating physician should provide the same information to assure that the individual providing a second opinion does not do so on incomplete or inaccurate information. Physicians asked to provide a second opinion should communicate with the treating physician directly to ensure that they have all the appropriate information, and to ensure that their recommendations are conveyed accurately. The initial treating team has an ongoing relationship with the family and has an obligation both to consider second opinions and to advise on their assessment of the applicability of the advice of the second opinion.

THE CHILD'S NEEDS

The burden imposed by relapse may be felt as intensely by the child as by the parents, particularly by the older child who has better appreciation of the implications. The difficulty of providing appropriate information at this time is complicated by the need to respect parental wishes. For the older child, however, full disclosure, in terms that are understandable, is necessary. If it is possible to convey the information in a way that allows congruence between the parents' and the child's understanding, then identifying the goals of therapy after relapse will be easier. Optimally, decisions affecting older children and adolescents will be made together by parents and child, with the input and advice of the treating team. In the event of dissent between parents and a competent child, the treatment team is placed in a very difficult situation. Under these circumstances, it is crucial to ensure that all parties have accurate information and that the advice resulting from second opinions, if sought, is provided to both the child and the parents.

INFORMATION ADDRESSING SUPPORT AND COPING, AND OTHER SOURCES OF INFORMATION

In early and ongoing phases of management, the need for practical assistance in maintaining home functions and financial viability, and for strategies to enable coping with the burden of illness, are addressed by hospital-based social workers or equivalent professionals. Counseling, provision of resource material, referral to community agencies, and provision of information concerning available practical support from government agencies, formal volunteer organizations such as cancer societies, and other support groups will usually be provided. Psychological services on an individual or family basis may be provided, and hospital-based support groups often exist. In skilled hands, these group settings may provide invaluable assistance. Some limited literature suggests that group interventions such as sibling support groups and parent support groups may have substantial benefit.[9,10]

One of the roles of the extended treatment team is to guide families to sources of information, support, and assistance in dealing with the burden of the illness. Resources from within the hospital or community treating team are invaluable, but they necessarily view illness through an institutional lens. The experiences of individuals who have traversed a similar path, or of an objective group not involved with direct care of the particular child, will add to the richness of supportive resources and expand the range of sources substantially.

Resource books

A substantial proportion of parents will prefer to have hard copy to refer to. Many excellent resource books, some oriented to childhood cancer in general, and some to childhood brain and spinal cord tumors, are available.[7,11–14] Some resource books are best used in conjunction with the Web or with other aids.

The Internet

The Internet has become the fastest adopted means of electronic communication in history, outpacing the adoption of the telegraph, telephone, television, and video. The estimated global audience for 2002 was 500 million users, with the fastest-growing community now being the Asian continent after a slowdown in growth after saturation (>50 per cent population access) in Europe and North America.[15] However, these developed countries are now experiencing acceleration in upgrading to high-speed (broadband) Internet connection.

CANCER INFORMATION ON THE INTERNET

Inevitably, health information has been distributed on the Internet. Its growth has been unplanned and unregulated, which has raised concerns for both patients and healthcare professionals.[16] Exceptions to this uncontrolled development have been the CancerNet,[17] Oncolink,[18] and National Cancer Institute (NCI) websites, which have provided the standard for oncology information. Currently, there are very few data on Internet usage in the area of pediatric oncology; most data come from adult studies.[19] A Canadian survey questioned both adult cancer patients and their oncologists about health information and the Internet:[20] 86 per cent of 191 patients surveyed wanted as much information as possible, 54 per cent reported receiving insufficient information from their healthcare team, and 50 per cent had used the Internet to search for cancer information, with the majority stating a positive experience. In contrast, 70 per cent of the 420 oncologists reported paying some attention to cancer-related information in the media and on the Internet as a whole, and the majority (85 per cent) felt that the information was only sometimes or rarely accurate. This difference in opinion between healthcare professionals and their patients about the quality of information has been reported in other studies and is now a topic of some debate about how to ensure quality health information on the Internet.[21]

INFORMATION QUALITY ON THE INTERNET

Suggested mechanisms for regulating consumer health information include codes of conduct (e.g. the American Medical Association[22]), self-applied quality labels (e.g. Hi-Ethics code), quality filters (e.g. OMNI gateway[23]), third-party quality rating (e.g. MedCERTAIN accreditation[24]), and user scoring systems (e.g. the DISCERN rating tool[25]). A number of studies in oncology have looked at the quality of cancer website information in specific cancers. One group concluded that information in Ewing sarcoma was inaccurate in only six per cent of websites, but the quality of content was of concern in many sites evaluated.[26] Another group looked at melanoma websites; they found an inaccuracy rate of 14 per cent and again a lack of basic information/quality in a significant number of sites.[27] Interestingly, a study looking at breast cancer sites found that popularity with health consumers was related not to quality but rather to type of site.[28]

INTERNET INFORMATION PROJECT: CHILDHOOD BRAIN TUMORS

We have preliminary pilot data on rating the quality of Internet health information in childhood medulloblastoma and ependymoma.[29] We used the validated DISCERN rating tool, which has been developed by Oxford University, the National Health Service (NHS) executive, and the British Library to assist health consumers in judging the quality of health information.[30] We also looked at content for 13 headings (e.g. "treatment," "staging," "prognosis," etc.). We searched the Internet using the simple terms "medulloblastoma" and "ependymoma" in the top six US search engines and evaluated the top 30 links in each condition for each of the six searches. Many links (>60 per cent) were duplicates of each other. If a site gave general information on the topic, then it was evaluated independently by two pediatric oncologists. There was excellent agreement between the observers (DISCERN kappa score 0.82, content kappa score 0.92). The sites were categorized into five groups (excellent to very poor) based on content and the score generated by the DISCERN tool. Half the sites were academic in origin, 13 per cent were charity-based, 12 per cent were hospital sites, and the rest comprised commercial, support group, or personal pages. We found a median inaccuracy rate of eight per cent and a median 53 per cent inclusion rate for basic cancer content (i.e. diagnostic process, treatment, etc.). No site was categorized as excellent, eight per cent were good, 23 per cent were fair, 57 per cent were poor, and 12 per cent were very poor. There was no correlation with type of site (i.e. some good commercial/support group sites and some poor academic/ hospital sites existed, and vice versa). The main failings were omission of basic information and lack of referencing or identification of authors, date of production of material, and other sourcing deficiencies. Although not evaluated formally, poor Web design, lack of child-appropriate information, and absence of multilingual sites were noted. Another concern was that several well-known, good-quality cancer websites were not found by our simple Internet search, and this needs to be considered in advising patients/ families on Internet search strategies.[31]

Future studies will expand the rating exercise to other pediatric brain tumors and compare the ability of parents in rating sites with that of health care professionals. In addition, a comprehensive Internet survey of usage in pediatric oncology will be completed. The role of rating/regulation is much debated, and an excellent comprehensive review in a theme issue of the *British Medical Journal* can be consulted for further information.[32]

INTERNET INFORMATION PROJECT: ADULT CANCER

Some innovative projects have aimed to use an Internet-based system to assist patients with cancer and to evaluate these as interventions in randomized controlled trials. The University of Wisconsin developed a project called the Comprehensive Health Enhancement Support System (CHESS), which provides not only evidence-based health information (text, graphics, audio and video clips) but also online support groups, ask-an-expert message boards, personal health record journals, and assisted decision-making tools.[33] In a population of breast cancer patients, several randomized controlled trials have identified better social support, greater information competence, greater participation in care, and, interestingly, shorter and more organized out-patient clinic attendance for those women using the system compared with a control group not using CHESS.[34,35] Online support groups (message boards/chat rooms/list serves) are a popular and widely used area of Internet communication; if incorporated into part of a health team community project, they may well assist in positive ways in providing emotional and practical support for individuals and families.[36,37]

FUTURE DIRECTIONS

A new academic subspeciality has emerged, variously termed e- (electronic), i- (Internet), or tele-health. It aims to look at how modern electronic communication can help in all aspects of healthcare.[38,39] This currently includes provision of health information, communication/time management (email use), use of videoconferencing for consultations, and Web-based remote data entry for multicenter clinical trials. In the future, it may include online electronic health records, remote tele-pathology, online central radiological review, and even remote real-time robotic surgery.

CONCLUSIONS

The great strength of the Internet is its potential weakness, i.e. the ability to easily produce and disseminate information and to make this available to a global audience. We need to evaluate scientifically the usage pattern, the quality and ratings of sites, and the capabilities of our patients and families before rushing to censor the Internet (an unrealistic option). Only by doing this can we, as healthcare professionals, provide our patients and families with the quality of information they deserve. Rather than focus our concerns on possibly inaccurate and misleading information on the Internet, we would serve our population better by providing them with evidence-based, understandable,

Table 28.1 *Childhood brain and spinal-cord tumors: Web-based resources for patients and their families*

Description	Website
General brain tumor sites	
National Cancer Institute (NCI)	www.cancer.gov/cancer_information/cancer_type/brain_tumor
American Brain Tumor Association	www.abta.org
Childhood Brain Tumor Foundation	www.childhoodbraintumor.org
Pediatric Brain Tumor Foundation of the USA	www.pbtfus.org
National Brain Tumor Foundation	www.braintumor.org
Brain Tumor Foundation of Canada	www.btfc.org/
The Brain Tumor Society	www.tbts.org
The Central Brain Tumor Registry of the USA	www.cbtrus.org
ASCO – People Living with Cancer	www.plwc.org/plwc/MainConstructor/1,47544,_12|001816|00_21|008|00_04|0060|00_17|001029,00.html
CancerBACUP (in association with UKCCSG)	www.cancerbacup.org.uk/info/child-brain.htm
Hospital sites	
St Jude Children's Research Hospital	www.stjude.org/diseasestudies/brain.html
Royal Marsden Hospital	www.royalmarsden.org/clinicalservices/clinicalunits/paediatric/paediatric.asp
Children's Hospital, Boston	http://web1.tch.harvard.edu/cfapps/CHprogDisplay.cfm?Dept = Neurology&Prog = Brain%20Tumor%20Program
The Children's Hospital of Philadelphia	www.chop.edu/consumer/your_child/condition_section_index.jsp?id = -8682
Children's Brain Tumour Research Centre	www.nottingham.ac.uk/~pdzmgh/cbtrc/
Specific CNS tumor sites	
Acoustic neuromas	
Acoustic Neuroma Association	http://anausa.org
ANA listserv	http://groups.yahoo.com/group/AcousticNeuroma_Awareness
Astrocytoma	
eMedicine – astrocytoma page	www.emedicine.com/ped/topic154.htm
NCI – cerebellar astrocytoma	www.cancer.gov/cancer_information/doc_pdq.aspx?version = patient&viewid = 8cf09a72-e55d-4ad2-b3d5-8bcc8b57dbaa
NCI – cerebral astrocytoma	www.cancer.gov/cancer_information/doc_pdq.aspx?version = patient&viewid = e8fba67f-e7b7-45b5-bc13-814cb10588c8
Astrocytoma listserv	http://groups.yahoo.com/group/astrocytoma
Brainstem tumor	
eMedicine – brainstem tumors	www.emedicine.com/NEURO/topic40.htm
Childhood Brain Tumor Foundation	www.childhoodbraintumor.org/brain.htm
NCI – brainstem tumors	www.cancer.gov/cancer_information/doc_pdq.aspx?viewid = E25F1930-600E-4016-A261-4ED3EC8BB01D
Brainstem listserv	http://groups.yahoo.com/group/brainstem-glioma
Ependymoma	
eMedicine – ependymoma 1	www.emedicine.com/ped/topic693.htm
eMedicine – ependymoma 2	www.emedicine.com/med/topic700.htm
NCI - ependymoma	www.cancer.gov/cancer_information/doc_pdq.aspx?version = patient&viewid = bdf371b6-bc60-43e3-95ac-4cbb4002c1f6
Ependyparents listserv	www.braintrust.org/services/support/othergroups/index.html#ependyparents
Medulloblastoma/PNET	
eMedicine – medulloblastoma 1	www.emedicine.com/neuro/topic624.htm
eMedicine – medulloblastoma 2	www.emedicine.com/ped/topic1396.htm
NCI medulloblastoma	www.cancer.gov/cancer_information/doc_pdq.aspx?version = patient&viewid = 09f49586-80cf-4610-a4d5-64ed410d3565
Supratentorial PNET	www.nci.nih.gov/cancer_information/doc_pdq.aspx?version = patient&viewid = c974f5fd-f977-4b80-85fa-474c96cea157
Childhood Brain Tumor Foundation	www.childhoodbraintumor.org/med.html
Medulloblastoma listserv	http://groups.yahoo.com/group/Medulloblastoma/

(continued)

Table 28.1 (*continued*)

Description	Website
Optic glioma	
eMedicine – optic glioma	www.emedicine.com/radio/topic486.htm
NCI optic glioma	www.nci.nih.gov/cancer_information/doc_pdq.aspx?version = patient&viewid = bc373014-ab82-4987-959c-8a8423ec236e
Optic glioma listserv	http://groups.yahoo.com/group/optic-glioma
Pediatric oncology	
ACOR – pediatric oncology resources	www.acor.org/ped-onc
Children's Cancer Web	www.cancerindex.org/ccw/
CancerBACUP (UKCCSG)	www.cancerbacup.org.uk/info/refer/fact-child.htm
National Childhood Cancer Foundation	www.nccf.org/
General listservs	
Pediatric brain tumor listserv	http://groups.yahoo.com/group/Pediatricbraintumors
Cerebellar mutism and posterior fossa syndrome listserv	http://groups.yahoo.com/group/cerebellarmutism
BRAINTMR mailing list	www.braintrust.org/services/support/braintmr/
Evaluating websites	
DISCERN rating tool	www.discern.org.uk/
NCI 10 Things to Know about Evaluating	www.cancer.gov/templates/doc.aspx?viewid =
Medical Resources on the Web	C68637AF-2AEB-479D-AB60-228118D9674E
American Medical Association Guidelines for Health Websites	www.ama-assn.org/ama/pub/category/1905.html

PNET, primitive neuroectodermal tumor.

age-appropriate material, and multilingual, engaging, well-designed sites that are updated regularly and accessed easily from common search engines. We can then harness the full potential of the Internet to help our patients and their families through the tremendous burden that a diagnosis of a brain or spinal cord tumor imparts.

Table 28.1 lists some useful websites for children/adolescents and their families with CNS tumors.

REFERENCES

1 Freeman K, O'Dell C, Meola C. Issues in families of children with brain tumors. *Oncol Nurs Forum* 2000; **27**:843–8.

2 Kai J. Parents' difficulties and information needs in coping with acute illness in preschool children – a qualitative study. *Br Med J* 1996; **313**:987–90.

3 Pyke-Grimm KA, Degner L, Small A, Mueller B. Preferences for treatment decision-making and information needs of parents of children with cancer. *J Pediatr Oncol Nurs* 1999; **16**:13–24.

4 Leonard A. *Right From the Start*. London: Scope, 1994.

5 Baile WF, Buckman R, Lenzi R, Glober G, Beale EA, Kudelka AP. SPIKES – a six-step protocol for delivering bad news: application to the patient with cancer. *Oncologist* 2000; **5**:302–11.

6 American Brain Tumor Association. *A Primer of Brain Tumors*, 5th edn. Des Plaines, IL: American Brain Tumor Association, 2001.

7 Shiminski-Maher T, Cullen P, Sansalone M. *Childhood Brain and Spinal Cord Tumors. A Guide for Families, Friends and Caregivers*. Sebastopol, CA: O'Reilly, 2002.

8 Nesbit TW, Shermock KM, Bobek MB, *et al.* Implementation and pharmacoeconomic analysis of a clinical staff

pharmacist practice model. *Am J Health Syst Pharm* 2001; **58**:784–90.

9 Hinds PS, Oakes L, Furman W, *et al.* Decision-making by parents and healthcare providers when considering continued care for pediatric patients with cancer. *Oncol Nurs Forum* 1997; **24**:1523–8.

10 Hinds PS, Oakes L, Quargnenti A, *et al.* An international feasibility study of parental decision-making in pediatric oncology. *Oncol Nurs Forum* 2000; **27**:1233–43.

11 Keene N. *Your Child in the Hospital: A Practical Guide for Parents*. Sebastopol, CA: O'Reilly, 1999.

12 Barr RD. *Childhood Cancer: Information for the Patient and Family*. Hamilton: Dekker, 2000.

13 McKay J, Hirano N. *The Chemotherapy and Radiation Survival Guide*. Oakland, CA: New Harbinger, 1998.

14 O'Connell A, Leone N. *Your Child and X-rays: A Parent's Guide to Radiation, X-rays and Other Imaging Procedures*. New York: Lion Press, 1988.

15 NUA Internet Surveys. How many on line? www.nua.com/surveys/how_many_online/index.html. Accessed 2002.

16 Mazzini MJ, Glode LM. Internet oncology: increased benefit and risk for patients and oncologists. *Hematol Oncol Clin North Am* 2001; **15**:583–92.

17 Quade G, Far F, Puschel N. Long-term evaluation of the CancerNet WWW service. *Medinfo* 1998; **9**:327–33.

18 Buhle EL, Jr, Goldwein JW, Benjamin I. OncoLink: a multimedia oncology information resource on the Internet. *Proc Annu Symp Comput Appl Med Care* 1994; 103–7.

19 Jenkins V, Fallowfield L, Saul J. Information needs of patients with cancer: results from a large study in UK cancer centres. *Br J Cancer* 2001; **84**:48–51.

20 Chen X, Siu LL. Impact of the media and the internet on oncology: survey of cancer patients and oncologists in Canada. *J Clin Oncol* 2001; **19**:4291–7.

21 Roberts JM, Copeland KL. Clinical websites are currently dangerous to health. *Int J Med Inf* 2001; **62**:181–7.

22 Winker MA, Flanagin A, Chi-Lum B, *et al.* Guidelines for medical and health information on the Internet: principles governing AMA websites. *J Am Med Assoc* 2000; **283**:1600–6.

23 Norman F. Organizing medical networked information (OMNI). *Med Inform (Lond)* 1998; **23**:43–51.

24 Eysenbach G, Kohler C, Yihune G, Lampe K, Cross P, Brickley D. A framework for improving the quality of health information on the world-wide-web and bettering public (e-)health: the MedCERTAIN approach. *Medinfo* 2001; **10**:1450–4.

25 Charnock D, Shepperd S, Needham G, Gann R. DISCERN: an instrument for judging the quality of written consumer health information on treatment choices. *J Epidemiol Community Health* 1999; **53**:105–11.

26 Biermann JS, Golladay GJ, Greenfield ML, Baker LH. Evaluation of cancer information on the Internet. *Cancer* 1999; **86**:381–90.

27 Bichakjian CK, Schwartz JL, Wang TS, Hall JM, Johnson TM, Biermann JS. Melanoma information on the Internet: often incomplete – a public health opportunity? *J Clin Oncol* 2002; **20**:134–41.

28 Meric F, Bernstam EV, Mirza NQ, *et al.* Breast cancer on the world wide web: cross-sectional survey of quality of information and popularity of websites. *Br Med J* 2002; **324**:577–81.

29 Hargrave D, Bouffet, E. Quality of health information on the internet in paediatric neuro-oncology: medulloblastoma and ependymoma websites. Presented at the International Society of Pediatric Neurooncology meeting, London, 2002.

30 Wu G, Li J. Comparing Web search engine performance in searching consumer health information: evaluation and recommendations. *Bull Med Libr Assoc* 1999; **87**:456–61.

31 Gustafson DH, Bosworth K, Hawkins RP, Boberg EW, Bricker E. CHESS: a computer-based system for providing information, referrals, decision support and social support to people facing medical and other health-related crises. *Proc Annu Symp Comput Appl Med Care* 1992; 161–5.

32 *Br Med J* 2002, **324**.

33 Gustafson DH, McTavish F, Hawkins R, *et al.* Computer support for elderly women with breast cancer. *J Am Med Assoc* 1998; **280**:1305.

34 Gustafson DH, Hawkins R, Pingree S, *et al.* Effect of computer support on younger women with breast cancer. *J Gen Intern Med* 2001; **16**:435–45.

35 Han HR, Belcher AE. Computer-mediated support group use among parents of children with cancer – an exploratory study. *Comput Nurs* 2001; **19**:27–33.

36 Larkin M. Online support groups gaining credibility. *Lancet* 2000; **355**:1834.

37 Eysenbach G, Jadad AR. Evidence-based patient choice and consumer health informatics in the Internet age. *J Med Internet Res* 2001; **3**:E19.

38 Eysenbach G. What is e-health? *J Med Internet Res* 2001; **3**:E20.

39 D'Alessandro DM, Dosa NP. Empowering children and families with information technology. *Arch Pediatr Adolesc Med* 2001; **155**:1131–6.

29

Future challenges

DAVID A. WALKER, GIORGIO PERILONGO, JONATHAN A. G. PUNT AND ROGER E. TAYLOR

As the last chapter is edited and dispatched to the publishers, the references are tidied and the images and figures numbered and located in the text, we realize that this book has brought together the editors and authors in a single project linking people, organizations, clinical practice, science and technology, psychology and education, methods of communication, nations, languages, cultures, and continents in the interests of children and their families. These pages have thrown down the gauntlet to the neuro-oncologists of tomorrow to introduce these ideas into their health systems, to integrate their growing knowledge of adjuvant treatments and their toxicities, so that they effectively complement the operative skills of the neurosurgeon in the multidisciplinary meeting, the operating room, and the clinical trials meeting.

CHALLENGES IN PEDIATRIC NEUROSURGERY

The challenges for neurosurgeons over the next few years will be organizational, technological, and scientific. Over the past 30 years, it has been an uphill struggle for pediatric neurosurgery to be recognized as a valid subspecialty within neurosurgery. The neurosurgical establishment has often been resistant to the concept, for reasons that may be less than noble. However as the timelines in Chapter 2 show, there has been progress, and in most countries with any developed medical services there is some level of pediatric subspecialization. In France, the UK, North America, Spain, Japan, Korea, Taiwan, and South America, there are pediatric neurosurgery groups that may consider issues such as training and service provision as well as scientific aims. In the European Union, the Union Européenne des Médecins Specialistes (UEMS) recognized pediatric neurosurgery in 1998, the first neurosurgical subspecialty to be given this recognition.

Those embracing the true ethos of pediatric practice appreciate that pediatric neurosurgical practice is not just a matter of providing a service for operative technology but demands a commitment to the ongoing, integrated care of children and young people, many of whom will have disabilities and health needs that they will carry into their lives as adults. Willingness to work in multidisciplinary groups is an essential requisite, and the truly committed pediatric neurosurgeon of the future will work within such teams. There is an urgent requirement to ensure that there is seamless care when the young person moves on to live as an adult. This may best be addressed by formal arrangements for linking services for children and adults, as occurs in some other areas, such as epilepsy and diabetology.

There will be issues around staffing. In adult practice, it is an accepted requirement that there is a 24-hour service for patients with ruptured intracranial aneurysms. There can be no reason, therefore, why an equivalent standard of service should not be available for the specialized management of children presenting as an emergency with a highly specialized tumor problem, such as an intracranial germ-cell tumor. Similarly, it will be necessary to ensure that children have the same access to technological advances at the same time as they come on stream for adults. Too often in the past there has been a deplorable lag time. This has been a particular problem for freestanding children's hospitals, often because of the considerable expense involved. We hope that stories of children being taken across major cities in arms, in taxis, and out of hours, in order to circumvent adult-centered funding arrangements, will be images of the past.

These very real staffing and technology issues will almost certainly need to be addressed by reducing the number of services to a smaller number of institutions that can meet all of the requirements all of the time. Whatever service arrangements are devised, it is axiomatic that they must be centered on the needs of the young patient rather than on the ambitions of the doctors.

The pediatric neurosurgeon dealing with children with central nervous system (CNS) tumors must be involved in research. It will be important to integrate robust structures for assessing the value and toxicity of surgery into clinical trial protocols. The emergence of the power of complete resection in posterior fossa ependymoma, and the morbidity of radical excision in craniopharyngioma, signal this imperative. It will be important to develop programs for the evaluation of new technology at an early stage after its introduction, rather than to use the new techniques assuming their benefit in children. The pediatric neurosurgeon will need to understand the importance of exploring the value of interactions between therapeutic modalities, as has been so successful in childhood cancers in other sites. There is a realization that disease-free remission is not the only aim: strategies are required to discover ways of minimizing neurological, neuropsychological, and neuroendocrine morbidity. The pediatric neurosurgeon will need to recognize that they have a special responsibility to play a central role in the harvesting of samples for biological studies; this will require an understanding of the ethical as well as the technical issues.

These aims will be realized only through a cohort of neurosurgeons who are not only collaborators but are also engaged fully with, and integrated into, the service and research processes. The nature of the presentation of many childhood CNS tumors will continue to place the neurosurgeon who encounters a newly diagnosed case of childhood CNS tumor in a unique position to influence the management that may affect not only outcomes but also the whole experience of the illness for the child, the family, and society. This is a heavy responsibility, and one that cannot be ignored.

TUMOR TYPES AND NEW TREATMENT STRATEGIES

Although CNS tumors account for approximately 20–25 per cent of malignancies in children, a wide variety occur, with extremely varied biological behaviour, clinical manifestations, and outcome. Institutional experience in the management of most individual tumor types is limited. Therefore, a pediatric CNS tumor textbook must include detailed analyses of tumors arising in these individual sites, and the histological types. Survival outcome for individual tumor types ranges widely from excellent (e.g. intracranial germinoma, cerebellar pilocytic astrocytoma) to extremely poor (e.g. atypical teratoid/rhabdoid tumor, diffuse pontine glioma). These differences have led to varied priorities for clinical research.

In the past ten to 15 years, a better understanding of the natural history of low-grade glioma has led to management strategies based on the appropriate use of surgery, radiotherapy, and chemotherapy, with the aim of maintenance of the good survival outcome, but with reduced long-term effects of therapy. As for adults with high-grade glioma, the outcome for children following "conventional" treatment with radiotherapy and chemotherapy remains poor, and an important priority is the identification of better chemotherapeutic agents, usually in up-front "window studies."

For ependymal tumors, the most important modality is surgical excision, which should be complete or as near-complete as possible. A priority is to identify the precise role of chemotherapy, possibly with the aim of achieving tumor response to facilitate second-look surgery. Radiotherapy has an established role, but there is a need to clarify the optimum dose, fractionation, and volume.

Embryonal tumors are characterized by their radio-sensitivity, chemosensitivity, and propensity for leptomeningeal spread. Current policies for the management of medulloblastoma are based on series of collaborative group randomized studies, and further trials need to clarify the optimum scheduling of radiotherapy and chemotherapy as well as the role of altered radiotherapy fractionation and high-dose chemotherapy.

The management of infants poses particular problems because of the relatively poor outcome combined with the significantly greater long-term consequences of therapy. In the late 1980s and early 1990s, infant tumors were lumped together and treated in generic infant studies, whereby chemotherapy was used to try to delay or avoid radiotherapy, with varying success. We are now in a new era whereby treatment policies for infants are appropriate for the histological type but modified for age.

Historically, for craniopharyngioma there have been few collaborative group studies. However, long-term consequences of therapy may be considerable, and national and international collaborative studies are needed. Intradural spinal tumors are rare, with a paucity of data on which to judge the value of the various therapy modalities, with generally small series of highly selected patients treated over a long timescale. It is important to recognize that the group of brainstem gliomas comprises a heterogeneous mix of diseases and sites of origin, with very different outcomes. Having explored the role of altered radiotherapy fractionation and "conventional" chemotherapeutic agents for diffuse pontine glioma, there is a need to identify effective novel therapies through research. For rare tumors, we have to make the best of small case series and case reports. It is important to collate information in editions such as this in order to provide a resource for clinicians faced with a child with a rare tumor.

HEALTH SYSTEMS' RESPONSES TO NEW TECHNOLOGIES

In developed countries, the incidence of CNS tumors seems to be rising. It is not clear why this is the case. Fortunately, in the same countries the survival rates are starting to rise as well. Making the diagnosis of children with these diseases is a challenge for health systems, requiring high levels of clinical aptitude and skill of individual medical and allied professionals, and supported by a balanced educational approach to undergraduate and postgraduate trainees, and advice through clinical protocols and reasonable access to resources for imaging. The current focus of clinical advances in practice through translational research within surgery and imaging is predominantly technology-driven, whether through the enhancements in anatomical imaging using computerized tomography (CT) or magnetic resonance scanning, functional imaging with magnetic resonance spectroscopy (MRS), or positron-emission tomography (PET). Linking information from these imaging techniques to the management of raised intracranial pressure, tumor debulking or biopsy, and the application of minimally invasive neurosurgical techniques, such as image-guided stereotaxy and neuroendoscopy, are clear examples of the application of technological advances that have revolutionized clinical practice in the past decade. Definition of the biological nature of tumors is being enhanced by the application of molecular techniques with increasing sophistication, microarray chips being the most recent examples of applied molecular technology. However, morphological descriptions amplified by antibody and genetic markers at the microscopic level remains as the bedrock of diagnostic classification. It is anticipated that molecular profiles of genetic or physiological information, expressed mathematically, will develop and ultimately determine treatment selection and therefore prognosis for survival as well as quality of survival.

Advances in the delivery of radiotherapy by improvements in focusing beams, enhanced fractionation of doses, and improved methods for immobilization of the young child can maximize anti-tumor effects whilst minimizing the toxicity to the normal brain. Implementation of these new, more complex technologies places greater demands on the multidisciplinary team, and compared with conventional techniques, higher degrees of accuracy of planning and delivery are essential. During the past decade, we have seen the development of radiation oncology discipline groups associated with national or international pediatric oncology organizations such as the Société Internationale de Oncologie Pédiatrique (SIOP). These groups provide an important forum for discussion, standard-setting, and education. In North America, these groups have taken a further step forward, and the Children's Oncology Group (COG), Radiation Oncology Discipline Committee (RODC), has close links with the Quality Assurance Review Center (QARC), which is responsible for radiotherapy quality assurance and protocol development in many pediatric and adult trials. Radiotherapy quality assurance will have to take on an increasingly important role as the new technologies such as conformal radiotherapy and intensity modulated radiotherapy (IMRT) are implemented more widely.

NEW BIOLOGICAL ERA

We hope that the greater biological understanding of these tumors will lead to the identification of new targets for treatment. The story of the Philadelphia chromosome and chronic myeloid leukemia (CML) has been a triumph of technology over cancer. We hope to repeat this story in CNS tumors (see Chapter 2). The early steps have already been taken by defining some of the common biological abnormalities within the CNS tumor groups. Hopefully, this will identify targets that will be vulnerable to manipulation and alter the biological nature of these tumors.

Drug development is progressing at a rapid rate. The hunt is on for new molecular targets within specific tumor types. The success of this will inevitably be determined by understanding the difference in function of target molecules between tumor and normal brain tissue. Advances in neuro-oncology at a scientific level will be limited by the rate of advances in understanding the very complex neurobiological environment. In the brain, the additional difficulties of delivering existing and new drugs across the blood–brain barrier, directly into the brain/tumor bed, or via the cerebrospinal fluid (CSF) requires special approaches if the new agents are to be effective in the most resistant tumors.

REHABILITATION

Neurosurgeons are the specialists in neuroscience in the neuro-oncology multidisciplinary team. They are familiar with the difficulties of neurological and neurocognitive rehabilitation in all their patient groups. Their links to community-based rehabilitation teams must be developed

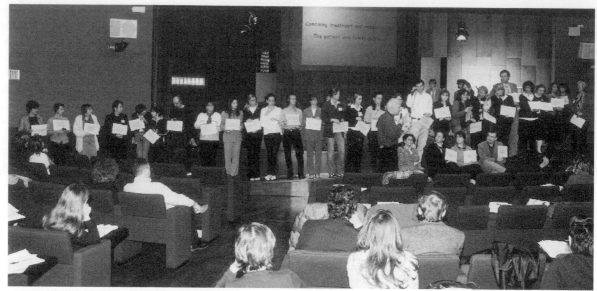

Figure 29.1 *The number of professional roles involved in the care and rehabilitation of a child with a brain tumor. The four people in the foreground represent the child and family, while those standing in the background represent each role in the full hospital- and community-based multiprofessional team.*

strongly as the children acquire neurological disability not only from surgery but also from the radiotherapy and chemotherapy approaches that attempt to eradicate residual disease.

Rehabilitation is lifelong. Hypothetically, its childhood age range is focused on achieving independence by the end of childhood and adolescence. This is inevitably a lengthy process requiring considerable commitment from people beyond the central hospital-based team who are involved in the diagnosis and initial management. The key to its success is communication. The communication must be with the family and child in the first instance, but it must go beyond them to the team supporting their local community if independence by adulthood is to be achieved. Figure 29.1 and Table 29.1 demonstrate the number of professional roles involved in the care and rehabilitation of a child with a brain tumor.

MEASURING OUTCOMES FOR TRIALS AND HEALTH PLANNING

The current research looking at directing gene therapy in adult gliomas is leading to a greater understanding of how to overcome the difficulties of drug delivery. We hope to learn from this so that the drugs directed at new targets will achieve their true potential. If the tumor is finally conquered, either by its eradication or its biological neutralization, then the key factor for the child and family is what cost has been paid for this success and what adaptations to the child's environment or education are needed to allow them to take part fully in their subsequent life. An essential component of this is the need to

Table 29.1 *Health professionals involved in the comprehensive care of children and young people with brain and spinal tumors*

Primary and secondary healthcare team
General practitioner
District nurse
Health visitor
School nurse
Educational psychologist
Pediatrician working in hospital and community
Pediatric nursing teams working in hospital and community
Audiometrist
Speech and language therapist
Dietitian
Pediatric radiographers (diagnostic)

Tertiary healthcare team
Pediatric oncologist
Pediatric neurosurgeon
Pediatric radiotherapist supported by radiotherapy team skilled in the care of children and young people and their families
Neuropathologist
Neuroradiologist
Pediatric neurosurgical and oncology nursing team
Specialist liaison nurses
Specialized chemotherapy pharmacy support
Specialist play therapist
Specialist rehabilitation team (pediatric physiotherapists and occupational therapists)
Specialist social worker
Educational liaison worker
Pediatric endocrinologist
Pediatric neurologist
Pediatric ophthalmologist
Neurophysiologist
Paediatric surgeon
Pediatric surgical specialists in ENT, orthopedics, maxillofacial, and plastic surgeries
Child psychiatrist
Clinical psychologist

establish means that can be used to measure quality of life within populations and trials cohorts, as it is only by demonstrating improvements in both of these aspects of survival for this group that governments can be expected to allocate scant resources for this group as well as the many other survivors of chronic illness in childhood.

THE LAST WORD

The editors have enjoyed the process of the collection and collation of this material with the help of their friends and colleagues. What started off being inspired by Belgian beer was supported further by the consumption of the products of grapes from Italy, grown in Argentina, and vinified by Tuscan enologists. This demonstrated our commitment to international biological science at every level and holds great hope for the expansion of collaboration to other parts of the world, where growing expertise will produce new leaders in this field of pediatric practice.

Pediatric neuro-oncology is an expanding and specialized field that needed a new book. A better book? Well, we are already working on it.

Index

Bold page numbers refer to figures and *italic* page numbers indicate tables.